Applied Veterinary Histology

Second Edition

Applied Veterinary Histology

Second Edition

WILLIAM J. BANKS, D.V.M., M.S., Ph.D.

Professor and Head
Department of Veterinary Anatomy and Fine Structure
School of Veterinary Medicine
Louisiana State University
Baton Rouge, Louisiana

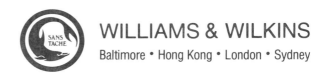

WILLIAMS & WILKINS
Baltimore • Hong Kong • London • Sydney

Editor: George Stamathis
Associate Editor: Carol Eckhart
Copy Editor: Shelley Potler
Design: Joanne Janowiak
Illustration Planning: Lorraine Wrzosek
Production: Anne G. Seitz

Copyright ©, 1986
Williams & Wilkins
428 East Preston Street
Baltimore, MD 21202, U.S.A.

Made in the United States of America

First Edition, 1981

Library of Congress Cataloging in Publication Data

Banks, William J.
    Applied veterinary histology.

    Includes bibliographies and index.
    1. Veterinary histology. I. Title.
SF761.B327 1985   636.089'1018   84-19535
ISBN 0-683-00411-5

90   10 9 8 7 6 5

DEDICATED TO
DR. ROBERT A. KAINER
PROFESSOR OF ANATOMY—
VALUED TEACHER,
RESPECTED COLLEAGUE
AND TREASURED FRIEND.

Preface to the Second Edition

Embarking upon the original edition of this textbook about 14 years ago was the initiation of a quest to fulfill a long-standing desire to write a textbook of veterinary histology. The completion of the project was as gratifying as envisioned originally. My feelings of gratification, however, were gradually but continually eroded and replaced by a growing awareness of the shortcomings and ephemeral nature of the book. The need to modify, to improve, and to update—to maintain pace with the burgeoning wealth of knowledge—became the ultimate responsibility and source of satisfaction.

The encouragement of my veterinary colleagues and veterinary medical students has been a continual source of motivation. Students, especially, have always been willing to share their thoughts about the utility, clarity (or lack thereof) and appropriateness of various materials. Their feedback has had a profound influence on this book. Their positive comments have been a source of great personal satisfaction; their negative but constructive comments have become the grist of the mill of improvement. That seems appropriate! This book is for them.

The approach used in this textbook reflects clearly my personal philosophy about educational experiences in a medical curriculum. Disciplinary information, histology notwithstanding, should be coherent, integrated, and relevant. Indeed, the author is fortunate to be teaching in a professional veterinary medical curriculum that permits the expression of this philosophy. The knowledge and insights of veterinary histology must afford students the opportunity to expand their clinical problem-solving ability. Just as importantly, the integration of histology with other bodies of knowledge demonstrates the existence, ultimately, of one body of knowledge viewed through the perspective of different disciplinary windows. These are the principles that have governed the generation of the content of this book.

Students of veterinary medicine seem to have less and less time to learn more and more about the expanding body of knowledge encompassed by their profession. A teaching-type textbook becomes a valuable vehicle in maximizing their learning and minimizing the amount of time spent in the process. Opinions expressed by first-year students who have used the textbook at Colorado State University and other institutions indicate that this book complements their learning. Their complimentary statements about the book are gratifying. Too often, however, books purchased for a course do little else than collect dust on an obscure portion of a bookshelf upon completion of the specific course. Worse yet, such books may be doomed to being recirculated through a second-hand book dealer. The most gratifying comments about this textbook have been from juniors, seniors, and graduates. They have related to me their continual use of the textbook throughout their education. If the book can become an "old friend" and help periodically throughout the total learning process, then the effort has been truly worthwhile.

The expansion of the knowledge base of a discipline is usually sufficient justification for expansion of textbooks. The broadening of the author's perspectives is also a reasonable justification. Both are operable in this situation. Although the new edition of this textbook has expanded, the inclusion and exclusion of new information has been approached judiciously. Moreover, the author has diligently edited every word, phrase, sentence, and concept to determine the suitability of inclusion in this edition. The problem for most authors, this one notwithstanding, is not what to include—definitive tomes are usually heavier than they are useful—but what to exclude and still achieve the utilitarian goals of the textbook. The primary goals, however, remain being a book that students can use to learn microanatomy, to integrate that knowledge base with functional correlates, and to view the application of this knowledge to clinical medicine and surgery.

The pertinent histology has been updated and expanded; however, the author has resisted the temptation of wholesale inclusion of ultrastructural information and electron micrographs. When included, it was done to enhance understanding and add to the coherence of a particular subject. Similarly, functional information has been expanded selectively and updated.

Histology is a visual science; the student learns the subject while looking through a microscope. The cryptic puzzles of tissue architecture are best deciphered when comparisons are possible. For this reason, the textbook is replete with illustrations. Numerous light and electron micrographs are complemented by many scientific illustrations, diagrams, and flow charts. The new edition contains almost 1000 illustrations, of which 109 are in color. Over 150 illustrations have been changed from the first edition. About half of them are new illustrations; the remainder are replacements for illustrations that needed updating or improvement. Many of the illustrations are classic, visually describing features of microscopic architecture. Some are speculative and represent attempts by the author and artists to present a visual story of some topics about which our knowledge is incomplete. Finally, flow charts have been used to show relationships and integrate the visual knowledge into a coherent story. The illustrative materials should facilitate the learning process.

The use of color micrographs in this edition has not changed from the previous edition. All of the color micrographs are grouped on plates after Section III. Although the use of color has many advantages, its use is not essential for learning histology. (Color-blind individuals have always performed well in my histology classes.) The grouping of color micrographs and their minimal use within the textbook are simply cost-saving devices. If color were used throughout this book, then neither of us could afford the book.

Magnifications, as stated within each caption, are original magnifications that the author used to photograph various histological structures. The original magnifications are reported for light micrographs, because that is what the student should see when examining a specimen through a microscope at a comparable magnification. Photographic enlargement factors do not translate readily during use of the microscope. Generally, most negatives of light microscopic materials for the text have been enlarged four to five times. Final magnifications of electron micrographs are reported, because that is the typical stage of examination—after photographic enlargement.

Every chapter in this edition has been subjected to careful scrutiny. Three chapters have been added. The information for one chapter is new; whereas, the information for the other two chapters was extracted from larger chapters in the previous edition. All the chapters have been reorganized in an attempt to facilitate identification and retrieval of specific information.

The basic organization of the textbook has not changed. Functional and clinical applications are interwoven throughout the histological story. The textbook is organized into five sections: Introduction to Histology, Cell Biology, Histology, Comparative Organology, Introduction to Exfoliative Cytology. Some of the particulars relating to changes in this edition follow.

Section I, Introduction to Histology, has been updated, reorganized and expanded. This section is intended to provide perspective for the new student of histology. Understanding most of the content of this section will complement the information in the remainder of the text and enhance learning.

Section II, Cell Biology, has been enlarged and many parts have been updated and rewritten. Most students entering a veterinary medical curriculum have an adequate background in cell biology. The inclusion of Chapter 4 in this textbook completes the story about cells and provides the necessary background for the remainder of the text materials. Mastery of the subject matter within this section is essential.

Section III, Histology, encompasses the classical tissues. Chapter 6, Extracellular Matrix, is new and the material included affords a comprehensive treatment of extracellular substances, including interstitial fluids. All of the other chapters in this section have been modified and reorganized. Most parts have been rewritten.

Section IV, Comparative Organology, still remains the bulk of the endeavor. Structure and function have been expanded, rewritten, and reorganized. Every chapter in this section has been altered.

Section V, Introduction to Exfoliative Cytology, has been improved, but the substantive materials have not been changed.

Exhaustive attempts have been made to integrate structural and functional considerations within the construct of being applicable to clinical medicine and surgery. The book, however, is still a textbook of histology. Some of the information will add to general knowledge about the biomedical sciences without much apparent application to the practice of medicine directly. Hopefully, the book will continue to provide the necessary information in a comprehensible and enjoyable manner while enhancing learning. Also, I hope that students will continue to use it long after their initial exposure to histology has been completed.

The input of many colleagues and students has been invaluable. I respectfully request that they continue to comment about the book to me. Notification of errors, inaccuracies, or inadequate discourse would be appreciated greatly.

Finally, the textbook is not intended to be a definitive tome on the subject. Rather, it is simply one person's perceptions of a rapidly expanding, vast, dynamic, and exciting body of knowledge.

William J. Banks
Baton Rouge, Louisiana

Preface to the First Edition

The original edition of this textbook, *Histology and Comparative Organology: A Text-Atlas*, was an attempt to present the elements of histology that are applicable to veterinary medicine. Structure and function, integrated throughout the text, were presented in a succinct format. This parochial and concise approach, although affording a foundation in microscopic organization, did not consider the application and relevancy to clinical endeavors. Similarly, functional considerations were limited in scope. In confidence that histology is a fundamental and relevant component of medical education, the revision of this original text was undertaken to broaden the scope and utility of the book.

The elements of histology have been retained in a concise format but have been expanded as necessary and selectively to maintain pace with the recent remarkable expansion of knowledge of microscopic structure. The histophysiology of cells, tissues, and organs has been expanded and broadened but remains integrated with structural considerations. Numerous examples of the applicability of histology and histophysiology to medicine and surgery have been interwoven throughout the text. The principles of renewal and repair of all tissue and most organs have been included with the microanatomical and physiological considerations. The text has been thoroughly revised, rewritten, and updated to present an applied approach to histology for veterinary medical students.

The basic organization of the book is unchanged. The text, now divided into five sections, proceeds from principles of histology to cytology, histology, organology, and exfoliative cytology. The first section consists of three new chapters that are designed to give the student a perspective of the scope of histology as a basic medical science, an appreciation of the methods of histology and insights into the interpretation of histological specimens. The chapter on cytology, which comprises the second section, has been expanded to include chemical, physical, and biological properties of cells. A concerted attempt has been made to correlate the ultrastructural features of cells to those features visible with light microscopy, thus bridging the "conceptual gap" between ultrastructural cytology and histology. Section III presents the basic tissues. The morphology has been updated, while the histophysiology has been expanded to afford the student a better appreciation of the role of the basic tissues in the structural and functional complexity of the animal body. The majority of the text is devoted to comparative organology. An introductory chapter on organology presents the the organizational schemes that characterize tubular and parenchymatous organs. Subsequent chapters present the morphological features of specific and/or unique organs that characterize the major domestic species, including carnivores, herbivores, and birds. Histophysiology is expanded and integrated with morphology of each of the organs. The last section in the text consists of a chapter on clinical cytology. The normal exfoliative cytology of various organs, tissues, and body cavities is compared and contrasted with abnormalities associated with these structures.

The new approach of this textbook has been influenced by the authors's experience in teaching functional anatomy to first- second-, and third-year veterinary students. The constructive comments of these students, relating to veterinary histology in general and the original edition of the textbook specifically, have had a profound impact upon the revision process. Similarly, the comments of colleagues and reviewers have been influential. All have expressed the desirability and need for a text that integrates histological and functional properties as well as demonstrating the applied significance of these principles. This text is an attempt to satisfy that need and is consistent with the author's educational philosophy.

Visual aids are essential components of the educational armamentarium of the effective teaching histologist. Because the text is replete with illustrative materials, it should serve as a valuable teaching and learning aid. The textual material is complemented by 883 black and white figures. Although the majority of the original light and electron micrographs have been retained, many have been replaced, improved, and supplemented with new micrographs. Electron micrographs of selected tissues and freeze-fractured specimens, as well as some scanning electron micrographs of selected organs, have been added to clarify or complement specific presentations of certain structures. Over 240 medical illustrations, diagrams, and flow charts complement the micrographs and text. Additionally, eight color plates have been added to assist the learning process. All of the illustrative materials should serve to improve the comprehension of structural and functional principles.

The text is not intended to be a definitive tome for the rapidly expanding field of veterinary histology. Rather, it is envisioned as a positive step in the integration of histological and physiological principles that are applicable to veterinary medicine and surgery.

William J. Banks
Fort Collins, Colorado

Acknowledgments

Many colleagues, students, and friends have made numerous and significant contributions to this edition of the text. Indeed, the author is indebted to many individuals who have contributed directly and indirectly to its improvement. Direct criticisms, subtle suggestions, intense discussions, and even blatant disagreements have been the basis for improving the second edition of this textbook.

Again, Mrs. R. Colter of the Histology Preparation Laboratory, Department of Anatomy, College of Veterinary Medicine and Biomedical Sciences, Colorado State University was most helpful. She was always willing to assist the author with numerous and varied tasks related to the generation of new histological specimens for inclusion in this edition. The vast histological specimen library of the Department was always available to me through her. Her patience in producing "just one more section" was most appreciated. Also, the many hours she devoted to the perfection of the glycol methacrylate technique were appreciated.

Various chapters were subjected to the scrutiny of generous individuals who gave willingly of their time, expertise, and interest. Dr. M. J. Burke, veterinarian, past graduate student, current junior human medical student, respected colleague, and treasured friend was a constant source of encouragement. His critical evaluations and our lively discussions were always a source of satisfaction.

Of the many veterinary students over the past three years at Colorado State University who have offered helpful suggestions for the improvement of the text, the author is especially indebted to D. Michael Davis and Flavia Zorgniotti. Both these students proffered useful insights in an enthusiastic and constructive manner. Ms. Zorgniotti scrutinized most of the chapters in her usual zestful, caring, and expert manner.

The micrographs, negatives, or samples that were supplied by colleagues for the first edition of this text were used again for this edition. My appreciation is expressed to: Drs. M. Carry, C. J. Connell, D. L. Eisenbrandt, J. J. England, G. P. Epling, R. A. Kainer, D. E. Kelly, J. W. Newbrey, H. D. Nornes, R. W. Norrdin, J. E. Rash, J. Storz, M. A. Thrall, W. Todd, and Ms. A. Sheppard. Additional materials were obtained from colleagues for this edition, too. Their willingness to permit various materials to be included in this edition was most helpful. The author is grateful to Dr. F. Al-Bagdadi (Louisiana State University), Dr. R. P. Amann, Dr. R. A. Kainer and Dr. T. Spurgeon (Colorado State University), and Drs. N. J. Wilsman and Dr. C. Farnum (University of Wisconsin). The permission granted by other authors and publishing companies to use selected copyrighted materials was appreciated. The cooperation of Dr. A. Peters (Boston University) is acknowledged gratefully.

The critical review of Chapter 20 by Dr. M. H. Fallding (University of Guelph) is acknowledged gratefully. Her in-depth comments about the integument were most helpful.

The excellent assistance of the art and photography staff of Biomedical Media, College of Veterinary Medicine and Biomedical Sciences, Colorado State University was invaluable in the generation of this edition. The author is especially indebted to Mr. John Daugherty for his artistic expertise and enthusiasm for this project. He completed the project in a timely and expert manner. The assistance of Ms. Laurie O'Keefe and Mr. Dave Carlson with the art and graphics is appreciated. Additionally, the assistance of Ms. Theresa Cermak with the graphics is acknowledged gratefully. All of the medical illustrations, diagrams, and flow charts are the result of the efforts of these talented, dedicated, and gracious individuals. The photographic support work of Mr. Charles Kerlee is appreciated, also. His assistance with the photomicrography and his expeditious processing of film was invaluable to the timely completion of the project.

Two colleagues deserve a special note of appreciation. The cooperation and encouragement of Dr. L. R. Whalen were especially valuable. He was always willing to discuss various aspects of this textbook that are of mutual interest. His comments about the neurology sections of the textbook were most helpful. The continual input of Dr. R. A. Kainer into this textbook was valuable and appreciated. His broad knowledge base of comparative histology and many years of experience are valuable resources. His willingness to share this knowledge and to discuss problems of mutual concern is appreciated. Our many hours of discussion were an especially enjoyable part of this project. The dedication of this edition to this fine scholar is the author's attempt to acknowledge his varied and on-going contributions.

The inventors of the microcomputer and the authors of the word processing software used for this project deserve the author's praise. Eventually, this technology became a marvelous tool in the generation of this textbook. The assistance of the author's brother, Mr. Thomas Banks, President of Santiago Data Systems, Inc., with some of the customary interfacing problems between novices and computers was valuable and appreciated. Similarly, the timely assistance and suggestions of Ms. Kay Brittingham of Waverly Press, Inc. are acknowledged gratefully.

Once again, the bulk of the typing was accomplished by my able, conscientious, organized, and extremely patient wife, Brenda F. Banks. Her mastery of the microcomputer culminated in the timely completion of this book. Her ability to dedicate herself to this task amid the usual distractions associated with a growing family is unbelievable. Her adeptness at interpreting cryptic syntax, deciphering and interpreting editorial and scientific hieroglyphics, and organizing the mass of paper and disks was an invaluable and appreciated contribution to this book. Her willingness to share the responsibilities contributes to the fun associated with this effort. Expressing my appreciation adequately for her enthusiastic participation is virtually impossible.

The assistance with varied tasks involved in the generation of this textbook became the responsibility of my daughters, Victoria and Kristin. The knowledge they gained from the experience far surpassed that which comes from an appreciation of manuscript production alone. They learned negotiation skills and some of the rudiments of finance. Their assistance was appreciated and enjoyed.

The completion of this edition would not

have been possible without the assistance, patience, support, encouragement, unselfishness, and understanding of my marvelous spouse, Brenda, and our wonderful children, Victoria and Kristin.

The able staff of Williams & Wilkins continues to make the project an enjoyable and gratifying experience. The generous and expert assistance of Carol Eckhart and Anne G. Seitz is acknowledged gratefully. The cooperative and supportive assistance of Ms. Seitz was especially appreciated. Our interactions were always delightful and productive. Her energy and enthusiasm on behalf of this book were truly appreciated. The author is especially indebted to George Stamathis, Editor, for his support, encouragement, and enthusiasm for all aspects of the project. His patience and friendship are especially valued. He has continued the fine tradition of professional expertise that has become the hallmark of my interactions with this publishing organization.

To my numerous students, teachers and colleagues, from whom I have learned so much, my sincerest appreciation is expressed.

William J. Banks
Baton Rouge, Louisiana

Contents

PREFACE TO THE SECOND EDITION vii

PREFACE TO THE FIRST EDITION ix

ACKNOWLEDGMENTS x

LIST OF COLOR ILLUSTRATIONS xvii

SECTION I: GENERAL PRINCIPLES OF HISTOLOGY

Chapter 1:
Insights Into Histology **2**
Introduction   2
Tissues—The Elements of
    Organization   2

Chapter 2:
Methods of Histology **4**
Introduction   4
The Paraffin Technique   5
Principles of Staining   7
Selected Preparation Techniques .   7

Chapter 3:
Microscopy and Interpretation   **12**
Introduction   12
Microscopy   12
Interpretation   15

SECTION II: CELL BIOLOGY

Chapter 4:
Cells—Structure and Function   **22**
General Cellular Characteristics . . .   22
    Chemical and Physical Properties   22
    Biological Properties   23
    Morphological Features   24
Nucleus   24
Cytoplasm   28
    Cellular Membranes   29
    Structure and Function   29

Transport Functions   32
Membranes as Receptors   32
Calmodulin, cAMP, and Cellular
    Activities   32
Cytoplasmic Membranous
    Compartments   32
Ribosomes and Rough Endo-
    plasmic Reticulum   32
Agranular Endoplasmic
    Reticulum   34

Golgi Apparatus   34
Mitochondria   36
Lysosomes   36
Peroxisomes   38
Cytoplasmic Skeleton and
    Inclusions   38
Microtubules   38
Cytoskeletal Components   43
Cytoplasmic Inclusions   43
Cell Division   45

SECTION III: HISTOLOGY

Chapter 5:
Epithelia **52**
General Characteristics   52
Simple Epithelia   54
Stratified Epithelia   55
Transitional Epithelium   58
Glandular Epithelia   59
Special Epithelia   66
Surface Specializations of Epithelia   68
Regeneration and Repair of
    Epithelia   73

Chapter 6:
Extracellular Matrix **76**
Extracellular Components   76
    Fibers   76

Collagen   76
Reticular Fibers   82
Elastic Fibers   82
Ground Substance   83
Tissue Fluid   86
    Body Fluids and Ground
        Substance   86
    Hydrostatic and Osmotic
        Relationships   86
    Alterations to Fluid Exchange . .   89

Chapter 7:
Proper Connective Tissues
    and Adipose Tissue . . .   **92**
General Characteristics   92
Resident Cell Populations   94

Transient Cell Populations   99
Embryonal Connective Tissues . . .   100
Proper Connective Tissues   101
Special Connective Tissues   104
Adipose Tissue   105
Macrophage System   106
Regeneration and Repair   106

Chapter 8:
Supportive Tissue—Cartilage   **108**
General Characteristics   108
Matrical Components   109
    Fibers   109
    Ground Substance   109
    Staining of Cartilage   110
    Ultrastructure of Cartilaginous
        Matrices   111

Types of Cartilage 113
  Hyaline Cartilage 113
  Elastic Cartilage 113
  Fibrous Cartilage 114
Maintenance and Repair of
  Cartilage 115

Chapter 9:
Supportive Tissues—Bone .. **119**
General Characteristics 119
Matrical Components 119
Envelopes of Bone 121
  Periosteum 121
  Endosteum 121
Cellular Components 122
  Relationships of Cells 122
  Mesenchymal Cells 122
  Osteoprogenitor Cells 122
  Osteoblasts 123
  Osteocytes 126
  Osteoclasts 129
Types of Bone 129
  Woven Bone 129
  Lamellar Bone 131
Configurations of Bone 131
  Cancellous Bone 131
  Compact Bone 131
Organization of Bone 131
  Lamellae of Bone 131
  Osteonal Bone 131
Bone Remodeling 135
  General Features 135
  Basic Metabolic Unit 139
  Histological Evidence of
    Remodeling 139
Bone-Endocrine Relationships 142
  Calcium Regulatory System .. 143
  Mechanisms of Action 143
  "In Concert" Influences of
    Hormones 144

Chapter 10:
Osteogenesis **146**
Development of Bone 146
Mechanisms of Development 146

Intramembranous Ossification .. 146
Endochondral Ossification 149
  Model Formation 153
  Model Growth 157
  Modeling Activity 159
Hormones and Bone
  Development 161

Chapter 11:
Blood **164**
Peripheral Blood 164
  General Characteristics 164
  Mammalian Blood Cells 166
    Erythrocytes 166
    Granulocytes 168
    Agranulocytes 169
    Platelets 171
  Formed Elements—Species
    Variations 171
  Avian Blood Cells 173
    Erythrocytes 173
    Granulocytes 174
    Agranulocytes 174
    Thrombocytes 174
Hemostasis 175
  Coagulation 175

Chapter 12:
Hematopoiesis **179**
Development of Blood 179
  General Characteristics 179
  Bone Marrow 180
  Erythropoiesis 181
  Granulocytopoiesis 181
  Thrombocytopoiesis 182
  Agranulocytopoiesis 182
Kinetics of Blood 183
  Erythrokinetics 184
  Granulokinetics 185
  Kinetics of Agranulocytes ... 186
Evaluation of Blood and Bone
  Marrow 186

Chapter 13:
Muscle Tissue **188**

General Characteristics 188
Smooth Muscle 188
  Histological Structure 188
  Ultrastructure 189
  Functional Correlates 190
Skeletal Muscle 190
  Histological Structure 190
  Ultrastructure 193
  Myofibrillar Organization ... 193
  Contractile Mechanism 193
  Relaxation/Contraction
    Morphology 193
  Types of Muscle Fibers 200
  Functional Correlates 200
Cardiac Muscle 204
  Histological Structure 204
  Ultrastructural Features 204
  Functional Correlates 206
  Purkinje Fibers 206
Repair and Regeneration 206

Chapter 14:
Nervous Tissue **208**
General Characteristics 208
Neurons 208
  General Properties 208
  Classification 208
  Neuronal Components 209
    Cell Bodies 209
    Dendrites 211
    Axons 211
Information Transfer 211
  Focal Sites of Transmission .. 211
    Electrotonic Transmission .. 211
    Synapses 211
  Neurochemical Transmission .. 213
    Presynaptic Components .. 213
    Postsynaptic Components .. 215
Neuroglia 217
  Central Glial Elements 218
  Peripheral Glial Elements ... 219
Cellular Investments of Neurons .. 219
  Cell Bodies 219
  Neuronal Processes 219

Color Plates **233**

SECTION IV: COMPARATIVE ORGANOLOGY

Chapter 15:
Organization of Organs **252**
Introduction 252
  Parenchyma and Stroma 252
Tubular Organs 252
  General Form 252
  Tunica Mucosa 252
  Tunica Submucosa 253
  Tunica Muscularis 253
  Tunica Adventitia and Tunica
    Serosa 253
  Surface and Glandular
    Modifications 254
Organization of Solid Organs 254
  Form and Function 254
Membranes as Simple Organs ... 254
  Mucous Membranes 254
  Serous Membranes 258

Chapter 16:
Musculoskeletal System **259**
General Characteristics 259
Bone as an Organ 259
  Physical Properties of Bone ... 259
  Biomechanical Properties of
    Bone 260
  Biological Properties of Bone ... 262
Fracture Repair 264
  General Features 264
    Influential Factors 264
    Stages of Fracture Repair ... 265
    Types of Repair Mechanisms . 266
  Primary Intention Healing 266
    Contact Repair 266
    Gap Repair 266
  Second Intention Healing 267
    Impact Stage 267

  Induction Stage 267
  Inflammatory Stage 267
  Reparative Stage 267
  Remodeling Stage 268
  Circumstances of Repair 269
Articulations 269
  General Characteristics 269
  Types of Articulations 270
  Fibrous, Cartilaginous, and Osseous
    Joints 270
  Synovial Joints 270
  Synovial Fluid 272
Muscle as an Organ 276
  Muscle-Tendon Relationships .. 276
    Muscle 276
    Tendons 276
  Muscle-Nerve Relationships 278

Chapter 17:
Nervous System **285**
General Characteristics 285
Anatomical Considerations 285
Physiological Considerations 286
   Functional Organization 286
    Reflex Arc 288
Peripheral Organizational
    Components 290
   Ganglia 290
    Sensory Ganglia 290
    Motor Ganglia 291
   Neuronal Processes 291
    Nerve Trunks 291
    Histological Organization 292
    Afferent Terminals 293
    Efferent Terminals 294
Central Organizational
    Components 294
   Meninges 294
    Pachymeninx 294
    Leptomeninges 296
   Cerebrospinal Fluid 296
    Choroid Plexus 296
    Dynamic Relationships 297
   Brain-Associated Barriers 300
    Blood-Cerebrospinal Fluid
     Barrier 300
    Blood-Brain Barrier 300
   Specific Organs 302
    Spinal Cord 302
    Brain Stem 303
    Cerebrum 303
Autonomic Nervous System 304
   Organization 304
    System Characteristics 304
   Sympathetic and Parasympa-
    thetic Divisions 306
    The Sympathetic Nervous
     System 306
    The Parasympathetic Nervous
     System 306
   Functional Correlates 306
   Synaptic Relationships 308
    Transmitters 308
    Cholinergic Receptor Sites . . . 308
    Adrenergic Receptors 309
   Adrenal Medulla 310
   Pharmacological Considerations . 311
    Parasympathetic System . . . 311
    Sympathetic System 312
Neuronal Response to Injury 312

Chapter 18:
Cardiovascular System **314**
General Characteristics 314
Mural Organization 314
Exchange System 314
High Pressure System 315
Low Pressure System 322
High and Low Pressure Systems
    Compared 322
Heart 323
   Mural Organization 323
   Cardiac Activity 325
    Regulatory Mechanisms 325
    Specialized Chemoreceptors . 325
    Specialized Baroreceptors . . . 326
    Neuroregulation 326

    Autonomic Reflex Activity 327
    Hormonal Influence 328
Lymphatic Vessels 328

Chapter 19:
Lymphatic System and
   Immunity **330**
General Characteristics 330
Diffuse Lymphatic Tissue 330
Dense Lymphatic Tissue 330
Lymphatic Organs 331
   Lymph Node 331
   Hemal Nodes and Hemolymph
    Nodes 334
   Spleen 334
   Thymus 337
   Bursa of Fabricius 341
Immunity 341
   Nonspecific Immunity 341
   Specific Immunity 341
   Hypersensitivity Reactions 345
   Type I Hypersensitivity 345
   Type II Hypersensitivity 346
   Type III Hypersensitivity 346
   Type IV Hypersensitivity 347
   Autoimmunity 347

Chapter 20:
Integumentary System **348**
General Characteristics 348
Mammalian Integument 348
   Typical Skin 348
   Organization of the Skin 349
   Specialized Skin Regions 350
   Hairs 350
   Special Skin Cells 355
   Glands of the Mammalian Skin . . 357
    Sebaceous and Tubular
     Glands 357
   Special Skin Glands 358
    Glands of the Perianal Region . 358
    Mammary Gland 361
    Miscellaneous Glands 365
Hooves and Claws 365
   Equine Foot 365
    Structure of the Hoof 365
    Corium of the Foot 371
   Ruminant and Porcine Claws . . . 371
   Claws of Carnivores 371
Integumentary Appendages 371
Repair of the Skin 372
Avian Integument 378

Chapter 21:
Digestive System I—Alimen-
   tary Canal **380**
General Characteristics 380
Oral Structures 380
   Buccal Cavity Proper 380
   Lip 381
   Cheek 381
   Hard and Soft Palates 381
   Tongue 382
Teeth 383
   Development 386
   Cellular and Matrical
    Components 388
   Associated Structures 389
   Types of Dentition 390
Pharynx 390

Esophagus 390
Glandular Stomach 393
   Structure 393
    Glandular Regions 395
    Histophysiology 398
Compound Stomach 400
   Histophysiology of Ruminant
    Digestion 404
Small Intestine 405
   Structure 405
   Regions of the Small Intestine . . 405
   Histophysiology of the Small
    Intestine 408
Large Intestine 409
   Structure 409
   Regions of the Large Intestine . . 409
   Histophysiology of the Large
    Intestine 410
Avian Digestive System 412
   Specific Components 412

Chapter 22:
Digestive System II—Extra-
   mural Organs **417**
Salivary Glands 417
Liver 419
   Histological Organization 420
   Liver Units 423
   Histophysiology of the Liver . . . 424
Gallbladder 428
Exocrine Pancreas 429

Chapter 23:
Urinary System **431**
Kidney 431
   General Features 431
   Nephron 433
    Renal Corpuscle 433
    Tubular Components 435
   Collecting Duct System 437
   Stromal Elements 438
Juxtaglomerular Complex 439
Histophysiology of the Kidney . . . 441
Urinary Passages 445

Chapter 24:
Respiratory System **447**
General Characteristics 447
Respiratory Tract 447
   Conductive Components 447
    Nasal Cavity 447
    Nasopharynx 449
    Larynx 449
    Trachea 449
    Extrapulmonary Bronchi . . . 450
Lung 450
   Conductive Components 450
    Intrapulmonary Bronchi . . . 450
    Bronchioles 452
   Transitional Components 453
    Respiratory Bronchioles . . . 453
   Exchange Components 455
    Alveolar Ducts, Saccules, and
     Alveoli 455
    Blood-Air Barrier 459
    Stromal Elements 459
   Histophysiology of the Lung . . . 460
    Exchange of Gases 460
    Regulation of Respiration . . . 462
Avian Respiratory System 462

Chapter **25:**
Endocrine System **467**
General Characteristics 467
Hypophysis Cerebri 467
Adenohypophysis 469
   Pars Distalis 469
     Chromophobic Cells 469
     Chromophilic Cells 469
   Pars Tuberalis 471
   Pars Intermedia 471
   Histophysiology of the
      Adenohypophysis 471
   Regulation of the
      Adenohypophysis 472
Neurohypophysis 472
Epiphysis Cerebri 473
Thyroid Gland 474
Parathyroid Glands 476
Adrenal Glands 478
   Adrenal Cortex 479
   Adrenal Medulla 483
Endocrine Pancreas 484
Miscellaneous Endocrine Glands . . 485

Chapter **26:**
Male Reproductive System . . **489**
General Characteristics 489
Testes 489
Genital Ducts 492

Spermatogenesis 495
Testicular Secretions 498
Accessory Glands 500
Urethra 502
Copulatory Organ 504

Chapter **27:**
Female Reproductive System **506**
General Characteristics 506
Ovary 506
Ovarian Cycle 507
Uterine Tubes 512
Uterus 513
Vagina 514
Vulva 514
Cyclic Changes 515
Species Differences 516
Comparative Placentology 517
   Distribution of Chorionic Villi . . . 519
   Extraembryonic Membrane
      Contributions 519
   Degree of Implantation 519
   Configuration of Chorionic
      Attachments 522
   Fetal and Maternal Contributions 522
Avian Reproductive System 523

Chapter **28:**
Eye and Ear **527**

General Characteristics 527
Eye 527
   Fibrous Tunic 528
     Sclera 528
     Cornea 529
   Vascular Tunic 532
     Choroid 532
Ciliary Body and Process 534
     Iris 535
   Compartments of the Eye 537
     Anterior Compartment 537
     Posterior Compartment 537
   Lens 537
   Nervous Tunic 539
     Organization of the Retina . . . 539
     Ocular Fundus 541
     Photoreceptor Cells 541
     Retinal Blood Supply 543
   Ocular Adnexa 543
     Eyelids 543
     Nictitating Membrane 544
     Lacrimal Apparatus 544
Ear 545
   External Ear 545
   Middle Ear 545
   Inner Ear 546
   Vestibular Apparatus 547
   Auditory Apparatus 549

SECTION **V: EXFOLIATIVE CYTOLOGY**

Chapter **29:**
**Introduction to Exfoliative
   Cytology** **554**
Introduction 554
Cytology of Selected Organs and
   Systems 554
   Nervous System 554

Hemic-Lymphatic System 554
Integumentary System 556
Digestive System 556
Urinary System 556
Respiratory System 557
Glandular Organs 558
Reproductive System 558

Body Cavities 559
Cytology of the Eye 561
Cytology of the Musculoskeletal
   System 561

Index **563**

List of Color Illustrations

(appears after Chapter 14)

Plate I. Various Stains of Selected Tissues and Organs 234

Plate II. Characteristics of Selected Cells 236

Plate III. Surface and Glandular Epithelia 238

Plate IV. Connective Tissue 240

Plate V. Muscular, Nervous, and Adipose Tissue 242

Plate VI. Peripheral Blood 244

Plate VII. Peripheral Blood and Exfoliative Cytology 246

Plate VIII. Exfoliative Cytology 248

SECTION I:

GENERAL PRINCIPLES OF HISTOLOGY

1: Insights into Histology

Introduction

As the study of a new discipline is initiated, the placement of the knowledge to be acquired into the proper perspective is often difficult. Questions concerning the nature, scope, depth, and relevance of such information often arise. Certainly, these questions are justifiable. The intent of the following short discourse is to answer a number of these questions.

The ultimate goal for the student of the biomedical sciences is an understanding of the organism in health and disease. The living organism is the sum of its constituent parts and much more. Thus, the study of the constituent parts is essential to gain some insights about the whole organism. Histology is one of those relevant biomedical disciplines that affords insights through an in-depth approach to the structure and function of the constituent parts.

Classically, *anatomy* is that branch of biomedical science that deals with the external and internal structure of the organism. Although classically considered to be a descriptive science exclusively, the objectives of this discipline are multiple and far exceed the limits of mere description. Descriptions of basic architectural patterns of cells, tissues, organs, and organisms are fundamental to the discipline. But, an understanding of the structural basis of function and mechanistic correlates is an essential component of anatomy. It is customary and didactically expedient to subdivide the science of anatomy into subdisciplines based upon the nature of the component parts and the methods by which they are studied. Accordingly, *gross anatomy* includes all those structural features that are studied by direct visual inspection, palpation, and/or dissection, whereas *histology* encompasses the study of structures that are not visible to the unaided eye.

If the student were to consult a medical dictionary, then he (she) would find that the terms *histology* and *microscopic anatomy* are synonyms. Unfortunately, the synonymous definition of these terms gives little insight into the evolution of this anatomical subdiscipline. Although it began as a simple descriptive science of subgross anatomic organization, histology has evolved into a hybridization of anatomy, physiology, chemistry, and physics. Whereas the classical definition of histology implies a purely descriptive science, the modern histology, microscopic anatomy, is a sophisticated science concerned with tissue structure and function from broad and multidisciplinary approaches.

Organology is the study of the structure and function of the numerous and varied component organs of an animal. Although studies of these organs may be approached from different perspectives, organs are studied commonly with a microscope. Thus, this branch of science falls within the purview of histology. *Comparative organology* emphasizes the organizational and functional differences and/or similarities of organs between and among various groupings of animals. The knowledge base encompassed by this discipline is essential for the student of Veterinary Medicine.

The expansion of any discipline, histology notwithstanding, is linked inexorably with the technical achievements of many disciplines. Advances in physics and engineering led sequentially to the development of various optical instruments used in histology: the light microscope, the transmission electron microscope, the scanning electron microscope, and other sophisticated optical instruments. The transmission and scanning electron microscopes are the tools of *ultrastructural cytology*, a body of knowledge encompassed by histology. Similarly, insights from inorganic chemistry, organic chemistry, and biochemistry have been applied to cells and tissues. Histology, then, includes the specialized subdisciplines of *histochemistry* and *cytochemistry*. Numerous other methodologies and subdisciplinary approaches have contributed to the broad and integrated body of knowledge that is histology: autoradiography, fluorescence techniques, immunocytochemistry, and culture techniques. These varied approaches require some type of microscope for observation. These are some of the tools of modern histology.

Finally, the discipline of histology is an integral component of a medical education. Not only does the subdiscipline afford insights into normal structure and function at the microscopic level of organization, but histology serves as the basic building block for understanding disease processes. The responses of cells and tissues to the insults associated with disease processes are the purview of *histopathology*.

Tissues—The Elements Of Organization

The term *histology*, derived from the Greek terms *histos* (web) and *logos* (study), means the study of tissues. The etymological derivation of the English word *tissue* is from the French *tissu*, which means *texture* or *weave*. This word was introduced into the medical sciences by a French gross anatomist and physician, Marie F. X. Bichat, in the late 18th century. He became fascinated by the various textures and weaves of the numerous structures that he noted during his detailed gross dissections. His observations resulted in the publication of a book in which he described more than 20 different tissues. It is interesting to note that this brilliant anatomist, considered by most to be the Father of Histology, did not use a microscope to found this discipline. Shortly after his death at the turn of the 19th century, the term histology was coined.

The original concept of 20 tissues comprising the body was useful in establishing the discipline. Today, most histologists recognize four basic tissue types with each type consisting of a number of subtypes. Some histologists, believing that the uniqueness of adipose tissue warrants a separate classification as a tissue, support the concept of five basic tissues. All of the diverse organs of the body result from the unique aggregation, association, and interdependence of these basic tissue types. The tissues, then, are the building blocks upon which the organs are constructed in a logical, orderly, and consistent manner. A thorough understanding of the tissues, their morphology and function, is essential for a comprehensive grasp of organ structure and function. Just as the organism is the sum of its organ components, so are the organs the sum of their tissue components. Similarly and logically, the tissues of the body are the products of their cellular and extracellular constituents. This logic can be extended to a more elementary level, because the cells and extracellular substances are the consequence of their biochemical composition.

A logical approach to histology is one that begins with biochemistry, progresses to the cells, continues to the tissues, and culminates with a study of the organs. Most students will have been exposed to biochemistry and cytology by this stage of their scientific growth and development. It is essential, therefore, to discuss the next order of organization—the tissues.

A tissue is a group of similar, identical, or dissimilar cells and their extracellular products that perform a specific function or a spectrum of related functions. This is a workable definition, but it does present some problems. In those instances in which the cells are identical, the recognition of a single tissue is obvious. In some tissues, the cells may be similar. In this circumstance, the identification of a single tissue may be accomplished easily. In others, cellular dissimilarity may imply multiple tissues incorrectly. In all of these situations, however, the functional relationships of the constituent cells unify them as cellular contributors to specific tissue types. Some tissues are characterized by scant amounts of extracellular materials, whereas others have tremendous amounts of these materials. Again, their functional relationships satisfy the definition. Extremes in structural and functional characteristics still satisfy the basic definition. Any artificial scheme of grouping biological entities is prone to interpretive problems, because **man classifies, nature doesn't.**

The *basic* or *simple tissues* of the body are: epithelia, connective tissues, muscular tissues, nervous tissues, and perhaps adipose tissue. The organs of the body consist of various quantities and types of these tissues in specific architectural patterns. Although the basic tissues are covered in detail in Section III, it is appropriate to place them in proper perspective now.

The first of these basic tissues is the *epithelium* (*epi*—upon, *thele*—nipple). Epithelia cover all of the external body surfaces, line all of the internal tubes of the body and form glands. Most of the epithelial tissues are derived from either the *ectoderm* (the external covering) or the *endoderm* (the internal covering); however, some epithelia are derived from the *mesoderm* of the embryo.

Characteristically, epithelial tissues have a high cellular density. The cells, usually quite similar and sometimes identical, are the predominant features. Little extracellular material is associated with these cells.

Protection is one of the prime functions of these tissues, but it is just one of a multiplicity of vital functions performed. Numerous morphological modifications to epithelia permit this functional diversity.

The nature of the epidermis of the skin affords protection from mechanical, bacterial, and dessicative damage. The epithelial tissue of the skin, the stratified squamous epithelium of the epidermis, is essential for locomotion (claws and hooves), protection (claws), heat conservation (hairs), and behavioral displays (feathers). The selective absorptive properties of the intestines permit entry of valuable metabolites while affording protection against the absorption of microorganisms, toxins, and other potentially toxic materials. Similarly, various materials (microorganisms, particulate matter, debris) are transported along epithelial surfaces by the action of cilia. Such modifications of the epithelia of the respiratory system also afford protection to the organism.

Secretory activity is a major function of epithelia. Special glandular modifications of epithelia represent vital functional adaptations. Sebaceous glands of the skin elaborate an oily material that softens the hairshafts and outermost layer of the skin. This secretory product keeps the skin pliable and impermeable to the movement of various materials in either direction. Mucous glands of various types secrete a viscous material that serves to moisten and lubricate many of the internal tubes of the body. Other glands elaborate materials such as saliva and digestive juices.

Many types of epithelial cells perform essential absorptive functions. Examples would include the cells of the respiratory, gastrointestinal, and urinary systems. Essential digested materials are absorbed by the gastrointestinal epithelium. Oxygen and carbon dioxide pass through the lining epithelium of the lung, whereas essential metabolites are absorbed by the tubular lining cells of the kidney.

Because the epithelial tissues are in contact with the animal's external environment (even the contents of internal tubes are external to the organism), much information concerning this environment can be sensed by these cells. Therefore, sensory functions are important homeostatic adaptations. These include cellular sensory modifications of the skin, gustatory organs, olfactory epithelium, and others.

Lastly, the gonads are composed of epithelial cells whose function is the perpetuation of the species.

Epithelial cells perform a diversity of functions. It will become apparent in Section III that corresponding morphological adaptations exist that permit this functional diversity.

The *connective tissues*, derivatives of the mesoderm, constitute one of the most diverse groups of the basic tissues. Although they are well named on the basis of their connective and binding properties, they subserve a variety of other functions. A

partial list of these varied functions includes: support, protection, mobility, insulation, thermoregulation, energy storage, repair, and nutrition.

Characteristically, connective tissues consist of groups of cells, in some cases quite dissimilar, that are separated by large quantities of extracellular materials, most of which are secreted by the constituent cells. These extracellular materials (*intercellular substance*) consist of various fibers and other biochemical compounds that impart specific structural and functional characteristics to these tissues. This intercellular material is suited ideally to the binding and connecting properties of some of these tissues. Similarly, the dense intercellular materials of cartilage and bone suit them ideally for their primary functions of support and mobility. *Adipose tissue* is a unique tissue that subserves protective, insulative, thermoregulatory, and metabolic functions. Blood, with its varied formed elements and plasma, is a unique connective tissue that affects, directly or indirectly, every cell of the body. The nutritive and defensive functions of this tissue are of vital importance to the organism.

The *muscular tissues* are derived from the mesoderm also. The cells of these tissues are modified uniquely for contraction. The movement of materials through the internal tubes of the body is accomplished primarily by smooth muscle. This movement includes the expression and transport of glandular secretions, the peristaltic movement of food through the digestive tract and the movement of blood through the vascular system. The movement or translocation of the organism within its environment is a function of the skeletal muscle of the body. The continuous movement of blood within the vascular system is the function of the cardiac muscle mass. The continuous demands made upon this organ are phenomenal. That it responds successfully for so long is even more remarkable. Throughout the course of the 70-year human life-span, the heart will have beaten approximately 2.58×10^9 times and will have pumped about 1.84×10^8 liters of blood.

Nervous tissue is derived from ectoderm and includes the brain, spinal cord, ganglia, and nerves. This tissue is organized uniquely to receive, transmit, integrate, and associate various stimuli from the animal's external and internal environment. The essence of these combined activities is the initiation of a response that maintains the well-being of the organism.

The basic tissues, then, are the building blocks of a complex organizational heirarchy—the organs. A comprehensive understanding of these tissue components is not only essential but simplifies the study of comparative organology.

2: Methods of Histology

Introduction

The technological progress in various disciplines of science affords the histologist a multiplicity of approaches for the study of cells and tissues. The type of information desired usually dictates the suitability of one approach over another or the use of a combination of approaches. The maximal information that is attainable with any particular technical approach requires a complete familiarity with the technique, an understanding of the nature and limitations of the informational output, and a comprehensive appreciation of its advantages and disadvantages. The following is an attempt to acquaint the student with the diversity of techniques that are available to examine living cells, dead cells, and components of cells. Any combination of these methods may be integral components of a comprehensive approach to histological problem solving.

Cell culture is a means of direct observation of living cells. Antibiotics have made this approach almost a matter of simple routine. Culturing techniques permit the continual observation, manipulation, and testing of explanted cells without any jeopardy to the donor (Figs. 2.1 and 2.2). Cellular differentiation, cellular transformations, cytogenetics, cellular metabolism, cell-to-cell interactions, host/parasite relationships, and other biological processes have been studied by this technique. Cell culture is indispensible in diagnostic virology (Figs. 2.3 and 2.4), vaccine development, and vaccine production.

Implantation of *transparent viewing chambers* and the *exteriorization* and *transillumination* of organs and tissues complements direct observation. Although the exteriorization technique imposes a limited time frame for observation, valuable insights concerning microcirculation and the response of various tissues and organs to chemotherapeutical agents have been obtained. Transparent viewing cham-

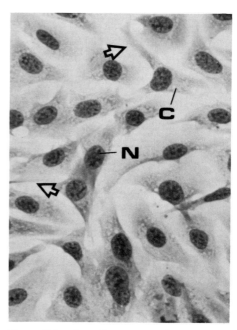

Figure 2.2. A medium-power micrograph of a monolayer of normal bovine fetal spleen cells. The nuclei *(N)* are vesicular and the foamy and granular cytoplasm *(C)* has processes *(open arrows)* that impart a stellate or spindle appearance. ×100 (Giemsa stain) (Courtesy H. Storz).

bers permit an extended period of observation. Neovascularization, cellular differentiation and movement, and other vital processes are studied by these techniques. The anterior chamber of the eye is a naturally occurring viewing chamber that is used in this approach.

The selective uptake of *vital* and *supravital stains* has added appreciably to our understanding of the function of some cells, cellular organelles and inclusions, and extracellular matrical materials. These stains have a low toxicity; they may be injected into a living organism (vital) or applied to living cells extirpated from the organism (supravital).

Oxytetracycline, a broad-spectrum antibiotic, may be used as a vital stain also. At therapeutic dosages this drug is deposited selectively at all surfaces upon which bone and similar tissues are being formed (Figs. 2.5 and 2.6). Insights concerning rates of

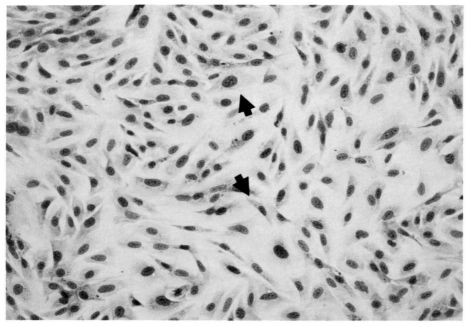

Figure 2.1. A low-power micrograph of a monolayer of normal bovine fetal spleen cells. Contact inhibition results in the formation of a monolayer of stellate- and spindle-shaped cells *(arrows)*. ×40 (Giemsa stain) (Courtesy H. Storz).

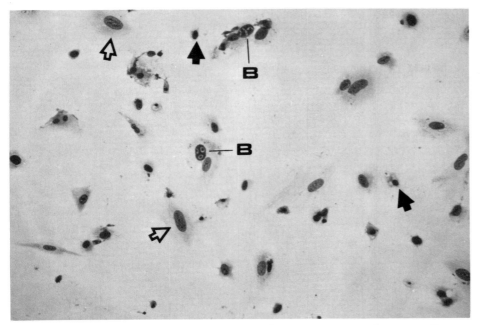

Figure 2.3. A low-power micrograph of a monolayer of bovine fetal spleen cells 48 hours postinfection with a parvovirus. The cells have been altered from the infection. The even distribution of cells as a monolayer is not apparent. Most of the cells are round and have withdrawn their cytoplasmic processes. Some nuclei are normal *(open arrows)*, whereas others are pyknotic *(solid arrows)*. Some cells contain nuclear inclusion bodies *(B)*. ×40 (Giemsa stain) (Courtesy H. Storz).

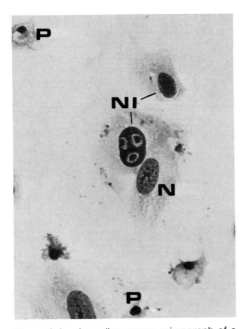

Figure 2.4. A medium-power micrograph of a monolayer of bovine fetal spleen cells 48 hours postinfection with a parvovirus. Pyknotic nuclei *(P)*, normal nuclei *(N)*, and nuclei with inclusion bodies *(NI)* are apparent. Note the altered cell shapes. Compare with Figure 2.2. ×100 (Giemsa stain) (Courtesy H. Storz).

bone formation, turnover, and maintenance have been obtained through carefully timed, spaced, serial administration of the drug.

Lithium carmine and trypan blue are vital dyes that are utilized to study phagocytosis. These dyes are phagocytized selectively by certain protective cells of the body.

Janus green B and neutral red are supravital stains used to study mitochondria and lysosomes.

The separation and purification of subcellular fractions through *differential centrifugation* and *density gradient centrifugation* are invaluable aids for the study of biochemical and metabolic phenomena.

The simplest method for the direct observation of living cells is to remove them from the organism, place them on a slide and examine them with a *phase-contrast microscope* (Fig. 3.4) or *dark-field microscope.*

Living cells and tissues are difficult to examine microscopically, because they are relatively transparent and thick. The indices of refraction of cellular constituents are sufficiently similar to preclude easy identification and differentiation of them. Superimposition artifacts and excessive absorption of light limits the amount of useful and reliable information that can be obtained from these unprocessed components. These problems are reduced when thin sections of tissues are obtained, stained, and examined. Such an approach requires extensive handling and processing of tissues; however, this approach is the standard for histological studies.

Tissues and cells for microscopic examination are usually killed by careful fixation to minimize alterations of in vivo mor-

phology. Subsequent processing ends with the tissues being embedded in a material that facilitates thin sectioning. Although a variety of techniques is used, the procedure used most commonly is the paraffin technique.

The Paraffin Technique

This technical approach to the preparation of samples for histological examination is a simple and reliable procedure. Although modification of cells and tissues does occur as a consequence of the treatments encompassed by this technique, the results are reliable and permit inferences to the in vivo situation. Unquestionably, the paraffin technique is the most common method used for the preparation of specimens for histology courses, diagnostic histopathology, and morphological research at the light microscopic level.

Acquisition. The acquisition of the sample is probably the most critical step in the process. Obtaining the sample requires that the histologist knows gross anatomy. Once the desired sample is identified, its removal must occur atraumatically. Most living tissues are fragile entities, the morphology of which changes with excesssive handling and poor extirpation techniques. **A "tissue conscience" is as important to the histologist as it is to the surgeon.** The use of dull and dirty scalpels or scissors and excessive pressure or traction applied with thumb forceps during sampling can induce drastic alterations to the components.

Most cells and tissues begin to undergo degenerative changes as soon as they are separated from their ideal microenvironments. Autolytic changes can be minimized by reducing the amount of time that the tissues are out of their normal microenvironments. Tissues must be removed rapidly and deftly; they should reach the fixative in the shortest time possible to inactivate the enzymes responsible for autolysis.

Fixation. Chemical fixation is used on histological specimens for the primary purpose of stopping *postmortem autolysis.* Because these agents denature protein, they inactivate the enzymes through which autolytic changes are mediated. Generally, the action of fixatives is sufficiently broad to react with most of the biochemical components of the cells. The frequently used chemical fixatives are formaldehyde, glutaraldehyde, paraformaldehyde, ethyl alcohol, acetic acid, picric acid, potassium dichromate, mercuric chloride, chromic acid, and osmic acid. Each has specific properties that result in various advantages and disadvantages of use.

Some chemical agents are *coagulative fixatives.* They induce changes in cells similar to those that occur when heat is applied to an egg. The conformation of macromolecules is altered markedly by such coagulative fixatives as ethanol and methanol. Others are described as *additive fixatives*. These achieve fixation by chemically react-ing with the biochemical components of the cell. They do not induce the marked morphological changes characteristic of the coagulative fixatives. The aldehydes (form-aldehyde, paraformaldehyde, and glutaral-dehyde) are additive fixatives that can be used in histological studies. **A 10% solution of neutral-buffered formalin is the most common fixative.** It consists of 10 volumes of commercial formalin (40% formalde-hyde in water) and 90 volumes of phos-phate-buffered water.

The action of most fixatives is multiple:

1) *prevent postmortem autolysis by inacti-vating hydrolytic enzymes*;
2) *facilitate sectioning of the tissues by hardening them*;
3) *enhance staining by acting as a mor-dant*;
4) *minimize the leaching of many constit-uents that results from subsequent proc-essing*;
5) *stabilize structural components in as near in vivo conditions as possible*;
6) *protect the histologist through the anti-septic properties of these substances.*

Immersion of the sample into the fixative must be accomplished immediately upon removal from the organism. Trimming of the block of tissue in fixative should result in a sample that is only a few millimeters thick. This permits thorough penetration (and fixation) of the entire sample. **The most ideal ratio of fixative volume to tissue volume is about 30:1.**

The actual time required for complete fixation to occur varies with the diffusion properties of the fixative, the concentration of the fixative, and the density of the tissue. Most formaldehyde fixation is achieved within a 24-hour period.

Dehydration and Clearing. Various sub-stances are used for this portion of the procedure. If paraffin or a similar substance is to be infiltrated into a sample to permit sectioning, then "something" must first be removed. That something is the 75% water that occurs in most tissues. After the exten-sive washing in water that functions to remove excess fixative, the sample is de-hydrated as a preparatory stage to embed-ding.

Many *dehydrating agents* are used (ethanol, butanol, dioxane, isopropanol), but the most common agent is ethanol. Tissue samples are subjected to increasing concentrations of alcohol until total dehy-dration is achieved with absolute ethanol. The use of this substance requires that the samples be processed through a clearing substance. Commonly employed *clearing agents* are xylene, toluene, and benzene. Generally, dehydrating and embedding agents are not miscible in each other. Clear-ing agents are substances that are miscible in dehydrating and embedding agents; thus, the clearing agent replaces the dehydrating fluid and the embedding agent replaces the clearing substance.

Embedding. This step is the one that

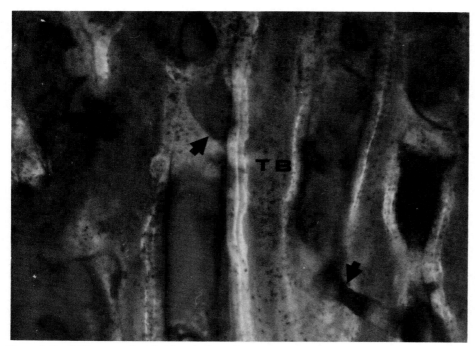

Figure 2.5. A 50-μm section of trabecular bone from an equine third carpal bone undergoing repair. Tetracycline at therapeutic dosages (5 mg/#) was administered at 10-day intervals and the sample was obtained 20 days after the initial injection. Two bright bands of fluorescence within trabecular bone *(TB)* indicate the uptake of tetracycline at the times of injection. The interval between the two labels indicates the amount of bone formed during the 10-day interim. *Solid arrows* are for orientation and comparison of this micrograph with Figure 2.6. ×40 (oxytetracycline-labeled, fluorescence microscopy).

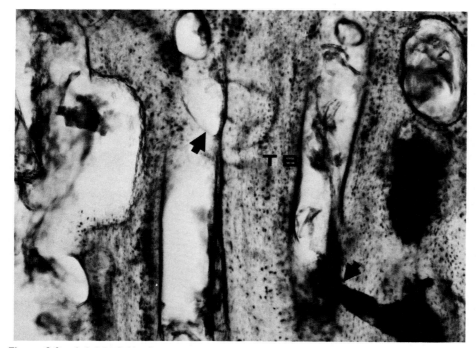

Figure 2.6. A bright-field micrograph of the same tissue field in Figure 2.5. The coupling of fluorescence and bright-field microscopy affords valuable insights about the morphological and dynamic changes that accompany fracture repair. ×40.

ultimately permits the specimen to be sectioned sufficiently thin to allow microscopic examination. The cleared specimens are processed through solutions containing increasing concentrations of paraffin. The pure embedding reagents must be maintained at their melting points (50–68°C) throughout the infiltration process, but the heat required to maintain the melted paraffin may induce some morphological changes in the tissues. Commercial mixtures of purified paraffin and plastic polymers are available. They are effective embedding materials. The infiltrated samples are placed into molds, surrounded with paraffin, and cooled. The blocks are then ready for sectioning.

Sectioning. After the paraffin has hardened, the molds are removed and the blocks are trimmed to expose the embedded tissue. They are then mounted on a *microtome* and thin shavings *(sections)* are removed from the cutting surface. The tendency of these sections to form a ribbon—the trailing edge of one section adhering to the leading edge of the subsequent section—facilitates the collection of the samples. Because some compression is associated with the sectioning process, ribbons may be floated on a warm water bath, subsequently stretched, and picked up on slides. Alternatively, portions of the ribbons may be put on slides. Placement of these slides on a warming table helps to minimize compression artifacts.

The *rotary microtome* permits the precision cutting of thin sections in 1μm (micron, micrometer) increments. Most specimens for routine histological examination, however, are sectioned between 5–7μm.

Staining and Mounting. The section and/or sections of paraffin-embedded materials affixed to glass slides simplify the remaining steps of staining and mounting. Most tissue stains are soluble in water or alcohol; therefore, the paraffin must be removed before staining. The reverse order of the previous procedures is used. Then the slides are stained. Once again the specimens are dehydrated, cleared, and covered subsequently with a mounting medium that is miscible with the clearing agent. A coverslip is applied to produce a permanent preparation.

Principles of Staining

General Features

Most observations of histological sections are achieved with a bright-field microscope. Cellular and tissue components are sufficiently similar optically that study is impossible without some enhancement of their optical properties. Stains accomplish this enhancement. Many stains and stain combinations are available and used in the histology laboratory (Plate I). The reactivity of stains with cells and tissues varies. Some stains are very selective, having a high specificity for certain cellular and/or tissue components. Other stains selectively stain cellular components and extracellular materials. Some stains are not selective and generally stain cellular and extracellular tissue components. Hematoxylin (H) and eosin (E) are examples of general stains that are used frequently in histology in combination with each other.

Stains are especially useful, and the information obtained is maximized, when the mechanisms governing their staining properties are understood. Unfortunately, the detailed chemical reactions for all stains is not understood completely; however, numerous and diverse stains exist for which the staining mechanisms are known. These afford the histologist the additional advantage of some chemical insights concerning cellular and tissue constituents.

Basic and Acidic Stains. Most of the stains used in histology are salts that dissociate in water. They are described as *acidic stains* or *basic stains.* If the coloring component is in the acidic radical, then the stain is designated an acidic stain. If the coloring component is in the basic radical, then the stain is designated a basic stain.

Acidic and basic staining is predicated upon the distribution of anionic and cationic charges associated generally with proteins and conjugated proteins in cells and tissues. The net charge on these substances is a function of the total number and nature of their ionizable radicals and the pH of their environment.

Basic cellular components react with acidic stains through the *neutralization* reaction that results in the formation of a (colored) salt and water. The basic components of the cells and tissues are *acidophilic*; they have an affinity for the acidic dyes. Acidic components of cells and tissues react with basic stains through the neutralization reaction. These biological components are *basophilic*; they have an affinity for the basic dyes.

Hematoxylin and Eosin. Neutralization is the staining mechanism of the H and E staining combination. The basic dye, hematoxylin, is applied first. Hematoxylin imparts a bluish purple color to acidic cellular components such as chromatin, ergastoplasm, and some secretory products. Eosin, the acidic dye, imparts a pink to red color to basic cellular components such as cytoplasm and numerous extracellular products.

Romanowsky Stains. The *modified Romanowsky stains* are useful dye combinations that contain methylene blue and eosin. Methylene blue is oxidized readily to form azure dyes. Combinations of methylene blue and the azure dyes (azure A, azure B, azure C) are called *polychromed methylene blue.* This stain has a broad staining range for acidic components. Eosin is the acidic counterstain. This combination of stains is used commonly to study peripheral blood smears and bone marrow samples (Plate VI).

Periodic Acid-Schiff Stain. The *periodic acid-Schiff (PAS)* reaction is a commonly employed and useful tool for histological studies. The procedure involves two steps to achieve the characteristic reactivity. The first reaction involves the oxidation of α-amino alcohols and/or 1,2 glycol groups to aldehydes by periodic acid. These aldehydes are then subjected to the Schiff reagent. The Schiff reagent consists of basic fuchsin that has been decolorized from its original red-violet color by the addition of sulfurous acid. The subsequent reaction of the aldehydes with the reagent forms a complex that restores the magenta color. Hematoxylin is the usual counterstain. Many carbohydrates and carbohydrate-protein complexes give a positive reaction with PAS (Plate I.12).

Selected Preparation Techniques

The amount and kind of information that can be obtained in histological studies is limited only by the number of approaches that can be utilized. If structural relationships are the only concern, then the paraffin technique is a useful method. Numerous shortcomings, however, are related to various factors:

1) *fixation employed*;
2) *heat required during subsequent processing*;
3) *use of organic solvents that have harsh effects upon the cells*;
4) *necessity for thick sections (5–7μm) to facilitate observation*;
5) *time required to complete the procedure.*

Many technical approaches are available that provide a variety of different information.

Cytological Studies. Cytological studies are useful adjuncts to histology when tissue architecture is a minimal concern. These techniques are discussed in Chapter 29.

Freezing Techniques. A concern for the alteration of morphology and function that may result from fixation and subsequent processing has been a strong impetus for the development of techniques less harsh than those employed routinely. The reduction of processing time has been an impetus also. Freezing techniques have been developed to satisfy these and other concerns. Frozen sections may be processed rapidly for examination. Biopsy samples obtained during surgery are usually prepared by this technique.

The *freeze drying technique* is one in which freshly extirpated samples are frozen to liquid nitrogen temperatures (−170°C) while under vacuum. The resulting sublimation of water precludes the necessity of fixation, dehydration, and clearing. Sam-

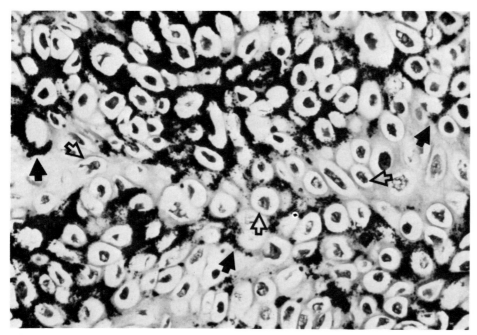

Figure 2.7. A section of developing cervine antler. The antler contains cartilage. The cartilage consists of chondrocytes *(open arrows)* surrounded by the matrix secreted by the cells. Mineralization of the cartilage *(solid arrows)* occurs before bone formation is initiated. The individual foci of mineralization *(solid arrows)* coalesce during development *(dark-staining areas)*. ×80 (von Kossa stain).

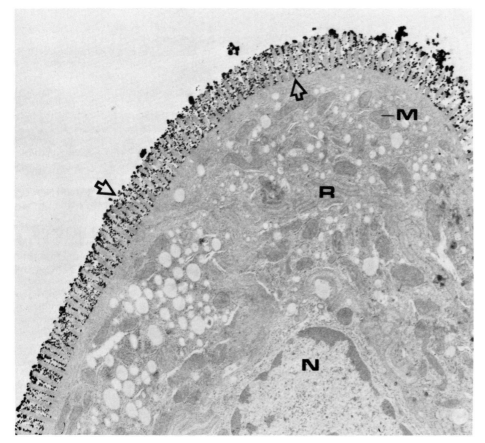

Figure 2.8. An electron micrograph of a murine intestinal lining cell. The dense granules *(open arrows)* associated with the microvilli represent reaction foci for the enzyme alkaline phosphatase. *M*, mitochondria; *R*, rough endoplasmic reticulum; *N*, nucleus. ×6000 (modified Gomori technique).

ples are subsequently embedded, sectioned, and stained. Of special interest is the ability to conduct chemical studies on such tissues. Valuable insights concerning the localization and activity of many enzymes have been obtained. Importantly, tissues prepared by this technique have fewer artifacts than those prepared by conventional chemical fixation.

Samples prepared by the *frozen section technique* afford advantages similar to the previously described technique; however, some damage occurs in the sample due to ice crystal formation, and section thinness is limited. Tissue samples are frozen rapidly to −40°C and are cut within an apparatus that maintains this temperature. This device, a *cryotome*, is a rotary microtome contained within a closed, cold environment.

Histochemistry and Cytochemistry. These techniques are attempts by histologist to localize and characterize various chemical substances within intact cells and tissues that chemists readily characterize in test tubes. The procedures range from simple to complex, but the principle that governs this technology is simple. If a chemical constituent can be complexed with a stain to enhance its visualization, then it lends itself to study. Naturally, the precision of the visualization and interpretation is a function of the specificity of the staining reaction, the localization and stability of the component being studied, and the degree to which the substance being examined is altered by processing techniques.

Virtually all chemical constituents of cells and tissues can be examined by histochemical and cytochemical methodologies: minerals (Fig. 2.7), carbohydrates, fats, proteins, and enzymes (Fig. 2.8).

The term *histochemistry* is usually confined to studies conducted at the light microscopic level of investigation, whereas *cytochemistry* is applicable to electron microscopic endeavors; however, the terms may be used synonymously. In enzyme studies, the effects of chemical fixation and the denaturation of enzymes is an important consideration. Freezing techniques and/or moderate chemical fixation are used. Electron microscopic studies of cytochemical phenomena require additionally that the trapped end-products are electron dense in order for visualization and localization to occur (Fig. 2.8).

Methacrylate Techniques. The paraffin technique affords a quick, easy and reliable method for histological inquiry. Despite these advantages, some significant disadvantages exist. The resolution of fine detail is not possible with specimens that must be sectioned between 5 and 7 μm. Also, the heat and harsh organic solvents required of the paraffin technique induce artifactual changes in the cells and tissues.

Electron microscopy offers the microscopist the advantage of greatly improved resolution. This enhanced resolution accrues from the electron beam characteristics and the ability to cut plastic-embedded specimens approximately 40 nm and less. Unfortunately, harsh chemicals must be used during the processing techniques. A definite morphological gap existed between the cytological features demonstrable with light microscopy and the paraffin technique and those features demonstrable with electron microscopy and plastic embedding/sectioning techniques.

Glycol methacrylate (GMA) is a water-soluble plastic embedding medium that permits the avoidance of the many harsh chemicals (dehydration and clearing agents) and heat required of the paraffin technique. Accordingly, the introduction of artifacts through processing methods is reduced. The use of glycol methacrylate represents a hybridization of techniques between light and electron microscopy that helps to bridge the gap between these methods of observation. Additionally, glycol methacrylate-embedded specimens can be sectioned in the 0.5- to 4.0- μm range. **Thin sectioning enhances the cytological detail that can be observed with the light microscope.**

Glycol methacrylate embedding is useful in various histochemical and cytochemical techniques. Determination of the activity of specific enzymes is enhanced when harsh chemicals are avoided. By avoiding or minimizing the exposure to water, water-soluble substances such as glycosaminoglycans are retained within the cells and tissues.

The glycol methacrylate techniques will not replace the standard techniques of light microscopic evaluation, but they do complement these methodologies.

Autoradiography. This technique is useful for histological studies of dynamic cellular processes. Sections of tissues are incubated with substances that have radioactive labels. Most generally these markers are soft β emitters. The sections are then coated with a photographic emulsion that is exposed by the radiation. The latent image in the photographic emulsion is developed routinely. Staining of the sections allows the visualization of the silver grains superimposed upon the section (Fig. 2.9). Because the silver grains are black and electron dense, these specimens may be examined with light or electron microscopes. Insights concerning cellular synthesis, secretion, and mitosis have resulted from these light and electron microscopic methods.

Immunocytochemistry. This technique is useful at the light and electron microscopic levels of investigation for the identification and localization of potentially antigenic substances (proteins, mucosubstances). A purified extract of the desired substance is prepared and injected as an *antigen* (Ag) into another animal. The animal develops an immune response and *antibodies* (Ab)

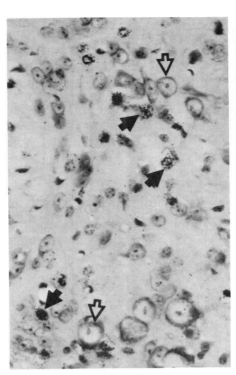

Figure 2.9. An autoradiograph of the substantia gelatinosa of the developing spinal cord of a mouse. The nuclei of some neurons *(open arrows)* are unlabeled, whereas the nuclei of other neurons *(solid arrows)* are labeled with tritiated thymidine. The electron-dense, dark-staining, silver grains are positioned over the nuclei that have been labeled. ×100 (Courtesy M. Cary and H. O. Nornes).

are produced. The antibodies are subsequently isolated and purified. The type of subsequent treatment is determined by the nature of the specific immunochemical technique utilized. In the *direct fluorescent antibody technique*, a fluorescent dye, usually fluorescein isothiocyanate (FITC), is complexed with the antibody. The Ab-FITC complex is allowed to interact with the specimen. Subsequent washing removes all of the reagent except that which has formed an Ag-Ab-FITC complex. Examination with an ultraviolet light source demonstrates fluorescence and localization of the antigen (Fig. 2.10). In the *indirect fluorescent antibody technique* an additional step is required to produce an *antiglobulin* (An) to the originally-produced antibody. The fluorescent tag is attached to the antiglobulin. The sample is incubated as described previously with a resultant Ag-AB-An-FITC complex being formed. This technique has the advantage of increasing the intensity and sensitivity of the reaction by allowing more complexes to form.

The markers used in this technique are not confined to fluorescent dyes. The enzyme *peroxidase* may be conjugated to the Ab or to the An. The visualization of the reactive complex is achieved by the histo-

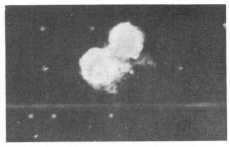

Figure 2.10. Direct fluorescent antibody reaction of bovine lung cells for IBR virus. Both cells are positive for the virus as evidenced by the bright fluorescence associated with them. ×400 (Courtesy J. J. England).

chemical demonstration of peroxidase activity. Similarly, *ferritin* may be complexed with the Ab or An. Ferritin contains 23% iron, is electron dense and permits visualization of the reaction with the electron microscope.

Investigations employing these techniques are not confined to substances considered to be classical antigens. Any substance of the body capable of inducing a humoral Ab response in another animal may be localized via this technology.

Transmission Electron Microscopy. The preparation of biological materials for electron microscopy is similar to those procedures described for the paraffin technique.

The sample must be acquired as atraumatically as possible. Any careless handling and/or introduction of contamination during this phase is observed readily at the levels of magnification used. Fixation, usually achieved with aldehydes (paraformaldehyde, glutaraldehyde) and/or osmic acid, must be excellent, and it is usually achieved at 4°C. Dehydration is similar to light microscopic preparations. Clearing agents are used in the manner described previously to permit the embedding of specimens in plastics. Plastic embedding, the precision of the cutting instruments, and the use of glass or diamond knives facilitate the acquistion of very thin specimens (30–60 nm thick). Thin sections are essential to allow the electron beam to pass through the specimen. If specimens are too thin, then insufficient scatter occurs, whereas excessively thick specimens absorb too much of the electron beam. Heavy metal stains (osmic acid, lead, uranium) are used to stain cellular and extracellular constituents selectively. These heavy metals, dispersed differentially throughout the specimen, account for the differential scattering of the electon beam and subsequent image formation (Fig. 2.11).

During the sectioning process, 1–2 μm sections of tissue are often examined for purposes of orientation. These thick sections are useful for histological study (Fig. 2.12).

Scanning Electron Microscopy. The

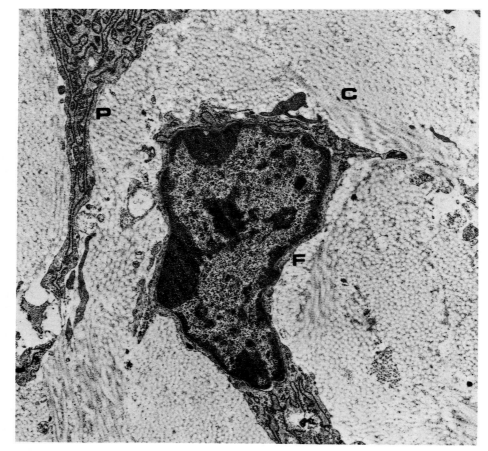

Figure 2.11. An electron micrograph of a section of cervine dermis. The fibroblast *(F)* is surrounded by collagenous fibers *(C)* cut in longitudinal and cross section. *P,* cytoplasmic processes of another fibroblast. ×6000.

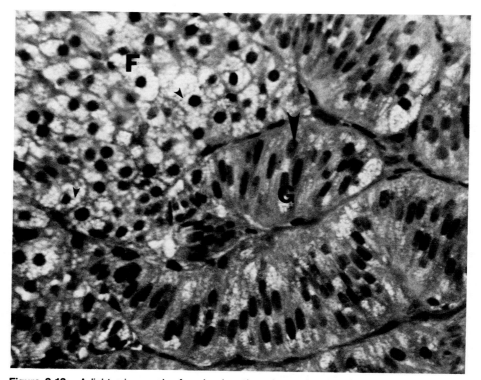

Figure 2.12. A light micrograph of a glycol methacrylate-embedded, 2-μm section of a canine adrenal gland. The sample is a section of the adrenal cortex. The cells of the zona fasciculata *(F)* and zona glomerulosa (G) have excellent detail. Note the foamy appearance of the spongiocytes *(small arrowheads)* and the nuclear detail *(large arrowheads)* of the cells of both zones. Although this preparation was made for light microscopy specifically, similar plastic sections are valuable for orientation purposes prior to studies with the electron microscope. ×100.

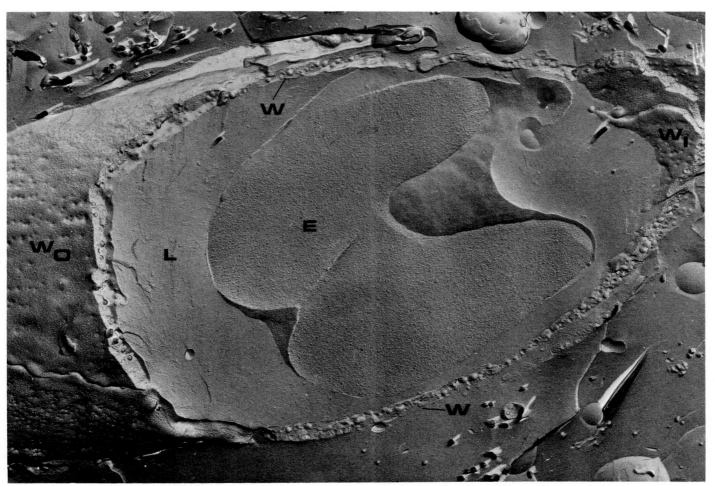

Figure 2.13.   An electron micrograph of a freeze fractured capillary. An erythrocyte *(E)* occupies the lumen *(L)* of the capillary. The wall of the capillary has been fractured in longitudinal *(W)* and cross section. The inner *(Wᵢ)* and outer *(Wₒ)* surfaces of the capillary wall are apparent. ×20,500 (Courtesy J. E. Rash).

preparation techniques for this type of microscopy are similar to those of transmission electron microscopy; however, sectioning and staining are not required. Specimens used in this technique are those that afford a natural or artificially induced surface. Specimens are acquired, fixed, and dried by *critical point drying* techniques to minimize surface tension distortion of their three-dimensional surface topography. They are then coated with a conductor, usually gold, that will backscatter secondary electrons to a collector. Such specimens require minimal treatment, yet they afford phenomenal insights into three-dimensional morphological relationships (Fig. 15.8.)

Freeze Fracturing. This technical approach utilizes the rapid freezing of samples with liquid nitrogen (or Freon) and bypasses the need for chemical fixation and dehydration. Frozen samples are mounted to plates within a special apparatus. The plates are moved slightly and the specimen is fractured. Metals, which are vaporized from a heated source, coat the fractured surfaces and form ultrathin metallic replicas of the fracture-induced surfaces. The metallic replicas are removed from the fractured tissues and are used as the sample that is examined with the transmission electron microscope. This technique affords high resolution insights into the architecture of real and induced surfaces—plasmalemma, cytomembranes, other organelles, matrical components, and inclusions (Fig. 2.13).

References

Baker, J. R.: *Cytological Techniques: The Principles Underlying Routine Methods.* 5th edition, John Wiley & Sons, Inc., New York, 1966.

Davenport, H. A.: *Histological and Histochemical Techniques.* W. B. Saunders, Philadelphia, 1960.

Gahan, P. B.: *Autoradiography for Biologists.* Academic Press, New York, 1972.

Gomori, G.: *Microscopic Histochemistry: Principles and Practice.* The University of Chicago Press, Chicago, 1952.

Hayat, M. A.: *Basic Electron Microscopy Techniques.* Van Nostrand Reinhold Company, New York, 1972.

Hayat, M. A.: *Principles and Techniques of Scanning Electron Microscopy: Biological Applications.* Vol. I, Van Nostrand Reinhold Company, New York, 1974.

Hearle, J. W. S., Sparrow, J. T. and Cross, P. M.: *The Use of the Scanning Electron Microscope.* Pergamon Press, New York, 1972.

Humason, G. L.: *Animal Tissue Techniques.* 3rd edition, W. H. Freeman and Company, San Francisco, 1972.

Koehler, J. K. (ed.): *Advanced Techniques in Biological Electron Microscopy.* Springer-Verlag, New York, 1973.

Koss, L. G.: *Diagnostic Cytology and Its Histopathologic Bases.* 2nd edition, J. B. Lippincott Company, Philadelphia, 1968.

Lillie, R. D.: *H. J. Conn's Biological Stains.* 9th edition, Williams & Wilkins Company, Baltimore, 1977.

Pearse, A. G. E.: *Histochemistry: Theoretical and Applied.* Vols. I and II, 3rd edition, Williams & Wilkins Company, Baltimore, 1968.

Pease, D. C.: *Histological Techniques for Electron Microscopy.* 2nd edition, Academic Press, New York, 1964.

Wischnitzer, S.: *Introduction to Electron Microscopy.* 2nd edition, Pergamon Press, 1970.

3: Microscopy and Interpretation

Introduction

The approach to the study of histology not only requires an appreciation of preparation techniques but also an understanding of the numerous ways by which cells and tissues can be examined. Both aspects dictate and/or limit the type of information that can be obtained from histological specimens. Preparation and examination are complemented by the ability to interpret that which is observed. The histologist, therefore, must combine these three facets of study to obtain a comprehensive understanding of structure and function.

Microscopy

The new student of histology is confronted with the interesting challenges of being able to conceptualize this new realm of structure and to appreciate the functional and dimensional relationships of the histologic components of the organism. The accompanying table and figure present dimensional considerations (Table 3.1 and Fig. 3.1), whereas the remainder of the text is devoted to the interpretive challenges.

Table 3.1.
Linear Measurements

Unit	Abbreviation	Relationships
Centimeter	cm	1 cm = 10^1 mm, 10^4 μm, 10^7 nm, 10^8 Å
Millimeter	mm	1 mm = 10^{-1} cm, 10^3 μm, 10^6 nm, 10^7 Å
Micrometer (Micron)	μm	1 μm = 10^{-4} cm, 10^{-3} mm, 10^3 nm, 10^4 Å
Nanometer (Millimicron)	nm	1 nm = 10^{-7} cm, 10^{-6} mm, 10^{-3} μm, 10^1 Å
Angstrom	Å	1 Å = 10^{-8} cm, 10^{-7} mm, 10^{-4} μm, 10^{-1} nm

The ability of the microscope to magnify objects is an important consideration in its usefulness to histology; however, the ability to display points that are approximated closely to each other as separate images is the most significant consideration. **The display of closely spaced objects as separate images is the resolving power of a lens or lens system.** Resolution is defined mathematically as R + 0.61 λ/NA. The resolving power (R in Å) is determined by the wavelength (λ in Å) of the illuminating source and the numerical aperture (NA) of the objective lens. The numerical aperture for a lens, n sin α, is the refractive index (n) multiplied by the sine of the half angle formed between the specimen and the maximal opening of the lens. This mathematical expression is a description of the light gathering properties of the lens. Wavelengths of about 5000 Å are used commonly in light microscopes, and the numerical aperture of good oil-immersion objective lenses is about 1.4. The resolving power for a system with these values would be approximately 2200 Å. Any components closer than 2200 Å would not be seen as separate objects. A reasonable estimate of the theoretical resolving power of an optical system is λ/2.

Spherical aberration, the inability of a curved surface to bring monochromatic light to a single focus, can affect resolution. Similarly, *chromatic aberration*, the manifestation of multiple focal points based upon the differential refraction of polychromatic light, can affect image quality. Generally, these aberrations are not significant in good light-optical systems, because the lenses are corrected for them.

Bright-Field Microscopy. The bright-field microscope is the instrument most commonly used in histology (Fig. 3.2). The limit of resolution of the compound microscope is approximately 2200 Å. Because of the transparency of living tissues, stained sections are necessary for maximal effectiveness of this type of microscopy.

Theoretically, the resolution of bright-

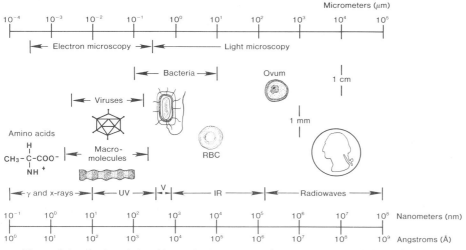

Figure 3.1. Scalar relationships and relative sizes of biological and nonbiological entities.

field microscopy can be increased by using an illumination source with a shorter wavelength. Wavelengths shorter than 4000 Å, however, are not transmitted through glass lenses. The ultimate limitation to resolution with this microscope, therefore, is a function of lens characteristics, not wavelength.

Ultraviolet Microscopy. This type of microscope utilizes an ultraviolet radiation source that emits radiation with wavelengths between 1000 Å and 3000 Å. An estimate of resolution of this system is between 500 Å and 1500 Å. Quartz lenses are necessary to allow this short wave radiation to enter the optical system. Ultraviolet radiation cannot be seen; therefore, photographic techniques must be employed.

Also, these wavelengths are damaging to the retina and living specimens. The primary application of this type of microscopy is in microspectrophotometry as an adjunct to histochemical studies.

Fluorescence Microscopy. This is a form of visible light microscopy in which an ultraviolet emitter is used as the light source. This monochromatic light serves as an excitatory illumination source to molecules that absorb the light and re-emit wavelengths in the visible range of the spec-

trum (Plate I.10). Barrier filters prevent the shorter wavelengths from reaching the retina. This is the type of microscopy used in the fluorescent antibody techniques described in Chapter 2.

Dark-Field Microscopy. This type of microscopy is achieved by slightly modifying a bright-field microscope. The usual condenser is replaced by one that causes light to strike the image at an oblique angle without any direct illumination reaching the objective lens. The light reaching the

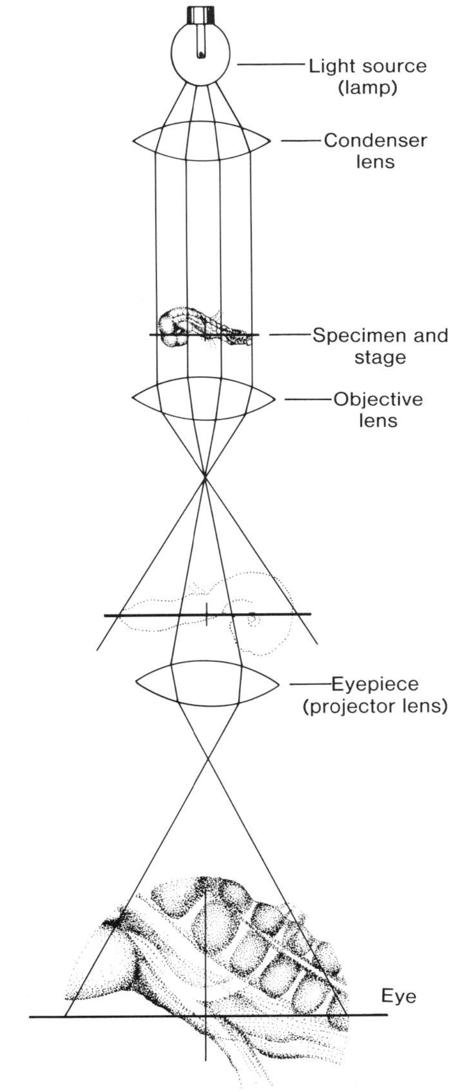

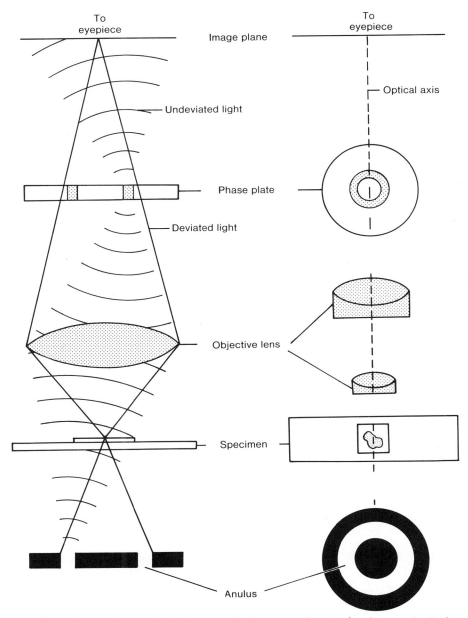

Figure 3.2. Diagram of the optical pathway in a bright-field microscope. The light source passes through glass lenses and the specimen before forming an image within the eye on the retina. Compare with Figure 3.8.

Figure 3.3. Diagram of the optical pathway and primary constituents of a phase-contrast microscope. The anulus and phase plate are the unique components of the microscope. The anulus presents an anular ring of light to the objective lens, thus separating the undeviated and deviated light rays from each other. The phase plate, built into the back focal plane of the objective lens, retards the central (undeviated) beam by ¼ λ and absorbs about 75% of this central light. The retardation is manifested as interference at the image plane and accounts for the contrast enhancement.

objective lens results from the scattering of light that occurs at the boundaries (interfaces) between components with different refractive indices. Cells and other tissue components appear bright against a dark background. The limits of resolution are similar to the bright-field microscope. Dark-field microscopes enable the microscopist to examine living, unstained specimens.

Phase-Contrast and Interference Microscopy. The phase-contrast microscope is a modified conventional microscope that requires a special condenser *(Zernike condenser)* and a *phase plate* positioned behind the objective lens. The alignment of optical components is achieved with a *focusing telescope.* As living or unstained specimens are transilluminated, the various constituents transmit phase-altered light as a function of their slightly different refractive indices and thicknesses. This *phase-altered (deviated) light* interacts with the *normophasic (undeviated) light* to produce an image. The image created through constructive and destructive interference results in an alteration of intensity that is visible. **The essence of the phase-contrast microscope, therefore, is the conversion of undetectable phase differences to amplitude difference that are visible to the human retina** (Fig. 3.3). This type of microscopy is especially useful for the study of living and unstained specimens (Fig. 3.4).

The same principles govern the Normarski interference phase microscope. Its sin-glemost advantage is the three-dimensional imaging of cells and tissues (Figs. 3.5 and 3.6).

Polarizing Microscopy. Some substances contained within or secreted by cells have a highly ordered molecular organization. When a beam of polarized light is passed through such substances, the transmitted light is split into two rays that are perpendicular to each other. An *ordinary ray* follows the laws of refraction, whereas the *extraordinary ray* undergoes a velocity change. This phenomenon is called *birefringence.* Birefringence is the property of having more than one refractive index. The indices are dependent upon the plane of polarized light vibration relative to the molecular orientation. Such substances are *anisotropic.* Substances that possess a single refractive index independent of the plane of polarized light vibration are *isotropic.*

This type of microscope is simply a bright-field microscpe to which a polarizer and an analyzer have been added with the specimen located between them. It is useful in studying such cellular constituents as the A (anisotropic) and I (isotropic) bands of muscle, and the orderly nature of bone (Fig. 3.7).

Transmission Electron Microscope (TEM). Although the general principles that govern light optical systems are applicable to electron microscopy, electron microscopes possess a number of unique features and characteristics because of the nature of the illumination source—the elec-

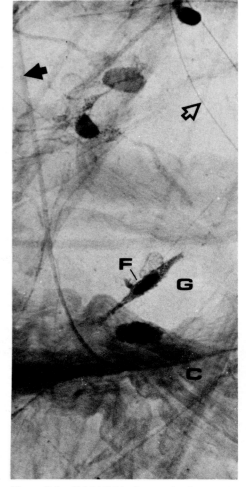

Figure 3.5. Bright-field micrograph of a stretch preparation of loose connective tissue. *F*, fibroblast; *solid arrow*, collagenous fiber; *open arrow*, elastic fiber; *C*, mass of collagenous fibers; *G*, ground substance. Compare with Figure 3.6. ×160.

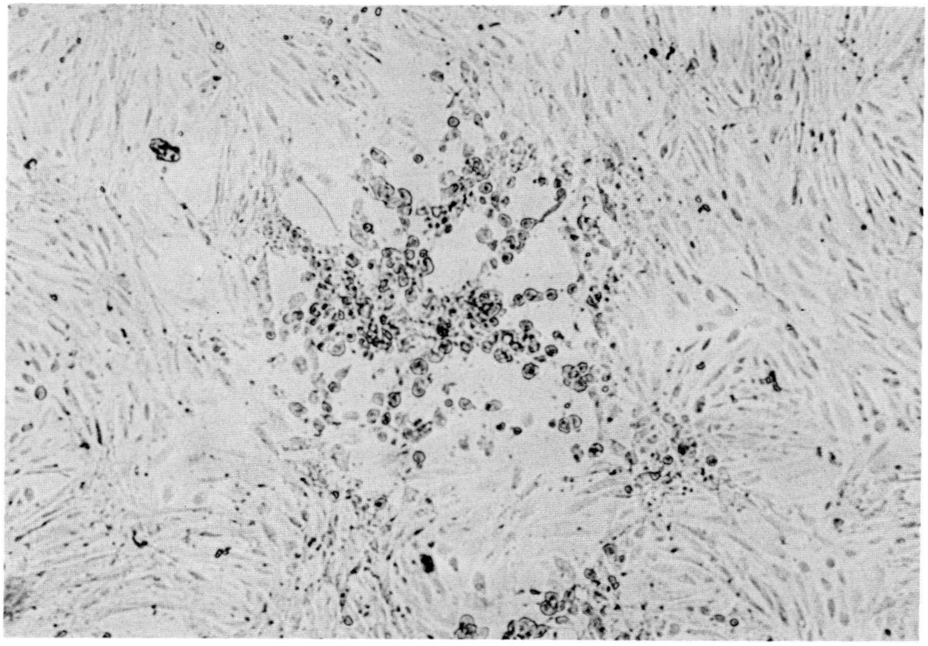

tron (Fig. 3.8). The massive, inverted column of the TEM consists of a source of electrons, a means of accelerating electrons, electromagnetic lenses to control them, a vacuum system, and an image translation system.

The light source is a triode in which the heated tungsten filament *(cathode)* is the source of electrons. Electrons are accelerated away from the cathode by the high potential of the *anode plate,* while the *grid (gun cap)* controls the amount of electon flow. The wavelength of the electrons is a function of the accelerating voltage, as expressed by de Broglie as: $\lambda = 12.3/V^{1/2}$. The wavelength at 50,000 volts would be 0.05 Å, whereas at 100,000 volts it would be 0.04 Å. A theoretical approximation of resolution ($\lambda/2$) would be 0.025 Å and 0.02 Å, respectively. This improved, theoretical resolution represents a potential 110,000-

Figure 3.4. Phase-contrast micrograph of bovine embryonic lung cells in culture. The culture was infected with IBR virus particles. The clumped cells in the center of the field are undergoing cytopathic changes as a consequence of the viral infection. ×16. (Courtesy J. J. England).

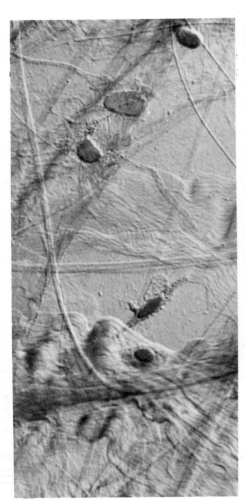

Figure 3.6. Nomarski interference phase micrograph of the same tissue field as that of Figure 3.5. The three-dimensional relief is a distinct advantage of this type of optical system. ×160.

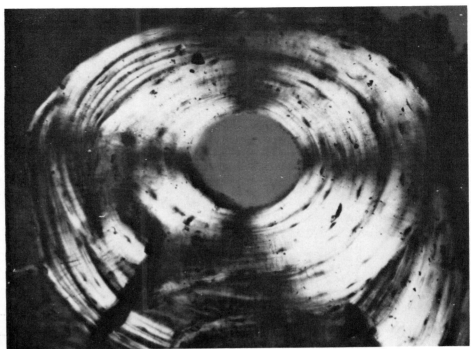

Figure 3.7. A canine osteon of bone photographed with polarizing microscopy. The four light bands radiating from the center of the osteon are indicative of the anisotropic properties of lamellar bone. ×40.

fold improvement over the theoretical resolution of conventional, light optical systems. Practically, this has not been achieved because of the imperfections (spherical aberration) of the lenses used. Most modern TEMs permit 3- to 5-Å resolution, but the nature of most biological specimens limits the average routine resolution to greater than 20 Å. This still represents an approximate 110-fold improvement of the resolution possible with bright-field microscopy.

Electromagnetic lenses control the path of the electrons through the condenser, objective, and projector lenses to the phosphorescent viewing screen. The invisible electrons strike the fluorescent screen causing emission of light in the visible spectrum; the electron-depleted beam is converted to a visible image. The visible image is used for locating desired morphological features and for focusing. Photographs are used routinely to study morphology revealed by the TEM.

Inasmuch as the mean free path of electrons in air is small, all of the events associated with electron microscopic imaging must occur within a vacuum.

The nature of the illuminating beam requires that the specimens are thin (<1000 Å) and stained with materials sufficiently dense to scatter electrons. The "depleted" beam that is projected to the viewing screen, in all simplicity, can be considered a shadow of the specimen.

Scanning Electron Microscopy (SEM). The optical system of the SEM is simpler than that of a TEM and its principles of operation are different (Fig. 3.9). The SEM consists of an electon source (cathode, grid and anode), condenser lens, and objective lens. The beam is focused on the surface of a coated specimen; however, the beam is not stationary. A scan generator moves the beam across the surface of the specimen in an orderly manner—a raster pattern. The scan generator also synchronizes the raster pattern of a cathode ray tube (CRT) with that of the beam raster. Electrons are backscattered from the surface of the specimen and picked up by an electon collector. The synchronized scan of the beam raster with that of the CRT permits a point for point display of the backscattered electrons on the CRT. The various angles of the specimen determine, point for point, the number of electrons that will reach the collector. This accounts for the variable intensity on the display screen. Magnification in this microscope is a function of the CRT raster scan length divided by the beam raster scan length. Because the CRT scan is constant, the progressive decrease in beam raster scan length results in an increased magnification.

The SEM does not replace the TEM. The biggest advantage of the SEM is its depth of field. This permits the display of three-dimensional images.

Interpretation

The interpretive skills required of the histologist are numerous and varied. The approach to interpretation demands a comprehensive appreciation of the limitations and advantages of the varied preparatory techniques that may be employed. If an histologist were interested in observing and/or staining various lipid components of cells, then the paraffin technique would probably be of little value. Many lipids are soluble in the chemicals (alcohol, xylene, chloroform) used for processing tissues by this methodology. Similarly, accurate indications of glycogen content are difficult to obtain if cells and tissues are exposed routinely to water during processing. Free glycogen molecules, being water soluble, are leached from cells during processing. A consideration of the type of fixation is important to the enzyme histochemist, because complete or partial denaturation of proteins affects enzyme catalysis dramatically.

Similarly, the type of microscope chosen to examine cells and tissues is linked to the preparatory processes required. Also, the type of information that can be obtained from a specified type of microscopy is limited. In many instances, the use of different types of microscopes is necessary and advantageous for the solution of histological problems.

Notwithstanding the significance of the previously discussed factors, the most important aspect of interpretive skills is an understanding of structure. This understanding must be sufficiently comprehensive to enable the histologist to translate the two-dimensional and static, structural and functional representations of sections into the three-dimensional and dynamic relationships that characterize the living organism. The remainder of this discussion is directed toward the skills requisite for the examination and interpretation of histological sections prepared by the paraffin technique.

Examination of the Specimen. Most histological studies are initiated at the time the sample is obtained. The histologist knows the organ from which the sample was obtained and probably noted its gross structural features (normal or abnormal). Most histologists do not have to worry about the gross anatomical origin of the sample at the time of evaluation. They either know the organ of origin or recognize the histological features that permit identification of the organ. **The study of histology without benefit of gross anatomical integration creates an artificial didactic situation, especially during examinations, that requires the student histologist to rely upon microscopic features to identify cells, tissues and organs.**

The initial step in the examination of sections, whether in the teaching or research laboratories, does not begin with the microscope. **All sections of known or unknown origin are best examined first with the unaided eye.** Many features of histological structure are evident through the use of this cursory yet effective first step. The distribution of staining properties (basophilia, acidophilia), the presence or absence of hollow spaces (lumina), and other architectural features may serve to direct attention to certain regions of the section. More-

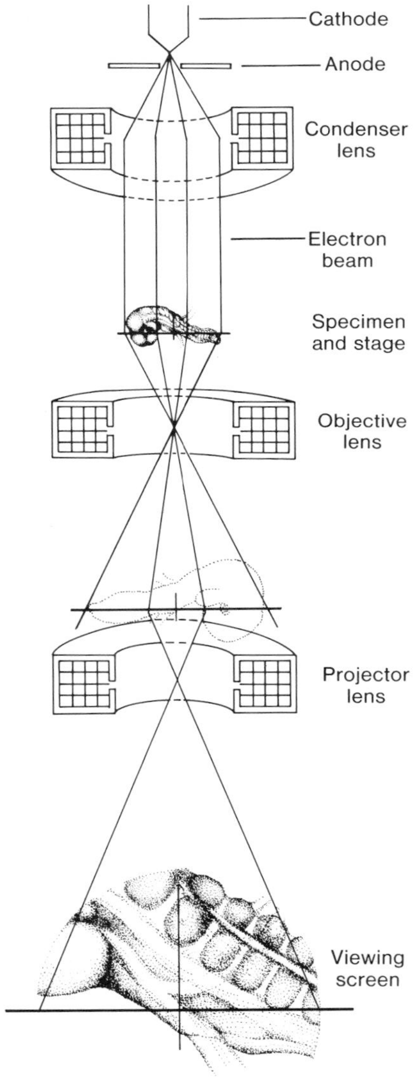

Figure 3.8. Diagram of the electron pathway in a TEM. The illumination source emits electrons that are refracted by magnetic lenses. Whereas the optical components are the same as a compound microscope, the TEM is many times larger that its bright-field counterpart. Compare with Figure 3.2.

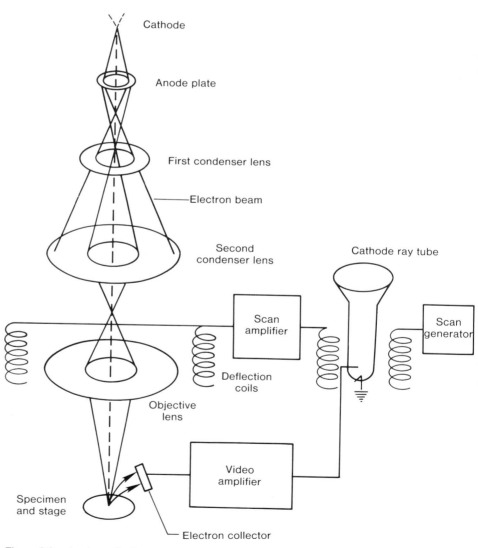

Figure 3.9. A schematic diagram of a SEM. The electrons pass through the column to the objective lens. The objective lens focuses the electron beam on the specimen. The deflection coils move the beam back and forth across the specimen. The detector picks up backscattered electrons. The signal is converted to an image on a CRT. Micrographs are obtained by photographing the display face of the CRT.

over, such an examination, if conducted carefully, limits the number of interpretive possibilities that exist.

The tendency "to want to see more" by going directly to the highest magnification usually results in a lack of orientation for the novice. Each incremental increase in magnification is always accompanied by a progressively narrower field of vision. It is best to progress through each stage of magnification noting the specific architectural features, cellular components, extracellular materials, and other structural features that characterize each field. The microscopist, literally, gets more and more information about less and less tissue with each increase in magnification. A routine examination may culminate with use of the oil-immersion lens. Often, however, the desired information about tissues is obtainable without the use of this lens.

Color and Morphology. The most important features to learn initially about cells and tissues are their morphological characteristics. If morphology is learned, understood and appreciated, then the color really does not matter. Color should be an aid to learning and study, not a crutch. Electron micrographs are an important part of the study of histology; they are black and white.

The sooner the student can learn to rely on morphology independent of tinctorial properties, the sooner the student will make the transition from histology, per se, to ultrastructural cytology. This text will assist in that transition. The judicious use of color in the text is intended as an aid to study.

Sectioning and Morphology. The first challenge in histology is to realize that the fixed, processed, stained, and sectioned piece of the body truly represents a reasonable sample of body constituents. The structural and functional relationships that are visible on the slide are a captured moment in the life of the organism or a part of the organism. The cells and tissues may not have had the exact same structural or functional characteristics the moment before section acquistion nor the moment later, if the life of that sample had progressed beyond the sampling point. Because the sample is representative, reasonable inferences about the organism and/or its constituent parts can be made.

The second challenge relates to the rellability of a section of tissue. Does a section of tissue from the spleen, liver, kidney, lung, or any other organ truly represent the entire organ? Admittedly, the student is forced to accept on faith, or conduct extensive self-inquiry, that the sample does represent something from within the organism. All the student needs to do is to accept that the small samples are representative and then proceed mentally to convert these biplanar and static samples into three-dimensional and dynamic pictures.

The last challenge is the ability of converting biplanar sections into a three-dimensional whole. Such a transition is necessary. Scientists do not work with sections for the sake of the sections. The use of sections is simply an expeditious way of gaining insights about the constituent parts, and thus the organism, without examining every milligram of the organism. The ability to convert these biplanar images to a three-dimensional whole is a function of familiarity and exposure.

Those items with which we are most familiar in our everyday existence are easily conceptualized. The word "chair" evokes a mental image of a chair without much difficulty. What, however, is the mental image of a chair if a person were shown this item in various planes of section (view)? The drafting student may have the advantage. Being familiar with top, side and front views (sections), this student may construct

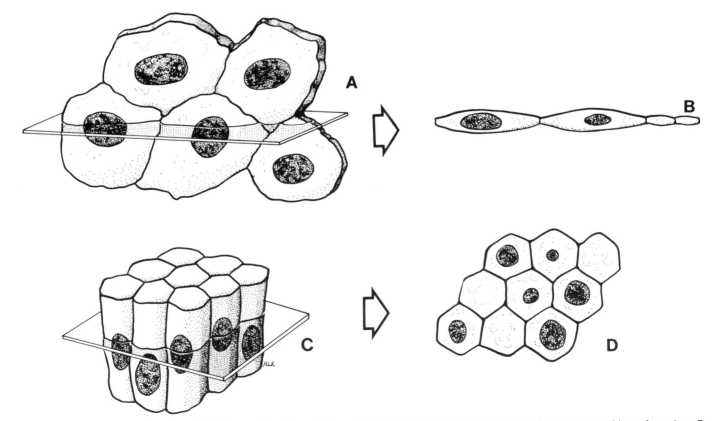

Figure 3.10.   The apparent alteration of cell shape with different views. *A.* The flattened or pancake-shaped cells appear round in surface view. *B.* After sectioning in a plane perpendicular to the surface, the cells appear flattened and elongated. The cells are a variable length, the nuclei are different sizes, and two of the cells appear to be devoid of nuclei. *C.* Some cells appear as columns when viewed from the side. *D.* After sectioning in a plane parallel to the surface, the cells appear more like those in *A* than *C.* Whereas their hexagonal shape is obvious in section, it would not have been obvious in a true side view. The uniform cells now appear to have nuclei of different sizes, and some cells appear to be devoid of nuclei.

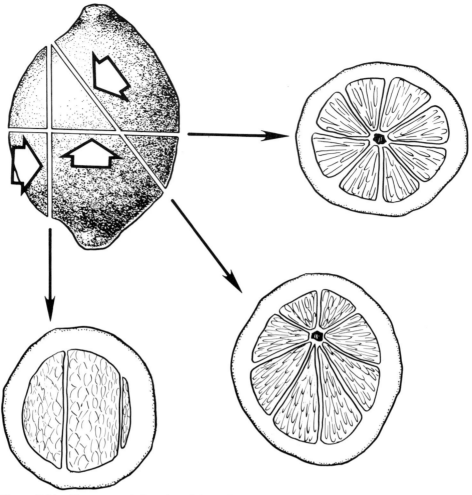

Figure 3.11. The apparent alteration of the architectural subdivisions of a lemon as a function of different planes of section. Cross sections, oblique sections, and parasagittal sections of this familiar fruit afford different perspectives of its internal organization.

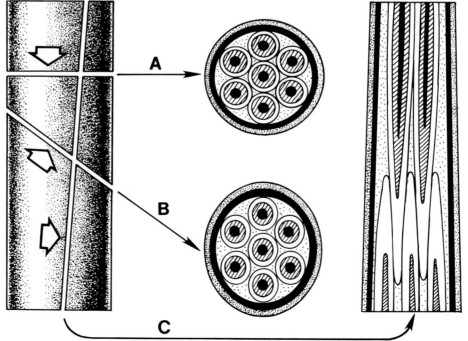

Figure 3.12. The apparent alteration of internal constituents of a coaxial cable as a result of different planes of section. (Redrawn and modified after Ham, A. W.: *Histology*. 6th edition, J. B. Lippincott, Philadelphia, 1969.)

the orthographic projection (three-dimensinal image) quite readily. Others of us may take longer but arrive at the same point—

a three-dimensional image of a chair. In many instances in histology, however, the student must be prepared to think three-

dimensionally from a single point of view or plane of section. A section normal to the long axis of pancake-shaped or flattened cells gives misleading information about cell shape (Fig. 3.10). In both instances, the third dimension must be considered.

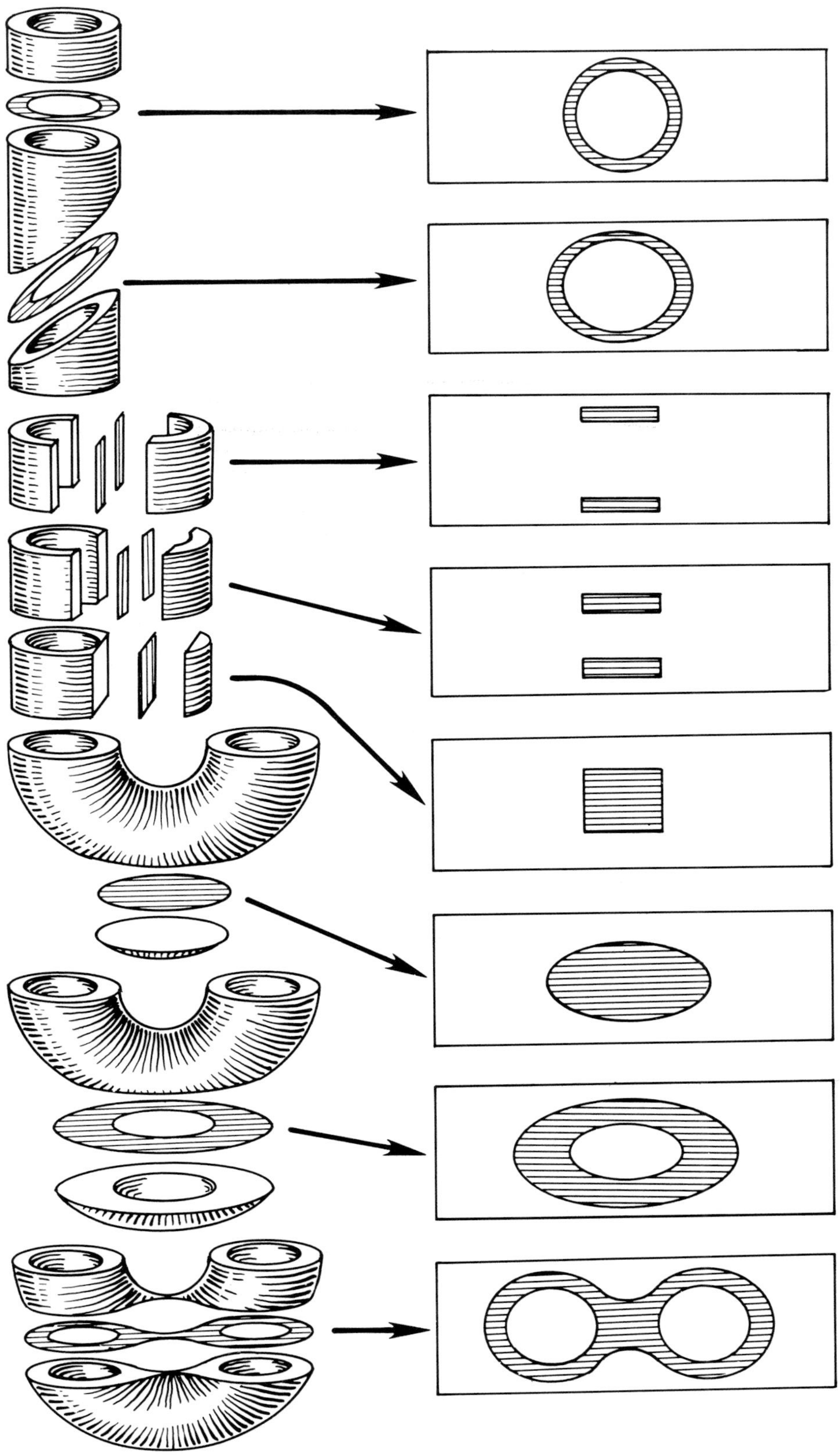

The correlation of three-dimensional structure with biplanar representations of familiar items is useful. The first slice perpendicular to the long axis of a hard-boiled egg rarely causes concern about the absence of a yolk. Progressive sectioning, also, will eventually "lose" the yolk. The three-dimensional relationship of the yolk to the white accounts for its sectioned structure. Similar problems are encountered in sections of tissues. Although all cells have nuclei, not all of the nuclei will be encountered in a single section (plane) of a given tissue (Fig. 3.10). The student can be as confident about the presence of a nucleus as he (she) was confident about the presence of a yolk. Importantly, misinterpretations of three-dimensional structure and components can occur with sectioning of an egg. Similar misinterpretations can occur in histology. The following considerations help to minimize such interpretive errors: familiarity with that which is sectioned, increasing the number of sections, and faith in the accumulated knowledge of histology relating to three-dimensional structure.

The tissue components of many organs are disposed generally in a pattern that affords various architectural subdivisions. The section of the familiar lemon demonstrates aptly the alteration of appearance associated with a specific slice or section of this fruit (Fig. 3.11). Sections of organs also will appear differently as a function of the plane of section. The student must be aware of these different representations when slides are being examined.

Some organs of the body are arranged as solid, tubular structures. Often, they are cut in simple, longitudinal or cross sections. Sometimes, these organs are sectioned obliquely. Their representation is best compared with different planes of section of a coaxial cable (Fig. 3.12). The altered appearance of the cable, especially in the oblique section (Fig. 3.12C), gives the misleading impression of discontinuity between the components.

Many organs of the body are arranged three-dimensionally as elongated, hollow, tubular structures (Fig. 3.13). The accompanying diagram demonstrates that such structures may assume various shapes in section. These shapes, if not carefully examined and interpreted, can give false impressions of the real nature of these structural entities.

Histological Artifacts. There is no doubt that processing tissues for histological examination induces many changes in cells and tissues. The student must learn to distinguish between changes that are constant

Figure 3.13.   The appearance of a hollow, tubular structure in various planes of section. (Redrawn and modified after Ham, A. W.: *Histology*. 6th edition, J. B. Lippincott, Philadelphia, 1969.)

and predictable and those alterations that result from capricious handling and/or processing of samples—*artifacts.*

Excessive shrinkage and/or swelling can alter the biplanar relationships of tissue components. Incomplete embedding often results in the complete loss of a region of a tissue during the sectioning process. Incomplete removal of the stain can be manifested as an excessive tissue precipitate. Improper knife angles during sectioning can impart a wavy (alternating thick and thin) characteristic to the tissue. The thick portion will appear more dense because of superimposition artifacts. Similarly, poorly sharpened knives will nick and scratch the paraffin block during sectioning. If the section is not stretched onto the slide, then folds or wrinkles will become apparent. Excessive stretching of the paraffin section can distort spatial relationships, too.

References

Brachet, J. and Mirsky, A. E.: *The Cell: Biochemistry, Physiology and Morphology.* Vol. I, Academic Press, New York, 1959.

Bullivant, S.: Freeze-etching and freeze-fracturing. *In:* Koehler, J. (ed.), *Advanced Techniques in Biological Electron Microscopy,* pp. 66–112. Springer-Verlag, New York, 1973.

Causey, G.: *Electron Microscopy: A Textbook for Students of Medicine and Biology.* Williams & Wilkins Company, Baltimore, 1962.

Cosslett, V. E.: *Modern Microscopy or Seeing the Very Small.* Cornell University Press, Ithaca, 1968.

Elias, H.: Three-dimensional structure identified from single sections. Science, *174:*993, 1971.

Elias, H. and Pauly, J. E.: *Human Microanatomy.* 3rd edition, F. A. Davis Company, Philadelphia, 1971.

Grivet, P.: *Electron Optics.* Vols I and II, 2nd edition. Pergamon Press, New York, 1972.

Hall, T., Echlin, P. and Kaufmann, R.: *Microprobe Analysis as Applied to Cells and Tissues.* Academic Press, New York, 1974.

Hayat, M. A.: *Principles and Techniques of Scanning Electron Microscopy: Biological Applications.* Vol I, Van Nostrand Reinhold Company, New York, 1974.

Needham, G. H.: *The Practical Use of the Microscope Including Photomicrography.* Charles C Thomas Co., Springfield, 1958.

Pollister, A. W. (ed.): *Physical Techniques in Biological Research.* 2nd edition, Vol. III, Academic Press, New York, 1966–1969.

Sjostrand, F. S.: *Electron Microscopy of Cells and Tissues: Instrumentation and Techniques.* Vol. I, Academic Press, New York, 1967.

Weibel, E. R.: Stereological principles for morphometry in electron microscopic cytology. *In:* Bourne, G. H., et al. (ed.), International Review of Cytology, pp. 235–302, 1969.

Wischnitzer, S.: *Introduction to Electron Microscopy,* 2nd edition, Pergamon Press, New York, 1970.

Woldseth, R.: *X-Ray Energy Spectrometry.* Kevex Corporation, Burlingame, 1973.

Wren, L. A.: *Understanding and Using the Phase Microscope.* Unitron Instrument Co., Newton Highlands, MA, 1963.

SECTION II:
CELL BIOLOGY

4: Cells—Structure and Function

General Cellular Characteristics

Chemical and Physical Properties

Protoplasm. The cell is a complex aggregation of chemicals. This aggregation, *protoplasm*, is a regulated, integrated, dynamic, balanced, and maintained accumulation of biochemical substances, salts, and water. Although the molecular components of protoplasm vary, some generalizations about its chemical constituents are possible. The diversity of components, however, is the basis for cellular variability.

Water, constituting approximately 75% of the protoplasmic mass, occurs in two forms—*bound water* and *free water*. Bound water constitutes less than 10% of the total water and is involved intimately in the structural integrity of the chemical components. Free water is that which is involved actively in the chemical events characteristic of protoplasm. Free water is also the solvent in which all of the miscible substances are dissolved, as well as the phase throughout which other substances are suspended. This suspension of particles imparts colloidal properties to protoplasm.

A *colloid* is an aggregate of atoms or molecules that is dissolved in but separated from the solvent phase. A colloid contains particles of a size sufficient to prevent their passing through a semipermeable membrane. Proteins possess colloidal properties and may exist in protoplasm as *sols* or *gels*. Sols are colloidal suspensions that have fluidlike properties, whereas gels are semisolid; both, however, are viscous, having gelatinous or mucinous characteristics. Protoplasmic proteins, as sols or gels, account for many of the significant structural and morphological properties ascribed to cells.

Crystalloids are substances that pass through semipermeable membranes when dissolved in water. Important crystalloids include glucose and numerous ions. Potassium is the primary protoplasmic cation, whereas phosphate, bicarbonate, and sulfate are the primary protoplasmic anions. Sodium and chloride are the primary extraprotoplasmic ions.

Nucleic acids, proteins, carbohydrates, and lipids are the most commonly occurring biochemical substances of protoplasm. These can occur as *macromolecules* that are composed of smaller monomeric subunits.

Nucleic Acids and Nucleotides. Nucleic acids are considered the repository of information essential for life. They contain the genetic code and serve as blueprints for the synthesis of the most important products of cells—proteins. The nucleic acids are macromolecules that consist of repeating monomeric units, *nucleotides*. Nucleotides are composed of a *pentose sugar, phosphoric acid*, and a *nitrogenous base*. The nitrogenous bases are either a *purine (adenine, guanine)* or *pyrimidine (cytosine, thymine, uracil)*.

Based upon the constituent sugar, nucleic acids are classified into two groups. *Deoxyribonucleic acid (DNA)* contains the sugar *deoxyribose*, whereas *ribonucleic acid (RNA)* contains the sugar *ribose*. The bases that occur in DNA are adenine, cytosine, guanine, and thymine; whereas, in RNA uracil replaces thymine.

DNA is primarily the nucleic acid of the nucleus; small quantities of DNA occur in mitochondria. RNA, however, occurs in both, especially the cytoplasm. Both nucleic acids are complexed with proteins to form *nucleoproteins*.

The quantity of DNA is a constant. This quantity must double before mitosis to ensure that the daughter cells receive the species-specific amount. Similarly, this amount must be halved in the gametes (via meiosis) to ensure that the species-specific amount is restored as a result of fertilization.

Different types of RNA have been identified in cells. *Ribosomal RNA (rRNA)* comprises approximately 85% of the cytoplasmic RNA and is complexed with protein as *ribonucleoprotein. Messenger RNA (mRNA)*, which is *encoded (transcribed)* by a single strand of DNA, carries the sequencing information for protein synthesis to the ribosomes and attaches to rRNA. *Transfer RNA (tRNA)* complexes with cytoplasmic amino acids and carries them to mRNA to effect the synthesis of proteins *(translation)*.

The acidic nature of these compounds generally assures that they will stain with a basic dye. Many of the basophilic components of cells contain nucleic acids. Moreover, the basic nature of some proteins with which nucleic acids are associated impart an acidophilia. The nucleolus of cells is a good example.

Although nucleotides are essential components of nucleic acids, not all nucleotides are confined to these macromolecules. *Adenosine triphosphate (ATP)* is a high energy storage compound that releases energy for cellular processes when a phosphate bond is broken and the compound is converted to *adenosine diphosphate (ADP)*. The conversion process, $ADP \rightleftharpoons ATP$ is the means of energy storage and release upon demand.

Cyclic adenosine monophosphate (cAMP) is an important free nucleotide and is considered a second messenger within the cell. Upon stimulation of specific receptors on cell membranes, *adenyl cyclase* activity increases and causes an increased formation of cAMP from ATP. The increased levels of cAMP stimulate enzymatic reactions. Also, studies of cAMP in bacteria have demonstrated that this compound may be a factor in gene regulation.

Proteins. Proteins, as the primary structural and functional components of cells, are essential for the architectural and metabolic integrity of living systems. These macromolecules are composed of repeating amino acid units joined covalently to each other. This *peptide linkage* is formed by the carboxyl group ($-COOH$) of one amino acid being joined to the amino group ($-NH_2$) of another amino acid. The particular sequence of amino acids in a protein is called the *primary structure*. If the number of amino acids produces a molecular weight greater than 10,000 then the molecule is a protein; less than 10,000 it is a *polypeptide*.

The regular, coiled conformation of peptide chains is the *secondary structure*. This is especially the characteristic of the α-helix of fibrous proteins. Some peptides, however, are folded sufficiently to impart a globular configuration called the *tertiary structure*. The *quarternary structure* results from the association of a number of globular and/or fibrous proteins. The fibrous proteins of cells include fibrinogen, myosin, tropocollagen, and keratin. The globular proteins include enzymes, some hormones, and the structural proteins of membranes.

Proteins occur as *simple (native)* or *conjugated* proteins. Simple proteins yield only amino acids upon hydrolysis, whereas conjugated proteins yield amino acids and nonproteinaceous prosthetic groups. Examples of simple proteins include the albumins, globulins, and histones. *Nucleoproteins* are those macromolecules that consist of a nucleic acid and a protein. *Chromoproteins* contain a metal that imparts pigmentation to the protein. Hemoglobin is a good example. *Glycoproteins* or *mucoproteins* contain a carbohydrate prosthetic group. Examples are mucin and some of the organic matrical components of cartilage and bone. *Lipoproteins* are characterized by a lipid prosthetic group. The components of cellular membranes are common examples of these macromolecules. *Phosphoproteins* contain a phosphorus prosthetic group; milk casein is an example.

Proteins will stain with the conventional acidic and basic stains used in histology. These large, nondiffusible, and charged colloids are stabilized with most fixatives to permit visualization (staining) with minimal denaturation (alteration to their tertiary structure).

Carbohydrates. Carbohydrates are classified as *monosaccharides, oligosaccharides,* and *polysaccharides*. Monosaccharides conform to the formula $(CH_2O)_n$. The pentose sugars (n = 5) are characterized by ribose and deoxyribose. Glucose, fructose, and galactose are hexose sugars (n = 6). The monosaccharides are important because they serve as immediate sources of energy (glucose) and as the building blocks of complex molecules. These polymers may consist of unaltered monosaccharides, amino sugars, uronic acids, or a combination of these monomers. *Amino sugars* are characterized by the replacement of one of the hydroxyl groups with a primary amine. Such a replacement on glucose results in glucosamine. These forms of the monosaccharides occur in many polysaccharides associated with connective tissue matrices.

The union of two monosaccharides via a glycosidic linkage results in the formation of a *disaccharide*. Examples are maltose and sucrose. Progressive addition of monomeric units results in the formation of longer chain saccharides. Arbitrarily, a chain of 10 or more monosaccharides is called a polysaccharide.

Glycogen is a polysaccharide that is the storage form of energy for the cell. Other polysaccharides include the glycosaminoglycans: hyaluronic acid, heparin, chondroitin sulfates, dermatan sulfate, and keratan sulfate. Many polysaccharides, beside those listed, occur as prosthetic groups of conjugated proteins. These complexes, referred to as mucoproteins or glycoproteins, are important structural or functional components or products of cells. Glycosaminoglycans complexed with core proteins are called *proteoglycans*, significant components of the ground substance of connective tissues.

Most carbohydrates can be stained for visualization with the light microscope.

Lipids. Lipids comprise a heterogeneous group of compounds that subserve a variety of functions. *Neutral fats* are esters of fatty acids and glycerol that are stored within cells as sources of high energy. Hydrolysis of fats yields the previously esterified components. The fatty acids may undergo β-oxidation with the acetyl groups (two-carbon chains) becoming activated as acetyl-coenzyme A. Acetyl-coenzyme A, then, can enter the tricarboxylic acid cycle (TCA cycle) by condensing with oxaloacetic acid.

Phospholipids are fats in which one of the fatty acids has been replaced by a phosphoric acid and a nitrogen-containing compound, such as choline, ethanolamine, or serine. Lecithin, cephalin, and sphingomyelin are examples, respectively. These compounds, with structural proteins, are important constituents of cellular membranes and the myelin sheath. Because these compounds are characterized by polar (hydrophilic) and nonpolar (hydrophobic) ends, they are an effective means of achieving chemical and physical compartmentalization of the cell.

Sterols comprise a group of lipids with the basic structure of the cyclopentanoperhydrophenanthrene ring. Cholesterol may be considered the prototype compound. Cholesterol, itself, is an important component of cell membranes. Many sterols function as hormones. These include estrogen, testosterone, progesterone, glucocorticoids, and mineralocorticoids.

A large group of lipids is complexed with sugars as *glycolipids*. These are the cerebrosides and gangliosides, essential components of cell membranes. *Waxes* are similar to the neutral fats, except they consist of longer chain fatty acids. They are cellular products that serve protective functions. Lipids can be demonstrated in histological specimens; however, lipid solvents must be avoided. Commonly employed lipid dyes are osmium tetroxide and the Sudan stains.

Biological Properties

Cellular Activities. The unique aggregation of the previously described molecular components imparts the varied properties to protoplasm that are ascribed to living entities. Whereas free-living unicellular organisms are required to be totally self-contained and conduct all living processes, the metazoan organism is a complex array of numerous cells that are dependent upon one another for a variety of functions. Significantly, these cells are not only interdependent but interact in such a way as to maintain an ideal internal environment in which all constituent cells may flourish. This interdependence or *division of labor* requires that some cells perform specific functions beyond those simply essential for survival. The following activities are characteristic of cells:

Metabolism, as a process that is basic to all cells, is the sum of all chemical reactions that occur within the cell. Reactions resulting in the synthesis of new molecular components that are essential for growth, maintenance, and repair are termed *anabolic*. Those reactions that result in the degradation of cellular components or products with a release of energy are termed *catabolic*. *Internal respiration*, or the chemical utilization of foodstuffs for the production of heat and energy, is the classical example of catabolism. Not all cells are characterized by the same metabolic activity or requirements. The bases for the similarities and differences are the molecular constituents of the protoplasm.

Irritability is that property of cells enabling them to respond to stimuli in their environment. It is this property of reactivity to stimuli that accounts for the biological behavior of cells. A unique aspect of irritability is that of *conductivity*, which is the special property of some cells (nerve, muscle) to transmit waves of excitation along their cellular membranes—information transfer.

A special form of the reactivity of cells is that manifested as *contractility*. Most cells are capable of changing shape, but muscle cells are adapted uniquely to change shape by shortening along their long axes. This characteristic enables them to accomplish work.

Endocytotic and exocytotic processes are essential for the *homeostasis* of all cells. *Endocytosis* is that process characterized by the movement of materials into the cell. Some fluids and dissolved substances therein may diffuse through the plasmalemma. Other fluids may gain entry via vacuoles formed in the cell membrane that eventually are "pinched-off" within the cytoplasm. These events are characteristic of *pinocytosis*. The engulfment and uptake of particulate matter is a special form of endocytosis called *phagocytosis*. The exit of materials from the cell is *exocytosis*. The egress from the cell of the waste products of metabolic processes is termed *excretion*, whereas the movement out of the cell of some special products synthesized by it is termed *secretion*.

Growth, maintenance, and *reproduction* of the protoplasm are universal characteristics. New molecular components are added, while others are replaced continually.

Morphological Features

The division of labor and specialization that characterizes the component cells of metazoans results in functionally diverse and interdependent cellular populations. This specialization is so precise that functional inferences can be made from structure alone; the converse is true also. Despite the degree of specialization, most cells have numerous characteristics in common (Fig. 4.1).

Cellular Shape. The shape of an animal cell is often described as spheroidal; this is a misleading and poor generalization. Specialization has a profound influence on cell shape. Cellular contact and pressure, as well as the inherent ability to alter shape, are determinants of morphological configuration. Thus, cells may be round (Fig. 4.2), stellate (Fig. 4.3), spindle-shaped (Fig. 4.4). elongated (Fig. 4.5), columnar (Fig. 4.6), squamous (Fig. 4.7), cuboidal (Fig. 4.8), and myriad other shapes.

Cellular Spatial Organization. Despite the diversity of cellular shape, the constituent organelles generally are positioned spatially in an organized and predictable manner. The nuclei of round, spheroidal, cuboidal, or spindle-shaped cells are usually rounded and located centrally (Fig. 4.2). Other shapes may characterize the nuclei of round cells (Fig. 4.9). The nuclei become ovoid and oriented parallel to the long axis as cells become elongated (Figs. 4.10 and 4.11). Nuclear position and shape may be correlated with the position of other organelles, as well as with the shape of the cell.

The Golgi apparatus is located generally in a juxtanuclear position, whereas the position of other organelles (rough endoplasmic reticulum, smooth endoplasmic reticulum, mitochondria) and inclusions (secretory droplets, fat) varies with the specific cell type considered.

Many cells (especially epithelial cells) are spatially polarized (Fig. 4.12). The nuclei of such cells are usually positioned eccentrically, and a corresponding orderly spatial relationship of other organelles and inclusions exists. Such organizational patterns are usually associated with secretory activity.

Cellular Size. Cells vary not only among the various groups of animals *(interspecific)*

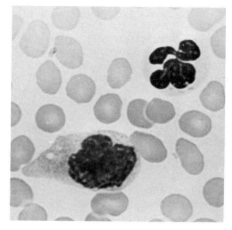

Figure 4.2. Round cells. The round cell with the lobulated nucleus *(top)* is a feline leukocyte. The elongated cell with the round nucleus *(bottom)* is also a leukocyte. ×400. The background cells are erytrocytes that are devoid of nuclei.

but even within the body of a specified organism *(intraspecific)*. No correlation exists, however, between the size of the organism and the size of its cells. Some cells are *macroscopic* (visible with the unaided eye), whereas others have a wide range of *microscopic sizes* (visible only with the aided eye). The *perikaryon* of a microgliocyte may be a few micrometers in diameter; the red blood corpuscle (RBC) ranges from 4–7 μm in diameter depending on the species, whereas the ovum may be as large as 300 μm in diameter. **(Incidentally, because red blood cells appear in most histological sections that are examined, they are effective built-in micrometers.)** The length of a striated muscle cell may be in inches, although the length of a nerve cell extending from the ventral horn of the spinal cord to the tip of an appendage may be several feet long. Even within the narrow limits of microscopic observation, a wide diversity of sizes may exist in at least one dimension. Giant cells, such as megakaryocytes, are appreciably larger than developing red blood corpuscles (Fig. 4.13). Similarly, striated muscle cells are much larger than the fibroblasts associated with them. Generally, most mammalian cells range between 10 and 30 μm.

Nucleus

The nucleus is responsible for the control and mediation of cellular activities. The information necessary for the control of cellular activity is encoded in the DNA macromolecules. This information is the basis for all generalized cellular form and function, because all nuclei contain the same genetic information. The unique features of specialized cells is a manifestation of the differential utilization of the genetic information by the repression or derepression of specific gene loci. Some functional

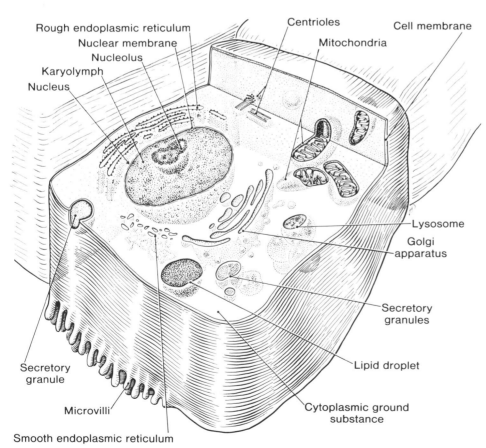

Rough endoplasmic reticulum
Nuclear membrane
Nucleolus
Karyolymph
Nucleus
Centrioles
Mitochondria
Cell membrane
Lysosome
Golgi apparatus
Secretory granules
Lipid droplet
Secretory granule
Microvilli
Smooth endoplasmic reticulum
Cytoplasmic ground substance

Figure 4.1. Schematic diagram of a typical cell. The major cellular components are included and labeled.

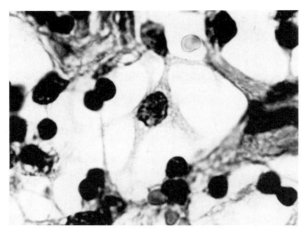

Figure 4.3. Stellate cell. A reticular cell from a canine lymph node is in the center of the field. The elongated cytoplasmic processes impart a star-shaped appearance to the cell. ×160.

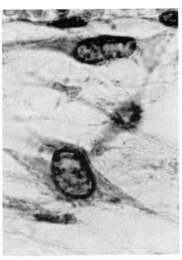

Figure 4.4. Spindle-shaped cells. The elongated and flattened cells are mesenchymal cells from a sample of bovine loose connective tissue. These cells may appear stellate in a different plane of section. The definitive identification of this cell is difficult. ×400.

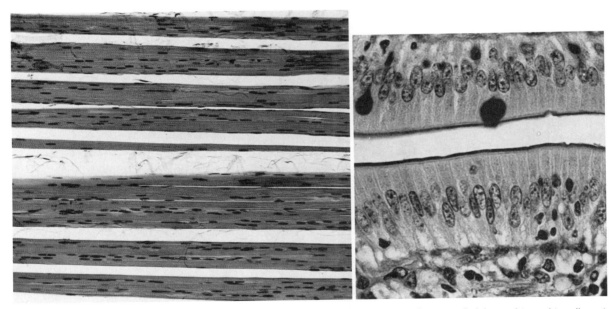

Figure 4.5. Elongated cells. The elongated, multinucleated cells are skeletal muscle cells. Each of these cells joins end-to-end to adjacent cells. ×40.

Figure 4.6. Columnar cells. These lining cells are longer than they are wide. The shape of the nuclei typically matches the shape of the cells. Compare this micrograph with the drawing of columnar cells in Figure 3.10. ×160.

correlations with nuclear morphology are possible. The most distinguishable of these are the morphological criteria associated with dividing *(mitotic)* and nondividing *(intermitotic, interphase,* or *vegetative)* cells.

In the interphase nucleus, four distinct components may be identified: *nuclear membrane, karyolymph, chromatin* and *nucleolus* (Fig. 4.14).

Numbers, Shape, and Position. Most often a cell will be mononucleated (Figs. 4.2–4.4, 4.6, and 4.8–4.10). Some, however, may be *binucleated*, whereas others may be

multinucleated (Fig. 4.15). Other extremes may range from enucleation, as in the mammalian erythrocyte (Figs. 4.2 and 4.9) and certain cells of the lens, to the case of the spermatozoon, in which the bulk of the cell is composed of a nucleus.

Nuclear morphology varies with the shape of the cell. Round to oval cells usually possess a similarly shaped nucleus (Figs. 4.3, 4.8 and 4.10). Elongated cells usually possess an elongated nucleus (Figs. 4.5, 4.6, and 4.11). Others, however, may possess nuclei that are crescent-shaped or

lobulated (Figs. 4.2, 4.9). A myriad of nuclear shapes exists. Identical cells within a specific cellular population are usually characterized by identical nuclear shapes.

The nuclei may be central, paracentral, or eccentrically-positioned. Specific cell types, however, are characterized generally by similarly or identically positioned nuclei. Definite spatial relationships are identifiable between the nucleus, cytoplasmic organelles, and inclusions. These are apparent especially when a cell has a distinct polarity (Fig. 4.12).

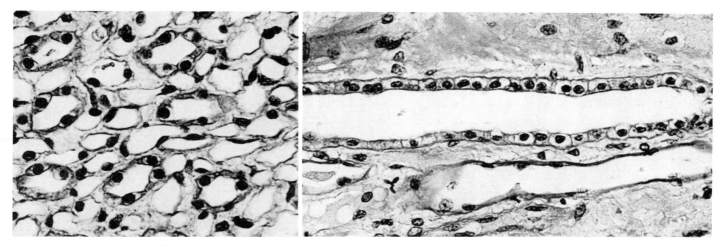

Figure 4.7. Squamous cells of the tubules of the canine kidney. The tubules are lined by flattened cells with a prominent nucleus. The cytoplasm appears as thin rims of dark-staining material. The perikaryon is the only obvious cytoplasmic region in most of the cells *(center)*. Cytoplasmic processes are obvious in some of the cells *(lower left and lower center)*. ×160.

Figure 4.8. Cuboidal cells. These cuboidal cells line the lumen of a tubule from a canine kidney. Although the cells appear as squares in biplanar section, the cells have a cuboidal shape in three dimensions. ×100.

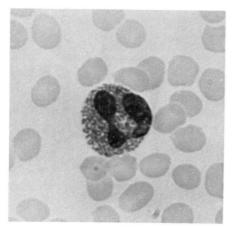

Figure 4.9. A round cell with a lobulated nucleus. The nuclear configuration is typical for this feline eosinophil. ×400.

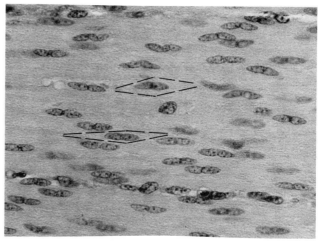

Figure 4.11. Smooth muscle cells from the intestine of a dog. The approximate margins of the cells are indicated by *dashed lines*. The elongated nuclei are oriented along the long axes of the cells. ×160.

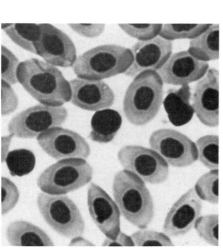

Figure 4.10. Avian erythrocytes. The slightly elongated cells contain elongated nuclei oriented parallel to the long axis of the cells. ×400. Compare with Figure 4.6.

In some cells, the nucleus may be the only dominant feature (Fig. 4.4). Stellate or squamous cells may possess small quantities of cytoplasm that are difficult to resolve with light microscopy (Fig. 4.7).

Nuclear Envelope. A dark, basophilic line of demarcation between the nucleus and surrounding cytoplasm is apparent in light microscopic section (Figs. 4.2– 4.4). This limiting membrane is a condensation of nuclear and cytoplasmic components, as well as stain, on either side of the *nuclear membrane* or *nuclear envelope*. The electron microscope (Fig. 4.16) reveals two membranes comprising the nuclear envelope, the *inner* and *outer nuclear membranes*. Each of these measures approximately 7.5 nm, and they are separated from each other by a *perinuclear space* or *cisterna* that varies from 40–70 nm wide. The

perinuclear space, and thus the outer nuclear membrane, is continuous with profiles of the rough endoplasmic reticulum RER (Fig. 4.17). *Ribonucleic protein* or *ribosomes* are often attached to the outer nuclear membrane. The intimate relationship of RER profiles to the nuclear membrane is especially apparent near the termination of mitosis. RER forms the nuclear envelope. The inner nuclear membrane is sometimes associated with filaments that form a *fibrous lamina* along its nuclear (inner) margin. The inner and outer nuclear membranes are discontinuous and reflected at certain points. Points of discontinuity or fusions between the inner and outer membranes are manifested as openings or *nuclear pores* (Fig. 4.18). The nuclear pores are approximately 70 nm in diameter. When sectioning perpen-

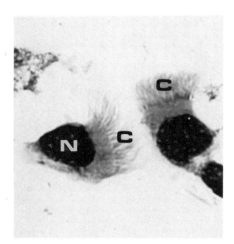

Figure 4.12. Polarized cells. These ciliated cells were exfoliated from the epithelial lining of the trachea. The nuclei *(N)* are displaced basally. The apical borders have cilia *(C)*. Polarization of cellular components, as evidenced by basal displacement of the nuclei, is a typical epithelial characteristic. ×160.

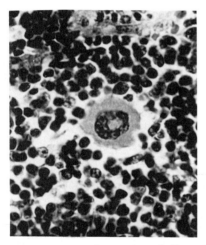

Figure 4.13. A megakaryocyte and other cells of the bone marrow. The megakaryocyte in the center of the field is many times larger than the cells surrounding it. ×100.

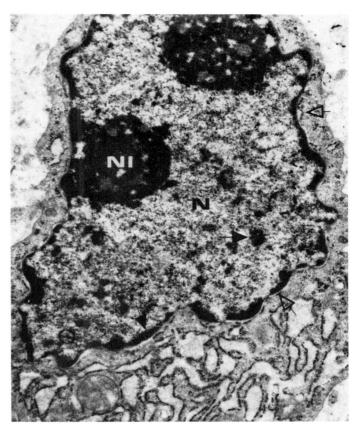

Figure 4.14. An electron micrograph of a fibroblast of loose connective tissue. The nucleus *(N)* contains two nucleoli *(NI)*. Heterochromatin *(solid arrows)* is interspersed with euchromatin. The nuclear envelope *(open arrows)* surrounds the nucleus. The condensation of heterochromatin along the peripheral margin of the nucleus precludes the visualization of the inner nuclear membrane at this magnification. ×16,000.

dicular to the nuclear membrane is accomplished, they appear to be covered by a septum or diaphragm that is thinner than the membranes that limit the margins of the pore (Fig. 4.16). On face view, these structures have a more complex architecture than is visible in the perpendicular plane (Fig. 4.18). Filamentous material contributes to a centrally positioned *anulus*. This morphology is indicative of open communication between the nucleus and cytoplasm. Unfortunately, little is known of the biochemical compositon and physiological properties of this complex. The degree of architectural organization, however, implies that nuclear pores may form a highly selective and specialized complex for the passage of materials between the

nucleus and cytoplasm. The distribution and number of nuclear pores may vary with the functional state of the nucleus. A schematic representation of a nuclear pore is depicted in Figure 4.19. The architecture of the pore is not unique to the nuclear envelope. Similar morphological complexes have been observed in cytoplasmic cisterns of the endoplasmic reticulum, either as stacks that are rich in pore complexes *(anulate lamellae)* or as isolated structures in RER. Such pore complexes have been demonstrated within intranuclear anulate lamellae, also.

Nuclear Matrix. The aforementioned limiting membrane encloses the *matrix of the nucleus*. This *nuclear sap* or *karyolymph* is the soluble phase of nuclear material. The terms *nuclear matrix* and *nuclear ground substance* have been used to describe this material.

Chromatin. *Chromatin* is contained within the confines of the nuclear envelope and is suspended in the nuclear matrix. The term chromatin is used to describe any area in the nucleus that contains DNA. Different types of chromatic materials are recognizable during the interphase. *Heter-*

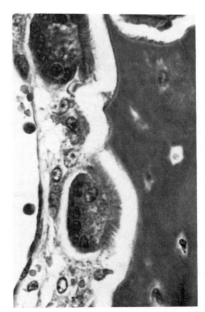

Figure 4.15. Multinucleated cells of bone. The osteoclasts contain a variable number of nuclei. The multinucleations result from cellular fusion rather than nuclear division without cytoplasmic division. ×100.

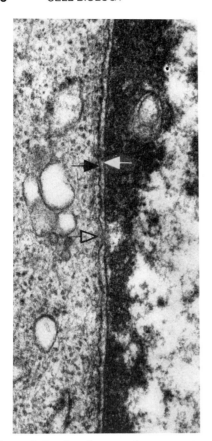

Figure 4.16. An electron micrograph of the nuclear membrane of a fibroblast. The outer nuclear membrane *(black arrow)* is separated from the inner nuclear membrane *(white arrow)* by the nuclear cistern. Heterochromatin obliterates portions of the inner nuclear membrane. A nuclear pore *(open arrow)* is apparent. ×52,000.

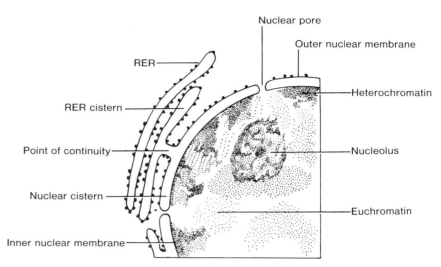

Figure 4.17. A schematic representation of a portion of the nucleus and RER as visualized with the electron microscope. The perinuclear space or cistern is continuous with the cistern of the RER. Ribosomes are attached to the outer nuclear membrane.

ochromatin is chromatic material that stains intensely with basic dyes and is condensed (Figs. 4.12 and 4.14). It is metabolically inert. *Euchromatin* stains lightly, is dispersed and is the metabolically active form of DNA (Figs. 4.14 and 4.20). Various ratios of heterochromatin/euchromatin appreciably alter the appearance of a nucleus from *condensed* (much heterochromatin) to *open* or *vesicular* (little heterochromatin). These nuclear features are aids for the identification of specific cell types. The spatial distribution of one to the other is a diagnostic feature of some cell types. Most significantly, the amount of euchromatin is an indicator of the potential protein-synthetic activity of a cell. The more heterochromatin, the less active the cell; the more euchromatin, the greater the potential protein synthesis (Figs. 4.14 and 4.20).

Some of the hetereochromatin is distinguishable as *Barr bodies*. These bodies consist of a condensation of one of the X chromosomes. The female of a species contains two X chromosomes; one is condensed, inactive, and visible as a Barr body (Plate VI.23). The other one is active in

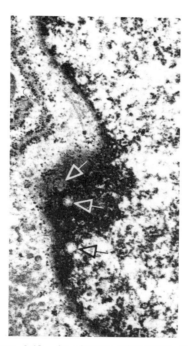

Figure 4.18. An electron micrograph of the face view of a nuclear membrane. The nuclear pores *(open arrows)* are not simple openings between the nucleus and the cytoplasm. An anulus *(upper arrow)* and particulate matter *(middle arrow)* characterize the apertures. ×23,000.

metabolic processes and part of the euchromatin of the nucleus.

Nucleolus. The *nucleolus,* or "little nucleus," is a prominently staining, highly refractive, smooth-surfaced body that occurs in the nucleus (Fig. 4.20). Single or multiple nucleoli may characterize specific nuclei. A nucleolus is readily identifiable in those cells involved in protein synthesis. Also, it is a prominent characteristic of blastoid and malignant cells.

Examination of electron micrographs reveals this structure as a discrete body that is not membrane-bound (Fig. 4.21). It occurs freely in the nucleus or may be attached to the inner nuclear membrane. It is composed of filamentous *(pars fibrosa)* and granular *(pars granulosa)* materials, both of which contain RNA. Chromatic material surrounds or extends into the nucleolus. The *nucleolus-associated chromatin* represents specific regions on specific chromosomes called *nucleolus organizers.*

The filamentous and granular components form thread-like and anastomotic strands called the *nucleolonema* (Fig. 4.21). Densely packed filaments form a centrally positioned and rounded mass called the *pars amorpha.*

The nucleolus is the center for the synthesis of ribosomal RNA. The ribosomal subunits may be formed in the pars fibrosa, mature in the pars granulosa, and subsequently assembled into functional ribosomes in the cytoplasm.

Cytoplasm

General Characteristics. The cytoplasm is present in varying amounts in all living cells. The types, kinds, and numbers of morphologically and biochemically identifiable components are responsible for the specializations that contribute to histological identification.

The bulk of the cytoplasm, or *ground substance,* is an admixture of water, protein, carbohydrates, organic salts, and inorganic salts. The physical properties of the cytoplasm are in a constant state of flux. Thus, sol-gel properties are apparent. Although this is not generally apparent in somatic cells, some cells (egg cells, amoeboid cells) possess a clear, peripheral *ectoplasm* and an internal, granular *endoplasm.* The former is more viscous (gel-like) and

consists of the fluid phase within which numerous substances are contained that are essential to the cell and its metabolism.

Structure and Function

Membranes and Glycocalyx. The *plasma membrane (plasmalemma, cell membrane)* encloses the entire cytoplasm and is that portion of the cell exposed to the extracellular environment. It is approximately 8.0 nm thick. The 200-nm limit of resolution of the white light microscope precludes resolving the plasmalemma as a distinct entity with the bright-field microscopy. Despite this, *cellular limits* are discernible within the aforementioned limits of resolution. This is due to a condensation of structural protein, addition of stain and the condensation of contiguous materials at the interfaces, as well as the presence of a *cell coat*.

Despite the ability of the electron microscope to resolve the plasmalemma, no concise and definitive structure has been determined for this entity. It appears as a trilaminar structure composed of two *osmiophilic* bands separated by an *osmiophobic* band (Fig. 4.22). Each band is approximately 2.5 nm wide. This is supposed to correspond to a sandwich-like relationship in which two layers of protein are laid upon a layer of lipid (protein-lipid-protein). This structural design comprised the *unit membrane concept*. This structure was supposed to be applicable to the structural configuration and biochemical composition of all membrane systems. Too many structural and chemical variations have been observed to consider this concept applicable to all membranes (Fig. 4.23).

Various technology has contributed to the current knowledge of membrane structure. All seem to confirm that the most reasonable representation of membranes is the lipid-globular protein, mosaic model (Fig. 4.24). The basic model is a bimolecular leaflet of phospholipids with their hydrophilic (polar) groups directed outwardly and their hydrophobic (non-polar) groups directed inwardly. Proteins are embedded within the lipid bilayer and project variously from either surface. Polysaccharides project from the outer surface. These are attached to proteins (glycoproteins) and lipids (glycolipids). The positions of the protein constituents are not constant. Instead, the changing properties and protein constituents (enzymes, receptor sites, antigenic sites, permeability sites) impart a fluid nature *(fluid mosaic model)* that appears to correspond to dynamic physiological activities. **The hydrophilic, globular proteins can account for the selective permeability of certain water-soluble substances and may function as pores, whereas the lipid components explain the relative ease of passage of lipid-soluble substances.**

The periphery of the plasma membrane

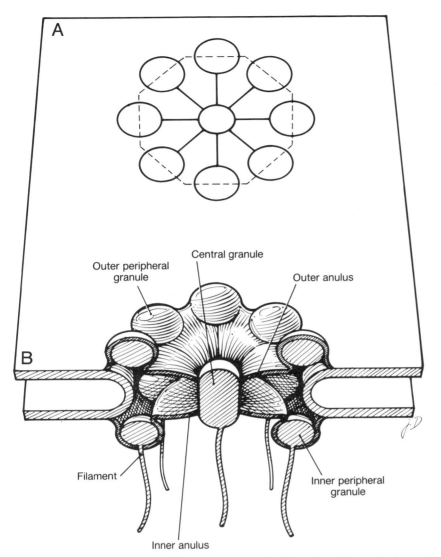

Figure 4.19. An artist's conception of a nuclerar pore. *A.* Face view. The nuclear pore has octagonal symmetry. *B.* Cross section. The nuclear pore consists of inner and outer anuli that are joined by a central granule. Peripherally positioned granules are associated with both anuli. Nuclear filaments radiate from the central and peripheral granules.

In figure labels: Outer peripheral granule, Central granule, Outer anulus, Filament, Inner anulus, Inner peripheral granule

relatively free of organelles compared to the more fluid, granular (sol-like) and organelle-rich endoplasm.

The cytoplasm of mature somatic cells is generally *acidophilic*; however, it may be totally or focally *basophilic*, as well as totally or focally *chromophobic* or *neutrophilic*. Numerous cytoplasmic components contribute to the general characteristics of a cell.

Cellular Membranes

Compartmentalization. The boundary layer between the protoplasm and its surrounding environment is the *plasma membrane*. This membrane circumscribes the protoplasmic mass and defines the limits of this living entity. The *nucleus* is membrane-bound within the protoplasm and contains protoplasm that is called *nucleoplasm* or *karyoplasm*.

The plasma membrane and nuclear membrane are complex structures whose biochemical components impart gel characteristics. Proteins are significant contributors to this important characteristic. As *hydrophilic* (water-loving) *colloids*, **proteins permit the movement of crystalloids and water to and from the cell,** as well as between the two major compartments of the cell—nucleus and cytoplasm. Furthermore, **lipid components of membranes permit the movement of lipid-soluble substances through them.**

The cell consists of numerous, orderly aggregations of macromolecules that compartmentalize it and effectively divide it into regions characterized by specific form and function. These compartments are the *organelles* that consist of cytomembranes with specific proteins (enzymes) or nucleic acids. The remainder of the protoplasm

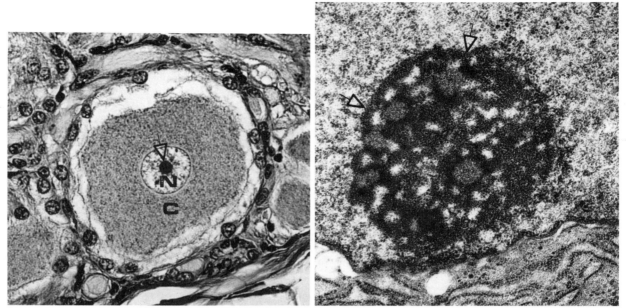

Figure 4.20.   A ganglion cell. The cytoplasm *(C)* contains a vesicular nucleus *(N)* in which euchromatic material predominates. A prominent nucleolus *(arrow)* is present. ×100.

Figure 4.21.   An electron micrograph of a nucleolus. The nucleolonema *(arrows)* is the prominent feature in this section. ×25,000.

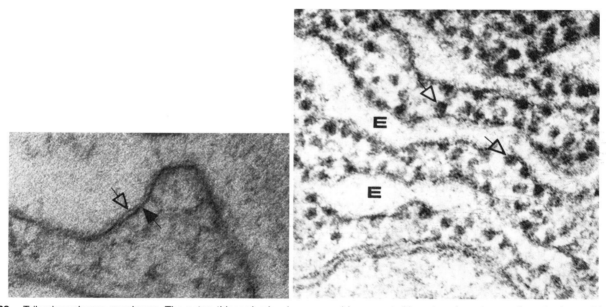

Figure 4.22.   Trilaminar plasma membrane. The outer, thinner lamina *(open arrow)* is separated by a translucent space from the inner, thicker lamina *(solid arrow)*. ×215,000.

Figure 4.23.   Globular cytoplasmic membranes. The cisterns *(E)* of the granular endoplasmic reticulum are membrane-bound and studded with ribosomes *(open arrows)*. The trilaminar appearance is not evident. Rather, the membrane components appear to be globular. ×156,000.

is covered by a layer of material that is rich in carbohydrates. The *glycocalyx (cell coat)* probably occurs on all cells and is well developed on some. The glycocalyx appears as "fuzzy" material with the electron microscope (Fig. 4.25). The glycocalyx is attached to and is integrated intimately into the structural components of the plasmalemma as glycoproteins and glycolipids. The polysaccharides of the cell coat ac-

count for its positive reaction with periodic acid-Schiff (Fig. 4.26).

The functions of the cell coat vary. *Cellular recognition* may be achieved between cells based upon specific biochemical components contained within it. Cells in cultural monolayers maintain this relationship by *contact inhibition*. Cell-to-cell *adhesion* and attachment to associated connective tissue is achieved through this cellular com-

ponent. *Absorption* of some materials involves the glycocalyx. Finally, *antigenicity* is associated with it.

Lipid and protein constituents, as described for the fluid mosaic model of the plasmalemma, occur in the cytomembranes that are components of the organelles.

Properties and Functions. Continuing research on membrane structure is one of the

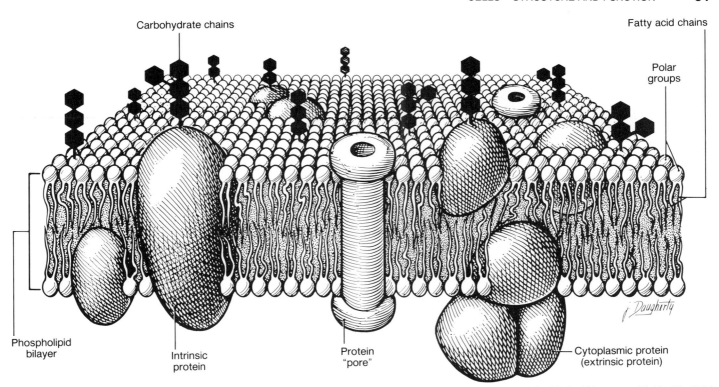

Figure 4.24. An artist's conception of the fluid mosaic model of the plasma membrane. Intrinsic proteins are embedded within a sea of lipids. The lipid bilayer consists of phospholipids whose hydrophilic heads project outwardly and hydrophobic tails project inwardly. Carbohydrates, as components of glycoproteins and glycolipids, project above the membrane as components of the glycocalyx. Conformational changes of intrinsic proteins may account for the pore characteristics associated with membranes.

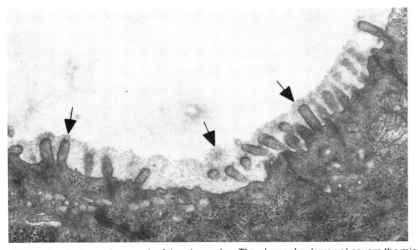

Figure 4.25. An electron micrograph of the glycocalyx. The glycocalyx (arrows) covers the microvilli and apical surfaces of these murine intestinal cells. ×14,000. (Courtesy A. M. Sheppard.)

primary thrusts of modern cell biology. Studies of the erythrocyte membrane, gap junctions, purple membrane of *Halobacterium halobium*, and others have broadened basic understanding, but a clear definition of membrane structure is still elusive. All biological membranes contain a lipid bilayer, but the specific constituents of proteins, lipids, and carbohydrates vary. The lipids are primarily phosphatidylcholine, phosphatidylethanolamine, phosphatidylserine, sphingomyelin, and cholesterol.

The membrane carbohydrates are those complexed to proteins as constituents of the glycocalyx.

Membrane proteins are classified into two groups—*peripheral proteins* and *integral (intrinsic) proteins*. Peripheral proteins are defined as those that are removed easily by ionic manipulation. These proteins are attached to the outer or inner portions of the membranes. The intrinsic proteins are those requiring manipulation with detergents before removal is accomplished.

These proteins are hydrophobically bonded to membrane components and are predominantly located in the polar regions of the bilayer. They may extend from the outer surface through the membrane to the inner surface. The following are broad spectrum functions that relate to membranes generally or their protein constituents specifically: *selective permeability, differential transport, compartmentalization, energy conversions, structural integrity, carrier molecules, pores or channels, enzymes, receptor molecules, adhesion, cellular recognition,* and *transmission.*

As the name fluid mosaic model implies, components within a membrane have the ability to move. *Membrane fluidity* involves various types of movements by constituents. Short chain, unsaturated fatty acids increase fluidity due to the rotational movement possible at C=C bonding. Long-chain, unsaturated fatty acids decrease membrane fluidity. Cholesterol tends to decrease membrane fluidity. Lateral movement of lipid components is also possible. Aggregates of lipids may diffuse as units either as free domains or in asociation with their protein constitiuents. Fluidity of membranes is responsible, in part, for the dynamic changes associated with specific membrane foci.

Transport Functions

Passive Transport. Various mechanisms have been described for the passive trans-

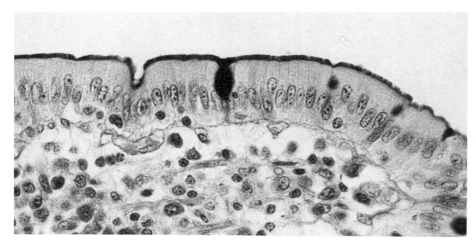

Figure 4.26. The glycocalyx as visualized with light microscopy and special staining. The apical, striated border of these intestinal lining cells is covered by a dark-staining glycocalyx. ×160 (PAS).

port of substances across the plasma membrane. Despite the diversity of processes, **all passive transport mechanisms are dependent upon concentration gradients (diffusion).** *Facilitated diffusion* is also called *carrier-mediated transport.* A carrier molecule (membrane protein) is used to facilitate the transport of sugars and amino acids.

Na-dependent facilitated diffusion is a transport mechanism for certain amino acids and sugars that is dependent upon a sodium transport system.

Active Transport. *Active transport* is an energy-requiring process that moves substances against their concentration gradients or electrochemical potential gradients. The process may also augment the spontaneous "downhill" movement of molecules. The relative external/internal concentration gradient for sodium dictates that equilibrium would be reached eventually. Cells need a sodium pump to move sodium out of the cell constantly. The energy is supplied by a Na-dependent ATPase.

Membranes as Receptors

Receptors. Proteins serve as receptor molecules on cellular membranes. These receptors are located on the plasmalemma as well as within the cytoplasmic membranes. The receptors function to unite with various substances that serve as messengers between cells. The union of the messenger with the receptor is usually associated with measurable changes in cellular behavior. The union could induce, among other events, alterations in carrier molecules that alter transport functions.

Receptors (and carrier molecules) are plastic substances; i.e., their numbers and distribution are alterable. An increased amount of a messenger (or a transported substance) may increase the number of receptor (and carrier) molecules. This is an example of *up regulation.* The same increases under a different set of circumstances could cause the number of receptor (and carrier) molecules to decrease—*down regulation.*

The alteration of transport functions in response to the union of a messenger molecule with a receptor is called *chemical gating.* The precise mechanisms by which pore alterations are achieved are not clear; such alterations may be dependent upon conformational changes in the proteins. Changes in electrical potential have profound effects upon the orientation of molecules within membranes. Such electrically induced changes are able to alter transport functions within membranes. Pore or channel alterations that result from potential changes are called *electrical gating.*

Cellular Messengers. Communication between cells is achieved with *primary messengers.* Their union with appropriate receptors usually initiates a cascade of subsequent intracellular events. The subsequent events are dependent upon informational transfer by *second messengers* or *intracellular messengers. Calcium, cAMP,* and *cyclic guanidine monophosphate (cGMP)* are second messengers. The influence of calcium as an intracellular messenger is mediated through *calmodulin,* a receptor protein for calcium.

Many primary messengers mediate their effects through cAMP. The initiating event is the activation of *adenyl cyclase.* This enzyme converts ATP to cAMP. The cAMP then mediates its influence by activating a *protein kinase.* A protein kinase phosphorylates some other effector proteins (enzymes), rendering them active or inactive. The effector protein, then, is responsible for the stimulation or inactivation of a specific biological behavior. The activation of a specific *phosphodiesterase* degrades cAMP to 5′-AMP. The degradation of cAMP activity terminates the activ-

ity of the protein kinase and returns the specific activity to the prestimulation level. Cyclic AMP is known to affect numerous cellular activites that include: altered membrane permeabilities, release of stored products, modifications in the rate of enzyme reactions, and induction of enzyme synthesis.

The functions of cGMP are not well understood. This messenger may require calcium and calmodulin.

Calmodulin, cAMP, and Cellular Activities

The major cellular receptor for calcium is *calmodulin,* a globular protein that seems to mediate and modulate most of the activities associated with calcium. Calmodulin has been demonstrated in virtually every kind of eukaryotic cell. Calcium influx into a cell raises the calcium concentration to a threshold level, beyond which four calcium ions become bound to calmodulin within the membrane. Upon binding calcium, calmodulin changes shape and becomes activated. The activated calmodulin influences the formation of cAMP. As more calcium enters the cell, calcium combines with cytoplasmic calmodulin. Activated cytoplasmic calmodulin then mediates the activation of a specific phosphodiesterase required to inactivate cAMP. Calmodulin then activates a Ca-dependent ATPase that pumps the calcium out of the cell. Calmodulin not only transmits the message to specific receptor proteins, but it actually modulates the amount of calcium within the cell. Calcium and calmodulin mediate the activation of cAMP, which subsequently influences various types of cellular behavior.

Enzyme phosphorylation is often a key phase of the intracellular regulatory process that requires the activation of a *kinase.* Calcium and calmodulin are known to influence various kinase activities.

Cytoplasmic Membranous Compartments

Ribosomes and Rough Endoplasmic Reticulum

Morphology and Function. The cytoplasm of many cells possesses either a total or focal basophilia. These areas contain high quantities of RNA and protein, *ribonucleoprotein (RNP).* Although tRNA and mRNA are present in the cytoplasm, the primary contributor to this staining property is rRNA. *Ribosomes* are small granules in the cytoplasm that consist of approximately 60% RNA and 40% protein. These structures occur in the cytoplasm as single units, *free ribosomes,* or as multiple units, *polyribosomes* or *polysomes* (Fig. 4.27). **The free ribosomes and polysomes are responsible for the synthesis of proteins for intracellular use.** These free granules are

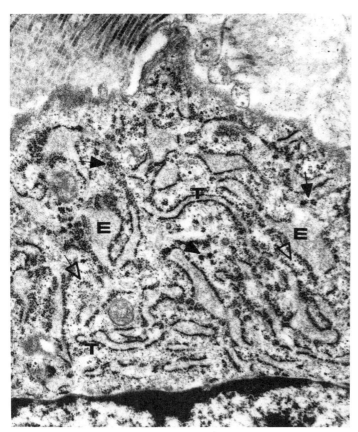

Figure 4.27. An electron micrograph of a fiber-forming cell. The cytoplasm contains numerous profiles of granular endoplasmic reticulum. Some are tubular *(T)* configurations, whereas others are cisternal *(E)* profiles. Ribosomes *(open arrows)* and polyribosomes *(solid arrows)* are abundant. ×20,000.

characteristic features of differentiating and growing cells.

An extensive network of tubules, flattened vesicles, and cisternae extends throughout the cytoplasm of many cells. When ribosomes and polysomes are attached to this network (reticulum), the organelle is called the *granular (rough) endoplasmic reticulum (RER)* (Figs. 4.23, 4.27 and 4.28). (Recall that this organelle is also continuous with the outer nuclear membrane.) In many cells, this organelle is scattered randomly throughout the cytoplasm. The distribution of this organelle in the plasma cell imparts a total cytoplasmic basophilia. In others, its distribution is associated with cellular polarity. The pancreatic acinar cell is an example of a cell characterized by a basally positioned basophilia due to the polarized position of RER (Fig. 4.29). **The proteins synthesized on the ribosomes of the RER are primarily for extracellular use. A cell with a vesicular nucleus, prominent nucleolus, and cytoplasmic basophilia usually has a high potential for protein synthesis.**

Protein Synthesis. The process of protein synthesis is summarized graphically in Figure 4.30. The *transcription* of the mRNA

occurs on the euchromatic DNA and requires the enzyme *RNA polymerase*. The ribosome consists of subunits of rRNA that are synthesized in the nucleolus, transported to, and subsequently assembled within the cytoplasm. The two *subunits* of unequal size form a groove at their point of contact. A slender strand of mRNA attaches to the smaller subunit of the ribosomes at this groove.

The messenger leaves the nucleus encoded with the proper information relating to amino acid sequence. The initiating event of transcription is the binding of the 5′ end of the mRNA to the smaller ribosomal subunit. This information is vested in *codons*, which are various triplet combinations of the nucleotides. Transfer RNA is synthesized in the nucleus and is active in the cytoplasm. A specific tRNA exists for each of the naturally occurring amino acids. Specific amino acids are transferred from the cytoplasmic pool to the appropriate tRNA by the acitivity of at least one of 10 specific *aminoacyl-tRNA synthetases*. The enzyme activity causes the activation of one amino acid and joins it to tRNA as an *aminoacyl-tRNA* complex. The different aminoacyl-tRNAs that are necessary to

form a polypeptide are selected individually and sequentially by specific codons of the mRNA. Attachment of the tRNA to an *initiator codon* of mRNA initiates polypeptide synthesis. Two tRNA binding sites exist on the ribosome—the *acceptor (A) site* and the *peptidyl (P) site*. The aminoacyl-tRNA binds initially to the A site, moves to the P site and carries the mRNA with it exposing the next codon. The vacated A site now becomes occupied with another aminoacyl-tRNA complex. A peptide linkage forms between the two amino acids. The aminoacyl-tRNA complex advances again, releases the initial tRNA, carries the mRNA with it and exposes another codon. This cycle of attachment, advance, peptide linkage formation, tRNA release and attachment continues until the 3- end *(terminal codon)* of the messenger is reached. The lengthening polypeptide is always attached to the new aminoacyl-tRNA complex that joins the A site. The ribosomes contribute actively to the translation process by catalyzing the peptide linkage formation.

The tRNA is subsequently released from the messenger and the ribosome moves along the mRNA. Another tRNA is then ready to read the next mRNA codon. Released tRNA is available for the transfer of another specific amino acid, whereas the released ribosomes are available for repeated nonspecific utilization. The specificity for the protein resides in the mRNA. This assembly process of amino acids into polypeptides is called *translation*. Assembly is a rapid process; some experimental data indicate approximately 10 msec per amino acid.

The length of the mRNA determines the number of ribosomes associated with it and thus the length of the polypeptide chain. Secretory proteins gain access to the tubules or cisterns of the RER, are translocated to the Golgi apparatus, and emerge as *condensing vacuoles* that are converted to *secretory granules*.

Signal Hypothesis. The mechanisms that govern the fate of newly formed polypeptides—intracellular use or extracellular transport—are explained by the *signal hypothesis*. According to this hypothesis, mRNAs for secretory proteins have a *signal codon* sequence. The translation process begins on the free ribosomes within the cytosol. The *signal sequence (signal peptide)* emerges from the free ribosomes and interacts with *ribosomal receptor proteins* that are located within the membrane of the RER. The larger subunits of the ribosomes attach to the receptor proteins. The receptor proteins are believed to be *ribophorin I* and *ribophorin II*, which are protein constituents of RER membranes but not smooth endoplasmic reticular membranes. The interaction of the signal sequence, receptor proteins and ribosomes

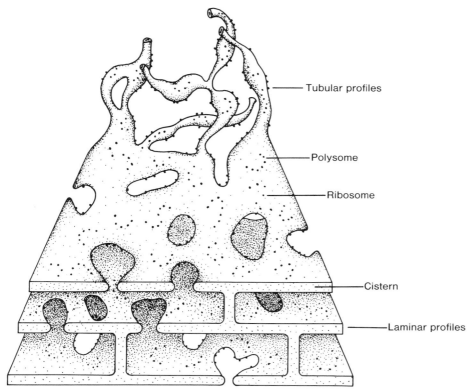

Figure 4.28. Schematic representation of the RER. The anastomotic plates and tubules may be scattered randomly or placed in an orderly array throughout the cytoplasm.

mation of various substances. The SER, through its drug metabolizing enzymes, is responsible for the biotransformation of numerous endogenous and exogenous substances. The involvement of this organelle in lipid metabolism is varied. In intestinal lining cells, the resynthesis of fatty acids back into fats and their transport to the basal or lateral cellular borders occur within the SER. The synthesis of steroid hormones and lipoproteins occurs within this organelle.

The sarcoplasmic reticulum represents a special type of SER. This organelle of muscle cells is used as the site for the sequestration and subsequent transport of calcium during excitation-contraction coupling.

Golgi Apparatus

Structure. The *Golgi apparatus* or *Golgi complex* is an organelle that may be visualized with light microscopy. Special stains such as silver or osmium can be used to impregnate or stain the organelle as a positive image. The organelle appears as a network of tubules and vacuoles scattered throughout the cell, sometimes in more than one focus, or is juxtaposed to the nucleus and confined to a discrete region. With routine staining (H and E), however, an extensive Golgi complex appears as a negative image because of its chromopho-

occurs in such a way that the large ribosomal subunits and receptor proteins form a channel across the membrane. The nascent polypeptide enters the cisterns of the RER. Upon entry into the cisterns, the signal peptide is cleaved by a *signal peptidase* located on the cisternal side of the RER membrane.

Agranular Endoplasmic Reticulum

Morphology and Function. The *smooth (agranular) endoplasmic reticulum (SER)* is not as extensive as its granular counterpart, except in certain types of cells. SER is not associated with ribosomes and polyribosomes; the organelle consists simply of "undecorated" anastomosing tubules (Fig. 4.31). Although the SER is an organelle that is structurally and functionally distinct from RER, the two sets of reticular profiles are connected to each other.

Functionally, the smooth endoplasmic reticulum is a more diverse organelle than its morphology would imply: *glycogen synthesis, lipid synthesis and transport, biotransformation, and ion storage and transport*. Glycogen and SER profiles are usually intimately associated with each other. The enzyme *glucose-6-phosphatase* is a component of this organelle in liver cells. Hepatocytes are involved in the biotransfor-

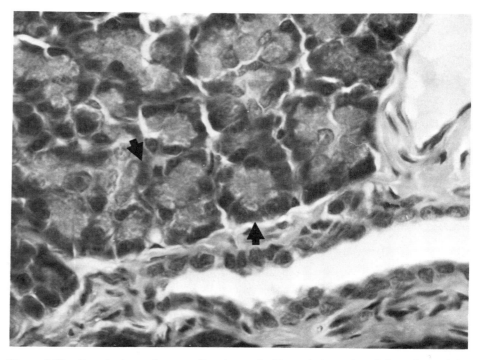

Figure 4.29. Ergastoplasm of pancreatic acinar cells. The apical margins of the cells are light-staining (acidophilic). The basal portions *(arrows)* are dark-staining (basophilic). The pancreatic acinar cells are polarized cells, and the distribution of basophilic and acidophilic materials from bases to apices, respectively, reflects the polarization of cellular components. ×40. Compare this light micrograph with the electron micrograph in Figure 4.48.

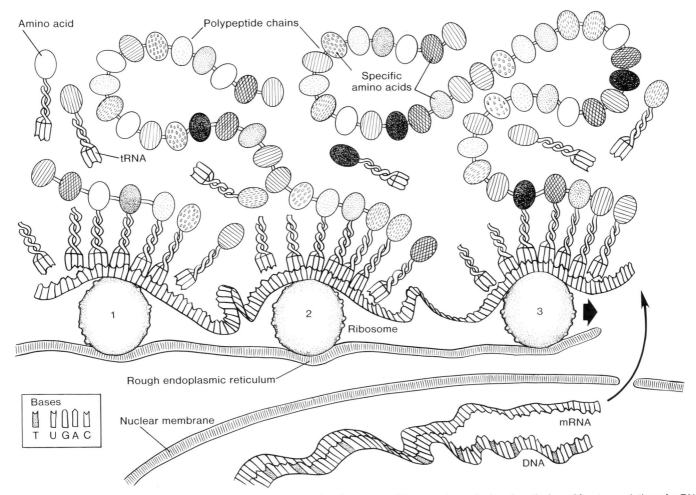

Figure 4.30. Schematic representation of protein synthesis upon the ribosomes of the granular endoplasmic reticulum. After transcription of mRNA upon DNA within the nucleus, the messenger enters the cytoplasm and becomes attached to ribosomes. The mRNA fits in the groove between the two subunits of the ribosome. The activation of specific tRNA occurs after its linkage to the appropriate amino acid in the cytoplasm. The nature of the message, codon, of the mRNA determines which tRNA attaches at the codon site, and therefore, which amino acid is used in the sequence. As the mRNA moves along the ribosomes, the tRNA molecules with attached amino acids translate the code, and the appropriate amino acids are deposited in the proper sequence that is characteristic for a specific protein. The tRNA molecules are released and made available, therefore, to attach to other free amino acids. The length of the mRNA determines the number of amino acids in the chain, thus the length of the protein that is assembled. Each ribosome is responsible for the synthesis of a complete chain of amino acids. As the mRNA moves from point 1 to point 3, the protein chain lengthens. Upon reaching the end of the mRNA at point 3, the ribosomes are released, the amino acid chain is freed and the ribosomes are available to attach to another mRNA. The bases involved in the codon include uracil (U), adenine (A), cytosine (C), and guanine (G). Thymine (T) occurs in DNA.

bic staining properties. In those cells in which polarity is apparent, such as epithelial cells, the position of the Golgi apparatus reflects this polarization; it is supranuclear, located between the nucleus and the apical or luminal surface of the cell.

Electron microscopy has contributed significantly to an understanding of the morphology of this organelle (Fig. 4.32). The Golgi apparatus consists of a parallel array of smooth surfaced membranes that are disposed as flattened saccules with dilated cisternae at their peripheral margins. The entire complex assumes a semilunar configuration of polarity. The *convex face* is associated with and ultimately fuses with *transfer vesicles* from the RER. Numerous fenestrations characterize this surface. The *concave face* is associated intimately with

numerous *secretory vesicles* in various stages of condensation and maturation (Fig. 4.33).

Function. The Golgi apparatus was considered to be functionally uniform because of the uniformity of its membrane morphology. But special staining and histochemical techniques have demonstrated a distinct polarity. A few saccules of the immature face stain with osmium tetroxide and contain *transferases* for sugars. The saccules of the mature face do not stain with osmium and contain the enzyme *thiamine pyrophosphatase (TPP)*. The function of TPP is unknown. Hydrolytic enzymes are associated with the middle saccules. Also, different types of secretory granules may be formed on the inner (concave) and outer (convex) face. This experimental ev-

idence is interpreted as being indicative of functional specialization within the complex.

The membranes of the Golgi stack are in a constant state of flux. "New membrane" is added constantly by the incorporation of transfer vesicles and "old membrane" is lost at the mature face through secretory vesicles. Exocytotic processes involve membrane-bound vesicles derived from the Golgi apparatus being incorporated into the plasmalemma. The translocation of membranes from the immature face through the Golgi stack to the surface of the mature face ultimately contributes to the plasmalemma and the glycocalyx.

The Golgi apparatus is responsible for the alteration and packaging of secretory units for intracellular and extracellular use.

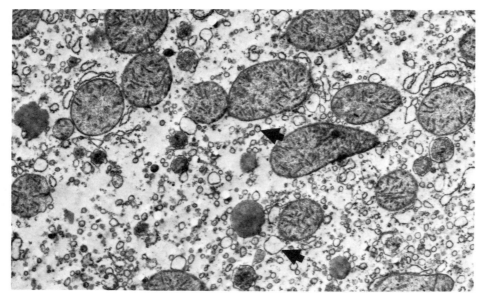

Figure 4.31. An electron micrograph of smooth endoplasmic reticulum of an hepatocyte. Although the cell has been ruptured, the tubular profiles *(arrows)* of the organelle are obvious. Mitochondria and rough endoplasmic reticular profiles are present also. ×11,400.

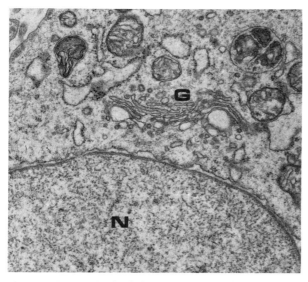

Figure 4.32. An electron micrograph of a Golgi apparatus. The Golgi apparatus *(G)* is positioned close to the nucleus *(N)*. ×20,000.

Protein transferred to the stack is condensed. Glycosylation of glycoproteins and collagenous precursors is one of the major post-translational functions of the Golgi apparatus. The addition of sugars to lipids is also a significant contribution in the synthesis of glycolipids. Sulfation of glycosaminoglycans also occurs in this organelle. Post-translational proteolysis occurs commonly in the Golgi apparatus converting prosecretory proteins into secretory proteins. The complex is also responsible for the synthesis of glycosaminoglycans. Additionally, the Golgi complex is important in the formation of lysosomes.

Mitochondria

Structure and Function. *Mitochondria* appear as threads or granules with various staining techniques at the light microscopic level. Special staining techniques, however, stain them specifically; e.g., the supravital stain, Janus green B. Their shape is varied; even within a specific cell type they are pleomorphic, ranging from round to oval or from elongated to filamentous. The number of mitochondria in a cell varies with the energy requirements of the cell. The size of mitochondria is also varied. Although most may be 2–3 μm long, mitochondria may exceed a length of 10 μm.

Mitochondria are demonstrable as a double-membrane system (Fig. 4.34) at the electron microscopic level. The *outer mitochondrial membrane* has a smooth contour, is approximately 7.0 nm thick and defines the peripheral limits of the organelle. The *inner mitochondrial membrane* is approximately 8.0 nm thick and is modified into plate-like or tubular folds *(cristae mitochondriales)*. The cristae are separated by a *mitochondrial matrix* that is homogeneous and finely granular but of varying density. Electron-dense granules, *mitochondrial granules*, occur within the matrix (Fig. 4.35).

In vitro studies have determined that mitochondria are capable of changing shape. A change in shape or conformation has been linked with *coupled* or *uncoupled oxidative phosphorylation*. The *orthodox conformation* is associated with coupled oxidative phosphorylation and is represented morphologically by the "typical" picture of mitochondria (Fig. 4.34). The *condensed conformation* is associated with an uncoupled oxidative phosphorylation and is represented by mitochondria with enlarged cristae and a condensed mitochondrial matrix (Fig. 4.36).

The inner mitochondrial membrane and mitochondrial matrix contain all the enzymes of the citric acid cycle and those involved in oxidative phosphorylation, as well as those involved in fatty acid oxidation. The primary role of mitochondria, therefore, is the production of energy. Mitochondria, however, also contain DNA and RNA. They possess, therefore, some genetic and protein-synthetic potential. As such, they are capable of replication, although the exact method (budding or division) is yet to be determined.

Lysosomes

Structure. *Lysosomes* are membrane-bound particles that are rich in *hydrolytic enzymes*. They are represented morphologically by numerous shapes and sizes. Except in a few instances, the histochemical demonstration of specific hydrolases *(acid phosphatase, arylsulfatase)* is necessary for the absolute identification of these organelles. At the light microscopic level, some of the granules of basophils, eosinophils, and neutrophils are lysosomes and clearly demonstrate the range of structure and staining properties associated with these particles (Fig. 4.37).

Lysosomes are particles in various stages of formation, maturation, and activity. This continuum is represented by particles of varying morphological configuration. Primary lysosomes are generally believed to form in a manner similar to secretory granules. The hydrolytic enzymes are synthesized in the RER, whereas the segregation and packaging occur within the Golgi apparatus. The lysosomes, therefore, are "secretory granules for intracellular use."

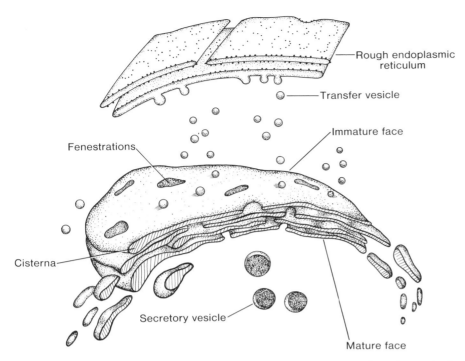

Fenestrations

Cisterna

Rough endoplasmic reticulum

Transfer vesicle

Immature face

Secretory vesicle

Mature face

Figure 4.33. Diagram of the Golgi apparatus and its relationship to the RER. Transfer vesicles bud from the RER and fuse with the immature face. Materials enter the stack at the immature face, traverse the stack, and emerge as presecretory vesicles. The vesicles mature into secretory vesicles.

point, the primary lysosome and engulfed pinocytotic vesicles are referred to as a *multivesicular body*. After the completion of the digestive process, it is assumed that the multivesicular body is converted to a primary lysosome for future functioning or, as in the case of phagocytosis, a residual body is formed.

Autophagocytosis. In *autophagocytosis*, a sequence of events occurs that is similar but not identical to that associated with phagocytosis. Various organelles, as well as insoluble portions of cytoplasm, tend to degenerate or become functionless. These granules or regions are represented as *foci of cytoplasmic degeneration*. The degenerative or functionless cytoplasmic components are engulfed by primary lysosomes and are referred to as *autophagic vacuoles* or *cytolysosomes*. The fate of cytolysosomes is similar to the fate of phagolysosomes.

Function. The complexity and diversity of lysosomal function accounts for the heterogeneity of these particles. Moreover, these particles are part of a continually dynamic process. Lysosomes are extremely important organelles; they should not be considered simply the "garbage dumps" of the cell. Not only are they responsible for

Some researchers believe that lysosomes are formed in the GERL (*G*olgi *E*ndoplasmic *R*eticulum *L*ysosome), a portion of the RER associated with the mature face of the Golgi apparatus.

The adjoining scheme represents the relationship of lysosomal particles in various stages of activity (Fig. 4.38). Vacuoles bud from the Golgi complex and are transformed into *dense bodies (primary lysosomes, inactive lysosomes)*. The fate of these primary lysosomes is dependent upon the subsequent activity with which they are associated. Two distinct types of activity are associated with lysosomes, *endocytosis* and *autophagocytosis*. Endocytotic activity may be further subdivided into *phagocytosis* or *pinocytosis*.

Endocytosis. In *phagocytosis*, particulate matter is engulfed by the cell in the form of membrane-bound vesicles *(phagosomes)*. The union of a primary lysosome with a phagosome produces a *secondary* or *active lysosome*, often referred to as a *phagolysosome*. Upon completion of the digestive activity of this newly formed structure, or during an arrest in the activity, a resulting *residual body* is formed. The latter, upon completion of the digestive function, is extruded from the cell.

In *pinocytosis*, fluid material is engulfed by the cell in *pinocytotic vesicles*. These vesicles fuse with primary lysosomes, but their integrity is not lost; i.e., they appear within a dense body as vesicles. At this

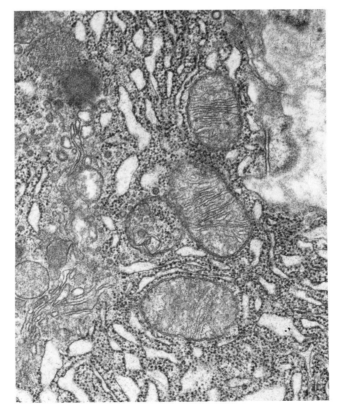

Figure 4.34. Typical mitochondria. The mitochondria are in the orthodox conformation. The cristae are prominent, because the mitochondrial matrix is not very dense. ×27,000. Compare the density of the mitochondrial matrix in this figure with that of Figure 4.36.

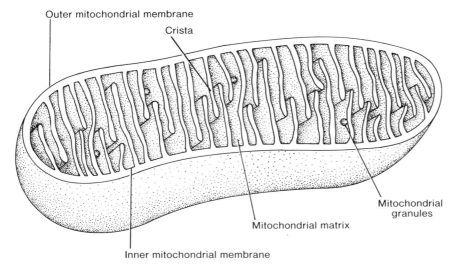

Figure 4.35. Diagram of a typical mitochondrion. The typical components of the organelle are labeled.

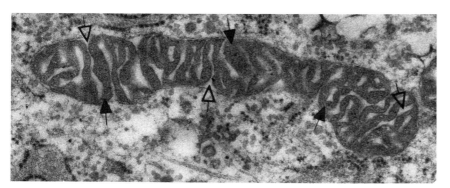

Figure 4.36. An electron micrograph of a mitochondrion in the condensed conformation. The cristae *(open arrows)* are separated from each other by a condensed mitochondrial matrix *(solid arrows)*. ×48,000.

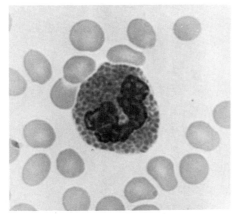

Figure 4.37. A feline basophil. The small, specific granules scattered throughout the cell are lysosomes. ×400.

the routine digestive properties of cells, but they are also important organelles through which protective functions of cells are mediated. The identification of lysosomes was based originally on the presence of acid phosphatase. Lysosomes are now known to contain approximately 50 *acid hydrolases*, including *phosphatases, nucleases, proteases, sulfatases, peptidases, glycosidases,* and *lipases*.

The hydrolyzed products, once released from the lysosomes, are available for reutilization by the cell. This intracellular function has led to the general misconception of their being exclusively refuse factories—scavenging, digesting, and sequestering various materials throughout the life cycle of the cell. Lysosomal enzymes also function outside the cell. Collagenases, proteases, and other hydrolases can destroy extracellular matrices. Lysosomes are responsible for protecting the body against foreign materials by digesting this particulate material. The organelle is responsible for destroying cells also. These organelles account for *autolytic processes*. Under normal conditions, routine cellular death *(necrobiosis)* is mediated through autolysosomal function *(autolysis)*. In pathological conditions, lysosomes can account for abnormal cell death *(necrosis)* via autolytic processes as well.

Lysosomes function in the degradation of biologically active molecules that regulate cellular activities related to growth, nutrition, metabolism, and differentiation. Receptor mediated endocytosis is significant in the flow of internalized substances to various organelles. Some of these substances are delivered to lysosomes for degradation, whereas others are not. The basis for this selective sorting of compounds to various cellular compartments is a subject of current research.

Peroxisomes

Structure and Function. *Peroxisomes* or *microbodies* are spherical or ovoid organelles that are smaller than mitochondria. Special staining techniques are required for their demonstration at the light microscopic level. They can be identified on the basis of the presence of certain enzymes. They are distinct organelles, the specific functions of which are being elucidated.

At the electron microscopic level of examination, microbodies are bound by a single membrane that encloses a matrix, the granularity and homogeneity of which have been compared to the mitochondrial matrix. A central density, core, or crystalloid particle (nucleoid) may be present within the matrix. The size, shape, and nature of these particles, as well as the presence or absence of same, is species-dependent. Cells with altered lipid metabolism have an increased number of peroxisomes. Peroxisomes have been identified in liver cells, the epithelial lining cells of the proximal convoluted tubules of the kidney, macrophages, and other cell types. They are, however, of variable occurrence in other cells of various animals.

The various enzymes that occur within peroxisomes—*catalase, flavin oxidases, d-amino oxidase, enzymes of the glyoxylate system (isocitrate lyase, malate synthetase, β-oxidation enzymes)*—are indicative of the diverse metabolic functions performed by peroxisomes. Some generalizations about their functional significance are possible. The pathways are catabolic, but some products (those of the glyoxylate pathway) may be used for anabolic purposes. The enzyme content and the function of peroxisomes vary from tissue to tissue. Catabolic pathways through peroxisomes represent an alternative mechanism for substrate metabolism. The unique peroxisomal enzymes—flavin oxidases and catalase—are associated with oxygen uptake.

Cytoplasmic Skeleton and Inclusions

Microtubules

Structure and Function. *Microtubules* occur in a variety of cells and subserve various functions. Except in the case of the mitotic spindle apparatus, microtubules are difficult to identify at the light microscopic level. Even then, they appear as fibers rather than being resolved as tubules.

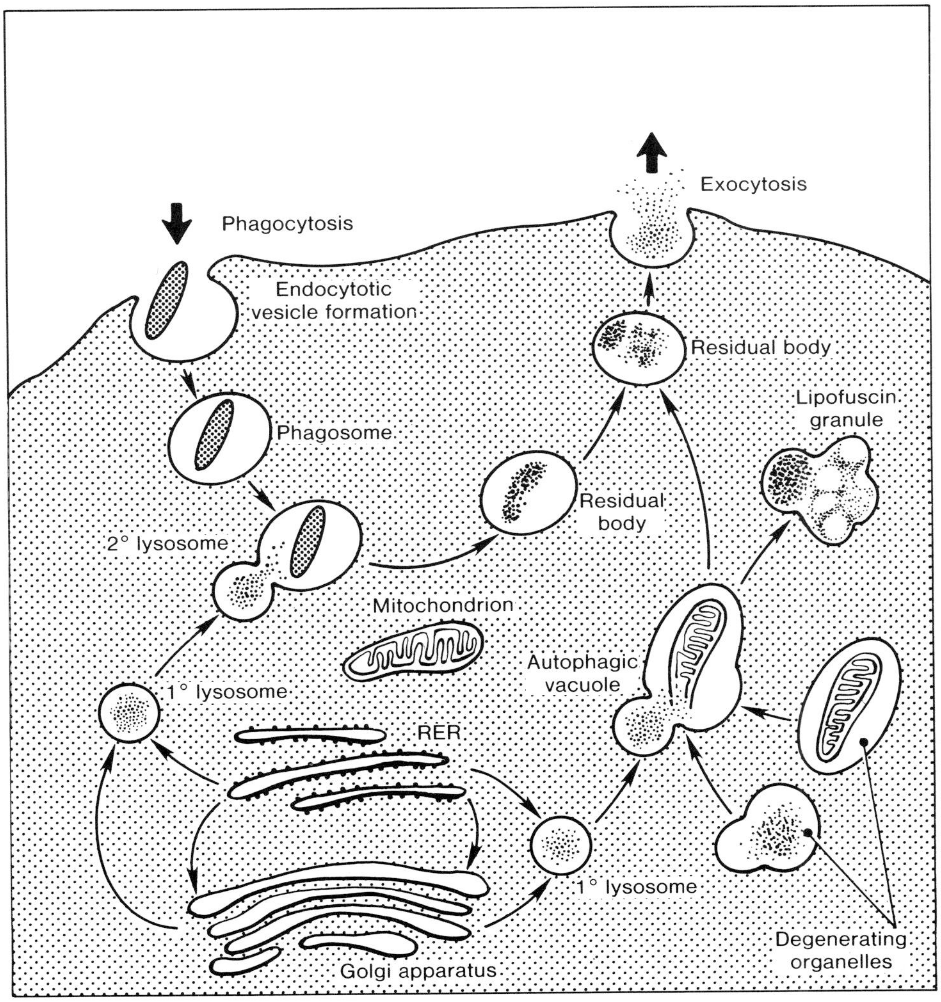

Figure 4.38. Diagram of lysosomal activity during phagocytosis and autophagocytosis. Particulate matter engulfed by the cell in endocytotic vesicles enters the cytoplasm within phagosomes. Primary lysosomes produced by the Golgi apparatus and/or the RER fuse with the phagosomes to form activated or secondary lysosomes. The digestion of the particulate matter culminates in the formation of a residual body that may be retained within the cell or extruded by the cell through exocytosis. Foci of degenerating organelles may be engulfed initially by membranes of the RER. Fusion with primary lysosomes forms autophagic vacuoles (secondary lysosomes). Residual bodies and/or lipofuscin granules result from autophagocytosis.

With the electron microscope, they are resolved as hollow, rod-like organelles with an outside diameter of 20–26 nm and a wall 5-7.0 nm thick (Fig. 4.39). Microtubules may be several micrometers in length. Microtubules occur scattered throughout the cytoplasm of many cell types, as well as being preferentially distributed throughout the cytoplasm in certain cells. Because microtubules are believed to be significant contributors to the maintenance of cell shape, they may be considered a part of the cytoplasmic skeleton. Microtubules occur in cilia, in flagella and in the manchette of spermatids. The organelles are significant, therefore, in the development of motility associated with these structures. Also, they are longitudinally oriented along the axoplasm of neurons, wherein they serve as a transport medium for various secretory products. Microtubules are an integral component of the spindle apparatus during mitosis.

Microtubules consist of smaller units called *tubulin*. This microtubular protein is a heterodimer of subunits called α- and β-tubulins, each with a molecular weight of 60,000 daltons. The dimers are arranged in series to form a *protofilament* (Fig. 4.40). Initial assembly of mictotubules appears to occur as coiled tubular protofilaments in association with the centrioles. Protofilamentous growth is accompanied by sequential polymerization at the ends or *nucleation sites* of the tubule.

Centrioles. The *centrioles* of resting cells are two small bodies contained within an area of gelatinous material referred to as the *centrosphere*. Although these bodies are usually inconspicuous in resting cells, special staining techniques can be utilized to demonstrate them at the light microscopic level.

The two small dots or bodies shown by the light microscope are resolved with the electron microscope as cylindrical units that are 150 nm in diameter and approximately 500 nm long (Fig. 4.40). They are oriented perpendicular to each other. Each of three cylinders is composed of groups of protofilaments. Although cylindrical, the groups of tubules are oriented eccentrically to each other. Fibrous material connects the terminal tubules of each group to the terminal tubules of adjacent groups. Also, fibrous material connects the peripherally located groups to the center of the centriole.

Centrioles play a significant role in the mitotic process, at which time they duplicate themselves and are associated with the microtubules of the spindle apparatus. A dense cytoplasmic region adjacent to the centrioles within the centrosphere has been associated with microtubule formation. This dense region has been implicated as a *microtubular organization center*.

Cilia and Flagella. *Cilia* and *flagella* are surface modifications of cells generally uti-

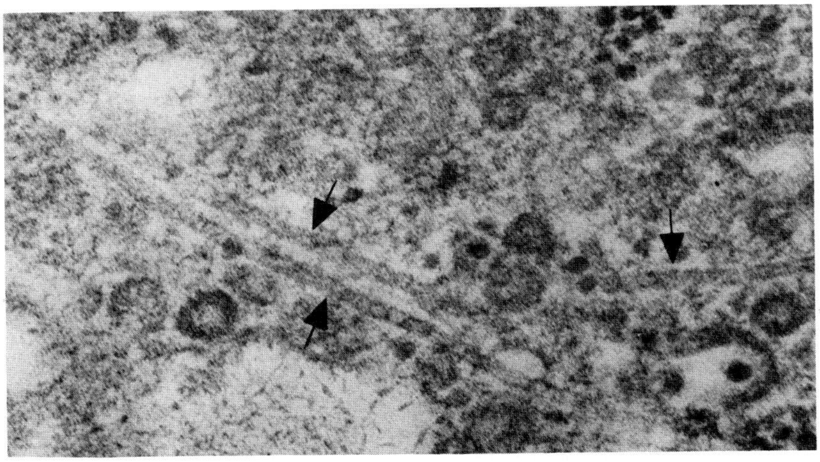

Figure 4.39. An electron micrograph of microtubules. The microtubules *(arrows)* are scattered throughout the cytoplasm. The distribution of microtubules is very specific and/or highly organized in some cells and in certain stages of the mitotic cycle.

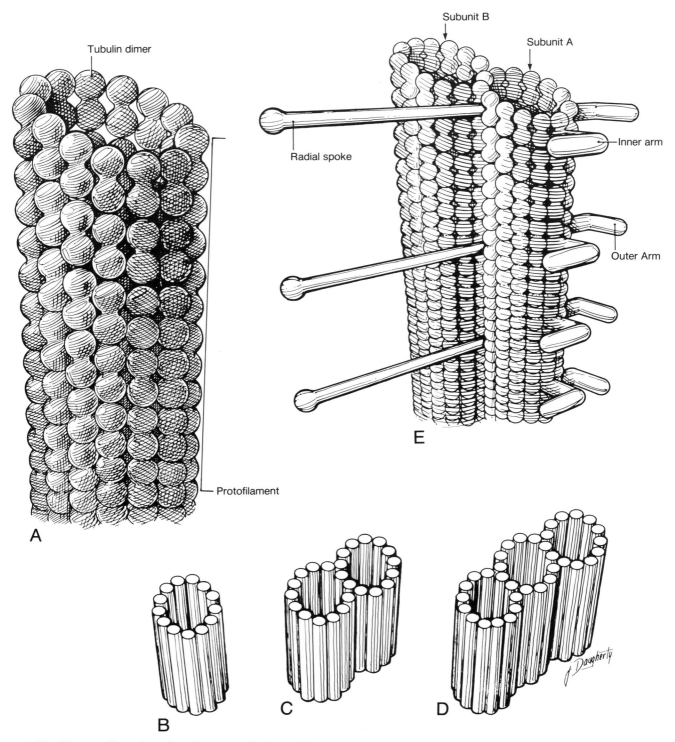

Figure 4.40. Diagrams illustrating microtubular organization. *A.* Microtubules consist of dimeric units called tubulin. Tubulin dimers are organized as linear arrays called protofilaments. *B.* Dimeric units are represented as protofilaments. Thirteen protofilaments comprise a mictotubule. *C.* Pairs of microtubules as occur in cilia and flagella. Protofilaments are shared by constituent microtubules. *D.* Microtubular triplets as occur in centrioles. Protofilaments are shared by microtubules in this configuration also. *E.* Mictotubular doublets as occur in cilia. Subunit A consists of 13 protofilaments. Inner and outer arms and radial spokes are attached to this subunit. Subunit B is incomplete and shares some of the protofilaments of subunit A.

lized for motility. An exception to this generalization exists. Two types of cilia are identified. *Stereocilia* are nonmotile processes of cells that are long and branched (Fig. 4.41); they lack the complex organi-

zation associated normally with cilia. These structures may be considered to be long microvilli. *Kinocilia*, often simply called cilia, are the motile, cellular processes.

Kinocilia are characteristic of many

types of epithelial cells wherein they serve functions related to movement. Some cells use cilia as sensory receptors. Typical ciliated cells have numerous cilia that range in length from 2 – 10 μm (Fig. 4.42). Flag-

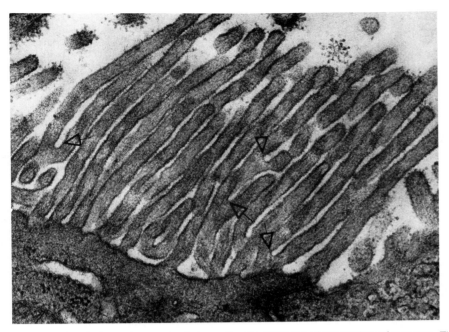

Figure 4.41. An electron micrograph of stereocilia of a lining cell of the trachea of a mouse. The stereocilia are branched *(arrows)* and lack the internal organization of kinocilia. (×46,000).

ellated cells (male gametes) normally have a single flagellum that ranges between 100 and 200 μm in length. Ciliary and flagellar diameters range between 0.3 and 0.5 μm.

The array of tubules, organized in a typical 9 + 2 pattern, is called the *axoneme* (Fig. 4.43). Nine peripheral pairs of microtubules surround two centrally positioned mictotubules. The components of the doublets share some protofilaments (Fig. 4.44). Microtubular *subfiber A* is essentially a complete microtubule with 13 protofilaments. *Radial spokes* and projecting arms *(inner* and *outer arms)* are attached to this subfiber. ATPase activity is localized to the inner and outer arms of subfiber A. The enzyme was named *dynein* (force protein) for its role in the mechanochemical transduction of energy necessary for ciliary motility. *Subfiber B* is an incomplete microtubule attached to subfiber A. Adjacent peripheral doublets are joined to each other by protein bridges called *nexins*. Similarly, peripheral doublets are joined by the radiating spokes to the central sheath that surrounds the central pair of microtubules (Fig.4.45). (The same organization is characteristic of flagella.)

Basal bodies form as centrioles within cells that develop cilia (and flagellae). The new centrioles migrate to the periphery of the cell subjacent to the plasmalemma.

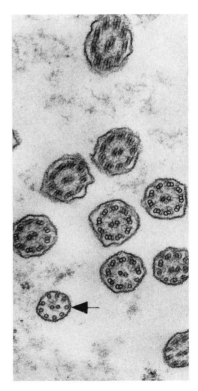

Figure 4.43. An electron micrograph of cross sections of cilia. The doublets and central pair of microtubules are apparent. The configuration of the peripheral microtubules is altered at the tip of the cilium *(arrow).* ×44,000.

Figure 4.42. A low magnification scanning electron micrograph of cilia from the trachea of a 9-month-old dog. (Courtesy of N. J. Wilsman and C. E. Farnum).

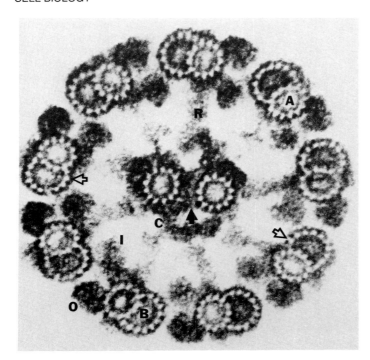

New dimers are added progressively at the distal nucleation sites and the nascent axonemes grow into a sheath of plasma membrane and cytoplasmic matrix to form the new cilia. *Rootlets* develop in association with the proximal ends of the basal bodies to anchor these structures in the cytoplasm. Also, a striated structure, the *basal foot*, develops and attaches laterally to the basal bodies.

Ciliary Motility. Movement of cilia is essential for the transport of materials across an epithelial surface. As such, these structures are essential components of the *mucociliary apparatus*—the combination of mucous secretion and ciliary motility that protects the underlying epithelial lining. The cilia of a cell may beat in synchrony with each other (isochronal rhythm) or out of synchrony with each other *(metachronal rhythm)*. In a metachronal rhythm, all of the cilia within a particular row beat in synchrony, whereas those in successive rows are slightly asynchronous with those in adjacent rows. The result is a wave of activity similar to the response of a field of grain to a gentle breeze.

A ciliary beat cycle consists of two phases—an effective stroke and a recovery stroke. During the *effective stroke*, the cilium is rigid and beats generally in the di-

Figure 4.44. A high magnification transmission electron micrograph of a normal ciliary axonemic profile following demembranization and tannic acid staining. *R*, radial spoke; *A*, subunit A; *B*, subunit B; *C*, central sheath; *solid arrow*, bridge; *open arrows*, protofilaments; *O*, outer arm; *I*, inner arm. Compare this micrograph with Figure 4.45. (Courtesy of N. J. Wilsman and C. E. Farnum).

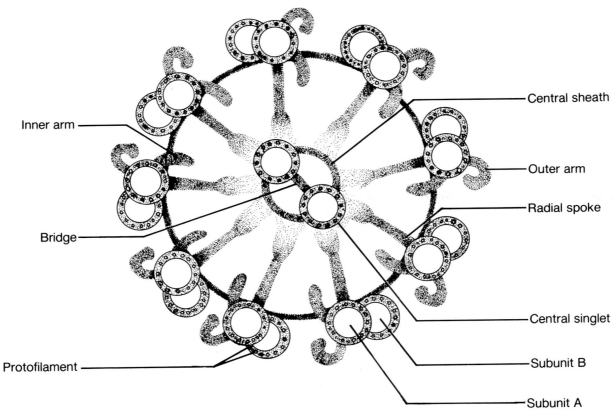

Figure 4.45. A diagram of an axoneme. Compare with the actual micrograph in Figure 4.44.

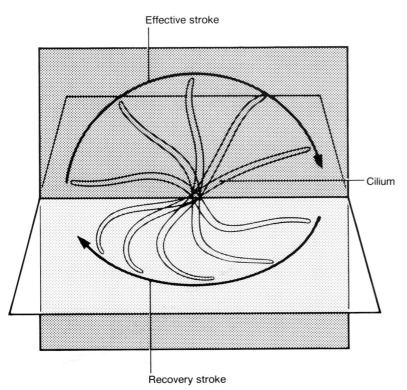

Effective stroke

Cilium

Recovery stroke

Figure 4.46. A diagram illustrating the two-phase ciliary beat. The cilium is rigid during the effective stroke. The structure relaxes, bends and returns to the starting point during the recovery phase.

rection of the cross-sectional axis between the pair of central microtubules (Fig. 4.46). During the *recovery stroke*, the cilium relaxes, bends, and returns to the starting position.

Cytoskeletal Components

Filaments. Various terms have been used to describe the long, thread-like structures that form networks or bundles of these structures in the cytoplasm. Common terms have included cytofilament, filament, tonofilament, microfilament, tonofibril, fibril, and fiber. These terms are confusing and they connate little more than a structure being elongated.

Three types of *cytofilaments* have been identified. *Microfilaments* are composed of *actin* and have a 5 – 6 nm diameter (Figs. 13.5 and 13.26). *Troponin* and *tropomyosin* are proteins associated with actin. These three proteins interact with the second type of filament, a *myosin filament* to mediate contraction (Fig. 13.15). Myosin filaments are 10 nm in diameter.

Intermediate filaments are 10-nm diameter filaments that are noncontractile. They form the supportive network of the cytoplasm (Fig. 4.47). Some intermediate filaments are involved in slow axoplasmic transport in neurons, cell spreading, and junctional complexes. These types of intermediate fibers are also called *tonofilaments*. Tonofilaments are especially prominent in a zone, the *terminal web*, that is subjacent

to the plasmalemma in some epithelial lining cells.

Cytoplasmic Inclusions

Secretory Inclusions. The secretory products of cells are varied and include such substances as enzymes, acids, proteins, and mucosubstances. The morphological configurations of the secretory products are as diverse as the products themselves. Lysosomes, as secretory products for intracellular use, have been described previously. *Zymogen granules*, membrane-bound packets of enzyme precursors for extracel-

lular use, typify many protein-secreting cells. As in the case of the pancreatic acinar cell, these secretory products appear as granules in a subluminal position. The granules are derived from the mature face of the Golgi complex, mature as they move toward the lumen and are secreted individually at the apical cell surface (Fig. 4.48).

Some cells that secrete *mucosubstances* are characterized, as in the case of the *goblet cell* depicted (Fig. 4.49), by a very foamy cytoplasm. The cytoplasm is basophilic and the nucleus is displaced basally. The foamy appearance is attributed to packets of mucous precursor materials contained within the cytoplasm (Plate II.9).

The secretion of lipid materials is associated normally with cells that possess a foamy but acidophilic cytoplasm. In these cases, however, the foamy appearance is a result of lipids having been leached from the cytoplasm. Cells from the cortex of the adrenal gland exemplify this type of secretory inclusion product (Fig. 4.50 and Plate II.3).

Some cells secrete various products that are not visible at the light microscopic level. Among these are the numerous active cells of the connective and supportive tissues. They secrete proteoglycans, glycosaminoglycans, and glycoproteins without any definitive, routine, and readily identifiable light microscopic evidence of this activity.

In some cells, a watery or *serous* secretion is accompanied by attendant alterations at the secretory surface. The accumulation of light microscopically visible products is not evident. The serous cells of some glands, characterized as cells with a finely granular and acidophilic cytoplasm and centrally or paracentrally located nuclei, exemplify another variation in cellular secretory activity and resulting products (Fig. 4.51 and Plate II.8).

Nutritive Inclusions. Most cells possess the ability to store various products that subserve a nutritive function. The most common substances that are readily visible

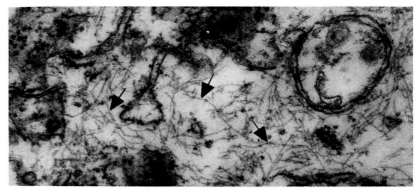

Figure 4.47. An electron micrograph of cytofilaments. The cell was ruptured during processing. Because much of the normal cytoplasmic matrix was lost during processing, the cytofilaments *(arrows)* are observed easily. ×52,000.

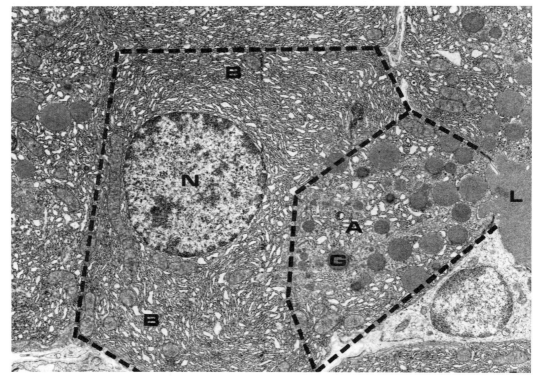

Figure 4.48. An electron micrograph of pancreatic acinar cells. The approximate limits of one cell *(outer dashed line)* are indicated. The apex *(A)* of the cell borders the lumen *(L)*. The apical portion of the cell *(inner dashed line)* contains numerous zymogen granules *(G)*. The basal portion *(B)* contains the nucleus *(N)*, RER, and mitochondria. ×7,000. Compare this electron micrograph with the light micrograph in Figure 4.29. Note that the distribution of acidophilic and basophilic staining corresponds to the distribution of specific organelles and inclusion bodies.

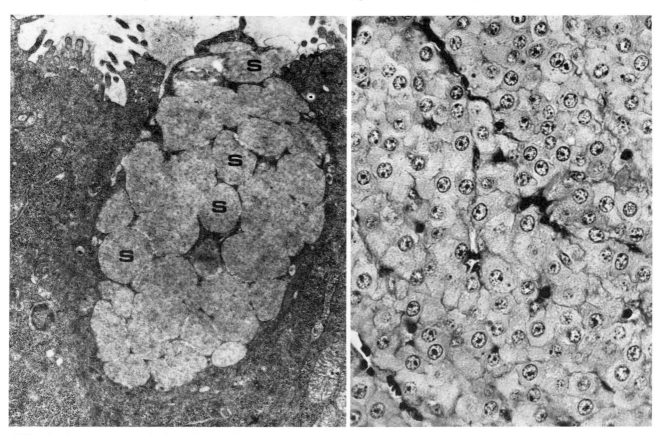

Figure 4.49. An electron micrograph of a goblet cell from the epithelial lining of a murine intestine. The cytoplasm has been displaced peripherally by the numerous secretory droplets (S). The nucleus is not in the plane of section. ×14,000. Compare this figure with the diagram in Figure 5.19. (Courtesy of A. M. Sheppard.)

Figure 4.50. Lipid-containing cells from the adrenal cortex. The pyramidal cells have a foamy appearance due to their content of lipid. Because the lipids were actually removed from the cells during processing by the paraffin technique, the foamy appearance is imparted by the spaces that remain. ×160.

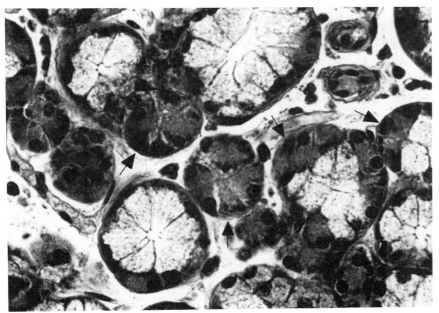

Figure 4.51. Serous cells from a salivary gland. The dark-staining cells *(arrows)* are the serous cells. The light-staining, pyramidal cells are mucous cells. ×160.

Cell Division

Cell Cycle. The *replacement* of old or dead cells with new ones is a continual but variable occurrence. Some cells, such as those of the skin, are replaced at regular intervals; others, such as the muscle cells of the heart, are not replaced. Generally, however, the body has the means to replace most cells. Besides the ability to replace worn out cells, the body must retain the ability to replace a given cell with an identical cell. The mechanism responsible for this faithful replication is *mitosis.*

This built-in replacement mechanism implies that cell lives are finite; however, the longevity of a cell is variable and specific for different cell types. Within the framework of a finite existence for various cell types, a definitive *cell cycle* can be defined. The cell cycle is the passage of a cell through the interphase and mitosis; the *generation time* is the time period required to complete one cycle (Fig. 4.55).

Although routine histologica¹ staining

at the light microscopic level are *glycogen* and *lipids.* Glycogen is especially apparent in the liver, skeletal muscle, and cells of cartilage. At the electron microscopic level, glycogen may appear as single particles that range from 15.0–30.0 nm in diameter with an irregular outline *(β particles)* (Fig.4.52). Accumulations in the form of *rosettes (α particles)* are also demonstrable (Fig. 4.53).

Lipid droplets within cells are the storage packets of triglycerides. Various cells store these lipids to varying degrees. The ultimate storage of lipids is manifested in adipocytes. At the electron microsopic level, lipid inclusions appear as osmiophilic bodies of varying density (Fig. 4.54). The degree of dark staining (uptake of osmium) is a function of the lipid composition of the droplet. Although they appear to be membrane-bound, they actually occur free in the cytoplasm. In specific instances, however, triglycerides in intestinal lining cells are membrane-bound.

Miscellaneous Inclusions. Numerous types of other inclusions occur within a large variety of cells. The most notable of these are the *pigment granules. Melanin* is the brown pigment responsible for that coloration in a variety of foci scattered throughout the body. *Lipofuscin* is a gold-brown pigment, the origin of which has been debated. Current thought is that this pigment occurs in residual bodies as a terminal inclusion of lysosomal activity. The accumulation of this pigment progresses with age; thus, it is often referred to as the "wear and tear" pigment. Altered cellular function is generally associated with its accumulation in nerve cells and cardiac muscle cells. *Hemosiderin* is a red-brown pigment resulting from the degradation of hemoglobin.

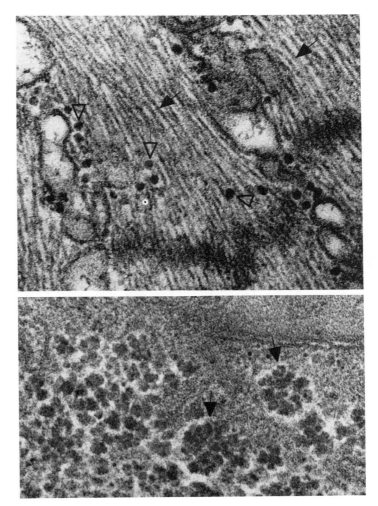

Figure 4.52. An electron micrograph of glycogen particles. The beta particles *(open arrows)* are scattered among the myofilaments *(solid arrows)* of a striated muscle cell. ×51,000.

Figure 4.53. An electron micrograph of glycogen particles. *Arrows*, α particles. ×133,000.

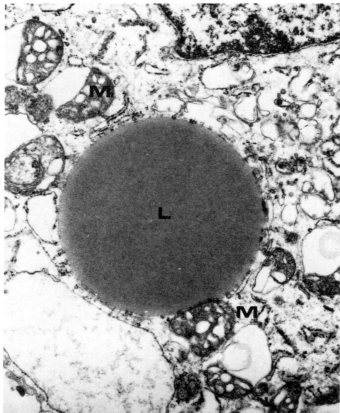

Figure 4.54.   An electron micrograph of a lipid droplet from a murine ascites tumor cell. The lipid droplet *(L)* is not membrane-bound. Condensed mitochondria *(M)* are present also. ×20,000.

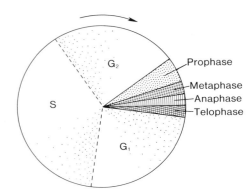

Figure 4.55.   Diagram of the cell cycle. The generation time of mammalian cells is variable but may average about 20 hours. The mitotic phase is the shortest, approximately 2 hours. The *S* phase is the longest, about 7 hours. Specific generation times characterize specific cells of the body.

cation of the chromosomes and a doubling of the DNA complement.

The *postduplication phase (postsynthetic phase)* is the G_2 stage. The naming of this phase refers only to the termination of DNA replication. Much synthetic, and therefore duplicative, activity characterizes this stage. The synthesis of histones, as well as that of RNA, occurs in this stage.

The interphase of the cell cycle is an extremely active phase responsible for a variety of cellular functions and events: increase in the total mass of a cell, increase

techniques allow only for the recognition of interphase and mitotic cells, autoradiographic techniques add valuable insights relating to other stages of activity during the cell cycle. Through the use of tritiated thymidine (a DNA precursor), subdivisions of the interphase are apparent. The *preduplication* or *presynthesis phase* (G_1) represents the period before the uptake of the labeled thymidine. This phase may be referred to as the *vegetative phase*. It is the stage during which time a cell conducts its "routine functions." Also, if a cell has a potential for mitosis, it is during this stage that the metabolites necessary to support mitosis are accumulated. **Most of the cells or accumulations of cells examined in histology will have been in the vegetative phase of the cell cycle.** The G_1 phase may be protracted in somatic cells. Such protracted phases of vegetative activity are referred to by some authors as the G_0.

The *duplication phase* (S) is the stage during which time DNA replication occurs, as evidenced by the nuclear uptake of labeled thymidine. Not all the chromatic material is labeled (or duplicated) simultaneously. *Telomeric* (near the chromosome ends) replication occurs before *centromeric* (near the middle of chromosomes) replication. The end result, however, is the dupli-

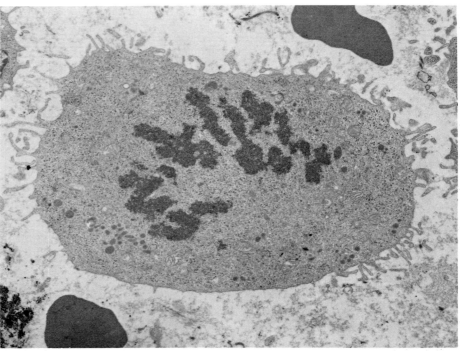

Figure 4.56.   An electron micrograph of a dividing mesenchymal cell from the connective tissue space. The cell is in prophase. The chromosomes have condensed, the nuclear membrane has disintegrated, but the spindle fibers have not yet formed. The mesenchymal cell has a high mitotic potential. ×2000.

in nuclear and nucleolar mass, duplication of chromatic material, synthesis of RNA and proteins, and conduction of routine cellular functions. In comparison with the interphase, the mitotic phase of the cell cycle is an extremely short, single-focus event.

Much valuable information concerning the cell cycle has been obtained from studies of cultured cells, especially synchronized cell cultures. Cells in these types of systems grow rapidly and have a rapid doubling time. This type of growth is encountered rarely in the cells of the adult body.

Differentiation and Mitotic Potential. During early stages of embryonic and fetal growth, most of the cells of the body have a high potential for division as well as the potential to become a variety of cells. As development ensues, the *differentiation* of varied cellular populations is apparent. A consequence of this *specialization* (differentiation) is the *reduction or loss of cellular potentiality* and a *reduction or loss of reproductive capacity (mitotic potential).*

Generally, highly specialized cells possess a low capacity for or an inability to duplicate themselves. Neurons (Fig. 4.20) and cardiac muscle cells (Fig. 13.23) are examples of these.

Specialized cell populations usually have specific cells associated with them from which other members of their populations differentiate. These are generally called *stem cells.* The basal layer of cells of the epidermis (stem cell or germinative cell layer) is an example of a residual cellular population within a community of specific cells that retains the ability to replace cells desquamated from the skin surface. These stem cells are capable only of forming "epidermal" cells. Other examples are included in subsequent sections.

The *mesenchymal cell* of the body is a cell similar to the aforementioned. It is a stem cell. This cell, however, possesses a high potentiality and reproductive capacity. It is an undifferentiated cell capable of specializing into a variety of cell types: muscle cells, bone cells, cartilage cells, fat cells, etc. It is scattered throughout the body in association with numerous cell populations wherein it retains this ability for mitosis and multiple expression. It may be apparent around small blood vessels in the *perivascular space.* The mesenchymal cell is a stellate or fusiform cell with a scant cytoplasm and a large, vesicular nucleus. Its ultrastructural features conform to the relationships discussed regarding euchromatin, ribosomes, polyribosomes, and RER. This cell, however, is difficult to identify positively in section.

Some cells, despite their high degree of differentiation, still retain a high reproductive capacity under certain conditions. One example of this apparent paradox is the *hepatocyte.* The cells of the liver become highly mitotic after an injury.

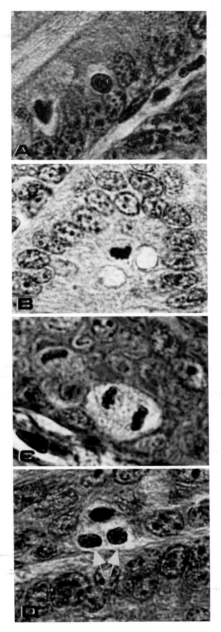

Figure 4.57. Mitosis of the lining cells of an intestinal crypt. The prophase *(A)* is initiated and the chromosomes migrate to the equitorial plane during the metaphase *(B).* During the anaphase *(C),* the chromosomes migrate toward the poles. During telophase *(D),* daughter cells *(arrows)* are formed. The cell above the daughter cells has entered prophase.

In order to maintain the reproductive capacity described, the dividing cells commit one daughter cell to the differentiation process and retain the other in an undifferentiated condition for future division.

Divisional Sequence. The continuum of the divisional process has been arbitrarily divided into five stages: *interphase, prophase, metaphase, anaphase,* and *telophase.* The last four stages actually comprise *mitosis;* however, the significance of

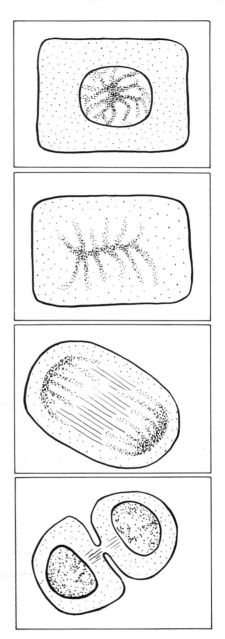

Figure 4.58. Diagrams of the phases of mitosis. The diagrams match the events in Figure 4.57. The daughter cells remain connected for a short period of time via the midbody.

the interphase cannot be neglected and has been elaborated upon previously.

During the *prophase* (Figs 4.56 and 4.57), the chromatic material undergoes a progressive condensation that culminates with the chromosomes becoming distinct entities in late prophase. The nuclear membrane disintegrates during the latter part of the prophase. At the same time, the nucleolus disappears. The *centrosphere* divides in the cytoplasm, each part containing a pair of *centrioles,* and the centrioles move toward opposite poles of the cell. *Spindle fibers,* composed of microtubules, are apparent between the migrating centrospheres.

During the *metaphase* (Figs. 4.57 and 4.58), the chromosomes migrate toward and align themselves along the *equatorial plane* of the cell. Microtubules attach themselves to the *centromere* and each chromosome is composed of two *chromatids* attached at the centromere. The alignment along the equatorial plane is random; *homologous chromosomes* do *not* align themselves one next to the other as pairs. This is an important distinction between *mitosis* and *meiosis*.

With the splitting of the two chromatids at the centromere, daughter chromosomes begin to migrate to the opposite cellular poles. These events mark the initiation of the *anaphase* (Figs. 4.57 and 4.58). Thus, the anaphase is characterized by the initiation of *karyokinesis*.

The reconstitution of the nuclear membrane marks the initiation of the *telophase* (Figs. 4.57 and 4.58). The chromosomes become dispersed while the nucleus enlarges. *Cytokinesis*, initiated peripheral to the equatorial plane, is completed and two identical daughter cells result.

References

General References

Bloom, W. and Fawcett, D.W.: *A Textbook of Histology.* 9th edition, W. B. Saunders, Philadelphia, 1968.
Brachet, J. and Mirsky, A.E.: *The Cell: Biochemistry, Physiology and Morphology.* 6 Vols. Academic Press, New York, 1959–1964.
Bresnick, E. and Schwartz, A.: *Functional Dynamics of the Cell.* Academic Press, New York, 1968.
DeRobertis, E.D.P., Nowinski, W.W. and Saez, F.A.: *Cell Biology.* 4th edition, W.B. Saunders, Philadelphia, 1965.
DuPraw, E.J.: *Cell and Molecular Biology.* Academic Press, New York, 1968.
Fawcett, D.W.: *Atlas of Fine Structure: The Cell, Its Organelles and Inclusions.* W.B. Saunders, Philadelphia, 1967.
Ham, A.W. and Cormack, D.H.: *Histology.* 8th edition, J. B. Lippincott, Philadelphia, 1979.
Lentz, T.L.: *Cell Fine Structure: An Atlas of Drawings of Whole-Cell Structure.* W. B. Saunders, Philadelphia, 1971.
Matthews, J.L. and Martin, J.H.: *Atlas of Human Histology and Ultrastructure.* Lea and Febiger, Philadelphia, 1968.
Porter, K. R. and Bonneville, M.A.: *Fine Structure of Cells and Tissues.* 3rd edition, Lea and Febiger, Philadelphia, 1968.
Sandborn, E.B.: *Cells and Tissues by Light and Electron Microscopy.* Academic Press, New York, 1970.

Nucleus

Bennett, H.S.: Fine structure of cell nucleus, chromosomes, nucleoli and membrane. Rev. Mod. Phys. *31:*297, 1959.
Dalton, A.J. and Haguenau, F.: *Ultrastructure in Biological Systems. The Nucleus.* Vol. 3. Academic Press, New York, 1968.
Monneron, A. and Bernard, W.: Fine structural organization of the interphase nucleus in some mammalian cells. J. Ultrastruct. Res. *27:*266, 1969.
Moses, N.J.: Studies on nuclei using correlated cytochemical, light and electron microscopic techniques. J. Biophys. Biochem. Cytol. *2:*397, 1956.
Wischnitzer, S.: The submicroscopic morphology of the interphase nucleus. Inter. Rev. Cytol. *34:*1, 1973.

Nuclear Envelope

Abelson, H.T. and Smith, G.H.: Nuclear Pores: The pore-annulus relationship in thin sections. J. Ultrastruct. Res. *30:*558, 1970.
Barnes, B.G. and Davis, J.M.: The structure of nuclear pores in mammalian tissues. J. Ultrastruct. Res. *3:*131, 1959.
Fawcett, D.W. and Chemes, H.: Changes in distribution of nuclear pores during differentiation of male germ cells. Tiss. Cell. *1:*147, 1979.
Franke, W. Isolated nuclear membranes. J. Cell Biol. *31:*619, 1966.
Franke, W. and Kartenbeck, J.: Structure of nuclear membranes isolated from brain cells. Experientia. *25:*396, 1969.
Franke, W.W., Scheer, U. and Krohne, G. and Jarasch, E.-D.: The nuclear envelope and the architecture of the nuclear periphery, J. Cell Biol. *91:*39s, 1981.
Kessel, R.G.: Fine structure of the pore-annulus complex in the nuclear envelope and the annulate lamellae of germ cells. Z. Zellforsch. *94:*441, 1969.
Maul, G.C.: On the octagonality of the nuclear pore complex. J. Cell Biol. *51:* 558, 1971.
Maul, G.C.: The nuclear and cytoplasmic pore complex: Structure, dynamics, distribution and evolution. Int. Rev. Cytol. *Suppl. 6:*76, 1977.
Wiener, J., Spiro, D. and Lowenstein, W.R.: Ultrastructure and permeability of nuclear membranes. J. Cell Biol. *27:*107, 1965.
Yoo, B.Y. and Bailey, S.T.: The structure of pores in isolated pea nuclei. J. Ultrastuct. Res. *18:*651, 1967.

Chromatin

Barr, M.L.: The significance of sex chromatin. Inter. Rev. Cytol. *19:*35, 1966.
Bujard, H.: Electron Microscopy of single stranded DNA. J. Molec. Biol. *49:*125, 1970.
Dales, S.: A study of the fine structure of mammalian somatic chromosomes. Exp. Cell Res. *19:*577, 1960.
Osgood, E.E., Jenkins, D.P., Brooks, R. and Lawson, R.K.: Electron micrographic studies of the expanded and uncoiled chromosomes from human leukocytes. Ann. N.Y. Acad. Sci. *113:*717, 1963.
Priest, J.H. and Shikes, R.H.: Distribution of labeled chromatin. J. Cell Biol. *47:*99, 1970.
Watson, J.D.: *Molecular Biology of the Gene.* W.A. Benjamin, Inc., New York, 1965.

Nucleolus

Bernhard, W. and Granboulan, N.: Electron microscopy of the nucleolus in vertebrate cells. *In:* Dalton, A.J. and Haguenau (eds.) *Ultrastructure in Biologic Systems: The Nucleus.* Vol. 3. Academic Press, New York, p 81, 1968.
Vincent, V.S. and Miller, O.J., Jr. (eds.): The nucleolus, its structure and function. Nat. Cancer Inst. Monogr. *23:* 1965.

Cellular Membranes

Bolis, L. and Pethica, B.A.: *Membrane Models and the Formation of Biological Membranes.* North Holland Publishing, Amsterdam, 1968.
Dalton, A.J. and Haguenau, F. (eds.): *Ultrastructure in Biological Systems: The Membranes.* Vol. 4. Academic Press, New York, 1968.
Davson, H.: Growth of the concept of the paucimolecular membrane. Circulation *26:*1022, 1962.
Finean, J.B.: The molecular organization of cell membranes. Progr. Biophys. *16:*143, 1966.
Hendler, R.W.: Biological membrane ultrastructure. Physiol. Rev. *51:*66, 1971.
Korn, E.D.: Structure of biological membranes. Science *153:*1492, 1966.
Robertson, J.D.: The ultrastructure of cell membranes and their derivatives. Biochem. Soc. Sympos. *16:*3, 1959.
Rothman, J.E. and Lenard, J.: Membrane asymmetry. Science *195:*743, 1977.
Singer, S.J. and Nicolson, G.L.: The fluid mosaic model of the structure of cell membranes. Science *175:*720, 1972.
Sjostrand, F.S.: A comparison of plasma membranes, cytomembranes and mitochondrial membrane elements with respect to ultrastructural features. J. Ultrastruct. Res. *9:*561, 1963.
Sjostrand, F.S.: A new repeat structural element of mitochondrial and certain cytoplasmic membranes. Nature *199:*1262, 1963.
Vanderkooi, G. and Green, D.E.: New insights into biological membrane structure. Bioscience *21:*409, 1971.

Ribosomes and Granular Endoplasmic Reticulum

Alfrey, V.G.: Nuclear ribosomes, messenger RNA and protein synthesis. Exp. Cell. Res. *9:*183, 1963.
Blobel, G. and Dobberstein, B.: Transfer of proteins across membranes. II. Reconstitution of functional rough microsomes from heterologous components. J. Cell Biol. *67:*852, 1975.
Haguenau, F.: The ergastoplasm: Its history, ultrastructure and biochemistry. Int. Rev. Cytol. *7:*425, 1958.
Kreibich, G., Ulrich, B.L. and Sabatini, D.D.: Proteins of rough microsomal membranes related to ribosome binding. I. Identification of ribophorin I and II, Membrane proteins characteristic of rough microsomes. J. Cell Biol. *77:*64, 1978.
Palade, G.E.: A small particulate component of the cytoplasm. J. Biophys. Biochem. Cytol. *1:*59, 1955.
Palade, G.E.: Intracellular aspects of the process of protein systesis. Science *189:*347, 1975.
Porter, K.R.: Observations on a submicroscopic basophilic component of the cytoplasm. J. Exp. Med. *97:*727, 1953.
Rich, A.: Polyribosomes. Sci. Amer. *209:*44, 1963.
Siekevitz, P. and Zamecnik, C.: Ribosomes and protein systhesis. J. Cell Biol. *91:*53s, 1981.
Spirin, A.S. and Gavrilova, L.P.: *The Ribosome.* Springer-Verlag, New York, 1969.

Agranular Endoplasmic Reticulum

Cardell, R.R.: Smooth endoplasmic reticulum in rat hepatocytes during glycogen deposition and depletion. Int. Rev. Cytol. *48:*221, 1977.
Christensen, A.K.: Fine structure of testicular interstitial cells in the guinea pig. J. Cell Biol. *26:*911, 1965.
Christensen, A.K. and Fawcett, D.W.: The fine structure of the interstitial cells of the mouse testis. Amer. J. Anat. *118:*551, 1966.
DePierre, J.W. and Dallner, G.: Structural aspects of the membrane of the endoplasmic reticulum. Biochim. Biophys. Acta *415:*411, 1975.
Ito, S.: The endoplasmic reticulum of gastric parietal cells. J. Biophys. Biochem. Cytol. *11:*333, 1961.
Remmer, H. and Merker, H.J.: Effects of drugs on the formation of smooth endoplasmic reticulum and drug metabolizing enzymes. Ann. N.Y. Acad. Sci. *123:*79, 1965.

Golgi Complex

Beams, H.W. and Kessel, R.G.: The Golgi apparatus: Structure and function. Int. Rev. Cytol. *23:*209, 1968.
Berlin, J.D.: The localization of acid mucopolysaccharides in the Golgi complex of intestinal goblet cells. J. Cell Biol. *32:*760, 1967.
Caro, L.G. and Palade, G.E.: Protein synthesis, storage and discharge in the pancreatic exocrine cell. An autoradiographic study. J. Cell Biol. *20:*473, 1964.
Farquhar, M.G. and Palade, G.: The Golgi apparatus (complex)—(1954–1981)—from artifact to center stage. J. Cell Biol. *91:*77s, 1981.
Hodge, A.J., McLeon, S.D. and Mercer, F.V.: A possible mechanism for the morphogenesis of lamellar systems in plant cells. J. Biophys. Biochem. Cytol. *2:*597, 1956.
Jamieson, J.D. and Palade, G.E.: Intracellular transport of secretory proteins in the pancreatic exocrine cell. I. Role of the peripheral elements of the Golgi complex. J. Cell Biol. *34:*597, 1967.
Neutra, M. and Leblond, C.P.: Synthesis of the carbohydrate of mucus in the Golgi complex as shown by electron microscope radioautography of goblet cells from rats injected with glucose-H³. J. Cell Biol. *30:*119, 1966.
Neutra, M. and Leblond, C.P.: The Golgi apparatus. Sci. Amer. *220:*100, 1969.

Mitochondria

Ashwell, M. and Work, T.: The biogenesis of mitochondria. Ann. Rev. Biochem. *39:*251, 1970.

Claude, A. and Fullom, E.F.: Electron microscopic study of isolated mitochondria. J. Exp. Med. *81:*51, 1945.

Fernandez-Moran, H., Oda, T., Blair, P.V. and Green, D.E.: A macromolecular repeating unit of mitochondrial structure and function. J. Cell Biol. *22:*63, 1964.

Green, D.E. and Young, J.H.: Energy transduction in membrane systems. Amer. Sci. *59:*92, 1971.

Hackenbrock, C.R.: Ultrastructural basis for metabolically-linked mechanical activity in mitochondria. I. Reversible ultrastructural changes in metabolic steady state in isolated liver mitochondria. J. Cell Biol. *30:*269, 1966.

Hackenbrock, C.R.: Ultrastructural basis for metabolically-linked mechanical activity in mitochondria. II. Electron transport-linked ultrastructural transformations in mitochondria. J. Cell Biol. *37:*345, 1968.

Hall, D. and Palmer J.: Mitochondrial research today. Nature *221:*717, 1969.

Lehninger, A.L.: *The Mitochondrion.* Benjamin, New York, 1964.

Munn, E.A.: *The Structure of Mitochondria.* Academic Press, New York, 1974.

Wagner, P.: Genetics and phenogenetics of mitochondria. Science *163:*1026, 1969.

Weber, N.E. and Blair, P.V.: Ultrastructural studies of beef heart mitochondria. I. Effects of adenosine diphosphate on mitochondrial morphology. Biochem. Biophys. Res. Commun. *36:*987, 1969.

Lysosomes

Bainton, D.F.: The discovery of lysosomes. J. Cell Biol. *91:*66s, 1981.

DeDuve, C.: Lysosomes. Sci. Amer. *208:*5, 1963.

Gahan, P.B.: Histochemistry of lysosomes. Int. Rev. Cytol. *21:*1, 1967.

Gordon, G.B., Miller, L.R. and Bensch, K.G.: Studies on the intracellular digestive process in mammalian tissue culture cells. J. Cell Biol. *25:*41, 1965.

Novikoff, A.B., Essner, E. and Quintana, N.: Golgi apparatus and lysosomes. Fed. Proc. *23:*1010, 1964.

Centrioles and Basal Bodies

Randall, J. and Hopkins, J.M.: Studies on cilia, basal bodies and somes related organelles. II. Problems of genesis. Proc. Linnean Soc. London. *174:*37, 1963.

Szollosi, D.: Centrioles, centriolar satellites and spindle fibers. Anat. Rec. *148:*343, 1964.

Wolfe, J.: Basal body fine structure and chemistry. Adv. Cell Mol. Biol. *2:*151, 1972.

Yamada, E.: Some observations on the fine structure of the centriole in the mitotic cell. Kurume Med. J. *5:*36, 1958.

Microbodies

Hruban, Z. and Rechcigl, M., Jr.: Microbodies and related particles: Morphology, biochemistry and physiology. Int. Rev. Cytol. Suppl I., 1969.

Microtubules, Filaments, and Fibrils

Behnke, O.: Studies on isolated microtubules. Evidence for a clear space component. Cytobiol. *11:*366, 1975.

Brody, I.: The ultrastructure of the tonofilaments in the keratinization process. J. Ultrastruct. Res. *4:*265, 1960.

Franke, W.W., Schmidt, E., Osborn, M. and Weber, K.: Different intermediate sized filaments distinguished by immunofluorescence microscopy. Proc. Nat. Acad. Sci. *75:*5034, 1978.

Gibbons, I.R.: Cilia and flagella of eukaryotes. J. Cell Biol. *91:*107s, 1981.

Haimo, L.T. and Rosenbaum, J.L.: Cilia, flagella and microtubules. J. Cell Biol. *91:*125s, 1981.

Huxley, H.E.: Electron microscopic studies in the structure of natural and synthetic protein filaments from striated muscle. J. Molec. Biol. *7:*281, 1963.

Inoue, S. and Stephens, R.E. (eds.): *Molecules and Cell Movement.* Raven Press, New York, 1975.

Ledbetter, M.C. and Porter, K.R.: Morphology of microtubules of plant cells. Science *144:*872, 1964.

Sandborn, E., Koen, P.F., McNabb, J.D. and Moore, G.: Cytoplasmic microtubules in mammalian cells. J. Ultrastruct. Res. *11:*123, 1964.

Slatterback, D.B.: Cytoplasmic microtubules. I. Hydra. J. Cell Biol. *18:*367, 1963.

Soifer, D. (ed.): The biology of cytoplasmic microtubules. Ann. N. Y. Acad. Sci. *253:*1, 1975.

Wessels, N.K.: How living cells change their shape. Sci. Amer. *225:*76, 1971.

Inclusions

Billingham, R.E. and Silvers, W.K.: The melanocytes of mammals. Quart. Rev. Biol. *35:*1, 1960.

Bjorkerud, S.: The isolation of lipofuscin granules from bovine cardiac muscle. J. Ultrastruct. Res. *5:*5, 1963.

Napolitano, L.: The differentiation of white adipose cells. An electron microscope study. J. Cell Biol. *18:*663, 1963.

Revel, J.P.: Electron microscopy of glycogen. J. Histochem. Cytochem. *12:*104, 1964.

Cell Division

Flemming, W. Contributions to the knowledge of the cell and its vital processes. J. Cell Biol. *25:*3, 1965. (A translation of the 1880 work).

Mazia, D. How cells divide. Sci. Amer. *105:*101, 1961.

Mazia, D.: Fibrillar structure in mitotic apparatus. In: Warren, K.B. (eds.). *Formation of Cell Organelles.* Academic Press, New York, 1967.

SECTION III:
HISTOLOGY

5: Epithelia

General Characteristics

Form. Epithelial tissues consist of aggregations of cells that cover or line the surfaces of the body and organs. Epithelia are composed generally of similar cells, or cells closely related structurally and/or functionally. They are in intimate contact with each other with little *intercellular substance* between them; therefore, these tissues have a *high cellular density*. Their close contacts and junctional complexes form effective barriers between the underlying connective tissue and the external environment or the environment characteristic of the tubular contents of the organs of which they are a part.

One margin of the cell is free, in contact with the environment (external or internal), and is termed the *apical* or *luminal border*. The *basal border* contacts the underlying connective tissue, whereas the *lateral surface* affords contact between adjacent cells. These cells possess apical/basal modifications that generally impart a distinct *cellular polarity*. Although cellular polarity is not a feature unique to epithelial cells, this characteristic is well-developed in them. The distribution of their constituent organelles reflects this polarity.

Epithelia are separated from the underlying connective tissues by a *basement membrane*. Epithelial tissues are avascular and are dependent upon the underlying connective tissue for the movement of metabolites and waste products.

The apical, lateral, and basal borders of epithelial cells have numerous modifications: *microvilli, kinocilia, stereocilia, desmosomes, basal lamina*, and various *junctional alterations*.

Functional Correlates. Epithelial cells are modified to subserve various functions essential to the organism. *Protection* from various insults—mechanical, microbial, desiccative, ultraviolet radiational—is achieved in various ways by these tissues. The body is protected from the aforementioned insults by virtue of its thickened and pigmented epithelial covering—the epidermis. The lining of the body tubes (digestive, respiratory and genitourinary systems) are subjected to mechanical injury, microbial invasion, and other insults to these surfaces. *Transport* of particulate matter along epithelial surfaces affords protection.

Secretion of various materials is an indispensable epithelial function. Waxy secretions of epithelial cells lubricate the covering epithelium and its associated structures—hairs and feathers. Also, secretions of epithelial cells moisten and protect lining epithelia. Other cells elaborate voluminous quantities of a watery secretion. During a 24-hour period, the secretory cells of the salivary glands of herbivores may secrete 10–15 gallons of this watery product. In some animals, the formation of sweat subserves a role in *thermoregulation* by providing a mechanism for evaporative cooling of the body. In the dairy cow, specific epithelial cells of the udder are responsible for the formation of 50–100 pounds of milk per day. Some epithelial cells are modified to synthesize and secrete digestive enzyme precursors. These examples of secretion characterize cells that elaborate their products onto a lining or covering epithelium. These are cells of *exocrine glands* or *glands of external secretion*.

Absorption of various materials occurs through the epithelial cells of the lungs, gastrointestinal tract, and renal tubules. Absorptive functions are highly selective and specific.

Epithelia subserve *sensory functions* in a diversity of ways. The entire nervous system is derived from epithelial cells, specifically the epithelial cells of neurectodermal origin. These cells secondarily lose their typical epithelial characteristics acquiring new ones that suit them ideally for intercellular communication. Epithelial cells that serve as sensory receptors are energy transducers.

Endocrine cells secrete their hormones into the surrounding microenvironment; however, these hormones cross endothelial cells and are transported to target cells via the blood.

Other epithelial cells, such as those that line the vascular and lymphatic systems, ensure that *functional exchange* occurs between the blood and lymphatic channels and the rest of the somatic (body) cells. Other similarly shaped cells line the body cavities (celomic spaces) and facilitate the movement of the visceral organs over smooth, lubricated surfaces.

Lastly, specific cells are reserved for the perpetuation of the species. These epithelial cells of the gonads perform the important *reproductive function* of gamete production.

Not all epithelial cells perform all the aforementioned functions. Some of them, however, perform a variety of these functions simultaneously. Most importantly, **the lining cells of epithelia form an effective barrier or interface that prevents the free outward movement of vital tissue fluid components, while simultaneously preventing the ingress of certain materials into the underlying fluid compartment.** Some epithelial cells are effective barriers; others characteristically permit some leakage across the lining.

Origin of Epithelia. During the early course of development, the embryo differentiates into three distinct germ layers—*ectoderm, mesoderm,* and *endoderm*. The outer covering (ectoderm) is separated from the inner lining (endoderm) by an intermediate packing layer, the mesoderm. Most of the epithelia are derivatives of the ectoderm and endoderm; a few are derived from mesoderm.

Diverse epithelial structures result from the development and differentiation of the ectoderm. The epithelium of the skin (epidermis) and its derivatives (hair, feathers, claws, hooves, horns, combs, wattles) are formed from the ectoderm. Invagination of the epidermis into the associated mesoderm results in the formation of sweat glands, sebaceous glands, mammary glands, and hair (feather) follicles. The ectoderm also differentiates into the epithelial cells of the: nasal cavity; paranasal sinuses and part of the buccal cavity; terminal portions of the digestive tract; genitourinary system; dental laminae; adenohypophysis and Rathke's pouch; lens of the eye and conjunctiva; outer layer of the tympanic membrane; organs responsible for auditory, olfactory, and gustatory sensations; nervous system.

The endoderm differentiates into numerous epithelial derivatives that line the inner aspect of the developing organism. This simple endodermal lining is characterized by numerous invaginations into the associated mesoderm. The epithelial derivatives of the endoderm include the following: lining of the digestive tract, except its initial and terminal portions; parenchyma of the liver, pancreas, and other digestive glands; glands of internal secretion (thyroid, parathyroid, adrenal cortex); thymus; trachea and lungs; urinary bladder; accessory sex glands and portions of the sex organs; portions of the oropharynx and nasopharynx; lining of the pharyngotympanic tube, middle ear cavity, and the inner lining of the tympanic membrane.

The mesoderm differentiates into the remaining tissues and organs of the body, including the adrenal cortex and part of the kidney. Additionally, this packing layer forms two kinds of epithelial cells. One population of cells, called *mesothelium*, lines the body cavities. **The name mesothelium means squamous cells derived from mesoderm that line the body cavities.** The lining cells (*endothelium*) of the heart, arteries, veins, capillaries, and lymphatic vessels comprise the other population. **The term endothelium means squamous cells derived from mesoderm that line the vascular and lymphatic channels.**

The *mesectoderm* consists of mesenchyme derived from neural crest cells. These primitive cells give rise to many cell types. One type, *mesenchymal epithelium*, lines certain spaces of the body. Mesenchymal epithelial cells comprise the leptomeninges (pia mater and arachnoid membrane), perilymphatic lining of the inner ear, and the iridial lining.

Unique Relationships. Epithelial tissues are avascular. They are dependent totally upon the underlying connective tissue for all of their nutrients. Similarly, waste products pass into this space for removal by the component vessels. This functional dependency upon the connective tissue is a requirement of all tissues. For those tissues that are "embedded within" or "surrounded by" the connective tissue space, the dependent relationship is less obvious than that noted in epithelia. Any separation of epithelia from the underlying connective tissue may have disastrous effects upon the integrity of this cellular boundary.

The intimate relationship between epithelia and their underlying connective tissues requires some sort of "glue" to hold them together. This is achieved by the *basement membrane*. This structure varies in thickness but is usually visible with the light microscope. Although the basement membrane is difficult to visualize with routine hematoxylin and eosin (H and E), it is demonstrable with silver stains and periodic acid-Schiff (PAS). It is a consistent modification associated with the basal border of epithelial cells.

The *glands of internal secretion (endocrine glands)* secondarily lose their association with a surface lining. One surface (usually basal), however, is still associated with the connective tissue. The other surface (usually apical) becomes associated intimately with the vasculature.

Classification. The classification and naming of epithelial tissues is based upon the number of cells layered upon each other and the predominant or surface cell shape (Fig. 5.1). An epithelial lining is either *simple* (one cell layer), *stratified* (more than one cell layer), *pseudostratified* (one cell layer appearing as more than one), or *transitional* (layers subject to change).

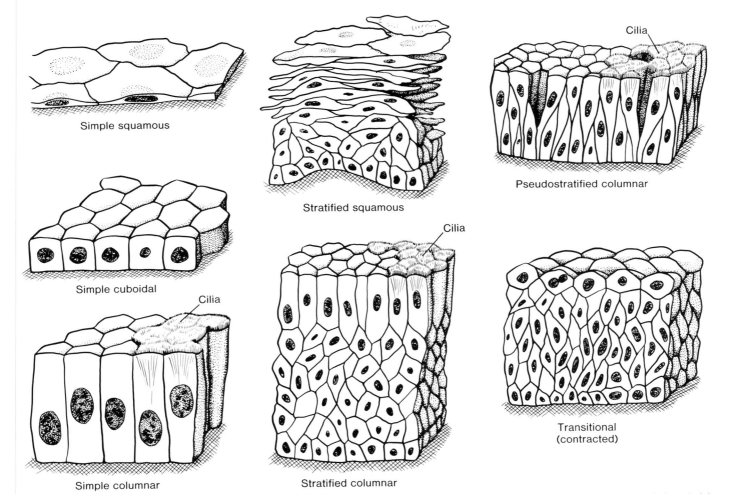

Simple squamous

Stratified squamous

Pseudostratified columnar

Simple cuboidal

Cilia

Simple columnar

Cilia

Stratified columnar

Cilia

Transitional (contracted)

Figure 5.1. Diagram of types of epithelial tissues. Simple, stratified, pseudostratified, and transitional epithelia are shown in relation to their underlying connective tissues. Simple cuboidal, simple columnar, stratified columnar, and pseudostratified columnar epithelia may be ciliated.

Simple epithelia are named according to the predominant cell type accordingly: *squamous, cuboidal, or columnar.* Pseudostratified epithelia consist predominantly of columnar cells, all of which touch the basement membrane. The pseudostratified epithelia are simple linings. Stratified epithelia, however, are named on the basis of the shape of the apical or luminal cell type accordingly: *squamous, cuboidal,* or *columnar.* Transitional epithelium is capable of varying the number of layers that are apparent.

Simple Epithelia

Simple Squamous Epithelium. This type of tissue is characterized by extremely thin cells, the cytoplasm of which is barely visible with light microscopy (Fig. 5.2). Often a prominent bulge into the free surface is apparent at the location of the nucleus. The cytoplasm is expansive, and nuclei of contiguous cells are generally separated from each other by long cytoplasmic processes. In many instances the cytoplasm, although expansive, is thin and gives the appearance of being absent. Electron micrographs, however, verify its presence and nature (Fig. 5.3). In surface view, the cells of this tissue are polygons, but they appear spindle-shaped when cut perpendicular to the free surface or basal border (Figs. 3.10*A* and *B*).

The morphology of these epithelial cells is suited ideally for the transport of materials across an attenuated cytoplasmic mass (Figs. 5.50 and 5.51). The endothelial lining of blood vessels permits the movement of fluids, crystalloids, and some colloids. Similarly, this type of epithelium in the lung contributes to the blood-air boundary. Thin segments of the loop of Henle in the kidney, lined by simple squamous epithelium, are involved in fluid exchange. The mesothelium of the celomic space permits the passage of tissue fluid into the body cavities. Mesothelium also serves as smooth, moistened surfaces for the movement of visceral organs over each other.

OCCURRENCE: **Lining of celomic spaces (mesothelium); lining of the heart blood and lymphatic vessels (endothelium); functional lining of lung; small ducts of numerous glands; specific portions of renal tubules and Bowman's capsule; membranous labyrinth of the inner ear.**

Simple Cuboidal Epithelium. The general shape of the cells of this tissue is described as cubes. In actuality, the cells appear as squares in sections perpendicular to the apical border (Fig. 5.4). From surface views they may appear as squares or hexagons. Nuclei are usually located in a *central* or *paracentral* position. Lateral cell borders may or may not be distinct.

This epithelium is associated generally with secretion and absorption; however, some of these cells may comprise nonsecretory or nonabsorptive linings of tubules.

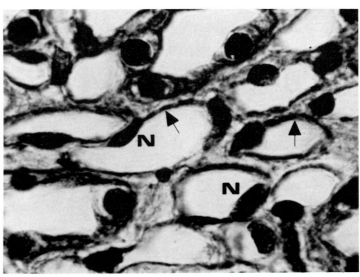

Figure 5.2. Simple squamous epithelial lining of canine kidney tubules. The dark nuclei *(N)* are the obvious components of the cells. The cytoplasm, which is barely visible *(arrows)*, appears as thin rims or cytoplasmic processes. The lining cells are actually pancake-shaped cells that are folded upon themselves and adjacent cells as tubules. ×160.

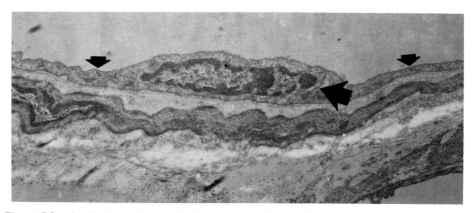

Figure 5.3. An electron micrograph of a simple squamous epithelial lining cell of a pulmonary alveolus. The nucleus *(large arrow)* protrudes into the lumen. The attenuated lateral projections of cytoplasm *(small arrows)* comprise the major lining component of the alveolus through which gaseous excahnge occurs. ×120,000. (Courtesy G. P. Epling.)

OCCURRENCE: **Secretory and ductal portions of numerous glands; certain tubules of the kidney; specific portions of the respiratory tree; surfaces of the lens and iris; surface epithelium of the ovary; specific tubules of the testis; pigmented epithelium of the retina (Plate III.1).**

Simple Columnar Epithelium. These cells are taller than they are wide (Fig. 5.5). The nuclei are elongated and generally displaced toward the basal border. A distinct cellular polarity is obvious. Usually, the nuclei are registered within a distinct row; occasionally, they may form two rows due to a crowding of cells.

The characteristic shape of these cells is associated typically with secretory processes. Most of the exocrine glands of the body are composed of these types of cells. Absorption is another important function accomplished by these columnar cells. Various apical border modifications suit columnar cells ideally for these functions.

OCCURRENCE: **Lining of glandular stomach, small intestine and large intestine; middle portions of the respiratory tree; lining of the uterus and uterine tubes; lining of the secretory and conducting portions of many glands; lining of the cholecyst (Plates III.2, III.3, and III.4).**

Pseudostratified Epithelium. All of the cells of this epithelium reside upon the basement membrane. Not all of them, however, reach the free or apical surface; only the columnar cellular constituents reach the luminal surface. In section, this epithelial type—based on the number of nuclei per unit area—appears to be overcrowded with cells (Figs. 5.6 and 5.40). The basal and middle parts of the lining are congested with the nuclei of the three cell types that

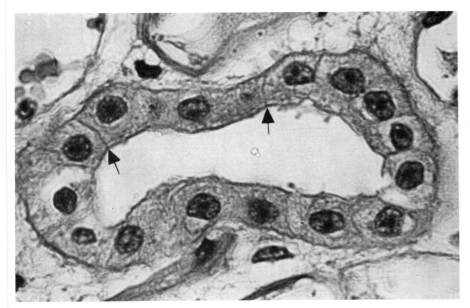

Figure 5.4. Cuboidal epithelial lining of a collecting tubule from the equine kidney. The nuclei occur within a homogeneous cytoplasm. The cellular limits of some cells are apparent *(arrows)*. Although these cells appear as squares in histological sections, the cells are actually cubic structures when viewed three-dimensionally. ×320.

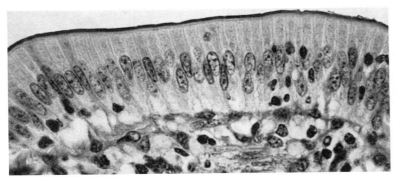

Figure 5.5. Columnar cells from the duodenum of a bird. The elongated and basally positioned nuclei accentuate the cellular polarity. The lining cells depicted are absorptive cells. ×320. Compare with Figure 3.10.

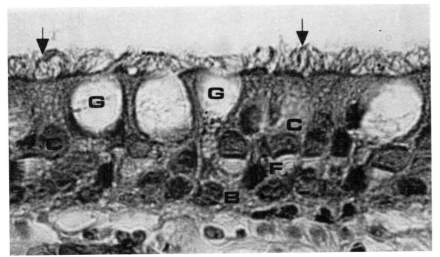

Figure 5.6. Pseudostratified ciliated columnar epithelial cells from an ovine trachea. All cells of this epithelial lining are in contact with the basement membrane, but not all of the cells reach the luminal surface. Compare with Figure 5.1. The apparent "stratification" is evident because of the arrangement of the nuclei of the basal *(B)*, fusiform *(F)* and columnar cells *(C)*. Cilia *(arrows)* occur along the luminal border. Goblet cells *(G)* are present. ×320.

constitute this epithelium—basal, fusiform, and columnar cells. A fourth type of cell, a *goblet cell*, is present in certain loci. Surface modifications, *cilia*, occur frequently on the luminal surfaces of the columnar cells. This epithelium is most precisely termed a *pseudostratified columnar* or *pseudostratified ciliated columnar epithelium.*

Often, this epithelium is confused with simple columnar epithelium that has been cut on a plane oblique to the surface (Fig. 5.7). Careful examination of the sections, however, will demonstrate that, even in an oblique plane, simple columnar epithelia do not possess the degree of nuclear congestion characteristic of pseudostratified columnar epithelium.

The primary function of this epithelium is to line certain tubular organs. Significant alterations to their apical surfaces, cilia, expand the function to that of surface transport. Surface transport facilitates the movement of particulate matter; thus, this property becomes protective. Surface transport within the uterine horns, however, facilitates fertilization. Numerous goblet cells, single-celled mucous glands, supply a viscous protective layer. Particulate matter contained within the mucous layer is moved by the cilia toward the exterior. The mucus and cilia constitute a protective mechanism called the *mucociliary apparatus.*

Pseudostratified epithelium also serves as an interface between simple and stratified epithelia, permitting a gradual increase in the thickness of a lining. These relationships are usually apparent within an excretory duct of a gland destined to open upon a stratified epithelial lining. Similarly, this tissue provides a gradual transition for those simple lining epithelia of ductal components that open upon a pseudostratified lining.

OCCURRENCE: **Lining of upper respiratory tract (Plate III.7); lining of specific regions of urogenital system; ducts of glands at points of transition between simple/stratified and simple/pseudostratified epithelia.**

Stratified Epithelia

Stratified Squamous Epithelium. Stratified squamous epithelium is characterized by many cellular layers that are derived from a single basal layer. This epithelium occurs at foci requiring protection for the underlying tissues (Fig. 5.8). This tissue type varies in thickness. It may be thin and consist of a few cellular layers as in the stratum lamellatum of the equine hoof. The tissue may be thick and consist of numerous cellular layers as in the bovine muzzle.

The basal layer of cells *(stratum basale)* consists of a single layer of pyramidal, cuboidal, or columnar cells (Fig. 5.9). This cellular layer resides upon the basement membrane. Stem cells comprise this layer of the tissue.

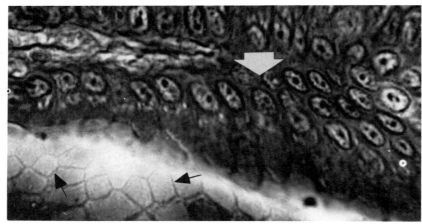

Figure 5.7. Oblique section of simple columnar epithelial cells from the duodenum of a bird. The cells to the left of the *white arrow*, cut normal to their long axes, appear as typical columnar cells. Those to the right of the *white arrow*, cut obliquely to their longitudinal axes, give the impression of stratification. This occurs because of the obliquity of the section, the length of the nuclei, and the unevenness of nuclear location within individual cells. *Solid arrows* are cross sections of the same cells. Note the uneven registration of nuclei in Figure 5.5 that contributes to the impression of stratification when the tissue is sectioned obliquely. ×320.

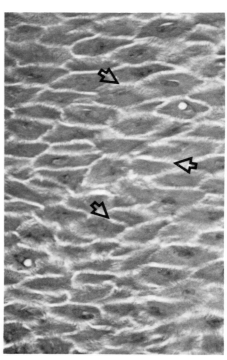

Figure 5.10. Stratified squamous epithelium of the canine muzzle. The stratum spinosum is depicted. Spinous processes *(arrows)* are apparent between contiguous cells. ×400.

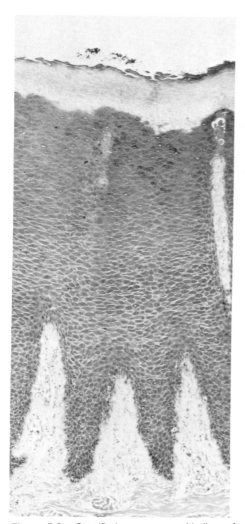

Figure 5.8. Stratified squamous epithelium of the canine muzzle. The epithelium, intimately associated with the underlying connective tissue, is keratinized *(light-staining material at the top of the field)*. ×25.

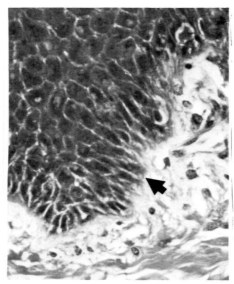

Figure 5.9. Stratified squamous epithelium of the canine muzzle. The stratum basale *(arrow)* is depicted. ×400. Figures 5.9 – 5.12 were obtained from different regions of the same epithelial lining.

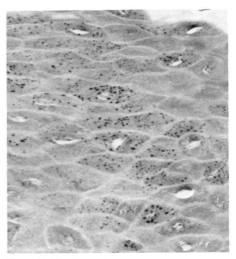

Figure 5.11. Stratified squamous epithelium of the canine muzzle. The stratum granulosum is depicted. This layer is the region of transition between the stratum spinosum and the stratum corneum. ×400.

The cells of the *stratum spinosum* have a lighter staining affinity than those of the basal layer and are progressively more flattened toward the luminal surface. Shrinking of cells by processing techniques demonstrates intercellular spaces in which numerous cellular processes from adjacent cells are in contact with one another (Fig. 5.10). These processes (*spines* or *prickles*) are not actually intercellular bridges but represent two cellular processes of contiguous cells joined by a *desmosome*. The desmosomal contacts remain, but the rest of the cellular margins shrink away from each other. This configuration is responsible for naming this layer the *spinous cell* or *prickle cell layer*. The cells of this layer also contribute to the stem cell population of this tissue.

The combined *stratum basale* and the *stratum spinosum* are called the *stratum germinativum*. Mitoses within the germinal layer are responsible for the replacement of cells desquamated at the luminal surface.

The *stratum granulosum*, depending upon the specific location of the epithelium, may be several cell layers thick or may be totally absent. The granularity of the spindle-shape cells of this layer is attributable to the basophilic *keratohyalin* granules (Fig. 5.11). These are precursor substances to *keratin*. Degenerative changes in the cells, as evidenced by pyknotic nuclei, are also characteristic of the cells of this layer.

The *stratum lucidum* is not a typical and prominent feature of the epidermis of domestic animals. When present, as in the canine digital pads, the cells are extremely flattened, pale-staining, or slightly acidophilic. This layer represents dead or dying cells. Nuclei are either indistinct or missing, and the cytoplasm is agranular. Occasionally, granules of *eleidin* are present. The closely packed cells of this region may be several layers thick.

The *stratum corneum* (Fig. 5.12) is a well-developed layer of closely packed dead cells in those regions typified by a high degree of *keratinization*, such as the canine digital pads and the equine hoof. The remainder of the skin is less keratinized, but this stratum is still present. The cells that are sloughed comprise a *stratum disjunctum*. Lesser degrees of keratinization or a total absence thereof are characteristic of the oral and aboral portions of the digestive tube, as well as portions along its length (esophagus, nonglandular portions of the ruminant stomach). The degree of keratinization is dependent upon the amount of pressure and abrasion to which the epithelium is subjected.

Not all of the typical layers of this tissue are present at all foci of occurrence (Fig. 5.13). Specifically, the transition from basal cellular layer to stratum corneum may oc-

cur rapidly without the intervening layers being apparent. The stratum basale is the constant and distinct layer. The layers are sometimes referred to as the *basal, parabasal, intermediate and superficial layers*. These terms are used frequently by cytologists when evaluating cells exfoliated from this tissue. When all the layers are present, the following correlations occur: **basal layer—stratum basale, parabasal layer—stratum spinosum, intermediate layer—stratum granulosum, superficial layer—stratum corneum**. If one or more of the layers are missing, then the terms are strictly positional.

Stratified squamous epithelium, in most locations, is a thick epithelial lining. The interface between the basal cell layer and the associated connective tissue is usually smooth but may be characterized by numerous interdigitations. The interdigitated morphological relationship affords a large

surface area for diffusion, as well as a large surface area for adhesion.

The protective function of this tissue is manifested in varied ways. The keratinized layer protects against dessicative and mechanical damage. The significance of this function is best considered in the epidermis. Even those epithelia that are not keratinized, or only minimally keratinized, afford protection from mechanical damage. The dental pad of ruminants also permits mastication with minimal damage from the abrasive action of foodstuffs. The upper digestive tract of ruminants is protected from the abrasiveness of roughened foodstuffs by this epithelium. Significantly, this epithelium also serves an absorptive function in ruminants.

OCCURRENCE: *(keratinized)*— General body surface; buccal cavity; anal region; ruminant forestomach (Plate III.5). *(nonkeratinized)*—Vestibular region of respiratory system; oral, esoph-

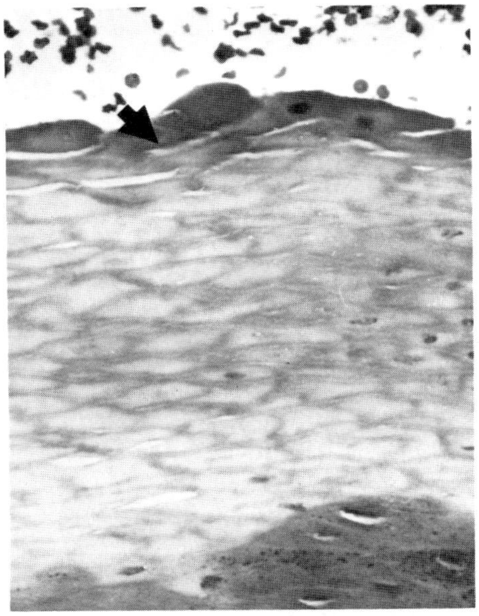

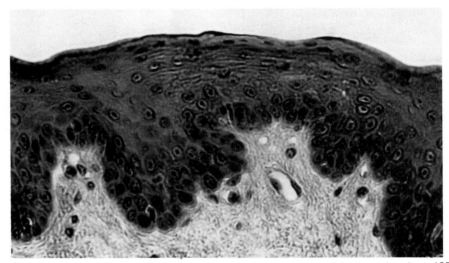

Figure 5.13. Nonkeratinized stratified squamous epithelium from the feline buccal cavity. ×125.

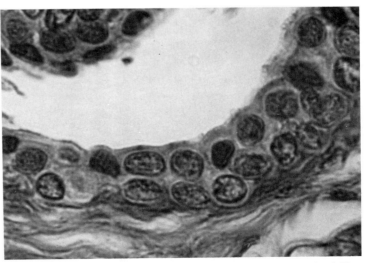

Figure 5.12. Stratified squamous epithelium of the canine muzzle. The stratum corneum comprises the majority of the micrograph. A portion of the stratum granulosum is visible *(bottom)*, and the stratum disjunctum is apparent *(arrow)*. ×400.

Figure 5.14. Bistratified cuboidal epithelium of a duct from a feline salivary gland. The occurrence of this tissue is limited generally to points of transition from simple to stratified epithelia and simple to pseudostratified epithelia. ×400.

ageal, and anal portions of digestive system; cornea of eye; conjunctiva; portions of the male and female urogenital systems (Plate III.6).

Stratified Cuboidal Epithelium. This epithelium consists of two layers of cells (Fig. 5.14). The basal layer consists of polygonal cells responsible for the regeneration of lost cells. The superficial or luminal layer consists of cuboidal cells. This epithelium is limited to a few loci; however, it is encountered frequently in regions of transition from simple to stratified or pseudostratified epithelia wherein it provides a gradual transition from one tissue type to another.

OCCURRENCE: **Specific portions of the genital system; ducts of various glands; zones of transition between simple and stratified or pseudostratified epithelia.**

Stratified Columnar Epithelium. This tissue may consist of two, three, or more layers of cells (Fig. 5.15). The basal and luminal cells are sometimes separated from each other by intermediate cell types. The basal cells are normally cuboidal; the intermediate, polygonal; the apical cells, columnar. This tissue is sometimes difficult to distinguish from pseudostratified epithelium.

Stratified cuboidal and columnar epithelia are presumed to serve only a lining function. Their interdigitation between the simple epithelia of glands and the stratified or pseudostratified epithelia of lining surfaces affords a gradual transition from one type to the other.

OCCURRENCE: **Zones of transition between columnar or pseudostratified and stratified epithelia; portions of the upper respiratory tract; ducts of some glands.**

Transitional Epithelium

Transitional Epithelium. This tissue, normally considered a stratified type, may be pseudostratified. Whichever is the case, the tissue still deserves special attention because of its ability to change shape as a result of the pressure applied on it from the luminal surface. Because it is associated only with the urogenital system, it is sometimes called *urothelium*.

In the relaxed state, this tissue may consist of as many as six or seven layers (Fig. 5.16). The basal cells are very small and assume a polyhedral configuration. The cells of the intermediate region are polyhedral or pear-shaped. The cells at the luminal border are cuboidal and their apical borders bulge into the lumen. During distention, the thickness of the epithelium is reduced markedly (Fig. 5.17). As few as two or three layers may be apparent. In a state of distention, this tissue is sometimes mistaken for stratified squamous epithelium.

The epithelium functions as a lining capable of accommodating to the stretching that results from an increased luminal vol-

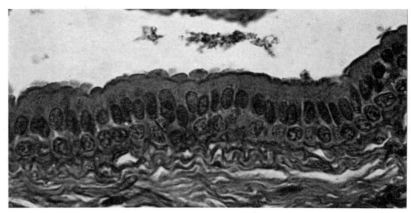

Figure 5.15. Bistratified columnar epithelium of a duct from a feline salivary gland. The function and distribution of this tissue is similar to bistratified cuboidal epithelium. ×400.

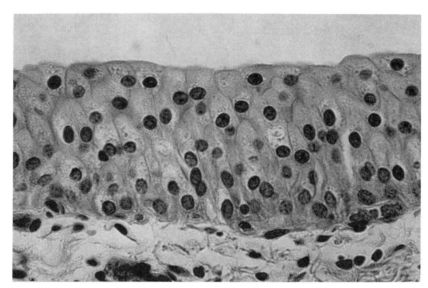

Figure 5.16. Transitional epithelium of the bovine bladder. The thickness of the tissue, as indicated by the number of "nuclear layers," indicates that the tissue is relaxed or contracted. ×160. Compare with Figures 5.1 and 5.17.

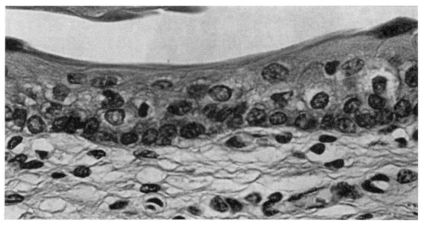

Figure 5.17. Transitional epithelium of the canine bladder. The reduced thickness of the tissue, as indicated by the reduced number of nuclear layers, indicates that the tissue is distended or stretched. Compare with Figures 5.1 and 5.16. ×160.

ume. More importantly, transitional epithelium is an effective barrier to the movement of water. Urothelium prevents the movement of water from the connective tissue space to the luminal space occupied by the hypertonic urine.

OCCURRENCE: **Lining of specific regions of the urinary system.**

Glandular Epithelia

General Features and Classification. Epithelia perform prominent secretory functions. Single cells and populations of cells produce a variety of products for extracellular use. Surface linings are modified to accomplish diverse secretory activities, and various mechanisms are used by these cells to accomplish these activities. Also, the relationships of glandular tissues to surrounding tissues are varied. Accordingly, numerous ways exist by which glandular tissue may be classified: number of cells constituting a gland; relationship to lining and surrounding tissue; configuration of multicellular glands; method of elaboration; type of secretory product.

Number of Cells in a Gland. Glands are either *unicellular* or *multicellular*. *Unicellular glands* are simply specialized cells that are scattered throughout an epithelial lining. Although varied modifications occur, the most common and representative unicellular gland is the goblet cell (Fig. 5.6). It is scattered commonly throughout the respiratory and digestive systems and occasionally in the urinary system (Plates III.3 and III.4). Until active, this cell cannot be distinguished from other columnar cells with which it is associated. When activity commences, droplets appear in the cytoplasm and eventually accumulate until the entire apical and middle portion of the cell is filled and swollen with *premucin* droplets (Figs. 5.18 and 5.19). These impart a foamy and basophilic appearance to the cytoplasm. The remainder of the cytoplasm and nucleus is displaced to the narrow basal region of the cell. Expulsion of the mucoid substances may be explosive or gradual. If explosive, the cell returns to a columnar configuration from which state the process will resume. If gradual, the continuing process does not alter the configuration of the cell.

Multicellular glands are diversified groups of secretory units. Entire sheets of epithelia may perform a secretory function, as in the lining of the glandular stomach. Intraepithelial glands, which are rare, represent accumulations of specialized secretory cells within an epithelial lining (Fig. 5.20). The glands occur in the lining of the upper respiratory system and male genital system. The greatest diversity of form and function is represented by those multicellular glands that assume an extraepithelial relationship to the epithelial lining. (Extraepithelial, in this context, implies that

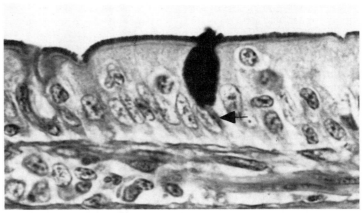

Figure 5.18. A goblet cell within the lining epithelium of the feline jejunum. The bulk of the goblet cell *(dark oval mass)* contains premucin droplets. The nucleus *(arrow)* is displaced basally. Note the extrusion of the secretory product upon the apical border of the cells. Compare with Figure 5.6. ×250. (Alcian blue and PAS).

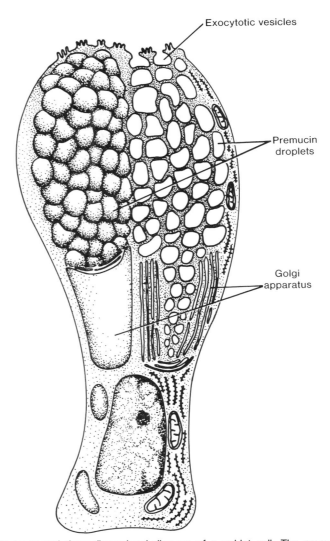

Figure 5.19. Biplanar and three-dimensional diagram of a goblet cell. The premucin droplets occupy the bulk of the cytoplasmic volume and displace other cytoplasmic components peripherally and basally. Premucin droplets fuse with the cytoplasmic face of the apical plasmalemma as exocytotic vesicles depositing mucinogen at the cell surface.

the glandular tissues, though continuous with the lining epithelium, are not in the same plane as the lining epithelium.) This type of gland represents most of those encountered in the body. Their true relationship to the epithelial lining is sometimes obscured by the morphological complexity they assume and the plane of section during observation. Their relationship to the lining is best understood by examining their developmental process (Fig. 5.21). Specific loci within the epithelial lining retain the potential for mitosis. The mitotic process is directed in such a way that a cord of cells invaginates into the underlying connective tissue space. These cells, however, do *not* actually invade the space but are separated from it by the basement membrane. A tube develops within the cord, whereas the remainder of the cells continue to proliferate and differentiate into secretory cells. The secretory cells as a unit are referred to as an *adenomere*. The tube connecting the adenomere to the epithelial surface is the duct of the gland. In some instances, portions of the duct may also become secretory.

Relationship to Lining and Surrounding Tissue. The persistence of the duct establishes that the gland will be of the *exocrine* variety. The growth of the adenomere and associated ducts is not limited to the simple example cited. Rather, very elaborate duct and secretory conformations may develop. Whether a simple or complex arrangement evolves, all these glandular types possess the common characteristic of cellular secre-

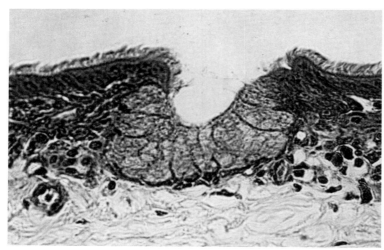

Figure 5.20.   Intraepithelial gland from the avian respiratory mucosa. ×200.

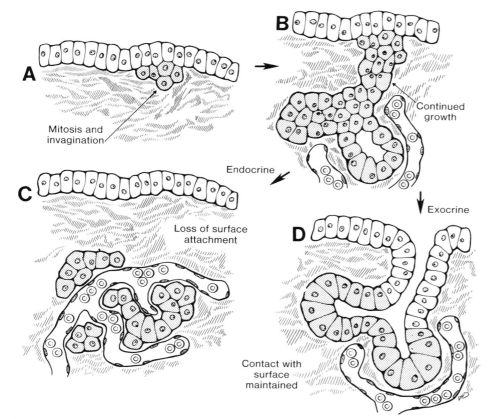

Figure 5.21.   Diagram of the development of exocrine and endocrine glands. Mitotic activity of the lining cells results in an invagination of the epithelium (and accompanying basement membrane) into the space occupied by the connective tissue (A). Continued mitotic activity and growth establishes a mass of cells (B) outside of the plane of the lining epithelium "within the connective tissue space." The mass of cells is attached to the surface lining epithelium (and is surrounded by a basement membrane). Subsequent disintegration of the surface attachment isolates the cord or clumps of epithelial cells within the connective tissue space as endocrine cells in close association with capillaries (C). The persistent attachment of lining and glandular cells to each other and the formation of a lumen establishes an exocrine gland (D).

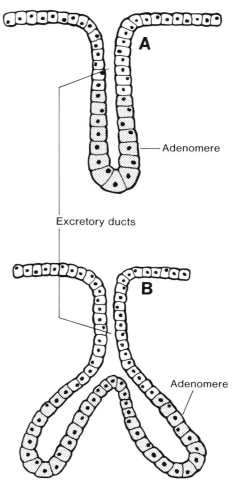

Figure 5.22.   Diagram of tubular glands. The adenomeres may be straight (A) or branched (B) tubules.

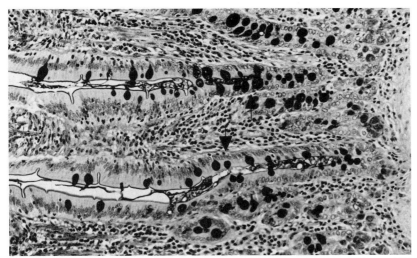

Figure 5.23.   Straight tubular glands from an equine duodenum. ×40. (Alcian blue and PAS).

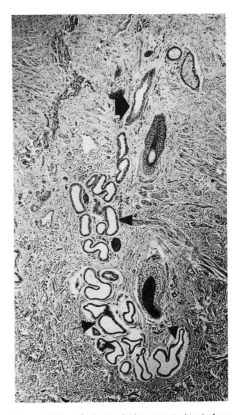

Figure 5.24.   Coiled, tubular sweat glands from ovine skin. The coiled nature of the gland is responsible for the discontinuities between glandular components that are apparent in section *(small arrows)*. The excretory duct *(large arrow)* eventually connects the adenomere to the surface. ×9.

tions being deposited into a system of ducts that eventually open at an epithelial surface.

In contrast to the aforementioned type, endocrine glands lose their connection to an epithelial surface (Fig. 5.21). The adenomeres do not assume tubular configurations. Rather, the secretory cells arrange themselves as cords or clumps of cells and deposit their secretory products into the vascular beds within the adjacent connective tissue space.

Configuration of Multicellular Glands. Various configurations are assumed by multicellular glands in extraepithelial positions. In a single section of these glands, the three-dimensional relationships can only be inferred. The following classification is based on serial sections and three-dimensional reconstructions of them. For this reason diagrams have been used. Multicellular exocrine glands may be either *simple* or *compound*. This classification is based upon the simplicity or complexity of the duct system associated with the secretory portions of the gland. The *secretory end-pieces (adenomeres)* may be *tubular* (a hollow cylinder), *alveolar* (globular or pear-shaped), or *tubuloalveolar* (combination of both) (Fig. 5.22).

In a *simple gland*, the adenomere deposits its products into an unbranched duct. The adenomeres may be *straight tubular* glands as are the intestinal glands (Fig. 5.23), *coiled tubular* glands as are the sweat glands (Figs. 5.24 and 5.25) or *alveolar* glands. The adenomeres may be branched and still deposit their products into a single duct system (Fig. 5.26). In this instance, they are referred to as *branched tubular* glands as in the submucosal glands of the intestine (Fig. 5.26) or *branched alveolar* glands as in the sebaceous glands (Fig. 5.27). The terms *alveolar* and *acinar* are used synonymously.

Numerous subdivisions of the duct sys-

tem and a variety of adenomeres occur in *compound* glands (Fig. 5.28). They may be *compound tubular* glands as in some of the salivary glands, *compound acinar* glands as in the pancreas or *compound tubuloalveolar* glands as in some of the salivary glands and the mammary glands.

The naming of the subdivisions of the duct system of compound glands is based upon the organizational pattern of the gland (Fig. 5.29). The *excretory duct* is the portion of the duct system that connects to the surface upon which the gland empties its secretion. It is the largest duct. Most glands are subdivided into smaller units

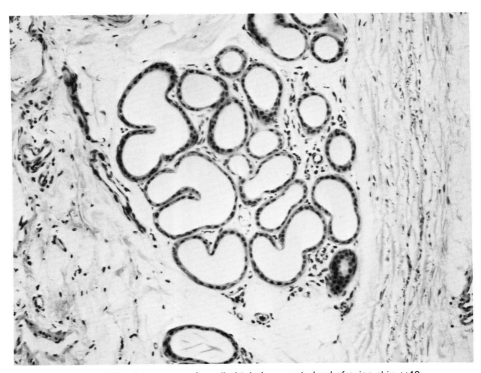

Figure 5.25.   Adenomere of a coiled tubular sweat gland of ovine skin. ×40.

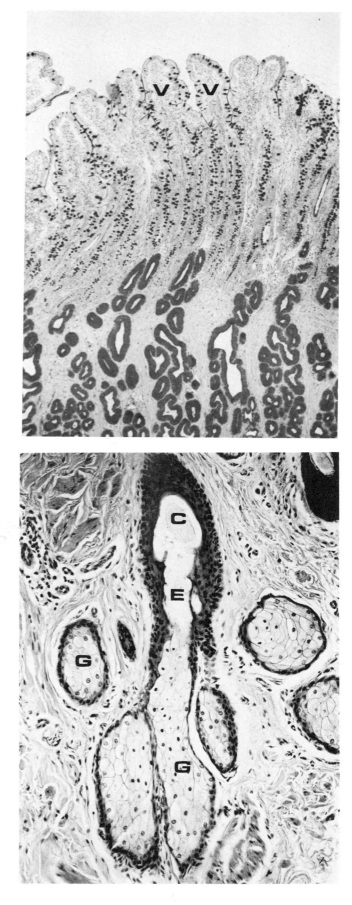

Figure 5.26. Submucosal glands of a canine duodenum. The branched tubular glands, *dark-staining*, are continuous to the surface *(top)* through the intestinal crypts. *V*, villi. ×16. (Alcian blue and PAS).

Figure 5.27. Alveolar gland from ovine skin. Sebaceous glands *(G)* are branched, alveolar glands. The glands are connected to the root canal *(C)* of a hair follicle through an excretory duct *(E)*. ×40.

called lobes. *Lobar ducts* drain the secretory products of lobes and are connected to the excretory duct. The large continuations of the lobar ducts within a lobe are referred to as *intralobar ducts*. Smaller subdivisional

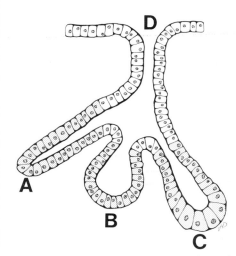

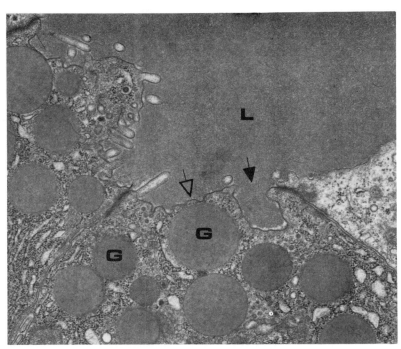

Figure 5.28. Diagram of the configurations of the adenomeres of compound glands. Tubular *(A)*, acinar or alveolar *(B)*, or tubuloalveolar *(C)* adenomeres open into a branched duct system *(D)*.

Figure 5.30. An electron micrograph of the luminal border of pancreatic acinar cells. The lumen *(L)* is filled with secretory material from the zymogen granules *(G)* that have emptied their contents onto the apical surface via exocytosis. A granule *(solid arrow)* may have fused with the cell membrane, while another granule *(open arrow)* is about to fuse with the cell membrane. ×22,000.

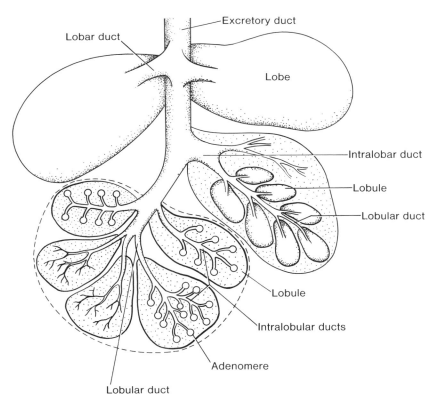

Figure 5.29. Diagram of the subdivisions of a compound gland. One lobe *(dashed line)* is enlarged to show the intralobular relationships. The flow of secretory product is from adenomere—intralobular duct—lobular duct—intralobar duct—lobar duct—excretory duct—surface. This pattern of organization or slight modifications of it typify many organs of the body (lungs, pancreas, kidneys) besides those described as typically glandular.

units of lobes are called lobules. Lobules are drained by *lobular ducts*. The continuation of the lobular duct within a lobe is called the *intralobular duct*. This duct is continuous with the secretory portion of the gland. Also, blood-vascular patterns of certain organs are named according to this scheme. This organizational scheme applies to numerous glandular organs, also.

Method of Elaboration. Not all of the secretory cells of the body elaborate their products in a manner identical to one another. Three secretory methods are recognized: *merocrine, apocrine,* and *holocrine*.

In the *merocrine* method of secretion, the cell contributes nothing more than the actual product it produced. The membrane surrounding the secretory droplet fuses with the plasma membrane; this fusion opens the product to the extracellular space (Figs. 4.48, 4.49, and 5.18). None of the cytoplasmic components along the secretory surface is lost, except the secretory product itself. This exocytotic method is typical of most of the glands of the body (Fig. 5.30).

In the *apocrine* method of secretion, the secretory product and a portion of the cytoplsm along the secretory surface are lost as the secretory end product. Characteristically, blebs or bulges along the secretory surface are observed during this exocytotic process (Fig. 5.31). The extent of the cytoplasmic contribution in this method has

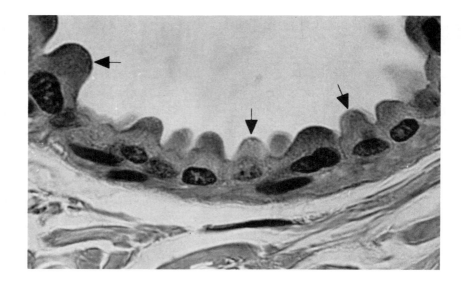

Figure 5.31. Apocrine tubular sweat glands of ovine skin. The apical blebs *(arrows)* indicate the apocrine method of secretion. ×500.

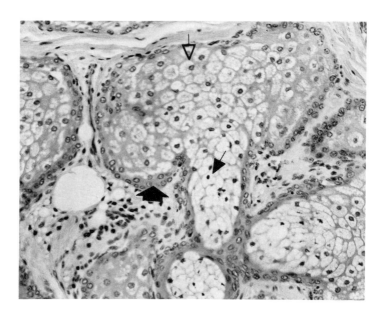

Figure 5.32. Sebaceous glands of an ovine orbital sinus. The cells that are located at the periphery of the adenomere *(large solid arrow)* are the stem cells for the adenomere. The stem cells divide and one of the daughter cells moves toward the lumen; the other remains at the base of the adenomere as another stem cell. As the cells move toward the lumen, they undergo degenerative changes that are characterized by the accumulation of lipids *(open arrow)* and pyknotic nuclei *(small solid arrow)*. The cells die and become the secretory product. The retention of one of the daughter cells as a future stem cell ensures continued activity of the gland. ×50.

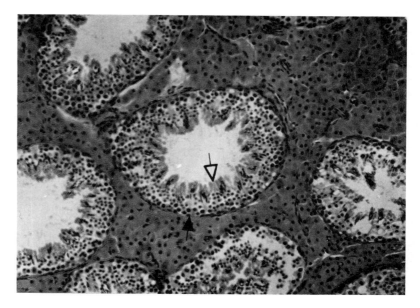

Figure 5.33. Seminiferous tubules of a porcine testis. Developing spermatozoa *(open arrow)* line the luminal surface of the seminiferous tubules. The developing germ cells constitute the "secretory product" of the tubules, whose stem cells are located at the periphery. ×40.

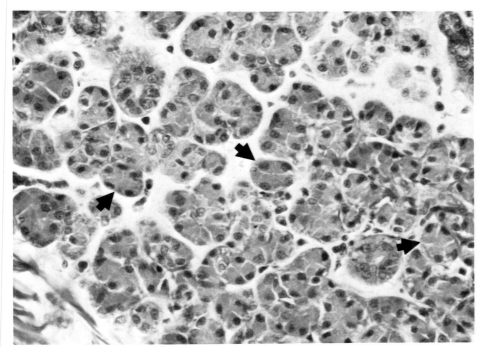

Figure 5.34. Serous cells of an adenomere from a salivary gland. The serous cells *(arrows)* are pyramidal cells with round, paracentrally positioned nuclei. The dark cytoplasm is granular and acidophilic. ×160.

along the basement membrane (Fig. 5.32). Mitotic activity of these cells forces cells into the interior of the adenomere at which time they begin to accumulate their lipid secretory product. The cells undergo necrobiosis and become the secretory product (Plate III.9). Other organs, the gonads and hematopoietic organs, elaborate cells that become the "secretory products" of these glands (Fig. 5.33).

Types of Secretory Units. Two distinct populations of secretory cells are recognized: *serous* and *mucous cells.* The serous cell secrete a clear, watery type of fluid that may contain enzymes; the mucous cells produce a viscous fluid that is rich in glycoproteins. Not all secretory cells can be included in this classification scheme. It is especially applicable to the digestive, respiratory, and reproductive glands.

The serous cell is a wedge-shaped or pear-shaped cell that usually possesses a finely granular, acidophilic cytoplasm (Fig. 5.34). The rounded nucleus is either central or paracentral in position. The lateral margins of the cell are usually indistinct. Some serous cells assume characteristics exemplified by the pancreatic acinar cells. A distinct polarity may be apparent; the apical portion of the cells is acidophilic, whereas the basal portion is basophilic due to the accumulation of ergastoplasm. Nuclear position and the lateral cell margins are as just described. The mucous cell is a pear-shaped cell with a foamy and basophilic cytoplasm (Fig. 5.35). A marked polarity is apparent; the hyperchromatic, flattened nucleus is positioned basally.

Mixed glands may be composed of these

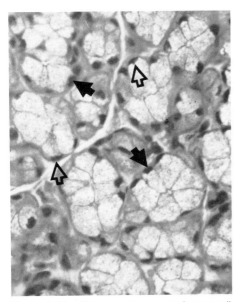

Figure 5.35. Mucous adenomeres from a salivary gland. The mucous adenomere *(solid arrows)* consists of mucous cells that are pyramidal. The cytoplasm of these cells is foamy, and the flattened nuclei *(open arrows)* are positioned basally. Note that some of the cells appear to be devoid of nuclei. ×100. (a glycol methacrylate, 2-μm section).

are shed continually by this method, glandular function would cease if cellular replacement were not accomplished. The continued function of holocrine glands is assured by the presence of a copious supply of stem cells.

In sebaceous glands, the stem cells are located at the periphery of the alveolus

been questioned recently. This method is typical of most of the sweat glands of domestic species, some of the sweat glands of man, and some products of the mammary gland (Plate III.8).

The *holocrine* method is characterized by the entire glandular epithelial cell becoming the secretory product. Because cells

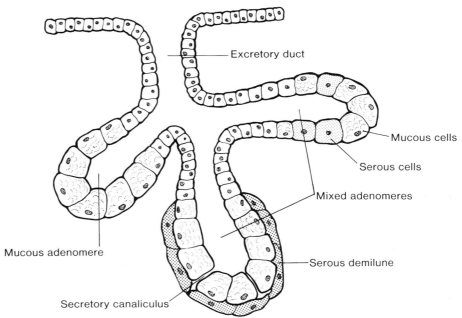

Figure 5.36. Diagram of different adenomeres of a salivary gland. Salivary glands may be serous, mucous, or mixed (seromucous) glands. The adenomeres of these glands, therefore, must be serous, mucous, or mixed. Mixed glands achieve this condition in various ways. The gland may consist of separate serous and mucous adenomeres. Mucous adenomeres may have serous demilunes associated with them. Also, serous and mucous cells may be intermingled within a single adenomere.

Excretory duct

Mucous cells

Serous cells

Mixed adenomeres

Serous demilune

Mucous adenomere

Secretory canaliculus

two cell types in various arrangements (Plate III.11 and Fig. 5.36). An entire gland may possess separate serous and mucous adenomeres (Fig. 5.37). Serous and mucous cells may be intermingled with each other and discharge their products at the luminal surface (Fig. 5.38). *Serous demilunes* may be attached to a mucous adenomere (Fig. 5.39). In this instance, small canals *(secretory canaliculi)* connect the serous cells with the luminal surface (Fig. 5.36).

Special Epithelia

Epithelial tissues are modified to perform highly specialized functions at certain loci. Among these epithelial tissues are *ciliated epithelium, sensory epithelium, pigment epithelium*, and *myoepithelium*.

Cilia are slender, cytoplasmic processes of the luminal surfaces of cells that are modified either for surface transport or secretory activity. *Kinocilia* are highly structured cytoplasmic processes that are usually associated with cells of pseudostratified columnar or simple columnar epithelia (Fig. 5.6). Isolated cells within the epithelial sheet or the majority of cells within the epithelial layer may be ciliated (Fig. 5.58). *Stereocilia* are long, unstructured, branched, protoplasmic structures from the luminal surface of cells that increase surface area for secretory activity (Fig. 5.40).

Certain cells of epithelial origin are modified to receive and transmit sensory information. These cells are associated with organs specialized to receive optic, olfactory, gustatory, auditory, and kinesthetic sensations. A *neurosensory epithelial cell (epitheliocytus neurosensorius)* is a nerve cell that is modified as a receptor and transmitter of information. The cells receive the information, transduce the stimulus and transmit the information along their axons. Photoreceptor and olfactory cells are examples of these types of epithelial cell. A *sensory epithelial cell (epitheliocytus sensorius)* is a non-neural cell that is the sensory receptor for gustatory, auditory, and vestibular sensations. These cells receive the stimuli, transduce the information, and transmit the information to neurons that are juxtaposed to them.

Various cells of the body typically possess various types of pigments. In one instance, however, an entire sheet of epithelium, the pigment epithelium of the retina of the eye (Fig. 5.41), is modified to contain large quantities of melanin.

Myoepithelial cells or *basket cells* are specialized epithelial cells associated with the adenomeres of most exocrine glands. They are spindle-shaped cells that surround the secretory end-pieces (Fig. 5.42). Although of epithelial origin, they contain myofibrils, are contractile, and are responsible for the expression of secretory products into ducts. They are associated with salivary, sweat, and mammary glands.

Cells of Endocrine Organs. These cells, uniquely modified to elaborate their protein or steroid secretory products *(hormones)* into the blood, assume varied morphological configurations. They are discussed in-depth with the endocrine organs.

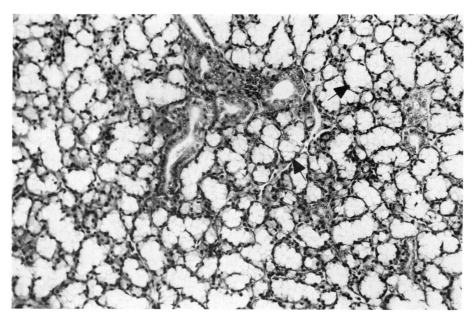

Figure 5.37. Canine salivary gland. The mucous adenomeres *(arrows)* comprise the bulk of the gland. ×40.

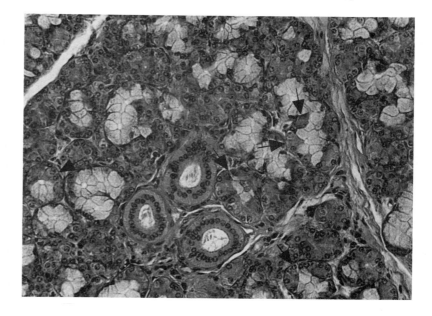

Figure 5.38. Porcine salivary gland. *Arrows* indicate regions within adenomeres in which serous cells are intermingled among mucous cells. ×63.

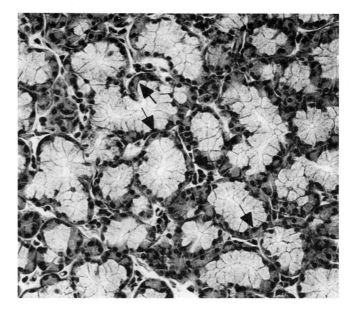

Figure 5.39. Equine salivary gland. The serous cells *(arrows)* are disposed as demilunes around the mucous adenomeres. ×63.

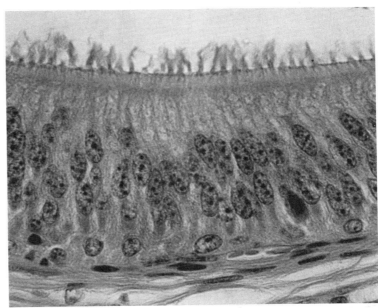

Figure 5.40. Stereocilia of the equine ductus epididymidis. ×200. (See Figure 5.51 also.)

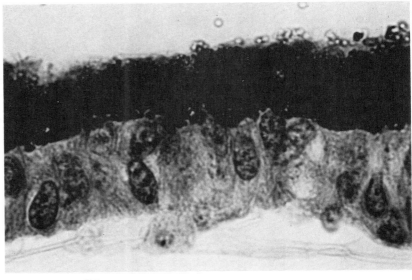

Figure 5.41. Pars ciliaris retinae of a canine eye. The pigment epithelium at the *top* of the micrograph is obscured by the pigment. The columnar cells in the *lower* portion of the micrograph comprise a separate layer. ×320.

Surface Specializations of Epithelia

Cell-to-Cell Modifications. The lateral surfaces of epithelial cells are modified to hold cells together, serve as diffusion barriers, facilitate diffusion between component epithelial cells, and permit intercellu-lar communication. The lateral surface modifications include alterations of the gly-cocalyx, lateral plasma membranes, and filamentous components of the cytoplasm.

The attachment points of epithelial cells to each other are visible with the light microscope. This apicolateral alteration of the cell surface was called the *terminal bar*. It appears as a continuous and collar-like al-teration around the entire cell. With the electron microscope, this modification is seen as a complex of different structural alterations that occurs at the junction be-tween adjacent cells. Thus, the name *junc-*

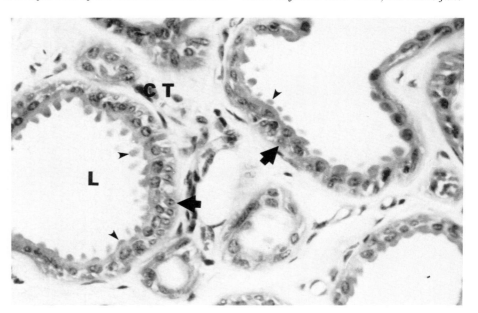

Figure 5.42. A section of apocrine tubular glands from an ovine inguinal pouch. The coiled adenomeres are separated by connective tissue *(CT)*. Apical blebs *(small arrowheads)* character-ize the luminal surface of these secretory cells. Myoepithelial cells *(large arrows)* surround the adenomeres and help to express the secretory product from the gland. *L*, glandular lumen. ×100.

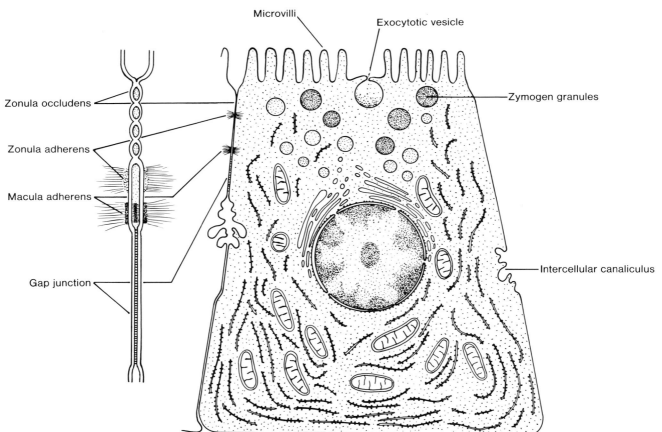

Figure 5.43. Drawing of a secretory cell as visualized with the electron microscope. Apical and lateral cellular membranous modifications are illustrated. (Redrawn and modified from Bloom, W. and Fawcett, D. W.: *A Textbook of Histology*, 10th edition, W. B. Saunders, Philadelphia, 1975.)

tional complex is applied more appropriately to this structure. The discrete units of junctional complexes may comprise continuous modifications along contiguous cell surfaces. Such bands of alteration are confined to distinct zones; thus, they are described as zonular (L. small zone). Others may be disposed as discrete patches or spots of alteration that are described as "spot welds" along contiguous surfaces. They are referred to as macular (L. a spot) alterations. Junctional complexes (Fig. 5.43) may consist of the following discrete components: *tight junction, intermediate junction, desmosome or gap junction.*

The *tight junction* or *zonula occludens* (Fig. 5.44) is the most commonly encountered component of junctional complexes.

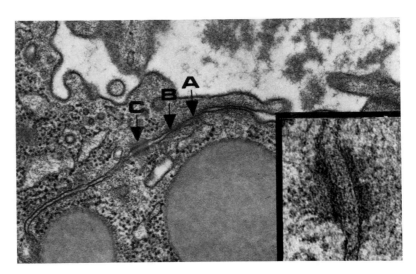

Figure 5.44. An electron micrograph of junctional complexes between contiguous pancreatic acinar cells. A tight junction *(A)*, intermediate junction *(B)*, and desmosome *(C)* are indicated. ×41,000. *Inset:* High magnification of a desmosome. ×146,000.

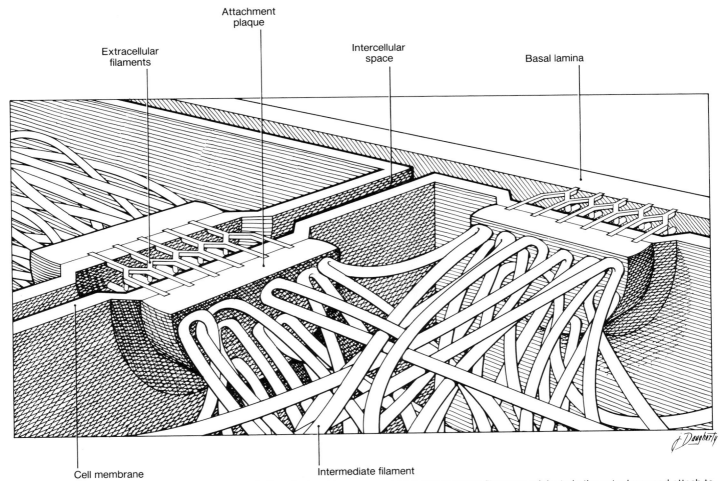

Figure 5.45. A diagram illustrating a desmosome *(left)* and a hemidesmosome *(right)*. Intermediate filaments originate in the cytoplasm and attach to the plaques. Extracellular filaments attach to contiguous cell membranes or basal lamina. These filaments pass through the cell membrane and attach in the plaques.

The outer and dense laminae of contiguous cell membranes are fused as one with a resultant obliteration of intercellular space. Cytoplasmic condensation may be apparent on either side of the junction. When this type of junction is well developed, the epithelium forms an effective barrier between the luminal and connective tissue spaces. The movement of extracellular materials is facilitated when these junctions are not well-developed.

The *intermediate junction (zonula adherens)* (Fig. 5.44) is usually associated with a tight junction and is characterized by the juxtaposition of adjacent cell membranes. They are not fused but are separated by a 20–90-nm space that is filled with a mucosubstance as the adhesive material. These junctions, too, extend around the apicolateral portion of the cell much like a belt. The adjacent cytoplasmic condensations contain numerous intermediate filaments that are continuous with those of the *terminal web*. The intermediate filaments are anchored to the membrane via electrondense plaques that are attached to the cytoplasmic side of the membrane. These intermediate junctions anchor the intermediate filaments of the terminal web thereby supplying a support for movement of microvilli. *Actin* filaments extend from the terminal web into the terminal portions of microvilli.

A *desmosome (macula adherens)* (Gr. bond + body) does not encircle the cell totally. These structures are scattered along the cell margins at discrete locations. They can be considered analogous to spot welds between cells (Fig. 5.44). Moreover, they are not confined to junctional complexes. The cytoplasmic margins of each contributing cell membrane is coated by an electron-dense plaque in which intermediate filaments are embedded (Fig. 5.45). These intermediate filaments originate in the cytoplasm, form loops in the dense material associated with the desmosomes, and return to the cytoplasm. Desmosomes, therefore, may play a significant role in the cytoskeletal architecture of the cell. A space of 25 nm between adjacent cell membranes is typical and a dense intermediate line may be apparent in this intercellular space. The presence of a sialic acid-rich material indicates that this is a modification of the glycocalyx for cellular adhesion.

The *gap junction (nexus, close junction, communicating junction)* appears similar to the tight junction but is separated by a 20-nm intercellular space (Fig. 5.46). Face views demonstrate that these areas are composed of an orderly array of hexagonal subunits. These hexagonal subunits consist of contiguous proteins that extend through the cell membranes and are in contact with each other.

The remaining 15-nm space between cells is occupied by the glycocalyx. The

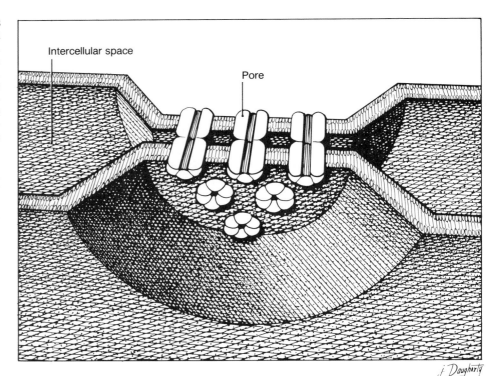

Figure 5.46. A diagram that illustrates the structure of a gap junction. Pores are cylindrical structures between contiguous cells that permit the movement of ions and small molecules such as cAMP between cells.

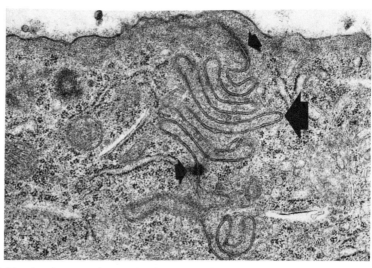

Figure 5.47. An electron micrograph of lateral surface modifications between adjacent murine intestinal lining cells. Lateral interdigitations *(large arrow)* are apparent. An intermediate junction *(small arrow)* is visible near the apical cellular surface. A desmosome is visible in the middle of the micrograph *(small arrow)*. ×25,000. (Courtesy of A. M. Sheppard.)

glycocalyx, as well as the aforementioned junctional alterations, are coupled with cellular interdigitations to ensure maximal cellular adhesion (Fig. 5.47).

Basal Border Modifications. The primary modifications associated with the basal border of epithelial cells are: *basal lamina, basal invaginations, caveolae, pinocytotic vesicles,* and *hemidesmosomes.*

Generally, all epithelial tissues are separated from the underlying or surrounding connective tissue by a boundary layer called the *basement membrane.* It is demonstrable readily with PAS staining or silver impregnation, but it is not observable with routine H and E staining (Figs. 5.48 and 5.49).

The ultrastructural detail of the basement membrane has been elucidated with the electron microscope (Fig. 5.50). The light microscopic entity actually includes the basal cell membrane, amorphous cell coat, some dense material, and associated connective tissue fibrils. With the electron microscope, some dense materials (50–70-nm wide) underlie the basal cell membrane and closely follow the contour of this membrane. This dense band *(lamina densa)* or *basal lamina* is separated from the cell membrane by a clear zone, the *lamina lucida*. The lamina densa contains glycoproteins and collagenous fibers as a fine feltwork. A thicker layer of collagenous fibers *(lamina fibroreticularis)* projects into the underlying connective tissue space. This light-staining zone, lamina lucida, represents the modified cell coat.

The basal lamina has been considered a condensation product of the connective tissue. Current immunological evidence indicates that the epithelial cells are probably the primary source of basal laminar materials. Type IV and V collagens are constituents of basal laminae. Type III collagen (reticular fibers) constitutes the fibroreticular lamina deep to the basal lamina or lamina densa. Laminin, a structural glycoprotein, is present also.

The basal cell membranes may be contoured regularly or may possess numerous infoldings (Fig. 5.51). The latter modification is especially apparent in cells involved in transport activities. In either case, small bulb-like invaginations of the cell membrane *(caveolae)* exist (Fig. 5.52). These pinch off from the membrane and form *pinocytotic vesicles* (Fig. 5.52). These two structures represent mechanisms for *endocytotic* and/or *exocytotic* activity (Fig. 5.53).

Hemidesmosomes (half-desmosomes) are encountered occasionally along the basal cell membrane (Figs. 5.45 and 5.54). These structures are the anchoring points for cytoskeletal elements to basal cell membranes, as well as the points of cellular adhesion to the underlying connective tissue through the basal lamina.

Apical Border Modifications. The primary apical border modifications of epithelia are *microvilli, caveolae, pinocytotic vesicles,* and *cilia.*

Microvilli occur on the surfaces of most cells. They vary in size, distribution, and organization. Their prime function is to increase the absorbing surface area of a cell. Microvilli achieve their highest degree of development in epithelia. They are slender, cylindrical, cellular processes that are oriented perpendicular to the apical, free, or luminal surface.

Microvilli of intestinal epithelial cells are organized on the apical borders to form a *striated* or *brush border* (Fig. 5.55). These processes are 1–1.5 μm long and approximately 0.1 μm in diameter. They are juxtaposed to each other in a parallel arrangement (Fig. 5.56). The cores of the microvilli are composed of actin microfilaments. These filaments attach to the cell membrane at the apex of the microvillus. Myosin filaments have been noted at the base of microvilli. These filaments are attached to the intermediate filaments of the terminal web. These relationships establish a mechanism for the controlled movement of the microvilli.

Certain lining cells of the kidney have microvilli on their apical borders. These, however, are not in as orderly an arrangement as those described previously (Fig. 5.57). In the past, this arrangement was referred to as a *brush border*, whereas the highly ordered array was called a *striated border*. Now these terms are used synonymously, because both represent modifications to increase the cell surface. The sur-

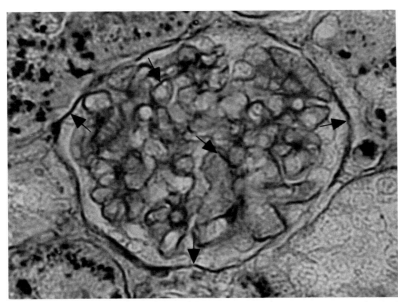

Figure 5.48. Glomerulus of a canine kidney stained with PAS. The basement membrane *(arrows)* is defined clearly. Compare with Figure 5.49. ×250.

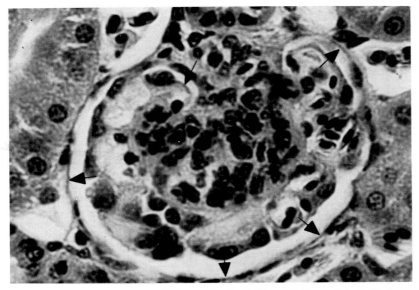

Figure 5.49. Glomerulus of a canine kidney stained with H and E. The cellular limits *(arrows)* are visible, but the basement membrane is not apparent. Compare with Figure 5.48. ×250.

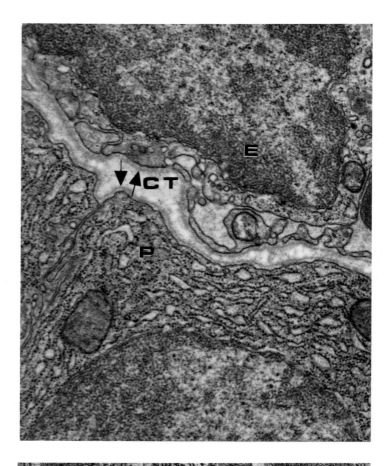

Figure 5.50. An electron micrograph of pancreatic acinar cells, associated connective tissue and capillary endothelium. The pancreatic acinar *(P)* and the endothelial cells *(E)* are underlaid by individual basal laminae *(arrows)*. The intervening space is connective tissue space *(CT)*. ×25,000.

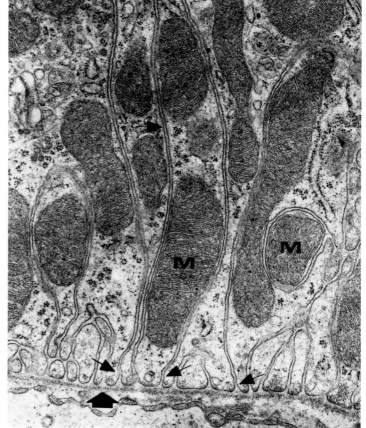

Figure 5.51. An electron micrograph of a lining cell of the proximal convoluted tubule of a canine kidney. Numerous basal cellular membranous infoldings are evident *(small arrows)*. Mitochondria *(M)* are contained within the cytoplasm between the membranes. The basal lamina *(large arrow)* is apparent. ×18,000.

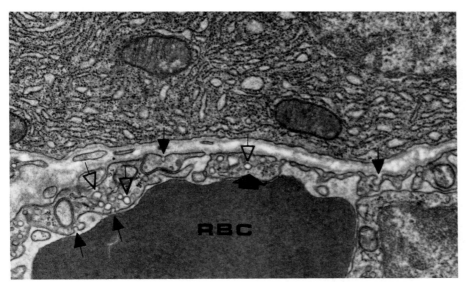

Figure 5.52. An electron micrograph of a capillary. An erythrocyte (RBC) is surrounded by capillary endothelium *(large solid arrow)*. Pinocytotic vesicles *(open arrows)* and caveolae *(solid arrows)* are apparent. ×18,000. Compare with Figure 5.53.

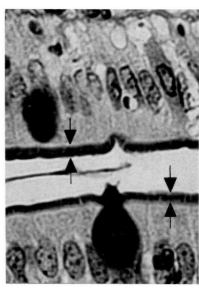

Figure 5.55. Striated border of equine jejunal lining cells. The striated border *(arrows)* results from the orderly arrangement of microvilli. The striated border appears prominent and dark because of the staining of the glycocalyx. ×250. (Alcian blue and PAS).

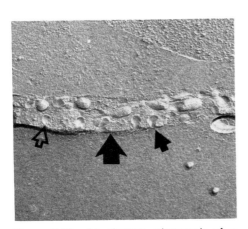

Figure 5.53. An electron micrograph of a freeze fractured capillary. The capillary endothelium *(large arrow)* contains pinocytotic vesicles *(open arrow)* and caveolae *(solid arrow).* ×43,000. Compare with Figure 5.52. (Courtesy of J. E. Rash).

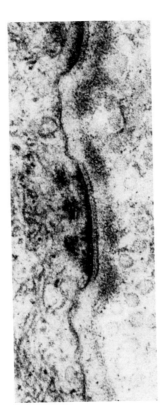

Figure 5.54. An electron micrograph of the basal border of a murine intestinal lining cell. A hemidesmosome is visible in the center of the field. ×91,000.

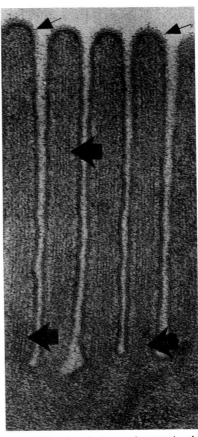

Figure 5.56. An electron micrograph of the striated border of a murine intestinal lining cell. The microvilli are arranged in an orderly manner, are covered by a glycocalyx *(small arrows)* and contain actin microfilaments *(large arrows).* ×70,000.

face coat or glycocalyx associated with microvilli is prominent.

Cilia, both *kinocilia* (Fig. 5.58) and *stereocilia* (Fig. 4.43) are typical apical modifications of specialized epithelial cells (Figs. 5.6, 5.20, and 5.40).

The *caveolae* and *pinocytotic vesicles* of the apical border are similar in structure and function to those structures associated with the basal border (Figs. 5.50 and 5.51).

Regeneration and Repair of Epithelia

Epithelia tissues in most locations are subjected to harsh environments that result in cells being damaged and lost. The lives of epithelial cells are finite; therefore, epithelial layers require renewal and replacement of lost components. In most instances, this need is satisfied by the presence of undifferentiated stem cells being included in the epithelial lamina. Various epithelial tissues accomplish this activity in different ways.

Simple epithelial membranes that are

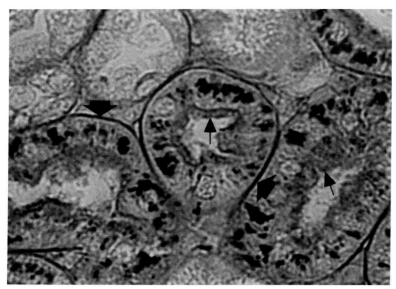

Figure 5.57. Brush borders of the lining cells of the proximal convoluted tubules of a canine kidney. The brush borders *(small arrows)* are indicated. The basement membranes are defined clearly *(large arrows)*. ×250. (toluidine blue and PAS).

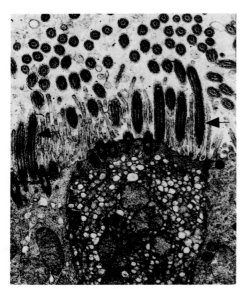

Figure 5.58. An electron micrograph of ciliated cells from a murine trachea. *Arrows,* cilia. ×8,000.

composed of squamous, cuboidal, and columnar cells that are not highly differentialted for secretory and/or absorptive functions retain a high mitotic potential. These cells serve as their own stem cells. This applies to typical epithelial lining cells as well as endothelial and mesothelial cells.

In those epithelial membranes characterized by columnar cells that are differentiated and specialized for absorptive or secretory functions (stomach, intestines), the specialization is accompanied by an attendant reduction in mitotic potential. Such cellular laminae are dependent upon stem cells for cellular replacement. The location of the stem cells in these simple epithelia varies. In the small intestine, epithelial lining cells of the villi are shed at the tips of these surface modifications. The stem cells are located some distance away from this locus in the depths of the intestinal crypts. Mitotic activity is characteristic of the cryptal cells. The daughter cells migrate along the glandular epithelium of the crypts, ascend the lateral shoulders of the villi and are shed at the apices of the villi.

The basal cells of stratified epithelia are the stem cells of these linings. The basal and fusiform cells of pseudostratified columnar epithelia are capable of differentiating into lining cells and goblet cells. Similar relationships are assumed to occur in the replacement of transitional epithelium.

The replacement of lost cells in stratified squamous epithelia is a necessity, because cells are shed constantly at the surface. Replacement through mitotic activity is the function of the stratum basale and stratum spinosum. Wound repair of the epidermis and underlying connective tissue (dermis) has been studied extensively. The nature of this process depends upon the nature and extent of the injury. After disruption of the epidermis, epidermal cells from the basal layers along the wound margin acquire ameboid activity and migrate to initiate coverage of the exposed connective tissue. Mitotic activity of these and contiguous germinal cells then occurs. Within 48 hours, the underlying connective tissue is covered by proliferative cells. This activity occurs beneath the scab. Proliferation continues, the epithelium is restored, and the scab of cellular and vascular debris is lifted from the replaced epidermis within 7 days.

References

Epithelium

Brody, I.: The keratinization of epidermal cells of normal guinea pig skin revealed by electron microscopy. J. Ultrastruct. Res. 2:482, 1959.

Dunn, J.S.: The fine structure of the absorptive epithelial cells of the developing small intestine of the rat. J. Anat. 101:57, 1967.

Fawcett, D.W.: *An Atlas of Fine Structure.* W. B. Saunders, Philadelphia, 1965.

Hackemann, M., Grubb, C. and Hill, K.R.: The ultrastructure of normal squamous epithelium of the human cervix uteri. J. Ultastrsuct. Res. 22:443, 1968.

Hicks, R.M.: The fine structure of the transitional epithelium of rat ureter. J. Cell Biol. 26:25, 1965.

Matthews, J.L. and Martin, J.H.: *Atlas of Human Histology and Ultrastructure.* Lea and Febiger, Philadelphia, 1971.

Porter, K.R. and Bonneville, M.A.: *Fine Structure of Cells and Tissues.* 4th edition, Lea and Febiger, Philadelphia, 1973.

Severs, N.J. and Hicks, R.M.: Analysis of membrane structure in transitional epithelium of rat urinary bladder. J. Ultrastruct. Res. 69:279, 1979.

Zelickson, A.S.: *Ultrastructure of Normal and Abnormal Skin.* Lea and Febiger, Philadelphia, 1967.

Glandular Epithelium

Bullough, W.S. and Ebling, F.J.: Cell replacement in the epidermis and sebaceous glands of the mouse. J. Anat. 86:29, 1952.

Ekholm, R. and Edlund, Y.: Ultrasrtucture of the human exocrine pancreas. J. Ultrastruct. Res. 2:453, 1959.

Gabe, M. and Arvy, L.: Gland cells.*In:* Brachet, J. and Mirsky, A.E. (eds.): *The Cell: Biochemistry, Physiology, Morphology,* Vol. V, pp1–88. Academic Press, New York, 1961.

Junqueria, L.C. and Hirsh, G.C.: Cell Secretion: A study of pancreas and salivary glands. Inter. Rev. Cyto. 5:323, 1956.

Parks, H.F.: Morphological study of the extrusion of secretory materials by the parotid glands of mouse and rat. J. Ultrastruct. Res. 6:449, 1962.

Scott, B.L. and Pease, D.C.: Electron microscopy of the salivary and lacrimal glands of the rat. Amer. J. Anat. 104:115, 1959.

Special Epithelia

Arstila, A. and Wersall, J.: The ultrastructure of the olfactory epithelium of the guinea pig. Acta Otolaryng. Stockholm. 64:187, 1967.

Edwards, E. and Duntley, S.: The pigments and color of living skin. Amer. J. Anat. 65:1, 1939.

Fitzpatrick, T.B. and Szabo, G.: The melanocyte; cytology and cytochemistry. J. Invest. Derm. 32:197, 1959.

Frisch, D.: Ultrastructure of mouse olfactory mucosa. Amer. J. Anat. 121:87, 1967.

Lundquist, P.G., Kimura, R. and Wersall, J.: Ultrastructural organization of the epithelial lining in the endolymphatic duct and sac in the guinea pig. Acta Otolaryng. Stockholm. 57:65, 1963.

Rhodin, J. and Dulhan, T.: Electron microscopy of the tracheal ciliated mucosa in rat. Z. Zellforsch. 44:345, 1956.

Travill, A.A. and Hill, M.F.: Histochemical demonstration of myoepithelial cell activity. Quart. J. Exp. Physiol. 48:423, 1963.

Surface Specializations

Barber, V.C. and Boyde, A.: Scanning electron microscopic studies of cilia. Z. Zellforsch. 84:269, 1968.

Claude, P, and Goodenough, D.A.: Fracture faces of zonulae occludentes from "tight" and "leaky" epithelia. J. Cell Biol. 58390, 1973.

Curtis, A.S.G.: Cell contact and adhesion. Biol. Rev. 37:82, 1962.

Farquhar, M. G. and Palade, G.E.: Junctional complexes in variouis epithelia. J. Cell Biol. 17:375, 1963.

Fawcett, D.W.: Physiologically significant specializations of the cell surface. Circulation 26:1105, 1962.

Fawcett, D.W.: Surface specializations of absorbing cells. J. Histochem. Cytochem. *13:*75, 1965.

Fawcett, D.W. and Porter, K.R.: A study of the fine structure of ciliated epithelia. J. Morph. *94:*221, 1954.

Goodenough, D.A.: The structure and permeability of isolated hepatocyte gap junctions. Cold Spring Harbor Symp. *40:*37, 1975.

Granger, B. and Baker, R.F.: Electron microscope investigation of the striated border of intestinal epithelium. Anat. Rec. *107:*423, 1950.

Hashimoto, K., Gross, B.G. and Lever, W.F.: Electron microscopic study of apocrine secretion. J. Invest. Derm. *46:*378, 1966.

Hudspeth, A.J. and Jacobs, R.: Stereocilia mediate transduction in vertebrate hair cells. Proc. Nat. Acad. Sci. USA. *76:*1506, 1979.

Ito, S.: The surface coat of enteric microvilli. J. Cell Biol. *27:*475, 1965.

Kelly, D.: Fine structure of desmosomes, hemidesmosomes and an adepidermal globular layer in developing newt epidermis. J. Cell Biol. *28:*51, 1966.

Kurtz, S.M. and Feldman, J.D.: Experimental studies on the formation of the glomerular basement membrane. J. Ultrastruct. Res. *6:*19, 1962.

Pierce, G.B.,Jr., Midgley, A.R.,Jr. and Sri Ram, J.: The histogenesis of basement membranes. J. Exp. Med. *117:*339, 1963.

Satir, P.: Cilia. Sci. Amer. *204:*61, 1961.

Sorokin, S.D.: Reconstruction of centriole formation and ciliogenesis in mammalian lungs. J. Cell Sci. *3:*207, 1968.

Staehelin, A.L.: Structure and function of intercellular junctions. Int. Rev. Cytol. *39:*191, 1974.

Susi, F.R., Belt, W.D. and Kelly, J.W.: Fine structure of fibrillar complexes associated with the basement membrane in human oral mucosa. J. Cell Biol. *34:*686, 1967.

Repair and Regeneration

Hunt, T.K. and Van Winkle, W.,Jr. (eds.): *Fundamentals of Wound Management in Surgery — Wound Healing: Normal Repair.* Chirurgecom, Inc., South Plainfield, New Jersey, 1976.

Leblond, C.P. and Walker, B.E.: Renewal of cell populations. Physiol. Rev. *36:*255, 1956.

Odland, G.F. and Ross, R.: Human wound repair. I. Epidermal regeneration. J. Cell Biol. *39:*135, 1968.

Peacock, E.E., Jr. and Van Winkle, W., Jr. (eds.): *Surgery and Biology of Wound Repair.* W.B. Saunders, Philadelphia, 1970.

Ross, R. and Odland, G.F.: Human wound repair. II. Inflammatory cells, epithelial-mesenchymal interactions and fibrogenesis. J. Cell Biol. *39:*152, 1968.

Weiss, P.: The biological foundations of wound repair. The Harvey Lectures, *55:*13, 1961.

6: Extracellular Matrix

Extracellular Components

Introduction. The *matrix* of a connective tissue is the amorphous ground substance and fibers that fill the space between the cells. The matrical components of the connective tissues are those constituents that impart the specific biomechanical properties by which these tissues are characterized. The pliability, elasticity and stretch characteristics of loose connective tissue relate to its constituent collagenous and elastic fibers, whereas the ability to bind water (and thereby resist compression) relates to its constituent glycosaminoglycans (GAGs). The elasticity of dense elastic tissue is a function of its elastic fibers. Similarly, the compressive and tensile properties of articular (hyaline) cartilage are related to its constituent GAGs and collagenous fibers, respectively.

Fibrous proteins are rod-like proteins with a high degree of secondary structure. The biological functions of these proteins are structural rather than metabolic. Many of these proteins are organized into helical arrays as supercoils embedded within amorphous sugar or protein matrices. The common fibrous proteins of the body are *collagen, elastin,* and *reticular fibers.* The fibrous proteins are characterized mechanically as substances with very high tensile strength.

Glycoproteins are macromolecules in which one or more saccharide chains (glucosamine, galactose, fucose, and others) and sialic acid are linked covalently to a polypeptide. The terminology applied to these and related substances is not standardized; some confusion exists. Many *enzymes, membrane proteins, receptors,* and *plasma proteins* are glycoproteins containing less than 50% carbohydrate. Salivary *mucins* are glycoproteins that consist of more than 50% carbohydrate. *Proteoglycans* are considered by some to be structural glycoproteins consisting of more than 95% carbohydrate; however, these substances may be distinguished on the basis of the amount of protein and the types of polysaccharide side chains. *Collagen* is a structural glycoprotein; however, this protein is considered a separate group on the basis of its short galactose and glucosylga-

lactose side chains. Also, sialic acid is not present. Other named structural glycoproteins include *fibronectin, chondronectin,* and *laminin.*

GAGs are polysaccharides that contain amino sugars. These polysaccharides become complexed to proteins as *proteoglycans.* Numerous proteoglycans and hyaluronic acid complex with each other in cartilaginous tissues to form *proteoglycan aggregates.*

Fibers

Collagen

General Properties. Collagen is the most ubiquitous and most abundant structural protein in the body. The liver contains about 4% collagen, whereas hyaline cartilage is composed of approximately 50% collagen. The dermis has 72% collagen; tendons and ligaments are predominantly collagen. Collagen contributes tensile strength to the body, since collagen itself is able to withstand high tensile forces, i.e., collagen resists stretching.

Collagenous fibers are the polymerized products of soluble precursor molecules that are secreted by fibroblasts, osteoblasts, chondroblasts, and other cells. In contrast

to its pure structural function in most loci, collagen has structural and optical functions in the eye.

The appearance of collagenous fibers varies in different types of tissues. In light microscopic sections stained with hematoxylin and eosin (H and E), the fibers are pink-staining. The degree of collagenous fiber staining, the three-dimensional orientation of the fibers, and their association with certain ground substance components alters their appearance. In the dermis, the highly polymerized fibers of the dense white fibrous connective tissue are thick, wavy, and oriented randomly. The random bundles of indefinite length have a diameter between 1 and 12 μm (Fig. 6.1). The length, thickness, and random orientation of the fibers are apparent in stretch preparations of the loose connective tissues (Fig. 6.2). The dense white fibrous connective tissue of tendons and ligaments consists of fibers that are difficult to resolve as individual units. The fibers are highly polymerized, packed tightly, and oriented in an orderly manner in response to the tensile forces exerted upon them. Collagenous fibers in loose connective tissue are oriented randomly and are thin. In the supportive tissues, the presence of collagenous fibers is not evident with routine preparation and

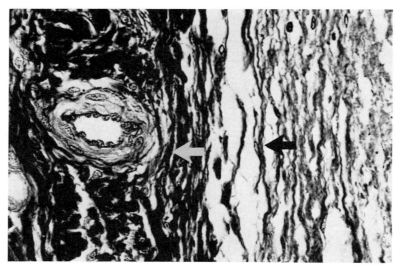

Figure 6.1. Collagenous fibers of the capsule of an adrenal gland. Coarse fibers *(white arrow)* and fine fibers *(black arrow)* comprise the capsule of the organ. ×160. (Azan.)

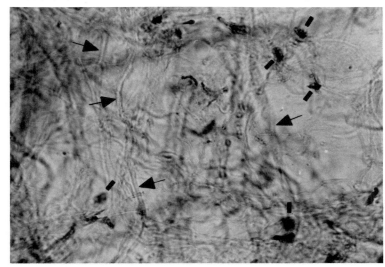

Figure 6.2. Stretch preparation of connective tissue from a murine subcutis. The collagenous fibers *(arrows)* are oriented randomly. The cells *(bars)* are out of the plane of focus.

examination techniques. The indices of refraction of collagen and intermingled ground substance are sufficiently similar to mask the collagen.

Chemical Characteristics. Electron microscopy and appropriate staining reveal unique features of this ubiquitous structural protein. Alternating dark- and light-staining patterns are apparent. One dark and one light band forms a 67-nm period that is repeated throughout the length of the fibers. This periodicity results from the precise registration of the monomers that polymerize to form collagen. This monomer, *tropocollagen*, consists of three smaller units called α-*chains*.

The protein is composed of three polypeptides, α-chains, that consist of approximately 1000 amino acids. Each α-chain has a molecular weight of about 95,000. Different types of α-chains have been identified and named on the basis of composition and sequencing of constituent amino acids. The α-chains have a repetitive amino acid sequence in which every third amino acid is glycine. Collagen has an unusually high quantity of proline. Proline and hydroxyproline occupy about every fourth position and account for 20–25% of the amino acid residues. Two hydroxylated derivatives of proline, *3-hydroxyproline* and *4-hydroxyproline*, only occur in collagen. Hydroxylysine, although not a common constituent of the α-chains, is significant because it is the site for the addition of sugars and the site of intermolecular cross linkages.

The α-chains of tropocollagen have an unique secondary structure. Each is a left-handed, integral residue helix in which there are three residues per turn. The occurrence of glycine at every third position facilitates the tight winding of the polypeptide. Hydrogen bonding does not contribute to the stability of the helix. Three α-chains are wound around each other to produce a right-handed, triple-helical molecule called tropocollagen. Hydrogen bonding does stabilize the helical pattern between associated α-chains. Short, nonhelical regions exist at the C- and N-terminus of the α-chains. These regions are important in intermolecular cross linkage.

Initial chromatographic studies of collagen derived from bone and the dermis of the skin determined that tropocollagen consisted of three α-chains. Two were identical; the third was different. This collagen, now designated *type I collagen*, has two α-chains designated α_1 and one α-chain designated α_2. The composition of type I collagen is designated as $[\alpha_1(I)]_2 \, \alpha_2(I)$. Since then, four additional collagens have been identified and their constituent α-chains have been characterized. These chains differ from the α_1 chains of type I collagen $[\alpha_1(I)]$ and the α_2 chains of type I collagen $[\alpha_2(I)]$. The accompanying table (Table 6.1) lists the types, occurrence and compositional differences of the collagens that have been characterized. *Types I, II, and III are interstitial collagens*, whereas *types IV and V are basement membrane collagens.*

Synthesis and Secretion. Not many years ago, the accepted dogma was that only the fibroblastic family (mesenchymal cell, fibroblast, chondroblast, osteoblast) was capable of the synthesis and secretion of collagen. Today, examples of cells from almost every tissue have been shown to secrete collagen (and GAGs) at some point in their life cycles. The collagen-producing cells are capable of the synthesis and secretion of more than one type of collagen. Also, these cells may change the type of collagen produced.

Current evidence indicates that the synthesis of collagenous precursors is similar to the synthesis of other proteins (Fig. 6.3). The generation of different types of collagen is contingent upon the ability to synthesize different polypeptide chains (α-chains). Numerous enzymes are involved in post-translational alterations to the collagenous precursors, including: "signal" peptidase, prolylhydroxylase, lysylhydroxylase, galactosylhydroxylysl-transferase, glucosylgalactosylhydroxylysl-transferase, procollagen carboxypeptidase, procollagen aminopeptidase, and lysyl oxidase. The extensive post-translational alterations to collagen, however, are unique. These alterations complicate synthesis and afford opportunities for errors in production that are recognizable as diseases.

The terminology relating to the naming of collagenous precursors and components needs some clarification and standardization. The terminology used in the following description is consistent with the majority

Table 6.1.
Types and Composition of Collagen

Type and Composition	Occurrence	Hylys/10³ Amino Acids	% Sugar
Interstitial			
I $[\alpha_1(I)]_2\alpha_2(I)$	Bone, loose and dense connective tissue, vascular media, G.I. tract wall, cornea	5	0.5–1.0
II $[\alpha_1(II)]_3$	Cartilage, cornea	20	5
III $[\alpha_1(III)]_3$	Reticular connective tissue, cornea	7	1
Basement Membrane			
IV $[\alpha_1(IV)]_3$	Basement membrane	45	10
V $[\alpha_1(B)]_2\alpha_1(A)$	Basement membrane	23–37	2–5

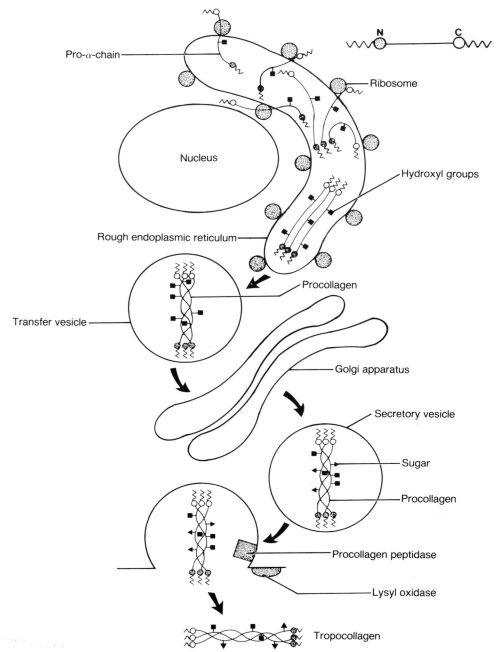

Figure 6.3. Synthesis and secretion of tropocollagen. The synthesis of tropocollagen is similar to the synthesis of other proteins. The mRNA for collagen is formed in the nucleus by transcription. The mRNA enters the cytoplasm and attaches to the ribosomes of the rough endoplasmic reticulum (RER). Translation results in the formation of *preprocollagen chains*. These are *pro-α-chains* to which a signal peptide is appended. The signal peptide is clipped from the polypeptide as the polypeptide enters the rough endoplasmic reticulum. Hydroxylation of proline and lysine occurs as the pro-α-chains enter the cisterns of the RER. Pro-α-chains become aggregated in triplets called procollagen. Transfer vesicles are incorporated into the immature face of the Golgi apparatus. Glycosylation within the Golgi stack results in the formation of stabilized procollagen molecules. The procollagen molecules leave the mature face of the Golgi apparatus within secretory vesicles. The secretory vesicles fuse with the plasma membrane as exocytotic vesicles. A procollagen peptidase, located either within the secretory vesicles or on the cell membrane, cleaves the tailpieces resulting in the formation of tropocollagen. Cross linkage between tropocollagenous molecules is achieved through the activity of lysyl oxidase. (Redrawn and modified from Hunt, T. K. and Van Winkle, W., Jr.: *Fundamentals of Wound Management in Surgery — Wound Healing: Normal Repair.* Chirurgecom, Inc., South Plainfield, NJ, 1976.)

of the literature on the subject. Also, some liberties were taken with names to present a coherent story (Figs. 6.3 and 6.4).

The initial translational product is a *pre-procollagen chain* that has a primary structure of (X–Y–Glycine)₃₃₃. Additionally, the amino-terminal and carboxy-terminal portions have propeptides attached that consist of 180 and 300 amino acids, respectively. The preprocollagenous chains have "signal peptides" attached to them. These signal sequences direct the transfer of the molecules from the polyribosomes across the membrane of the rough endoplasmic reticulum (RER) to the cisternae of this organelle. Membrane-bound enzymes (signal peptidases) remove the signal peptides on the luminal side of the membrane of the RER. The shortened chains are called *procollagen chains* (pro-α-chains); they are polypeptide chains devoid of their signal

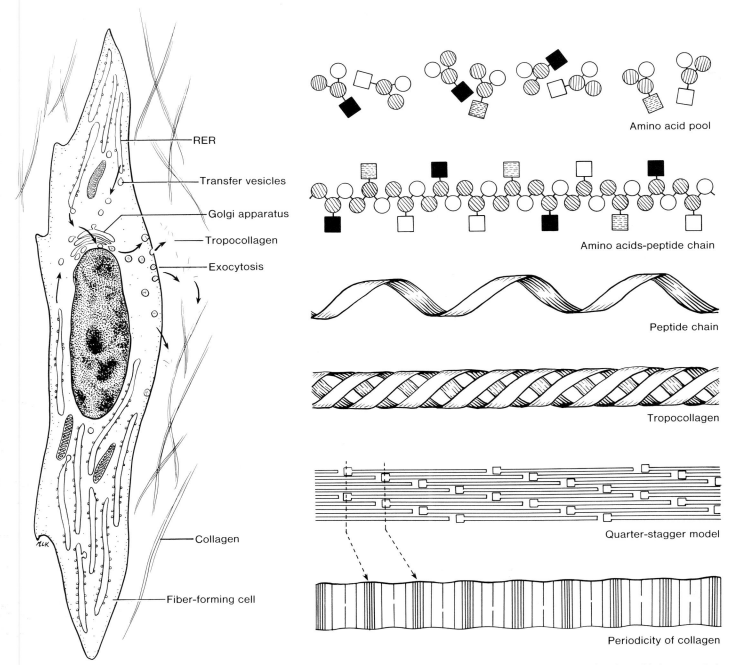

RER

Transfer vesicles

Golgi apparatus

Tropocollagen

Exocytosis

Collagen

Fiber-forming cell

Amino acid pool

Amino acids-peptide chain

Peptide chain

Tropocollagen

Quarter-stagger model

Periodicity of collagen

Figure 6.4. Synthesis, secretion, and polymerization of tropocollagen. Glycine, proline, and lysine comprise the majority of amino acids incorporated into tropocollagen. Hydroxyproline is a specific marker for collagen, because it does not occur in other biochemical substances in significant amount. The amino acids are sequenced during translation to produce typical polypeptide chains. Procollagen, the secretory product of fiber-forming cells (fibroblasts, osteoblasts, chondroblasts), polymerizes within the connective tissue compartment to form typical collagen. Although other models have been proposed to account for the 67-nm periodicity of collagen, the quarter-stagger model is widely accepted and is the model shown in this diagram. This model accounts for most of the repetitive features of collagen in relation to the 280-nm length of tropocollagen. The quarter-stagger model would be exact if the periodicity of collagen were 70 nm. Other models have been proposed to account for the discrepancy of 12 nm. Importantly, not all collagen has a 67-nm periodicity; it may range from 20–1000 nm in some tissues. (Redrawn and modified but based on descriptions by Goss, J. and Porter, K. R.: *Connective Tissue:Intercellular Macromolecules.* J. and A. Churchill Ltd., London, 1964.)

peptides. The pro-α-chains become associated with each other in a non-orderly array. The first modification to the pro-α-chains occurs as the polypeptides pass through the membrane of the rough endoplasmic reticulum. The amino acids 3-hydroxyproline, 4-hydroxyproline and hydroxylysine are characteristic of the collagenous fiber. Proline and lysine, however, are the amino acids incorporated into the chains during translation. *Prolylhydroxylase* and *lysylhydroxylase* are responsible for the hydroxylation of these amino acids as they pass into the lumen of the RER. The hydroxylation of these amino acids is essential for the proper transport of collagen out of the cell. Also, triple helix formation is dependent upon hydroxylation. When the hydroxylation step is interrupted, fiber-forming cells accumulate an abnormal form of collagen called *protocollagen*. The hydroxylation process progresses normally as the pro-α-chains aggregate and move through the cisternae of the RER.

Aggregation of the pro-α-chains within the cisternae of the RER results in the formation of *procollagen*. An important modification of procollagen is the formation of disulfide bonds within the amino and carboxy terminals. The amino terminal is involved in intrachain disulfide bonding, whereas the carboxy terminal is involved in interchain disulfide bonds.

Additonal modifications to procollagen involve some of the hydroxylysyl residues. Glycosylation, necessary for helical stabilization, transport and secretion, occurs within the RER and Golgi apparatus. *Galactosylhydroxylysl-transferase* uses *uridine diphosphate (UDP)-galactose* as a source of galactose to add to certain hydroxylysyl residues. *Glucosylgalactosylhydroxylysyl-transferase* uses *UDP-glucose* as a source of glucose to be added to galactosylhydroxylysyl residues. The resulting molecule, *procollagen*, is an hydroxylated and glycosylated macromolecule with disulfide bonds that is registered in a triple helical configuration. The molecule passes through the Golgi apparatus and is extruded from the cell.

Procollagen is the secretory product of collagen-producing cells. Additionally, these cells secrete the enzymes necessary for the completion of the synthetic process. Extracellular processing is a significant component in the generation of collagen.

Extracellular Alterations and Self-As-sembly. The first step in the extracellular processing of procollagen is the removal of most of the nonhelical extension peptides at the C- and N-terminus (Fig. 6.5). The role of these extension peptides is uncertain. They seem to assist with the formation of the helix, and they may facilitate intracellular and extracellular transport. Their fate after cleavage is uncertain also. Two enzymes are necessary to cleave the terminal peptides; *procollagen carboxypeptidase* cleaves the C-terminal peptide, whereas *procollagen aminopeptidase* removes the N-terminal peptide. The activity of these enzymes results in the formation of the insoluble *tropocollagen*, which is composed of three α-chains. Tropocollagen is a helical structure along 95% of its length; the remaining 5% is attributable to the residual, nonhelical C- and N-terminal peptides. The tropocollagen molecule is approximately 290 nm long by 1.5 nm wide.

Spontaneous self-assembly of tropocollagen into collagenous fibers follows removal of the terminal peptides. The primary structure of the constituent α-chains provides the necessary information for the proper registration of the components. The final step in the assembly process ensures

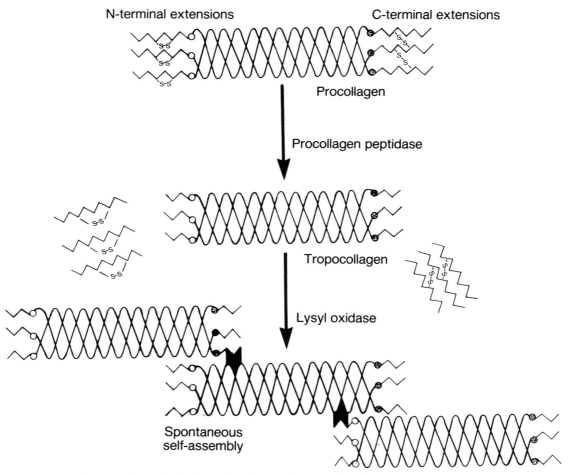

N-terminal extensions   C-terminal extensions

Procollagen

Procollagen peptidase

Tropocollagen

Lysyl oxidase

Spontaneous self-assembly

Figure 6.5.   Diagrams illustrating the formation of tropocollagen and its subsequent spontaneous self-assembly.

that the tensile strength of collagen is established. This requires the formation of intermolecular cross linkages occurring between the nonhelical components of constituent tropocollagens. Cross linkage is achieved through the oxidative deamination of lysyl and hydroxylysyl residues into aldehydes through the action of *lysyl oxidase*. Subsequent to this activity, aldol condensation and Schiff base formation with Amadori rearrangement results in stabilized intramolecular and intermolecular cross linkages.

Polymerization: Microfibrils to Fibers. Electron microscopic observations, extraction, and reconstitution techniques afforded insights into the architectural arrangement of the tropocollagenous monomers into the polymerization product—collagenous fibrils. The *quarter stagger model* was proposed as a reasonable explanation of the *axial periodicity* that characterizes collagen. According to this model, the tropocollagenous molecules overlap each other by one-quarter of their length. A 280-nm tropocollagenous molecule would be divisible, therefore, into 70-nm repetitive units. The model afforded valuable insights but was less than perfect. The length of tropocollagen is about 290 nm and the axial periodicity is 67 nm. The quarter stagger model was modified to include a hole region of about 40 nm between the linearly oriented tropocollagenous molecules (Fig. 6.6). The 67-nm axial periodicity results from the precise end-to-gap-to-end arrangement. All tropocollagens are

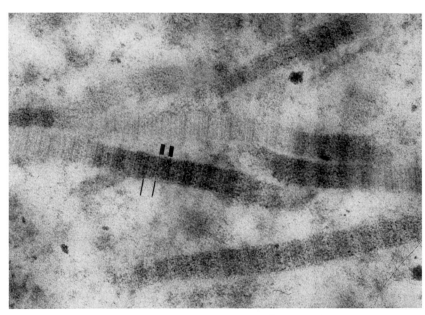

Figure 6.7. An electron micrograph of sectioned collagen. The periodic banding is obvious. The dark band *(thick bars)* and light band *(thin bars)* comprise the typical 67-nm period of collagen. ×94,000.

arranged in this manner. The N–terminal of a molecule overlaps the C–terminal end of an adjacent tropocollagen by 27 nm, not the entire 67-nm repetitive unit. Thus, the axial periodicity of collagen consists of *overlap zones* (27 nm) and *hole zones* (40 nm). The hole zone typically fills with stain in negatively stained preparations for electron microscopy and appears dark. The

overlap zone does not fill with stain in these types of preparations and appears light. Naturally, just the reverse staining pattern occurs with positively stained materials observed with the electron microscope (Fig. 6.7). Additionally, 12 bands (I–XII) are visible in sectioned and positively stained preparations.

Microfibrils less than 40 nm in diameter

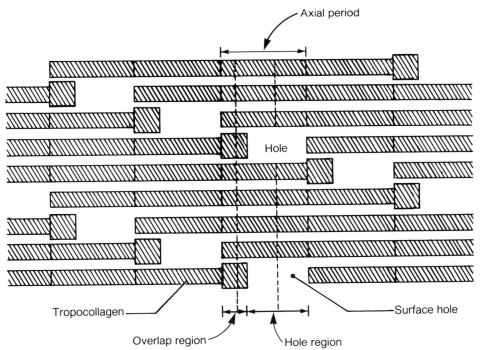

Figure 6.6. A diagram illustrating the overlap/hole modification of the quarter stagger model. (Redrawn and modified from Glimcher, M.: *Handbook of Physiology-Endocrinology* VII, Williams & Wilkins Co., Baltimore, 1976.)

are visible with the electron microscope. Further polymerization of bundles of microfibrils results in the formation of *fibrils* (approximately 0.5 μm in diameter) that are visible with the light microscope. Bundles of fibrils form the characteristic *fibers* of light microscopy.

Functional Correlates. Disruptions in the numerous post-translational events associated with the maturation of the collagenous precursors results in disease processes. Collagenous diseases result from: a deficiency of lysylhydroxylase (Ehlers-Danlos VI); inability to remove the amino terminal of one of the collagenous precursors (Ehlers-Danlos VII, dermatosparaxis of sheep and cattle); deficiency of lysyl oxidase (Ehlers-Danlos V). Lathyrism, either naturally occurring or experimentally induced, results from feeding excessive quantities of the sweet pea *(Lathyrus sp.)* or an extract from this plant, β-amino proprionitrile (BAPN). This lathyritic agent inhibits lysyl oxidase. Cross linkages are inhibited and the tensile strength of the collagen is reduced. The agent has been useful in elucidating the mechanisms involved in cross linkages.

Reticular Fibers

General Characteristics. The reticular fibers of light microscopy are impossible to demonstate with routine staining techniques. As such, these fibers are indistinguishable from collagenous fibers. Reticular fibers, however, are demonstrable with special staining techniques involving silver impregnation (Fig. 6.8). Because of their ability to be stained with silver, the fibers are referred to as being *argyrophilic*—silver-loving.

Reticular fibers were named on the basis of their forming a delicate, finely branched

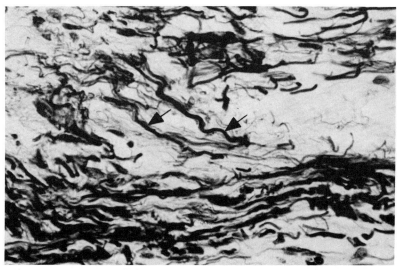

Figure 6.9. Elastic fibers of loose connective tissue. Although the elastic fibers *(arrows)* are difficult to demonstrate with routine stains, the fibers are demonstrable with special staining techniques. ×160. (Verhoeff's stain.)

network (L. *rete*, net) of fibers in close association with the individual cells of the parenchyma of various tissues and organs. These fibers occur frequently with basement membranes and are components of most tissues and organs. Reticular fibers form a delicate network around bundles of collagenous fibers in tendons and ligaments, around individual smooth muscular fibers, and form the stroma in a myriad of other loci. The organs of the hemic-lymphatic system use these fibers as the primary means of connective tissue support.

The arygyrophilic staining property of reticular fibers led to the belief that reticular fibers were unique, something distinct from collagenous fibers in chemical composi-

tion. Electron microscopy did not confirm this supposition. Rather, the fibers were demonstrated to have the same distinct collagenic property—an axial periodicity identical to collagen. Subsequently, type III collagen has been isolated biochemically and identified immunohistochemically from reticular connective tissue. The silver staining property of reticular fibers relates to their being coated with carbohydrates.

Fibroblasts secrete the collagenous fibers of the proper connective tissues. Reticular fibers in these tissues are probably the secretory products of fibroblasts also.

Elastic Fibers

General Characteristics. The elastic fibers of light microscopy are not demonstrated easily with routine staining. With H and E, however, the discerning eye will note that the elastic fibers stain a brighter pink than collagenous fibers. Elastic fibers are observed readily as long, thin, or wavy fibers with special staining techniques (Fig. 6.9). If they are broken, then they are wavy fibers that may have a corkscrew appearance (Figs. 6.10 and 6.11).

The elastic fibers consist of two distinct components that are visible with the electron microscope. The primary component is *elastin*. It forms an amorphous mass of electron dense material (Fig. 6.12). A glycoprotein is present that forms microfibrils associated intimately with the amorphous mass. The microfibrils surround and are embedded within the amorphous mass of elastin. Microfibrillar protein is secreted by elastin-producing cells as a supporting network to mold the amorphous mass into cylindrical structures. Absence of microfibrillar protein probably precludes elastin from assuming its fibrous nature. Neither of these components has an axial periodic-

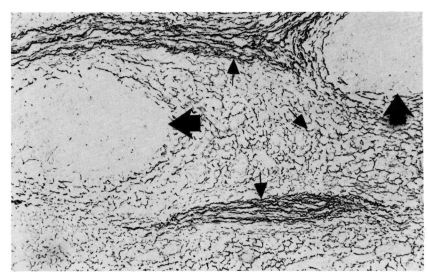

Figure 6.8. Reticular fibers within a canine lymph node. The argyrophilic fibers *(small arrows)* are arranged in dense and loose aggregates. Areas devoid of fibers *(large arrows)* are the germinal centers of the secondary lymph nodules that are characteristic of the lymph nodes of immune competent animals. ×40. (Snook's reticulum stain.)

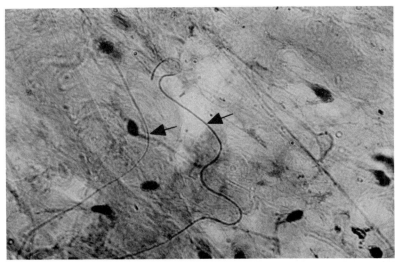

Figure 6.10. Elastic fibers in a stretch preparation of loose connective tissue from the subcutis of a mouse. The broken elastic fibers *(arrows)* appear wavy. Other cellular and fibrous components are out of the plane of focus. ×160.

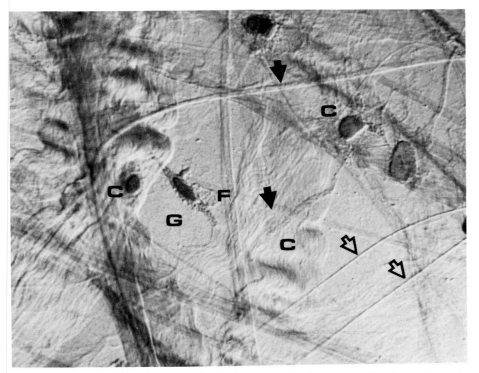

Figure 6.11. Nomarski interference contrast micrograph of the loose connective tissue of a murine subcutis. *F,* fibroblast; *G,* ground substance; *open arrows,* elastin; *solid arrows,* collagen; *C,* bundles of collagenous fibers. ×160.

cyclic products of amino acid alteration called *desmosine* and *isodesmosine*. These substances covalently link four tropoelastin chains to form elastin.

Elastin has a limited but significant distribution in the quadruped animal. The *nuchal ligament* is composed of dense elastic connective tissue. The aorta and other elastic arteries contain large quantities of elastic fibers within their walls. Elastic fibers also contribute to the compliance of the lung. Elastic fibers are constituents of cartilage in limited foci. Although scant, elastic fibers are present in other proper connective tissues.

Ground Substance

General Properties. The fibrous and cellular components of the proper connective tissues are demonstrable easily in routine preparations for light microscopy. That these components are bathed by an aqueous medium is a reasonable supposition. Aqueous continuity must (and does) exist between the vascular, extracellular, and intracellular spaces. The notion that amorphous materials occupied the intercellular and interfibrillar spaces and held water in place developed slowly, was difficult to appreciate, hard to characterize, and is easy to overlook. The cells, fibers and aqueous media *(tissue fluid, interstitial fluid)* are held by a viscous gel-like material called *amorphous ground substance*. The ground substance is the secretory product of the characteristic cells of the tissue—fibroblasts, osteoblasts, chondroblasts—and consists primarily of carbohydrates. The carbohydrates, the types and quantities of which differ in different tissues, comprise the viscous, gel phase of the interstitial space. The tissue fluid, with all of its dissolved substances, comprises the fluid phase of the interstitial space *(interstitium)*. The ground substance and the interstitial fluid, although distinct entities, are, in fact, inseparable.

The nature of the ground substance helps to characterize the properties of the tissues. The free and bound water of the interstitium ensures an ample supply for the cells. Also, all transport to and from the cells must occur through this aqueous medium. Not only must the tissue fluid be maintained, but it must be maintained in proper amounts. Too little (dehydration) and too much (edema) tissue fluid can have devastating effects upon the organism or parts thereof.

The ground substance, composed of components that are highly water soluble, is observed rarely with routine paraffin techniques. Special care (freezing techniques) must be used to preserve this material for staining. The obvious spaces between cells and fibers in proper connective tissue are artifacts of preparation. In the living organism, those "spaces" are oc-

ity that should be confused with that of collagenous fibers.

Although some of the biochemical characteristics of elastin are known, the actual conformation of the macromolecule has not been determined. Glycine and proline each comprise about one-third of the amino acid composition; however, the amount of hydroxyproline is scant. Elastin subunits do not form a polyproline-type helix that is typical of collagen. An elastin

precursor, *proelastin*, is synthesized and secreted by the cells in a manner similar to the production of procollagen. An extracellular enzyme appears to remove a portion of the molecule (tailpiece) in a manner similar to the mechanism of conversion of procollagen to tropocollagen. Another enzyme, lysyl oxidase, converts the ε-amino terminus of a lysine to an aldehyde, an *allysine*. Three allysines and a lysine react (aldol condensation) to form the hetero-

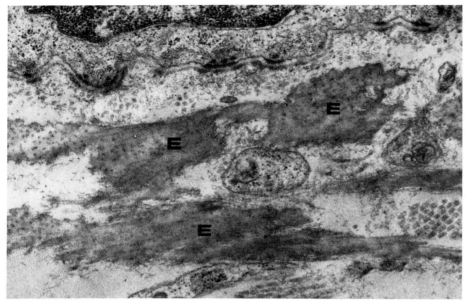

Figure 6.12. An electron micrograph of elastic fibers. The irregularly shaped elastic fibers *(E)* are scattered throughout the connective tissue. ×26,000.

cupied by carbohydrates. Materials must diffuse or filter through and/or around the ground substance materials. Large molecules have much difficulty moving through the ground substance. Similarly, microorganisms do not move through the ground substance of proper connective tissue easily. The virulence of bacteria is related to a number of factors, one of which is their ability to spread or invade the body beyond a particular site of entry. Many bacteria have developed the ability to produce *hyaluronidase.* This enzyme or *spreading factor* breaks down the ground substance and facilitates their spread. Some bacteria also produce *collagenase*; this enzyme aids their dispersion by degrading collagen.

GAGs. The viscous, semifluid, gelatinous ground substance of most connective tissues consists predominately of carbohydrates. The carbohydrates are *polysaccharides* that have been called *mucopolysaccharides.* Sulfated mucopolysaccharides were called *acid mucopolysaccharides*; nonsulfated mucopolysaccharides were called *neutral mucopolysaccharides.* All of these substances have been called *mucosubstances* collectively. Although new terminology has been adopted for these substances, some of the old terminology still remains. A group of diseases characterized by the inability to metabolize some of these substances appropriately is called the *mucopolysaccharidoses.*

The predominant carbohydrates of the ground substance are called *GAGs* currently. The term literally means an amino sugar (glycosamino-) polysaccharide (-glycan). GAGs are high molecular weight polymers of repeating disaccharide units. One of the monosaccharides in the disaccharide unit is an *amino sugar*—either *N-acetylglucosamine* or *N-acetylgalactosamine.* The other monosaccharide in the repeating unit is either a *uronic acid* or *galactose.* The GAGs are a heterogeneous group of carbohydrates that have some significant properties in common. They are *polyanions* capable of binding water in large quantities. The repeating units contain one hexosamine. The sugars are linked through β 1,3 or β 1,4 glycosidic linkages, but a β 1,6 linkage occurs occasionally. The compounds differ in various ways. The polyanionic nature depends upon sulfate groups, carboxylate groups, or both. Each of the repeating units differs, but a particular disaccharide repeating unit characterizes a particular GAG. The length of the polymers differ also. All of the GAGs, with the exception of hyaluronic acid, are complexed to proteins as proteoglycans. Also, the GAGs have a variable distribution throughout the connective tissues (Table 6.2). The GAGs include the following compounds: *hyaluronic acid, chondroitin-4-sulfate, chondroitin-6-sulfate, keratan sulfate, dermatan sulfate, and heparin.*

Hyaluronic acid (Fig. 6.13) is a long-chain polymer whose disaccharide units consist of glucuronic acid and glucosamine *(glucuronate β-1,3 N-acetylglucoasamine β-1,4).* This long, unbranched compound contains 2500 diasaccharide units and has a molecular weight of about 2×10^6. This substance is the most commonly occurring GAG in the connective tissues. Notably, it is the only GAG that is not sulfated. Also, it is the only GAG that is not complexed to proteins routinely. Secondary associations with proteoglycans form large aggregates that comprise cartilaginous matrices.

The *chondroitin sulfates* (Fig. 6.13) are polymers of repeating units of glucuronic acid and galactosamine *(glucuronate β-1,3 N-acetylgalactosamine β-1,4).* The position of the sulfate determines which isomer is formed—*chondroitin-4-sulfate* or *chondroitin-6-sulfate.* One form of this compound may not be sulfated. The significance of the positioning of the sulfates is not understood; however, these isomers do have a differential distribution relating to the tissue, age, and state of health of the organism. Each polysaccharide consists of 30–50 disaccharide units with a molecular weight between 15,000 and 25,000.

Dermatan sulfate (Fig. 6.13) differs from chondroitin-4- and -6- sulfates by iduronic acid being the predominant substitution for glucuronic acid. The chain lengths of this polysaccharide are approximately twice the lengths of the chondroitins and have molecular weights in the range of 20,000–50,000.

Keratan sulfate (Fig. 6.13) is the most heterogeneous GAG. The polymer consists of repeating disaccharide units of glucosamine and galactose *(N-acetylglucosamine β-1,3 galactose β-1,4).* The polysaccharide chains are short, each consisting of about 15 disaccharides. The molecular weight of this compound varies between 5000 and 10,000. The degree of sulfation of keratan sulfate is variable; the sulfation can exceed more than one sulfate per disaccharide unit. Two types of keratan sulfates have been isolated—*keratan sulfate I* and *II.* Keratan sulfate I is a corneal component, whereas keratan sulfate II is a skeletal tissue constituent. These GAGs are branched and use a β-1,6 glycosidic linkage to achieve the

Table 6.2.
Type and Distribution of Glycosaminoglycans

Type	Distribution
Hyaluronic acid	Synovial fluid, umbilical cord, vitreous humor, loose connective tissue
Chondroitin	Cornea
Chondroitin-4-sulfate	Cartilage, bone, cornea, aorta
Chondroitin-6-sulfate	Cartilage, nucleus pulposus, sclera, tendon, umbilical cord
Keratan sulfate	Cartilage, bone, cornea, nucleus pulposus
Dermatan sulfate	Aorta, cardiac valves, ligamentum nuchae, sclera, skin, tendon
Heparin	Mast cells
Heparin sulfate	Cell surfaces

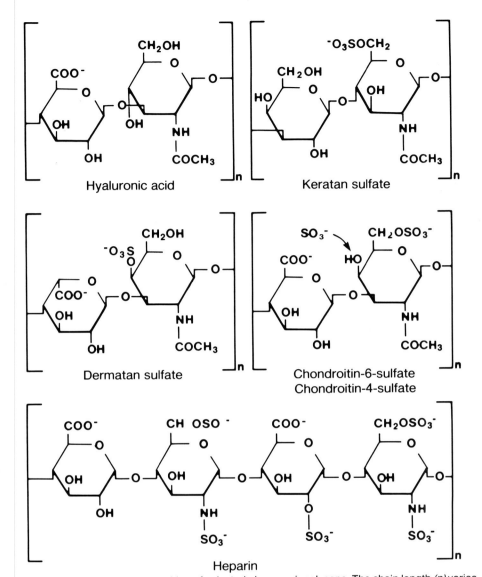

Figure 6.13. Chemical composition of selected glycosaminoglycans. The chain length *(n)* varies among these substances: hyaluronic acid, n = 2500; keratan sulfate, n = 10-20; dermatan sulfate, n = 120; chondroitin sulphates, n = 60; heparin, n = 15. The structure of heparin illustrates some of the structural features that characterize the molecule. The actual sequence depicted has been chosen arbitrarily. Iduronic acid may substitute for glucuronic acid. Also, Few of the NH groups are acetylated, but all of them are sulfated.

contains more acetylated groups and fewer sulfate groups than heparin. It has an extracellular distribution and has been associated with cellular surface coats.

Sialic acid, although not a GAG, is a constituent of them and is a contributor to the synthesis of GAG chains, especially as they occur in glycoprotein. Sialic acid consists of two components—N-acetylglucosamine complexed with lactic acid.

Proteoglycans. *Proteoglycans* are conjugates of GAGs and protein. Because these macromolecules contain at least 95% carbohydrate, they act more like sugars than proteins.

A typical proteoglycan has a *core protein* with a molecular weight of about 20,000 to which numerous GAGs are complexed (Fig. 6.14). Such a molecule, containing about 100 chondroitin sulfate chains, about 110 keratan sulfate chains and approximately 15 other oligosaccharides, would have a molecular weight of approximately 2.5×10^6. Specific regions of the core protein have been identified—*chondroitin sulfate binding region, keratan sulfate binding region*, and *hyaluronic acid binding region*. The keratan sulfate binding region is characterized also by the attachment of oligosaccharides. The hyaluronic acid binding site is involved in the formation of *proteoglycan aggregates*.

The polyanionic nature of the proteoglycans suits them ideally for their basic functions and biological significance. They are contributors to lubrication within the synovial fluid. They also absorb water readily. This property contributes significantly to the compressive properties of a tissue, provides for a depot when excessive water occupies the interstitial space (edema), and ensures a readily available source of water for the cells. So, proteoglycans contribute to the stability and support provided by connective tissues. Also, they help with the maintenance of water volume and electrolyte distribution throughout the body.

Proteoglycan synthesis requires many of the processes involved in glycoprotein syn-

branching. The keratan sulfates also contain additional monosaccharides such as mannose, fucose, sialic acid, and N-acetylgalactosamine.

Two types of heparins exist. *Heparin* is formed from repeating disaccharide units consisting of glucosamine and glucuronic acid or iduronic acid (Fig. 6.13). The linkages in heparin are α-glycosidic linkages. Few glucosamine groups are N-acetylated, but all have sulfate groups. The sulfate content per disaccharide is approximately 2.5 sulfates per unit. Heparin is a product of mast cells that is an anticoagulant and lipid-clearing agent with a molecular weight between 6000 and 20,000. *Heparin sulfate*

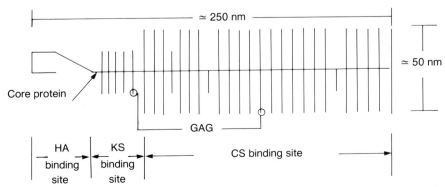

Figure 6.14. A simplified diagram of a typical glycoprotein. The oligosaccharides have not been included. *HA*, hyaluronic acid; *KS*, keratan sulfate; *CS*, chondroitin sulfate; *GAG*, glycosaminoglycan.

thesis. Core protein is synthesized within the RER and moves into the Golgi apparatus wherein polysaccharide attachment and elongation, and sulfation occur. The formation of polysaccharide chains is dependent upon the activity of six different *glycosyltransferases*, whereas sulfation occurs as a result of the sulfate donation from *3'-phosphoadenine 5'-phosphosulfate (PAPS)*. Although the linkage characteristics of GAGs to core proteins are known, the mechanisms that govern the quantitative and qualitative characteristics of the proteoglycans are not understood. Substrate specificity of constituent enzymes and specific core protein acceptor molecules seem to be important determinants in proteoglycan characteristics. Also, UDP sugar complexes are not only sources of the various sugars used in the synthesis process, but the strict regulation of these compounds subjects proteoglycan synthesis to the same regulatory mechanisms.

Degradation of proteoglycans within the connective tissue space is dependent upon the sequential action of *proteases, glycosidases, deacetylases,* and *sulfatases*.

Staining of GAGs. The biochemical characterization of the GAG content of tissues is an essential but difficult technique. Histochemical techniques are simple but not very precise; however, the demonstration of these substances in histological sections affords valuable insights about the tissues examined. The sulfated GAGs stain with the basic component of routine staining preparations. As acidic substances, they are basophilic; therefore, they stain blue with H and E. Since the GAGs are polyanions, cationic dyes, such as alcian blue (copper phthalocyanin) are effective stains. Alcian blue is used often with varying molar concentrations of magnesium chloride to characterize the family of GAGs. These polysaccharides also have the ability to bind certain stains whose color changes once binding is achieved. This property is called *metachromasia*. A typical metachromatic stain such as toluidine blue stains the GAGs purple.

PAS reactivity is not usually characteristic of GAGs and proteoglycans if typical oxidation times with periodic acid are used. However, the PAS procedure will demonstrate the glycoproteins, because the 1, 2 glycol groups of attached sugars are oxidized readily during the oxidation time period used normally for this stain.

Other Structural Proteins. *Fibronectin* (L. *fibro*, fiber; L. *nectere*, to tie) is a product of various cells in culture (fibroblasts, myoblast, some epithelial cells) with a molecular weight of approximately 230,000 daltons. This glycoprotein contains about 5% carbohydrate. Two types of fibronectin have been identified. A *plasma fibronectin* has been identified as a cold insoluble globulin. *Cellular* or *cell surface fibronectin* seems to subserve the biological role of tying cells to collagenous fibers and/or

GAGs. This glycoprotein appears early in the embryo and has been identified as a basement membrane component. Fibronectin occurs in most proper connective tissues, but the substance does not occur in supportive tissues. The precise relationships between fibronectin, connective tissue components, plasma membranes, and intracellular proteins have not been determined. Figure 6.15 is a diagram of a model that may explain these relationships.

Laminin is a large glycoprotein with a molecular weight of about 660,000 daltons. It is a component of basal laminae that attaches nonconnective tissue cells to collagenous fibers (Fig. 6.15).

Chondronectin is a large glycoprotein that attaches chondrocytes to collagenous fibers in a manner similar to that described for fibronectin.

Tissue Fluid

Body Fluids and Ground Substance

Body Water. The total volume of water is about 65% of the total body weight. This percentage, however, is related more directly to the mass of the lean tissues of the body rather than to total body weight. Lean animals contain a higher percentage of water than do obese animals. The distribution of the water volume is not equal, because tissues and organs of the body contain different but characteristic amounts of water.

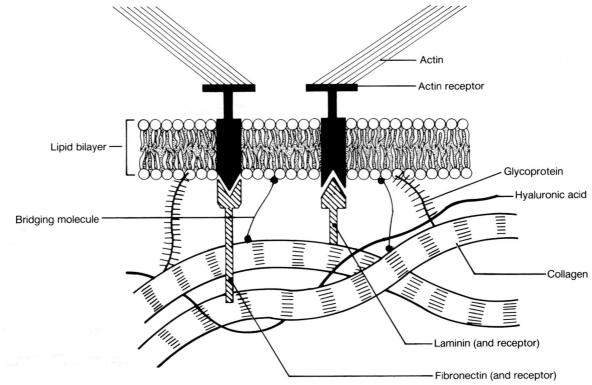

Actin
Actin receptor
Lipid bilayer
Glycoprotein
Hyaluronic acid
Bridging molecule
Collagen
Laminin (and receptor)
Fibronectin (and receptor)

Figure 6.15. A diagram illustrating the relationship of extracellular molecules with the cell membrane. This model is a theoretical composite of various models that have been proposed. It assumes that receptor molecules exist within the membrane for most if not all of the extracellular molecules.

This unequal distribution of water is divisible into two compartments—*extracellular fluid* and *intracellular fluid* (Fig. 6.16). The extracellular fluid comprises approximately 24% of the total fluid volume and includes the *plasma (4%), interstitial* or *tissue fluid (15%)* and *transcellular fluid (5%)*. The transcellular fluids are those that occur in the body cavities, hollow visceral organs, eye, and as secretory products of various glands. The remaining 41% of the fluid compartment is intracellular. These separate fluid compartments are exchangeable and are in a state of flux.

Plasma, Tissue Fluid, and Lymph. The *plasma* or intercellular fluid phase of the blood contains numerous and varied crystalloids as well as the plasma proteins (albumin, globulins, fibrinogen). The colloids do not leave the blood in any significant quantity under normal conditions; only the water and crystalloids freely gain access to the connective tissue space. *Tissue fluid*, then, is plasma devoid of most of its characteristic proteins. The tissue fluid that gains access to the lymphatic capillaries is called *lymph*. Lymph does contain significant quantities of proteins. Those plasma proteins that enter the interstitium are returned to the general circulation indirectly through the lymphatic vessels.

Ground Substance and Tissue Fluid. The unique characteristics of the connective tissues are attributable to the nature of the constituent GAGs. These substances, as proteoglycans, are capable of binding large quantities of water. Most of the interstitial fluid is bound to proteoglycans. Despite the interchangeability of all of the fluid of the body, large volumes of fluid do not leave

the vascular bed, traverse the interstitial space, and enter the cell as intracellular water. Actual flow of fluid through the interstitium does occur, but that is not the primary mechanism of movement of fluid and dissolved substances. Movement is achieved by diffusion, the movement of fluid and dissolved substances molecule by molecule down their concentration gradients through the intercellular space. If five molecules were to enter the interstitium from the vascular bed, then five molecules would leave the interstitium and enter the cells, vascular beds, or lymphatic capillaries. The five molecules leaving the interstitium would not be the exact same molecules that entered. Such movement is the result of a "domino" or cascade effect upon the tissue fluid and all dissolved ions within the interstitium. Diffusion is a rapid and efficient mechanism for transport of materials through the interstitial space.

Because dissolved substances and water are essential for normal cellular function, the interstitium assumes an important transport role. The integrity of this function is critically important to the well-being of all cells of the body. Unfortunately, routine preparations of proper connective tissue do not demonstrate the components except as spaces between constituent fibers and cells. Nevertheless, these spaces and the components they contained before processing are important to the organism.

Vascular and Tissue Fluids. Metabolites and oxygen must traverse the tissue fluid before the cells are reached. Metabolic waste products traverse the tissue fluid and are transported in the blood to their appropriate sites of excretion (kidneys) or exchange (lungs). Although a basal lamina and endothelial barrier separate the vascular compartment from the extravascular compartment (tissue fluid compartment), these spaces may be considered a continuum on the basis of the movement of fluids, crystalloids, and gases between these two compartments. These dissolved substances move down their concentration gradients *(diffusion)* randomly to or from the vascular compartment through spaces between endothelial cells or through fenestrations within endothelial cells. Pinocytotic vesicles, which may be apparent in the endothelial cells, do not account for the rapid movement of diffusable particles and water. Rather, they may assist in the transcapillary movement of macromolecules between the two fluid compartments. The selective permeability of the endothelial cells precludes, except for a minimal amount, the transport of macromolecules (proteins) across this barrier.

The movement of fluid and dissolved substances is governed by hydrostatic and osmotic pressure relationships that regulate the delicate fluid balance within the body. The hydrostatic pressure (HP) within the capillary beds continuously moves fluid and its dissolved substances into the connective tissue space. Continuous loss of fluid from the vascular space would occur were it not for the osmotic pressure of the plasma proteins of the capillary beds pulling fluid from the interstitial space back into the capillary space. Although these simple relationships represent the essence of the mechanism, the maintenance of fluid balance is more complicated than that.

Hydrostatic and Osmotic Relationships

The movement and distribution of fluid within the body depends upon the balance of four factors. These factors govern the direction and quantity of fluid that is moved and/or maintained in various loci. These factors are: *capillary HP, interstitial HP, capillary colloid osmotic pressure (COP)* and *interstitial COP*.

Capillary Pressures. Precise measurements of *capillary HP* are difficult to obtain. A reasonable estimate of *arterial capillary HP* is 25 mm Hg, whereas a similarly reliable estimate of *venous capillary HP* is 10 mm Hg. The arterial capillary HP is the result of the mechanical activity of the heart and the contributions of peripheral vascular elements. Vascular smooth muscle contributes actively to the maintenance of peripheral blood pressure. Collagenous and elastic fibers, based upon their physical characteristics (modulus of elasticity), contribute passively to the maintenance of peripheral blood pressure. The reduced HP on the venous side of the capillary bed is a consequence of fluid loss and the inability

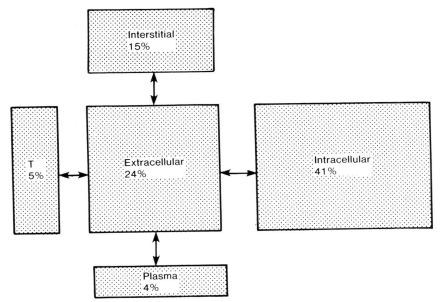

Figure 6.16. Distribution of fluids within the animal body. The percentages are based upon water comprising 65% of the body weight. The 24% extracellular fluid consists of transcellular fluids *(T)*, plasma, and interstitial fluid. The fluids move freely between all fluid compartments.

of the walls of the capillaries to contribute significantly to intravascular HP.

The *capillary COP* is from the proteins and ions dissolved in the plasma. The proteins contribute because these substances do not move readily across the semipermeable "capillary membrane." Also, the *Gibbs-Donnan equilibrium effect* essentially increases the osmotic pressure by approximately 50% more than exerted by the proteins alone. The negative charges of the proteins are balanced by the positive charges of the cations, predominantly sodium. This increase the number of particles and the osmotic pressure.

The COP of plasma is approximately 28 mm Hg. The plasma concentration and size of albumin dictate that this plasma protein contibutes about 70–75% of the osmotic pressure. Because very few plasma proteins diffuse into the interstitial space from the vascular bed, the COP on the venous side of the circulation stays the same. This pressure is the single significant factor influencing the return of fluid to the capillary bed.

Interstitial Pressures. The *interstitial HP* has been just as difficult to determine as the capillary HP. The interstitial HP referred to in this discussion results from the pressure exerted by the free fluid. The interstitial HP is −6.3 mm Hg. The negative or sub-atmospheric HP within the interstitial space can be explained on the basis of direct measurements, the mathematical necessity of balancing all pressures across the capillary wall and the suction effect of the lymphatic capillaries upon the interstitial space. The negative HP within the interstitium tends to "suck" fluids out of the capillaries and tends to hold elements of the tissues close together.

Although numerous proteins occupy the extracellular space, very little protein leaks from the vascular bed to be transported within the tissue fluid. Nevertheless, this small amount of protein makes the *interstitial COP* approximately 5 mm Hg, or approximately 18% of capillary COP.

Mechanisms of Exchange. The random movement of crystalloids and ions across the capillary wall is augmented by *filtration*. Filtration is the movement of fluids and dissolved solutes across the capillary boundary.

Capillary HP is initiated and maintained by the mechanical driving force of the heart, as well as by the active and passive contributions of the mural elements of blood vessels. Although capillary HP drops appreciably in the arterial side of the capillaries to 25.0 mm Hg, this pressure exceeds the interstitial HP, which is −6.3 mm Hg. The *effective HP (EHP)* in this region of the capillary bed is the sum of both pressures (31.3 mm Hg) (Fig. 6.17). The intravascular pressure tends to push fluid into the interstitium, while the negative

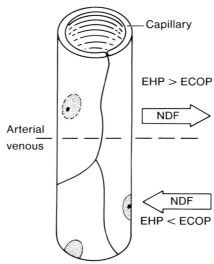

Figure 6.17. Filtration across the capillary bed. Movement of fluids and solutes from the capillary bed into the connective tissue space occurs on the arterial side of the capillary bed because the EHP is greater than the ECOP in this region. The net driving force *(NDF)* is reversed on the venous side of the capillary bed, because the ECOP is greater than the EHP in this region.

pressure of the interstitium tends to suck fluids into the interstitial space. Both combine to move fluids into the extracellular space.

The plasma proteins, principally albumin, contribute to the COP of the blood. This is approximately 28.0 mm Hg in the arterial side of the capillary bed; the COP of the tissue fluid is approximately 5.0 mm Hg. The *effective COP (ECOP)* in this part of the capillary bed is 23.0 mm Hg, favoring the movement of water into the capillary bed (Fig. 6.17). (Remember that water moves from an area of low osmotic pressure or low solute concentration to an area of high osmotic pressure or high solute concentration when separated by a semipermeable membrane.) The *net driving force* (EHP minus ECOP) in this part of the capillary is 8.3 mm Hg (Fig. 6.17). Therefore, the movement of fluids from the capillary bed to the connective tissue compartment occurs nomally under the influence of a *filtration pressure* of 8.3 mm Hg (Fig. 6.18).

The net outward driving force ensures that fluids are "pushed" into the tissue fluid space. A gradual change in the governing parameters assures that fluid is returned to the venous side of the capillary bed (Fig. 6.17). As fluids leave the capillary bed, the HP within the capillary on the venous side is reduced to 10.0 mm Hg, while the tissue HP is maintained at −6.3 mm Hg. The sum of these values is the EHP on the venous side of the capillary bed. The EHP (16.3 mm Hg) on the venous side of the capillary bed still favors the movement of

fluid into the interstitial space. The COP of the blood and tissue fluid remains relatively constant at 28.0 and 5.0 mm Hg, respectively. The ECOP in the venous portion of the capillary is the difference between these pressures or 23.0 mm Hg inward. A net driving force of 6.7 mm Hg *(reabsorption pressure)* favors the return of fluids to this portion of the capillary.

The filtration pressure (8.3 mm Hg) moves about 0.3% of the plasma fluid volume into the connective tissue compartment during a 24-hour period. The reabsorption pressure (6.7 mm Hg) moves about 90% of the filtered fluid from the connective tissue space back into the vascular bed. The remaining 10% of the fluid not returned to the vascular bed would destroy these filtration and reabsorption relationships were the fluid permitted to remain in the interstitium. Instead, the fluid and the small amount of protein are returned to the general circulation via the lymphatic vessels.

This mechanism of exchange accounts for the dynamic and continuous formation and turnover of fluids throughout the body. Although the numerical parameters vary slightly between specific loci, the relationships between HP and COP do not. Importantly, this mechanism ensures that the cells of the body are bathed continuously in a fluid environment conducive to their homeostasis. This mechanism is also important in the formation of urine.

Lymphatic Channels and Fluid Balance. All connective tissue spaces, directly or indirectly, contain lymphatic capillaries as blind-ended structures that originate within the interstitium. Most organs, but not even all lymphatic organs, have lymphatic capillaries. These vessels are the media through which potential residual fluid is returned to the cardiovascular system indirectly. Ninety percent of the filtered plasma fluid is returned to the cardiovascular system directly; the remaining 10% courses through the lymphatic vessels to be returned indirectly to the cardiovascular system. Even though the amount of protein that moves into the interstitium during a given short period of time is small, more than 50% of the plasma proteins leaks into the interstitium daily. Their return is essential for the maintenance of proper osmotic pressures within the vascular system and extracellular space.

The series of lymphatic channels are branching vessels that drain the majority of the body. The most peripheral portions are the lymphatic capillaries. Capillaries fuse to form larger venules; venules fuse to form larger veins; larger veins coalesce to form the cisterna chyli that is continuous with the thoracic duct. The thoracic duct returns lymph to the general circulation at the subclavian and external jugular veins (species variable).

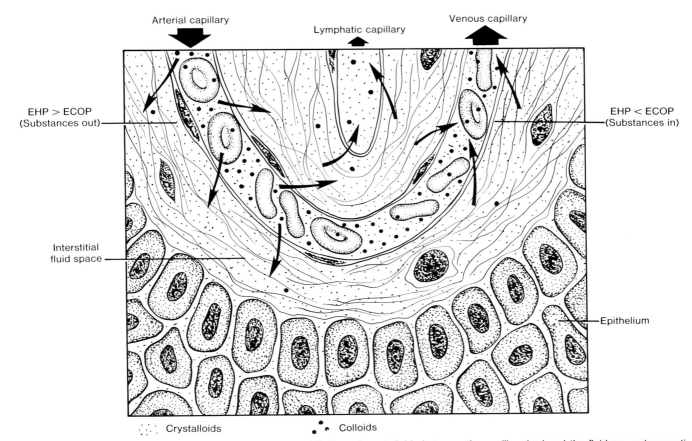

Figure 6.18. A diagram to demonstrate the normal movement of fluids and crystalloids between the capillary bed and the fluid space (connective tissue compartment). The basal lamina is not shown but separates the connective tissue from the nonconnective tissues. Substances move into the connective tissue compartment on the arterial side of the capillary bed and are returned to the capillary bed on the venous side. Very few colloids escape into the interstitial space. The labels used for this figure are applicable to Figures 6.17–6.22. (Figs. 6.18–6.22 were redrawn and modified from Ham, A. W.: *Histology*. 7th edition. J. B. Lipponcott Company, Philadelphia, 1974.)

Lymphatic capillaries are very permeable structures with gaps between adjacent endothelial cells. The gaps, however, are covered by cytoplasmic processes *(marginal folds)* that form one-way valves. The valves open inwardly to permit the ingress of fluid but close to prevent fluid from moving back into the interstitial space. Collagenous and reticular fibers serve as *anchoring filaments* that connect the endothelial cells to the connective tissue space. The sparse remnants of the basal lamina are the points of endothelial attachment for the anchoring filaments.

The unique morphology permits a one-way flow, but the flow itself is very slow. The amount of lymph flow in the thoracic duct of a nonruminant is approximately 2 ml/kg/hr. Despite this sluggish flow, this rate of lymph flow represents the entire plasma volume being transported during a span of 24 hours. Exercise can increase the flow of lymph as much as 15 times the normal flow rate at rest. The flow of lymph is influenced by various factors: interstitial fluid pressure, contraction of skeletal muscle, lymphatic vessel contraction, arterial pulsations, and body movements.

Fluid moves into the lymphatic capillaries despite the normal negative interstitial HP. As lymphatic capillaries expand, they create a suction that pulls fluid into their lumina. Similarly, periodic compression of the connective tissue space causes a transitory rise in pressure that propels fluid into the lymphatic capillaries. Any factor that causes an increased interstitial fluid pressure, except lymphatic obstruction, causes an increased flow of lymph. These factors include: increased capillary HP; decreased capillary COP; increased interstitial COP; increased capillary permeability.

Lymphatic vessels have numerous valves. These structures ensure a one-way flow (centrally) when the luminal volume of the vessel is reduced due to body movement, skeletal muscle contraction, or contraction of the smooth muscle that lines the wall of larger lymphatic vessels. Arterial pulsations can compress the fluid volume within the lymphatic vessels also, because these vessels are companions to each other. Decreased luminal volume in one segment propels the fluid centrally. Upon return to normal luminal size, the fluid is trapped in the adjacent segment by the closing of the

one-way valve. A progressive series of contractions, either intrinsic or extrinsic, causes the lymph to move continually in one direction.

The mechanisms that affect larger lymphatic vessels apply equally to lymphatic capillaries. Additionally, the transitory accumulation of plasma proteins in the interstitium aids in the pumping activity of lymphatic capillaries. Fluid return to the venous side of the circulation is accompanied by a progressive accumulation of plasma proteins in the interstitium. The accumulation increases the interstitial COP. The increased interstitial COP decreases tissue fluid being returned to the venous capillaries; thus, an increaed interstitial HP results. The increased pressure functions as a pump returning both fluid and protein to the lymphatic capillaries. The periodic washout returns essential plasma proteins and fluid to the general circulation indirectly.

Alterations to Fluid Exchange

Numerous factors can influence and alter the delicate balance that exists among the fluid components of the vascular system, lymphatic system, and connective tissue compartment. Alterations (excessive or inadequate water intake, electrolyte imbalances, protein deficiencies, inflammatory processes, systemic diseases) can be manifested as a localized or generalized disruption of fluid balance.

Edema. *Edema* is the retention and subsequent accumulation of tissue fluid resulting from the interstitial HP becoming positive. Systemic and/or regional edematous conditions do not occur readily. As a clinical manifestation, edema is usually the result of serious disease processes. Two specific mechanisms provide a safety margin for fluid accumulation. The ground substance is capable of absorbing about 30% more fluid than present normally. Lymph flow mechanisms provide an additional margin of safety. This flow is influenced by the negative interstitial HP, lymphatic capillary pumping, and interstitial protein washout mechanism. The lymph flow mechanisms provide a mechanism that requires a 70% increase in capillary HP before edema is observed. Also, an approximate 70% reduction of capillary COP is necessary before an edematous condition is achieved. Despite these safety factors, edema does occur. Four basic mechanisms account for the excessive formation of tissue fluid: *lymph vessel obstruction, increased capillary permeability, decreased concentration of plasma proteins,* and *increased capillary HP.*

Lymphatic Obstruction. Lymph vessel obstruction (Fig. 6.19) exerts its influence upon this process in two ways. First, lymph obstruction prevents the return of tissue fluid to the circulation, resulting in a gradual and continuous increase of fluids within the connective tissue compartment. This increases the tissue fluid HP. Also, a progressive accumulation of proteins occurs in the connective tissue compartment. The proteins increase the connective tissue COP, which results in the propensity to attract and hold more water. Certain parasitic diseases and metastatic tumors may result in lymphatic obstruction. Also, solid tumors may grow around and subsequently occlude major lymphatic channels.

Increased Capillary Permeability. An increased capillary permeability (Fig. 6.20) results in the leakage of plasma into the connective tissue compartment. The increased interstitial COP due to excessive proteins in the connective tissue compartment causes an increased amount of tissue fluid. Most significantly, the blood has a decreased ability to attract water back into the capillaries. Inflammatory processes, allergic reactions, toxic substances, and burns may cause edema due to increased capillary permeability.

Decreased Capillary Osmotic Pressure. A decreased vascular COP is associated with a decreased concentration of plasma proteins (Fig. 6.21). Such a deficiency results in a diminished ability to attract fluid

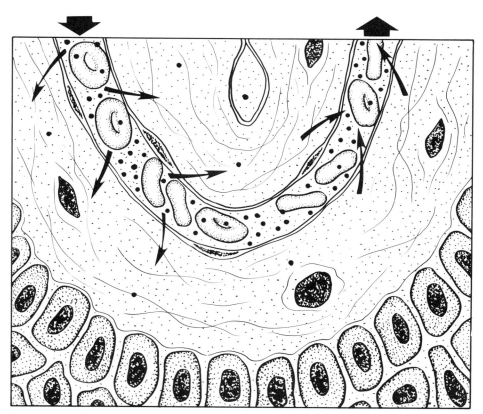

Figure 6.19. Altered tissue fluid formation and exchange resulting from lymphatic obstruction. Lymphatic obstruction causes excessive fluid and colloids to accumulate in the interstitial fluid space. The interstitial compartment swells and alters cellular and matrical component relationships.

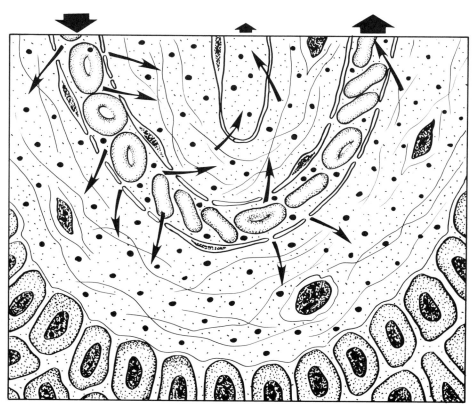

Figure 6.20. Altered tissue fluid formation and exchange resulting from increased capillary permeability. The movement of colloids into the interstitial space causes the space to swell.

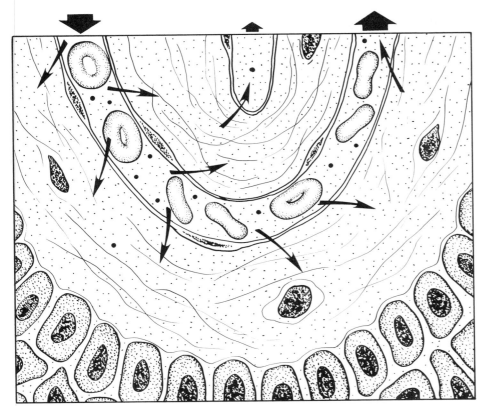

Figure 6.21. Altered tissue fluid formation and exchange resulting from decreased COP. The capillary bed has a diminished ability to attract fluids. The fluids accumulate in the interstitial space and swelling results.

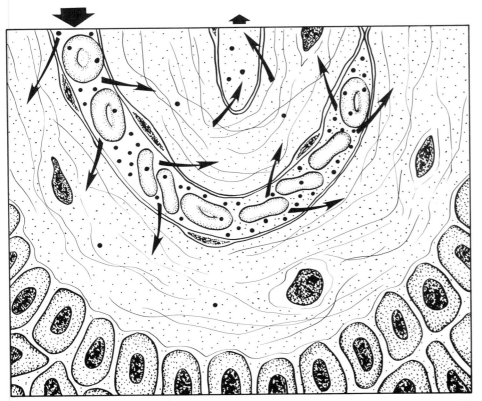

Figure 6.22. Altered tissue fluid formation and exchange resulting from an increased capillary HP induced by a venous obstruction. Capillary HP increases and fluids are retained within the interstitial space. Swelling results.

into the blood from the connective tissue. Hypoproteinemia may result from liver disorders, excessive protein loss in the urine, protein malnutrition, excessive protein loss through the digestive tract, and parasitism.

Increased Capillary HP. Venous obstruction (Fig. 6.22) results in an increased capillary HP. When the hydrostatic pressure exceeds the capillary COP, fluids are retained in the connective tissue compartment. Increased capillary HP may result from congestive heart failure, inflammation of veins, increased pulmonary resistance and tight bandages. Generally, any elevation in venous blood pressure can cause edema.

The real significance of the altered exchange associated with the aforementioned problems is not the swelling. The swelling expands the connective tissue compartment and may compromise the nutritional microenvironment of the cells. Diffusion distances for metabolites are increased and waste products of metabolism may accumulate.

References

Bensley, S.H.: On the presence, properties and distribution of the intercellular ground substance of loose connective tissue. Anatamy 60:93, 1934.

Chain, E. and Duthie, E.S.: Identity of hyaluronidase and the spreading factor. Brit. J. Exp. Path. 21:234, 1940.

Eyre, D.R.: Collagen: Molecular diversity in the body's protein scaffold. Science 207:1315, 1980.

Fahrenback, W.H., Sandberg, L.B. and Cleary, E.G.: Ultrastructural studies on early elastogenesis. Anat. Rec. 155:563, 1966.

Ghadially, F.N.: *Ultrastructural Pathology of the Cell and Matrix: A Text and Atlas of Physiological and Pathological Alterations in the Fine Structure of Cellular and Extracellular Components.* 2nd edition, Butterworths, London, 1982.

Ginsberg, V. and Robbins, P. (eds.): *Biology of Carbohydrates.* Vol. 1. John Wiley & Sons, New York, 1981.

Greenlee, T.K., Jr., Ross, R. and Hartman, J.L.: The fine structure of elastic fibers. J. Cell Biol. 30:59, 1966.

Gross, J.: Collagen. Sci. Amer. 204:120, 1961.

Hall, D.A.: *The Ageing of Connective Tissue.* Academic Press, New York, 1976.

Hay, E.D.: Extracellular matrix. J. Cell Biol. 91:205s, 1981.

Lillie, R.D.: Histochemistry of connective tissues. Lab. Invest. 1:30, 1952.

Mancini, R.E.: Connective tissue and serum proteins. Inter. Rev. Cytol. 14,193, 1963.

Miller, E.J.: Biochemical characteristics and biological significance of the genetically distinct collagens. Molec. Cell. Biochem. 13:165, 1976.

Petruska, A.J. and Hodge, J.A: A subunit model for the tropocollagen macromolecule. Proc. Nat. Acad. Sci. USA. 51:871, 1964.

Prockop, D.J., Kivirikko, K.I., Tuderman, L. and Guzman, N.A.: The biosynthesis of collagen and its disorders. N. Engl. J. Med. 301:13, 1979.

Schubert, M.: *A Primer on Connective Tissue Biochemistry.* Lea and Febiger, Philadelphia, 1968.

Snodgrass, M.J.: Ultrastructural distinction between reticular and collagenous fibers with an ammoniacal silver stain. Anat. Rec. 187:191, 1977.

Spicer, S.S., Horn, R.G. and Leppi, T.J.: Histochemistry of connective tissue mucopolysaccharides. *In:* Wagner, B.M. and Smith, D.E. (eds.). *The Connective Tissue.* pp. 251–303. Williams & Wilkins, Co., Baltimore, 1967.

Uy, R. and Wold, F.: Post-translational covalent modifications of proteins. Science 198:890, 1977.

7: Proper Connective Tissues and Adipose Tissue

General Characteristics

Form and Function. Connective tissues, derived from the mesoderm, are a diverse group of tissues. They consist of heterogeneous populations of cells that are separated from each other by copious amounts of *extracellular material (intercellular substance)*. The fibrous and amorphous components comprise the connective tissue *matrix*. The fibers may impart a feltwork or weave-like consistency to the matrix. The *ground substance* is the amorphous component and consists of *glycosaminoglycans* and *proteoglycans*. These substances fill the intercellular and interfibrillar spaces and form a three-dimensional framework that connects and supports other tissues and organs. The relative number and type of cells and the amount and type of matrical components of connective tissues vary throughout the organism in response to structural and functional needs. For these reasons, precise definitions, descriptions, and classifications of connective tissues are difficult. Classification schemes, however, have been devised (Fig. 7.1).

Connective tissues serve numerous functions. They *connect* one tissue or organ to another. Also, they *suspend* organs from the body wall or other organs. Various connective tissues *insulate* organs from mechanical damage, and they account for the *form* of the organs and the body. They are an important line of *defense*, because numerous protective cells are part of their cellular populations. Conversely, some connective tissues are the means by which infective agents spread throughout a region or to various parts of the body via established fascial planes. The connective tissues serve a *nutritive* function as well. Not only do vascular beds have to traverse connective tissues to reach other tissues, but metabolites also move through the connective tissue space to reach individual cells. *Heat regulation, water metabolism* and *food storage* are also important functions. They aid in *support* and *locomotion* in conjunction with other tissues. Some connective tissues also play an important role in *repair* and *regeneration*. Most connective tissues are

able to regenerate and/or repair themselves after injury. Some nonconnective tissues are unable to repair themselves and must rely upon certain connective tissues to replace damaged tissues.

Origin of Connective Tissue. All of the connective tissues are derivatives of mesoderm. This compartment of mesenchyme begins early in development as a well-defined, well-delineated, and continuous space bounded by the ectoderm peripherally and the endoderm internally. Many tissues develop within this space. The *mesenchymal cell* is the stem cell for all mesodermal derivatives, including all of the cells of the connective tissues (Fig. 7.2).

Progress in development is characterized by the continuous and progressive "invasion" of the connective tissue compartment by invagination of cells from the ectoderm and endoderm. Also, continuous development of cavities within the mesoderm (celomic spaces), the differentiation of vascular elements (endothelium), and the differentiation of muscles and supportive tissues all tend to infringe upon this compartment. The net result is the conversion of the connective tissue compartment into a tortuous, irregular, and "apparently" discontinuous array of spaces (Fig. 7.3). Nothing is further from the actual reality of the relationship. Those elements that invaginate into or are developed within the connective tissue never actually gain access to the connective tissue compartment. They are separated from it by the ever-present basal lamina, which is visible with the electron microscope. The relationship is similar to attempting to gain access to the air-filled space of a balloon by pushing a finger into it. The finger never gains access to the space but is always covered by the peripheral margin of the balloon. The basal lamina is analogous to the peripheral margin of the balloon.

As ectodermal and endodermal derivatives infringe upon the connective tissue compartment, they essentially "push" the basal lamina in front of them. Even nonconnective elements that develop within the mesenchyme secondarily develop a basal lamina. **The basal lamina separates**

all connective tissues from nonconnective tissues. A few noteworthy exceptions exist.

The basal lamina may be considered the peripheral limit of the connective tissue compartment. Cells of connective and supportive tissues are devoid of a basal lamina. Because all nonconnective tissues are covered by and separated from the connective tissue space by a basal lamina, what then is the proper classification of adipose tissue? Adipose tissue generally occurs in intimate association with the proper connective tissues. Isolated populations of fat cells or entire sheets, as adipose tissue, occur "in" the connective tissue compartment. Yet, these cells are covered by a basal lamina. Classically, adipose tissue was considered a connective tissue. The presence of a basal lamina, however, precludes its inclusion with these tissues. Also, adipose tissue is highly cellular with little intercellular matrix. As with muscle, adipose tissue may be considered a separate and distinct tissue.

Unique Relationships. The connective tissue compartment is associated intimately with all tissues. All metabolites carried by the vascular system must leave the capillaries, cross the basal lamina of the endothelial cell, traverse the connective tissue compartment and cross the basal lamina of a nonconnective tissue cell before being incorporated into a nonconnective tissue cell. Similarly, waste products of metabolism follow the reverse sequence from the nonconnective tissue cells back to the vascular beds. This sequence of flow applies equally to all tissues that are non-connective tissues. Connective tissue cells, however, are bathed continuously by the fluid (*connective tissue fluid* or *interstitial fluid*) that accounts for this two-way flow pattern. This fluid, also referred to as *extracellular fluid (ECF)*, comprises a vast ECF compartment. The peripheral limits of the ECF compartment correspond to the limits of the connective tissue space as delimited by the basal lamina.

The connective tissue space is the compartment within which the organism mounts specific (humoral antibodies, cell-mediated immunity) and nonspecific immune respones (phagocytosis). The resi-

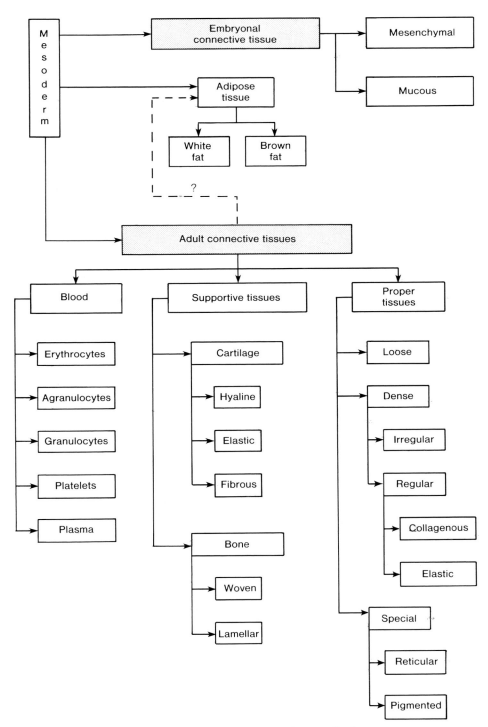

Figure 7.1.   Organizational scheme of connective tissue.

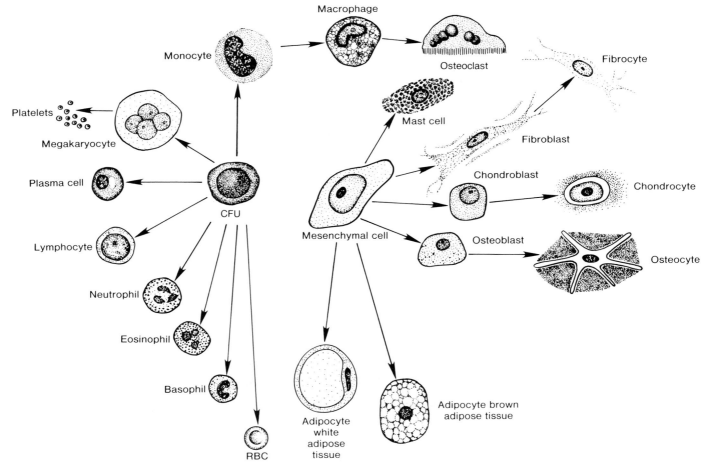

Figure 7.2. Connective tissue cell derivatives. All connective tissue cells are derived directly from mesenchymal cells, except the blood cells. The relationships of mature blood cells to the colony forming unit (CFU) are indicated. The relationship of the CFU to the mesenchymal cell is not clear. Detailed relationships among these cells is discussed in subsequent chapters.

dent populations of cells (macrophages and mast cells) and transient populations of cells (neutrophils, eosinophils, plasma cells) contribute to the protective significance of this compartment.

Classification. Despite the problems associated with a definitive classification scheme, the relationships outlined in Figure 7.1 are useful. Four criteria are used primarily for the classification of connective tissues: predominant cell type or types; type of fibrous components of the matrix; number of fibers in a unit volume of the matrix; orderliness of the matrical components

Resident Cell Populations

The cell population of any connective tissue will vary with the tissue, as well as the physiological state of the tissue at the time of observation. Nevertheless, some cells of connective tissues are encountered frequently. These may be called the *resident cell population* and include: *mesenchymal cells, reticular cells, fibroblasts (fibrocytes), macrophages, pericytes, fat cells, and mast cells.*

Mesenchymal Cells. The *mesenchymal cell* is the precursor of most connective tissue cells. It is a stellate or spindle-shaped cell with a high nuclear to cytoplasmic ratio. It has a large, vesicular nucleus that is rich in euchromatin (Fig. 7.4). The cytoplasm is acidophilic and scant. In most preparations the cytoplasm is indistinguishable from surrounding matrix components (Plate II.6). At the ultrastructural level, the predominant cytoplasmic organelle is the polyribosome (Fig. 7.5). The combination of prominent euchromatin and extensive free polyribosomes is indicative of the high protein synthesis potential of this cell. Few other organelles are apparent.

Although mesenchymal cells are scattered throughout the connective tissue space, the cells are usually difficult to identify. They may be most prominent in the perivascular region. These cells are probably the primary means though which *metaplasia* occurs.

Reticular Cells. The *reticular cell* is a stellate or spindle-shaped cell that occurs in myeloid tissue and lymphatic organs. It generally forms a *cellular reticulum* in association with a fibrous stroma of reticular

fibers. The nucleus is round to oval and vesicular (Fig. 7.6). The cytoplasm is extensive and slightly basophilic. The cytoplasmic processes of these cells are in contact with each other and account for the typical *cellular meshwork* or *reticulum.*

The reticular cells are attributed with diverse functional activities. Reticular cells, functioning like fibroblasts, form the fibrous stroma, reticular fibers, of the organs and tissues of which they are an integral part. Reticular cells have been attributed with phagocytic activity also. Light microscopic evidence supports the existence of *phagocytic reticular cells,* whereas evidence from electron microscopy refutes it. Similarly, *primitive reticular cells,* some sort of undifferentiated stem cell, were believed to be the stem cells for bone marrow elements and macrophages. Compelling evidence for this role of the reticular cell in blood cell development is lacking. The exact nature and potential of the reticular cell has not been defined clearly. The reticular cell occurs not only in association with reticular fibers but is the characteristic resident cell of reticular connective tissue.

Fibroblasts. The *fibroblasts,* or fiber-

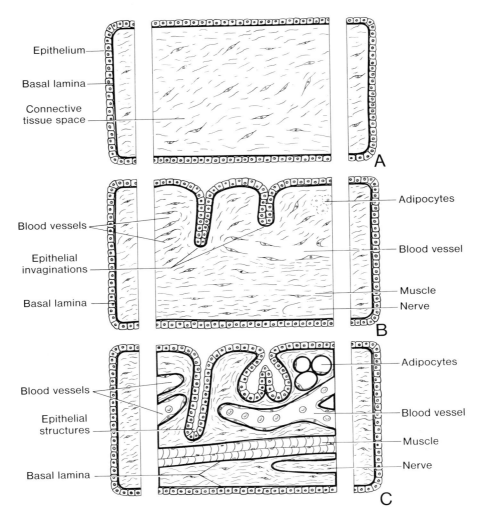

Epithelium

Basal lamina

Connective
tissue space

Adipocytes

Blood vessels

Blood vessel

Epithelial
invaginations

Muscle

Basal lamina

Nerve

Adipocytes

Blood vessels

Blood vessel

Epithelial
structures

Muscle

Nerve

Basal lamina

Figure 7.3. Schematic representation of the connective tissue space and basal lamina. Although the connective tissue space, as defined by the peripherally positioned basal lamina, is a single, vast, continuous space, it is represented as a discontinuous space in these diagrams to imply its vastness. A single closed compartment in a diagram does not do justice to it. *A.* Early in development, the connective tissue space may be visualized as a compartment that consists exclusively of connective tissue components—mesenchymal cells, fibroblasts, fibers, and amorphous matrix materials. The boundary of the compartment is defined by the basal lamina *(dark black line)*. *B.* As development progresses, various cells differentiate within or invade into the compartment. *C.* Complete development of components associated intimately with the connective tissue has been achieved. Although the connective tissue compartment has been reduced in volume and has become irregularly shaped, its integrity is still maintained. Nothing has actually gained access to the compartment. The basal lamina still separates connective tissue components from nonconnective tissue components.

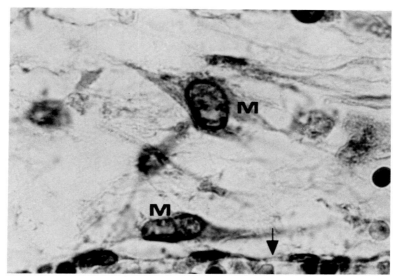

Figure 7.4.   Mesenchymal cells from a perivascular space within loose connective tissue. The mesenchymal cells *(M)* are typical and occur close to a capillary bed. The endothelial cells of the capillary are indicated *(arrow).* ×400.

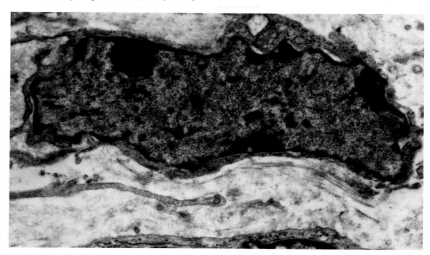

Figure 7.5.   An electron micrograph of a mesenchymal cell. The ratio of the nuclear/cytoplasmic volumes of the cell is large. ×12,000.

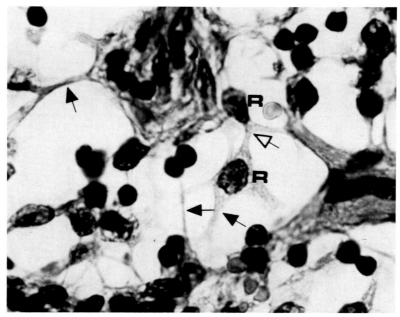

Figure 7.6.   Reticular cells of the medullary region of an canine lymph node. The reticular cells *(R)* extend cytoplasmic processes *(solid arrows)* that contact the cytoplasmic processes of other cells. These relationships form the cellular reticulum that characterize these organs. Points of contact between these stellate-shaped cells *(open arrows)* are apparent occasionally. ×320.

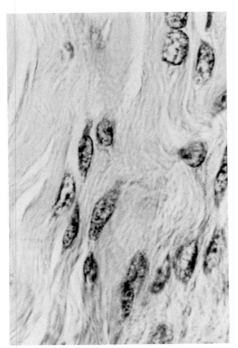

Figure 7.7. Fibroblasts of loose connective tissue. The cytoplasm is barely visible, whereas the vesicular nuclei are apparent. Collagenous fibers are oriented randomly throughout the section. ×340.

forming cells of the proper connective tissues, are the most frequently encountered cells. Young fibroblasts are stellate or spindle-shaped cells with long cellular processes. The large, oval or round nucleus is vesicular and has a prominent nucleolus (Fig. 7.7). Basophilic cytoplasm is abundant. This active form of the cell has an abundant granular endoplasmic reticulum and a well-developed Golgi apparatus (Fig. 7.8).

Inactive fibroblasts *(fibrocytes)* have nuclei that contain more heterochromatin than their active counterparts. Fibrocytes are spindle-shaped cells with a scant cytoplasm that is acidophilic, if it is visible. A corresponding reduction in their intracellular organelles is characteristic.

Fibrosis, the formation of fibrous connective tissue as a reaction to chronic insult, results from the activity of these cells. Similarly, repair of matrical components after injury (laceration, surgical incision, inflammation) results from the fibroblastic activity. Excessive quantities of fibrous connective tissue *(granulation tissue)*, especially characteristic of connective tissue repair in the horse, is the end product of fibroblastic activity.

The fibroblast is responsible for the secretion of procollagen. The precise role of the fibroblast in the process of polymerization and spatial orientation of the polymerized fibers has not been determined. The cell may contribute to precise spatial arrangements. Mechanical stress in the tissues may serve as the basis for spatial orientation also. Both mechanisms may occur.

Macrophages. *Macrophages* are the resident phagocytic cells of the connective tissue compartment. They may be either *fixed* or *wandering*. As fixed cells, they are most prominent in the pericapillary space. They may also be fixed along the length of collagenous fibers. They become *wandering* or *ameboid* upon activation by various stimuli.

Macrophages vary from spindle-shaped cells in the fixed configuration to round or oval cells with blunt cellular processes during their wandering activities. The nucleus is slightly smaller than the fibroblast nucleus and is darker because of a coarse heterochromatic pattern. Lastly, but most importantly, the nucleus is often indented; i.e., it is *bean-shaped* or *kidney-shaped* (Fig. 7.9). Usually, the cell is polarized. The concavity or indentation of the nucleus faces the bulk of the cytoplasm. The basophilic cytoplasm may possess a juxtanuclear, pale-staining region.

At the ultrastructural level, the prominent organelles in macrophages are the Golgi apparatus (in the nuclear indentation), rough endoplasmic reticulum (RER)

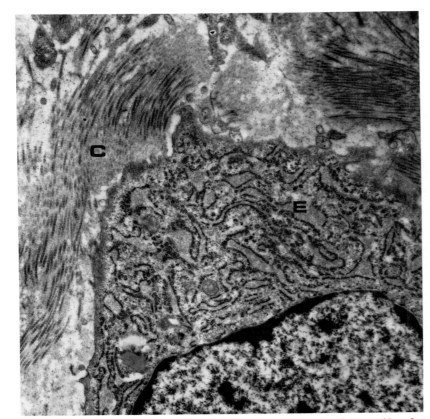

Figure 7.8. An electron micrograph of a fibroblast. The cell contains extensive quantities of granular endoplasmic reticular profiles *(E)* that are filled with a granular material. Collagenous fibers *(C)* are present in the connective tissue space. ×6000.

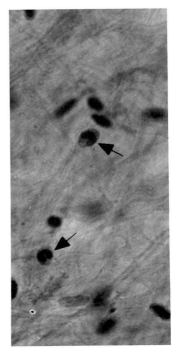

Figure 7.9. Macrophages in a stretch preparation of loose connective tissue. The nuclei of the macrophages *(arrows)* are typical. The other cellular and matrical components are out of the plane of focus. ×100.

and lysosomes (Fig. 7.10). At the light and electron microscopic level, ingested particulate material may be apparent if the cell is active.

Macrophages originate from monocytes. Within the confines of the blood vascular system *(intravascular)*, this cell is called a monocyte. Once it enters the connective tissue compartment *(extravascular)*, it is called a *histiocyte* or macrophage.

Macrophages are one of the prime cellular agents for defense against the invasion of particulate matter into the body. They also play a significant role in the phagocytosis and removal of cellular debris.

Additionally, macrophages fuse to form *giant cells.* Fusion of macrophages in response to foreign material seems to be an attempt to increase surface area for phagocytosis. These *foreign body giant cells* effectively wall off, enclose, or encircle foreign materials. Nodular inflammatory lesions *(granulomas)* consist of these cells encircling foreign matter.

Pericytes. Any cell that occurs around a capillary or small vessel may be a pericyte. In a more limited context, however, the *pericyte* is a specific cell or cell type. *Pericytes* or *cells of Rouget* intimately contact the endothelium of the small vessels with which they are associated (Fig. 7.11). They are invested with a basal lamina except at the point of contact with the endothelial cell (Fig. 7.12). Some of these cells have been shown to be contractile; thus, they may control the size of the vascular lumen. Others have not been demonstrated as contractile and their function is unknown.

Mast Cells. *Mast cells* are sometimes called *tissue basophils.* These cells occur variably in the connective tissue space but commonly reside along the pathway of small vessels. Usually, they occur in small clusters. These cells vary in size and shape in different species. Generally, they are ovoid cells with a small, pale, ovoid and centrally located nucleus. The prominent feature is the presence of basophilic granules in the cytoplasm (Fig. 7.13). It is not uncommon to observe these highly refractile granules surrounding the mast cell. The mast cells are fragile; they rupture readily during preparatory techniques. The granules are also highly water-soluble; thus, they are preserved rarely by routine techniques.

The granules of mast cells contain two substances of medical significance, *heparin* and *histamine*. The mast cells of some species also contain *serotonin.* Heparin is significant as an anticoagulant. Heparin ensures against the possible clotting of fibrinogen in the local environment. Heparin also acts as a *clearing agent* on blood, serving as a cofactor for the enzyme *lipoprotein lipase.* This enzyme is a secretory product of endothelial cells that promotes the clearance of chylomicrons from the blood. The mast cell also releases many substances that are involved in allergic responses (Chapter 19).

Although the mast cell is believed to be derived from the mesenchymal cell, very little information is available about its origin, cell cycle, and generation time. The cells seem to have a long life and long turnover time. They are sometimes referred to as tissue basophils; an unfortunate name, because the inference is that they are somehow related to the blood basophil (basophilic leukocyte). The basophil and mast cell are independent cell types.

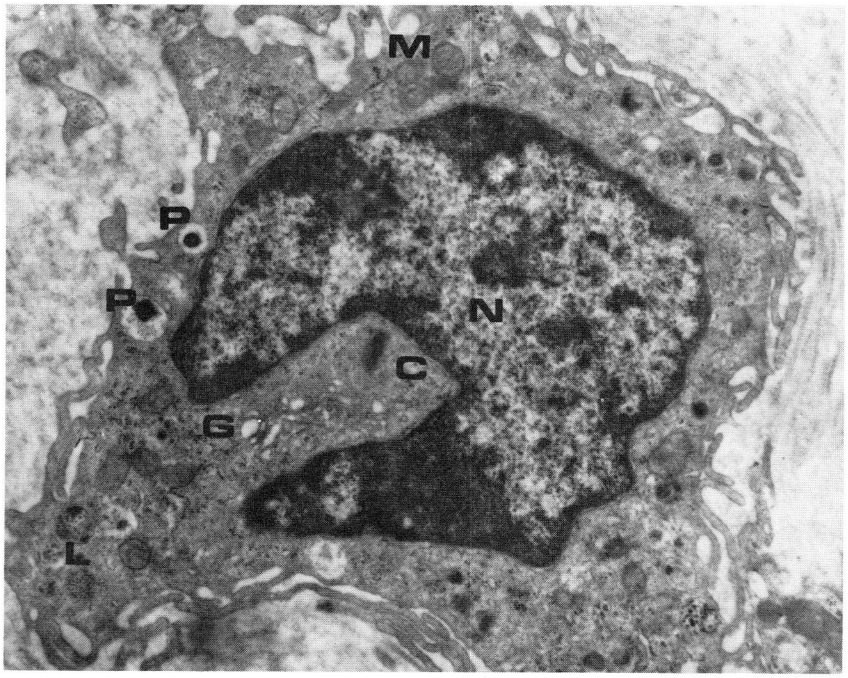

Figure 7.10.   An electron micrograph of a macrophage from loose connective tissue. The horseshoe-shaped nucleus *(N)* is typical. The Golgi apparatus *(G)* is well-developed and juxtanuclear. One of the centrioles *(C)* is visible. Mitochondria *(M)* are scattered throughout the cell. Phagosomes *(P)* and lysosomes *(L)* are typical features of active macrophages. ×26,000.

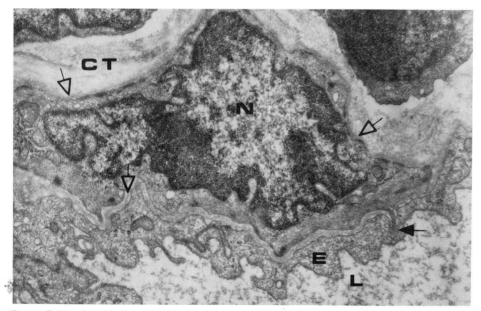

Figure 7.11.   An electron micrograph of a pericyte from a bovine lung. The nucleus *(N)* of the pericyte is prominent. The cell is in close association with an endothelial cell *(E)* that defines the lumen *(L)* of the capillary. The basal lamina *(open arrows)* surrounds the pericyte and separates it from the connective tissue *(CT)* and endothelium. The region indicated by the *solid arrow* is enlarged in Figure 7.12. ×17,000. (Courtesy of G. P. Epling).

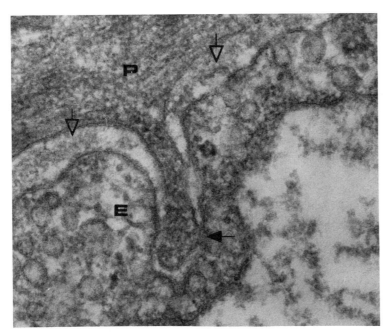

Figure 7.12. An electron micrograph of the contact between a pericyte and an endothelial cell within a bovine lung. The pericyte *(P)* and endothelial cell *(E)* are separated by a basal lamina *(open arrows)*, except at a single contact point *(solid arrow)*. ×125,000. (Courtesy of G. P. Epling).

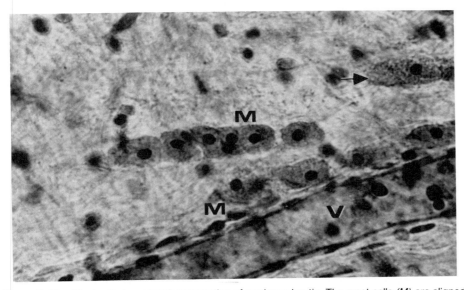

Figure 7.13. Mast cells in a stretch preparation of murine subcutis. The mast cells *(M)* are aligned along the course of a blood vessel *(V)*. A ruptured mast cell *(arrow)* has extruded its granules into the surrounding environment. Ruptured mast cells are observed frequently in histological preparations as a result of harsh handling during processing. ×160.

Fat Cells. *Fat cells, adipocytes,* occur as single cells, clusters of cells, or as massive sheets of cells associated with connective tissues, especially loose connective tissue. Because of their enigmatic relationship to connective tissues, these cells and adipose tissue are discussed in a subsequent section of this chapter.

Transient Cell Populations

Most of the transient cells are protective and may be considered residents in some connective tissue loci. In most instances their numbers vary. The *transient cell population* includes *plasma cells, melanocytes, lymphocytes, monocytes, neutrophils, eosinophils,* and *basophils.* Only the plasma cell and pigment cell are discussed here; the blood cells are discussed in Chapter 11.

Plasma Cells. *Plasma cells* perform an important function in the immediate and prolonged protection of the organism against antigens. These cells synthesize and secrete large quantities of *humoral antibodies (immunoglobulins)* that are part of the specific immunological responsiveness. These cells may occur in the connective tissue space but generally occur in those regions that are subjected continually to antigenic challenge. They may be considered part of the resident cell population of the connective tissues associated with the gastrointestinal, genitourinary and respiratory organs.

The plasma cell is easily demonstrated by routine techniques. It is a round cell with a definite polarity. The basophilic cytoplasm contains an eccentrically placed and round nucleus (Fig. 7.14). The nucleus contains extensive heterochromatin that is sometimes arranged as the spokes of a wheel. A juxtanuclear, pale-staining, Golgi region is often apparent. The basophilia of the cytoplasm is due to the extensive development of RER and free ribosomes (Fig. 7.15).

Melanocytes. Pigment-bearing cells are associated with various organs. Some pigment-bearing cells actively produce the pigment, whereas others acquire it passively. The primary pigment is *melanin. Melanoblasts* are cells derived from neural crest ectoderm. These cells migrate throughout the body and come to reside in or close to the basal layer of the epidermis. They possess the potential to produce melanin but do not do so until they have achieved their place of residence. When they begin to synthesize melanin, they are termed *melanocytes* (Fig. 7.16). Melancytes are able to spread throughout the epidermal layers and pass their pigmentation to other cells. The epidermal recipients of this pigment are morphologically indistinguishable from

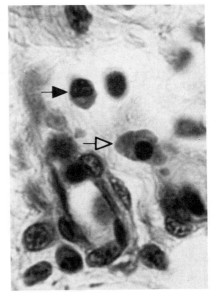

Figure 7.14. A plasma cell of loose connective tissue. The plasma cell *(solid arrow)* is typical. Note the position of the nucleus and the negative Golgi area. A macrophage *(open arrow)* is present also. Note the difference between these two cells. ×160.

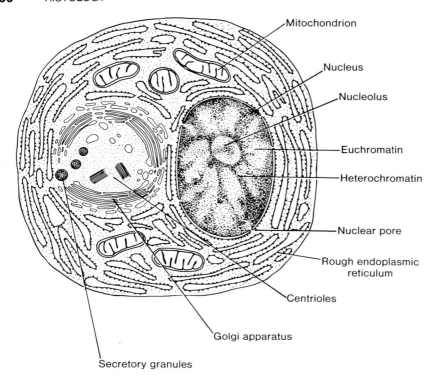

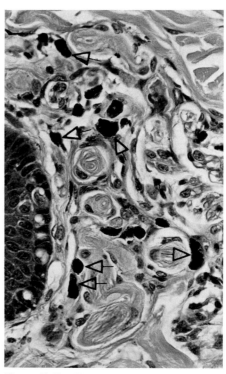

Figure 7.15. A diagram of a plasma cell as visualized with the electron microscope. The constituent organelles are indicated. Note the spoke-wheel configuration of the chromatin, extensive RER and well-developed Golgi apparatus.

Figure 7.16. Pigment-bearing cells *(open arrows)* of the connective tissue of the dermis. ×100.

melanocytes. These passive recipients of this pigment are termed *melanophores.* Melanocytes rarely occur in the connective tissue compartment. The pigmented cells of this compartment have either passively received the pigment or have phagocytosed the pigment. Thus, they are *melanophores* or *chromatophores.*

A simple histochemical test, the *dihydroxyphenylalanine (DOPA) reaction,* is used to determine which cells are melanocytes. Only melanocytes are capable of converting DOPA into melanin because of the presence of the enzyme *tyrosinase.* A *protyrosinase* is produced in the RER, passes through the Golgi apparatus, and is part of secretory vesicles *(stage I melanosome).* Internal changes in the contents of the vesicles convert them to particles called *premelanosomes (stage II melanosomes). Active tyrosinase* is demonstrable within these vesicles, and melanin begins to accumulate upon the matrix within the vesicles. Synthesis continues within the vesicles. Melanin accumulation obscures the vesicular substructure of these structures, now called *stage III melanosomes.* The mature vesicles are called *melanin granules (stage IV melanosomes).* The dense granule is filled with melanin but no tyrosinase activity is evident.

The primary function of these cells is to protect the body from excessive exposure to ultraviolet radiation. Of interest, melanoblasts and melanocytes can be involved in the formation of rapidly spreading and,

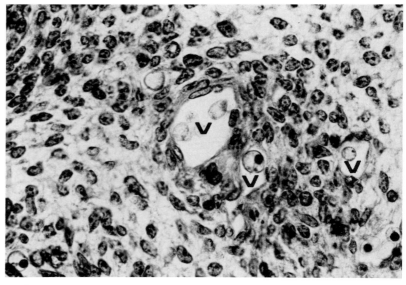

Figure 7.17. Mesenchymal connective tissue from a limb bud of a hamster. Vessels *(V)* are scattered among the mesenchymal cells. The mesenchymal connective tissue would have eventually differentiated into other tissues derived from the mesoderm. Mesenchymal connective tissue is a transitory connective tissue during development. ×160.

therefore, potentially dangerous cancerous growths.

Embryonal Connective Tissues

Mesenchymal Connective Tissue. This typical, unspecialized mesodermal tissue of the embryo is a transitory tissue that disappears rapidly from the developing organism as differentiation occurs (Fig. 7.17). The primary constituent of this tissue is the mesenchymal cell. These stellate or fusiform cells form numerous cellular contacts and give the appearance of a *cellular reticulum.* Pale-staining interstices contain a ground substance of glycosaminoglycans.

Delicate collagenous or reticular fibrils occur close to cells that are differentiating into fibroblasts. Also, mesenchymal cells are capable of producing small quantities of fibers and ground substance.

This tissue is derived from mesoderm and is the precursor for other tissues, such as *proper* and *special connective tissues, cartilage, bone, blood,* and *muscle.* In the adult, the mesenchymal connective tissue is reduced to isolated and scattered foci of mesenchymal cells in those tissues derived from it.

Mucous Connective Tissue. This connective tissue, a more advanced stage of the one described previously, is the characterisitic connective tissue of the umbilical cord, wherein it is referred to as *Wharton's jelly* (Fig. 7.18). It consists of a cellular reticulum of *fibroblasts* and a few scattered *mesenchymal cells.* The matrix is composed of mucin and contains delicate collagenous fibers. The ground substance appears granular with proper fixation.

In the developing embryo, this connective tissue occurs in the subepidermal regions as well as the umbilical cord. In the adult it is usually the transitory tissue deposited during the repair of supportive tissues. Also, it occurs normally in the comb and wattles of gallinaceous birds. It also occurs in specific portions of the lamina propria mucosae of the ruminant omasum.

Proper Connective Tissues

Areolar Connective Tissue. *Areolar connective tissue* is also called *loose* or *ordinary connective tissue.* It is the most ubiquitous connective tissue. It is composed of a loose array of randomly oriented *collagenous, reticular,* and *elastic fibers.* Collagenous fibers, however, are the predominant extracellular, fibrous elements. All of the cells previously described, except the reticular cell, may occur in this connective tissue. Normally, the predominant cell type is the fibroblast or fibrocyte (approximately 90%). The prevalent ground substance component is hyaluronic acid; however, some chondroitin sulfate and dermatan sulfate are also present. This combinatin of matrix components imparts a soft, pliable, and elastic quality to the tissue (Fig. 7.19).

The accompanying photomicrograph of a stretch preparation of subcutis serves as an example of loose connective tissue (Fig. 7.20). Randomly oriented collagenous and elastic fibers are apparent within the ground substance. Reticular fibers are present also. Numerous vessels and scattered fat cells are present. All the cells mentioned previously as part of the resident and transient populations may be encountered within this tissue.

In section, loose connective tissue assumes an appearance that differs from its stretch preparation characteristics (Fig. 7.21). Nevertheless, the interlacing and randomly oriented bundles of fibers with cells scattered between is typical. Most of these cells are fibroblasts. Examination at high magnification reveals the other cells.

In a section of loose connective tissue associated with the digestive tract a very different-appearing tissue is observed (Fig. 7.22). Although the fibers and fibroblasts are present, the predominant feature is the presence of defensive cells—lymphocytes, plasma cells, and macrophages. This appearance is typical in this and similar regions that are subjected to constant insult. The previous example of this tissue (Fig. 7.21) would appear similar in response to an insult (Plate IV.2).

MORPHOLOGICAL FEATURES: **A fine network of collagenous, reticular and elastic fibers loosely arranged in random array is apparent. Collagenous fibers and fibroblasts predominate. Large number of cells occur within a stroma of few**

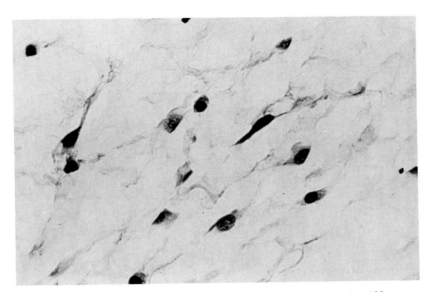

Figure 7.18.   Mucous connective tissue of the ovine umbilical cord. ×160.

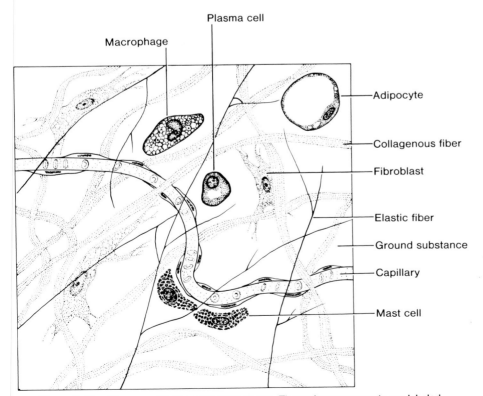

Figure 7.19.   Diagram of loose connective tissue. The major components are labeled.

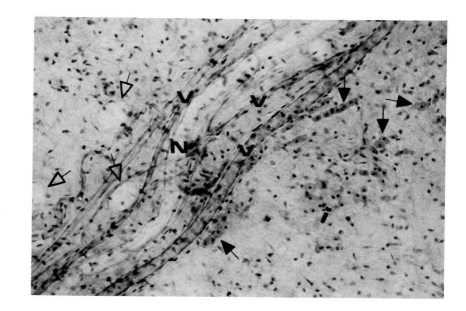

Figure 7.20. Stretch preparation of loose connective tissue from a murine subcutis. Vessels *(V)* and a nerve *(N)* traverse the tissue. Mast cells *(solid arrows)*, a macrophage *(bar)* and adipocytes *(open arrows)* are present. The remainder of the nuclei are those of fibroblasts. ×40.

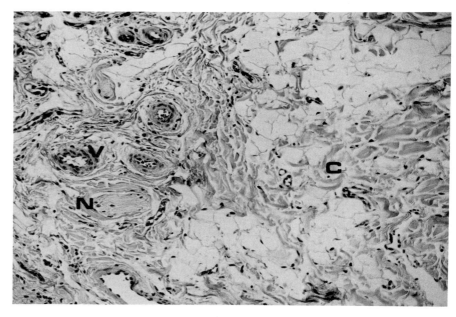

Figure 7.21. A section of loose connective tissue. Collagenous fibers *(C)*, nerves *(N)* and blood vessels *(V)* are scattered throughout the tissue. Fibroblasts and adipocytes are present also. ×40.

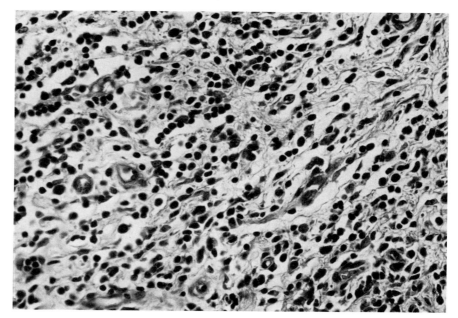

Figure 7.22. A section of loose connective tissue from the upper digestive tract. The basic components are similar to those of Figure 7.21. The numerous dark nuclei are those of mononuclear cells—lymphocytes, macrophages, plasma cells. The mononucleated cells impart a hyperplastic (hypercellular) appearance to the tissue. This cellular population of loose connective tissue is typical of that which occurs in regions that are subjected continually to antigenic insult. ×100.

fibrous components. Cellular constituents vary with location and physiology.

OCCURRENCE: Subepithelial connective tissue, mesenteries, between muscles and nerves, components of most organs (Plate IV.1).

Dense White Fibrous Connective Tissue—Irregular. This connective tissue, most often abbreviated as DWFCT, is closely related to areolar connective tissue. All of the fibrous and cellular elements of areolar connective tissue can occur in DWFCT. Usually, the fibroblast and collagenous fibers are the predominant features. The collagen appears as thick, wavy fibers (Fig. 7.23). The collagenous fibers form a coarse network within which few cells are located.

MORPHOLOGICAL FEATURES: A coarse network of collagenous fibers with some reticular and elastic fibers is apparent. The number of cells is reduced and the number of fibers is increased compared to loose connective tissue.

OCCURRENCE: Subepidermal connective tissue, capsules of organs (Plates I.3, and IV.3).

Dense White Fibrous Connective Tissue—Regular. The significant feature of this connective tissue is the orderly, parallel orientation of collagenous fibers (Fig. 7.24). Although distinct bundles of fibers are present, they do not appear as such in routine preparations. Rather, the fibers (with hematoxylin and eosin [H and E]) form a relatively homogeneous pink-staining background. The fibrocytes seem to delimit

the extent of individual bundles. The nuclei of these cells vary from oval to thin and elongated. They are dark-staining. Although present, it is rare that the thin processes of the cytoplasm will be distinct. The nuclei and fibers may appear wavy. Although other cell types may be present normally, they are extremely rare.

This connective tissue is the predominant type that forms *tendons* and *ligaments*. Individual bundles of these highly organized fibers, however, are held together by loose connective tissue. Also, the few blood vessels and nerves observed are surrounded by loose connective tissue. The ordered, collagenous fiber arrangement resists the great amount of tensile stress applied to tendons and ligaments.

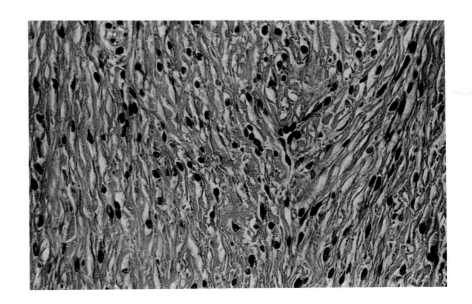

Figure 7.23. A section of DWFCT, irregularly arranged, from the tunica albuginea of a canine testis. Collagenous fibers and fibroblasts are the predominant elements. ×100.

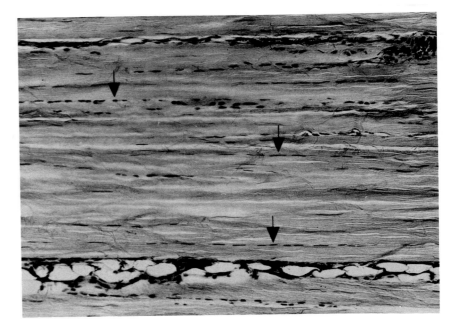

Figure 7.24. A section of DWFCT, regularly arranged, from a tendon. The fibrocytes *(arrows)* are oriented parallel to the collagenous fibers. ×40.

MORPHOLOGICAL FEATURES: Very few cells—mostly fibrocytes—are present. Heavy collagenous fibers that appear as a relatively homogeneous background matrix between cells predominate. Fibrocytes are arranged in a longitudinal orientation. Cells and fibers may appear wavy. Collagen stains a light pink with H and E.

OCCURRENCE: Tendons (attachments of muscle to bone), ligaments (attachments of bone to bone), aponeuroses (thin, sheet-like tendons) (Plates IV.5, and IV.6).

Elastic Connective Tissue. This type of connective tissue is a basic modification of the type previously discussed. The predominant fiber type is the elastic fiber, whereas the predominant cell type is the fibroblast (Fig. 7.25). The fibers are larger than col-

lagenous fibers, and they branch and anastomose with each other. Individual elastic fibers are surrounded by areolar connective tissue. The elastic fibers are ordered as evidenced by the orderliness of the fibroblasts. Without careful examination, this tissue is easily confused with DWFCT. Upon careful examination, however, the presence of bright, pink-staining fibers (with H and E) is apparent. With special staining, the elastic fibers are readily apparent (Fig. 7.26).

In cross section, note the large fibers and the extrafibrillar position of the nuclei (Fig. 7.27) of the fibroblasts.

MORPHOLOGICAL FEATURES: Elastic fibers in parallel and branched array predominate. Fibers

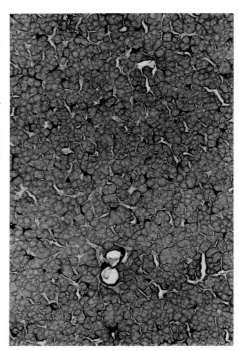

Figure 7.27. Cross section of the elastic connective tissue of a canine nuchal ligament. ×80.

stain intensely pink with H and E. Fibroblasts predominate; few other cell types are present.

OCCURRENCE: Nuchal ligament (ligamentum nuchae), some dorsal ligaments of spinal column, mural elements of arteries (Plate IV.4).

Special Connective Tissues

Reticular Connective Tissue. The predominant fiber in this tissue is the reticular fiber. The fibrous network is complemented by a cellular reticulum (network) of reticular cells. Because this type of tissue is associated with *cytogenic organs (cell-producing)*, careful examination is required to observe the cellular and fibrous reticulum through the mass of other cells normally present. Numerous cell *(stem cells, reticular cells, lymphocytes, agranulocytes, plasma cells, histiocytes)* may be present. In a section of spleen that has been flushed with physiological saline, the reticulum is apparent. With special staining techniques for reticular fibers, the fibrous reticulum is easily observed (Fig. 6.8). Ordinary staining does not demonstrate this tissue definitively; however, its association with certain cell types and organs is a reliable key to its identification.

Reticular fibers also constitute the finer interstitial connective tissue of many organs. In this instance, the defensive cells are absent or occur with a frequency similar to that expected in areolar connective tissue. In these regions, the predominant cell is the fiber-forming reticular cell.

MORPHOLOGICAL FEATURES: A fine reticulum of fibers and cells is apparent; the fibers are argy-

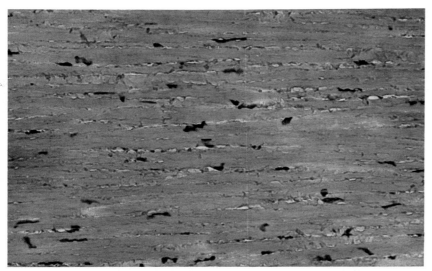

Figure 7.25. A longitudinal section of elastic connective tissue from a canine nuchal ligament. The dark profiles are nuclei of fibroblasts, some of which have been displaced from their interfibrillar positions. ×100.

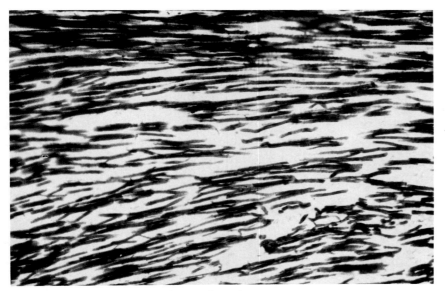

Figure 7.26. A longitudinal section of elastic fibers from a canine nuchal ligament. Only the elastic fibers are stained. ×40. (Verhoeff's stain).

rophilic. **The tissue is usually associated with cytogenic organs that produce defensive cells.**

OCCURRENCE: **Stroma (fibrous support) of lymphatic and hematopoietic organs; finer interstitial connective tissue of some organs.**

Pigmented Connective Tissue. This tissue is areolar connective tissue in which pigment-containing cells occur (Fig. 7.16). It is of limited but significant occurrence.

MORPHOLOGICAL FEATURES: **Pigment-bearing cells are present.**

OCCURRENCE: **Iris and choroid coat; connective tissue associated with pigmented skin.**

Adipose Tissue

Form and Function. Adipose tissue is composed of a homogeneous population of cells, *adipocytes* or *fat cells*, that may occur as single cells, groups of cells, or extensive masses of cells. Although this tissue consists of blood vessels, nerves, and elements of loose and/or reticular connective tissue, the predominant feature is the adipocyte. The tissue, therefore, is very cellular. Although adipose tissue may occur in association with all of the loose connective tissue of the body, predilection sites do occur: Adipose tissue may form an extensive subcutaneous sheet, the panniculus adiposus. Extensive quantities of this tissue often occur in association with the visceral, parietal and connecting mesothelial membranes of the celomic cavities. Adipose tissue occurs in regions otherwise devoid of other tissue components—the axillary region, inguinal region. Most organs contain some adipose tissue. Even the popular prime cuts of beef are a mixture of skeletal muscle, connective tissue, and adipose tissue (marbling).

This tissue is a readily available source of energy. The stored fats of adipose tissue contain more energy per gram than corresponding quantities of proteins or sugars. (Fats supply 9 calories per gram, whereas carbohydrates and proteins each supply 4 calories per gram.) Adipose tissue is an important contributor to thermoregulation. Its placement throughout the body aids in the conservation of heat. Adipose tissue is also an important mechanical insulator. Its proper placement in association with the visceral organs and greater omentum helps to protect these organs from mechanical damage. The rich deposit of adipose tissue within the digital cushion of the equine foot is an important devise in absorption of concussive forces. Also, adipose tissue associated with synovial membranes serves to absorb shock as well as afford some additional stability to diarthrodial joints.

Morphologically, two types of adipose tissue are identified—*white adipose tissue* and *brown adipose tissue.*

Origin of Adipose Tissue. The questions of the precise origin of fat cells and the relationship of white fat cells to brown fat

cells have not been answered satisfactorily. The special stem cell for adipocytes is probably the mesenchymal cell. This can account for specific predilection sites rather than adipocytes being spread ubiquitously throughout the body as a result of the fibroblastic accumulation of fat. Moreover, the presence of a basal lamina around individual adipocytes is difficult to explain if they are differentiated from fibroblasts. The occurrence of age and species differences relative to the propensity to accumulate fat, as well the anatomical sites in which the accumulation takes place support the idea of separate populations of fat cells.

White Adipose Tissue. This tissue is also called *white fat, unilocular fat,* and *ordinary adipose tissue* (Plate V.11). The cells of white adipose tissue are very large, ranging to about 130 μm. They are spherical cells that may appear polyhedral. *Unilocular fat cells,* the predominant cell of this tissue, have a signet-ring appearance (Fig. 7.28). The bulk of the cytoplasm is occupied by a single large fat droplet that is rimmed by a thin margin of cytoplasm. The nucleus, which is usually displaced to one side of the cell, accounts for the signet-ring configuration. In most planes of section, the nucleus is not apparent (Fig. 7.29). In routine

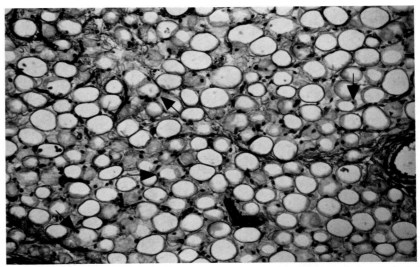

Figure 7.28. A section of yellow adipose tissue. *Arrows,* nuclei of those cells in a typical signet-ring configuration. ×40.

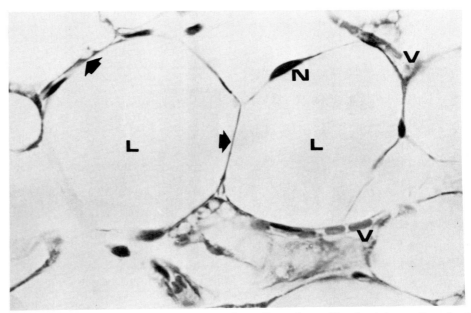

Figure 7.29. A section of adipocytes from yellow adipose tissue. The signet-ring configuration is obvious. The nucleus *(N)* is displaced to one side of the cell. The cytoplasm is reduced to a thin margin at the periphery of the cell *(arrows).* The spaces that had been occupied by the lipid droplets *(L)* are the predominant cytoplasmic features. Vessels *(V)* occur within the associated connective tissue. ×160.

paraffin sections of fat cells, the space that was occupied by the lipids is all that remains; the lipid solvents used in the process dissolved the fats. Special preparation techniques such as freezing and special stains (osmium tetroxide, Sudan stains) are required to demonstrate the lipids of fat cells (Fig. 7.30).

The lipids of these cells are triglycerides and certain fatty acids. They are mobilized through enzymatic hydrolysis by lipases, and free fatty acids enter the blood as an available source of energy.

White adipose tissue may be subdivided into smaller units (lobules) by loose connective tissue septa. Reticular fibers extend from these septa and surround individual fat cells. The extensive vascular supply and nerves of this tissue gain access via these connective tissues.

Brown Adipose Tissue. This tissue consists of *multilocular fat cells* (Plate V.12). The predominant feature of these cells is the presence of numerous small fat droplets within the cytoplasm (Fig. 7.31). The round nucleus is not displaced to one side of the cell but may assume any position. Unless the special preparatory precautions mentioned previously are taken, the lipids are leached from these cells also. This imparts an acidophilic and foamy appearance to the cytoplasm of these cells (Fig. 7.31).

The brown color of this tissue results from numerous mitochondria and the corresponding high quantities of the cytochrome oxidase system. Brown fat cells contain more mitochondria and the tissue is better vascularized and innervated than their white fat cell counterparts. A lobular organization is sufficiently extensive to impart a glandular appearance.

The metabolism of the stored lipids releases heat, warms the blood, and raises

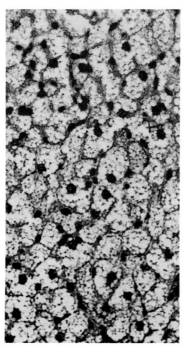

Figure 7.31. A section of multilocular adipose tissue. Spaces that had been occupied by individual lobules of lipids are apparent within the cells. ×100.

body temperature. Brown adipose tissue has a limited but specific distribution. It develops during the prenatal period and is confined generally to the axilla, interscapular region, mediastinum, mesenteries, and perirenal region. The tissue may assist young animals to resist postnatal cold extremes. Hibernating rodents, similarly, have brown adipose tissue deposits in the regions specified previously. These depots assist with body temperature maintenance during hibernating periods.

The lipid droplets of both types of fat cells are not membrane-bound. Rather, they are rimmed by a condensation of cytoplasm that may contain some cytofilaments.

Two types of fat cell tumors occur in domestic animals, especially the dog. The benign lipoma is difficult to distinguish from typical white adipose tissue histologically, whereas the malignant liposarcoma cells may look like multilocular fat cells histologically.

Macrophage System

Many cells of the body have the ability to ingest particulate matter (phagocytosis). Some cells, however, have an exceptional ability for phagocytosis. The *fixed* and *wandering macrophages* of the connective tissue compartment possess this ability and are important cellular defense components for the organism. The ability of macrophages to range "far and wide" within connective tissues affords a ready and mobile defense force that is associated with almost every tissue and organ of the body. Many organs of the body contain phagocytic cells that are integral parts of their tissue architecture and defense mechanisms. Unfortunately, it is easy to lose sight of their commonality of function—phagocytosis—because they are named differently in different loci—microgliocytes, blood monocytes, Kupffer cells, alveolar macrophages, littoral cells of sinusoids (Fig. 7.32).

This common function of phagocytosis was first recognized by Metchnikoff in the late nineteenth century. He looked upon these phagocytes as a diffuse cellular system of "big eaters" and coined the name *macrophage system*. Other cells, namely specialized endothelial lining cells and the cellular stroma ("phagocytic reticular cell") of certain organs, were believed to have well-developed phagocytic activity. The original system of phagocytes was expanded conceptually to include these reticular and endothelial cells. Thus, the name *reticuloendothelial system* was coined.

The bulk of evidence today controverts the reticular cell and endothelial cell contributions to the reticuloendothelial system. Reticular cells (fiber-forming cells) are not known to be phagocytic. Nor is the reverse true. Similarly, many endothelial cells, once considered to be phagocytic, are now considered to be specialized macrophages that have established residence as littoral cells in many epithelial membranes. For these reasons, the name reticuloendothelial system has fallen into disfavor. A more descriptive name that is gaining acceptance is the *mononuclear phagocyte system* or *macrophage system*, the latter having been proposed by Metchnikoff almost 100 years ago.

This system includes numerous mononuclear cells of different organs that function through phagocytosis to protect the body from foreign materials and microorganisms. They also serve to rid the body of dead constituent cells and matrical materials. They are involved in the processing of antigens.

Regeneration and Repair

The fibroblast is the primary cell responsible for regenerative and reparative processes within the proper connective tissue. Connective tissue is not a static entity. Old and/or damaged cells are removed and replaced by new fibroblasts. Similarly, matrical components that have been damaged or altered chemically are removed and replaced by new components. The macrophage is the key cell in this removal activity.

The ability of the fibroblast to mediate repair or regeneration is predicated upon a number of factors. This cell is capable of division. So, this cell is able to serve as its

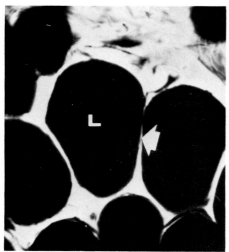

Figure 7.30. A special stain for lipids. The large lipid droplets *(L)* remain as dominant features of the cytoplasm. The cellular margins are indicated by the *arrow.* ×125. (Osmium tetroxide stain.)

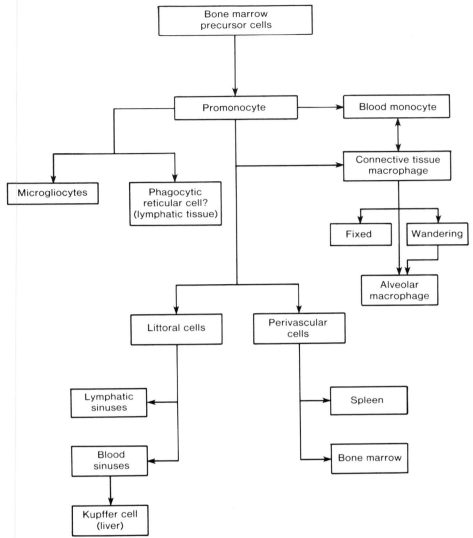

Figure 7.32. Diagram of the relationships of the component cells of the mononuclear phagocyte system. The origin, distribution, and relationships of the constituent cells are outlined. Littoral cells, not endothelial cells, of bone marrow and splenic sinuses may be phagocytic also. Conclusive evidence is lacking.

fibrous connective tissue, *fibrosis*. The formation of fibrous connective tissues in the repair process of other tissues may limit, reduce, or obliterate the normal function of the repaired tissue.

own "stem cell" in times of need. Additionally, mesenchymal cells are scattered throughout connective tissue, especially in a pericapillary position. Mitotic activity and subsequent differentiation of some of these cells serve to replenish the fibroblastic population.

Fibrous connective tissue may also mediate the repair of other tissues. After an acute myocardial infarction (heart attack), degenerative cardiac muscle is replaced by a scar of fibrous connective tissue. Skeletal muscle that has been injured severely is replaced similarly by a connective tissue scar. The result of chronic inflammation is the deposition of abnormal quantities of

References

Carpenter, J.C., Perrelet, A. and Orci, L.: Morphological changes of the adipose cell membrane during lipolysis. J. Cell Biol. *72*:104, 1977.

Chapman, J.A., Gough, J. and Elves, M.W.: An electron microscopic study of the in vitro trnasformation of human leucocytes. II. Transformation to macrophages. J. Cell Sci. *2*:371, 1967.

Cohn, Z.A., Fedorko, M.E. and Hirsch, J.G.: The in vitro differentiation of mononuclear phagocytes. IV. The ultrastructure of macrophage differentiation in the peritoneal cavity and in culture. J. Exp. Med. *123*:747, 1966.

Cohn, Z.A., Fedorko, M.E. and Hirsch, J.G.: The in vitro differentiation of mononuclear phagocytes. V. The formation of macrophage lysosomes. J. Exp. Med. *123*:757, 1966.

Downey, H.: The development of histiocytes and macrophages from lymphocytes. J. Lab Clin. Med. *45*:499, 1955.

Fawcett, D.W.: An experimental study of mast cell degranulation and regeneration. Anat. Rec. *121*:29, 1955.

Harrington, J.S.: Fibrogenesis. Environ. Health Perspec. *9*:271, 1974.

Hayward, J.S., Lyman, C.P. and Taylor, C.R.: The possible role of brown fat as a source of heat during arousal from hibernation. Ann. N. Y. Acad. Sci. *131*:441, 1965.

Hunt, T.K. and Van Winkle, W., Jr.: *Fundamentals of Wound Management in Syrgery—Wound Healing: Normal Repair.* Chirurgecom, Inc., South Plainfield, NJ, 1976.

Kolouch, F., Jr.: The lymphocyte in acute inflammation. Amer. J. Path. *15*:413, 1939.

Leibovich, S.J. and Ross, R.: The role of macrophages in wound repair. Amer. J. Path. *78*:71, 1975.

Litt, M.: Eosinophils and antigen-antibody reaction. Ann. N. Y. Acad. Sci. *116*:964, 1964.

Maximow, A.A.: The morphology of the mesenchymal reaction. Arch. Pat. Lab. Med. *4*:557, 1927.

Movat, H.Z. and Fernando, N.V.P.: The fine structure of connective tissue. I. The fibroblast. Exp. Molec. Path. *1*:509, 1962.

Movat, H.Z. and Fernando, N.V.P.: The fine structure of connective tissue. II. The plasma cell. Exp. Molec. Path. *1*:535, 1962.

Padawar, J. (ed.): Mast cells and basophils. Ann. N. Y. Acad. Sci. *103*:1, 1963.

Sheldon, H., Hellenberg, C.H. and Winegard, A.I.: Observations on the morphology of adipose tissue. Diabetes *11*:378, 1962.

Smith, R.E., Hock, R.J.: Brown fat: Thermogenic effector of arousal in hibernation. Science *140*:199, 1963.

Weinstock, A. and Albright, J.T.: The fine structure of mast cells in normal human gingiva. J. Ultrastruct. Res. *17*:245, 1967.

West, G.B.: Function of mast cells. J. Pharm. Pharmcol. *14*:618, 1962.

8: Supportive Tissue — Cartilage

General Characteristics

Form and Function. Cartilage consists of cells embedded within an amorphous, gel-like substance. The cells of cartilage secrete various substances and become embedded in their own secretory products. The secretory products of chondrocytes form a firm but resilient matrix. These qualities suit cartilage to its functional role in *weight-bearing, movement*, and *organ integrity*.

The mesenchymal cells from which cartilage cells arise are located at the periphery of the cartilage in a membrane referred to as the *perichondrium*. (The perichondrium may also be considered the capsule of the cartilage).

The chrondroblastic line of differentiation at a perichondral surface is the means by which new chondrocytes are added to cartilage. The new cells deposit matrix upon pre-existing cartilage. This type of growth is called *appositional growth*. Once the chondroblasts have become embedded in their own products as chondrocytes, growth does not cease. Rather, chondrocytes divide within the confines of their *lacunae*. This mitotic activity from within, *interstitial growth*, causes expansion of the resilient matrix. **Most cartilage utilizes both appositional and interstitial mechanisms for growth.**

Cartilage is an avascular tissue. Although large blood vessels pass through cartilage, there are no intracartilaginous capillaries that directly supply the nutritional needs of this tissue. All metabolites must diffuse from the periphery to the cells in the depths of the tissue. The solid ground substance of cartilage complicates the movement of fluid and dissolved substances to and from the cells. Despite the diminished diffusion and the increased distances over which it must occur, chondrocytes flourish in their environment. They are adapted to survive in an environment with diminished oxygen concentrations. The problem of movement of metabolites and waste products becomes more difficult with age. The natural fate of cartilage is to become mineralized. This increases the problem of percolation of metabolites through the matrix. The older cells die, the tissue is removed by phagocytic cells and bone is deposited in its place.

Sensory innervation of cartilage is achieved by neuronal terminals scattered within the fibrous portion of the perichondrium.

Cartilage is the primary support tissue of the fetus. Suppport structures of cartilage develop in association with the upper and lower respiratory tract, the pinna and external auditory meatus, and auditory tube. These cartilaginous structures continue to develop during adolescense and are maintained in the adult. Much of the cartilaginous mass of the fetus and neonatal organism is involved intimately with the developing musculoskeletal system. Certain structures, such as fibrocartilaginous intervertebral discs and fibrocartilaginous attachments of ligaments and tendons to bone, continue to develop and become integral parts of the supportive and locomotor structures of the musculoskeletal system. Much of the hyaline cartilage of the developing organism, however, is involved directly in bone development. The small amounts of cartilage in the growing postnatal and adult organisms do not reflect the importance of cartilage as a supportive tissue.

Origin of Cartilage. Sites within which cartilage is going to develop in the fetus are identifiable initially as sites of *mesenchymal cell condensation*. The mesenchymal cells withdraw their cellular processes, become round and form dense populations of cells. These presumptive sites of cartilage formation are called *chondrogenic centers*. The mesenchymal cells differentiate into chondroblasts. These cells enlarge and secrete their characteristic surrounding matrix. As the matrix or interstitial material increases, the cells become separated further from each other and each cell is surrounded by its own secretory products. The space occupied by each cell is called a *lacuna*. The space occupied by a chondrocyte is similar to the space occupied by a fibroblast. The relationships of all connective tissue cells to their surrounding matrices are similar. The lacuna associated with the chondrocyte is readily apparent in light microscopy because of the consistency of the matrix. The lacuna is an artifact of preparation and sectioning techniques.

Interstitial and appositional growth mechanisms, as the names imply, are most active during development and growth.

The potential for this type of activity is reduced in the adult. Nevertheless, this type of activity is a significant component of fracture repair processes in young and adult organisms.

Cells of Cartilage. Cartilage is composed of a homogeneous population of cells. Mesenchymal cells, either in a chondrogenic center of the embryo or in the perichondrium, differentiate into active cells that synthesize and secrete large quantities of matrix components. These *chondroblasts* envelope themselves with their own secretions and eventually become isolated within their lacunae. At this point, the cells are referred to as *chondrocytes*. They are the cells responsible for the maintenance and turnover of matrix materials. They perform the same functions as chondroblasts, but their level of activity is reduced compared to that of chondroblasts. The chondroblast/chondrocyte relationship is probably best considered as the same cell in a different stage of its life cycle. Different subpopulations of chondrocytes have been identified based upon matrical, ultrastructural and histochemical properties.

A third cell type may be observed in cartilage, especially during developmental stages. It is a multinucleated giant cell, the *chondroclast*. This cell is responsible for the removal of cartilage matrix and cells. Because of the morphological and physiological similarity of this cell to a cell of bone, the *osteoclast*, the chondroclast and the osteoclast are considered to be identical. Recent evidence clearly establishes that **osteoclasts, multinucleated giant cells, are fusion products of macrophages.** As chondroclasts "eat" their way through cartilage, chondrocytes are released from their lacunae. Whatever their fate (complete phagocytosis or recycling as members of new populations of cells), they are not incorporated into chondroclasts as contributors to the syncytium.

The chondroblastic and fibroblastic cell lines, as well as the osteoblastic cell line, are closely related populations of cells. All are derived originally from the mesenchymal cell. All secrete collagen and glycosaminoglycans (GAGs). Yet, each is associated with a matrix that imparts distinctive characteristics to its respective tissues. Under varying circumstances, these tissues (fibrous connective tissues, cartilage, and bone) occur in regions in which they are not expected. This abnormal transformation of a specific, adult, fully differentiated tissue into another differentiated type is called *metaplasia*. Cartilage and bone can form de novo in fibrous connective tissue; bone and fibrous connective tissue can form at sites occupied by cartilage; cartilage and fibrous connective tissue can form in sites occupied by bone. The stem cells associated with these tissues are responsive to subtle but significant changes in their microenvironment. Under such circumstances, stem cells of a perichondrium, which under normal conditions would differentiate into cartilage cells, may produce one or both of the other fiber-producing cells. Similarly, stem cells of the covering of bone (periosteum) may differentiate into all three cell types.

Classification. Three types of cartilage are identified on the basis of the relative amounts of amorphous matrix and the amount and types of fibers embedded within the amorphous material. They are *hyaline cartilage, elastic cartilage,* and *fibrocartilage.*

Matrical Components

Fibers

The predominant fiber of cartilage is the fine collagenous fiber. In hyaline cartilage, these fibers are scattered in a random pattern throughout the matrix. In routine preparations, they are observed rarely because their index of refraction is similar to that of the ground substance. In fibrocartilage, however, the collagenous fibers are observed easily because they are the primary constituents of the cartilage. The amount of ground substance is reduced greatly. This tissue has characteristics that are similar to cartilage and dense white fibrous connective tissue. The fibers of elastic cartilage include both collagenous and elastic fibers. Elastic fibers are visualized readily with normal preparatory techniques, as well as by special staining procedures.

Ground Substance

The primary constituents of the ground substance are the *GAGs*. Minor differences in the quantities of specific GAGs are related to age and location. Chondroitin-4-sulfate and chondroitin-6-sulfate are most abundant. Chondroitin-6-sulfate is more common in adult cartilage, whereas chondroitin-4-sulfate is more common in the cartilage of young animals. Small quantities of hyaluronic acid are present in cartilage. Keratan sulfate concentrations increase with age.

GAGs are complexed with *core protein* to form *proteoglycans*. Proteoglycans have the ability to form large aggregates once they've been secreted by the cells. These *proteoglycan aggregates* may achieve molecular weights in excess of 5.0×10^6. The aggregation phenomenon is dependent upon hyaluronic acid. Although hyaluronic acid occurs in low quantities in cartilage, its role in the structure of cartilaginous ground substance is significant (Fig. 8.1). Hyaluronate may comprise as little as 0.01 % of the proteoglycan aggregate, yet may bind with as much as 250 times its weight in proteoglycans.

Link proteins seem to stabilize the aggregates into large compounds with bottle brush-like configurations. The proteoglycan aggregates perform three significant functions in cartilage: *stability of the matrix, volume definition of the matrix,* and *compressive properties of the matrix.*

The *stability* of the matrix is achieved by the chemical linkage of proteoglycans to hyaluronic acid and collagenous fibers (Fig. 8.2). This ensures that the proper spatial orientation of the matrical constituents is achieved. Proper spatial orientation is essential for the proper binding of interstitial fluid. These macromolecules define spatial volumes by entrapping the surrounding interstitial fluid. The proteoglycans can absorb solvent volumes that are as much as 50 times their dry weight. This property contributes significantly to the *volume def-*

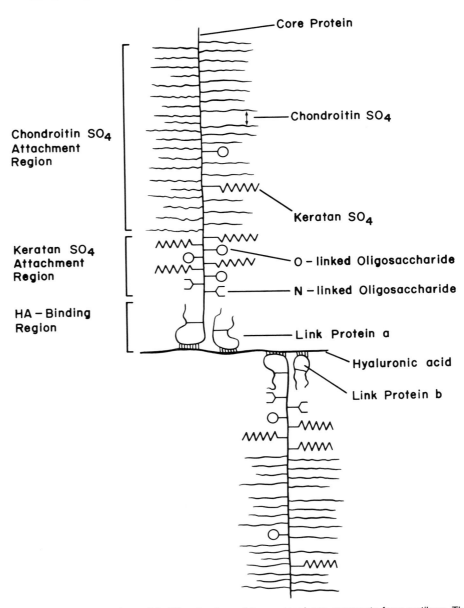

Figure 8.1. A schematic model of the structure of the proteoglycan aggregate from cartilage. The appropriate features are labeled. Oligosaccharides are linked to the core proteins either through oxygen *(O-linked)* or nitrogen *(N-linked)*. (Redrawn and modified from Hascall, V. C.: Proteoglycans: Structure and Function. *In:* Ginsberg, V. and Robbins, P. (eds.): *Biology of Carbohydrates.* Vol 1. page 7, John Wiley & Sons, New York, 1981.)

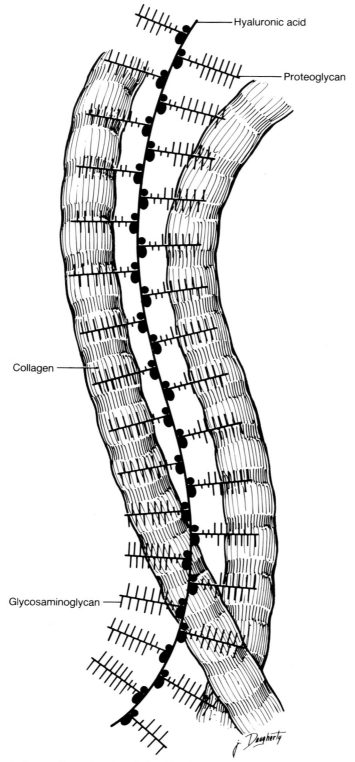

Figure 8.2. A diagram illustrating the relationship of proteoglycan aggregates to collagenous fibers in cartilage. The GAGs of constituent proteoglycans are linked electrostatically to the collagenous components. The collagen provides the tensile properties, whereas the proteoglycans provide the compressive properties of cartilage. The linkages between GAGs and collagenous fibers provide a rigid matrical framework for this tissue.

and replacement of cartilage during endochondral ossification. Alterations in bone development, as exemplified in *chondrodystrophy*, have been related to the synthesis of defective proteoglycans.

The absorption of water by proteoglycan aggregates imparts a vast hydrodynamic domain to them. Proteoglycan aggregates are reversibly resistent to compressive forces. Subjecting proteoglycan aggregates to centrifugal force decreases their volume in proportion to the applied force. Upon removal of the force, these macromolecules return to their original volume. Recall that these substances are polyanions. As the molecular domain of each proteoglycan decreases, the charge density and constraints on mobility within the molecule increases. These factors, coupled with the noncompressible property of water, account for the compressive properties of cartilaginous tissues. Weight-bearing on articular surfaces is contingent upon this physical characteristic. Loss of or inappropriate synthesis and aggregation of these compounds or their constituents decrease the hydrodynamic domain of the remaining or resulting proteoglycan aggregates. This decreases the amount of water contained within the cartilaginous matrix and increases its compressibility. Decreasing the ability to resist compression increases the possibility of damage to the tissue. Alteration to the tissue in this manner may be a contributing factor in the development of degenerative joint disease.

Staining of Cartilage

The presence of sulfate groups on these compounds imparts an acidic nature to the matrix. As such, the ground substance of cartilage is basophilic and stains appropriately with routine stains (hematoxylin and eosin [H and E]). The matrix of most cartilage, however, does not stain uniformly (Fig. 8.3). Young cartilage may be acidophilic, whereas the matrix of the perilacunar margin (*capsular* or *territorial matrix*) of old cartilage stains intensely basophilic. The region of the matrix between individual cells or groups of cells, the *interterritorial matrix*, stains less intensely basophilic than the territorial matrix. The staining properties relate to the number of sulfate and carboxylate groups (basophilic components) and the acidophilic nature of the collagen. In young cartilage with fewer sulfate groups, the acidophilia of the collagen dominates the staining. In the remainder of cartilage, the basophilic components dominate the stain reaction.

The metachromatic staining properties of cartilaginous matrical materials are dependent upon the constituent GAGs. Metachromatic stains such as toluidine blue are useful to demonstrate these substances, Safranin O and ruthenium red are nonspecific stains for GAGs that are useful with light

inition of the tissue. Defective GAG and proteoglycan synthesis, secretion and aggregation are associated with a decreased

tissue volume because of a diminution in the ability to absorb water. Bone length and shape are dependent upon proper growth

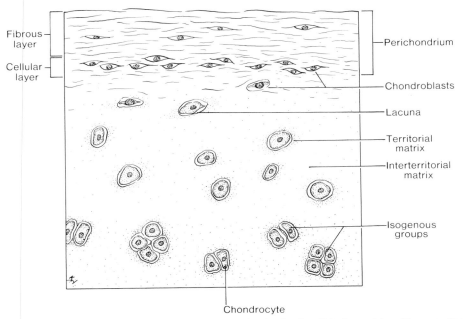

Fibrous layer

Cellular layer

Perichondrium

Chondroblasts

Lacuna

Territorial matrix

Interterritorial matrix

Isogenous groups

Chondrocyte

Figure 8.3. Diagram of typical hyaline cartilage. Mitosis of cells within the perichondrium results in appositional growth. Mitotic activity within the matrix results in the formation of isogenous groups (cell nests) and interstitial growth.

and electron microscopy. Magnesium chloride extinction coupled with alcian blue staining adds valuable information about the distribution of different types of GAGs in the matrices.

Not all cartilage stains the same. Tracheal, intervertebral disc and articular cartilage stains differently. Also, young hyaline cartilage of an articular surface stains differently than old cartilage of a similar surface. Hyaline cartilage of articular foci does not stain homogeneously with the MgCl$_2$ extinction technique. The homogeneous, blue-staining matrix at low concentrations of MgCl$_2$ is replaced by heterogeneous staining characteristics at high concentrations of MgCl$_2$. The heterogeneity is manifested as matrical *haloes* within the territorial matrices of some cells; i.e., the territorial matrix stains a lighter blue than the interterritorial matrix. Not all cells are associated with the haloes; the territorial and interterritorial matrices of some cells may stain identically. The territorial matrix may also stain more intensely than the interterritorial matrix of some cells. This and other information has led to the conclusion that different populations of chondrocytes exist within cartilage that are capable of producing different types of matrical components. Albeit the haloes are probably caused by a leaching of territorial matrical components, the materials within the territorial matrices that leach must be different than those in the interterritorial matrices that do not leach. An increased incidence of haloes has been associated with the onset of degenerative joint disease.

Although the sulfated glycosaminogly-cans of cartilaginous matrix are periodic acid-Schiff (PAS)-negative, cartilaginous matrix stains positively with PAS. All of the molecules responsible for this stain reactivity have not been determined, but they are probably collagen and other structural glycoproteins.

Ultrastructure of Cartilaginous Matrices

The homogeneous nature of the intercellular materials of hyaline cartilage appears differently when viewed with the electron microscope. Cellular/matrical relationships and the nature of the lacunar space also differ (Fig. 8.4). The chondrocytic lacunae are not apparent. Fibrillar and granular materials are adjacent to the cells. Some collagenous fibers are apparent also (Fig. 8.5). There is, then, a continuum of matrical materials from the cellular margin to the matrix proper.

Three matrical zones are visible with the electron microscope: *pericellular matrix, territorial matrix,* and *interterritorial matrix.* The pericellular matrix is immediately adjacent to the cell (Fig. 8.4). This matrix consists of granules and fibrillar materials. Characterization of the matrix at this cell/matrical interface is the subject of current research. The retraction of the cell and the exaggeration of this interface probably accounts for the lacunae of light microscopy. The *territorial matrix (capsular matrix, lacunar matrix)* consists of fibrillar and granular materials (Figs. 8.4 and 8.5). The granular materials, *matrix granules,* consist of proteogylcan aggregates. These granules typically stain with GAG-specific stains

(ruthenium red) and are removed by appropriate enzymatic digestions *(hyaluronidase, chondroitinase, keratinase).* Banded collagenous fibrils are not evident in this region. Fibrillar materials, *microfibrils,* probably represent a diversity of substances—nonbanded collagen, noncollagenous proteins (core proteins), and hyaluronic acid (Fig. 8.6). The *interterritorial matrix* is characterized by banded collagen. Type II collagen is typical. Components of this region of the matrix also include the fibrillar materials and the matrix granules described previously.

Matrix granules appear free in the matrix, in intimate association with microfibrils and juxtaposed to collagenous fibrils (Fig. 8.6). All of the matrix components are linked chemically to each other (Fig. 8.2). Additionally, cytoplasmic processes project from the cells and extend into the matrix. An additional component is present in certain foci of hyaline cartilage. These are membrane-bound vesicles, *matrix vesicles,* that are pinched off from the cells or cellular processes and are located in the matrix. They occur in the mineralization zones of the hyaline cartilage of the growth plate. They are the sites that may be utilized by the cartilage for the initiation of mineralization (Fig. 8.7).

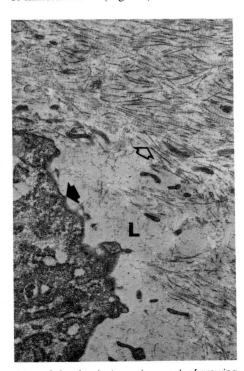

Figure 8.4. An electron micrograph of growing cartilage. The cellular margin *(solid arrow)* and lacunar margin *(open arrow)* are separated from each other by a lacunar *(L)* or territorial matrix. The territorial matrix is composed of granular materials (matrix granules), fibrillar materials and some cellular processes, but banded collagen is not evident. ×6800. (Courtesy of J. W. Newbrey.)

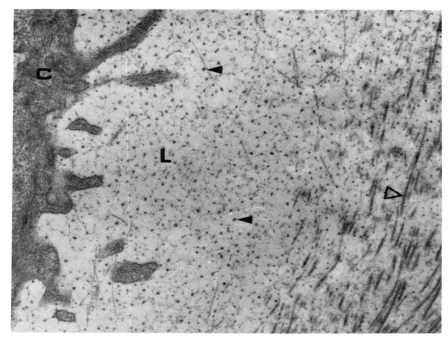

Figure 8.5. An electron micrograph of growing cartilage. The chondroblast *(C)* has cellular processes that extend into and through the lacunar *(L)* or territorial martix. Matrix granules *(solid arrowheads)* are evident in both the territorial and interterritorial matrices. The matrix granules within the territorial matrix occur in juxtaposition to microfibrils. The interterritorial matrix is characterized by matrix granules interspersed among banded collagenous fibers *(open arrowhead)*. The preparation was stained with ruthenium red, an electron-dense stain that stains GAGs effectively. ×15,000. (Courtesy of J. W. Newbrey.)

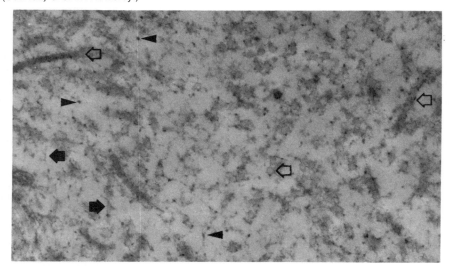

Figure 8.6. An electron micrograph of the matrix of growing cartilage. The sample was stained with ruthenium red, an electron-dense stain used to demonstrate GAGs. The intimate relationship of the biochemical matrical components is demonstrated. Matrix granules *(small solid arrowheads)*, microfibrils *(large solid arrows)*, and sectioned collagenous fibers *(open arrows)* are evident. Note the intimate juxtaposition of matrix granules to microfibrils and collagen. The microfibrils have been demonstrated to be hyaluronic acid. Some of the collagenous fibers are cut in longitudinal section, others are cut in cross section. Hyaluronic acid, other GAGs, and collagen are linked biochemically to each other within the matrix. ×36,000. (Courtesy of J. W. Newbrey.)

Types of Cartilage

Hyaline Cartilage

Grossly, hyaline cartilage has a white, glassy appearance (Gr. *hyalos*, glass). In histological section this avascular tissue is separated from the surrounding tissue by a *perichondrium* (Fig. 8.8), which is analogous to the capsule of other organs. The perichondrium consists of *fibrous* and *cellular* parts. The fibrous portion is dense white fibrous connective tissue (DWFCT) that usually blends insensibly with the surrounding connective tissue. The cellular portion contains *mesenchymal cells* that give rise to fibroblasts of the fibrous perichondrium as well as to chondroblasts (Fig. 8.9). The cellular constituent is a prominent part of the perichondrium in young growing cartilage only.

In young cartilage a definite gradation from *mesenchymal cells* to *chondroblasts* to *chondrocytes* is apparent (Fig. 8.10). As mesenchymal cells differentiate into chondroblasts, these cells secrete matrical components and surround themselves in their own secretory products. As a result, a small *lacuna* (lake) is formed. The cells reside within these spaces without any contact with other cells or the surface. The lacunae of cartilage being devoid of cells in some sections is an artifact of sectioning. The lacunae, as well as the cells within them, are flattened with their long axes parallel to the surface. The matrix of this region is generally acidophilic.

Maturation of the chondroblasts into chondrocytes is accompanied by cellular hypertrophy, an enlargement of the lacunae, and a change in lacunar shape to an ovoid or angular configuration (Fig. 8.11). Chondrocytes are also clustered as *isogenous groups* or *cell nests*. These cell nests represent the daughter cells of a single chondrocyte that underwent mitosis (interstitial growth). The isogenous groups of cells in this structure assume a columnated configuration (Fig. 8.12).

Chondrocytes appear as smooth-surfaced cells that are withdrawn from the lacunar margins (Fig. 8.13). With the electron microscope, numerous cellular processes are seen that intimately contact the matrix (Fig. 8.14).

The lacunar margins of individual chondrocytes or isogenous groups are more basophilic than other portions of the matrix. This marked basophilia delimits the *capsule* or *territorial matrix* of these cells, whereas the lighter region of basophilia marks the *interterritorial matrix*.

Although the perichondrium is generally a consistent feature of hyaline cartilage, **the hyaline cartilage of articular surfaces of bone secondarily loses its perichondrium** (Fig. 8.15).

MORPHOLOGICAL FEATURES: **A few cells are embedded within a gel-like matrix that appears afibrillar. The limits of the tissue are usually well marked by a perichondrium. The matrix generally stains with basic dyes.**

OCCURRENCE: **Most bone-forming sites of the fetus and young animal; articular cartilages; airways of the respiratory tree; support structures of the nose and larynx. (Plates IV.8, and IV.9).**

Elastic Cartilage

Grossly, this tissue is yellow and is more resilient than hyaline cartilage due to the

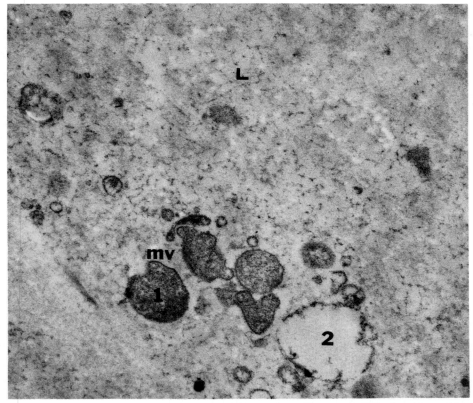

Figure 8.7. An electron micrograph of mineralizing cartilage. Two types *(1,2)* of matrix vesicles *(mv)* are present within the matrix. The matrix vesicles are foci for the initiation of cartilage mineralization. They usually occur within or close to the interterritorial matrix. The lacunar or territorial matrix *(L)* is indicated. ×34,000. (Courtesy of J. W. Newbrey.)

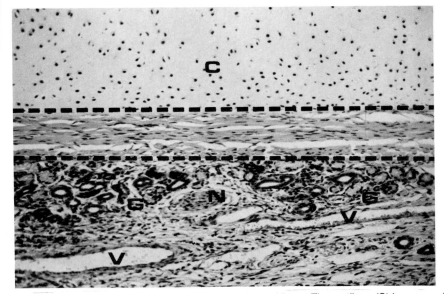

Figure 8.8. Cartilage and associated tissue of an ovine turbinate. The cartilage *(C)* is surrounded by a perichondrium *(dashed lines)*. The peripheral loose connective tissue *(below perichondrium)* contains nerves *(N)*, glands *(G)*, and blood vessels *(V)*. ×40.

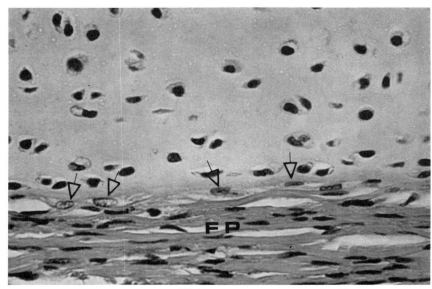

Figure 8.9. Perichondrium of cartilage. The fibrous perichondrium *(FP)* consists of collagenous fibers and fibroblasts. The cellular perichondrium *(arrows)* consists of mesenchymal cells and chondroblasts. The cellular layer of the perichondrium is most evident in a growing animal. ×160.

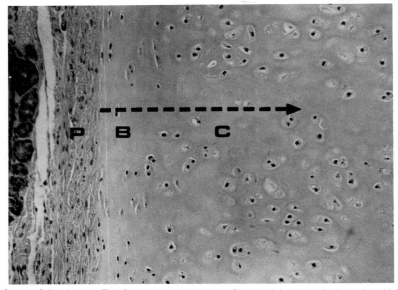

Figure 8.10. Growing cartilage from a feline larynx. The fibrous perichondrium *(P)* is peripheral to the layer in which chondroblasts *(B)* are evident. Enlargement of chondroblasts and their differentiation into chondrocytes *(C)* is apparent. *Dashed line,* progression of differentiation. ×40.

presence of elastic fibers. Other than the elastic fibers, this tissue is identical to hyaline cartilage. In some foci, more isogenous groups than those characteristic of hyaline cartilage may be apparent. The elastic fibers are demonstrable with H and E as pink-staining fibers scattered throughout the matrix (Fig. 8.16). They are easily demonstrated with special staining techniques (Fig. 8.17).

MORPHOLOGICAL FEATURES: **Identical to hyaline cartilage, except for the presence of elastic fibers. Isogenous groups may be observed more frequently.**

OCCURRENCE: **External ear (pinna); external auditory canal; auditory tube; parts of the laryngeal cartilages; epiglottic cartilage (Plate I.11, and IV.10).**

Fibrous Cartilage

This tissue, also called *fibrocartilage*, has a limited occurrence but imparts additional strength to cartilage and DWFCT. Fibrocartilage is an intermediate form between DWFCT and cartilage. Because visible collagenous fibers predominate, it may be considered a modified DWFCT. Also, features of cartilage and DWFCT are apparent at

the ultrastructural level of examination. Large collagenous *fascicles* (bundles) are oriented in an orderly array and are separated by isolated portions of cartilage (Fig. 8.18). The chondrocytes, which are located between the fascicles, secrete diminutive quantities of typical cartilaginous matrical materials. The classical appearance of this tissue is the *herringbone* configuration (Fig. 8.19) in which collagenous bundles are oriented to each other in the form of a V. Typically, however, the orientation of the fibers may not appear as orderly as described (Fig. 8.20).

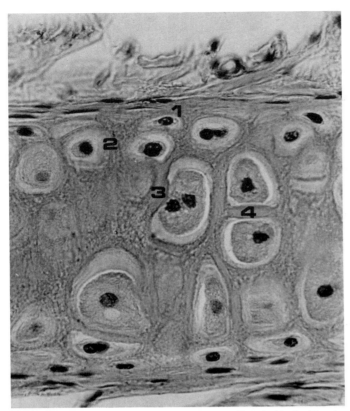

Interstitial growth potential is lost also. Repair of adult cartilaginous tissues is mediated generally by a fibrous connective tissue that may be derived from the perichondrium or the DWFCT of adjacent fascia. The newly added tissue, referred to as a granulation tissue by some authors, may be transformed gradually into cartilage. The new cartilage may retain a fibrocartilaginous character.

Fibrocartilage, however, reacts differently to injury. It is a dense tissue that is devoid of a perichondrium. The vascular supply to fibrocartilage is limited, especially in the menisci of the stifle joint and the intervertebral discs, to a few foci at its periphery. These vascular relationships coupled with a paucity of stem cells generally preclude good healing. Meniscal damage and intervertebral disc rupture usually compromise the vascular supply sufficiently to warrant the generalization that

Figure 8.11. Growing elastic cartilage of a porcine pinna. Chondroblasts *(1)* enlarge to become chondrocytes *(2)*. Chondrocytes may divide *(3)* to form isogenous groups *(4)*. Interstitial growth consists of new cells and matrix being added from within the mass of the cartilage. ×160.

Fibrocartilage is usually located at points of transition between DWFCT and cartilage and between DWFCT and bone. Fibrous cartilage imparts additonal strength to these points of transition and/or attachment. Also, this tissue is an important constituent of articulations. **This tissue does not have a perichondrium.**

MORPHOLOGICAL FEATURES: **Coarse collagenous bundles in parallel and/or V-shaped orientation predominate. Chondrocytes and limited amounts of matrical materials occur between the bundles.**

OCCURRENCE: **Intervertebral discs; attachments of certain tendons and ligaments to bone; menisci. (Plate IV.11).**

Maintenance and Repair of Cartilage

Because cartilaginous tissues are avascular, they are dependent totally upon diffusion of metabolites from capillary beds within the perichondrium. Nutritional compromise of the chondrocytes leads to degenerative changes that are apparent especially in thick cartilaginous masses of aged animals. Mineralization of the matrix is a common sequel to the aging process of cartilage.

The hyaline cartilage of the growth plate normally undergoes mineralization. This "normal" process may be perceived as an acceleration of the aging process. As the cells are displaced further away from their blood supply, they may be compromised nutritionally and mineralization of the matrix results.

The actual maintenance of the the cartilagnous matrix is the responsibility of the chondrocyte. These cells remove and replace fibrous and amorphous components. The intense basophilia of the capsular matrix reflects the ability of chondrocytes to add highly sulfated GAGs to the matrix.

Cartilage repair is not achieved to the same degree in all types of cartilage; nor, does the same type of cartilage achieve the same degree of repair in different locations. The age of the animals is a significant factor also.

The presence of a perichondrium ensures an ample and readily available supply of mesenchymal cells. The continued proliferation and differentiation of mesenchymal cells of the perichondrium is a characteristic feature of young, growing animals. This is complemented by interstitial growth. Damage to hyaline or elastic cartilage during this period is repaired readily by the appositional growth of the perichondrium and by interstitial growth. In the adult, however, the perichondrium is not active and some of its regenerative ability is lost.

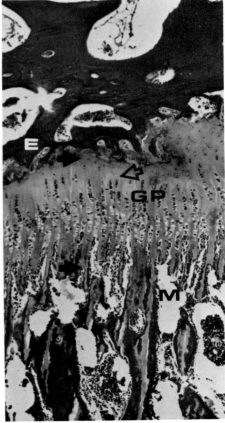

Figure 8.12. The growth plate of a developing bone. The growth plate *(GP)* consists of hyaline cartilage interdigitated between the bone of the epiphyseal endplate *(E)* and the complex tissues of the metaphysis *(M)*. The approximate limits of the physis are indicated by *solid arrows*. Stacks of young chondrocytes *(open arrow)* divide and form ordered columns of maturing cells. Each column represents a unique configuration of an isogenous group. The physis, therefore, grows by interstitial growth. ×16.

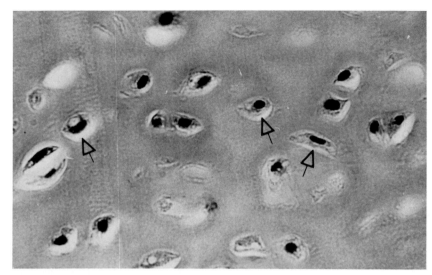

Figure 8.13. Mature chondrocytes within hyaline cartilage. The chondrocytes may occur as single cells or as components of isogenous groups. The lacunae *(open arrows)* are features of light microscopy, because the cellular limits artifactually shrink away from the margin of the matrix during processing. ×100.

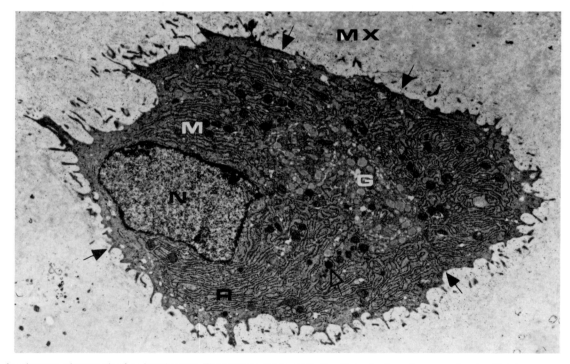

Figure 8.14. An electron micrograph of a chondrocyte. The nucleus *(N)* is vesicular. The cytoplasm has an extensive Golgi apparatus *(G)* and rough endoplasmic reticulum *(R)*. Mitochondria *(M)* and dense bodies *(open arrows)* are present also. The interface *(solid arrows)* between the cell and its matrix *(MX)* is intimate. Cellular processes extend into the matrix. Note that a lacunar space is not evident. ×5000.

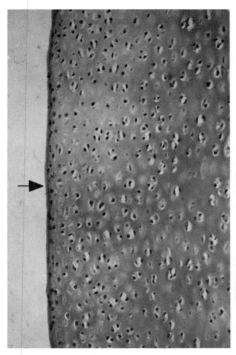

Figure 8.15. Articular surface of the proximal head of a canine humerus. The hyaline cartilage of the articular surface *(arrow)* is devoid of a perichondrium. ×38.

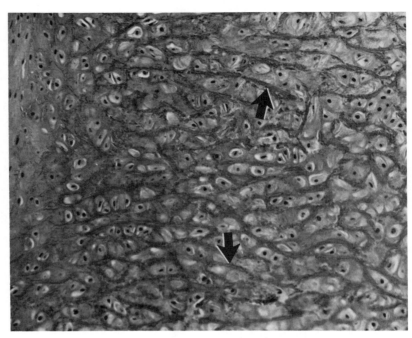

Figure 8.16. Elastic cartilage from a bovine epiglottis. The elastic fibers *(arrows)* are predominant features of the matrix. ×40.

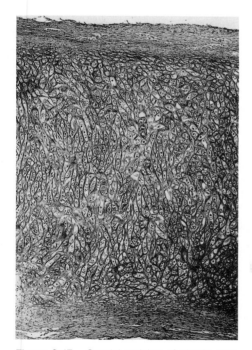

Figure 8.17. Special staining of elastic cartilage. The elastic fibers are stained black. ×13. (Verhoeff's stain.)

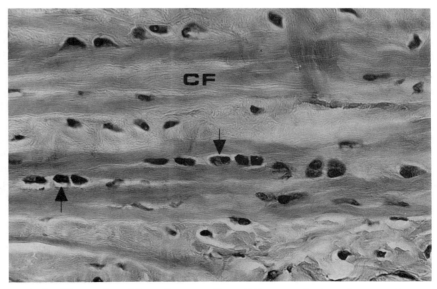

Figure 8.18. Fibrocartilage. The collagenous fibers *(CF)* are predominant features of this tissue. Chodrocytes within their lacunae *(arrows)* are spaced in an orderly manner between the fibers. ×100.

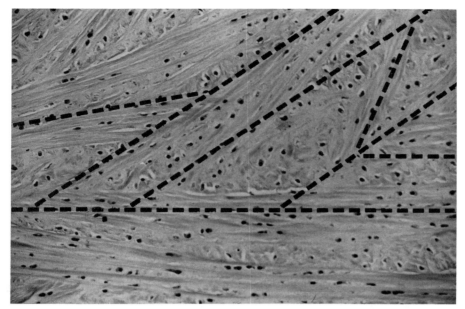

Figure 8.19. Fibrocartilage from a meniscus of a canine stifle. The herringbone configuration *(dashed lines)* is apparent readily in this section. ×40.

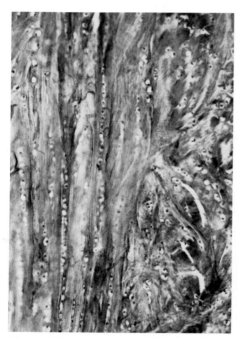

Figure 8.20. Fibrocartilage from an intervertebral disc. The herringbone configuration is not as apparent in this section as it is in Figure 8.19. ×39. (Verhoeff's stain.)

fibrocartilaginous repair potential is poor. This applies to the fibrocartilaginous interface at attachment points of ligaments and tendons to bone also.

The hyaline cartilage of the articular surface is a unique focus that is devoid of a perichondrium. The interstitial mechanism is active until adulthood is achieved. Superficial damage to the articular surface may be repaired by this mechanism. Any minor blemish to the matrix of the articular surface, in the young or adult animal, may be repaired by an increased secretion of matrix components. In the adult, articular cartilage repair varies with the extent and location of the damage. On the weight-bearing surface, superficial damage can only be repaired by compensatory secretion by the chondrocytes. If the damage were to extend through the cartilage to the subchondral bone (full-thickness defect), then a number of possibilities for repair exist. Stem cells associated with that region may differentiate into fibrous connective tissue, fibrocartilage, or bone. Under carefully controlled experimental conditions these stem cells may give rise to hyaline cartilage when subjected to continuous passive motion. Full-thickness defects of cartilage, however, may be repaired by transplanting autologous perichondral grafts over the damaged surface. The replacement of the hyaline cartilage by bone represents a degenerative change called *osteoarthrosis.*

Along the nonweight-bearing surface at the periphery of the articular cartilage, damage generally results in replacement with fibrocartilage.

The most ideal repair results in the re-placement of a particular tissue with an identical type of tissue. The repair of cartilage, especially that of the articular surface of the adult, is less than ideal or satisfactory. The replacement tissues do not have the same properties; therefore, structure and function are usually compromised.

References

Amprino, R.: On the incorporation of radiosulfate in the cartilage. Experientia *11*:65, 1955.

Anderson, H.C.: Vesicles associated with calcification of the matrix of epiphyseal cartilage. J. Cell Biol. *41*:59, 1969.

Cameron, D.A. and Robinson, R.A.: Electron microscopy of epiphyseal and articular cartilage matrix in the femur of the newborn infant. J. Bone Joint Surg. *40*:163, 1958.

Goodman, G.C. and Lane, N.: On the site of sulfation in the chondrocyte. J. Cell Biol. *21*:353, 1964.

Goodman, G.C. and Porter, K.R.: Chondrogenesis studies with the electron microscope. J. Biophys. Biochem. Cytol. *8*:719, 1960.

King, D.: The healing of semilunar cartilages. J. Bone Joint Surg. *18*:333, 1936.

Kuettner, K.E., Soble, L.W., Ray, R.D., Croxen, R.L., Passovoy, M. and Eisenstein, R.: Lysosome in epiphyseal cartilage. II. The effect of egg white lysozyme on mouse embryonic femurs in organ cultures. J. Cell Biol. *44*:329, 1970.

Lane, J.M. and Weiss, C.: Review of articular cartilage collagen research. Arthritis Rheum. *18*:553, 1975.

Larsson, S.E. and Kuettner, K.E.: Microchemical studies of acid glycosaminoglycans from isolated chondrocytes in suspension. Calc. Tiss. Res. *14*:49, 1974.

Maroudas, A.: Distribution and diffusion of solutes in articular cartilage. Biophys. J. *10*:365, 2970.

Meachin, G.: The effect of scarification on articular cartilage in the rabbit. J. Bone Joint Surg. *45(B)*:150, 1963.

Nemeth-Csoka, M.: The influence of inorganic phosphate and citrate anions on the effect of glycosaminoglycans during collagen fibril formation. Exp. Path. *14*:40, 1977.

Palfrey, A.J. and Davies, D.V.: The fine structure of the chondrocyte. J. Anat. *100*:213, 1966.

Pritchard, J.J.: A cytological and histochemical study of bone and cartilage formation in the rat. J. Anat. *86*:259, 1952.

Salter, R.B., Harris, D.J. and Clements, N.D.: The healing of bone and cartilage in transarticular fractures with continuous passive motion. Orthop. Trans. *2*:77, 1978.

Sheldon, H. and Robinson, R.A.: Studies on cartilage. I. Electron microscope observations on normal rabbit ear cartilage. J. Biophys. Biochem. Cytol. *4*:401, 1958.

Skoog, T. and Johansson, S.H.: The formation of articular cartilage from free perichondrial grafts. Plast. Reconstructr. Surg. *57*:1, 1976.

Sokoloff, L. (ed.): *The Joints and Synovial Fluid.* Academic Press, New York, 1978.

Spycher, M.A., Moor, H. and Ruettner, J.R.: Electron microscopic investigations on aging and osteoarthritic human articular cartilage. II. The fine structure of freeze-etched aging hip joint cartilage. Z. Zellforsch. *98*:512, 1969.

Svajger, A.: Chondrogenesis in the external ear of the rat. Z. Anat. Entwicklungsgesch. *131*:236, 1970.

Thyberg, J. and Friberg, U.: The lysosomal system in endochondral growth. Progr. Histochem. Cytochem. *10*:1, 1978.

9: Supportive Tissues—Bone

General Characteristics

Form and Function. Bone is a specialized connective tissue consisting of cells embedded within a gel-like substance that becomes mineralized. The method of secretion and the manner in which the cells become embedded in the matrix are similar to those phenomena observed in cartilage. The mineral phase is a distinctive feature of bone. The mineral component consists predominantly of *hydroxyapatite crystal (HAP)*. The organic matrix of bone is similar to cartilage.

Other characteristics distinguish bone from cartilage. Bone cells *(osteocytes)* are in contact with each other and surface cells (osteoblasts) through cellular processes located in small canals *(canaliculi)* in the matrix. The cellular processes are not only a means through which coordinated activities are mediated, but they and the canalicular space are significant in transport mechanisms through bone. Bone is an extremely vascular tissue. The cells of bone are rarely more than 2 mm from a supply of blood vessels. The mineralized matrix of bone is minimally expandable. Bone, therefore, is unable to grow by the interstitial mechanism. **Appositional growth is the only mechanism by which bone tissue can grow.** This requires a copious supply of *stem cells*.

The stem cells of bone, osteoblasts, and osteoclasts are located in covering membranes called the *periosteum* and *endosteum*. Because of the periosteal and endosteal relationships to bone, all surfaces of bone (except some in old age) are covered by cells.

Bone satisfies some important metabolic requirements by virtue of its labile nature. Once formed, the mineral of bone is not irreversibly sequestered in the body. Rather, the mineral may be mobilized by distinct mechanisms. Bone functions, therefore, as an important dynamic store (sink) of calcium and phosphate (and other bone-seeking substances). Bone is metabolically active and constantly changing. The extensive vascular supply to bone gives some insights to its viability and metabolic activity. The cells of bone are responsive to numerous and varied stimuli. Numerous hormones act "in concert" upon bone, influencing directly its cellular activity and, indirectly, its intercellular substance. Mechanical forces acting upon bone influence the amount of bone in the skeleton as well as its three-dimensional distribution.

To say that bone is not different than other tissues would be a definite overstatement. All of the essential physiological activities conducted by other tissues are conducted by bone. Bone cells must perform these activities within the confines of a mineralized matrix. This imposes some interesting features to bone.

One of the interesting features of bone as a tissue relates directly to its mineralized matrix. Whereas the turnover of matrical components in other connective tissues must be observed indirectly with various types of labels, the turnover of bone matrix may be evaluated by direct observation. Observations of the matrix, therefore, afford useful insights into the tissue as a whole. **The matrix of bone is a telltale record of the events that had occurred previously.**

Classification. Two types of bone tissue exist. Bone is either *woven (immature, fibrous)*, or *lamellar (mature).* Both of these tissues may be arranged differently into distinct *configurations*. These configurations, *cancellous (spongy, trabecular) bone* or *compact bone* (Fig. 9.1), are visible grossly, radiographically, and microscopically.

Remembering that bone is both a tissue and an organ is important. **Bone as a tissue can grow only by appositional growth; bone as an organ grows by appositional and interstitial growth.**

Matrical Components

Introduction. The matrical components of bone constitute a major portion of the tissue mass. The extracellular matrix, occupying between 92 and 95% of the tissue volume, consists of various organic and inorganic constituents: *collagen, sugars, glycoproteins, proteoglycans, glycosaminoglycans (GAGs), peptides, lipids, organic ions, inorganic ions, and water.* Many factors influence the types and quantities of the constituents—age, species, state of health, bone type, bone configuration. Although a pure sample of bone is difficult to obtain, chemical analyses of bone have been performed and reasonably reliable values for diaphyseal compact bone have been obtained. The organic matrix constitutes about 22% of the weight of a bone sample. The inorganic materials account for 69%, whereas bone contains about 9% water.

Organic Matrix. The organic *matrix* of bone, called *osteoid*, consists of a fibrous *stroma* and *amorphous ground substance.* *Collagen*, the predominant ingredient of the matrix, constitutes about 90% of the organic matrix. The remaining 10% of the organic material is the amorphous ground substance. Conjugated proteins, small amounts of proteoglycans, and very small amounts of lipids are components of the matrix. Interfibrillar substances may function as foci for the initiation of mineralization.

Various proteins, including *sialoproteins, glycoproteins*, and *phosphoproteins*, have been isolated from bone. Sialoproteins with a high calcium-binding capacity may contribute to the mineralization process. Phosphoproteins, too, have the ability to bind calcium; they may contribute to the mineralization process also. Other proteins, including plasma proteins (albumin, α_2HS-glycoprotein, γ-carboxyglutamic acid-containing proteins) have been isolated from bone, but their functional significance has not been determined.

Proteoglycans with chondroitin-4-sulfate and keratan sulfate are part of the osteoid. Also, hyaluronic acid is present. The onset of mineralization in bone is known to be accompanied by the removal of proteoglycans from the matrix. Proteoglycans may function as initiators and inhibitors of mineralization. Phospholipids may be involved in the mineralization process. Although the water content of bone is described as 9%, this value varies with the age of the animal and the degree to which the skeleton is mineralized.

Inorganic Matrix. The mineral phase of bone is about 69% of the weight of bone. About one-half of the maximal mineral-holding capacity of bone is deposited at the time of initial mineralization. With time, approximately a year, a given sample of bone will achieve 100% mineralization.

HAP crystal is the predominant salt

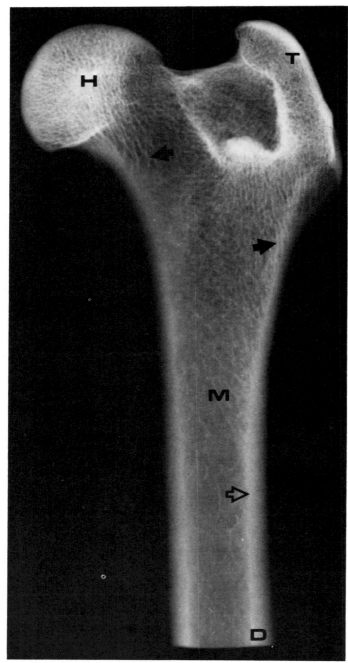

Figure 9.1. A radiograph of the proximal portion of a longitudinally sectioned canine femoral bone. Note the cancellous *(solid arrow)* and compact *(open arrows)* bone. *H*, head; *T*, greater trochanter; *M*, marrow cavity; *D*, diaphysis.

bones are loaded along their long axes. Such loading corresponds, generally, to the orientation of osteons within diaphyseal compacta and the general orientation of stacked laminae of collagenous fibers in osteons. **The tensile properties of bone relate directly to the tensile properties of its constituent collagenous fibers.** The ability of bone to resist tensile stress is about one-half its ability to resist compressive stress. **Compressive stress properties relate to the mineral content of bone.**

The collagen of bone is usually organized into highly ordered arrays. In *mature bones* this organizational pattern is manifested as layers of collagenous fibers deposited upon each other in a helical pattern; each layer of a helix is oriented at a different angle to the previous layer (Fig. 9.2). The angle of collagenous fiber orientation between successive laminae may be acute, 90° or obtuse. The pattern of fiber orientation, responsible partially for the tensile properties of bone, imparts a lamellar appearance to mature bone *(lamellar bone)* that is especially apparent with polarizing microscopy (Fig. 3.7).

The microcrystalline structure of HAP provides for a surface area of about 200 m^2/g of crystal. The three-dimensional array of the crystal provides an enormous surface area for absorption and exchange of materials between itself and the surrounding, metastable fluid of the extracellular compartment.

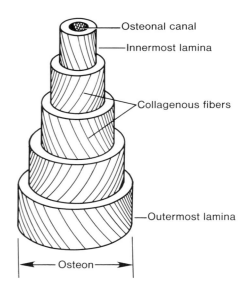

Figure 9.2. A diagram of an osteon. The concentric laminae of bone have been removed partially to show the orientation of collagenous fibers within each lamina. In this example, collagenous fibers within each laminae are oriented at approximately 90° to each other. The osteon is an elongated structure (cylinder) comprised of successive laminae of bone matrix. The relationship of the fibers to the apatitie crystals is not indicated.

within a sample of bone that has achieved mineralization maturity. Numerous salts are involved in the phase transitions from salts of initiation to salts of maturity. *Dicalcium phosphate dihydrate* progresses to an *octacalcium phosphate*; eventually the transition leads to the formation of *amorphous calcium phosphate*. Thermodynamic stability is achieved with the formation of the HAP crystal.

HAP has the chemical formula $Ca_5(PO_4)_3OH$. Numerous substitutions occur in vivo that reduce the theoretical calcium:phosphate molar ratio to less than the 1.66 expected. Among the numerous substituted elements and compounds are: Na^+, Mg^{++}, $CO_3^=$, F^-, Pb^{++}, Sr^{++}, citrate, phosphate esters, diphosphonates, pyrophosphates, and amino acids.

Functional Correlates. The tensile properties of bone, or the resistance to elongate when stretched (loaded), are greatest when

Preparation of Bone Samples. The histological study of bone may be approached by examination of either *demineralized* or *mineralized (ground)* sections. Demineralization is accomplished by two primary means, *chelation* or *acid hydrolysis*. Demineralization, sometimes referred to as *decalcification*, results in the removal of the mineral phase of bone. The organic material that remains after this type of treatment is called *osteoid*. Thin sections of bone may be obtained for study by this particular approach. Sections of bone prepared by this method retain near normal matrical relationships. Good cytological detail is retained also.

Mineralized samples must be cut with a diamond-tipped saw blade or ground on an abrasive material. Sample thickness of 50-100 μm can be obtained. Cytological detail is not retained with this method; however, the nature of the matrix supplies valuable information about cellular activity. Micrographs used in this chapter are of bone samples that have been prepared by both of these techniques. **Unless otherwise specified in the caption, micrographs of bone were obtained from demineralized sections.**

Envelopes of Bone

The cellular population of bone is distributed throughout the tissue in two distinct loci. The osteocytic subset is located within the osseous matrix. The other cells are located on bone surfaces within morphologically distinct envelopes called the *periosteum* and the *endosteum*. Morphologically, the cellular populations of these envelopes appear identical; however, they are not identical functionally. Differential cellular responsiveness of these subsets occurs during growth and aging. Differential responses to various types of stimulation occur in health as well as in disease.

Periosteum

The *periosteum* is the outer covering of a bone (Fig. 9.3). This envelope covers the entire bone, except for the articular surfaces. The covering must be incised or removed before the underlying osseous tissue is visible directly. The periosteum consists of fibrous and cellular layers. The fibrous layer is dense white fibrous connective tissue (DWFCT) considered to be the capsule of the organ (Fig. 9.4). Collagenous fibers of ligaments and tendons blend with and pass through this fibrous capsule before becoming anchored to the osseous tissue beneath it. The cellular layer of the periosteum consists of mesenchymal cells, osteoprogenitor cells, osteoblasts, and osteoclasts. The periosteum is well-vascularized.

During development, osteogenic cells of this envelope increase the diameter of the diaphysis. In the adult, the envelope is re-

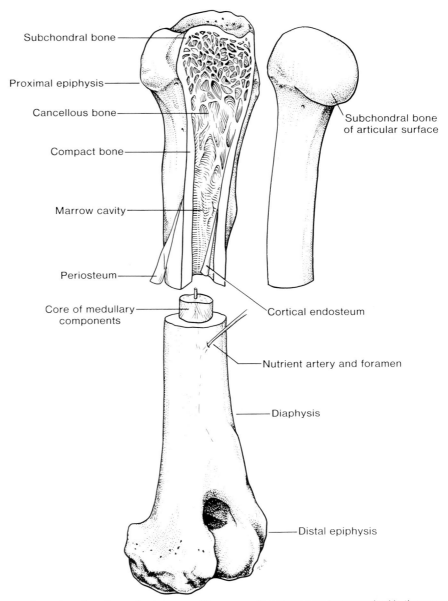

Figure 9.3. Drawing of a canine humerus. The preparation of the specimen resulted in the removal of the articular cartilage. The periosteum covers all external bone surfaces except those of the articulations. The endosteum covers all internal bone surfaces. Compare with Figure 9.6.

Labels in figure: Subchondral bone — Proximal epiphysis — Cancellous bone — Compact bone — Marrow cavity — Periosteum — Core of medullary components — Subchondral bone of articular surface — Cortical endosteum — Nutrient artery and foramen — Diaphysis — Distal epiphysis

sponsible for the maintenance of the associated bone surface. Bone remodeling and fracture repair activities are manifested at this surface also. This envelope is responsive to various insults that result in *periosteal new bone* formation.

Endosteum

The *endosteum* is the inner and internal covering of bone as an organ and tissue (Fig. 9.5). The compact bone adjacent to the marrow cavity, the trabecular bone of the marrow cavity and the osteonal canals within the substance of the compact bone are lined by elements of the endosteal envelope. Three subdivisions of the endosteum are named on the basis of their ana-

tomical distribution and differential functional responsiveness. The three subsets of the endosteum are: *cortical endosteum, trabecular endosteum, osteonal endosteum.* The cortical endosteum is the envelope that covers the compact bone and defines the peripheral limit of the marrow cavity (Fig. 9.6). The cortical endosteum is continuous with the trabecular endosteum covering the osseous trabeculae of the marrow cavity. In most long bones, the trabeculae and their associated envelopes are confined generally to the proximal and distal epiphyses and metaphyses (Fig. 9.6). The cortical and trabecular endosteal envelopes may be considered the inner lining of bone. The osteonal endosteum lines the osteonal canals (Figs.

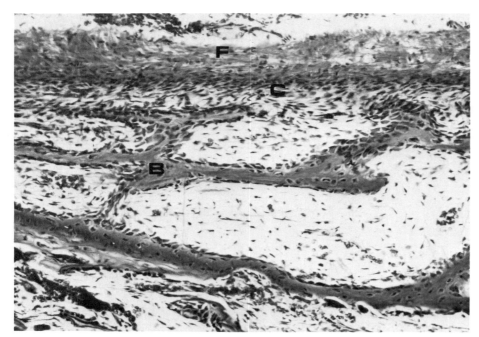

Figure 9.4. Periosteum of a developing long bone. The fibrous *(F)* portion of the periosteum consists of DWFCT, whereas the cellular *(C)* portion of the periosteum consists of different types of bone cells. The cellular component of the periosteum is evident especially during growth and fracture repair, as well as in response to insults other than fracture. Bone spicules *(B)* have formed as a result of periosteal activity. ×40.

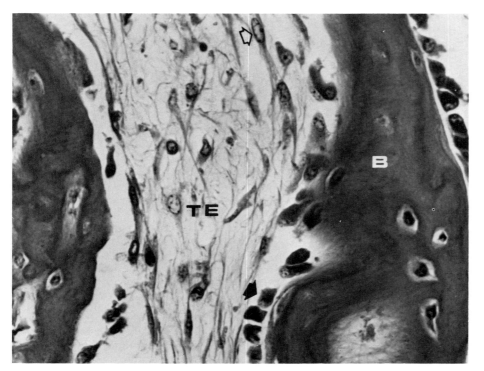

Figure 9.5. Trabecular endosteum within a bovine fetal jaw. The trabecular endosteum *(TE)* consists of loose connective tissue. Stem cells *(open arrow)* occur within the loose connective tissue of the endosteum; they are the source of cells for the loose connective tissue, as well as for the bone. Osteoblasts *(solid arrow)* occur at the interface between the connective tissue of the endosteum and the bone. Some of the spindle-shaped cells similar to that indicated by the *open arrow* could be osteoprogenitor cells. *B,* bone. ×100.

9.7 and 9.8). The osteonal endosteum may be considered the internal lining of bone. This envelope is continuous with the periosteal and cortical endosteal envelopes. The osteonal endosteum provides cellular continuity from the external surface through the substance of bone to the inner surface of gross bones.

The cellular layer of the endosteum consists of cells identical to those within the periosteum. The endosteum, however, is a loose connective tissue (Fig. 9.5). at the periphery of which are located the typical cells of bone.

Developmentally, the periosteum gives rise to and is continuous with all subdivisions of the endosteum. This continuity is apparent in the Volkmann's canals (Figs. 9.6 and 9.7).

Cellular Components

Relationships of Cells

Classically, the mesenchymal cells associated with bone have been described as differentiating into the specific cells of bone—osteoprogenitor cells, osteoblasts, osteocytes and osteoclasts. Moreover, these cell types have been described as being nonfixed, postmitotic cells, the products of mesenchymal cell modulation. Current evidence clearly establishes that two distinct lines of cells constitute the bone cell populations. The osteogenic cells are derived from mesenchymal cells. *Osteoprogenitor cells,* differentiating from mesenchymal cells, are mitotic and continue to differentiate into *osteoblasts.* Osteoblasts continue through their life cycle as *osteocytes. Osteoclasts* are *multinucleated giant cells* that form as fusion products of macrophages. Both cell lines are essential for the proper maintenance of the skeleton. The relationships of these cells are detailed in Figure 9.9.

Mesenchymal Cells

The morphology of this cell has been described elsewhere (Fig. 9.10). Although mesenchymal cells are present in osseous envelopes, there is evidence that the mesenchymal cells are not capable of differentiating into all of the typical mesenchymal cell derivatives. Rather, the mesenchymal cell seems to have a limited potency that is established early in development. Some mesenchymal cell populations are osteogenically competent and differentiate into osteoprogenitor cells.

Osteoprogenitor Cells

The *osteoprogenitor cell* is also called an *osteogenic cell.* These cells are similar morphologically to mesenchymal cells. They are identified on the basis of their location on bone surfaces or within the envelopes of bone as cells peripheral to osteoblasts, their

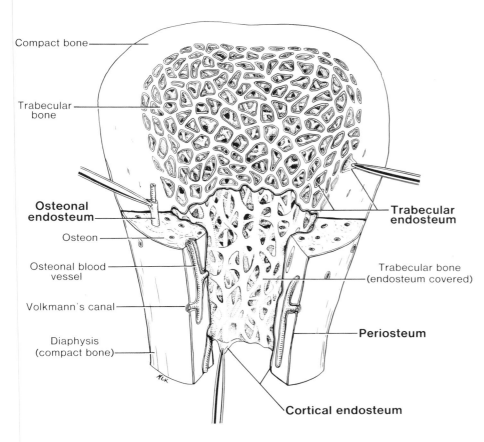

Compact bone

Trabecular bone

Osteonal endosteum

Osteon

Osteonal blood vessel

Volkmann's canal

Diaphysis (compact bone)

Trabecular endosteum

Trabecular bone (endosteum covered)

Periosteum

Cortical endosteum

Figure 9.6. Drawing of a sectioned long bone. The endosteum covers all internal bone surfaces. Compare with Figures 9.3 and 9.7.

ultrastructural features and their ability to incorporate tritiated thymidine (Fig. 9.10). The osteoprogenitor cell is the only bone cell that actively divides, as evidenced by the active uptake of tritiated thymidine. This marker subsequently appears in osteoblasts.

The presence of mitotically active osteoprogenitor cells ensures a plentiful supply of stem cells used in growth, maintenance, remodeling, and repair.

Osteoblasts

These cells are the bone-forming cells of the body. They are responsible for the secretion of procollagen and other organic matrical components. They are also the storage cells of the mineral used in mineralization.

Osteoblasts or osteoprogenitor cells cover most bone surfaces. During periods of inactivity, osteoblasts assume a spindle shape (Fig. 9.11). During inactive periods of their life cycles they are called *inactive osteoblasts.* Spindle-shaped cells, however, may also be osteoprogenitor cells, because active osteoblasts become apparent on these surfaces subsequently (Fig. 9.11). The cytoplasm is weakly basophilic and surrounds a single oval or round nucleus. During periods of activity the cells hypertrophy and become polarized (Fig. 9.12). They assume definite epithelioid characteristics. The single nucleus, with a prominent nucleolus, is

displaced to the end of the cell away from the bone surface. The cytoplasm is moderately basophilic due to the high content of ribosomal ribonucleic acid. A well-developed Golgi apparatus and numerous mitochondria are characteristic (Plate II.5).

Calcium is an essential ion for the proper operation of various cellular systems. The low but closely regulated levels of intracellular calcium favor the movement of this ion into the cell. Calcium exchange for sodium at osteoblastic plasma membranes and active transport mechanisms involving magnesium and adenosine triphosphate help to maintain appropriate levels of intracellular calcium. Excess intracellular calcium, which is cytotoxic, is sequestered by various organelles. Calcium-binding proteins aid in the sequestration process. Mitochondria assist with the calcium sequestration process. This mechanism is manifested morphologically as the appearance of calcium-laden *mitochondrial granules.* The sequestered calcium can move between the granules and the cytosol. Osteoblasts have numerous mitochondrial granules that may be part of the normal mineralization sequence. These cells may store calcium and release it on demand.

The activity of osteoblasts along a bone-forming surface is well-synchronized. The cells produce approximately 2 μm^3 of osteoid per day. This osteoid accumulates, layer upon layer, until a definitive *osteoid*

seam approximately 10–15 μm thick is apparent. This osteoid seam, which has never been mineralized, is a lighter pink (hematoxylin and eosin [H and E]) than the mineralized osteoid (Fig. 9.13). The osteoid seam is set apart from the remaining osteoid by a dark-staining *reversal band,* the region from which centripetal mineralization of the osteoid seam progresses. The osteoid seam is apparent with mineralized sections and special staining techniques (Fig. 9.14 and Plate I.9). Osteoid seam is organic matrix that has never been but ultimately will become mineralized.

The secretory activity of the osteoblast is biphasic. The first phase of activity involves the synthesis and secretion of organic materials. Tropocollagen polymerizes outside the cell and becomes oriented in an orderly manner (Fig. 9.2). Orientation of the collagenous fibers may result from osteoblastic influences, response to stress, or a combination of both factors. The first phase culminates in the formation of the osteoid seam. **The second phase of this activity is the mineralization of the osteoid seam.** Calcium ions that had been stored in the osteoblast, especially in the mitochondria, are released from the cell and react with the collagen. Mineralization occurs first on and subsequently within the collagenous fibers. The attachment of some GAGs to collagen may prevent mineralization of the osteoid seam during the first

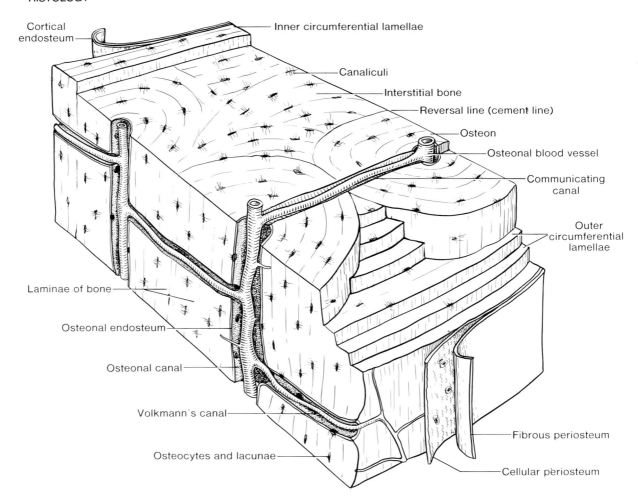

Figure 9.7. Diagram of a section of compact bone from a diaphysis. All typical structures have been included and labeled. Not all cross sections of diaphyseal bone, however, will consist of all these features.

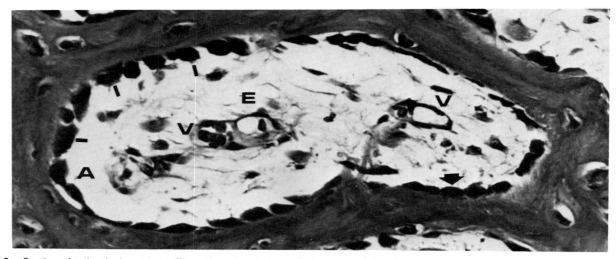

Figure 9.8. Section of a developing osteon. The osteonal endosteum (E) is surrounded by bone that was formed by the cellular components of the endosteum. Loose connective tissue and blood vessels (V) are components of the envelope. Active osteoblasts (bars) and inactive osteoblasts (or osteoprogenitor cells) are present (arrow). The endosteum was separated from the bone (A) as a result of sectioning. Continuous centripetal deposition of bone along the peripheral margin of the endosteum will increase the bone mass while reducing the mass of the endosteum. Compare with Figure 9.32. ×100.

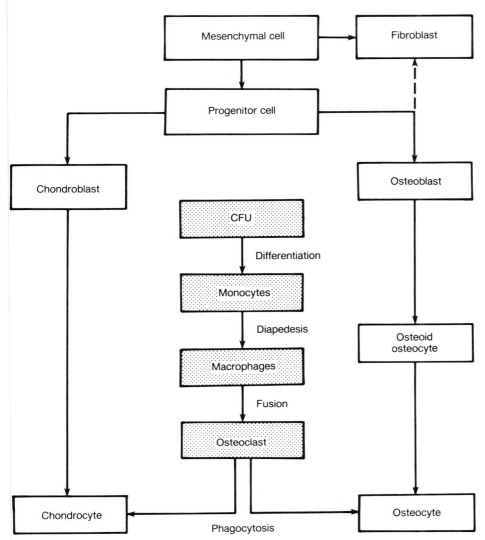

Figure 9.9. Diagram demonstrating the dual origin of the cells associated with bone and cartilage. The osteoprogenitor cell is an established cell in the differentiation sequence for bone cells. The same or a similar cell is presumed to be in the differentiation sequence for cartilage. The osteoclast is derived from monocytes.

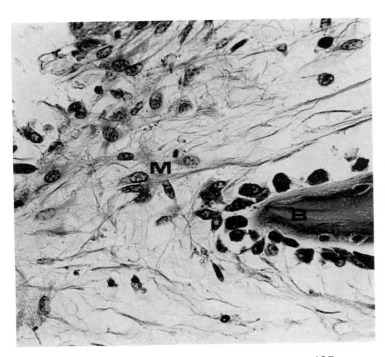

Figure 9.10. Stem cells of bone located within an endosteal envelope. The stem cells (M) of bone are considered to be the mesenchymal cells. The stem cells indicated in the micrograph may be mesenchymal or osteoprogenitor cells. A spicule of bone (B) is covered by osteoblasts. ×100.

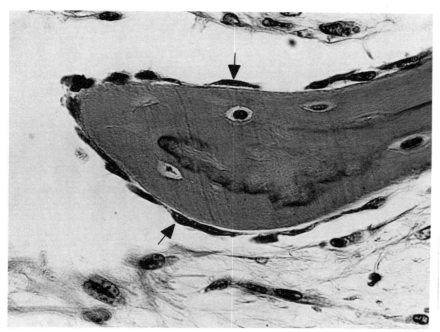

Figure 9.11. Lining cells upon a spicule of bone. The lining cells *(arrows)* may be inactive osteoblasts or osteoprogenitor cells. The empty space above and to the left of the bone is an artifact of processing. ×160.

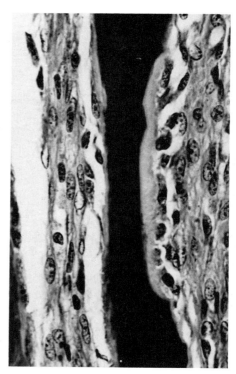

Figure 9.13. Osteoid seam in a demineralized section of bone. The light-staining region adjacent to and at the right of the black portion of the spicule is osteoid seam. ×140.

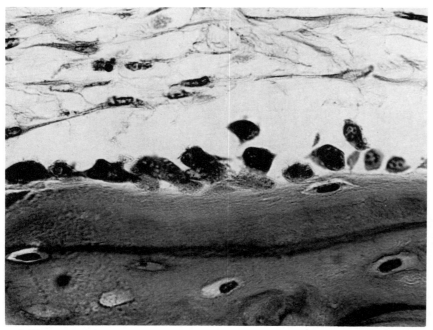

Figure 9.12. Active lining cells upon a bone surface. The cuboidal and columnar cells are active osteoblasts. Compare with Plate II.5. ×160.

phase. Subsequent removal of some of these substances, then, may facilitate the mineralization of the matrix. Initial mineralization accounts for approximately one-half of the total holding capacity of the matrix. Gradual and progressive addition of mineral occurs over several months at the expense of water.

The progressive formation and subsequent mineralization of osteoid seam accounts for the highly ordered and laminar characteristics of mature bone (Fig. 9.15). Disruptions and/or alterations in this orderly sequence alter the quantity and quality of bone formed. If the first phase does not occur, then continual osteoclasia without the balanced formation by osteoblasts results in a quantitative reduction in bone—a *quantitative osteopenia*. If the second phase of the osteoblastic acitivity does not occur, then the organic matrix does not become mineralized. This results in a qualitative change in bone—a *qualitative osteopenia*.

A quantitative osteopenia is a reduction in bone mass/unit volume. The bone present is normal; there just is not enough of it. Cushing's syndrome, disuse osteoporosis, and senile osteoporosis are diseases characterized by quantitative bone changes. **The qualitative bone changes result from too little mineral in the matrix.** There may be adequate to excessive amounts of matrix with insufficient amounts of mineral. Rickets, renal secondary hyperparathyroidism, and nutritional secondary hyperparathyroidism are examples of diseases associated with qualitative bone changes.

As the osteoblasts secrete their products and retreat before the advancing front of osteoid, a few of the cells (about one of 10) become embedded in their own secretory products. At this point the osteoblasts are called osteocytes.

Osteocytes

Osteocytes are osteoblasts that have become embedded in their own secretory products. Osteocytes are sometimes ob-

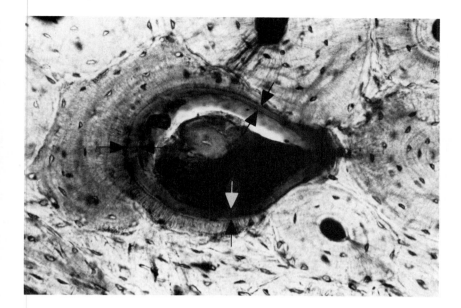

Figure 9.14. Osteoid seam in a mineralized sample of bone. The *arrows* delimit the osteoid seam. The centripetal formation of bone in this filling osteon by the progressive deposition and mineralization of osteoid seams would have reduced the diameter of the osteonal canal. A mature osteon *(lower right)* would have resulted. ×25 (ground bone section). Compare with Plate I.9.

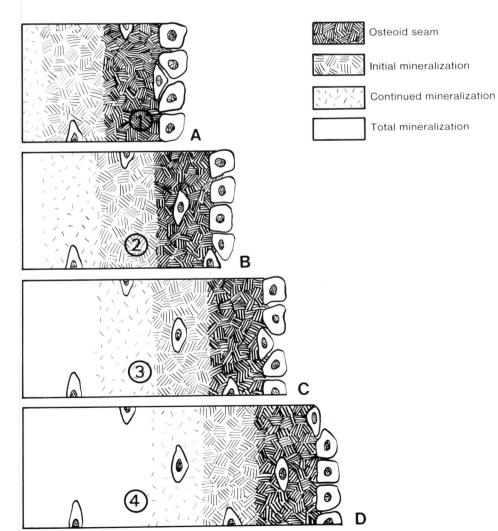

Osteoid seam

Initial mineralization

Continued mineralization

Total mineralization

Figure 9.15. Biphasic activity of osteoblasts during osteogenesis. Bone formation in an adult occurs on preexisting bone surfaces. The initial stage of osteoblastic activity culminates with the formation of osteoid seam upon a pre-existing bone surface *(A)*. Initial mineralization occurs within the most recent osteoid seam *(B)*. New osteoid seam forms, while older osteoid seams become progressively more mineralized *(C)*. This activity continues *(D)* until a specified amount of bone forms. Numbers *1–4* indicate the fate and relative position of the initial osteoid seam that had been formed in this diagram.

served shortly after they have become embedded in the osteoid seam as *osteoid osteocytes* (Fig. 9.16). Once the interstitial substance becomes mineralized, these cells are simply referred to as osteocytes.

Osteocytic processes are prominent features of these cells, and the cytoplasm is either weakly basophilic or acidophilic. The osteocyte is a less active form of the osteoblast. The *lacuna* and the contained cell may vary from round to lenticular. As a result of fixation, osteocytes are retracted from lacunar surfaces. Occasionally, lacunae may appear empty; this may be an artifact of sectioning or an indication of pathology.

The cellular processes of osteocytes are not readily seen with the light microscope. The *canaliculi* are easily observed in mineralized sections (Fig. 9.17). Visualization of canaliculi in paraffin sections is enhanced by reducing the quality of the illumination. Canaliculi form an extensive communicative network between osteocytes (Fig. 9.17). Each canaliculus is occupied by a cellular process of an osteocyte (Fig. 9.18). The osteocytic processes and associated canaliculi extend to and are in contact with the cells at the periosteal and endosteal surfaces (Fig. 9.19). These contacts between osteocytes facilitate coordination of their activities. Similar contacts

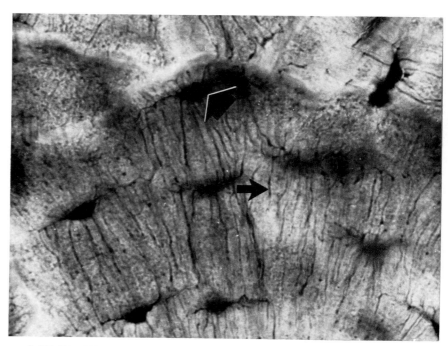

Figure 9.17. A portion of the canalicular system of bone. Osteocytic lacunae *(large arrow)* are continuous with canaliculi *(small arrow)*. The canaliculi form an extensive communication and transport network throughout the matrix of bone. ×200 (ground bone section).

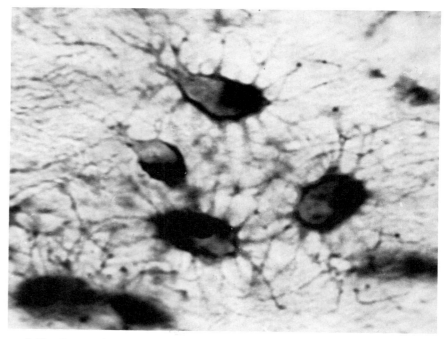

Figure 9.18. Osteocytic processes and canaliculi. The extensive canalicular system contains osteocytic processes of adjacent cells. The canaliculi are continuous with each other. The osteocytic processes contained therein from contiguous osteocytes are in contact with each other. ×320 (ground bone section).

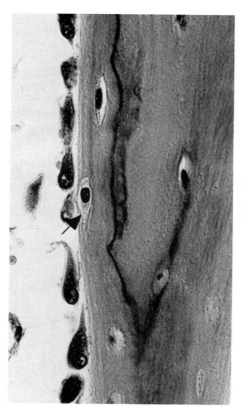

Figure 9.16. Osteoblasts and osteocytes. An osteoblast was recently incorporated into bone as an osteoid osteocyte *(arrow)*. ×160.

with surface cells—osteoblasts—ensures coordination with these cells also. These contacts provide for the coordinated activity of the *osteocyte-osteoblast pump*, a mechanism for the homeostatic maintenance of plasma calcium levels.

The osteocytes, once the "forgotten cells of bone," are responsible for the maintenance of the matrix. They synthesize and secrete matrical materials; however, their activity level is less than that of osteoblasts. Also, they are capable of removing matrix

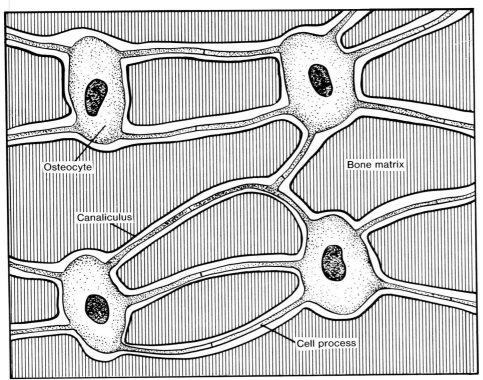

Figure 9.19. A diagram illustrating osteocytic relationships. Junctional complexes occur at the points of contact with each other. Also, osteocytic processes contact surface osteoblasts.

by a process termed *osteocytic osteolysis*. The ability of these cells to add and remove bone matrix is an important mechanism in the homeostatic maintenance of blood calcium level.

The functional duplicity of the osteocytes ensures the maintenance of skeletal volume and proper levels of calcium in the plasma. The 23,000 osteocytes/mm^3 of tissue affords an extensive lacunar surface upon which these cells are able to function.

Osteoclasts

Osteoclasts are *multinucleated giant cells* of the body responsible for the removal of bone. These cells possess the cellular mechanisms necessary for the dissolution of bone mineral as well as the digestion of the organic matrix. Their releasing organic acids (citrate, lactate) decreases the pH of the immediate microenvironment. The acids dissolve the bone mineral and enhance the activity of lysosomal enzymes that are released; acid hydrolases actively hydrolyze the organic matrix. The process of bone removal mediated by osteoclasts is termed *osteoclasia*. These cells have few to numerous nuclei contained within a foamy and acidophilic cytoplasm (Fig. 9.20). The cells are polarized; the nuclei are displaced to the cellular border away from the bone (Plate II.4). The cellular border adjacent to the bone is composed of numerous cellular processes—a *brush border* (Fig. 9.21). This

brush or *ruffled border* terminates at a smooth zone at the periphery that serves as a tight seal between the cell and bone surface. This confines the pH change to the region subjacent to the ruffled border.

Osteoclasts reside on the surfaces of bones in concavities called *Howship's lacunae* (Fig. 9.22). The cells may be artifactually separated from the surface by sectioning. Osteoclasts may be observed along a bone surface in which bone deposition is occurring (Fig. 9.23), or an entire surface

may be occupied by osteoclasts. Osteoclasts also develop within compact bone from macrophages within the osteonal endosteum. In this instance, Howship's lacunae are continuous with each other as a *resorption space* (Fig. 9.24). The resorption space is the cross-sectional representation of a cylindrical portion of bone that was being removed by osteoclasia. The serrated edges of Howship's lacunae are evidence that bone resorption was occurring.

Osteoclasts are derived from macrophages.

Types of Bone

All of the bones are composed of either woven or lamellar bone. They are the two types of osseous tissues (Fig. 9.25).

Woven Bone

This type of bone is called *immature bone*, *coarsely bundled bone*, or *woven bone*. It is very cellular, and the lacunae are very large and round (Fig. 9.26). The lacunae and their contained cells are dispersed randomly throughout the matrix. Bundles of collagenous fibers are arranged in a random pattern; thus, there is no regular birefringent pattern with polarizing microscopy. The organic matrix is basophilic, stains unevenly, and holds less mineral than mature bone.

Immature bone is the first bone that forms in ossification centers of the fetus and the primary spongiosa of developing adolescent bones. It is also the first bone that forms at the site of fracture repair. Certain types of bone tumors are characterized by this type of bone. Normally, it occurs in alveolar bone associated with teeth and at points of attachment of ligaments and tendons to bone.

Although this type of bone may vary in configuration from cancellous to compact, osteons are rarely composed of this tissue.

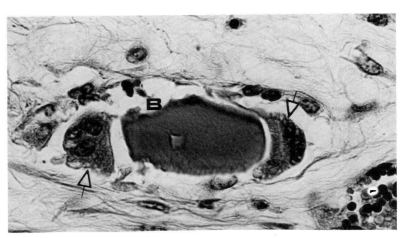

Figure 9.20. A spicule of bone and osteoclastic activity. A spicule of bone *(B)* is being removed by the activity of osteoclasts. Osteoclasts *(arrows)* are multinucleated giant cells derived through the fusion of macrophages. ×160.

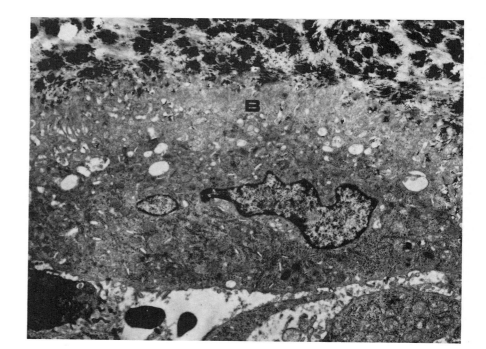

Figure 9.21. An electron micrograph of an osteoclast. The cell is multinucleated and polarized. The brush or ruffled border *(B)* is in contact with the bone surface. ×5000.

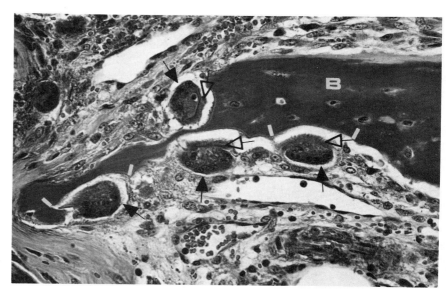

Figure 9.22. A spicule of bone and multiple foci of osteoclasia. A spicule of bone *(B)* is being removed and/or remodeled by numerous osteoclasts *(solid arrows)*. The boundaries of Howships's lacunae are indicated by the *white bars*. Note the brush or ruffled borders *(open arrows)* and their relationships to the serrated margins of the bone. ×100. (Masson's trichrome).

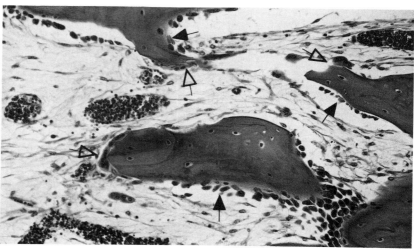

Figure 9.23. Simultaneous deposition and removal of bone. Osteoblastic *(solid arrows)* and osteoclastic activity *(open arrows)* are occurring at the same time. ×40.

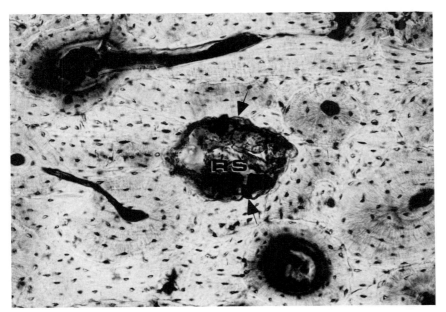

Figure 9.24. A resorption space in bone. The resorption space *(RS)* has serrated edges *(arrows)* due to the confluence of Howship's lacunae. ×40 (ground bone section).

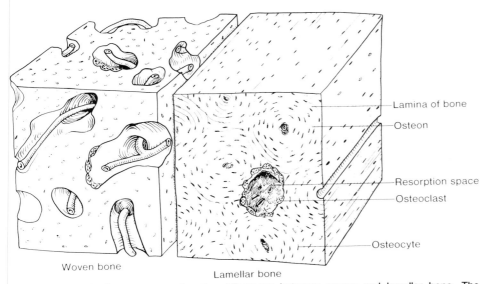

Woven bone

Lamellar bone

Lamina of bone

Osteon

Resorption space

Osteoclast

Osteocyte

Figure 9.25. A diagram comparing the differences between woven and lamellar bone. The organizational differences are marked. Especially note the difference in the disposition of osteocytic lacunae. Lamellar bone comprises the bulk of the adult skeletal mass, whereas woven bone is limited in occurrence in the adult skeleton.

Under normal circumstances, this bone is always replaced by lamellar bone. It is a temporary tissue that affords support for the developing organism.

Lamellar Bone

This bone is also called *mature bone.* It constitutes the bulk of the adult skeleton. The lacunae, and thus the cells of this bone, are more lenticular than in immature bone. Also, the lacunae are dispersed in an orderly fashion throughout the matrix in a pattern that reflects the ordered, lamellar arrangement of the collagen (Fig. 9.27).

The collagenous fibers are deposited in helical array at varying angles in successive lamellae; thus, a very ordered pattern of birefringence is apparent with polarizing microscopy (Figs. 3.7 and 9.2). The demineralized organic matrix of mature bone stains lightly and evenly with acidic dyes.

Configurations of Bone

Cancellous Bone

Cancellous bone is arranged into *spicules* or *trabeculae.* Many of these spicules are actually *plates* of bone when examined

three-dimensionally. These spicules may be either *woven bone* or *mature bone.* In the adult skeleton they are composed of mature bone.

The diagnostic feature of cancellous bone is the impression of more interosseous space than bone (Fig. 9.28). There are, however, numerous gradations of this type of configuration (Fig. 9.29). The degree of porosity is the basis of classifying bone as cancellous or compact. The *bone porosity* or amount of interosseous space in cancellous bone ranges from approximately 30 to 95%.

Compact Bone

Compact bone represents the extreme amount of bone in a given volume of tissue. Bone occupies more than 30% of the tissue volume in this configuration (Fig. 9.30); however, gradations exist. Compact bone may be organized into *laminae (lamellae)* or *osteons (Haversian systems).*

Organization of Bone

Lamellae of Bone

Bone deposition in a successive laminar pattern is typical of the bone-forming activity of the *periosteum* and *endosteum.* Successive *lamellae* or *laminae* of mature bone are deposited in extensive sheets of bone called the *outer circumferential lamellae* or *periosteal lamellae* (Fig. 9.31). The cortical endosteum also forms laminae of bone. This bone constitutes the *inner circumferential lamellae* or *endosteal lamellae* (Fig. 9.32). The inner lamellae may continue as part of the trabeculae of bone of the marrow cavity.

Osteonal Bone

Osteonal bone is the lamellar bone that comprises *osteons* or *Haversian systems* (Figs. 9.33 and 9.34). The bone is disposed in concentric laminae or sheets around an *osteonal canal* or *Haversian canal* (Fig. 9.35). The peripheral limits of the osteonal bone are marked by a *reversal line* or *cement line.* The osteonal canal contains blood vessels, vasomotor nerves, as well as cells of the osteonal endosteum.

Osteons are either primary or secondary. *Primary* osteons are formed on the periosteal surface. They are cylinders with small diameters that are composed of a few concentric laminae of bone. Their method of formation at the periosteal surface is depicted in Figure 9.36. They add strength to bone, smooth the surfaces at which they are formed and account for continuity of periosteal vessels with those of the compact bone. The formation of these structures demonstrates clearly the continuity of the envelopes and establishes that the origin of the osteonal endosteum is from the periosteum.

Secondary osteons are concentric lami-

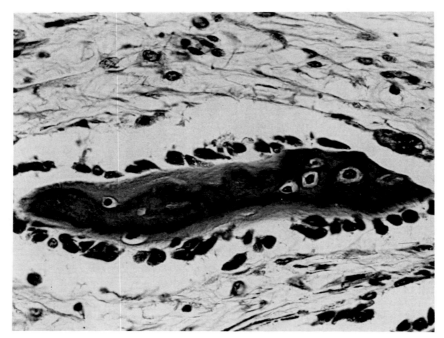

Figure 9.26.   Woven bone in a developing bovine mandible. Note the mottled appearance of the matrix, large osteocytes and the random orientation of the cells. ×100.

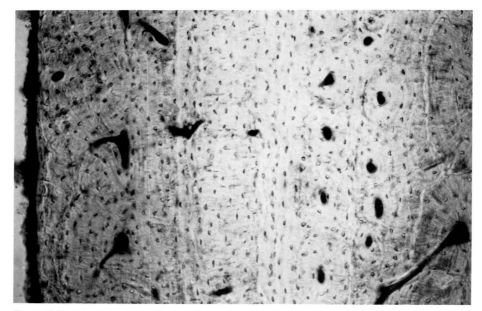

Figure 9.27.   Lamellar bone. The lamellar nature of the bone is indicated by the ordered disposition of the osteocytic lacunae within the circumferential, primary osteonal, and secondary osteonal bone. ×40 (ground bone section).

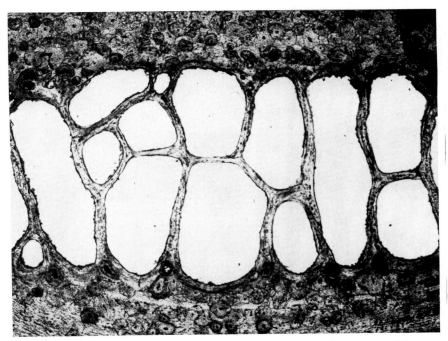

Figure 9.28. Cancellous bone within the marrow cavity of a cervine rib. The amount of interosseous space exceeds the amount of bone that is present. ×10 (ground bone section).

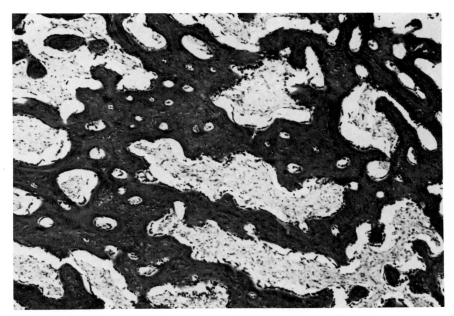

Figure 9.29. Dense cancellous bone of a developing canine humerus. The interosseous space is reduced and the amount of bone is increased. Compare with Figure 9.28. ×16.

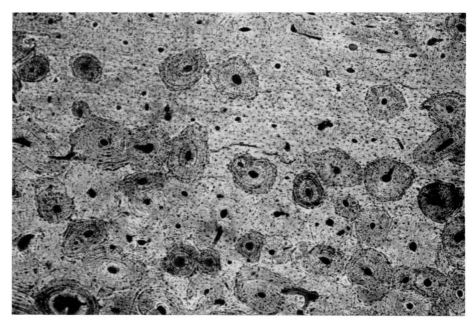

Figure 9.30. Compact bone of an adult canine humerus. The interosseous space is reduced appreciably and is confined to the osteonal and communicating canals. This section of bone consists of portions of outer circumferential lamellae, interstitial and osteonal bone. ×16 (ground bone section).

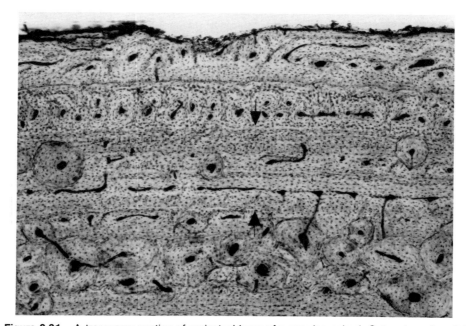

Figure 9.31. A transverse section of periosteal bone of a growing animal. Outer circumferential lamellae occur between the *arrows*. The lamellae alternate with layers of primary osteons. ×16 (ground bone section).

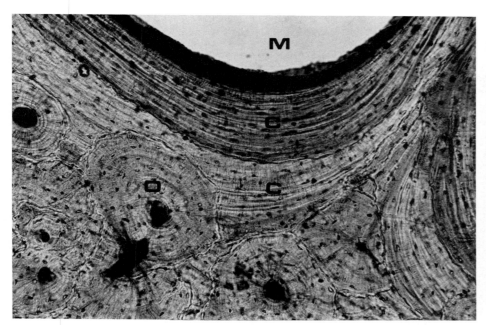

Figure 9.32. Inner circumferential lamellae. The marrow cavity *(M)* is bordered by the inner circumferential bone *(C)*. An osteon *(O)* has formed within part of the inner circumferential bone as a result of remodeling. ×40 (ground bone section).

nae of bone that form within compact bone. The only prerequisite for their formation is the existence of a tunnel within the bone. The most obvious tunnel is that of the primary osteon. The tunnel (osteonal canal) of these structures becomes the substrate upon which the osteoclasts function. Osteoclasts remove bone and expand the limits of the osteonal canal. The limit of this osteoclasia is defined by the *reversal line (cement line)*. **The reversal line, then, is the peripheral limit of bone removal and is the surface upon which new bone is deposited by osteoblasts once osteoclasia ceases in that region.** The centripetal deposition of successive laminae of bone results in the formation of new osteons, secondary osteons (Figs. 9.34, 9.35, and 9.37). This general term is applicable to all subsequent generations of osteons—secondary, tertiary, or quarternary. This type of bone resorptive and formative activity (remodeling) results in the destruction of previously formed osteons, the formation of new osteons, and the formation of remnants of osteonal and circumferential bone. The remnants are called *interstitial bone* (Figs. 9.7, 9.35, and 9.37). The secondary osteons may abut each other or may be separated by segments of interstitial bone. Also, secondary osteons may be isolated within circumferential bone.

Osteons are the structural units of bone. They are long cylinders with a hollow cavity, the osteonal canal. Osteons may be extensively branched. They usually occur in those regions of greatest bone stress. Thus, these morphological entities may be

likened to bundles of reinforcing rods in concrete, too.

The blood vessels of bone are entrapped during developmental stages. These vessels are connected with vessels at the periosteal or cortical endosteal surface through large *Volkmann's canals.* Osteonal vessels freely

communicate with each other through *communicating canals* (Fig. 9.38). Thus, the internal vascular supply is extensively anastomotic (Fig. 9.7).

Bone Remodeling

General Features

The biomechanical properties of the musculoskeletal system are dependent upon a number of integral associations between bone, muscle, cartilage, and fibrous connective tissue. The maintenance of the normal architectural features of each of the skeletal components is essential. Although the gross anatomical features of bones do not change appreciably throughout the adult life of the organism, changes occur constantly within the substance of bone as a tissue. The process is the means by which microscopic packages of bone are removed and replaced without an alteration to skeletal volume. The essence of the process is to accomplish the turnover while maintaining the architectural and physiological competence of individual skeletal units. This process is called remodeling.

This lifelong activity is not a unique feature of bone. All elements of the body undergo similar replacement phenomena; however, the tissue architecture and mineralized matrix impose unique temporal and spatial dependencies. The remodeling process involves the removal of packets of old lamellar bone and its replacement with new lamellar bone. Remodeling activity occurs

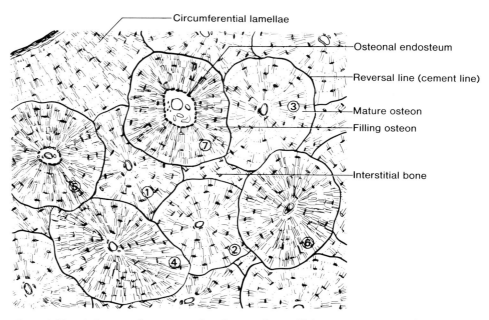

Figure 9.33. A diagram of a cross section of mature bone. All the osteons are secondary osteons; they formed as a result of remodeling activity. Interstitial remnants resulted from the formation of osteons *1, 2,* and *3,* the first generation of secondary osteons. Osteons *4, 6,* and *7,* second generation osteons, infringed during their formation upon osteons *1, 2,* and *3.* The formation of osteon *5,* a third generation osteon, infringed upon the first and second generation osteons.

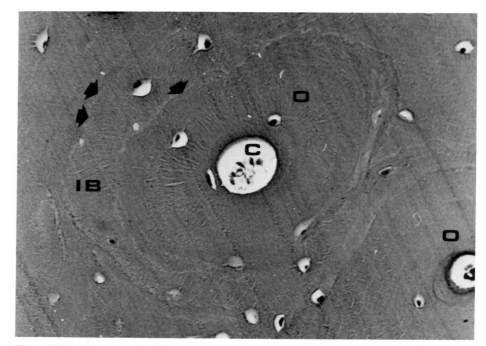

Figure 9.34. Cross section of compact bone. The limits of secondary osteons *(O)* are the reversal or cement lines *(solid arrow)*. A remnant of a previous generation osteon as interstitial bone *(IB)* is apparent. The reversal line of the old osteon is apparent *(double arrows)*. The osteonal canal *(C)* contains endosteum. ×100.

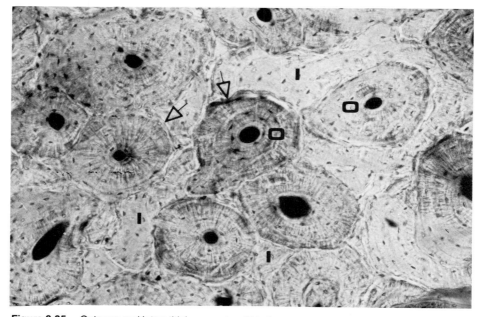

Figure 9.35. Osteons and interstitial remnants within the compacta. *I,* interstitial bone; *O,* osteons. All of the osteons in this section are mature. The osteonal canals, dark regions within the osteons, are small. *Open arrows,* reversal lines. ×40 (ground bone section).

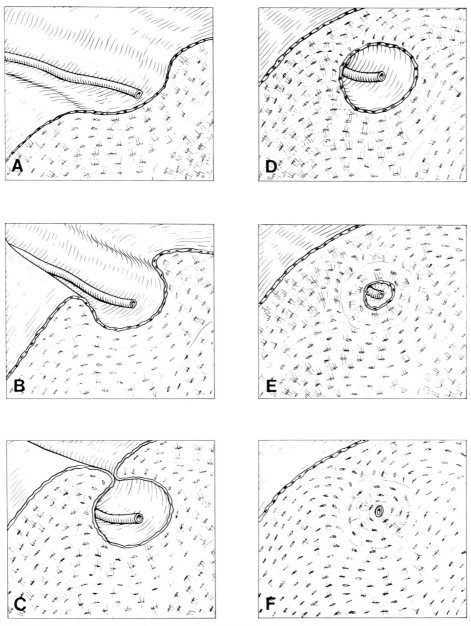

Figure 9.36.   A diagram of the development of primary osteons at the periosteal surface. Longitudinal depressions on the periosteal surface *(A)* become covered by bone *(B and C)* as a result of differential osteoblastic activity at that surface. Blood vessels and periosteal elements *(D)* become entrapped in the substance of the compact bone. Despite these elements being derivatives of the periosteum, they are subsequently referred to as osteonal endosteal elements. Centripetal growth *(E)* results in the formation of a primary osteon *(F)*. (Redrawn and modified from Ham, A. W.: *Histology*. 6th edition. J. B. Lippincott, Philadelphia, 1969).

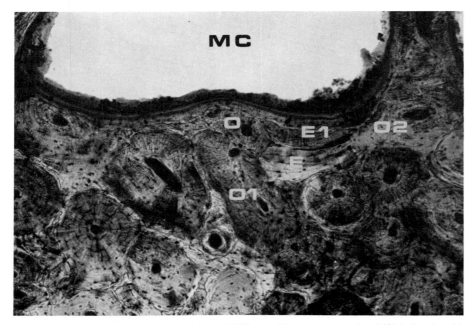

Figure 9.37. Secondary osteons and interstitial bone. The marrow cavity *(MC)* is bordered by remnants of inner circumferential lamellae *(E1)* that are interrupted by an osteon *(O)*. Osteons *(O1, O2)* also interrupt the endosteal bone *(E)*. Compare with Figures 9.32, 9.33, and 9.35. ×25 (ground bone section).

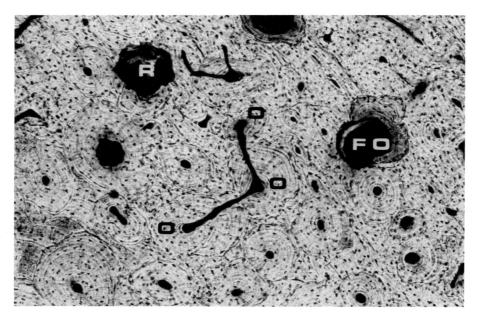

Figure 9.38. Section of compact bone. Communicating canals connect three osteonal canals *(O)*. A resorption space *(R)* and a filling osteon *(FO)* are present. ×25 (ground bone section).

on all bone surfaces; all of the envelopes of bone are involved. The osseous envelopes, then, are responsible for the turnover and maintenance of their contained volume of osseous tissue. Their effectiveness in maintaining the human skeletal mass throughout adulthood is not equivalent. Cortical and trabecular endosteal envelopes are associated with a skeletal loss (negative skeletal balance), while the activity of the osteonal envelope is in perfect balance. Periosteal activity is generally manifested as a positive balance. Although all of the envelopes contribute to skeletal balance, they do so differentially. Trabecular bone is more labile than osteonal bone; furthermore, the trabecular endosteal remodeling activity may be as much as three times greater than osteonal endosteal remodeling activity.

Numerous stimuli result in remodeling activity. Bone is responsive to all of the following diverse stimuli:

1. As the vascular supply moves away from osteocytes, some of them die. Repositioning of vessels within the bone substance to minimize osteocytic death is a consequence. Removal of dead bone becomes an essential stimulus.

2. Continual stress upon the skeleton results in the formation of microfractures that must be repaired.

3. Increased biomechanical stress upon bone necessitates the repositioning or reorientation of osteons. Also, stress may require the replacement of primary osteons and circumferential lamellar bone with secondary osteons.

4. As a reservoir for the storage of minerals, bone responds to dietary influences. Malabsorption of calcium or dietary deficiencies of this ion may result in increased remodeling activity.

5. Immobilization and the disuse attributed to convalescence during fracture repair is characterized by increased remodeling. **(Note that increased and decreased stress are stimuli for increased remodeling.)**

6. Remodeling activity is an integral component of the repair process.

7. Finally, altered endocrine signals, endocrine diseases and the prolonged use of certain chemotherapeutic agents increase the remodeling activity of the skeleton.

Importantly, **remodeling is a normal process.** This process can be increased in response to any, all or a combination of the previously described circumstances.

Basic Metabolic Unit

The evidence of remodeling, past or present, is recorded in the matrix. The histologist uses a number of keys to determine the extent of this process: primary and secondary osteons, interstitial bone, resorption spaces, and the amount of bone present at a specific locus of compact bone. These morphological features afford insights concerning the changes that occurred in the matrix, as well as the balance of activity between formative and resorptive processes.

The cells responsible for the formative and resorptive processes are the osteoblasts and osteoclasts. Together, these cells and their progenitors combine to form a functional unit called the *basic metabolic unit (BMU)* or *bone remodeling unit.* The events associated with the BMUs are considered to be part of the *ARF* sequence, where: *A* is *activation*, *R* is *resorption*, and *F* is *formation*. A new BMU begins its activity upon a bone surface in response to the translation of the previously described circumstances into a local stimulus. The precise nature of the *activation* has not been determined; however, it must be involved in the stimulation of macrophages or their progenitors within the osseous envelopes. In the normal adult skeleton, the amount of bone does not change. New bone is added only at the expense of old bone. *Resorption*, then, is accomplished by osteoclasts removing a discrete quantity of bone. These cells are able to remove approximately 5000–20,000 μm^3 of bone/day/osteoclastic nucleus. This is the equivalent of resorbing the amount of bone produced by 10 to 40 osteoblasts per each osteoclastic nucleus. Osteoclasia is the mechanism for "creating space" for the new bone. *Formation* is initiated in a local region by stimulating osteoprogenitor cells to differentiate into osteoblasts. Osteoblastic activity culminates in the formation of a new packet of bone serving as a *bone structural unit.*

Theoretically, the amount of bone in the skeleton should not vary throughout the adult life of the organism. Despite this stability, packets of the skeleton are removed continually. The amount of bone removed and subsequently replaced by a BMU is designated $\Delta B.BMU$. If the skeleton were in perfect balance, then $\Delta B.BMU = 0$. The amount of bone removed and replaced under this circumstance is equal, or resorption equals formation (R = F). A progressive loss of bone occurs when $\Delta B.BMU < 0$ (-$\Delta B.BMU$), or resorption exceeds formation (R > F). Finally, incremental accumulations of bone result when $\Delta B.BMU > 0$ (+$\Delta B.BMU$), or resorption is less than formation (R < F). **Two factors govern the absolute amount of bone loss or gain—the magnitude of the ΔB and the number of BMU's activated.**

The period of time required for a BMU to pass through the ARF sequence is termed σ (sigma). If $\Delta B.BMU = 0$ were to be considered the steady state, then the time required to pass through the ARF sequence in response to a stimulatory perturbation and return to the steady state is σ. Or, σ is the time required to remove and subsequently reform the same amount of bone that had been removed originally. Sigma is composed of two subperiods. The resorption period (σ_r) is the amount of time required to complete the osteoclasia, whereas the formative period (σ_f) is the time necessary to form the same amount of new bone. Therefore,

$$\sigma = \sigma_r + \sigma_f.$$

Immediate advantages accrue to the organism as a consequence of BMU activation. During the σ_r period, calcium is made available to the body generally. Even though skeletal volume is ultimately maintained ($\Delta B.BMU = 0$), the transitory availability of calcium through the activity of the BMU may satisfy a transitory need. Sigma values normally range in months but may extend to years in abnormal skeletons.

Histological Evidence of Remodeling

Remodeling phenomena occur in association with all of the envelopes of bone. The following descriptions of the remodeling activity of the osteonal endosteum apply equally to the other osseous surfaces; however, the three-dimensional spatial arrangements are different.

In any cross section of compact bone, resorption spaces, mature osteons, and filling osteons are apparent. The temporal and spatial relationships of these structures are more apparent when a longitudinal section is compared to cross sections (Figs. 9.39–9.41). Activation of macrophages to become osteoclasts occurs at a given point in an osteon in response to an activating stimulus. The osteoclasts proceed down the tunnel formed by the osteonal endosteal/bone interface and remove bone both longitudinally and centrifugally. This cavitation process expands the diameter of the osteonal canal, the peripheral limit of which becomes the *reversal line*. While osteoclastic activity progresses away from the point of activation via the *cutting cone*, osteoprogenitor cells differentiate into osteoblasts at the same origination point. So, formation follows resorption. Eventually, osteoclastic activity ceases, whereas the osteoblasts continue to form new bone by apposition from the original reversal line. This centripetal process results in the formation of a new osteon. **[Tetracycline labels may be given at timed intervals to determine bone apposition rates at a given locus (Figs. 2.5 and 9.43 and Plate I.10)].**

The resorption space is a cross-sectional representation of a sequence of events that resulted in the removal of an entire cylinder of bone (Fig. 9.40). *Filling osteons* are osteons in various stages of the formation process that eventually culminate in *mature osteons* (Figs 9.33, 9.35, 9.37, 9.38,

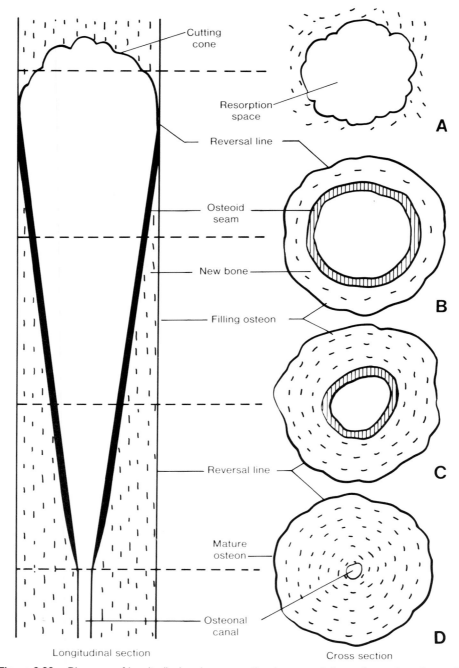

Longitudinal section   Cross section

Figure 9.39. Diagrams of longitudinal and cross sectional representations of an osteonal remodeling unit. The cutting cone, initiated at D, moved along the osteonal canal removing bone longitudinally and centrifugally. *Point A* represents the cutting cone. Gradual refilling with new bone *(points B and C)* resulted in the formation of a new osteon. Because the cavitation of the bone occurred initially at *point D*, the temporal relationships resulted in *point D* having more new bone as a mature osteon than the rest of the cross sectional representatives as filling osteons *(B and C)* Eventually, the filling osteons of *points B and C* would have been converted to mature osteons. The reversal line truly represents a reversal of function, and it is the point at which osteoblastic activity replaced ostoblastic activity. It is evident from the diagram that the reversal line forms the peripheral limit of the osteon.

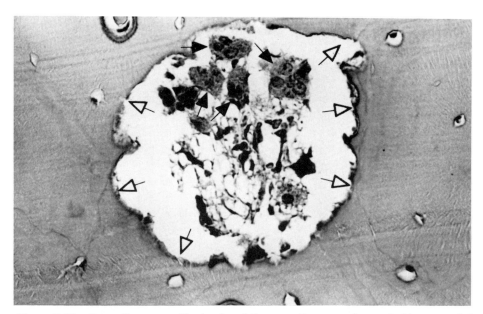

Figure 9.40.   Resorption space. The border of the resorption space is serrated because of the confluence of Howship's lacunae *(open arrows)*. Osteoclasts *(solid arrows)* are displaced from the lacunae by the sectioning techniques. ×125. Compare with Figures 9.22 and 9.38.

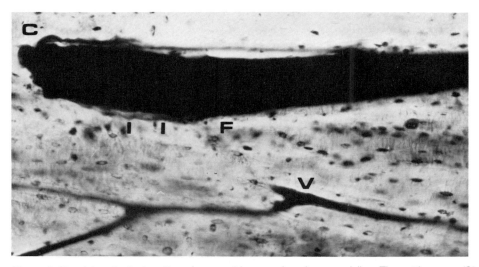

Figure 9.41.   A longitudinal section of compact bone undergoing remodeling. The cutting cone *(C)* *is the front of osteoclasia. The reversal line (bars)* is the peripheral limit of the newly forming osteon *(F)*. The vessel *(V)* and osteonal endosteal elements comprise a narrow osteonal canal before and after cavitation of the bone. ×40 (ground bone section).

and 9.42). The timing of these events from osteoclastic activation to mature osteon formation is measured normally in months. The activity of the BMU resulted in the formation and distribution of its numerous components—secondary osteons, mature osteons, filling osteons, resorption spaces, and interstitial bone.

Bone-Endocrine Relationships

Introduction. Calcium is involved in or regulates a diversity of functions within the organism. These include: *neuronal and muscular excitability, synaptic and neuromuscular junctional transmission, muscular contraction (activation-contraction coupling), exocytosis (activation-secretion coupling), membranous structure and permeability, cellular adhesion, coagulation, intracellular communication,* and *structure of the skeleton.* It is not surprising, therefore, that elaborate mechanisms evolved to control the amount of calcium available to the organism on a minute-to-minute basis. The physicochemical nature of the calcium/phosphorus system and the metabolic requirements of the cells demand that regulation be precise. The skeleton must provide a depot for storage of these ions during periods of excess and must provide a source of ions when intrinsic sources are reduced. The gastrointestinal and renal systems complement these important skeletal functions.

The total plasma calcium concentration of mammals is approximately 10 mg/dl (10 mg%). Because of the precise regulation of this ion within very narrow limits, blood calcium concentrations have been referred to as "nature's constant." Under normal conditions, this value does not change, is not species variable and is independent of diet and aging. The total calcium concentration of the plasma (10 mg/dl or 2.5 mM) is divisible into two distinct forms: nondiffusible, protein-bound calcium and diffusible calcium. *Non-diffusible, protein-bound calcium* accounts for an average 40% of the total calcium or 4 mg/dl (1.0 mM). Since plasma proteins remain relatively constant under normal conditions, the amount of bound calcium does not deviate significantly from this value. The *diffusible calcium* (6 mg/dl or 1.5 mM) is divisible into two subunits. *Free calcium* accounts for about 83% of the diffusible fraction (5 mg/dl or 1.25 mM), whereas the remaining 17% (1 mg/dl or 0.25 mM) is *complexed calcium* that is attached to citrate, bicarbonate, orthophosphate, and pyrophosphate.

Free calcium moves readily into the interstitial space. Accordingly, the calcium concentrations within the extracellular space are the same as within the plasma. Similar concentrations characterize the fluid spaces within the osseous tissue. The

intracellular concentration of calcium is in the range of $10^{-6} - 10^{-7}$ M.

Most of the calcium within the body, approximately 99%, is in the skeleton as HAP crystal. Despite the surface exposure and potential physicochemical exchange, only 1% or less is exchanged in this manner. This does not mean that the rest of the mineral is irreversibly sequestered in the skeleton. Cellular mechanisms used by the body make virtually every milligram of "sequestered bone mineral" available for exchange. Minor deviations from 10 mg/dl are compensated by physicochemical mechanisms. Major perturbations to this parameter require cellular responsiveness

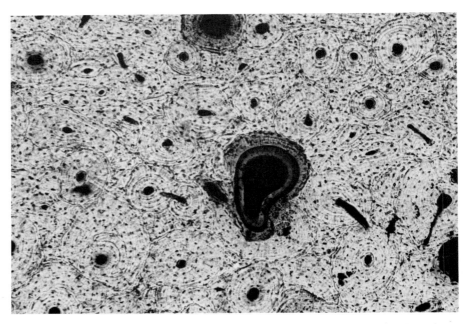

Figure 9.42. Refilling osteon. The osteon in the center of the field is filling. Compare its morphology with the osteon in Figure 9.14. The osteon at the top of the field is immature and inactive. (An osteoid seam is not apparent.) The remaining osteons are mature. ×25 (ground bone section). Compare with Plate I.9.

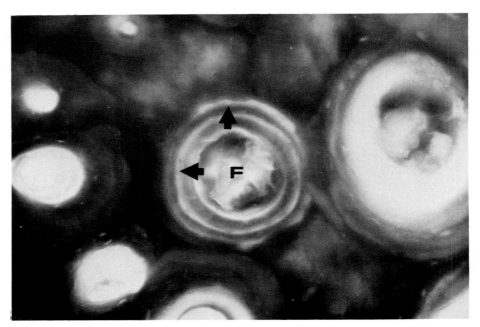

Figure 9.43. A 50-μm section of the cortex of a canine bone. The successive layers of fluorescence *(arrows)* indicate the active deposition of bone in a filling osteon (F). (Courtesy of R. W. Norrdin). Compare with Plate I.10.

to the appropriate hormones. These mechanisms ensure that the organism maintains a continual normocalcemic state rather than ranging from hypercalcemia after a meal to hypocalcemia before the next meal.

Phosphorus is an abundant ion in all biological systems, but the plasma concentration of this substance is subject to more variation than calcium. Generally, plasma phosphorus concentrations are about one-half that of plasma calcium, about 5 mg/dl. A useful but abridged relationship is that the solubility products of calcium and inorganic phosphorus (P_i) equal a constant ($k = [P_i] \times [Ca^{++}]$).

Calcium Regulatory System

Control Substances. *Parathormone (PTH)* is a polypeptide secretory product of the *chief cells* of the parathyroid glands. Parathormone is the *hypercalcemic factor*. Release of this hormone in response to *hypocalcemia* (low plasma calcium) causes an elevation of plasma calcium concentration. The normal range of plasma calcium concentration is called *normocalcemia*, whereas the elevation of plasma calcium concentration above normal is called *hypercalcemia*.

Calcitonin (CT) is the secretory product of the *parafollicular cells* of the thyroid gland. Calcitonin is the *hypocalcemic factor*. The release of the hormone from the parafollicular cells in response to elevated levels of plasma calcium causes a depression of the plasma calcium concentration.

Vitamin or *hormone D* is the third major substance involved in the regulation of calcium. As a vitamin, it is required in the diet, but hormone D is also synthesized by the body.

Vitamin D_3 or cholecalciferol is ingested in small amounts and can be synthesized in the sebaceous glands of the skin. The synthesis of hormone D from *7-dehydrocholesterol* requires the photoactivation of the substance by ultraviolet radiation. Hormone D_3 is then transported to the liver wherein the first of a series of hydroxylations occurs to create a compound called *25-hydroxycholecalciferol (25-HCC or 25-(OH)D_3)*. The hydroxylated substance has biological effects in high concentrations; however, it serves primarily as a precursor for the formation of more active metabolites of D_3. This circulating metabolite is transported to the kidney. The fate of 25-HCC within the kidney is dependent upon the need for calcium at the time. If a calcium demand exists, then 25-HCC is converted to *1,25-dihydroxycholecalciferol (1,25-DHCC, or 1,25-(OH)_2D_3)* within the mitochondria of renal tubular epithelial cells. If the organism does not have a need for calcium at the time, then 25-HCC is converted to *24,25-dihydroxycholecalciferol (24,25-DHCC, or 24,25-(OH)_2D_3)*

within the mitochondria of renal tubular epithelial cells. Eight different metabolites are produced in the metabolism of D_3. The functions of these numerous substances, as well as their type and sites of action, are the subjects of intensive research efforts.

Vitamin D_2 (calciferol) is formed by the irradiation of *ergosterol*, a plant sterol. This compound, once ingested and absorbed, undergoes transformations similar to those described for D_3. Vitamin D_2 is active in mammals but is inactive in birds.

Mechanisms of Action

Effects of Hormones. PTH is the principle hormone responsible for the minute-to-minute, homeokinetic maintenance of the plasma calcium concentration. The most important biological effects of this hormone include:

1. elevation of plasma calcium with a corresponding decrease in plasma phosphorus
2. increasing the urinary excretion of phosphorus (phosphaturia)
3. increasing the urinary conservation of calcium
4. increasing the rate of skeletal remodeling
5. increasing the rate of osteocytic osteolysis
6. facilitating the formation of 1,25-dihydroxyvitamin D_3 by exerting a trophic effect upon the 1-hydrolase system
7. increasing the calcium and phosphorus absorption from the small intestine by having a direct effect upon the formation of 1,25-DHCC.

PTH release results in the elevation of plasma calcium. The effects upon the skeleton result in the release of 1.66 moles of calcium for each mole of phosphorus. Calcium and phosphorus are absorbed from the small intestine in equimolar concentrations. So, two of the mechanisms cause both ions to be elevated in the blood. These mechanisms do not satisfy the relationship dictated by the equation $[Ca^{++}] \times [P_i] = k$. The parathyroid/renal axis is responsible for the necessary adjustments to elevate calcium while reducing phosphorus. The renal tubular reabsorption of calcium is enhanced, while the renal tubular reabsorption of phosphorus is blocked under the influence of PTH.

The effects of calcitonin upon osteoclastic and osteocytic cells is antagonistic to the action of PTH. The effect of calcitonin upon the kidney complements the action of parathormone. Calcitonin also manifests an inhibitory effect upon the intestinal absorption of calcium and phosphorus. The effects of calcitonin within the regulatory system include:

1. the reduction of plasma calcium and phosphorus
2. the inhibition of parathormone stimulated osteoclasia and osteocytic osteolysis
3. the indirect inhibition of calcium and phosphorus absorption from the small intestine
4. the short term stimulation of osteoblastic activity.

CT reduces of plasma calcium. The effects of CT upon the gut may be an indirect effect of CT upon the reduced synthesis of 1,25-DHCC. The precise and direct role of CT upon the kidney is not clear.

The dual regulation of calcium by PTH and CT results in more regulatory precision than possible with one hormone. PTH seems to protect against hypocalcemia, whereas CT seems to be an emergency-type of hormone that protects against postprandial hypercalcemia. As a polypeptide hormones, the effects of PTH and CT are mediated through cyclic adenosine monophosphate.

The active metabolites of hormone D represent another aspect of the dual regulatory mechanisms involved in calcium homeokinesis.

Increased calcium demand (need) favors the formation of 1,25-DHCC. The intestine responds by increasing the absorption of calcium and phosphorus. Osteoclasia and osteocytic osteolysis are increased by 1,25-DHCC. This metabolite is necessary for these cells to respond to PTH. The precise effects of 1,25-DHCC upon the kidneys need further clarification. The compound is inhibitory to the parathyroid glands. The specific functions of 24,25-DHCC need to be clarified. The metabolite has a negative influence upon the production of PTH, and 24,25-DHCC may facilitate the deposition of calcium in bone. The mechanisms by which these active metabolites mediate their effects are typical of the steroid hormones.

Target Organ Responses. The target organs for these hormones are the small intestine, kidneys, and bone. The integrated functions of the target organs in this regulated system are the essential mediators of calcium homeokinesis.

The small intestine is responsible for the absorption of calcium and phosphorus. The 1,25-DHCC metabolite enhances this activity by two mechanisms: activation of absorptive cells and the synthesis and secretion of calcium-binding proteins (CaBPs).

Diets with reduced calcium enhance the synthesis of caBPs; thus, calcium absorptive efficiency is increased. This relationship may serve as part of the rationale for the dietary reduction of calcium in dairy cows just before parturition. Such reductions decrease the incidence of *milk fever (parturient paresis)* by inducing the cow to increase absorptive efficiency just before the increased demands imposed upon her by milk letdown. Additionally, the PTH/bone axis is activated.

The effects of CT upon this target organ are not clear. The inhibitory effect of this hormone upon gut absorption may be through its negative influence upon the synthesis of 1,25-DHCC. PTH exerts its influence on this target organ through its positive effect upon the synthesis of 1,25-DHCC.

The renal component of the regulatory system is responsible for the conservation and/or excretion of calcium and phosphorus. The differential activity of the renal tubular epithelial cells is the essential contributor to the elevation of plasma calcium levels. Receptors for PTH occur within the basilar membrane of the lining cells of the proximal and distal convoluted tubules. Enhancement of distal convoluted tubular reabsorption under PTH influence seems to be an important mediator of the homeokinetic maintenance of calcium. Phosphorus is usually reabsorbed from the filtrate within the proximal convoluted tubule; selective resecretion occurs within the distal convoluted tubule. PTH stimulation of proximal convoluted tubular lining cells blocks the reabsorption of phosphorus from the filtrate within this segment of the nephron. The resulting *phosphaturia* elevates urinary phosphorus, decreases plasma phosphorus, and tends to favor the elevation of plasma calcium.

The physiologic functions of CT upon the kidney, however, are not clear. CT receptors have been demonstrated in the epithelial cells of the ascending limb of Henle's loop and the distal convoluted tubule.

PTH has a trophic effect upon the 1-hydroxylase system within the renal tubular lining cells. Although these active metabolites of hormone D—1,25-DHCC and 24,25-DHCC—are synthesized within the kidney, their effects upon the kidney need clarification.

Bone not only serves as a mineral sink to prevent excesses in plasma calcium levels, but this tissue must function as a source of minerals to prevent hypocalcemia. Osteoblasts and osteocytes function to form and maintain bone, respectively. They also function together to remove bone. Similarly, osteoclasts augment the pool of circulating metabolites through their lytic activity. All of the cells of bone contribute to the homeokinetic maintenance of plasma calcium.

The osteocytes and osteoblasts are linked structurally through their cellular processes within the canaliculi. Functionally, they are linked as an *osteocyte-osteoblast pump*. The immediate effect of PTH stimulation is the activation of this pump. The activated pump mobilizes mineral from the "depths" of bone and transport it to the surface whereupon the mineral enters the circulating pool. The initial action is *osteocytic osteolysis*. Osteocytes secrete organic acids and various hydrolases (proteases, collagenases) into the lacunar environment. The subsequent enlargement of lacunae is associated with released organic and inorganic materials from the lacunar surfaces. The calcium may move down its concentration gradient to the surface cells through canaliculi. Or, the calcium may be transported actively through the cellular processes to the osteoblasts. Each osteocyte does not mobilize much mineral, but their cellular density insures that enough mineral is mobilized to alter blood calcium levels. **Osteocytic osteolysis and the osteocyte-osteoblast pump are the rapid, minute-to-minute, PTH-responsive mechanisms for increasing the concentration of plasma calcium.**

Osteoclastic participation in mineral mobilization is an adjunctive mechanism that is stimulated by PTH. Hours are required to measure the responsiveness of these cells to PTH. Accordingly, osteoclasts probably contribute to long-standing calcium deficiencies, not minute-to-minute corrections for minor perturbations. Osteoclasts are capable of mobilizing large quantities of mineral from beneath the "sealed" microenvironment of the ruffled border. The mechanism by which this mobilization is achieved is similar to that described for osteocytes. Organic acids and hydrolases are essential secretions. Degraded materials are ingested by the osteoclasts, processed further, and ultimately moved to the extracellular environment.

CT manifests its effect upon bone by blocking both osteoclasia and osteocytic osteolysis. This effect, however, is transitory. Also, bone formation is an initial response to calcitonin. The active metabolite 1,25-DHCC is necessary for bone cells to respond to parathormone.

Various disorders exist in which abnormalities of mineral metabolism are manifested as clinical disease entities. Hypocalcemic tetany *(eclampsia)* in the bitch associated with parturition and milk letdown is a life-threatening situation. Similarly, *parturient paresis (milk fever)* is a serious complication of birth and milk letdown in the cow.

Hypercalcemia can be a complication of various metabolic bone diseases. One of the consequences is the *metastatic calcification* of normal tissues. The response of this system to hypocalcemia and hypercalcemia is illustrated in Figure 9.44.

"In Concert" Influences of Hormones

Specific Hormones and Influences. The elaborate *PTH-CT-vitamin D regulatory system* is a precise mechanism for calcium homeostasis. The complexity of this regulatory scheme is compounded by the "in concert" effect of numerous other hormones. The mechanisms by which numerous and varied hormones exert their influences, for the most part, have not been elucidated. Interaction with the calcium regulatory system is an attractive choice.

The *gonadal hormones* exert numerous effects upon the mature skeleton that are species-variable. The removal of the ovaries or their dysfunction with age results in an estradiol deficiency. This deficiency, notable in the human female with the onset of menapause, is associated with a reduction of skeletal mass. This *osteoporosis* results from an altered remodeling. *Estrogen* and the other *sex steroids (testosterone)* probably exert an inhibitory influence upon osteoclasia. Removal of the inhibition causes and increased remodeling characterized by a $-\Delta$B.BMU in which resorption is increased, whereas formation is normal. Some experimental evidence has shown that the administration of sex steroids interfaces with the conversion of 25-HCC to 1,25-DHCC. The sex steroids may mediate their effect through the metabolic pathways for vitamin D.

The relationship of the *glucocorticosteroids* to bone is well established. Osteoporosis is often a complication of Cushing's syndrome or the improper use of these hormones therapeutically. The *adrenocorticoids* also have an inhibitory effect upon calcium absorption from the small intestine and calcium conservation by the kidneys. The osteoporosis of this syndrome is characterized by an inhibition of osteoclastic activity that is less than the inhibition of osteoblastic activity. The ΔB.BMU still results in skeletal loss. The precise mechanisms are not known; some evidence suggests that interference of vitamin D metabolism may be involved. Also, the inhibition of protein synthesis may be a factor.

The *thyroid hormones (T_3 and T_4)* are known to influence bone remodeling and metabolism. *Hyperthyroidism* is associated with hypercalcemia and increased skeletal remodeling. *Thyrotoxicosis* may interfere with the generation of circulating levels of 25-HCC.

The *somatotropin-somatomedin* axis is the important mechanism for *growth hormone (somatotropin)* to exert its influence upon the growing and repairing skeleton. These hormones may mediate their effects and satisfy the increased demand for calcium by stimulating the production of 1,25-DHCC.

A reduced skeletal mass has also been associated with diabetes mellitus. This defect may result from a calcium malabsorption problem in the small intestine. Experiments with animals show that a defect in the generation of 1,25-DHCC may be part of the disease process. *Insulin*, then, may influence vitamin D metabolism also.

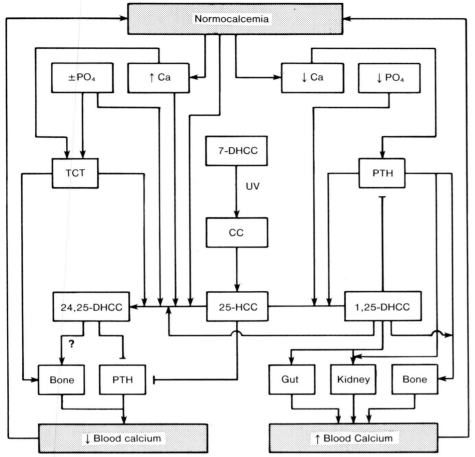

Figure 9.44. Diagram of the relationships of various substances in the regulation of calcium. *Arrows*, stimulation; *bars*, blockage or inhibition.

Prolactin has been shown to increase circulating levels of 1,25-DHCC. Also, the *prostaglandins (A, B, E* and *F)*, especially *prostaglandin E₂ (PGE₂)*, are strong promoters of bone resorption. It is interesting to speculate that this effect may be mediated through vitamin D metabolism.

The "in concert" effects of the hormones upon the skeleton have been known for years. The mechanisms by which these effects are mediated remain speculative. The calcium regulatory system of PTH/CT/vitamin D provides a functional substrate upon which all of the other hormones exert their influence. Even more simply, though speculative, the vitamin D/target organ axes may constitute the basic mechanism upon which all of the hormones exert their effects. These axes may be the *final com-* *mon pathway* for skeletal balance generally and calcium regulation specifically.

References

Amprino, R. and Engstrom, A.: Studies on x-ray absorption and diffraction of bone tissue. Acta Anat. *15*:1, 1952.
Ascenzi, R., Bonucci, E. and Bocciarelli, D.S.: An electron microscope study om primary periosteal bone. J. Ultrastruct. Res. *18*:605, 1967.
Belanger, L.F., Robichon, J., Migicovsky, B.B., Copp, D.H. and Vincent, J.: Resorption without osteoclasts (osteolysis). *In*: Sognnaes, R.F. (ed.). *Mechanisms of Hard Tissue Destruction.* AAAS, Washington, D. C., 1963.
Bourne, G.H. (ed.): *The Biochemistry and Physysiology of Bone.* Volumes I–III, Academic Press, New York, 1972.
Cohen, J. and Harris, W.H.: The three dimensional anatomy of Haversian systems. J. Bone Joint Surg. *40a*:419, 1958.

Cooper, R.R., Milgram, J.W. and Robinson, R.A.: Morphology of the osteon: An electron microscopic study. J. Bone Joint Surg. *48A*:1239, 1966.
Christakos, S. and Norman, A.W.: Interaction of the vitamin D endocrine system with other hormones. J. Mineral Electrolyte Metab. *1*:231, 1978.
DeLuca, H.F.: The kidney as an endocrine organ for the production of 1,25-dihydroxyvitamin D₃, a calcium-mobilizing hormone. N. Engl. J. Med. *289*:359, 1973.
Fischman, D.A. and Hay, E.D.: Origin of osteoclasts from mononuclear leukocytes in regenerating newt limbs. Anat. Rec. *143*:329, 1962.
Frost, H.M.: *Bone Remodelling Dynamics.* Charles C Thomas, Springfield, 1963.
Frost, H.M.: *The Physiology of Cartilaginous, Fibrous and Bony Tissue.* Charles C Thomas, Springfield, 1972.
Gonzales, F. and Karnovsky, M.J.: Electron microscopy of osteoclasts in healing fractures of rat bone. J. Biophys. Biochem. Cytol. *9*:299, 1961.
Gothlin, G. and Ericsson, J.L.E.: The osteoclast. Clin. Orthop. *120*:201, 1976.
Hancox, N.M.: *Biology of Bone.* University Press, Cambridge, 1972.
Heller-Steinberg, M.: Ground substance, bone salts, and cellular activity in bone formation and destruction. Amer. J. Anat. *89*:347, 1951.
Hobdell, M.H. and Boyde, A.: Microradiography and scanning electron microscopy of bone sections. Z. Zellforsch. *94*:487, 1969.
Jee, W.S.S. and Nolan, P.D.: Origin of osteoclasts from the fusion of phagocytes. Nature *200*:225, 1963.
Jotereau, F.V. and LeDouarin, N.M.: The developmental relationship between osteocytes and osteoclasts: A study using quail-chick nuclear marker in endochondral ossification. Dev. Biol. *63*:253, 1978.
Kincaid, S.A. and VanSickle, D.C.: Bone morphology and postnatal osteogenesis: Potential for disease. Vet. Clin. N. A. *13*:3, 1983.
Little, K.: *Bone Behavior.* Academic Press, New York, 1973.
Martin, J.H. and Matthew, J.L.: Mitochondrial granules in chondrocytes, osteoblasts and osteocytes. Clin. Orthop. *68*:273, 1970.
Mathews, J.L.: Bone structure and ultrastructure. *In:* Urist, M.R. (ed.). *Fundamental and Clinical Bone Physiology.* pp 4–44, J.B. Lippincott, Philadelphia, 1980.
Nichols, G., Jr. and Wasserman, R.H. (eds.): *Cellular Mechanisms for Calcium Transfer and Homeostasis.* Academic Press, New York, 1971.
Owen, M.: Histogenesis of bone cells. Calc. Tiss. Res. *25*:205, 1978.
Parfitt, A.M.: Mechanisms of calcium transfer between blood and bone and their cellular basis: Morphological and kinetic approaches to turnover. Metabolism *25*:809, 1976.
Queener, S.F. and Bell, N.H.: Calcitonin: A general survey. Metabolism *24*:555, 1975.
Rasmussen, H. and Goodman, D.B.P.: Relationships between calcium and cyclic nucleotide in cell activation. Physiol. Rev. *57*:421, 1977.
Sumner-Smith, G. (ed.): *Bone in Clinical Orthopaedics: A Study in Comparative Osteology.* W.B. Saunders, Philadelphia, 1982.
Urist, M.R. (ed.): *Fundamental and Clinical Bone Physiology.* J.B. Lippincott, Philadelphia, 1980.
Walker, D.G.: Experimental osteopetrosis. Clin. Orthop. *97*:158, 1973.
Walker, D.G.: Spleen cells transmit osteopetrosis in mice. Science *190*:785, 1975.
Walker, D.G.: Bone resorption restored in osteopetrotic mice by transplant of normal bone marrow and spleen cells. Science *190*:784, 1975.

10: Osteogenesis

Development of Bone

General Characteristics. Osteogenic processes begin in the fetus and continue throughout the life of the animal. Although the actual cellular mechanism of bone deposition is the same in all osteogenic processes, the differentiation of mesenchymal cells into osteoblasts normally occurs in two different microenvironments. For this reason, two types of normal ossification processes are described—*intramembranous ossification* and *endochondral ossification*.

Ossification vs. Mineralization. *Ossification* is a process in which a complex sequence of spatially and temporally linked events leads to the formation of bone. Two distinct yet related stages characterize this process. The *morphogenetic phase*, involving complex movements and interactions of cells, determines the basic shape of the skeleton. The *cytodifferentiation phase* is the period in which cellular and tissue differentiation occur.

Mineralization, a part of the ossification process, is the process by which the organic matrix of bone acquires its usual complement of inorganic components.

Occasionally, bone formation occurs in foci not normally occupied by osseous tissue. This *pathological (metaplastic) ossification* may be observed in otherwise normal tissues of cicatrices, tracheal and laryngeal cartilage, lateral cartilages of the equine foot, and other organs. *Calcification* or *mineralization* of normal tissues, occurring in association with persistent hypercalcemia, is termed *metastatic calcification*. The calcification of degenerative or dead tissues is termed *dystrophic calcification*. The concentrations of calcium and phosphorus exceed their solubility product and precipitation occurs.

Developmental Modeling and Remodeling. The cellular mechanism of bone formation is identical in intramembranous and endochondral ossification. Moreover, bone formation in the adult results from the same cellular mechanism. The essence of the process is the biphasic activity of the osteoblast. Intramembranous ossification is responsible for the attainment of the definitive shape of a limited number of bones that are not preformed in cartilage.

Endochondral ossification is responsible for various activities relating to the morphogenesis of skeletal components. Elongation of the diaphyses and the shape and size of epiphyses are two easily observed consequences. The elongation process is complemented by mechanisms that increase the transverse diameters of developing diaphyses. Both ossification processes are used separately and in combination with each other in certain circumstances to achieve the skeletal end products. The achievement of the definitive, adult, recognizable gross architecture is the result of *modeling*.

After the initial deposition of bone in a membranous or cartilaginous environment, subsequent bone formation occurs on pre-existing bone surfaces by appositional growth. Continued deposition naturally leads to bone growth. The modeling of bones, however, is the combined result of osteoblastic and osteoclastic activity. The balance of these combined activities favors the deposition of bone during periods of growth.

Although osteogenic processes most noticeably occur during adolescence, they are not confined to this period. The deposition and removal of bone, without any significant alteration of the gross form of the structure, occur throughout life. This *remodeling* process complements the adolescent modeling of bones. Remodeling activity is an essential feature of skeletal development and growth. As the mass of the body increases, the skeleton compensates to carry the additional load effectively. Formation of new osteons, repositioning of secondary osteons and the proper placement of trabecular bone are the integral components of development and growth that are contributed by the remodeling process.

Mechanisms of Development

Intramembranous Ossification

Sequence of Histogenesis. The bones destined to form, either totally or partially in this manner, are the bones of the skull, mandible, and clavicle, which are not weight-bearing structures.

The first recognizable stage of skeletal development during the embryonic period is *mesenchymal condensation*. Initially, these regions are characterized by mesenchymal cells within a homogeneous, fluid ground substance. The subsequent development of a *fibrocellular* tissue results from the differentiation of some *fibroblasts* from mesenchymal cells. *Collagenous fibers* are randomly scattered among the numerous fibroblasts and mesenchymal cells. Many of these cells are destined to become *osteoprogenitor cells*.

The next identifiable step in the differentiation process is the recognition of osteoblasts (Fig. 10.1). Although bone matrix is not always visible during early stages of differentiation, subsequent secretory activity of these cells results in recognizable osteoid (Figs. 10.2 and 10.3) within early ossification centers (Fig. 10.4).

Progressive development and differentiation produces identifiable spicules of bone (Fig. 10.5). A fibrocellular connective tissue with numerous blood vessels surrounds the developing bone. As osteoblasts deposit bone appositionally, some cells remain entrapped in their own secretory products as osteocytes (Figs. 10.5 and 10.6). The bone being deposited in these ossification centers is the *woven* type (Fig. 10.6).

Woven bone serves as a temporary structure during development. Woven bone production decreases with time, while lamellar bone formation increases progressively. Osteoclasia accounts for the removal of woven bone as the temporary tissue (Fig. 10.6). Ultimately, only lamellar bone remains.

Osteoblastic and osteoclastic activities are integral components of bone formation (Fig. 10.7). The necessity for active osteoblasts is obvious. Osteoclasts remove woven and lamellar bone. The combined activity results in the movement of osseous spicules through space (Fig. 10.7). Spicules of bone form, move through space, coalesce, and convert the ossification center into a recognizable osseous structure. Areolar and dense connective tissues develop as integral components of periosteal and endosteal envelopes. Similarly, the characteristic vascular beds of bone develop within the mesenchyme of the ossification center.

The covering envelopes associated with developing spicules are typical. These en-

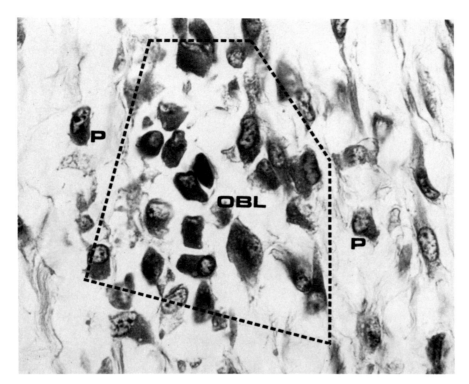

Figure 10.1. Differentiation of osteoblasts within an intramembranous ossification center of a bovine fetal jaw. The *outlined area* is an ossification center that contains osteoblasts *(OBL)*. The light-staining cells at the periphery may be osteoprogenitor cells *(P)*. ×160

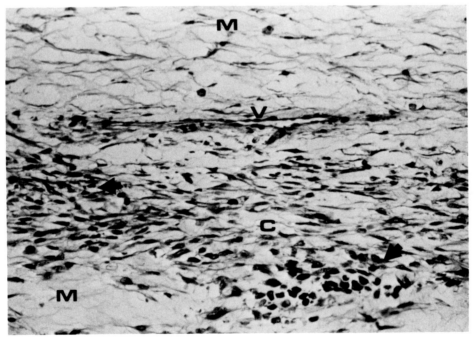

Figure 10.2. Presumptive ossification center in a bovine fetal jaw. The mesenchyme *(M)* surrounds an area of mesenchymal condensation *(C)*. Dark-staining cells *(arrows)* are osteoblasts. Bone matrix has not been formed at these sites yet. A blood vessel *(V)* has developed in association with the ossification center. ×40.

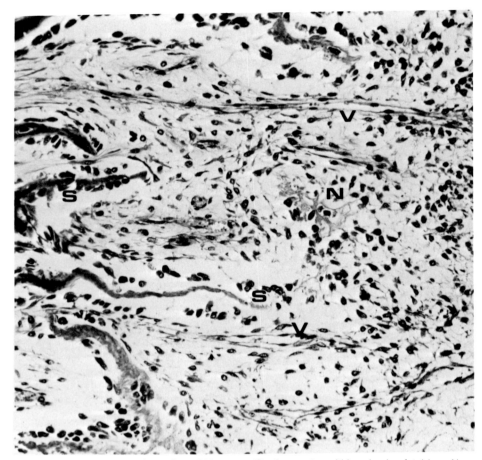

Figure 10.3. Bone matrix formation within an ossification center within a bovine fetal jaw. New matrix formation *(N)* is evident. Continued activity of osteoblasts forms progressively larger spicules *(S)* of bone. An extensive vascular bed *(V)* is developing also. ×40.

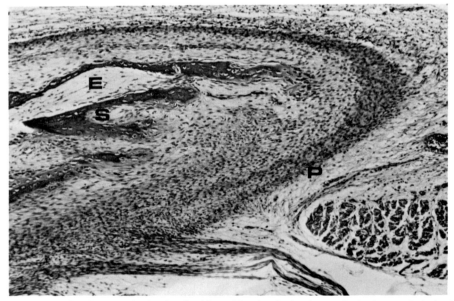

Figure 10.4. Ossification of a bovine fetal jaw. The developing bone site is demarcated clearly from the surrounding mesenchyme by the condensation of mesenchymal cells that have formed a periosteum *(P)*. Bone spicules *(S)* and endosteal elements *(E)* are apparent within the ossification center.

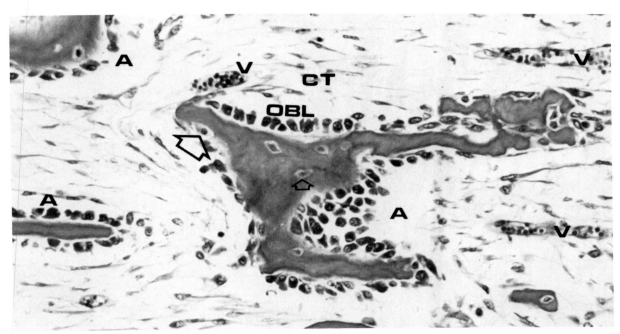

Figure 10.5. Spicules of bone within an ossification center of a bovine fetal jaw. Spicules of bone are surrounded by endosteum consisting of fibrocellular connective tissue *(CT)*. Blood vessels *(V)* are evident. The endosteum is separated artifactually from the bone *(A)*. Osteoblasts *(OBL)* become entrapped in bone *(large arrow)* and are recognized eventually as typical osteocytes *(small arrow)*. ×63.

velopes develop simultaneously within the ossification center, naturally, coincident with the appearance of bone. Most of the osseous coverings could be called trabecular endosteal envelopes by virtue of their association with spicules of bone. The peripheral covering becomes the periosteum. Complete distinction of the various envelopes is possible when some definitive organ shape is apparent.

Progressive expansion of the ossification center (increased size of the developing bone) is accompanied by an alteration of the configuration of the constituent osseous tissue. Isolated foci become more typically cancellous bone (Fig. 10.8). Osteons also may form in the cancellous bone as some of it becomes compact bone. The cancellous nature of the bone within the forming marrow cavity is retained throughout adulthood. The periosteum, however, continually deposits laminae of bone in a compact configuration that serves to strengthen the bone and increase its diameter. The osteoclasts of the cortical endosteum continually remove bone, effectively expanding the marrow cavity while maintaining the essential thickness of the compact bone. During growth, then, the bone formed by the osteogenic activity of the periosteum eventually will be removed by the osteoclastic activity of the cortical endosteum until the definitive diameter of the structure is achieved.

The essence of this ossification mechanism is the de novo formation of bone in mesenchyme. Subsequent appositional bone growth on the recently formed spi-

cules increases the mass of the ossification center. Continual addition of bone results in the achievement of a definitive shape characterized by the appropriate distribution of cancellous and compact bone.

Endochondral Ossification

General Features. *Endochondral ossification, enchondral* and *intracartilaginous ossification* are descriptive terms; the development of bone by this process occurs initially within a mass of hyaline cartilage. The models are actually miniature versions of the future definitive bones (Fig. 10.9). The cartilage is removed gradually and is replaced continuously by bone. Endochondral ossification encompasses all of the activities responsible for the formation of the weight-bearing bones. Elongation is achieved in such a way that the animal is able to bear weight while growing.

The premature termination of endochondral ossification is considered an abnormality in most species. In certain breeds of dogs, the early cessation of endochondral ossification results in shortened bones that are the normal standard for the breed. *Achondroplasia (chondrodystrophy, chondrodysplasia)* describes a premature termination of the endochondral ossification process. Achondroplasia is generalized in bulldogs and the Pekingese, localized to the head in Boxers and Boston Bull Terriers and localized to the limbs of Dachshunds and Bassett Hounds.

Functions. The functions of endochondral ossification are: *elongation of the skel-*

etal mass; contribution to the shape, size, and spatial orientation of articulations; formation of most of the cancellous bone.

Endochondral ossification provides for the elongation of most of the skeletal mass during growth. This function is initiated before and during actual weight-bearing. The rate at which growth progresses, the duration of the process and the direction of the process in three-dimensional space is affected by numerous factors—genetic, nutritional, metabolic, and mechanical. The majority of the definitive height of the organism is attained through the activity of the growth plate. The continuous addition of cartilage and the subsequent replacement of it by bone is the essence of the elongation process.

Endochondral ossification contributes to the shape, size, spatial orientation, and alignment of the articulations between bones. Normal locomotor function is related directly to the modeling activity of this ossification process. Most of the long bones of the body are characterized by epiphyses whose diameters are generally larger than diaphyseal diameters. Endochondral ossification activity within secondary ossification centers and differential bone cell activities within the periphery of the metaphyses are essential for the attainment of proper epiphyseal shape and size. The morphological features of the epiphyses afford biomechanical advantages.

Endochondral ossification forms the majority of the cancellous bone of the body. Cancellous bone reduces the skeletal mass without compromising the ability to bear

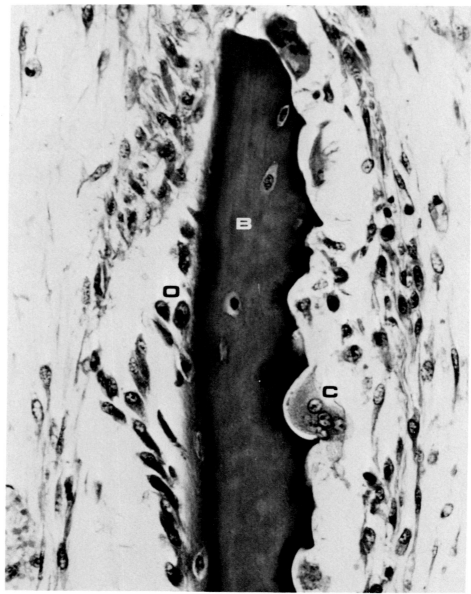

Figure 10.6. Bone spicule in an intramembranous ossification center within a bovine fetal jaw. Osteocytes have been incorporated into the bone spicule *(B)*. Osteoblastic *(O)* and osteoclastic *(C)* activity is evident. Both types of cells are always associated with bone developmental processes. The spicule is composed of woven bone. ×100.

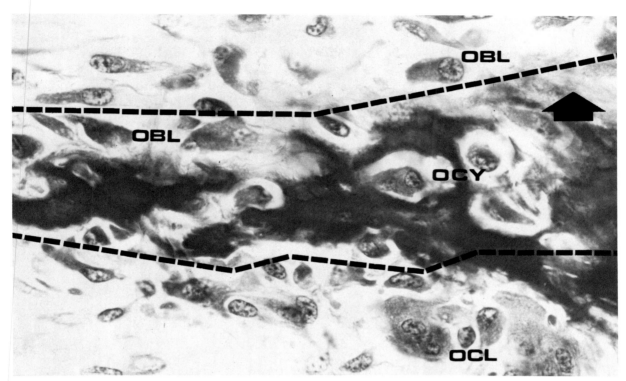

Figure 10.7. Progressive development and activity of the ossification center within a bovine fetal jaw. The osetoblasts *(OBL)* on the upper portion of the spicule are active, as evidenced by their columnar-like shape. Those osteoblasts on the lower portion of the spicule are inactive, based upon their spindle shape. Osteoclasts *(OCL)* are present also. If the same relative cellular activity were to progress beyond the stage depicted, then the spicule would be altered as outlined. The spicule would thicken in the left portion of the micrograph and appear to move upward *(arrow)* in the right portion of the micrograph. Osteocytes *(OCY)* are oriented randomly in this immature bone. ×160.

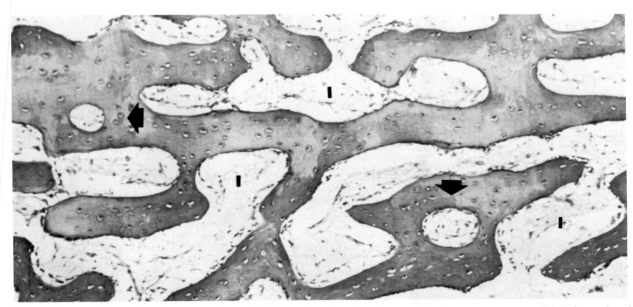

Figure 10.8. An increased amount of bone within the ossification center of a bovine fetal jaw. The interosseous space *(I)* is being replaced by bone. Continued centripetal deposition of bone at the *arrows* may be the initiation of the formation of osteons. ×63.

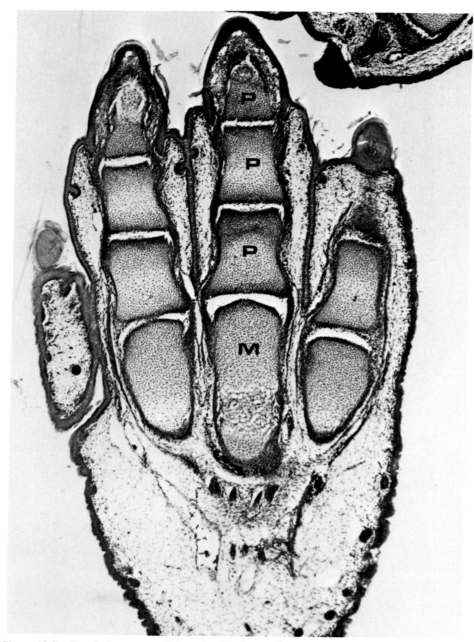

Figure 10.9.   Developing manus of a hamster. The bones of the manus (phalanges and metacarpals) are preformed in cartilage. The metacarpal bones *(M)* and phalanges *(P)* are miniature versions of the adult structures. Note that the metacarpal-phalangeal joints and the interphalangeal joints appear early in development. ×10.

weight, because the trabeculae are positioned for maximal mechanical advantage.

The events of endochondral ossification are summarized diagrammatically in Figure 10.10.

Model Formation

Chondrogenic Centers. *Mesenchymal cell condensation* characterizes regions in which bones develop by endochondral ossification (Figs. 10.10*A* and 10.11). The newly developing matrix contributes to the differentiation of mesenchymal cells. Early stages of matrical prodution are characterized by the presence of hyaluronic acid, which may be required for the aggregation of mesenchymal cells. As cytodifferentiation continues, chondroitin sulfates increase as hyaluronate is removed. The condensation, resulting from aggregation

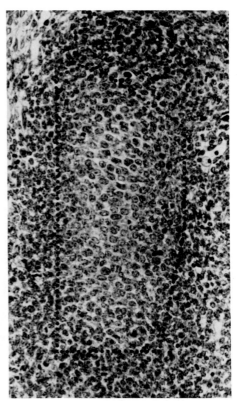

Figure 10.11. Mesenchymal condensation in a presumptive bone-forming site, a fetal hamster humerus. The mesenchymal condensation is outlined. A perichondrium will differentiate at the periphery of the condensation. ×60. (Periodic acid-Schiff.)

and the mitotic activity of the cells, produces a hypercellular region. The relationships of future bones are apparent in the presumptive bone-forming sites. The cells eventually differentiate into chondroblasts and form a *chondrogenic center* referred to as the *cartilaginous model* (Fig. 10.12). Commensurate with the differentiation of the cartilage, mesenchymal cells at the periphery of the model condense and form a *perichondrium* that encloses the entire model. Appositional growth activity of the perichondrium lengthens and thickens the model. Interstitial growth complements the appositional growth of the model. As adjacent bone-forming sites lengthen, the perichondrium at the promimal and distal ends degenerates, forming a synovial cavity between the developing bones (Fig. 10.12). These denuded sites eventually become the articular surfaces. After these events, the model is dependent upon interstitial growth exclusively.

The progressive lengthening and thickening of the model is associated with the maturation of the cartilage cells. Those that differentiate first occupy the center of the model. The young cells, which are located proximally and distally, mature toward the center. Young cells and their lacunae be-

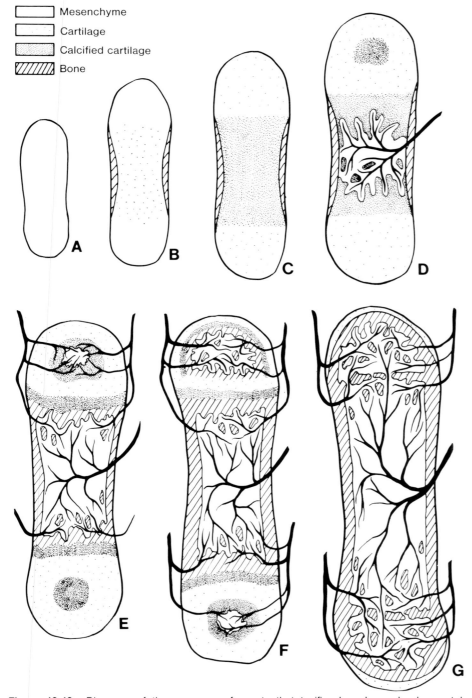

Mesenchyme
Cartilage
Calcified cartilage
Bone

Figure 10.10. Diagrams of the sequence of events that typifies long bone development by endochondral ossification. Refer to the text for a complete description of the process.

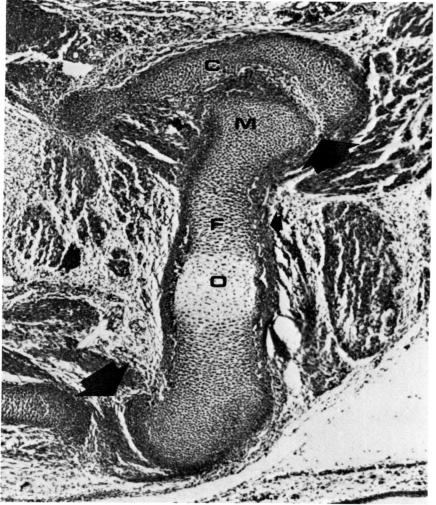

Figure 10.12. Developing model of the os coxa and femur of a canine fetus. The general forms of the femur *(F)* and os coxa *(C)* are apparent at this early stage of development. The majority of the model is composed of mesenchymal cells *(M)*. The center of the model *(O)*, composed of cartilage, is the early ossification center. The model is surrounded by a perichondrium *(small arrows)*. The mesenchyme has disintegrated in the regions of the acetabulum and stifle, thus, these joints are evident at this early stage of development also *(large arrows)*. ×16.

come progressively larger with maturation. Eventually, the lacunae of contiguous cells become sufficiently large to reduce the intervening matrix to a thin separating rim. Such older cells are hypertrophic (excessively enlarged). At the same time these maturation events are occurring, the perichondrium in the middle of the model (presumptive diaphysis) is invaded by blood vessels, and some of the cells in this envelope begin to differentiate into osteoblasts and osteoclasts; thus, the *periosteum* is formed (Fig. 10.10*B*). This envelope forms woven bone that circumscribes the chondrogenic model *(collar* or *sleeve bone).* This bone is the newly forming diaphysis. The *diaphyseal ossification center* has been established (Fig. 10.10*C*).

Primary Ossification Center. The continued latitudinal expansion and development of the *primary ossification center*

(diaphyseal ossification center) is contingent upon the continued osteogenic activity of the periosteum. The continued elongation is dependent upon the continued production of cartilage and its replacement within the confines of the surrounding sleeve bone (Fig. 10.10*C*). The matrix associated with hypertrophic chondrocytes in the center of the primary ossification center eventually becomes calcified. The hypertrophic chondrocytes participate in the calcification process. Although some of the chondrocytes die, speculation exists about the ultimate fate of those that survive. Chondrocytes released from their lacunae may give rise to other populations of osteoblasts. Some evidence exists that supports the belief that modulation of chondrocytes to osteoblasts is possible. In other foci (articular cartilage), chondrocytes appear to be fixed postmitotic cells; modulation of

chondrocytes to different and/or more primitive cells seems unlikely.

The cartilaginous model is avascular. Although blood vessels are located at the periphery as part of the periosteum, none are located within the cartilaginous model. Also, *the cartilaginous model is devoid of stem cells.* All of the mesenchymal cells that formed the chondrogenic center were differentiated into chondrocytes. Continued developmental progress of the cartilaginous model is contingent upon neovascularization and repopulation of the model with stem cells.

Periosteal Bud Formation. A reasonable presumption is that the calcified cartilage is dead tissue. As such, this tissue must be removed from the expanding ossification center. Macrophages, the cells responsible for the formation of osteoclasts, invade the center of the calcified cartilage from the perivascular region of the periosteum. This cavitation process creates spaces within the calcified cartilaginous mass. These spaces become filled with blood vessels and perivascular cells (Fig. 10.10*D*). Many *periosteal buds* penetrate the model after the wave of osteoclastic activity. One of these buds will eventually become the *nutrient artery.*

Periosteal buds invading into the chondrogenic model result in three events that are essential for the continuation of appropriate development: *removal of calcified cartilage; neovascularization of the model; repopulation of the model with appropriate stem cells.*

The essence of the endochondral ossification process is the formation of bone within cartilage. The osteoclastic removal of the calcified cartilage by osteoclasts creates spaces and new surfaces within the cartilaginous model. These surfaces become the ones upon which woven bone is deposited, replacing the cartilage that had been removed. **Bone replaces cartilage; cartilage is not converted into bone.** The newly formed bone at the periphery of the cartilaginous model is continuous with the collar bone that surrounds the model. The repopulation of the model with stem cells establishes the endosteal envelopes. The periosteum, therefore, gives rise to all of the endosteal envelopes. The marrow cavity, which is an expansion of the coalesced spaces formed by osteoclastic activity, and the development of the myeloid tissue contained therein are integral parts of bone development.

Sleeve Bone Formation. The deposition of bone at the periphery of the chondrogenic model as a consequence of the perichondrium being converted into a periosteum has been described as intramembranous ossification. It seems to be didactically useful to make a distinction between intramembranous ossification and the circumstances associated with sleeve bone formation. Intramembranous ossification is the de novo formation of bone within the "membranous" environment described previously. Once a spicule of bone has formed, the continued growth of osteogenic centers is dependent upon two factors: the continued de novo development of new bone; and, the continued growth of the spicules by the simple formation and apposition of new bone to pre-existing bone. The essence of the process is bone formation in a "membrane" followed by appositional growth.

The first spicules of sleeve bone are the products of the newly formed periosteum. The new bone is formed upon the chondral model within a vascularized microenvironment. The de novo formation of these spicules of bone upon cartilage is followed by the apposition of new bone to pre-existing bone. The essential difference between this pattern of ossification and intramembranous ossification is the use of cartilage upon which bone formation occurs initially. It seems prudent to distinguish the mechanism of sleeve bone formation as *epichondral ossification*.

Continued Growth—Primary Center. Chondrocytes continue to divide at the proximal and distal ends of the model, accounting for the continual increase in length (Fig. 10.13). The periosteum continues to add new bone to the diaphysis to maintain the longitudinal relationship with the growing cartilage. Continued apposition of new bone also accounts for an increased diaphyseal diameter. The cells progress through the maturation stages described previously, and their matrices ultimately calcify. *Capillary loops* from the periosteal bud, with their pericapillary populations of bone cells, continue to advance into the calcified matrix removing cartilage by osteoclasia and creating new surfaces for bone formation (Fig. 10.14).

Osteoclastic activity at the apex of the capillary loop is accomplished by mononucleated cells. Multinucleated giant cells are not observed often in these foci. The macrophages have not fused at this point in the process, but osteoclasts are apparent away from the advancing front of chondroclasia toward the center of the ossification center. The chondrocytes are arranged into columns, each column representing isogenous groups or cell nests. The chondroid material between each chondrocyte is a *transverse septum*. Successive removal of transverse septa results in the demise of the chondrocytes and confluence of contiguous chondrocytic lacunae. The remaining intercolumnar matrix, *longitudinal septa*, becomes the calcified cartilaginous surfaces upon which new woven bone is deposited. The longitudinal septa appear as spicules of calcified cartilage separated by spaces that are filled with capillary loops and perivascular cells. In actuality, the longitudinal

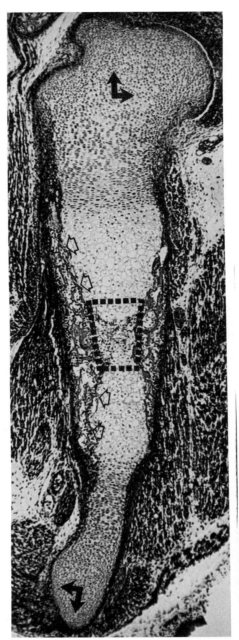

Figure 10.13. Progressive development of the primary ossification center of a fetal hamster humerus. *Outlined area*, primary ossification center. Periosteal collar bone has developed *(open arrows)*. The bone continues to grow in the directions indicated *(solid arrows)*. ×7.

septa are the walls of tunnels upon which bone deposition occurs. (Push a blunt object into a mass of clay. Continue doing so until numerous holes are separated by thin rims of clay. The tubular profiles of clay-lined tunnels are analagous to the relationships described between the longitudinal septa and intervening spaces.) Cartilage is removed to create surfaces upon which bone deposition may occur.

Some bones develop from a single ossi-

fication center. In these instances, the expanding osseous replacement reduces the growing cartilage to a zone that underlies the articular cartilage. This zone of growth *(growth cartilage)* supplies new chondrocytes to the maturation sequence that culminates in osseous replacement within the primary ossification center. Spicules of calcified cartilage and woven bone are used for the deposition of lamellar bone. The region of the ossification center that contains these three tissues (calcified cartilage, woven bone, lamellar bone) is called the *primary spongiosa* (Fig. 10.15). Gradually,

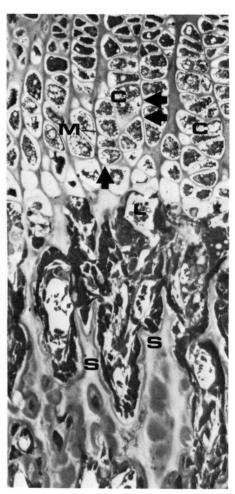

Figure 10.14. Removal of calcified cartilage within the primary ossification center of a murine femur. The chondrocytes *(C)* within their lacunae are separated from each other by thin rims of cartilaginous matrix *(M)*. Transverse septa *(arrow)* do not mineralize in most animals, whereas longitudinal septa *(double arrows)* undergo mineralization. Capillary loops *(L)* are surrounded by numerous perivascular cells. The lacunae are opened by osteoclasts that remove the transverse septa. The contiguous lacunar surfaces and intervening matrix become the surfaces *(S)* or longitudinal septa upon which woven bone depostion occurs. ×160. (plastic-embedded, 1-μm section.)

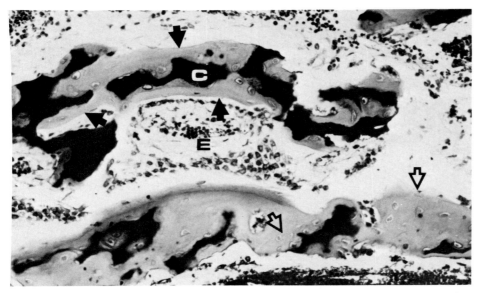

Figure 10.15. Tissues of the primary spongiosa. Spicules of bone contain cores of calcified cartilage (C). Woven bone (open arrows) comprises the bulk of the osseous tissue. Lamellar bone formation is apparent upon the spicules (solid arrows). Elements of the endosteum and myeloid tissue fill the interosseous spaces. ×40. (Aldehyde fuchsin).

calcified cartilage and woven bone (as well as some lamellar bone) are removed by osteoclasia and are replaced totally by lamellar bone. The *secondary spongiosa* is the region of the ossification center in which replacement by lamellar bone is accomplished completely.

In some bones, trabeculae of the primary spongiosa extend from proximal cartilage through the marrow cavity to the distal growth cartilage. In these bones, the secondary spongiosa, characterized by trabeculae of lamellar bone, expands longitudinally toward the growth cartilage. Upon cessation of growth, cancellous bone is continuous from both epiphyses through the marrow cavity. In other bones, the secondary spongiosa is a narrow zone of lamellar bone, because osteoclastic activity removes all trabeculae of bone from the marrow cavity. Upon cessation of growth, the secondary spongiosa is confined to the proximal and distal epiphyses as trabecular bone, whereas the marrow cavity is devoid of bone.

While progressive elongation has been

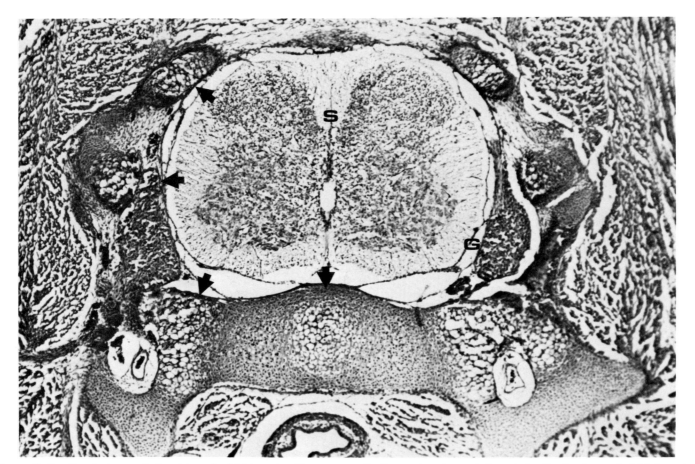

Figure 10.16. Developing cervical vertebra of a fetal hamster. Numerous ossification centers (arrows) characterize the development of this irregular bone. The developing spinal cord and a dorsal root ganglion (G) are apparent within the spinal canal. ×10.

occurring, the periosteum has been increasing the length and diameter of the organ. The increase in bone diameter is accompanied by an increase in marrow cavity diameter. Simultaneously, the trabecular endosteum forms bone at the point of metaphyseal osseous replacement and may remove bone if the marrow cavity is to be hollow.

These events lead to a definitive structure in those bones that develop from a single ossification center. Most bones, however, develop from more than one ossification center.

Model Growth

Secondary Ossification Centers. Most of the long bones have at least three ossification centers. The primary ossification center forms the diaphysis, whereas *proximal* and *distal ossification centers* form the proximal and distal epiphyses. These are referred to as *secondary ossification centers* (Figs. 10.10D and E). All ossification centers that develop subsequent to the primary ossification center are called secondary ossification centers. Irregularly shaped bones have numerous ossification centers, each one responsible, generally, for a single irregularity (Fig.10.16). Developmentally, each of the secondary ossifications centers may be considered the development centers for "separate bones" that must fuse secondarily with the the primary ossification center to form the definitive structure. Sometimes the fusion does not occur. Elbow dysplasia, as an example, can result from the nonunion of the anconeal ossification center (ununited anconeal process) with the rest of the ulna.

Some of the temporal and spatial relationships within the secondary centers, however, differ from those within the primary centers. At some point in time, branches from epiphyseal vessels either actively invade or are incorporated into the cartilage of the presumptive epiphyses. These vessels occur within a network of tunnels called *cartilage canals* (Fig. 10.17). The cartilage canals contain arterioles and venules that are connected by a terminal glomerulus. The vessels and terminal capillary bed are ensheathed in perivascular connective tissue. The periglomerular cartilaginous matrix undergoes calcification. Osteoclasts and their precursor macrophages initiate the removal of the calcified cartilage. The margins of the spaces thus formed serve as the surfaces upon which woven bone formation occurs. Continued radial chondroclasia and complementary osteogenesis occur within the coalescing marrow cavity of the secondary ossification center. Myeloid tissue develops within this center.

The morphological features and timing sequence of the events of the secondary ossification center are a variation of the events of the diaphyseal ossification center.

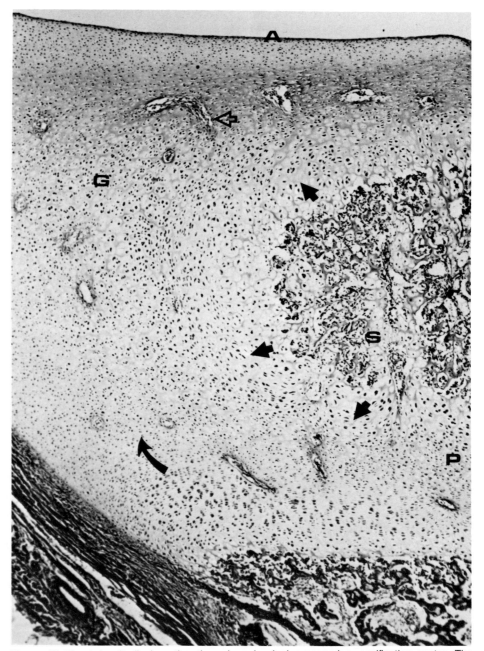

Figure 10.17. A longitudinal section through a developing secondary ossification center. The cartilage of the epiphysis includes the articular cartilage *(A)*, growing cartilage *(G)*, and presumptive growth plate cartilage *(P)*. The continuity of the growth plate cartilage *(curved arrows)* with the articular cartilage often is maintained throughout development. The secondary ossification center expands progressively *(solid arrows)* reducing the epiphyseal and growth plate cartilage to narrow zones. *Open arrow*, cartilage canal. The band of cartilage beyond the extent of the cartilage canals is destined to become articular cartilage. For reasons yet to be determined, the cartilage canals do not invade into the presumptive articular cartilage. ×10.

The cascade of events associated with vascular invasion are postponed, presumably until the appropriate stimulatory signal. Despite these differences, the results are the same—an ossification center is formed. The new ossification center defines the growing limits of the epiphyseal cartilage and a band of cartilage interposed between the primary and secondary ossification centers (Fig. 10.17). The formation of this band or *growth plate* is a consequence of secondary ossification center formation.

Growth Plates. Cartilage remains as an articular surface and cartilage remains as a disc or plate between the bone forming in the epiphyseal center and the bone forming in the diaphyseal center (Fig. 10.17). This plate of cartilage between the primary and secondary centers of ossification is called the *growth plate (epiphyseal plate, epiphyseal disc, physis)*. Cartilage is added continuously to the secondary ossification center by the interstitial growth of the cells from the subarticular cartilage and the epiphyseal side of the growth plate. These zones of proliferative cells are continuous with each other at the peripheral margin of the cartilage of the epiphysis. The proliferative zone of the growth plate adds new cartilage cells to the diaphyseal and epiphyseal ossification centers simultaneously for a variable but short amount of time. Eventually, epiphyseal osseous replacment adjacent to the growth plate overrides the proliferative capacity of the cartilage on this side of the growth plate. This results in the formation of an *endplate* of epiphyseal bone juxtaposed to the cartilage (Figs. 10.18 and 10.19). *Two direct consequences result from end-plate formation:*

1) the growth and shaping of the epiphysis then becomes the exclusive function of the proliferative activity of the subarticular cartilage of the epiphysis;
2) the growth plate only contributes cartilage to the diaphyseal ossifiction center.

The formation of the growth plate occurs as a consequence of the development and expansion of a secondary ossification center (Figs. 10.10*E* and *F*, 10.17 and 10.19). The continued elongation of the diaphysis is a consequence of the interstitial growth of the cartilage within the growth plate. Mitotic activity within the reserve chondrocytic zone adds new cells constantly and moves the epiphysis further from the center of the diaphysis. This addition tends to thicken the growth plate; however, the growth plate maintains a relatively constant thickness throughout its functional existence. The thickness is maintained because the rate of proliferation of the reserve chondrocytic zone equals the rate of metaphyseal osseous replacement. Accordingly, the elongation of the diaphysis is coincident with the movement of the growth plate through space. Cessation of growth is achieved and the growth plate becomes progressively thinner and eventually closes when the rate of cartilage proliferation is exceeded by the rate of metaphyseal osseous replacement. Growth plates close at different times in different bones in different species. Closure times for specific growth plates in specific bones of a given

species occur in a given time period. At closure, the trabecular bone of the metaphysis becomes continuous with the trabecular bone of the epiphysis (Figs. 10.10*F* and *G*).

Zones of the Growth Plate. The histological organization of the growth plate is similar to that of the ossification center before plate formation. The events within the growth plate are identical to those described for the primary ossification center. The growth plate is the limit of the expanding primary ossification center.

Five zones of cartilage cells are identifiable within the growth plate (Figs. 10.19 and 10.20): resting chondrocytes, proliferative chondrocytes, maturing chondrocytes, hypertrophied chondrocytes, and calcified cartilage.

The *zone of resting chondrocytes* is juxtaposed to the epiphyseal end-plate. These cells do not divide. Their primary function seems to be to weld the growth plate to the epiphysis.

The zone of *proliferative chondrocytes* is characterized by stacks of thin, wedge-shaped cells that are actively mitotic. The stacks of cells are isogenous groups. The activity of this zone is responsible for elon-

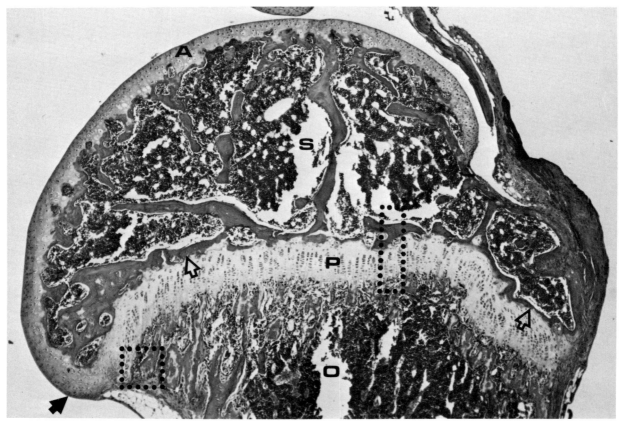

Figure 10.18.   The ossification centers and growth plate of the proximal humerus of a growing gerbil. The growth plate *(P)* separates the primary ossification center *(O)* from the secondary ossification center *(S)*. The growth plate is continuous with the articular cartilage *(arrow)*. Spicules of bone, calcified cartilage and myeloid tissue fill both ossification centers. The spaces are artifacts of sectioning. The end-plate *(open arrows)* resides upon the proximal margin of the physis. The presence of the end-plate indicates that the growth plate no longer contributes to the formation of the epiphysis. Rather, continued growth and expansion of the secondary ossification center is dependent upon growing cartilage that is deep to the articular cartilage. The square area is enlarged in Figure 10.25; the rectangular area, Figure 10.19. Compare with Plate IV.9. ×10.

with *matrix vesicles* and is confined generally to the longitudinal septa. In some species, however, portions or all of the transverse septa may be mineralized also.

Perivascular cells of the capillary loops in this region of calcified cartilage remove the transverse septa (Figs. 10.21 and 10.22). Chondrocytic lacunae become confluent and their contiguous surfaces are those upon which woven bone is deposited. These surfaces actually are the longitudinal septa. In longitudinal section they appear as finger-like projections into the metaphysis (Plate I.8). In actuality, they are tunnels the inner surfaces of which are used for bone deposition (Fig. 10.23).

The relationships of the *primary spongiosa* and *secondary spongiosa* in association with the growth plate are identical to those relationships described with the primary ossification center (Fig. 10.23).

Modeling Activity

These activities combine to produce the definitive shapes that characterize all of the bones. Modeling activities are complemented by remodeling.

Diaphyseal Growth. The attainment of

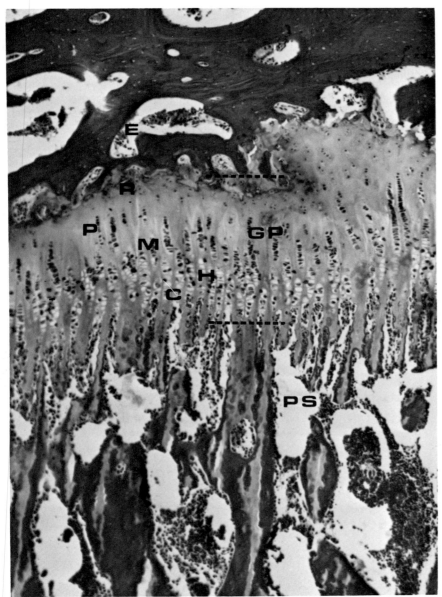

Figure 10.19. Definitive growth plate. The end-plate *(E)* has formed on the epiphyseal side of the growth plate, thus ending the physeal contribution to the shape and growth of the epiphysis. The approximate limits of the growth plate *(GP)* are indicated by the *dashed lines*. The growth plate maintains a relatively constant thickness until closure begins. The cells within the growth plate are columnated and are divisible into distinct yet related groups or zones. *R*—resting chondrocytes; *P*—proliferative chondrocytes; *M*—maturing chondrocytes; *H*—hypertrophied chondrocytes; *C*—zone of calcified cartilage. The primary spongiosa *(PS)* is just below the physis. ×50.

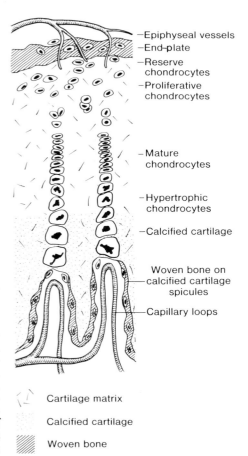

Figure 10.20. Diagram of a physis. Compare this drawing with the micrograph in Figure 10.19. The morphological features of the physis are labeled.

gation as well as adding new cells to replace those lost to metaphyseal osseous replacement (Fig. 10.21).

The *zone of maturing chondrocytes* is the region in which various cellular characteristics may be observed. Cell and lacunar size increase progressively and lacunae become more rounded than in the proliferative and resting zones. The columnation of these cells is obvious. Mechanical influences upon the growth plate probably account for this columnation.

The *zone of hypertrophied chondrocytes* is a narrow zone adjacent to the maturation

zone. The cells are large and the intercellular substance is reduced progressively. *Transverse septa*, the matrical material separating contiguous cells within a column, are especially thin. The *longitudinal septa*, the cartilage matrix between adjacent columns of cells, eventually undergo calcification. This zone is the weakest region of the growth plate. Fractures of growth plates *(epiphysiolysis)* generally occur through this zone.

The *zone of calcified cartilage* consists of cells, the matrix of which undergoes calcification. This calcification is associated

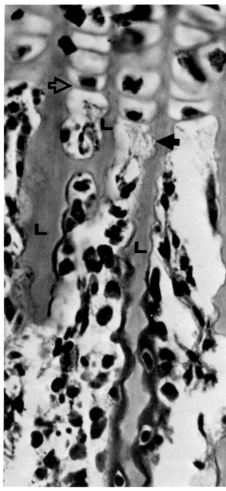

Figure 10.21. Osseous replacement within the primary spongiosa. Chondrocytes are released from their lacunae *(solid arrow)* after removal of the transverse septa *(open arrow)* by osteo-clasts. The fate of these cells is not clear. Cells removed in this region of the growth plate are replaced by the mitotic activity of the proliferative chondrocytes. Some chondrocytes have been displaced from their lacunae by the sectioning techniques. The remaining longitudinal septa *(L)* have scalloped borders that correspond to the confluent lateral margins of the lacunae of con-tiguous chondrocytes. The dark material depos-ited on the longitudinal septa is woven bone. Compare with Figure 10.20. ×100.

definitive length is primarily the function of the growth plate. Although some length is achieved before the formation of a growth plate, the greatest amount of length results from the interstitial growth of the growth plate cartilage.

The continual apposition of bone by os-teoblastic activity of the periosteum in-creases the diameter of the diaphysis (Fig. 10.24). The increased outside diameter is accompanied by an increase in the diame-ter of the marrow cavity. To accomplish this, the periosteal envelope must form bone, while the cortical endosteal envelope

removes bone. The net effect of this com-bination of cellular activity is the cortical compacta of the animal being derived pri-marily from the periosteum. Most of the diaphyseal circumferential bone and pri-mary osteons are formed by the perios-teum.

The marrow cavity of most long bones is filled with myeloid tissue, but very little bone is present. The primary and secondary spongiosa are removed during develop-ment. Metaphyseal osseous replacement of cartilage is accomplished within the pri-mary spongiosa by the trabecular endosteal envelope. The same envelope removes woven bone and adds lamellar bone within

the primary spongiosa. Ultimately, lamel-lar bone totally replaces calcified cartilage within the secondary spongiosa. In a typical long bone, the secondary spongiosa may be difficult to observe, because trabecular en-dosteal osteoclastic activity removes these spicules of bone. This removal process re-sults in a marrow cavity devoid of osseous tissue.

The differential activity of these three envelopes during growth is one of the rea-sons that the envelopes are distinguished from one another functionally. The osten-sible morphological similarities of these en-velopes is contrasted to their functional individuality. The periosteum forms bone,

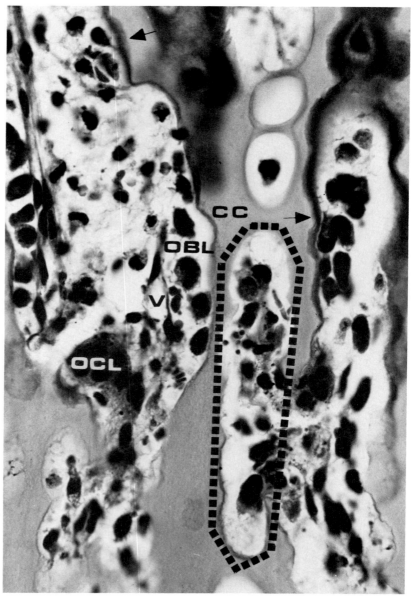

Figure 10.22. Osteoblastic and osteoclastic activity adjacent to the growth plate. Confluent lacunae and their remaining longitudinal septa *(outlined region)* are the surfaces upon which osteoblasts *(OBL)* deposit woven bone *(arrows)*. Osteoblasts and osteoclasts *(OCL)* comprise a major portion of the perivascular cell populations associated with numerous vascular loops *(V)*. ×160.

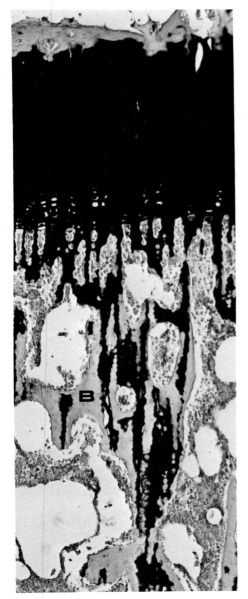

Figure 10.23. Growth plate and primary spongiosa. Finger-like projections of dark-stained material, calcified cartilage, extend from the growth plate into the primary spongiosa. The progressive deposition of bone *(B)* is coupled to the continual removal of calcified cartilage. ×16. (Aldehyde fuchsin.)

while the cortical endosteum removes bone. The trabecular endosteal envelope of the primary spongiosa forms bone, while the same envelope within the secondary spongiosa removes bone to form a marrow cavity devoid of bone.

The peripheral aspect of the growth plate is joined to the cylindrical diaphysis by the spicules of bone that covers the cores of calcified cartilage (Fig. 10.25). This margin is the only point of contact and union between these two structures. As new bone is deposited upon calcified cartilage, the osseous tissue is also deposited upon spic-

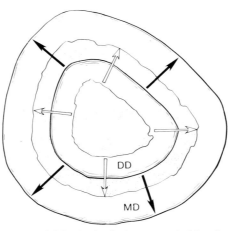

Figure 10.24. Latitudinal movement of the diaphysis during growth. The developing diaphysis *(DD)* grows in width through the osteogenic activity of the periosteum *(solid arrows)*. As periosteal bone is added, the cortical endosteum removes bone via osteoclastic activity *(open arrows)*. The net result is a diaphysis with an increased diameter and an increased marrow cavity diameter *(MD—mature diaphysis)*. Also, these related activities result in most of the diaphysis of a long bone being derived from the periosteum.

ules that constitute the forming diaphysis. The two structures are essentially welded to each other. The spicules of bone, which in reality are tunnels of bone, serve as the surface upon which layers of bone are deposited (Fig. 10.26). This provides for osseous continuity from the growth plate to the diaphysis also.

Epiphyseal Growth. The epiphysis of a bone is, by definition, a part of a long bone that develops from an ossification center distinct from that used by the shaft (Fig. 10.17). Furthermore, the epiphysis is initially separated from the shaft by a growth plate. In the adult, an epiphysis consists of bone (with contained marrow elements) that is covered by articular cartilage. In the developing organism, three distinct cartilaginous zones are apparent within the epiphysis. The *presumptive articular cartilage* has a mitotically active zone positioned deeply. An *acidophilic cartilage* zone is subjacent to the presumptive articular cartilage zone. The acidophilic cartilage is underlaid by the *growth cartilage* that feeds chondrocytes into the endochondral ossification process of the epiphysis. A zone of mitotically active cells is a peripheral component of the growth cartilage. The developing *chondroepiphysis*, then, consists of the following from superficial to deep:

1. *presumptive articular cartilage*
   a. *maturing*
   b. *dividing*
2. *acidophilic cartilage*
3. *growth cartilage*
   a. *dividing*
   b. *maturing*

The activity of these zones is responsible ultimately for the definitive characteristics of the adult epiphysis

The ends of long bones generally are larger than the diaphysis (Fig. 10.27). The epiphyses and metaphyses are characterized by a distinct flare. After the formation of the epiphyseal end-plate, the growth of the epiphysis occurs independently of the events of the diaphyseal ossification center. The growing cartilage subjacent to the articular cartilage contributes to the expanded epiphysis. Naturally, the growing diaphysis must maintain a proper relationship with the enlarged epiphysis. This is achieved by selected modeling activities in the metaphyseal region. During growth, bone is resorbed on the periosteal side of the metaphysis, and bone is added to the trabeculae (tunnels) of the metaphysis as these join the endosteal side of the diaphysis. This facilitates a gradual flaring of the proximal and distal aspects of the bone.

Perichondral Ring. The point of transition between the periosteum and articular cartilage is called the *perichondral ring*. The second name is especially descriptive, because the structure is a ring of perichondrium covering the periphery of the growth plate. Appositional growth of the growth plate is achieved by the cells within this envelope. The envelope is responsible for the latitudinal expansion of the growth plate to maintain pace with the expanding diaphysis and epiphysis.

Hormones and Bone Development

Specific Hormones and Effects. Differentiation, mitosis, carbohydrate synthesis and secretion, protein synthesis and secretion, calcium metabolism, and phagocytosis are integral functions of the cellular populations of the connective, cartilaginous, osseous, and vascular tissues that are essential components of this developmental process. All of these events are regulated and influenced by numerous factors.

The effects of *estrogens* upon endochondral ossification are diverse, complex, and species-specific. Generally, the estrogens inhibit linear growth by favoring the closure of the growth plates. This involves an acceleration of metaphyseal osseous replacement and an inhibition upon the proliferative chondrocytes.

Testosterone exerts an effect similar to the estrogens. Skeletal maturation is dependent upon the presence of this hormone, because it favors bone formation. Its presence is important in the achievement of normal growth plate closure.

Excessive quantities of *glucocorticoids* inhibit skeletal growth and retard the development of secondary ossification centers. A decreased proliferation and hypertrophy of chondrocytes is a consistent developmental problem with excessive quantities of these substances. The phenomenon

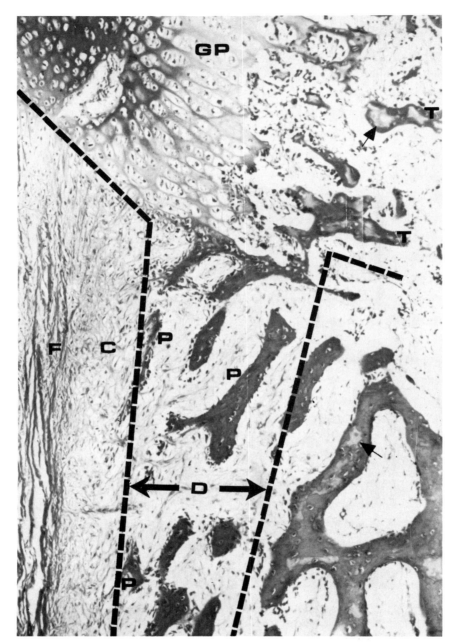

Figure 10.25. Union of the growth plate to the diaphysis. The peripheral aspects of the growth plate *(GP)* are united to the diaphysis *(D)* by the walls of the tunnels *(T)* of calcified cartilage and bone that comprise the primary spongiosa. The periosteum, fibrous *(F)* and cellular *(C)* components, covers the bone at this point of union (metaphysis). The periosteum may form bone *(P)* as well as remove it from the region. Removal of the bone at this focus results in the epiphyseal flaring that is characteristic of long bones. ×25.

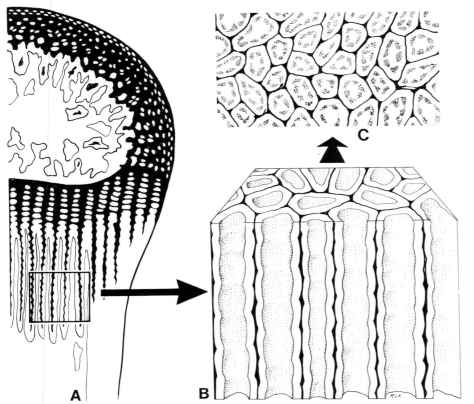

Figure 10.26. Diagrams of the morphological relationships of components of the primary spongiosa. The retained longitudinal septa of calcified cartilage with woven bone deposited on their surfaces appear as spicules or finger-like projections in longitudinal section *(A)*. The spicules are actually the peripheral margins of tunnels when viewed in three dimensions *(B)*. The walls of the tunnels are formed of bone deposited upon a peripheral core of calcified cartilage. The tunnels become filled progressively with bone at their points of union with the diaphysis *(C)*. (Redrawn and modified from Ham, A. W.: *Histology*, 7th edition, J. B. Lippincott, Philadelphia, 1974.)

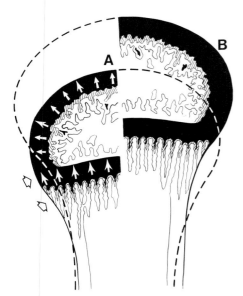

Figure 10.27. A diagram of the activity associated with the modeling of epiphyses. The ends (epiphyses) of long bones are generally larger than the diaphyses. The growth plate and growth cartilage subjacent to the articular cartilage are

may be explained by the inhibitory effects of glucocorticosteroids upon protein synthesis. Osteoblastic activity within the primary and secondary spongiosa is reduced also. Similarly, they decrease the osteoblastic activity of the periosteum and endosteum of growing bones.

Growth hormone mediates its effect upon the growing skeleton by regulating the rate of mitosis of the proliferative chondrocytes. Excesses of growth hormone before growth plate closure result in *pituitary gigantism*. After growth plate closure, excesses result

responsible for the longitudinal movement of epiphyses through space. Interstitial growth of these components *(white arrows)* moves the epiphyses and articular surface from A to B. The epiphyseal flaring is accomplished by bone being resorbed by periosteal osteoclasts *(open arrows)*, while deposition along the inner surface of the bone is accomplished via the trabecular endosteum associated with the tunnels of the primary spongiosa that are continuous with the diaphysis. (Redrawn and modified from Ham, A. W.: *Histology*, 7th edition, J. B. Lippincott, Philadelphia, 1974.)

in a pronounced periosteal new bone formation called *acromegaly*.

Although the *thyroid hormones* (T_3 and T_4) affect the cellular metabolic activity of most cells, their effects upon the developing skeleton are manifested primarily in the cartilage. Thyroxine (T_4) is necessary for the proliferation and maturation of the chondrocytes. It also affects the proliferation and modulation of osteogenic cells of the primary and secondary spongiosa.

References

Ascenzi, A. and Bendetti, L.: An electron microscope study of the foetal membranous ossification. Acta Anat. (Basel) *37*:370, 1962.

Anderson, C.E. and Parker, J.: Electron microscopy of the epiphyseal cartilage plate. Clin. Orthop. *58*:225, 1968.

Bassett, A.L.: Current concepts of bone formation. J. Bone Joint Surg. *44A*:1217, 1962.

Bonucci, E. Fine structure of early cartilage calcification. J. Ultrastruct. Res. *20*:33, 1967.

Boskey, A.L.: Current concepts of the physiology and biochemistry of calcification. Clin. Orthop. *157*:225, 1981.

Brighton, C.T.: Structure and function of the growth plate. Clin. Orthop. *136*:22, 1978.

Brookes, M.: Cortical vascularization and growth in foetal trabecular bones. J. Anat. *97*:597, 1963.

Clark, E.R. and Clark, E.L.: Microscopic observations on new formation of cartilage and bone in the living animal. Amer. J. Anat. *70*:167, 1942.

Crelin, E. and Koch, W.: An autoradiographic study of chondrocytic transformation into chondroclasts and osteocytes during bone formation in vitro. Anat. Rec. *158*:473, 1967.

Farnum, C.E. and Wilsman, N.J.: The pericellular matrix of growth plate chondrocytes: A study using post-fixation with osmium ferrocyanide. J. Histochem. Cytochem *31*:765.

Frost, H.M.: Tetracycline-based histological analysis of bone remodeling. Calc. Tiss. Res. *3*:211, 1969.

Frost, H.M.: *Bone Remodeling and Skeletal Modeling Errors*. Charles C Thomas, Springfield, 1973.

Haines, R.: Cartilage canals. J. Anat. *68*:45, 1933.

Holtrop, M.E.: The ultrastructure of the epiphyseal plate. II. The hypertrophic chondrocyte. Calc. Tiss. Res. *9*:140, 1972.

Kincaid, S.A. and Van Sickle, D.C.: Bone morphology and postnatal osteogenesis: Potential for disease. Vet. Clin. N. A. *13*:3, 1983.

Kuettner, K.E., Sobel, L.W., Ray, R.D., Croxen, R.L., Passovoy, M. and Eisenstein, R.: Lysozyme in epiphyseal cartilage. J. Cell Biol. *44*:329, 1970.

Matthews, J.L., Martin, J.H., Lynn, J.A. and Collins, E,J,: Calcium incorporation in the developing cartilaginous epihysis. Calc. Tiss. Res. *1*:33, 1968.

Odegaard, J.: Growth of the manidible studied with the aid of metallic implants. Am. J. Orthop. *57*:145, 1970.

Schenk, R.K., Spiro, D. and Wiener, J.: Cartilage resorption in the tibial epiphyseal plate of growing rats. J. Cell Biol. *34*:275, 1967.

Schenk, R.K., Weiner, J. and Spiro, D.: Fine structural aspects of vascular invasion of the tibial epiphyseal plate of growing rats. Acta. Anat. *69*:1, 1968.

Scherft, J.P.: The ultrastructure of the organix matrix of calcified cartilage and bone in embryonic mouse radii. J. Ultrastruct. Res. *23*:333, 1968.

Weinmann, J.P. and Sicher, H.: *Bone and Bones*. C.V. Mosby, St. Louis, 1955.

Wilsman, N.J., Farnum, C.E., Hilley, H.D. and Carlsen, C.S.: Morphological evidence of a functional heterogeneity among physeal chondrocytes in growing swine. Amer. J. Vet. Res. *42*:1547, 1981.

Young, R.W.: Cell proliferation and specialization during endochondral osteogenesis in young rats. J. Cell Biol. *14*:357, 1962.

11: Blood

Peripheral Blood

General Characteristics

General Considerations. Blood consists of a large volume of fluid matrix and numerous formed elements (Table 11.1). A fibrous component *(fibrin)* is also present during blood clotting.

The fluid phase of the blood is called *plasma*. Varied cells and/or fragments of cells are suspended within the fluid phase. Upon removal of *fibrinogen* and *fibrin*, the remaining fluid is termed *serum*.

The functions of blood are numerous. The *transport* of oxygen and carbon dioxide is an important complement to pulmonary (external) and cellular (internal) respiration. Several important *buffer systems* occur in blood: carbonates, phosphates, hemoglobin, and proteins. All food substances must pass through the blood; thus, *nutrition* is an important function. An *excretory* function is obvious through the removal of metabolic waste products. The *maintenance of the fluid volume* of the body is accomplished through a balance between the blood-vascular system, tissue fluid space, intracellular fluid space, and lymphatics. The water content of the body is a medium for *heat regulation*. Also, the transport of hormones gives the blood a *regulatory* function. These hormones may be transported free in the plasma and/or be attached to specific transport proteins. The blood is also an important *protective device* for the body through its cells and various suspended materials (antibodies, antitoxins, etc.).

Plasma. *Plasma* is the straw-colored and transparent fluid matrix of blood. The plasma is apparent when a blood sample with an anticoagulant added has been centrifuged or the formed elements have been allowed to settle to the bottom of a collection vial. Generally, the fluid phase comprises about 35–50%. Numerous other factors (age, degree of hydration, disease, athletic conditioning) affect this percentage.

Plasma consists of approximately 90% water and 10% dissolved substances and solids. Dissolved inorganic ions (Na^+, K^+, Cl^-, HCO_3^-, Ca^{++}, and others) constitute about 1% of the plasma. Plasma proteins (albumins, globulins, fibrinogen) comprise approximately 7% of the total plasma. Other organic substances (urea, uric acid, amino acids, fatty acids, glycerol, and others) constitute 1%. Additionally, plasma normally contains various quantities of hormones, enzymes, pigments, vitamins, and dissolved gases.

Many of the characteristics attributed to plasma are a function of its protein components, which help in the maintenance of intravascular osmotic pressure (colloid osmotic pressure), the transport of various plasma constituents (hormones, waste products), the clotting mechanism, and the protection of the body by humoral antibodies (immunoglobulins). Electrophoretic separations are used commonly to characterize the protein constituents of plasma (or serum). Such characterizations demonstrate that plasma proteins consist of: albumin, α-globulins (α_1, α_2), β-globulins (β_1, β_2), γ-globulins and fibrinogen (Fig. 11.1). The globulin components are subject to species variations.

The albumin and fibrinogen fractions of the plasma proteins are produced by the liver. About three-quarters of the globulins are produced there as well. The rest of the globulins are produced in cells of the lymphatic system. The plasma is the immediate source of proteins when tissue proteins are depleted. Plasma proteins in the tissue fluid space are imbibed by macrophages via pinocytosis. The proteins are digested into their constituent amino acids, secreted, and used locally or transported to the blood for distribution throughout the body. The amount of available amino acids in the blood is in dynamic equilibrium with circulating plasma proteins and tissue proteins.

Albumin is a small protein with a molecular weight of about 70,000. It accounts for approximately one-half of the total protein

Table 11.1.
Blood Parameters of Selected Domestic and Laboratory Species*

| Species | Parameter | | | | | | | | | |
	Packed Cell Vol. PCV, %	Hb gm %	RBC × 10⁶/mm³	Total Protein†	Platelets × 10³/mm³	MCV‡ × 10¹⁵ L	RBC μm	MCHC gm/dl	M/E Ratio	WBC × 10³/mm³
Dog	45	15	6.8	6.0–7.5	550	70	7.0	34	1.2	11.5
Cat	37	12	7.5	6.0–7.5	450	45	5.9	33	1.6	12.5
Horse	42	15	9.5	6.0–8.0	330	46	5.4	35	1.6	9.0
Ox	35	11	7.0	6.0–8.0	500	52	5.7	33	0.7	8.0
Sheep	38	12	12.0	6.0–7.5	400	33	4.5	34	1.1	8.0
Goat	35	10	13.0	6.0–7.5	450	27	4.1	32	0.7	9.0
Pig	42	13	6.5	6.0–7.0	520	63	6.0	32	1.8	16.0
Rabbit	48	12	5.6	6.0–7.2	500	61	6.8	32	1.0	7.9
Rat	45	15	8.5	6.1–7.1	532	60	6.9	32	1.6	11.5
Guinea pig	40	14.5	5.6	5.1–6.3	500	65	7.5	30	1.5	10.8
Domestic fowl	36	10.3	2.8	4.0–5.2	27.6	127	10.7 × 7.1	29		16.6

* These average parameters vary with age, sex, strain, and breed of animal.
† Range of values.
‡ MCV—mean corpuscular volume, MCHC—mean corpuscular hemoglobin concentration, and M/E—myeloid/erythroid ratio.

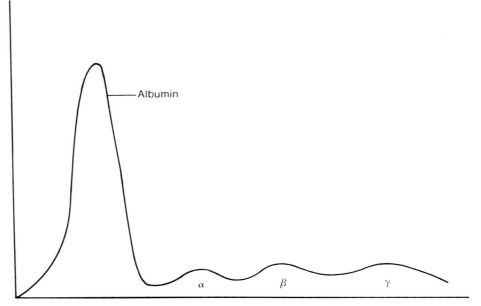

Figure 11.1. An idealized electrophoretic pattern of a serum sample. Relative and absolute alterations in the components are valuable in diagnostic evaluations.

Albumin

α β γ

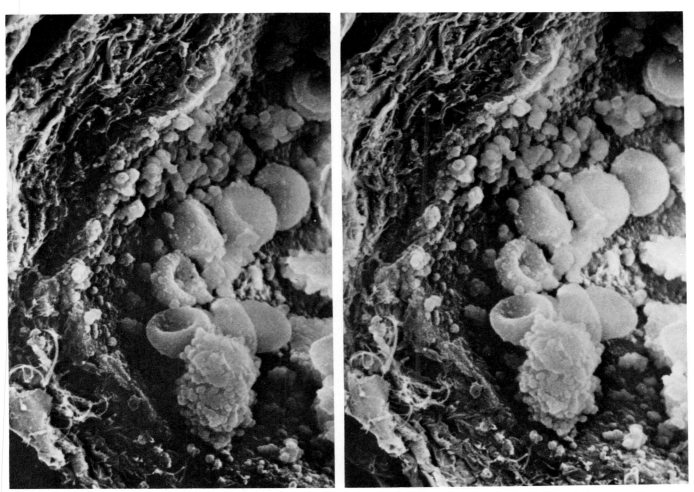

Figure 11.2. A scanning electron micrograph of canine erythrocytes. The freeze fractured sample is from the testis. The micrograph, a stereo pair, is comprised of one photograph with a specimen normal (perpendicular) to the beam. The second photograph was taken with the specimen tilted 6° from the beam axis. The three-dimensional quality of the photographs is apparent when viewed with stereo glasses. The large, globular structure with numerous processes is a white blood cell. Note the central depression in the erythrocytes. Some of the erythrocytes are bowl-shaped. ×4,000. (Courtesy of C. J. Connell).

of the plasma and about 70% of the intravascular osmotic pressure. Albumin contributes to the concentration gradient between blood and extracellular fluid. Also, it binds and transports hormones (thyroxine), metabolites (bilirubin) and drugs (barbiturates).

The *α-globulins* contribute to the osmotic pressure of the vascular bed as well as serving as carriers for various substances: copper by *ceruloplasmin*, hemoglobin by *haptoglobin*, thyroxine by *thyroxine binding globulin, cortisol by transcortin*. Lipoproteins of this fraction also transport triglycerides, fatty acids, vitamins, and other substances. Additionally, this fraction contains cholinesterase, alkaline phosphatase, lactic dehydrogenase, and factors involved in coagulation (factors V, IX, and X).

The *β-globulins* contribute to osmotic pressure and serve as transport substances; iron is transported by *transferrin* and hemin by *hemopexin*. Lipoproteins, complement, fibrinogen, and coagulation factors (VII, VIII) are present also.

The *γ-globulins* consist of the immunoglobulins (Chapter 17), blood group globulins, and the cryoglobulins.

The staining properties for the subsequent cells are described in terms of the use of Wright's or Giemsa stain.

Mammalian Blood Cells

Erythrocytes

Form and Function. The *erythrocytes* are also called *red blood cells (RBCs), red blood corpuscles*, and *rubricytes*. The erythrocyte is an anucleated, biconcave disc that is round in most mammalian species (Fig. 11.2). It is, however, oval in the members of the Camelidae (camel, dromedary,

llama, and alpaca). The diameter range is 3.5–7.5 μm in different species.

In smear preparations the biconcavity may be apparent because of the differential light transmission from the periphery to the central part of the corpuscle (Figs. 11.3 and 11.4). The RBCs may swell in hypotonic media or shrink in hypertonic media. All cells respond in this manner to varying tonicity, but it is most easily demonstrated in the erythrocyte.

In sections stained by routine procedures, the RBCs will stain pink. Within the capillary beds, larger vessels and even as

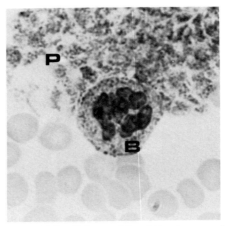

Figure 11.4.   Feline peripheral blood smear. A basophil *(B)* is surrounded by aggregated platelets *(P)* and erythrocytes. Variations in central pallor within this small population of erythrocytes is apparent.

extravasated blood, erythrocytes may become stacked one upon the other in a typical *rouleaux* formation. This formation is indicative of the manner by which they move through the smallest blood vessels (capillaries). The occurrence of the RBCs outside the vascular bed is usually an artifact of preparation techniques in normal tissues.

The RBC is modified uniquely to perform its primary function, carrying oxygen to the tissues in the form of *oxyhemoglobin* and carrying some carbon dioxide away from the tissues in the form of *carboxyhemoglobin*. Most of the cellular organelles (nucleus, Golgi, mitochondria, etc.) are lost during cytodifferentiation and the bulk of the corpuscle is composed of *hemoglobin*. The structural modification as a biconcave disk also facilitates the movement of this entity through the capillary bed (Fig. 11.5).

Erythrocytic Variants. Numerous variations occur in the morphology of the RBC. Some are attributable to improper processing of samples, whereas others are the result of disease processes. Some changes in morphology, however, cannot be explained. During the examination of peripheral blood smears from different species, many of the following changes will be observed.

Many erythrocytic variants are noted in the peripheral blood in a condition called *anemia*. A *regenerative anemia* is characterized by the bone marrow attempting to compensate by producing new erythrocytes. In *nonregenerative anemia*, the bone marrow is not responsive to the peripheral need for more RBCs.

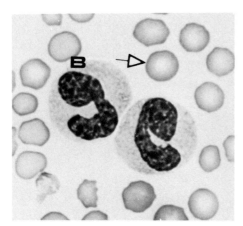

Figure 11.3.   Feline peripheral blood smear. The large cells in the center of the field are immature neutrophils—neutrophilic band cells *(B)*. Central pallor is apparent in some red blood corpuscles *(arrow)*. The concavity and, therefore, the central pallor are neither equally developed nor equally apparent in all species. ×400.

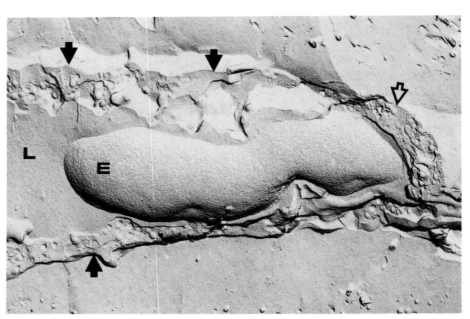

Figure 11.5.   An electron micrograph of a freeze fractured capillary and erythrocyte. The collapsed capillary is defined by its endothelial lining in longitudinal section by the *solid arrows*; in cross section, by the *open arrows*. The capillary lumen *(L)* contains a single erythrocyte *(E)* that conforms to the shape of the capillary. Erythrocytes are capable of adjusting their shape to that of the capillary. Compare with Figure 2.13. ×25,600. (Courtesy of J. E. Rash).

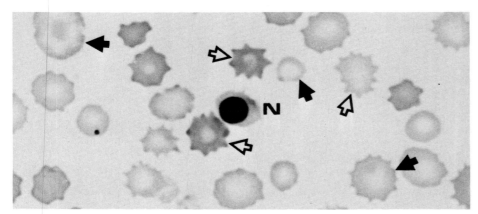

Figure 11.6. Peripheral blood smear from a young piglet with a regenerative anemia. A nucleated erythrocyte, metarubricyte, occupies the center of the field *(N)*. Acanthocytes *(open arrows)* are present. Note the different sizes of the erythrocytes *(solid arrows)*. This condition is called anisocytosis. ×400. (Giemsa stain).

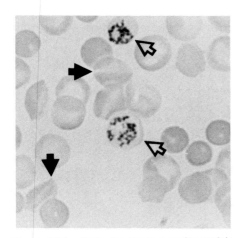

Figure 11.7. Reticulocytes in a canine peripheral blood smear. The reticulocytes *(open arrows)* are surrounded by large erythrocytes (macrocytes) and small erythrocytes (microcytes). The range of sizes in erythrocytes is called anisocytosis. Note the leptocytes *(solid arrows)*. ×400. (new methylene blue stain).

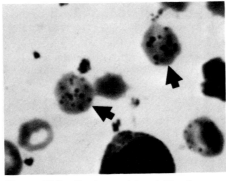

Figure 11.8. Bovine peripheral blood smear. Basophilic stippling *(arrows)* is apparent. ×400. (Giemsa stain).

Immature RBCs, usually confined to the bone marrow, may gain access to the peripheral circulation. One of these immature forms is a *metarubricyte* (Fig. 11.6). Normally, the nuclei are extruded from the cells before their entry into the vascular bed. Metarubricytes in the peripheral circulation usually indicate regeneration.

Immature cells containing remnants of ribosomal material also gain access to the peripheral circulation. These corpuscles, characterized by a diffuse cytoplasmic basophilia, are called *reticulocytes* (Fig. 11.7). Positive identification of these cells requires seeing basophilic granules or a fibrillar network with supravital stains such as new methylene blue. *Polychromatophilic erythrocytes* are immature cells whose cytoplasm has a mixed affinity for the acid and basic dyes of Romanowsky stains. *Polychromasia* describes the condition of the blood

sheep, but it can also indicate heavy metal poisoning that results in defective RBC formation. Moreover, basophilic stippling is not observed with new methylene blue.

Howell-Jolly (HJ) bodies are nonrefractile, nuclear remnants within RBCs that may be positioned eccentrically. Although HJ bodies indicate increased erythrocyte production, they are observed routinely in 1% of the RBCs of feline and equine blood.

Erythrocyte refractile (ER) bodies are demonstrable in unstained wet mounts as highly refractile bodies near or protruding from the periphery of the RBCs. The bodies appear as small circular pale areas at the periphery of the erythrocytes with Wright's stain (Fig. 11.9). They may be observed in 10% of normal feline RBCs. *Heinz bodies* are peripherally-positioned intracytoplasmic masses of altered hemoglobin that appear as pale areas with Romanowsky stains and as refractile blue-black spheres with new methylene blue. Heinz bodies and ER bodies are the same structures. They result from the oxidation of hemoglobin by certain agents; feline hemoglobin is more susceptible to oxidation than other species.

Although the size of erythrocytes varies, this parameter is constant for a given species. RBCs of normal size and hemoglobin content are called *normocytes* (Figs. 11.3 and 11.4). Any alteration to this normal size is referred to as *anisocytosis* (Fig. 11.10). Cells that are larger than normal are called *macrocytes*; cells that are smaller than normal, *microcytes*. Anemias in domestic animals are classified sometimes on the characteristic cell size as normocytic anemia, macrocytic anemia or microcytic anemia. *Normocytic anemia* is commonly a secondary disorder associated with various chronic diseases (infections, malignancies, nephritis). The most common cause of *macrocytic anemia* in domestic animals is the increased production and subsequent release of reticulocytes into the peripheral blood in response to crises resulting from blood loss or blood destruction. Because the anemia corrects itself once the crisis is

when these entities are present (Plate VII.4). The reticulocyte and the polychromatophilic erythrocyte are the same cell stained differently. Polychromasia is indicative of regeneration and should not be confused with the *basophilic stippling* of erythrocytes that are stained with a Romanowsky stain (Fig. 11.8). The latter indicates regeneration in cats, cattle and

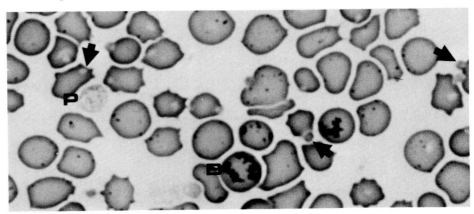

Figure 11.9. Feline peripheral blood smear. Basophilic stippling *(B)* and Heinz bodies *(solid arrows)* are evident. *P*, platelet. ×400. (Wright's stain).

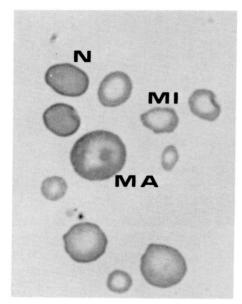

Figure 11.10. Anisocytosis in a porcine peripheral blood smear. Macrocytes *(MA)*, normocytes *(N)*, and microcytes *(MI)* are evident. The microcytes are hyperchromatic. ×400. (Giemsa stain).

met, this type is referred to as a *transitory* or *pseudomacrocytic anemia*. True *macrocytic anemia* results from a maturation arrest in the bone marrow in which immature (large) cells gain access to the peripheral blood. The most common cause of a *microcytic anemia* is an iron-deficiency. Chronic blood loss is one of the most common causes of iron-deficiency.

The constant size of the RBC under normal conditions, as well as their presence in most tissue sections, affords the microscopist a "built-in micrometer." The RBCs are generally about 5–6 μm in diameter.

The number of RBCs/mm³ generally varies inversely with the size of the blood corpuscles. An increase in the numbers of RBCs/mm³ is called *polycythemia*, whereas a decrease is called *oligocythemia*.

Any deviation from the normal shape of the RBC is termed *poikilocythemia*. There are numerous alterations to shape that are associated with many disease processes and/or faulty processing techniques. *Acanthocytes* have spine-like or blunt processes protruding from their surfaces. These cells can result from various diseases (Fig. 11.6). Similar morphological changes can result during processing in which slow-drying fluids create a hypertonic solution. Then the cells are called *crenated cells*. Bowl- or cup-shaped erythrocytes appear to have "punched-out" centers when observed in stained smears. Red blood cells normally assume a parabolic shape as they pass through capillaries (Fig. 2.13). Some type of cytoplasmic stromal defect does not permit these cells to return to their normal biconcave configuration. *Leptocytes* are

RBCs with a decreased volume and a normal to increased surface area (Fig. 11.11). Leptocytes are either target cells or folded cells. A *target cell* has a dense central zone surrounded by a clear zone with another dense zone at the periphery of the cell. These altered densities are generally attributed to a heterogeneous distribution of hemoglobin. *Folded cells* have a folded membrane across the cell. *Ovalocytes* are eliptical erythrocytes that may be encountered periodically. They are normal in avian, piscine and cameline blood. *Poikilocytes* are erythrocytes with a variety of abnormal shapes. Most commonly they may have a "tear drop" shape. They can indicate disease as well as slow drying problems during processing. *Schistocytes* are erythrocytic fragments with irregular shapes (Fig. 11.12). A spheroid cell with a decreased volume compared to its diameter and without a central region of pallor is called a *spherocyte*. Although it may be associated with other disease processes, it occurs commonly in autoimmune problems. *Stomatocytes* have a linear region of central pallor (Fig. 11.13). These cells are associated with hereditary erythrocytic membrane defects.

The homogenous staining of RBCs, except for the area of central pallor, is a function of the amount and distribution of hemoglobin. The normal amount and dis-

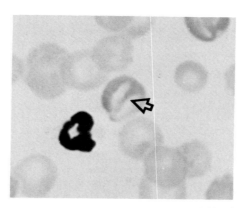

Figure 11.11. A fold cell in a peripheral blood smear of canine blood. A fold of membrane *(arrow)* crosses the central area of pallor. ×400.

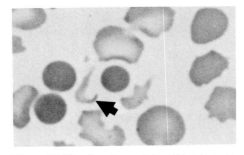

Figure 11.12. A canine peripheral blood smear. *Arrow*, schistocytes. ×400. (Wright's stain).

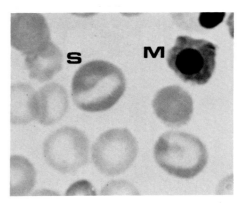

Figure 11.13. A canine peripheral blood smear. *S*, stomatocyte; *M*, metarubricyte. ×400.

tribution of hemoglobin is termed *normochromic*. A decrease in the hemoglobin content is *hypochromasia*. The release of reticulocytes from the bone marrow and iron deficiency results in the appearance of hypochromasia. Reticulocytes contain hemoglobin, but the cells are larger than normal. A *macrocytic hypochromic anemia* is characteristic of a regenerative anemia in all domestic animals except the horse, which does not release immature erythrocytes from the bone marrow. A *microcytic hypochromic anemia* results from an iron deficiency that is commonly associated with chronic blood loss (ectoparasites, endoparasites, gastric ulcers).

Granulocytes

Granulocytes are *white blood cells (leukocytes)* with specific granules and lobed or segmented nuclei. They are important protective cells that function within the vascular bed as well as within the extravascular tissues (Table 11.2).

Neutrophilic Granulocytes. The *neutrophil, heterophil,* or *polymorphonuclear leukocyte (PMN)* is the most frequently encountered granulocyte (Plates VI, VII). The cell is about twice the size of the RBC (9–12 μm) and is characterized by a segmented nucleus that may have from three to five lobes connected by a strand of nucleoplasm (Figs. 11.14–11.16). The specific granules may vary from light pink to purple depending upon the stain used; thus, the term *heterophil*. In some species (rabbit, guinea pig) these particles stain with acid dyes and the cells are usually referred to as *pseudoeosinophils*. In some cases, due to preparatory techniques, the particle may not be apparent.

Neutrophilic granulocytes contain two types of granules. *Primary granules (azurophilic granules)* are lysosomes. They contain the typical complement of lysosomal enzymes. *Specific granules*, however, do not contain lysosomal enzymes. Instead, they contain a bactericidal substance and alkaline phosphatase. After the phagocyto-

Table 11.2.
Differential Counts for Selected Domestic and Laboratory Species*

Species	Cells†					
	Mature Neutrophils	Immature Neutrophils‡	Lymphocytes	Monocytes	Eosinophils	Basophils
Dog	70	3	20	5.0	4.0	Rare
Cat	60	3	32	2.8	5.2	Rare
Horse	52	2	39	4.4	4.1	0.5
Ox	28	2	57	5.0	8.8	0.5
Sheep	30	Rare	62	2.5	5.0	0.5
Goat	36	Rare	56	2.5	5.0	0.5
Pig	37	3	53	5.0	3.5	0.5
Rabbit	43	2	42	9.0	2.0	4.0
Rat	28	1	62	5.0	2.0	1.0
Guinea pig	42	3	45	7.0	5.0	1.0
Domestic fowl	26		64	6.0	2.0	2.0

* These average parameters vary with age, sex, strain and breed of animal.
† Values are percentages of total WBCs.
‡ Values represent upper limits of normalcy.

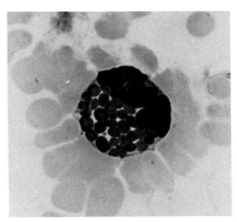

Figure 11.18. An equine peripheral blood smear. An eosinophil occupies the center of the field. Note the characteristic shape of the specific granules of the eosinophils of this species. ×400.

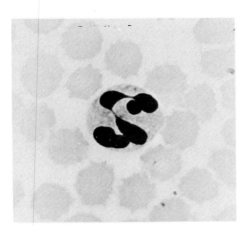

Figure 11.14. A canine peripheral blood smear. A neutrophil (PMN) occupies the center of the field. ×400.

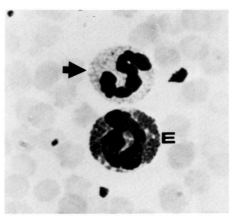

Figure 11.16. An ovine peripheral blood smear. An eosinophil (E) and a neutrophil *(arrow)* are present. ×400.

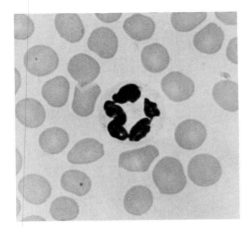

Figure 11.15. A feline peripheral blood smear. A neutrophil occupies the center of the field. Compare with Figure 11.3. ×400.

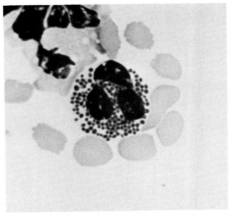

Figure 11.17. A bovine peripheral blood smear. An eosinophil occupies the center of the field. ×400.

sis of certain bacteria, the specific granules fuse initially with phagosomes containing bacteria and subsequently with primary granules.

Thus, the primary function of the neutrophil is phagocytosis of various particles, bacteria, and other microorganisms. This activity is especially apparent in acute local inflammation during which time great numbers of these cells are present in the connective tissue.

Eosinophilic Granulocytes. The *eosinophil* or *acidophil* is the next most frequently encountered granulocyte (Plate VI). Its diameter is approximately 12–14 μm. Usually, the nucleus is bilobed, but it may be polymorphic (Fig. 11.17). The acidophilic granules are the distinguishing feature. They are uniform within a cell, but they do vary from species to species (Fig. 11.16). They are especially large in equids (Fig. 11.18). These granules are lysosomes (Fig. 11.19).

The exact function of the eosinophil is not understood completely. They increase in numbers during allergic reactions (type I hypersensitivity), during parasitic infections and become especially numerous in the extracellular space at sites of antibody/antigen reactions. They are phagocytic cells but to a lesser degree than the neutrophils.

Basophilic Granulocytes. The *basophil* or *basophilic leukocyte*, the least numerous of the granulocytes (Plate VI), is about the same size as the neutrophil (9–12 μm). The nucleus is bilobed, although more lobes may be present. The *specific granules* are round, coarse, variable in size, basophilic, and metachromatic (Figs. 11.20 and 11.21). They usually stain much darker than the nucleus and may partially obscure it.

The function of these cells is obscure. They may increase in certain types of parasitism (canine heartworm disease). These cells are phagocytic and contain large quantities of histamine. Their histamine content is released in response to allergic stimulation.

Agranulocytes

The *agranulocytes* are white blood cells that do not contain specific granules; however, granules may be present. They are

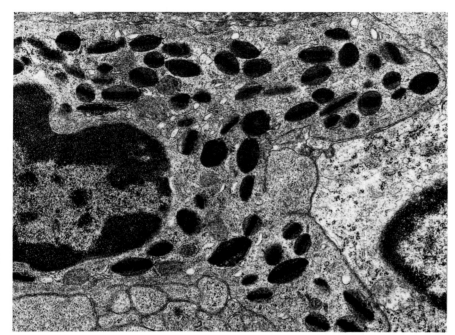

Figure 11.19. An electron micrograph of an eosinophil. The dark bodies are the specific granules of the cell. ×17,000. (Courtesy A. M. Sheppard).

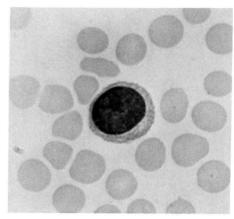

Figure 11.22. A feline peripheral blood smear. A lymphocyte occupies the center of the field. ×400.

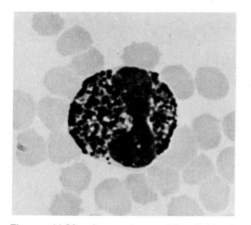

Figure 11.20. An equine peripheral blood smear. A basophil occupies the center of the field. ×400.

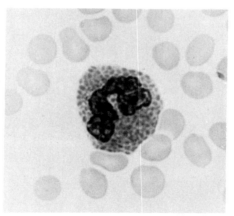

Figure 11.21. A feline peripheral blood smear. A basophil occupies the center of the field. Note the light-staining specific granules that characterize this species. ×400.

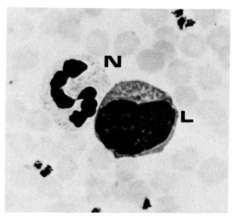

Figure 11.23. An ovine peripheral blood smear. A lymphocyte (L) is adjacent to a neutrophil (N). ×400.

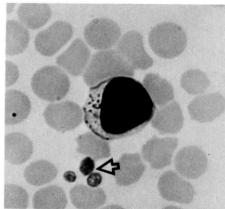

Figure 11.24. An equine peripheral blood smear. A lymphocyte occupies the center of the field. Note the azurophilic granules within the cytoplasm. Arrow, platelets. ×400.

round cells with more or less rounded nuclei.

Lymphocytes. The *lymphocytes* are usually the most frequently encountered agranulocytes (Plate VI). They are characterized by a high nuclear/cytoplasmic ratio (Fig. 11.22). The nucleus is usually round and sufficiently dense to obscure the nucleolus. A nuclear indentation may be seen (Fig. 11.23). The clear basophilic cytoplasm may contain some nonspecific, azurophilic granules (Fig. 11.24). Their occurrence, however, is variable (Plate VII.2). Generally, the nucleus is outlined by a peripherally condensed heterochromatin that readily diffracts light through the minimally granulated cytoplasm. The predom-

inant cytoplasmic organelles are ribosomes, polyribosomes, and rough endoplasmic reticulum. The Golgi apparatus and mitochondria are scant.

Lymphocytes vary in size. *Small lymphocytes* have a diameter of 5–10 μm and are the predominant lymphocytes in the circulating blood. *Medium-sized lymphocytes* range from 10–18 μm. The medium-sized lymphocytes are sometimes difficult to distinguish from monocytes. *Large lymphocytes* typically occur in lymphatic tissue.

Immunological techniques permit an evaluation of lymphocytes based on function. Two populations have been defined— *B lymphocytes* and *T lymphocytes*.

B lymphocytes (B cells) are responsible for the production of *antibodies (immunoglobulins)* in response to antigenic stimulation. They are the basis for the blood-borne or *humoral antibody immunity* (Chapter 19). Their cell surfaces have specific receptors for antigen, immunoglobulin Fc and C3b. They occur in bone marrow, bursa of Fabricius (in birds), and the germinal centers of lymphatic nodules and splenic follicles.

The *T lymphocytes (T cells)* are a functionally diverse population of cells. They are responsible for *cell-mediated immunity.* In response to antigenic stimulation (Chapter 19), this population of cells may become cytotoxic T cells, T helper cells, T suppressor cells, memory cells or may produce transfer factors and lymphokines.

Transfer factors are extracts of lymphocytes that confer specific cell-mediated reactivity on a normal recipient of the extract. These factors may be a ribonucleoprotein. *Lymphokines* are nonantigen-specific, low molecular weight proteins (25,000–75,000 daltons) that are biologically active. These substances are synthesized and secreted by activated T cells primarily, although B cells may produce them in response to nonspecific stimulation. Over 90 different lymphokine-mediated activities have been characterized. Lymphokines influence cellular populations (macrophages, lymphocytes, granulocytes) by changing their biological behavior. Some of the lymphokines are: *MIF—Migration Inhibition Factor, MAF—Macrophage Aggregating Factor, MCF—Macrophage Chemotactic Factor, MF—Mitogenic Factor, IFN—Interferon.* MIF prevents the migration of macrophages; MAF causes macrophages to aggregate; MF stimulates lymphocytes to divide; MCF attracts macrophages; IFN prevents the replication of viruses.

The surfaces of T cells generally have a Thy-1 or τ antigen. There are other surface differences and stimulation responses that distinguish T cells from B cells. T cells occur in the thymus, paracortical zones of lymphatic nodules, and the periarteriolar zone of splenic corpuscles.

Most of the circulating lymphocytes in most species are T cells. The life-span of lymphocytes may vary from hours to years. The long-lived B and T lymphocytes are believed to be the *memory cells.*

Monocytes. *Monocytes* are consistently the largest of the blood vascular elements (Plate VI). They range from 16–25 μm in diameter. The nucleus is kindey-shaped or bean-shaped, but it may be round as well as trilobed (Fig. 11.25). The nuclear chromatin is lighter and more reticulated than the lymphocytic nuclear material (Fig. 11.26). The cytoplasm is generally gray. The even distributuion of clear granules imparts a ground-glass appearance to the cytoplasm. Scattered azurophilic granules are contributory to this staining quality. The nuclear configuration is an excellent and definitive diagnostic feature.

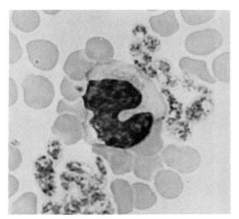

Figure 11.25. A feline peripheral blood smear. A monocyte occupies the center of the field and is surrounded by erythrocytes and aggregated platelets. The monocytic nucleus is described as having a "spaghetti and meatball" appearance. ×400.

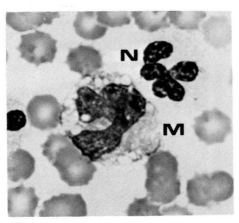

Figure 11.26. A canine peripheral blood smear. A monocyte *(M)* and neutrophil *(N)* are apparent. ×400.

Monocytes are phagocytic cells that become macrophages once they have gained access to the extravascular space. Subsequent to their access to the connective tissue space and under appropriate stimulation, these cells may fuse to form *foreign body giant cells* and *osteoclasts.*

Plasma Cells. The morphology and general function of *plasma cells* was discussed in Chapter 7. Their origin and relationship to B cells is discussed in Chapter 12 *(Agranulocytopoiesis)*, whereas their immunological function is discussed in Chapter 19.

Platelets

Blood platelets are small protoplasmic discs that are about 2–4 μm in diameter (Fig. 11.27). They are cytoplasmic fragments of a large cell, the *metamegakaryocyte.* The platelets are membrane-bound, round to oval fragments that contain a central, basophilic region *(chromomere)*

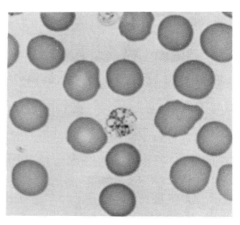

Figure 11.27. A canine peripheral blood smear. A platelet is apparent in the center of the field. ×400.

and a pale, homogeneous peripheral zone *(hyalomere).* The chromomere contains mitochondria, endoplasmic reticular profiles, and granules (Figs. 11.28 and 11.29). The hyalomere may contain some glycogen, but it is usually characterized by a homogeneous cytoplasmic matrix and microtubules.

Platelets are functionally significant in hemostasis. Although their role in the cessation of bleeding may be their most prominent function, they subserve a variety of other functions. By virtue of their serotonin content, they are important mediators of vasoconstriction. By combining with bacteria, they aid phagocytosis by serving as *opsonins.* They may serve a similar function by combining with viral particles.

Mammalian platelets are called thrombocytes occasionally.

Formed Elements—Species Variations

The blood cells of various domestic species are compared in color on Plates VI and VII.

Canine Blood Cells. The average size of the canine erythrocyte is 7.0 μm. These large cells usually have a well-defined central pallor. Occasionally, leptocytes are present. Although HJ bodies and nucleated erythrocytes are seen occasionally, they are not considered to be normal for the species. Reticulocytes normally should comprise less than 1% of the erythrocytes in an adult dog. Rouleaux formation occurs in canine erythrocytes.

The canine neutrophil contains an irregularly lobed nucleus, the lobes of which are usually joined by a narrow strand of nucleoplasm rather than a true filament. The cytoplasm stains faintly a pink-gray color and contains fine, diffuse granules. The eosinophil of canine blood consists of granules that vary in number and size. Also, these granules stain faintly with the acid

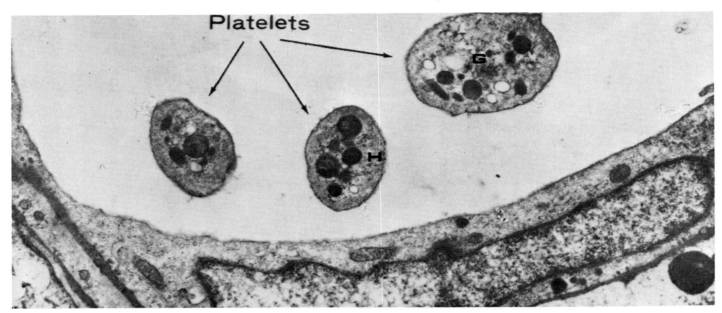

Figure 11.28. An electron micrograph of platelets within a capillary. *G*, granulomere; *H*, hyalomere. (Reprinted with permission from Bloom, W. and Fawcett, D. W.: *Textbook of Histology*, 10th edition, W. B. Saunders, Philadelphia, 1975.)

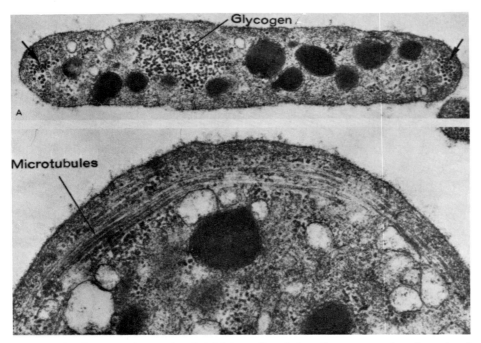

Figure 11.29. Electron micrographs of platelets sectioned along the narrow surface *(upper)* and parallel to the flat surface *(lower)*. Glycogen granules are obvious within the granulomere, whereas microtubules *(arrows)* are apparent within the hyalomere. Upper, ×31,000; lower, ×45,600. (Reprinted with permission from Bloom, W. and Fawcett, D. W.: *Textbook of Histology*, 10th edition, W. B. Saunders, Philadelphia, 1975.)

dye (eosin). Usually, part or all of the nucleus is seen, because the granules are localized to a small part of the cytoplasm. The shape of this cell is variable. The canine basophil contains granules that vary in size and number also. The intensity of the staining properties of the granules is variable. The number of granules is rarely sufficient to cover the nucleus or fill all of the cytoplasm. Because basophilic granules are water-soluble and easily removed during processing, this cell could be confused with a monocyte.

The small lymphocyte is the predominant cell in the peripheral blood. Azurophilic granules occur rarely in these cells.

Canine monocytes contain fine azurophilic granules and large nuclei. The nucleus is described typically as C-shaped with large blunt ends; however, the cell and nucleus are usually pleiomophic.

Feline Blood Cells. The average size of feline RBCs is 5–9 μm. These corpuscles stain uniformly, and the central pallor is not usually as prominent as in canine erythrocytes. HJ bodies may occur in 1% of normal feline erythrocytes. Nucleated erythrocytes may be encountered in the peripheral blood. Rouleaux formation is a prominent feature of feline RBCs.

The neutrophil of the cat contains a large nucleus that is usually coiled. Nuclear lobes may be connected by filaments or thin strands of nuclear materials. The fine, pink granulations are contained within a gray cytoplasm. The granules of the feline eosinophil are rod-shaped, refractile, and numerous. They generally cover the nucleus. Basophils are rarely encountered in the peripheral blood. They contain numerous, small, round, light-staining, lavender granules with occasional large dark granules.

The small lymphocyte is the predominant lymphocyte in the peripheral blood. Azurophilic granules are rare. The monocyte has a dull, blue cytoplasm that appears granular. Azurophilic granules are rare but cytoplasmic vacuoles may occur.

Equine Blood Cells. One of the most significant features of equine blood is the rapidity with which rouleaux formation occurs. Although single erythrocytes with a slight central pallor may be observed in blood smears, many cells will overlap in rouleaux formation. HJ bodies may occur in normal erythrocytes. One of the most striking features of equine peripheral blood is the absence of immature erythrocytic forms. Reticulocytosis, even in anemia, is extremely rare.

The neutrophilic nucleus contains numerous foci of clumped heterochromatin. Interlobar filaments are rare. The gray cytoplasm contains fine, pink granules. The eosinophil is the identifying feature of equine blood. The granules are large, round to oval, stain a bright red-orange and generally obscure most of the nucleus. The contour of the cell is defined by the granules. The basophilic granulocyte contains purple granules that are scattered throughout the cytoplasm. Their shape and size are irregular; they may cover the nucleus.

Most of the peripheral lymphocytes are small. Large lymphocytes, however, may be as large as monocytes. Azurophilic granules are seen occasionally. The monocytic nucleus, most typically, is kidney-shaped. Small azurophilic granules may be scattered throughout the cytoplasm; small vacuoles may be present also.

Bovine Blood Cells. The small size of bovine erythrocytes and the absence of rouleaux formation is the reason bovine blood does not sediment readily. Anisocytosis is normal in this blood. The smallest RBC may be one-half of the diameter of the largest RBC. Normally, a central pallor is difficult to observe. Also, reticulocytes occur rarely in the peripheral blood of this animal.

The neutrophilic leukocyte has a lobed nucleus that generally has one lobe connected to the main part of the nucleus by a filament. Usually nuclear lobation is simply a partial constriction of the nucleus. The numerous, small granules may vary in staining properties from light pink to red. Neutrophils are the second most common white blood cell of bovine blood. The eosinophil contains numerous, small, round, red granules that may fill the cytoplasm and partially cover the nucleus. Although the nucleus may be lobed, it is usually a C-shaped structure. The basophil, although rare, is typical.

The lymphocyte is the primary leukocyte of bovine blood. Small, medium, and large lymphocytes occur in the peripheral blood. The large lymphocytes are confused easily with monocytes. Although the small and medium lymphocytes are typical, the large lymphocytes have a light-staining and eccentrically positioned nucleus that is kidney-shaped, pale blue cytoplasm, and numerous azurophilic granules. Cytoplasmic vacuolations may be apparent. The morphology of monocytes is difficult to characterize; they vary in size, and their nuclear morphology is variable. A clover-leaf nucleus may be observed occasionally. The cell may be confused with large and medium lymphocytes; however, monocytic cytoplasm stains more darkly and is more

granular than that of lymphocytes. The rare occurrence of azurophilic granules in the cytoplasm of monocytes is a useful distinguishing feature.

Ovine Blood Cells. The RBCs of sheep are smaller than those of bovids. A faint central pallor is observed, as well as a limited amount of rouleaux formation. All other characteristics of ovine erythrocytes are similar to those of the bovid.

The neutrophil is typically multilobed, and these lobes are connected by fine filaments. The faintly staining, pink cytoplasm contains diffuse small granules. A few large granules occur also. As in bovine blood, these cells do not occur as frequently as in other nonruminant species. The eosinophil contains red-orange granules that are equal in size, oval, and refractile. These granules fill the cytoplasm and partially cover the nucleus. The basophil has granules that are dark with a red halo.

The lymphocytes vary from small to large but are difficult to categorize by size. All lymphocytes have nuclei with a smooth chromatin network that may stain with a red tint. Although the single nucleus is usually round, or oval and smooth, binucleated cells are encountered occasionally. The cytoplasm stains blue. Azurophilic granules may be observed also. The monocytes have nuclei that may be oval, indented, or even trilobed. Strands of dark-staining chromatin impart a lacy texture to the nucleus. The ground-glass-appearing cytoplasm stains more intensely than that of the large lymphocytes. Azurophilic granules are rare.

Caprine Blood Cells. The caprine erythrocytes are the smallest RBCs of domestic animals. They are round or triangular and devoid of a central pallor. Anisocytosis and rouleaux formation is not a common observation in adult blood. The blood of young goats, however, is characterized commonly by anisocytosis and poikilocytosis.

The neutrophil of the goat is similar to that of the sheep, except fewer lobes occur. The number of neutrophils is similar to other ruminants. The eosinophil of the goat contains a nucleus that may vary from C-shaped to mono-, bi-, or trilobed. The blue-stained cytoplasm contains numerous, small, round granules that stain an intense red. The basophil is typical; however, the purple granules have a red halo that imparts a red tint to the cytoplasm.

The caprine lymphocytes are small, medium, and large. The nuclei are generally round to oval, but an occasional kidney-shaped nucleus is observed. The chromatin pattern in the nuclei of large lymphocytes is an important feature in differentiating these cells from monocytes. Large lymphocytes have coarsely clumped heterochromatin, and nucleoli or nucleoli-like structures are present. Azurophilic granules of

various sizes may be present. The monocytes of the goat are similar to those of the sheep.

Porcine Blood Cells. Crenation and rouleaux formation occur, whereas the occurrence of central pallor is variable.

The neutrophil is characterized by an intensely stained nucleus that may be coiled. The lobes are connected by strictures; filaments are present rarely. The pale blue cytoplasm is filled with pale-staining, small granules. The eosinophil contains orange granules that fill the cytoplasm, obscure the cellular margin, and partially obscure the nucleus. The basophil is characterized by red-purple granules that assume coccoid or dumbell shapes.

The small lymphocytes of the pig are typical. The nucleus fills the cell and may be surrounded by a thin rim of pale blue cytoplasm. Large lymphocytes have a nucleus that is more vesicular than the smaller types. Azurophilic granules occur variably, tend to be rod-shaped and distributed along the cellular margin. The monocyte is typical, but azurophilic granules are not a conspicuous feature.

Avian Blood Cells

Erythrocytes

Morphology. The normal mature erythrocytes of avian blood are oval cells with oval nuclei (Fig. 11.30). These cells range from 10–13 μm long and from 6–7 μm wide. The elongated nucleus is about one-half of the dimensions of the cell. Nuclear heterochromatin may appear uniformly distributed in an oval nucleus. A nucleolus is not present. The cytoplasm may vary from orange-pink to red with routine blood stains. Numerous artifactual changes may alter the configuration and staining affinity

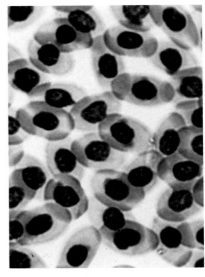

Figure 11.30. Erythrocytes in an avian peripheral blood smear. ×400.

of these cells. Erythrocytes of fishes and amphibians are morphologically similar to those of birds.

Granulocytes

Heterophils. The *heterophil* of birds is the equivalent of the neutrophil in other species. The heterophil has a diameter of 6–9 μm. Despite its ameboid properties, it is usually seen as a round cell in blood smears. The multilobed nucleus may have as many as five lobes and the heterochromatin is coarsely clumped. The distinguishing feature is the presence of brightly stained, eosinophilic rods with a fusiform configuration (Fig. 11.31). These specific inclusions are randomly scattered throughout the cell. They are easily dissolved in aqueous media and all that may remain is a red-stained *central body* or *vacuole*. As a result of this dissolution, the normally clear cytoplasm usually becomes acidophilic. Under these conditions the heterophils are easily confused with eosinophils.

Eosinophils. The avian *eosinophil* has a diameter between 5 and 9 μm. It has a multilobed nucleus with coarsely clumped heterochromatin. The cytoplasm, although usually obscured by tightly packed granules, stains a pale clear blue (Fig. 11.32). This characteristic is of diagnostic significance in distinguishing eosinophils from heterophils in which the rods have been partially dissolved. The granules of some eosinophils may appear as homogeneous bodies. In larger cells, the granules appear to be composed of three or four subunits that are combined in such a manner that a vacuity or clear space appears in the center of the complex. The eosinophilic granule is more refractile than that of the heterophil.

Basophils. The *basophil* of birds is similar to that of mammalian species.

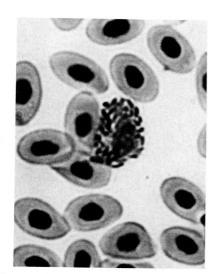

Figure 11.31. An avian peripheral blood smear. A heterophil occupies the center of the field. ×400.

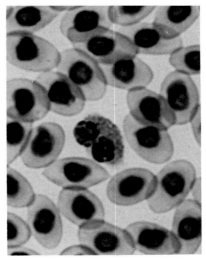

Figure 11.32. An avian peripheral blood smear. An eosinophil occupies the center of the field. ×400.

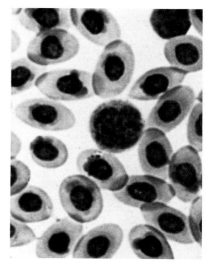

Figure 11.33. An avian peripheral blood smear. A lymphocyte occupies the center of the field. ×400.

Agranulocytes

Lymphocytes. Avian *lymphocytes* are about the same size as comparable mammalian cells. Small, medium, and large lymphocytes have been described. The cell is generally round with an even contour (Fig. 11.33). Cytoplasmic blebs, however, may be apparent. The nucleus is usually centrally located, but some cells may be polarized. Coarsely clumped heterochromatin is characteristic of this structure. Also, the nuclear/cytoplasmic ratio is high. A sharp indentation in the nucleus may also be apparent. Cytoplasmic characteristics are variable. The cytoplasm may stain faintly and be homogeneous, or it may stain intensely and be flocculated with basophilic material. The flocculation may be fine and slightly reticulated or heavy and coarsely reticulated. Some magenta-staining granules may be evident.

The previous discussion of the B cells and T cells of the mammal is applicable to the bird.

Monocytes. The avian *monocyte* is the largest cell of the mature elements of the agranulocytic series. Usually, the average lymphocyte diameter approximates the diameter of the monocyte nucleus. Although the monocyte is usually round, numerous other configurations attest to its ameboid characteristics (Fig. 11.34). The nuclear/cytoplasmic ratio is smaller than that of the lymphocyte. The bean-shaped or kidney-shaped nucleus contains a fine reticulum of heterochromatin. The region of the cytoplasm associated with the nuclear indentation is characteristic for the monocytes. This juxtanuclear region contains orange granules or it may be tinged orange. The ground-glass appearance of the cytoplasm, azurophilic granules, and the juxtanuclear

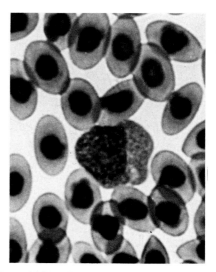

Figure 11.34. An avian peripheral blood smear. A monocyte is apparent in the center of the field. ×400.

characteristics are diagnostic features for the monocyte.

Thrombocytes

The *thrombocytes* of birds and other submammalian vertebrates are nucleated cells. These cells are somewhat smaller than erythrocytes and have average dimensions of 5 × 9 μm. The centrally located, elongated nucleus is coarsely granular with heterochromatin (Fig. 11.35). The cytoplasm is finely reticulated and basophilic and may contain a number of azurophilic, specific granules.

Besides functioning in hemostasis in a manner similar to mammalian platelets, the avian thrombocytes have been shown to be *trephocytic* and *phagocytic*.

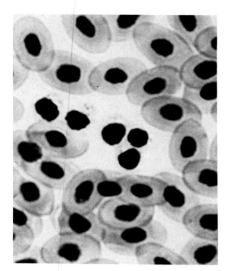

Figure 11.35. An avian peripheral blood smear. Thrombocytes are apparent in the center of the field. ×400.

Hemostasis

Hemostasis is a process in which a complex series of interactions culminate in the termination of blood loss after vascular injury.

Response of Vasculature. Vasoconstriction immediately follows the rupture or cutting of a vessel, and this may be due to any one or a combination of factors: *localized spasm (contraction) of intramural smooth muscle, reflex activity involving vasomotor nerves of the sympathetic nervous system, the localized release of vasoconstrictor substances, especially serotonin.* Vasoconstricting compounds are able to maintain vasoconstriction for 20–60 minutes after injury. This reduces blood loss and facilitates the accumulation (aggregation) of platelets at the injury. The denuded or damaged endothelial surface exposes subendothelial collagen, while damaged cells release *adenosine diphosphate (ADP).* These events facilitate platelet aggregation by increasing the adhesiveness of their surfaces. The contact with the exposed collagen activates intrinsic coagulative mechanisms. *Plasminogen* is released at the site of vascular injury also.

Platelet Function. Platelets that aggregate at the injuries are transformed into sticky, irregularly shaped structures with pseudopodia that extend into the injury and between the individual platelets of the aggregate. The aggregation process causes a *release reaction* in which the platelets secrete some of the products stored within their granulomeres. The products include *ADP, serotonin, histamine, platelet phospholipids (PF3),* and enzymes that cause the formation of *thromboxane A* in the plasma. Thromboxane A and ADP activate other platelets causing them to adhere to the original aggregate. Platelet phospholip-

ids catalyze several reactions involved in the formation of thrombin. This release reaction is called *degranulation.* Platelets, then, contribute to continued aggregation of more platelets. Erythrocytes contain high concentrations of ADP. Their entrapment and rupture within the plug releases more ADP enhancing more aggregation of platelets. The reversible process of *platelet plug* formation stops blood loss from the injury. These temporary plugs can be washed away from the site; rebleeding can occur as a consequence. Additional mechanisms are required to transform this temporary plug into an irreversible aggregation of platelets.

Permanency is imparted to the platelet plug through the interaction of *viscous metamorphosis* of platelets and *fibrin* generation. Viscous metamorphosis is characterized by irreversible morphological changes of the platelets within the plug. Filaments that have contractile properties appear in the platelets. Soluble, contractile proteins, actin and myosin, polymerize and form definitive microfilaments within the platelets. The actual mechanisms by which contractile proteins, platelets, and fibrinous strands achieve clot retraction are not known. Fibrin attaches to platelet pseudopodia; contraction of actin/myosin complexes probably exerts tension on the fibrinous strands. This is one mechanism believed to account for *clot retraction.* Moreover, fibrin deposition on the platelet aggregate is believed to be the activation mechanism for viscous metamorphosis. Calcium is essential for clot contraction, whereas cyclic adenosine monophosphate (cAMP) has been implicated as the regulator of viscous metamorphosis.

The *platelet* or *hemostatic plug* formation may be limited or compromised in animals with coagulation disorders *(coagulopathies).* Mechanisms that normally limit plug formation at sites of vascular injury include: *dilution of activated clotting constituents by continued blood flow; endothelial cell release of prostaglandins that cause vasodilation and inhibit platelet aggregation; antithrombin III inactivation of coagulation factors.* These mechanisms, coupled with inadequate generation of fibrin, result in continuous bleeding from sites of vascular injury.

Coagulation

General Mechanisms. *Coagulation* is a complex series of interactions in which the blood loses its fluid characteristics and is converted to a semisolid mass. The formation of the "irreversible clot," resulting from the interaction of damaged tissue, platelets and fibrin, is an integral part of this process. The formation of fibrin results from a complex process that involves tissue and/or blood factors.

The blood and tissue factors, except factor IV, are proteins; most of them are prob-

ably produced by the liver. The activation of the fibrin-producing mechanism that originates in the tissues is called the *extrinsic pathway.* The activation of a fibrin-producing mechanism within the blood is called the *intrinsic pathway.* These two pathways converge upon the activation of factor X in the *common pathway* that leads ultimately to fibrin formation. The numerous factors that contribute to these pathways have many synonyms. The coagulation scheme is outlined in Fig. 11.36.

The sequence of events that leads to coagulation is considered to occur in three stages:

Stage I—the formation of a prothrombin-converting factor;
Stage II—the conversion of prothrombin to thrombin by the prothrombin-converting factor;
Stage III—the induction of fibrin formation from fibrinogen by thrombin.

Stage I may be achieved by either the intrinsic or extrinsic pathways. Stages I, II, and III constitute the common pathway.

Extrinsic Pathway. The *extrinsic pathway* is the means by which *prothrombin activator substance* is generated in response to blood contacting extravascular tissues. The achievement of coagulation by this pathway is rapid, occurring in less than a minute under circumstances of severe tissue trauma. Also, this pathway is not subject to inhibition by natural inhibitors that may influence the intrinsic pathway.

The initial contact of the blood with the extravascular tissues causes the release of *tissue phospholipids* (from cellular membranes) and *tissue thromboplastin (Factor III).* Factor III, calcium, and *Factor VII* form a complex that acts enzymatically in the presence of tissue phospholipids to convert *Factor X* to *activated Factor X.* The remainder of the process is the common pathway.

Intrinsic Pathway. The *intrinsic pathway* provides for the formation of *prothrombin activator substance* by blood being damaged directly or by blood contacting collagenous fibers or other subendothelial elements. The inherent ability of blood to clot is the basis for the name of this pathway. Perturbations to the blood cause the inactive *Factor XII* to change configuration converting this substance into a proteolytic enzyme called *activated Factor XII.* Kallikrein and high molecular weight *kinninogen* may function to modulate Factor XII activation. Concomitantly, the damage that initiates the activation of Factor XII also damages platelets. This damage results in the release of *platelet phospholipids,* a factor called *platelet factor 3 (PF3).* PF3 influences subsequent steps of the cascading intrinsic pathway. Activated Factor XII acts enzymatically to convert *Factor XI*

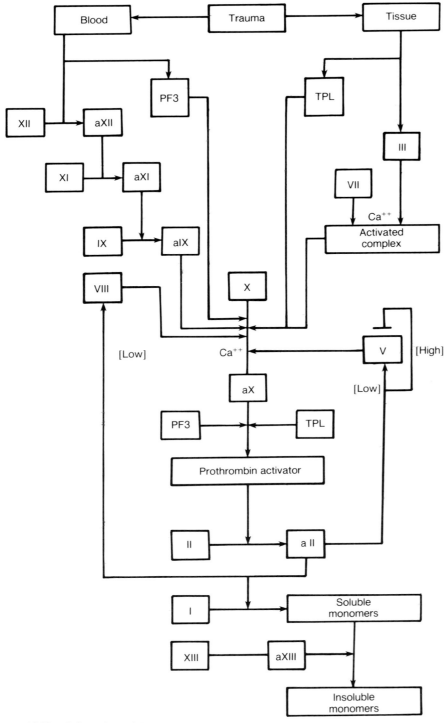

Figure 11.36. A flow chart of the coagulation schemes. The extrinsic pathway begins with tissue trauma and terminates with the activation of Factor X. The intrinsic pathway begins with blood trauma and terminates with the activation of Factor X. The common pathway begins with the activation of factor X. a—activated; TPL—tissue phospholipid; PF3—platelet factor 3

into *activated Factor XI*. This conversion step occurs rapidly. Activated Factor XI acts enzymatically upon *Factor IX* to convert it rapidly to *activated Factor IX*. Activated Factor IX with *Factor VIII* and PF3 act together to activate *Factor X*. Bleeding problems attributable to decreased numbers of platelets *(thrombocytopenia)* are manifested because of the inability to activate Factor X via the intrinsic pathway.

Common Pathway. The *common pathway* begins with the activation of Factor X.

Factor X may be activated through the combination of various substances (Factor III, calcium, Factor VII, and tissue phospholipids) involved in the extrinsic pathway. Similarly, PF3, Factor IX, and Factor VIII combine to activate Factor X through the intrinsic pathway.

Activated Factor X combines with *Factor V* and platelet and/or tissue phospholipids to form *prothrombin activator substance*. Prothrombin activator substance then initiates the activation of *Factor II (prothrombin)* to *activated Factor II (thrombin)*. The major role of thrombin is to convert *fibrinogen (Factor I)* to *soluble fibrin monomers*. Fibrin monomers are cross-linked by *activated Factor XIII* to form insoluble fibrin polymers. The polymerization process stabilizes the fibrinous clot. Trace amounts of thrombin also increase the activities of Factors V and VIII. High concentrations of thrombin cause digestion of Factor V. Thus, the production of thrombin both increases and subsequently decreases its own production.

Functional Correlates. The liver is an essential organ for the normal coagulation mechanisms to be operable. Most of the coagulation factors, except Factor VIII, are synthesized by the hepatocytes. Factor VIII is synthesized primarily by endothelial cells. Proper coagulation is dependent upon normal synthetic activity of the hepatocytes, because the half-lives of the coagulation factors vary from a few hours to a few days. The exocrine function of the hepatocytes is essential for normal coagulation, also.

Vitamin K is a fat-soluble vitamin that is produced by the intestinal flora. This vitamin is produced in sufficient quantities that vitamin K deficiencies should not occur. The absorption of vitamin K, however, is dependent upon bile salt production by the hepatocytes. Liver disease, therefore, can cause a malabsorption of vitamin K and subsequent deficiency. The synthesis of coagulation Factors II, VII, IX, and X are vitamin K-dependent. Without this vitamin, bleeding problems can result.

Regulation of the coagulation mechanism is necessary to prevent a positive feedback loop effect. The most important anticoagulants in the blood are those that remove thrombin. A natural inhibitor of coagulation is an α-globulin called *antithrombin III (ATIII)*. ATIII mediates its anticoagulant properties by complexing with the coagulation factors that are called *serine proteases*. The serine proteases, those coagulation factors with serine at their enzymatic site, are Factors II, VII, IX, X, XI, and XII. The complexes, such as ATIII-Factor II, are then removed from the blood by the liver. Heparin functions as an anticoagulant by enhancing the inhibition of coagulation through ATIII.

Clot Formation and Fibrinolysis. The

platelet is an essential component of clot formation and retraction. The necessity of fibrin in the formation of an irreversible platelet plug was discussed previously. Despite the so-called irreversibility of the platelet plug, blood clots are not permanent structures. The cascading effects of the clotting and coagulation mechanisms, once initiated, do not continue unregulated under normal circumstances. The devasting consequences of unchecked hemostatic mechanisms should be obvious. The fibrinolytic mechanism is outlined in Figure 11.37. Unfortunately, not all of the details of this mechanism are understood.

The cessation of clot formation assists with the ultimate removal of the clot. One of the limiting factors in the formation of clots is the ability of fibrin to absorb the thrombin that is generated. The absorptive process limits both the growth and spread of the clot.

The dissolution of the insoluble clot is dependent upon enzymatic digestion by a serine protease called *plasmin* or *fibrinolysin*. The precursor of this substance occurs as a plasma protein called *plasminogen* or

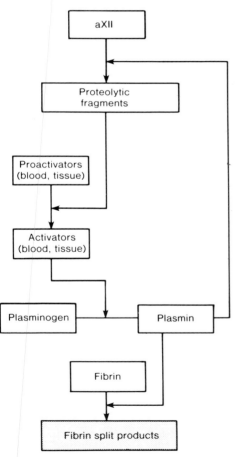

Figure 11.37. A flow diagram of the fibrinolytic mechanism. Plasmin degrades fibrin into fibrin split products and exerts a positive feedback influence upon activated Hageman factor.

prefibrinolysin. A delicate balance exists between plasmin activators and plasmin inhibitors. The precursor molecules, some of which become entrapped within forming clots, are activated by various substances: activators released from damaged endothelial cells, activated Hageman factor (Factor XII), thrombin, lysosomal enzymes from damaged tissues. Once generated, plasmin not only digests fibrin, but fibrinogen (Factor I), prothrombin (factor II), Factor V, Factor VIII, and Factor XII are subjected to digestion by this protease. Plasmin not only digests clots, but it interferes with the coagulation mechanism by digesting coagulation factors.

An α_2-globulin called *antiplasmin* inhibits the generation of plasmin normally. The incorporation of plasmin precursors into the forming thrombus may serve as a device to protect the plasmin-generation mechanism from inhibition by antiplasmin. Also, the generation of fibrinolysin within the thrombus limits the proteolytic activity to localized accumulations of fibrin. This localized entrapment precludes plasmin from digesting circulating factors, an effect that could compromise the ability to achieve subsequent coagulation.

Certain bacteria use the plasmin system to assist their spreading throughout the body. Streptococcal organisms release an activator enzyme called *streptokinase*. This enzyme activates plasmin. Plasmin, in turn, dissolves clots within blood, lymphatic fluid, and tissue fluid. This facilitates bacterial spreading throughout the fluid environment rather than their being confined within the semisolid or solid environment of a clot.

References

Erythrocytes

Baker, R. F.: Ultrastructure of red blood cells. Fed. Proc. 26:1785, 1967.

Fisher, J. W. and Gordon, A. S.: Conference: erythropoietin. Ann New York Acad. Sci. 149, 1968.

Hevesy, G. and Ottesen, J.: Life-cycle of the red corpuscle of the hen. Nature 156:534, 1945.

Hillman, R.S. and Finch, C.A.: *The Red Cell Manual.* 4th edition. F.A. Davis, Philadelphia, 1974.

Koehler, J. K.: Freeze-etching obervations on nucleated erythrocytes with special reference to the nuclear and plasma membranes. Z. Zellforsch. 85:1, 1972.

London, I.M.: Iron and heme: Crucial carriers and catalysts. *In:* Wintrobe, M.M. (ed.): *Blood, Pure and Eloquent.* McGraw-Hill Book Co., New York, 1980.

Marks, P and Rifkind, R. A.: Protein synthesis: Its control in erythropoiesis. Science 175:955, 1972.

Schalm, O. W.: Hematologic characteristics of autoimmune hemolytic anemia in the dog. Calif. Vet. 23:19, 1969.

Granulocytes

Archer, G. T. and Hirsch, J. C.: Motion picture studies of degranulation of horse eosinophils during phagocytosis. J. Exp. Med. 118:287, 1963.

Beeson, P.B. and Bass, D.A.: *The Eosinophil.* W.B. Saunders, Philadelphia, 1977.

Dolowy, W. C., Cornet, J. and Henson, D.: Particles in leukocytes of normal human beings after negative staining in electron microscopy. Nature 209:1358, 1966.

Dvorak, A.M. and Dvorak, H.F.: The basophil. Arch. Pathol. Lab. Med. 103:551, 1979.

Franklin, D. A.: Electron microscopic study of human basophils. 29:878, 1967.

Hamre, C. J.: Origin and differentiation of heterophil, eosinophil and basophil leucocytes of chickens. Anat. Rec. 112:339, 1952.

Hersh, I. G. and Cohn, Z. A.: Degranulation of polymorphonuclear leucocytes following phagocytosis of microogransims. J. Exp. Med. 112:1005, 1960.

Miller, F., DeHarven, E. and Palade, G. E. The structure of eosinphil leucocytes granules in rodents and in man. J. Cell Biol. 31:349, 1960.

Natt, M. P. and Herrick, C. A.: Variation in the shape of the rodlike granule of the chicken heterophil leucocyte and its possible significance. Poult. Sci. 33:828, 1954.

Agranulocytes

Elves, M. W.: *The lymphocytes.* Lloyd Luke Ltd., London, 1966.

Fiore-Donati, L. and Hanna, M. G., Jr.: *Lymphatic Tissue and Germinal Centers in Immune Response.* Plenum, New York, 1969.

Gowans, J. L.: The life history of lymphocytes. Brit. Med. Bull. 15:50, 1959.

Gowans, J. L.: The immunological activities of lymphocytes. Progr. Allerg. 9:1, 1965.

Greaves, M. R., Owen, J. J. T. and Raff, M. C.: *T and B Lymphocytes: Origins, Properties and Roles in Immune Responses.* North-Holland Publishers, New York, 1975.

Hoshino, T., Takeda, M., Abe, K. and Ito, T.: Early development of thymic lymphocytes in mice, studied by light and electron microscopy. Anat. Rec. 164:47, 1969.

Mackay, L. J., Jarrett, W. F. H. and Coombs, R. R. A.: Two populations of lymphocytes in a cat. Vet. Rec. 96:41, 1975.

Movat, H. Z. and Fernando, N. V. P.: The fine structure of the lymphoid tissue during antibody formation. Exp. Molec. Path. 4:155, 1965.

Tizard, I. R. : *An Introduction to Veterinary Immunology.* 2nd edition. W. B. Saunders, Philadelphia, 1982.

Tompkins, E. H.: The monocyte. Ann. N. Y. Acad. Sci. 59:732, 1955.

Zinkl, J.G.: The leukocytes. Vet. Clin. N. A. 11:237, 1981.

Platelets and Thrombocytes

Behnke, O.: Electron microscopic observations on the membrane systems of the rat blood platelet. Anat. Rec. 158:121, 1967.

Carlson, H. C., Sweeney, P. R. and Tokaryk, J. M.: Demonstration of phagocytic and trephocytic activities of chicken thrombocytes by microscopy and vital staining techniques. Avian Dis. 12:700, 1968.

Clarke, J. A., Hawkey, C. and Salisbury, A. J.: Surface ultrastructure of platelets and thrombocytes. Nature 233:401, 1969.

Rodman, N. F. and Mason, R. G.: Platelet-platelet interaction: Relationship to hemostasis and thrombosis. Fed. Proc. 26:95, 1967.

Simpson, C. F.: Ultrastructural features of the turkey thrombocyte and lymphocyte. Poult. Sci. 47:848, 1968.

Comparative Hematology

Afonsky. D.: Blood picture in normal dogs. Amer. J. Physiol. 180:456, 1955.

Archer, R. K.: *Haematological Techniques for Use in Animals.* Blackwell Scientific, Oxford, 1965.

Benjamin, M. M.: *Outline of Veterinary Clinical Pathology.* 3rd edition. Iowa State University Press, Ames, 1978.

Calhoun, M. L. and Brown, E. M.: Hematology and Hematopoietic Organs. *In:* Dunne, H. W. (ed.): *Swine Diseases* pp.33–75. Iowa State University Press, Ames, 1975.

Diggs, L. W., Sturm, D. and Bell, A.: *The Morphology of Human Blood Cells*, Abbott Laboratories, North Chicago, 1970.

Ferguson, L. C., Irwin, M. R. and Beach, B. A.: On variation in the blood cells of healthy cattle. J. Infect. Dis. *76:*24, 1945.

Holman, H. H.: A negative correlation between size and number of the erythrocytes of cows, sheep, goats and horses. J. Path. Bact. *64:*379, 1952.

Lucas, A. M.: A discussion of synonymy in avian and mammalian hematological nomenclature. Amer. J. Vet. Res. *20:*887, 1959.

Rich, L. J.: *The Morphology of Canine and Feline Blood Cells with Equine References*, Ralston Purina, St. Louis, 1974.

Schalm, O. W., Jain, N. C. and Carroll, E. J.: *Veterinary Hematology.* 3rd edition, Lea and Febiger, Philadelphia, 1975.

Winthrobe, M. M.: *Clinical Hematology.* 7th edition. Lea and Febiger, Philadelphia, 1974.

Wintrobe, M. M., Shumacker, H. B., Jr. and Schmidt, W. J.: Values for number, size and hemoglobin content of erythrocytes in normal dogs, rabbits and rats. Amer. J. Physiol. *114:*502, 1936.

Hemostasis

Bennett, B. and Douglas, A. S.: Blood coagulation mechanism. Clin. Haematol. 2.3, 1973.

Day, H. J.: Role of platelets in hemostasis and thrombosis. Ser. Haematol. *8:*23, 1975.

Dodds, W. J.: The diagnosis, management and treatment of bleeding disorders. I and II. Mod. Vet. Prac. *58:*680, *58:*756, 1977.

Hall, D. E.: *Blood Coagulation and Its Disorders in the Dog.* Bailiere, Tindall, London, 1972.

Kirk, R. W. (ed.): *Current Veterinary Therapy VI. Small Animal Practice.* pp. 421–492, 1977.

12: Hematopoiesis

Development of Blood

General Characteristics

Introduction. Blood cell replacement is achieved through the activities of stem cells that are confined to specific regions. These regions of *hematopoiesis* differ in the prenatal, postnatal, and adult animal. During early prenatal development, hematopoiesis begins in the mesenchyme as blood islands associated with the yolk sac. Hematopoietic activity becomes widespread in the fetus and includes the liver, spleen, thymus, lymph nodes, and bone marrow. Postnatal formation of erythrocytes, granulocytes, and platelets is confined primarily to the red bone marrow. The spleen also is involved to a lesser degree. A progressive reduction in red bone marrow occurs throughout adolescence. Ultimately, hematopoiesis in the adult is confined to the marrow cavities of the sternebrae, ribs, vertebrae, and cranial bones. This reduction in hematopoiesis is associated with a conversion of *red bone marrow* to *yellow bone marrow*.

During early development, the thymus is the primary organ of lymphocytopoiesis. The spleen and remaining lymphoid tissues then produce agranulocytes throughout the life of the organism.

Developmental Theories. Historically, three theories on the origin of blood cells have been popular. The *monophyletic* theory stated that *all* blood cells were derived from a single stem cell. The *diphyletic* theory stated that a separate stem cell existed for the agranulocytes and granulocytes/ erythrocytes. The *polyphyletic* theory proposed that separate stem cells gave rise to distinct blood cells. Ultimately, the concept of a pluripotent stem cell called a *colony- forming unit (CFU)* was developed (Fig. 12.1).

Colony-Forming Unit. The concept of a CFU being the pluripotent stem cell of blood evolved as the culmination of insights gained from numerous elegant experiments. The student should consult the references for details of these experiments. The transfusion of splenic cells into animals incapable of producing blood cells

results in the repopulation of the bone marrow with stem cells capable of producing blood cells. Concomitantly, the spleen of the recipient animals form nodules of new blood cells called *colonies*. The pluripotent stem cell responsible for the differentiation and proliferation of the colony (clone) was called a CFU. **CFUs are not confined to the classic hematopoietic tissues; they also circulate in the blood.** The CFU is responsible for the differentiation and proliferation of all blood cells.

The CFU is a small cell with a diameter between 7 and 10 μm and ultrastructural features similar to a small lymphocyte. The comparison is not meant to imply that the CFU is a small lymphocyte.

Developmental Determinants. The pluripotent stem cell, CFU, is a typical stem cell. Colonies of specific blood cells develop in culture in response to specific inducer substances. *Erythropoietin* is an inducer that influences the committed stem cell to produce morphologically identifiable

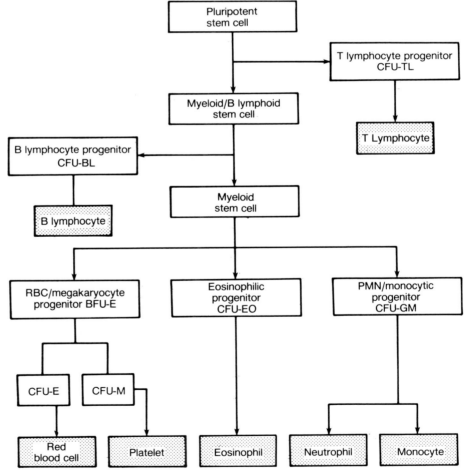

Figure 12.1. A flow diagram demonstrating the origin and differentiation of blood cells from a pluripotent stem cell.

179

erythrocytic precursors. A *burst-forming unit—erythropoietic (BFU-E)* is an early progenitor in the series that gives rise to committed stem cells. The committed progenitor for the series is the *CFU-E (colony-forming unit of the erythrocytic line of differentiation* or *CFU—erythrocytic)*. Various other factors, including *granulopoietin* and *thrombopoietin*, serve as the basis for identifying six distinctive lines of differentiation:

> *erythrocytic—CFU-E;*
> *megakaryocytic—CFU-M;*
> *granulocytic/monocytic—CFU-GM;*
> *eosinophilic—CFU-EO;*
> *B lymphocytic—CFU-BL;*
> *T lymphocytic—CFU-TL.*

Little is known about the origin of basophils.

Besides the influence of various inducer or regulatory factors, many of which are glycoproteins, the microenvironment, marrow cellular populations and cell-to-cell interactions seem to exert a significant influence upon the proliferation and differentiation of the stem cells. The *hematopoietic inductive environment (HIM)*, which differs within different hematopoietic organs, is not well understood. Reticular cells, macrophages, lymphocytes, and endothelial cells seem to interact in the differentiation of erythrocytes.

Trends in Development. The differentiation of mature red blood corpuscles and granulocytes is characterized by sequential changes that typify the developmental process (Fig. 12.2).

The early cells in the sequence are large and become smaller with maturation. In the erythrocytic series, the nucleus is extruded from the cell. The nucleus of early cells is light-staining and acidophilic. With maturation it becomes darker and basophilic. Similarly, the cytoplasm of early cells is basophilic and becomes progressively acidophilic with the matruation process. The nuclei of stem cells are round and light-staining. The chromatin is disposed in a fine reticulated distribution. With maturation, the nuclei become indented, lobed, or segmented and the chromatin stains more darkly and is clumped.

Early cells are devoid of granules. In the granulocytic series, early granules are nonspecific and are replaced or augmented by the specific, granulocytic, inclusion granules. Early cells have one or more nucleoli that are not apparent as development progresses toward the definitive cell type. Also, mitotic activity is high in more primitive cells in normal development.

Similar trends are characteristic of the agranulocytic series also.

Bone Marrow

The marrow tissue is a hypercellular and highly vascularized form of connective tissue. It is contained within the *medullary cavity (marrow cavity)* as interosseous tissue in all bones. During development and growth, all of the marrow is *red bone marrow*. By adulthood, the red bone marrow is confined to a limited number of loci: sternebrae, ribs, vertebrae, and cranial bones. The remaining loci will have been replaced with *yellow bone marrow*.

The peripheral limits of the marrow contain elements of the cortical endosteum, while trabecular endosteum may be contained within the substance of the marrow tissues. The acquisition of blood-cell formative and blood-cell destructive functions, although acquired secondarily, is maintained throughout life.

Red Bone Marrow. The red color of bone marrow results from the accumulation of erythrocytes, erythrocytic precursors, and their contained pigment. *Red bone marrow* is an hemopoietic tissue often called *myeloid tissue.* Erythrocytes, granulocytes, platelets, and agranulocytes are produced within this tissue.

The marrow consists of arteries, veins, sinuses, a reticular fiber framework, free cells of the blood cell lineages, macrophages, and some adipose tissue (Fig. 12.3). The marrow is divisible into two compartments: vascular and hematopoietic. The *vascular compartment* includes all of the vessels of the bone marrow. The sinuses are described as being lined by phagocytic cells, but the phagocytes are probably perivascular cells. The *hematopoietic compartment* constitutes the irregular islands of tissue between the vascular beds and includes fibroblasts, reticular fiber stroma, the elusive reticular cells, CFUs, phagocytic cells, intermediate and mature blood cell forms, adipose tissue, and other typical connective tissue cells (plasma cells, mast cells) (Fig. 12.4). The primary function of the red bone marrow is blood cell production.

Yellow Bone Marrow. The amount of active (red) bone marrow is reduced appreciably by the time adulthood is achieved. Adipose tissue replaces most of the blood cell-producing elements of the hematopoietic compartment. Under conditions of

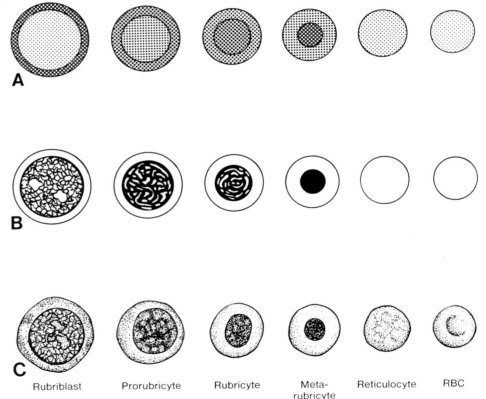

| Rubriblast | Prorubricyte | Rubricyte | Meta-rubricyte | Reticulocyte | RBC |

Figure 12.2. A series of diagrams depicting the cellular changes associated with the differentiation of blood cells. *A.* The large, pale-staining nucleus becomes progressively smaller with development. The nucleus is extruded in the erythrocytic series. The basophilic cytoplasm becomes progressively lighter as development progresses. *B.* Nuclear and cytoplasmic size is reduced during development, whereas more heterochromatin becomes obvious during the progress toward a mature cell. *C.* The stages of development of erythrocytes may be compared with the generalities of *A* and *B*. (Modified and redrawn from Diggs, L. W., Sturm, D. and Bell, A.: *The Morphology of Blood Cells.* Abbott Laboratories, North Chicago, 1954.)

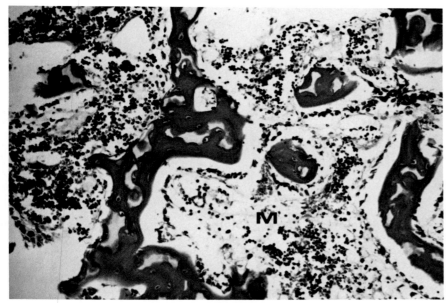

Figure 12.3. Red bone marrow within the medullary cavity of a developing bone. The bone marrow *(M)* occupies the interosseous spaces between the developing osseous and calcified cartilaginous spicules of the primary spongiosa. ×40.

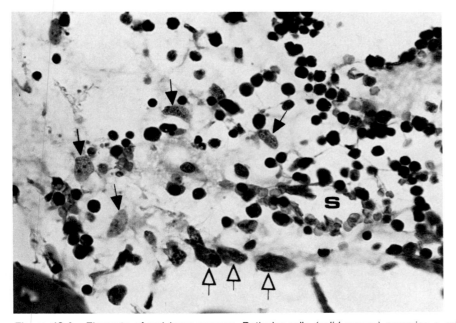

Figure 12.4. Elements of red bone marrow. Reticular cells *(solid arrows)* comprise a cellular reticulum. Numerous free blood cells are in various stages of development. A sinus (S) and osteoblasts *(open arrows)* are apparent. The osteoblasts were separated artifactually from their osseous surface. ×160.

stress (including disease), the *yellow bone marrow* can revert to an active hematopoietic tissue.

Erythropoiesis

Cytology of Differentiation. The following cells comprise the erythrocytic series: *rubriblast, prorubricyte, rubricyte, metarubrictye, reticulocyte, mature red blood corpuscle* (Figs. 12.1 and 12.2).

The *rubriblast (proerythroblast, pronor-* *moblast)* is the earliest recognizable form of this series. The nucleus of this cell is primitive, being vesicular with a prominent nucleolus. The thin rim of dark blue cytoplasm forms a narrow band around the nucleus. The nuclear/cytoplasmic ratio is high.

The *prorubricyte (basophilic erythroblast, basophilic normoblast)* is smaller than the rubriblast, has a coarsely distributed nuclear chromatin and an intensely basophilic cytoplasm. The nucleolus is

either poorly defined or absent. Mitotic activity is high.

The *rubricyte (polychromatophilic erythroblast, polychromatophilic normoblast)* is a small cell with a small, round, and dense nucleus. Nucleoli are not apparent. Various developmental stages of this cell are described on the basis of the progressive synthesis of hemoglobin. The cytoplasm begins with a mottled basophilia, becomes polychromatophilic, and finally has an acidophilic appearance. These changes are linked with a progressive increase in hemoglobin and a progressive decrease in ribonucleoprotein (Plates VII.2 and VII.22). Mitotic activity is high.

The *metarubricyte (orthochromatic erythroblast, normoblast)* has an acidophilic cytoplasm that is similar to the mature red blood cell (RBC) (Plate VII.5). The nucleus becomes condensed and eventually pyknotic. The nucleus is lost either by simple extrusion from the cell or by *karyolysis*. The resulting enucleated cell is the *reticulocyte (polychromatophilic erythrocyte, diffusely basophilic erythrocyte)*. The cytoplasm is diffusely basophilic, and with special staining techniques a fine cytoplasmic reticulum is demonstrable. Ribosomes, polyribosomes, and mitochondria are still present. Some reticulocytes occur normally in the peripheral blood.

The increased cytoplasmic basophilia represents the accumulation of ribonucleoproteins for cellular synthesis. Hemoglobin, first synthesized by the rubricyte, results in a mottled cytoplasmic appearance. Increased synthesis of hemoglobin and a reduction of the appropriate cellular organelles characterizes the metarubricytic stage. A continuation of this process results in the mature RBC. The circulating erythrocytes of the embryo are nucleated and probably represent metarubricytes.

Granulocytopoiesis

The general pattern of cytodifferentiation includes a reduction in size, a decreased nuclear/cytoplasmic ratio, a decreased cytoplasmic staining intensity and the appearance of specific granules.

Cytology of Differentiation. The following cells comprise the granulocytic series: *myeloblast, promyelocyte, myelocyte, metamyelocyte, band cell, mature granulocyte* (Figs. 12.1 and 12.2).

The *myeloblast* has a diameter of 15–20 μm. The basophilic cytoplasm is unevenly stained and is darker at the periphery than in the perinuclear region. The nucleus is large, finely reticular, and red-staining. Two or more nucleoli may be observed. The myoblast is larger than the rubriblast and has more cytoplasm than the rubriblast.

The *promyelocyte (progranulocyte)* is a large cell. The nucleus is round with coarsely distributed chromatin. Nucleoli are not readily observed. The cytoplasm, although basophilic, contains acidophilic regions. Granules are present and vary from acidophilic to basophilic. There is a gradual decrease in *nonspecific granules (primary granules)*. The primary granules or *azurophilic granules* are lysosomes. The synthesis of primary granules is initiated in the promyelocytic stage of development. These granules are formed in large numbers during this stage but decrease in numbers toward the mature granulocyte. Promyelocytic mitotic activity is high.

A promyelocyte becomes a basophilic, eosinophilic, or neutrophilic myelocyte when the specific granulocyte can be identified on the basis of the staining affinity, size, and shape of the specific granules. The nucleus is smaller and the chromatin is more coarse than the previous stages. A nucleolus is not present. Also, the nucleus is oval and a slight indentation may be apparent. The decreased cytoplasmic basophilia is complemented by an increase in the number of *specific granules*. Mitotic activity of these cells is high.

The nature of the specific granules varies with the specific granulocytes. The neutrophilic myelocyte and its mature progeny have two types of granules. The azurophilic granules are the lysosomes. The specific granules do not contain lysosomal enzymes; a bactericidal substance and alkaline phosphatase are present. The specific granules of eosinophilic myelocytes and their mature progeny are lysosomes. The specific granules of basophils are not lysosomes but contain glycosaminoglycans (heparin).

The *metamyelocyte (basophilic metamyelocyte, eosinophilic metamyelocyte, neutrophilic metamyelocyte)* is characterized by a bean-shaped or horseshoe-shaped appearance. The cytoplasm is slightly acidophilic and filled with specific granules. Progressive indentation results in the lobed nuclear appearance of the mature granulocytes.

Neutrophilic granulocytes are the most predominate granulocytes of the myeloid tissue and peripheral blood. Immature forms of neutrophils are commonly encountered in the peripheral blood. A *neutrophilic metamyelocyte* is also called a *juvenile*. The progressive indentation of the nucleus results in a neutrophil called a *neutrophilic band cell, neutrophilic stab cell, neutrophilic nonsegmented* (Plates VI.23, VII.1, and VII.3). The nucleus of this cell is horseshoe-shaped. The subsequent lobulation of the nucleus results in a mature cell called a *neutrophil, neutrophilic segmenter, PMN, polymorphonuclear neutrophilic granulocyte, neutrophilic filamented, or neutrophilic polymorphonuclear.*

Thrombocytopoiesis

Cytology of Differentiation. The cells that comprise the platelet formation series

are: *megakaryoblast, promegakaryocyte, megakaryocyte, metamegakaryocyte,* and *platelets* (Fig. 12.1).

The rare *megakaryoblast* has a lightly basophilic cytoplasm and a nucleus that stains red and is finely granular. The peripheral cytoplasm has pseudopodia and a few foamy vacuoles.

The *promegakaryocyte* is larger than the previous cell type and two nuclei may be present. The cytoplasm is slightly basophilic and contains numerous basophilic granules. Cytoplasmic blebs with a foamy appearance may be apparent at the periphery.

The *megakaryocyte* is larger than the previous cell type. Karyokinesis occurs and as many as 32 nuclei may form. These fuse to form the characteristic bulged and lobed nucleus of this cell. The cytoplasmic volume is large and acidophilic. Vacuoles and pale-staining areas are scattered among the evenly distributed, lightly basophilic granules.

The *metamegakaryocyte* is the largest cell in the series. Except for the aggregation of cytoplasmic granules and the appearance of platelets at the cellular periphery, it is similar to the megakaryocyte.

This series of cellular changes is characterized by an increase in size and number of nuclei per cell—the reverse of the general trend in the aforementioned series. Mitosis *(endomitosis)* occurs in which nuclear separation *(karyokinesis)* is not accompanied by a cytoplasmic separation *(cytokinesis)*.

Platelets form from metamegakaryocytes by an exocytotic process in which they pinch off from the cell surface.

Agranulocytopoiesis

General Characteristics. Agranulocytic development (lymphocytes, monocytes, macrophages, and plasma cells) occurs in the lymphoid organs and bone marrow. For this reason, some authors refer to these organs as *lymphomyeloid organs*. The development of these cells is not as clearly defined as they are for the previous series. Moreover, the location and nature of all stem cells, specific areas in which development occurs and the relationships of these mononucleated cells to each other need further clarification. Figure 12.5 represents a summary of the known relationships among these cells.

Lymphocytopoiesis and Plasma Cells. Current evidence establishes that the mononucleated leukocytes are derivatives of CFUs: CFU-GM—granulocytes and monocytes; CFU-BL—B lymphocytes; CFU-TL—T lymphocytes.

Lymphoblasts are the largest cells of this series. They have large, round vesicular nuclei with one or more prominent nucleoli, and have a basophilic cytoplasm. Progressive differentiation and mitosis results in a smaller cell with a nucleus that contains more coarsely clumped heterochromatin. These are *large lymphocytes* that may be called *prolymphocytes* or *medium lymphocytes* by some authors. The

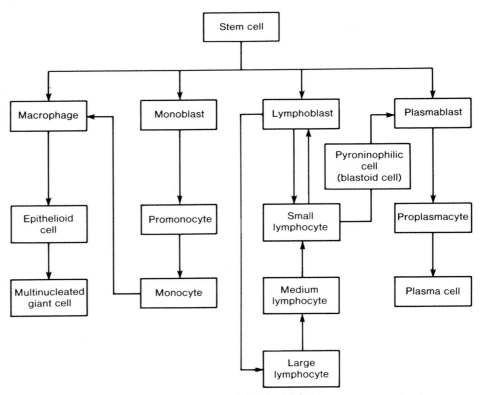

Figure 12.5. A flow diagram of the established relationships among agranulocytes.

subsequent division of these intermediate forms results in *small lymphocytes*. Any of these cells can enter the peripheral circulation.

Small lymphocytes are not fixed postmitotic cells. Under appropriate stimulation they can dedifferentiate into lymphoblasts that can subsequently give rise to more small lymphocytes. Also, with appropriate antigenic stimulation, the small lymphocyte is converted to a *pyroninophilic cell*. These cells contain large quantities of ribonucleic acid, which is stainable with pyronin, and are sometimes called *immunoblasts*. The cells are characterized by a blastoid transformation that permits them to become *plasmablasts*. *Plasmablasts* and *proplasmacytes* are not distinct and identifiable cytological intermediates in the differentiation of *plasma cells*.

Origin of Lymphocytes. During embryonic life, stem cells are produced sequentially in the yolk sac, liver, and spleen (Fig. 12.6). Lymphocytes differentiate in the liver and spleen. Stem cells then populate the bone marrow. The bone marrow functions as the major source for two distinct yet interrelated populations of lymphocytes.

One population of stem cells leaves the bone marrow and populates the thymus. These cells proliferate and differentiate within this organ. During *peripheralization* lymphocytes from the thymus, *T lymphocytes*, populate specific regions of lymph nodes and the *periarteriolar zone of splenic*

corpuscles. These cells are responsible for cell-mediated immunity and interact with B lymphocytes in an undetermined way to induce antibody formation (Fig. 12.6).

The organs involved in the development of *B lymphocytes* in the mammal have not been characterized completely. Stem cells leave the bone marrow and populate the bursal equivalent. In birds, these cells infiltrate the bursa of Fabricius and subsequently populate secondary lymphatic organs. Because mammals do not have a bursa of Fabricius, extensive research has been directed to defining a bursal equivalent. It was thought that *gut-associated lymphatic tissue (GALT)* was the bursal equivalent. It was conjectured that the bone marrow assumed the role of the bursa of Fabricius. Bursal functions in mammals may be the combined responsibility of intestinal lymphatic tissue and bone marrow. After populating the bursal equivalent, these cells populate the secondary lymphatic organs— *germinal centers of lymphatic nodules*. The B cells produced in these areas synthesize antibodies (humoral antibody response) and are capable of transformation into plasma cells (Fig. 12.6).

Monocytopoiesis. Although the precise nature and morphology of the stem cell for monocytes has not been clarified, it is clear that monocytes originate in the bone marrow. Immature monocytes in the bone marrow are larger than but similar to their mature counterparts. The large oval or round nucleus has numerous nucleoli.

These *promonocytes* are difficult to distinguish from granulocytic precursors.

Kinetics of Blood

The finite existence of the formed elements of the blood requires that old and/or damaged cells be removed from the circulation and new elements be added by the lymphomyeloid tissues. The rate at which these two processes occur normally accounts for the usual populations of cells that constitute the peripheral blood. Any alterations to the formative and/or removal processes can result in abnormal parameters. The dynamics of this balanced activity are referred to as *blood kinetics*. Many organs contribute to the formation and/or destruction of blood cells. The bone marrow, spleen, and other organs with macrophage populations are involved also in the destruction of cells. The liver contributes significantly to iron metabolism and retains its fetal potential for hematopoiesis. Portions of the gastrointestinal system contribute to erythrogenesis by their absorption of iron and production of *intrinsic factor*. Intrinsic factor exists in man but may not occur in domestic animals. The kidney is important in the regulation of erythropoiesis through its involvement in the generation of *erythropoietin*. The balance between production and turnover is affected readily by disruptions to the normal contributions by these numerous organs.

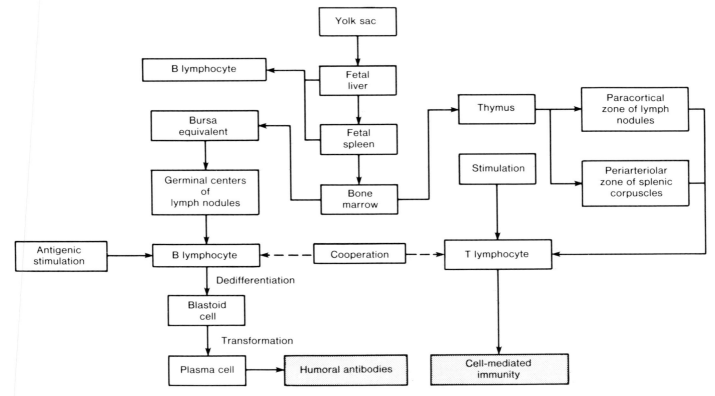

Figure 12.6. A flow diagram of the origin, fate and function of B and T lymphocytes.

Erythrokinetics

Life Cycle of Erythrocytes. The extrusion of its nucleus, the synthesis of hemoglobin, and its biconcave shape ensure that the RBC has a maximal oxygen-carrying capacity and a good volume to surface ratio. The ultimate stimulation for erythropoiesis is a reduced amount of oxygen in the tissues *(tissue hypoxia)* (Fig. 12.7).

The kidney and other organs respond to hypoxia by releasing *renal erythropoietic factor (REF), erythrogenin.* Renal hypoxia may cause the release of a prostaglandin (E_2) that sequentially activates cyclic adenosine monophosphate, a protein kinase, and the synthesis of renal erythropoietic factor. This factor reacts with a plasma α-globulin produced in the liver to produce *erythropoietin (EP).* Then EP stimulates stem cells, CFU-Es, to differentiate into rubriblasts. EP does not seem to influence the mitotic activity of BFU-Es, but the division of these cells gives rise to numerous CFU-Es. EP also induces rubriblasts, prorubricytes, and early rubricytes to increase their mitotic activity. EP stimulation also increases the amount of the enzyme *aminolevulinic acid synthetase,* an enzyme necessary for the synthesis of heme. Removal of the kidneys does not result in a loss of EP. Other organs, most likely the liver, are involved in the production of this regulatory substance also.

Although such stimulation is immediate, increased numbers of red blood cells are not noted in the peripheral circulation for about three days. The normal proliferation and differentiation cycle within the bone marrow takes about 3–5 days. Deleted mitoses and the early release of immature forms can occur, but the number of erythrocytes is not increased.

A progenitor cell (CFU-E) and its descendants undergo four mitoses in a span of five days to produce 16 erythrocytes. Mitotic activity ceases in the late rubricytic stage.

The BFU-Es circulate in the blood, whereas the CFU-Es seem to be confined to the hematopoietic tissues. The circulating levels of the BFU-Es is increased during severe anemia. The progenitor cells may be the means by which yellow bone marrow becomes repopulated with stem cells and becomes actively hematopoietic as red marrow.

The life-span of the erythrocytes of domestic animals is variable. Average life-spans are listed in Table 12.1. Reticulocytes occur rarely in normal blood of animals with an average RBC life-span that is greater than 100 days. As erythrocytes age, they are removed from the circulation by macrophages, especially those of the spleen. Although morphological alterations are not visible with normal erythrocytic aging, metabolic pathways are altered. Because the

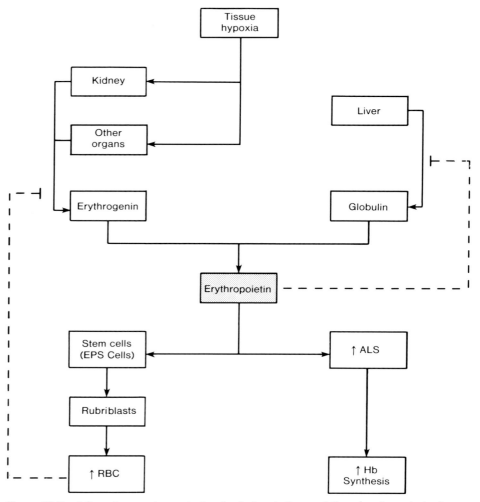

Figure 12.7. A flow diagram demonstrating the factors in the regulation of erythropoiesis. *Arrows* represent direction of flow and/or stimulation. *Bars* represent inhibition. *EPS* cells—erythropoietin-sensitive cells; *ALS,* amino-levulinic acid synthetase; *Hb*— hemoglobin.

number of erythrocytes is a homeostatic parameter of the blood, **erythropoiesis must equal erythroclasia.** A medium-sized dog will produce and destroy approximately 5×10^7 erythrocytes/minute.

Hemoglobin Synthesis, Destruction, and Reutilization. *Hemoglobin* is a *chromoprotein* (conjugated protein) that consists of a *heme* and *globin.* Heme is a protoporphyrin plus ferrous iron that is synthesized in mitochondria. Hemoglobin constitutes approximately 95% of the dry weight of the mature RBC. Variations in the amino acid sequence of the globin account for different types of hemoglobin (embryonic, fetal, and adult).

Old erythrocytes are removed from the circulation by the phagocytic cells of the macrophage system. Although the spleen is the primary organ for erythroclasia, it does occur in other organs (bone marrow, liver). Subtle membrane alterations and increased RBC fragility probably account for the phagocytic process. All components of the

hemoglobin molecule are reutilized by the body. The extravascular metabolism and reutilization of components are detailed in Figure 12.8.

Hemoglobin is split into its two components. The globin is hydrolyzed to its component amino acids, which become part of the body's circulating amino acid pool. Iron is removed from the heme, leaving the protoporphyrin. Iron, bound to plasma transferrin, is transported to the bone marrow for reutilization. Ferritin and hemosiderin are the storage forms of the iron in macrophages of the bone marrow and spleen. The protoporphyrin is converted to *biliverdin* and then *bilirubin.* Bilirubin is transported in the plasma bound to plasma proteins. Although it is bound, this is the *unconjugated* form of bilirubin. Bilirubin enters the hepatocytes and is conjugated to a glucuronide by the activity of the enzyme *glucuronyl transferase.* This conversion *(conjugation)* to *bilirubin glucuronide* is a biotransformation process that makes bili-

Table 12.1.
Average Life-Span of Erythrocytes

Species	Average Life Span—Days
Canid	120
Felid	73
Equid	145
Bovid	159
Ovid	110
Caprid	125
Porcid	67

rubin water-soluble. A small amount of this compound re-enters the circulation and is excreted by the kidney as *urobilinogen*. Most of the conjugated bilirubin is secreted by the hepatocytes as the major bile pigment in the bile. Bilirubin absorbed by the small intestine recirculates back into the liver via the *enterohepatic circulation*. Further alteration of bilirubin occurs in the intestines and the resultant compounds, *urobilin* and *sterocobilin*, are eliminated in the feces. These pigments impart the characteristic color to fecal material.

An excessive amount of bilirubin imparts a yellow color to the tissues. This condition, *jaundice (icterus)*, occurs under various circumstances. Excessive RBC destruction *(hemolytic jaundice)* is characterized by increased quantities of unconjugated bilirubin. Bile duct obstructions are characterized by increased quantities of conjugated bilirubin.

Granulokinetics

Neutrophils. Neutrophilic granulocytes proliferate and mature within the bone marrow (Fig. 12.9). Neutrophils released to the vasculature comprise a *circulating* and *marginal pool*. The cells leave the vascular compartment and enter the *tissue pool*. They do not return from the tissues to the circulating pool.

Five mitoses are characteristic of the developmental sequence of this cell. Myeloblasts and progranulocytes each divide once, whereas myelocytes divide three times. Five days are required for myelocytes to become mature, fully differentiated neutrophils. A 3-to-5 day lag-period occurs before an increased or decreased response from the bone marrow will be noted in the peripheral blood. However, an increase in circulating neutrophils can occur rapidly by mobilizing the neutrophils that comprise the marginal pool. The marginal pool consists of neutrophils that marginate along the walls of small vessels. This pool may equal the circulating pool (dog) or may be two to three times the circulating pool (cat).

The half-life of neutrophils within the circulating pool is approximately six hours. The circulating pool of neutrophils is replaced approximately every 10–12 hours. The replacement occurs directly from the

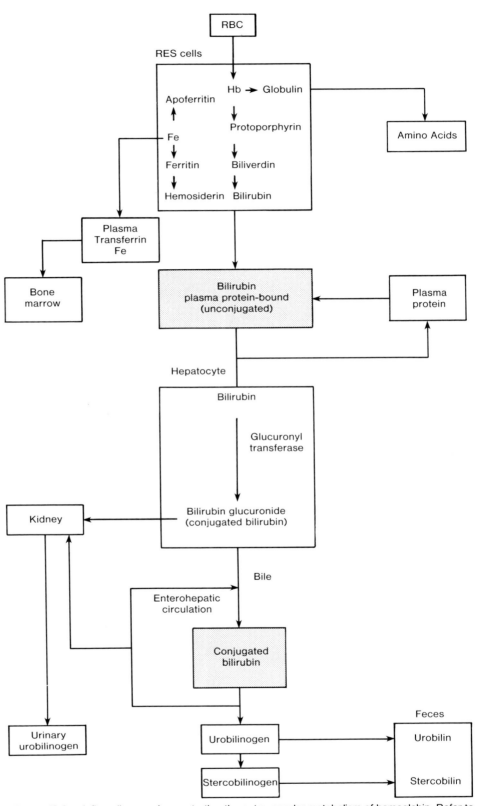

Figure 12.8. A flow diagram demonstrating the extravascular metabolism of hemoglobin. Refer to the text for a complete description of the process. *RES*—macrophage system.

maturation pool. Under normal conditions of peripheral neutrophil utilization, the re-

serve pool in the canine bone marrow contains about a 5-day supply of cells. Mature

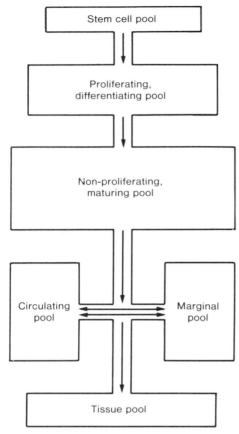

Figure 12.9. A diagram of the flow and distribution of neutrophils within various pools within the body. The proliferating, differentiating pool consists of myeloblasts, progranulocytes, and myelocytes. The nonproliferating, maturing pool consists of metamyelocytes, band cells, and mature cells.

cells are the first neutrophils that are mobilized from the maturation pool. As the demand for neutrophils increases, progressively younger cells are released from the bone marrow. Even neutrophilic myelocytes may occur in the circulation during periods of extreme demand and excessive depletion of the maturation pool.

Neutrophilia is an increased number of circulating neutrophils, whereas *neutropenia* is a decreased number of circulating neutrophils. A neutrophilia with a slight to moderate increase in the number of immature neutrophils (>3%) is called a *regenerative left shift*. A *degenerative left shift* is characterized by a low to slightly elevated neutrophil count in which the number of immature forms is greater than the number of mature neutrophils. A *right shift* is characterized by an increased number of older cells in which nuclear hypersegmentation is obvious.

Regulation of Neutrophils. Many factors involved in the specific and nonspecific immune response—complement fragments, bacterial products, and tissue en-

zymes—influence the production and migration of granulocytes. Additionally, a glycoprotein called *colony stimulating factor (CSF)* influences the mitotic activity of the CFU-GM and subsequent neutrophilic intermediates. This factor is released by macrophages in response to local inflammation, endotoxin, and some immunologic mediators. The release of prostaglandins by macrophages inhibits the proliferative activity of the CFU-GM. Also, neutrophils secrete a substance called *colony inhibiting activity (CIA)*, which limits the proliferative activity of the CFU-GM despite normal levels of colony stimulating factor being present. *Neutrophil releasing activity (NRA)* or *leukocytosis-inducing factor (LIF)* is a circulating substance that causes the release of immature neutrophils into the general circulation. Endotoxin induces an increased level of leukocytosis-inducing factor.

Eosinophils. The maturation pattern, production time, life-span and circulation of the eosinophil is similar to the pattern described for the neutrophil. The production time for the eosinophil is about 3–6 days. Although circulating numbers of eosinophils are low, approximately 300 cells to every circulating eosinophil constitute the maturation pool. About 100 cells for every circulating cell constitutes the proliferating pool.

The ultimate stimulation for an increased number of eosinophils is the release of histamine from degranulated mast cells. The local release of histamine serves as an eosinophilic chemotactic factor, but this is not always associated with an *eosinophilic leukocytosis (eosinophilia)*. Circulating histamine probably accounts for eosinophilia. Various factors associated with immune responsiveness are associated with increased numbers of eosinophils locally or in the circulation. Additionally, an *eosinophilopoietin* is believed to exist. Antigenic factors may influence eosinophils through this stimulatory factor.

Basophils. The small numbers of these cells within the body complicate kinetic studies of them. Their life-span is approximately 10–12 days. The functions of these cells are similar to the mast cell.

Kinetics of Agranulocytes

Lymphocytes. T lymphocytes are more numerous in the peripheral blood than B lymphocytes. T cells are long-lived cells that may remain in the body for months or years. Thymocytes, however, are short-lived (3–4 days) and most of them degenerate within the thymus. B cells that are responsible for the *primary immune response* are short-lived, whereas those responsible for the *secondary immune response* are long-lived. Accurate data concerning the life-span of lymphocytes are

difficult to obtain because of the recirculation of lymphocytes.

Large and medium lymphocytes of the bone marrow, spleen, and lymph nodes seem to generate in about 8 hours, whereas small lymphocytes within these organs may require at least 4 days. In the dog, a sufficient number of lymphocytes enters the vasculature from the thoracic duct to indicate that all lymphocytes may be replaced every 12 hours.

Except for thymocytes, the common stimulator for lymphopoiesis is the presence of antigen.

Circulating lymphocytes can gain access to lymph nodes by leaving the circulation through venules in the paracortical zones of lymph nodes. These venules are called *postcapillary venules*. Once inside the parenchyma of the lymph node, these lymphocytes may return to the vascular bed via the postcapillary venules. The lymphocytes may enter the lymph node within the circulation and exit the vasculature at the postcapillary venules, enter the efferent lymphatics and eventually be returned to the circulation through the thoracic duct. The *recirculation* phenomenon ensures that immunocompetent cells are distributed widely throughout the body and that numerous lymphocytes are exposed to a local antigen. Evaluation of lymphatic outflow from lymph nodes indicates that 95% of these lymphocytes may be of blood origin, whereas 5% are of nodal origin. T cells appear to recirculate as much as five times faster than B cells.

Lymphocytosis is an increase in the number of lymphocytes, whereas *lymphopenia* is a decrease in the number of lymphocytes. Certain types of disease processes cause a lymphocytosis (bacterial infection); others (viral) cause a lymphopenia.

Monocytes. Monocytes marginate in the vascular bed; this marginal pool may be five times as large as the circulating pool. Because young monocytes leave the bone marrow rapidly, the maturation pool is considered to be small. Once these cells gain access to the vascular compartment they enter the tissues randomly. The tissue pool of histocytes may be 400 times greater than the circulating pool of monocytes. Whereas the circulating half-life of human monocytes is about eight days, the life-span of histocytes probably exceeds 100 days.

The regulation of monocytic proliferation is not understood completely. Those factors that influence the CFU-GM and result in an augmented production of neutrophils influence the monocytes similarly.

Evaluation of Blood and Bone Marrow

Whole blood evaluations invariably involve the use of substances that inhibit coagulation. Such substances, *anticoagu-*

lants, include *EDTA (ethylenediamine tetraacetic acid), heparin, sodium citrate,* and various salts of oxalic acid *(sodium oxalate, potassium oxalate).* Heparin interferes with the generation of fibrin by functioning as an antithrombin and antithromboplastin. The other compounds arrest coagulation by forming insoluble salts with calcium. Often, hematological evaluation requires the use of a blood sample with an anticoagulant added, a clotted blood sample for serum evaluations, and a blood smear for qualitative and quantitative evaluations.

Peripheral Blood Parameters. *Erythrocyte and white blood cell counts* can be accomplished with automated systems, but the use of a *hemocytometer* is a quick, easy and inexpensive counting method. RBCs and total white blood cells are reported as the number of cells/mm³ of blood. Often, erythrocytes are not counted, but the *packed cell volume (PCV)* is determined. The PCV is a valuable parameter that is related to RBC numbers and size.

The *differential count* of white blood cells is accomplished on a stained blood smear. The count identifies the frequency of different white blood cells when 100 or 200 white blood cells are counted. Identification of mature and immature forms is an important part of this subjective evaluation. It is customary to note also other distinguishing characteristics of the cell (anisocytosis, polychromasia, toxicity), as well as the presence of nucleated RBCs and any other notable features. A differential leukocyte count generates *relative values* for white blood cell. The percentages are converted to *absolute values* by multiplying the total white cell count by the percentage of occurrence of each cell type, mature and immature.

The *mean corpuscular volume (MCV)* is used to determine the size of RBCs. The MCV is determined by multiplying the PCV by 10 and dividing by the RBC count. The MCV is expressed in femtoliters (1 × 10^{-15} liters).

Hemoglobin concentration is determined routinely with a *hemoglobinometer.* This simple technique is the determination of *oxyhemoglobin* by its light absorption. Although the values obtained by this method are less accurate (±10%) than wet chemical methods for *cyanomethemoglobin,* they are useful for clinical evaluations. The *mean corpuscular hemoglobin concentation (MCHC)* is used for distinguishing anemias as normochromic or hypochromic. The MCHC (g/dl) is determined by dividing the hemoglobin concentration (g/dl) by the PCV and multiplying by 100.

The *erythrocyte sedimentation rate* is determined by using a tube of blood to which an anticoagulant has been added and noting the amount of erythrocyte settling that occurs in a given time period.

Total protein determinations can be made on serum or plasma proteins by refractometry. *Electrophoresis* can be accomplished on the sample also. The *albumin/globulin ratio (A/G ratio),* normally 0.7–1.0, is a valuable diagnostic parameter that is determined by electrophoresis.

Bone Marrow Evaluation. Bone marrow evaluations can be used to offer more insights concerning peripheral blood observations. Different biopsy sites are used in different domestic animals. A bone marrow evaluation requires familiarity with the cytology of differentiation. A differential count of 500 cells is a valuable parameter. The *myeloid/erythroid ratio (ME ratio)* is determined by dividing the total number of granulocytic cells by the total number of nucleated erythrocytic cells of the marrow differential count.

References

Development of Blood

Ackerman, G. A.: Ultrastructure and cytochemistry of the developing neutrophil. Lab. Invest. *19*:290, 1968.

Barr, R.D., Whang-Peng, J. and Perry, S.: Hematopoietic stem cells in human peripheral blood. Science *190*:284, 1975.

Behnke, O.: An electron microscope study of the megakaryocyte of the rat bone marrow. I. The development of the demarcation membrane system and the platelet surface coat. J. Ultrastruct. Res. *24*:412, 1968.

Calhoun, L. M.: Bone marrow of horses and cattle. Science *104*:423, 1946.

Calhoun, L. M.: A cytological study of costal marrow. I. The adult horse. Amer. J. Vet. Res. *15*:181, 1954: II. The adult cow. Amer. J. Vet. Res. *15*:395, 1954.

Campbell, F. R.: Nuclear elimination from the normoblast of fetal guinea pig liver as studied with electron microscopy and serial sectioning techniques. Anat. Rec. *160*:539, 1968.

Chamberlain, J.K. and Lichtman, M.A.: Marrow cell egress: Specificity of the site of penetration into the sinus. Blood *52*:959, 1978.

Fedorko, M.: Formation of cytoplasmic granules in human eosinophilic myelocytes: An electron microscopic autoradiographic study. Blood *31*:188, 1968.

Johnson, F. R. and Roberts, D. B.: The growth and division of human small lymphocytes in tissue culture: An electron microscopic study. J. Anat. *98*:303, 1964.

Kaihotsu, N.: Electron microscopic studies on the maturation process of neutrophilic leucocytes. Kobe J. Med. Sci. *13*:47, 1967.

Kato, K.: Monophyletic scheme of blood cell formation for clinical and laboratory reference. J. Lab. Clin. Med. *20*:1243, 1935.

Loutit, J. F.: Transplantation of haemopoietic tissue. Brit. Med. Bull. *21*:118, 1965.

Metcalf, D.: Hematopoietic colonies—in vitro cloning of normal and leukemic cells. Recent Results in Cancer Research. Vol 61, Springer-Verlag, Berlin, 1977.

Mohandas, N. and Prenant, M.: Three-dimensional model of bone marrow. Blood *51*:633, 1978.

Moore, M.A.S.: Regulatory role of macrophages in hematopoiesis. J. Reticuloendothel. Soc. *20*:89, 1976.

Osoba, D.: Precursors of thymic lymphocytes. Ser. Haematol. *7*:427, 1974.

Pease, D. C.: An electron microscopic study of red bone marrow. J. Hemat. *11*:501, 1956.

Quesenberry, O. P. and Levitt, L.: Hematopoietic stem cells. N. Engl. J. Med. *301*:755, 1979.

Scott, R. E. and Horn, R. G.: Fine structural features of eosinophil granulocyte development in human bone marrow. J. Ultrastruct. Res. *33*:16, 1970.

Stanley, E. R., Hanson, G., Woodcock, J. and Metcalf, D.: Colony stimulating factor and the regulation of granulopoiesis and macrophage production. Fed. Proc. *34*:2272, 1975.

Tavassoli, M.: The marrow-blood barrier. Br. J. Haematol. *41*:297, 1979.

Wetzel, B. K., Horn, R. G. and Spicer, S. S.: Fine structural studies on the development of heterophil, eosinophil and basophil granulocytes in rabbits. Lab. Invest. *16*:349, 1967.

Wu, A. M., Till, J. E., Siminovitch, L. and McCulloch, E. A.: A cytological study of the capacity for differentiation of normal hemopoietic colony-forming cells. J. Cell Physiol. *69*:177, 1967.

Yamada, E.: The fine structure of the megakaryocyte in the mouse spleen. Acta Anat. *29*:267, 1957.

Kinetics

Everett, N. B., Caffrey, R. W. and Rieke, W. D.: Recirculation of lymphocytes. Ann. New York Acad. Sci. *113*:887, 1964.

Finch, C. A.: Some quantitative aspects of erythropoiesis. Ann. New York Acad. Sci. *77*:410, 1959.

Firth, J. L.: Life-span, recirculation and transformation of lymphocytes. Int. Rev. Exp. Pathol. *5*:1, 1966.

Giblett, E. R.: The plasma transferrins. Prog. Med. Genet. *2*:34, 1962.

Graber, S.E. and Krantz, S.B.: Erythropoietin and the control of red cell production. Ann. Rev. Med. *29*:51, 1978.

Greenwalt, T. J. and Jamieson, G. A.: *Formation and Destruction of Blood Cells.* J. B. Lippincott, Philadelphia, 1970.

Jamuar, M.P. and Cronkite, E.P.: The fate of blood granulocytes. Exp. Hematol. *8*:884, 1980.

Lajtha, L. G., Pozzi, L. V., Schofield, R. and Fox, M. Kinetic properties of hemopoietic stem cells. Cell Tiss. Kinet. *2*:39, 1969.

Leblond, C. P. and Walker, B. E.: Renewal of cell populations. Physiol. Rev. 36255, 1956.

Morley, A. A.: A neutrophil cycle in healthy individuals. Lancet *2*:1220, 1966.

Perutz, M. F.: The hemoglobin molecule. Proc. R. Soc. (London) (Biol.) Ser. B. *173*:1113, 1969.

Schalm, O. W.: Interpretation of leukocyte responses in the dog. J. Am. Vet. Med. Assoc. *142*:147, 1963.

Schalm, O. W., Hughes, J. and Hardy, D.: Dynamics of the neutrophilic leukocyte and a unique response in acute indigestion in the cow. Calif. Vet. *21*:20, 1967.

Weed, R. I.: The importance of erythrocyte deformability. Am. J. Med. *49*:147, 1970.

13: Muscle Tissue

General Characteristics

Form and Function. The structural element of muscular tissue is the *muscle cell* or *muscle fiber*. *Contractility* is a well-developed characteristic. Muscle comprises the majority of the "flesh" (*sarcos*, Gr., flesh) or "meat" of an organism. Muscle is also a primary mural element of tubular organs. Muscle fibers are elongated cells. They are enclosed by a *sarcolemma* (plasmalemma) and fine *reticular fibers*. The *sarcoplasm* (cytoplasm) contains typical organelles as well as contractile elements. These *myofilaments* are composed of the proteins, *actin* and *myosin*. The myofilaments are grouped as *myofibrils*.

The contractility of muscle is the means by which work is accomplished—locomotion, expression of secretions from glands, movement of blood through the cardiovascular system, movement of materials through the digestive system.

Functionally, muscle may be *voluntary* or *involuntary*. Structurally, it may be *smooth (nonstriated)* or *striated*. Through the combination of these characteristics, the following classification is derived: *Smooth muscle—nonstriated, involuntary; Skeletal muscle—striated, voluntary; Cardiac muscle—striated, involuntary.*

Smooth Muscle

Histological Structure

Smooth muscle fibers are elongated, spindle-shaped cells with finely tapered ends. The central region in which the nucleus is located is the widest part of the cell. These cells may be as short as 20 μm as mural elements of a small tubule or as long as 0.5 mm in the wall of a gravid uterus. This appearance is not always apparent in a single section. Often, the cells are packed tightly and appear to blend as a homogeneous mass (Fig. 13.1, Plates V.1. and V.2)). The elongated, cylindrical nucleus is rounded at the ends and contains a fine chromatin network with peripherally clumped heterochromatin. Two to several nucleoli may be apparent. The nuclei may be twisted and wrinkled or assume a helical configuration. This may be indicative of

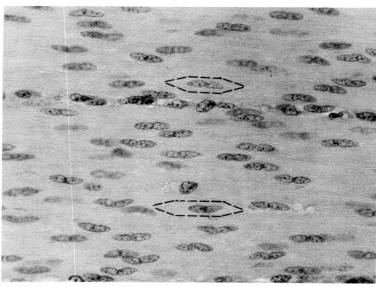

Figure 13.1. Longitudinal section of smooth muscle. *Dashed lines*, approximate cellular limits. The elongated nuclei are oriented parallel to the long axis of the muscle fiber. Cellular limits are difficult to discern in longitudinal sections of sheets of smooth muscle. Some of the torpedo-shaped nuclei appear to be twisted. This is an indication that the cells are contracted. ×160.

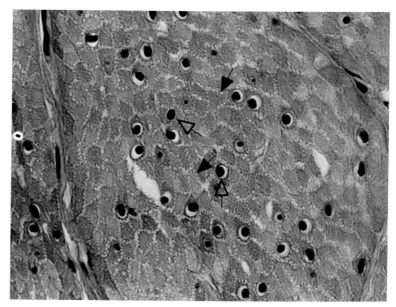

Figure 13.2. Cross section of smooth muscle. The nuclei *(open arrows)* and cellular limits *(solid arrows)* are apparent. Most of the nuclei are out of the plane of section. ×160.

active contraction at the time of fixation or a passive distortion due to agonal changes. The cytoplasm is homogeneous, bright-staining and acidophilic.

In longitudinal section, smooth muscle cells appear as described previously. Because of their shape, however, not all nuclei are included in any given section. The cells are staggered; the thickest portion of one is adjacent to the tapered portion of another.

In cross section, the cells are round to oval (Fig. 13.2). The nuclei are round and centrally located or slightly eccentric in position. Again, the nuclei are not seen in all cells sectioned.

Smooth muscle fibers are intimately associated with fine reticular fibers (Fig. 13.3). Each muscle fiber is surrounded by a basement membrane in which reticular fibers are embedded. Bunches of muscle fibers may be intimately associated with connective tissue as in the corium. In other regions, the muscle cells are arranged in extensive sheets, a few to many layers thick. In these instances, the fine reticular fibers are eventually continuous with the connective tissue surrounding the entire sheet. These sheets are often arranged so that the muscle fibers of one sheet are at "right angles" to the muscle fibers of another. In cross-sections through a tubular organ, such as the gut, one sheet ("circularly oriented" and inner) is sectioned longitudinally. The adjacent sheet ("longitudinal" and outer), at "90°" to the other, is cross sectioned (Fig. 13.4). Naturally, in longitudinal section of an organ the reverse occurs. (Generally, the inner layer of muscle is disposed as a tighter helix than the outer layer.)

MORPHOLOGICAL FEATURES: **A homogeneous, brightly acidophilic cytoplasm is apparent. Elongated nuclei have a fine chromatin network. Nuclei, dependent upon the degree of contraction, may be smooth-surfaced, wrinkled, twisted or helical. Cells are packed tightly and cellular boundaries may be indistinct.**

Ultrastructure

The ultrastructure of smooth muscle reflects its light microscopic appearance (Fig. 13.5). The nucleus is elongated and finely granular with peripherally clumped heterochromatin. The organelles are confined to the perinuclear regions of the cell, especially at the poles of the nucleus. Mitochondria, rough endoplasmic reticulum, free ribosomes, and a small Golgi apparatus are present. Parallel, discontinuous, spirally oriented bundles of myofilaments are present within the cytoplasm. These bundles vary in thickness and are oriented generally along the long axis of the cell. Dense, amorphous, round bodies are scattered throughout the cytoplasm and are associated with the plasmalemma. These bodies appear to be points of attachment for the myofila-

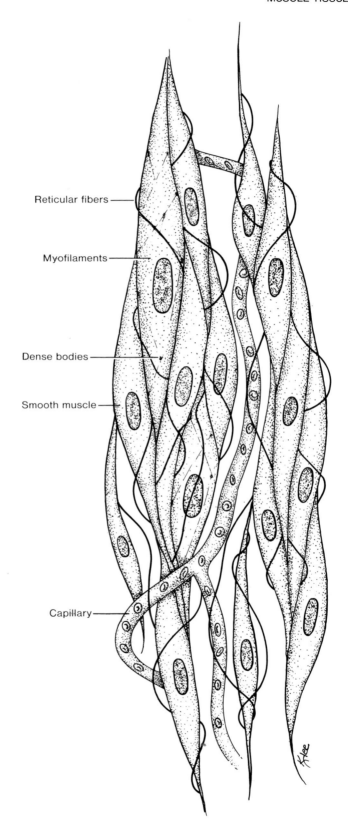

Reticular fibers

Myofilaments

Dense bodies

Smooth muscle

Capillary

Figure 13.3. Diagram of the three-dimensional relationships between smooth muscle cells and associated tissue. Myofilaments are scattered throughout the cytoplasm and are attached to the surface and within the cytoplasm by dense bodies.

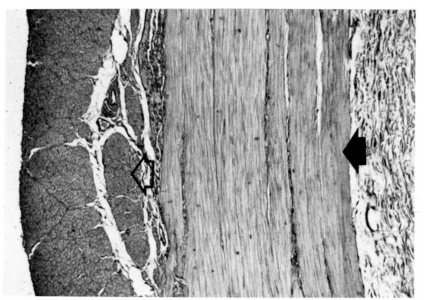

Figure 13.4. Tunica muscularis of the wall of the gastrointestinal tract. The inner circular muscle *(solid arrow)* is sectioned longitudinally; the outer longitudinal muscle *(open arrow)* is cross sectioned. ×40.

ments within the cytoplasm as well as at the cell surface (Fig. 13.5). *Dense bodies* are considered to be analogous to Z lines in skeletal muscle. The myofilaments consist of *actin* and *myosin.*

The plasma membrane contains numerous caveolae, and many pinocytotic vesicles are juxtaposed to the membrane (Fig. 13.5). The basal lamina covers the entire cell, except at points of cell-to-cell contact, the *nexi* (Fig. 13.5). A *nexus* or *gap junction* is an intimate contact point between adjacent cells that functions to facilitate the spread of excitation from one cell to another. These are regions of low electrical resistance.

Functional Correlates

Smooth muscle is slow to contract; it is characterized by a sustained contraction that is resistant to fatigue. The contraction mechanism is probably based upon the sliding filament mechanism. Upon contraction, the spindle-shaped, elongated, smooth-surfaced cell is converted to a shortened cell with numerous dimples on the surface. The dimples result from the bulging of cytoplasm between points of contact between the *anchoring plaques* and the plasma membrane. This imparts the characteristic thickening and twisting of the cell during contraction. The twisting and the absence of an orderly sarcomeric arrangement permits the smooth muscle cell to shorten more in proportion to its length than skeletal muscle.

Calcium is an essential ion for activating and sustaining smooth muscle contraction. Most likely, the influx and outward move-

ment of calcium is associated with the sarcoplasmic reticulum and caveolae.

Although neuronal stimulation can initiate smooth muscle contraction, not all smooth muscle cells are innervated. The spread of excitation occurs by nexi through which adjacent cellular contractile mechanisms are activated. The morphological distortion of cells can be transmitted to adjacent cells by the generation of forces through the connective tissue fibrous coverings. Also, smooth muscle is responsive to humoral agents. One of the most important stimuli to contraction of smooth muscle is its responsiveness to stretch. This local stimulus is important in the normal function of hollow visceral organs.

Smooth muscle may be considered a single morphological entity; yet, additional distinctions among this tissue type are possible on the basis of physiological and pharmacological properties. *Vascular smooth muscle* or *multiunit smooth muscle* has a high density innervation. Functionally, this smooth muscle type acts like skeletal muscle because of its dependency upon neuronal stimulation. Not all of the cells are innervated, and nexi are not observed between adjacent cells. The release of neurotransmitters from nondirected synapses probably accounts for the stimulation of adjacent cells that are not innervated. *Visceral smooth muscle* or *single unit smooth muscle* has a lower innervation density than multiunit smooth muscle. Visceral smooth muscle cells act as single units and the spread of excitation is dependent upon ephaptic conduction mechanisms. This smooth muscle type is characterized further by *rhythmic* and *tonic contractions.*

Rhythmic contraction is initiated by the spontaneous and periodic activation of "pacemaker cells" within the muscle mass. *Tonic contraction* accounts for the characteristic partial contraction or *tone* of smooth muscle. An *intermediate type* of smooth muscle exists. The intermediate type has an innervation density greater than that observed in single unit smooth muscle, and nexi are present.

Smooth muscle is also excited or inhibited by hormones secreted by the gastrointestinal tract. Uterine smooth muscle is responsive to the hormones associated with estrus, pregnancy, and parturition. Epinephrine has a significant influence on smooth muscle also.

Smooth muscle is an integral component of the walls of hollow visceral organs. The intramural mass of muscle contributes to the size of the lumen, the tone of the walls, and the movement of materials through the organs. Smooth muscle is not confined to the hollow viscera; it occurs also in the eye and orbit (iris, ciliary body, eyelid, third eyelid, periorbita) and capsules of the spleen and hemal nodes. In the vascular system the smooth muscle of the vessel wall actively contributes to peripheral resistance, which assists in the maintenance of blood pressure.

Skeletal Muscle

Histological Structure

The skeletal muscle fiber is an elongated cell that is slightly tapered or blunt at the ends. Most muscle fibers are between 1 and 40 mm. They vary from 10–100 μm in diameter. These cells are multinucleated and striated (Fig. 13.6). The oval nuclei have peripherally clumped heterochromatin. The nuclei are located at the periphery of the cells. Some nuclei appear to be centrally located. This, however, is usually an artifact of sectioning; i.e., the section may be close to the sarcolemma above or below the observation plane.

Cross-striations, or dark and light bands, are oriented perpendicular to the long axis of the muscle fiber (Plate V.3). Upon higher magnification the regularity of the banding is resolved (Fig. 13.7). The lighter *I bands* separate the darker *A bands.* Contained within the I bands are dense lines, the *Z lines* (Plate II.12). **A sarcomere, the unit of muscular contraction, includes the myofilaments contained between two adjacent Z lines.**

Individual muscle fibers are oriented in an unbranched, parallel array and are separated from one another by loose connective tissue. Naturally, a basement membrane separates the connective tissue compartment from the associated muscle fibers.

In cross section, the peripheral relationship of the nuclei to the muscle fibers is

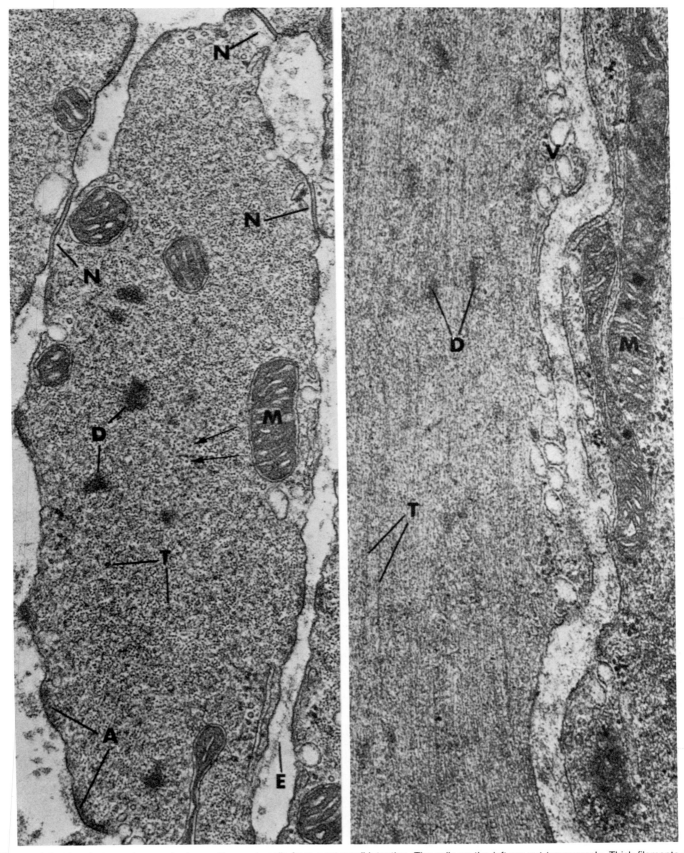

Figure 13.5. An electron micrograph of smooth muscle cells from a rat small intestine. The cells on the *left* are cut transversely. Thick filaments *(T)*, probably myosin, are scattered among numerous thin actin filaments. A third type of filament *(arrows)* are noncontractile intermediate size filaments. Attachment plaques *(A)* anchor the myofilaments to the cell membrane, and dense bodies *(D)* anchor the filaments within the cytoplasm. Nexi *(N)* between adjacent cells are apparent. Mitochondria *(M)* are present. The cells on the *right* are sectioned longitudinally. Pinocytotic vesicles *(V)* are evident along the cell membrane. *E*, basal lamina. ×89,600. (Reprinted with permission from: Copenhaver, W. M., Kelly, D. E. and Wood, R. L.: *Bailey's Textbook of Histology*, 17th edition, Williams & Wilkins, Baltimore, 1978.)

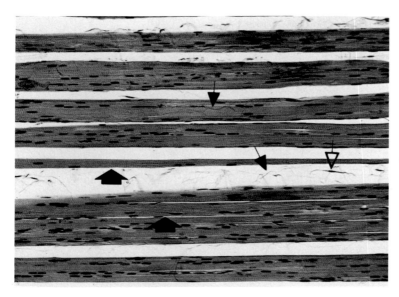

Figure 13.6. Longitudinal section of skeletal muscle. Individual muscle fibers *(large arrows)* are striated and multinucleated. Compare the muscle fiber size with the connective tissue cell *(open arrow)*. Endomyseal connective tissue *(solid arrows)* surrounds the muscle fibers. ×40.

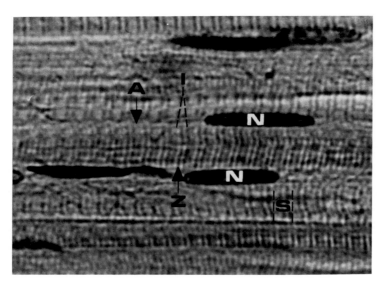

Figure 13.7. Striations of skeletal muscle. The nuclei *(N)*, A band *(A)*, I band *(I)* and Z lines *(Z)* are indicated. The sarcomeres are registered with each other. The sarcomere *(S)* below the S is outlined with *dashed lines*. The sarcomere extends from Z line to Z line. ×400.

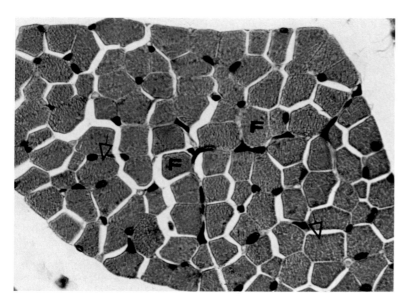

Figure 13.8. Cross section of skeletal muscle. The fibers *(F)* are grouped in bundles or fascicles. The grouping of myofibrils as Cohnheim's areas *(arrows)* is apparent. The nuclei are positioned peripherally. ×160.

observed more readily (Fig. 13.8). Also, the myofibrils are seen as clumps of acidophilic dots *(Cohnheim's fields)* (Plate V.4).

Ultrastructure

The detailed morphology of a sarcomere has been clarified with the electron microscope (Fig. 13.9). **One sarcomere extends between two adjacent Z lines in a myofibril and includes one-half of the I bands on either side of the A band (Fig. 13.10).** The only myofilaments contained within the I bands are the thin actin filaments. The A band, however, contains thin actin filaments and thick myosin filaments. Two separate actin filaments extend from each Z line through the A band. The gap between their ends within the A band is the H band. Upon contraction, the I band is shortened, the H band is obliterated, and a dense M line is formed in the space previously occupied by the H band.

A small and inactive Golgi apparatus is juxtaposed to many of the nuclei. Mitochondria are numerous, occurring at nuclear poles, beneath the sarcolemma, and interdigitated among the myofibrils. The intimate relationship between the mitochondria and the myofibrils is significant in the contractile mechanism.

The *sarcoplasmic reticulum* consists of an extensive network of cisterns and tubules *(sarcotubules)* that occur among and on the myofibrillar units (Fig. 13.11). This canalicular network corresponds to the smooth endoplasmic reticulum. Most of these tubular profiles are oriented longitudinally to the myofibrils. At specific loci within the cell, these tubules become confluent and form *terminal cisterns* that are oriented perpendicular to the long axis of the cell. At these specific loci, two terminal cisterns are separated from each other by a transversely oriented, slender *transverse tubule*. Transverse tubules are invaginations of the plasmalemma that comprise the *transverse sarcotubular system (T tubular system)*. Two terminal cisterns and a transverse tubule comprise a *triad* (Figs. 13.11 and 13.12). In the skeletal muscle of amphibians, the triads are located at Z lines. In mammalian skeletal muscle, triads are located a A-I junctions of a sarcomere, resulting in two triads per sarcomere.

Substances within the transverse tubules are actually outside of the cell, because these tubules are slender invaginations of the cell membrane. The relationships of the sarcoplasmic reticulum and transverse tubules to the cell and sarcomeres are depicted in Figure 13.13.

Myofibrillar Organization

Myofibrils are composed of two different kinds of myofilaments, *actin* and *myosin* (Fig. 13.14). The disposition and registration of the myofilaments within and between sarcomeres account for the typical striated pattern of skeletal muscle.

Myosin is a thick filament that is approximately 10 nm in diameter by 1.5 μm long. It is the principal component of the A band wherein these parallel filaments are separated by a distance of 45 nm. Thick filaments have a smooth and thick central portion that tapers toward each end. The slender portion of these filaments have radial projections. The isolation and dissociation of thick filaments yields *myosin*. Myosin is a cone-shaped molecule approximately 150 nm long with a globular portion or head at one end. The thick filaments of the A band are formed by the association of myosin molecules such that the elongated, rod-shaped part of the molecules projects toward the thicker central protion of the filament. The globular heads project in the opposite direction and account for the radial projections associated with the slender portions of the thick filaments of myosin. Digestion of myosin with trypsin yields two major fragments, *light meromyosin (LMM)* and *heavy meromyosin (HMM)*. The LMM fragment constitutes the rod-shaped portion of the molecule, whereas the HMM fragment constitutes the radially-projecting globular heads.

The thin *actin* filaments have a 5 nm diameter and a 1 μm length. They originate from the Z line, comprise the I band exclusively and extend into the A band between the thick myosin filaments. Each thin filament of actin consists of two strands of *fibrous actin (F actin)* disposed in a double helix. F actin is a polymer of about 200 *G actin (globular actin)* monomers. A fibrous protein, *tropomyosin*, occupies the space between the F actin, whereas *troponin*, a globular protein, occupies a specific locus at each half-turn in the helix. Tropomyosin and troponin are regulatory proteins in the contractile mechanism.

Contractile Mechanism

The contraction of skeletal muscle is initiated at the motor end-plate (Fig. 13.11). The action potential reaches the presynaptic region and *acetylcholine*, a cholinergic neurotransmitter, is released. The activation of cholinergic receptors culminates in the generation of end-plate potentials that result in an action potential spreading from this site along the cell membrane and into the depths of the cell via the transverse sarcotubular system. This inward movement of the wave of depolarization causes the release of calcium from the sarcoplasmic reticulum and initiates contraction (Fig. 13.15). These events comprise *excitation-contraction coupling*.

Calcium is sequestered within the sarcoplasmic reticulum bound to a calcium-binding protein called *calsequestrin*. The release of calcium from the sarcoplasmic reticulum into the sarcoplasm probably evokes a conformational change in troponin that detects the altered calcium levels and causes the movement of tropomyosin. Tropomyosin, which normally blocks the active sites of actin and myosin during relaxation, is displaced sufficiently to remove this inhibition and permit the interaction between the globular heads (HMM) of the myosin with the G actin monomers of actin. This interaction occurs as a result of the outward movement of the globular heads and is dependent upon the conversion of adenosine triphosphate (ATP) to adenosine diphosphate (ADP) with the release of energy. This occurs with each make and break event. ATPase, which is present in the globular heads, is responsible for this conversion and release of energy. The outward movement is facilitated by the flexibility of the neck region that connects LMM with globular heads (Fig. 13.16).

The thick and thin filaments may be visualized as two interacting worm gears. Contraction is envisioned as sequential connections, disconnections, and reconnections between the globular heads of myosin with G actin. Each reconnection at an adjacent G actin monomer site results in the incremental shortening of the sarcomere. The number of reconnections, each equivalent to the approximate 56 Å diameter of G actin, is summed as the total shortening of the sarcomere and the contraction of the muscle fiber.

ATP also supplies the energy for the active transport or pumping of calcium from the sarcoplasm to the sarcoplasmic reticulum where it is stored in the terminal cisterns. This event causes relaxation. The ADP is phosphorylated to ATP, troponin and tropomyosin assume their precontraction relationships, the globular heads of myosin swing back to their relaxed configuration, and the muscle fiber is ready for the next contraction.

Relaxation/Contraction Morphology

The previously described events represent the *sliding filament hypothesis* of muscle contraction. These events coincide with the morphology of the sarcomere as observed with the light and electron microscope. The ultrastructure of the sarcomere is schematically presented in Figure 13.17. At rest, the sarcomere appears as described previously with the ultrastructure.

The I band, consisting of actin thin filaments, is the light-staining region of the sarcomere. It is divided in half by the Z line. The A band, consisting of myosin thick filaments and actin thin filaments, is the dark-staining region of the sarcomere. Because the actin thin filaments do not extend through the entire width of the A

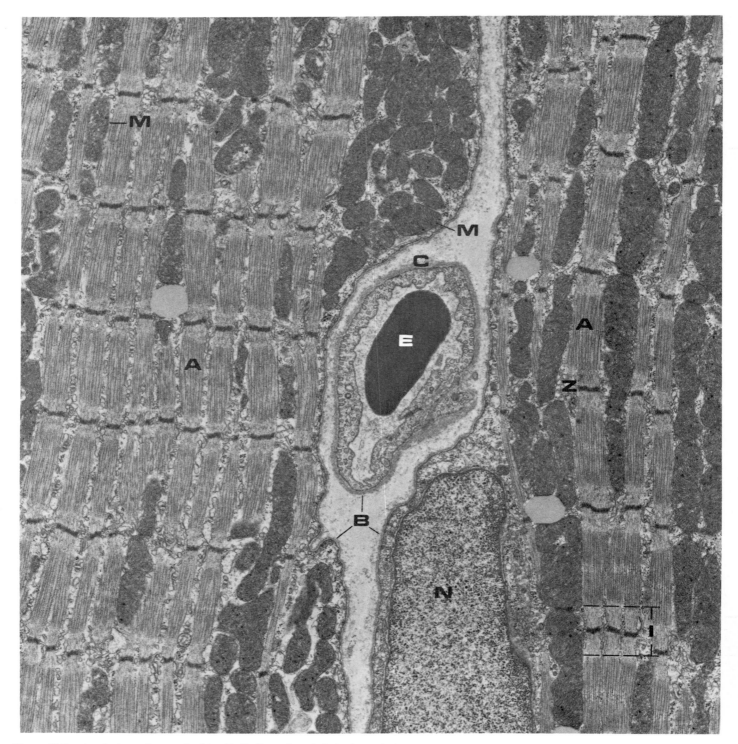

Figure 13.9.   An electron micrograph of longitudinally sectioned skeletal muscle from the extrinsic eye muscles of a slow loris. Two muscle fibers are separated by the endomyseal connective tissue space, which is bounded by a basal lamina (B). The connective tissue space contains a capillary (C) with an erythrocyte (E). Caveolae and pinocytotic vesicles are contained within the endothelial cell of the capillary. The A bands (A) or anisotropic bands are darker than the I bands (I) or isotropic bands. Z lines (Z) occur in the middle of the I bands. Mitochondria (M) occur between the myofibrils and beneath the sarcolemma (subsarcolemmal). A nucleus (N) of one muscle fiber is included in the section. ×14,600. (Courtesy D. E. Kelly and included with permission from Copenhaver, W. M., Kelly, D. E. and Wood, R. L.: *Bailey's Textbook of Histology*, Williams & Wilkins, Baltimore, 1978.)

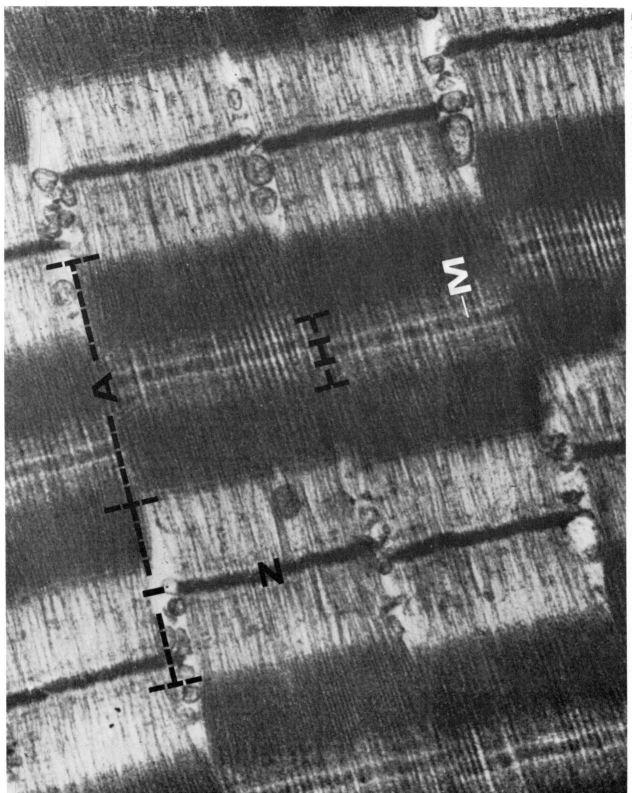

Figure 13.10. An electron micrograph of myofibrils from the psoas muscle of a rabbit. The dark A bands (*A*) contain a lighter H band (*H*). An M line (*M*) bisects the H band. The light I bands (I) contain a dark Z line (Z). ×52,000. (Reprinted with permission from: Copenhaver, W. M., Kelly, D. E. and Wood, R. L.: *Bailey's Textbook of Histology*, Williams & Wilkins, Baltimore, 1978.)

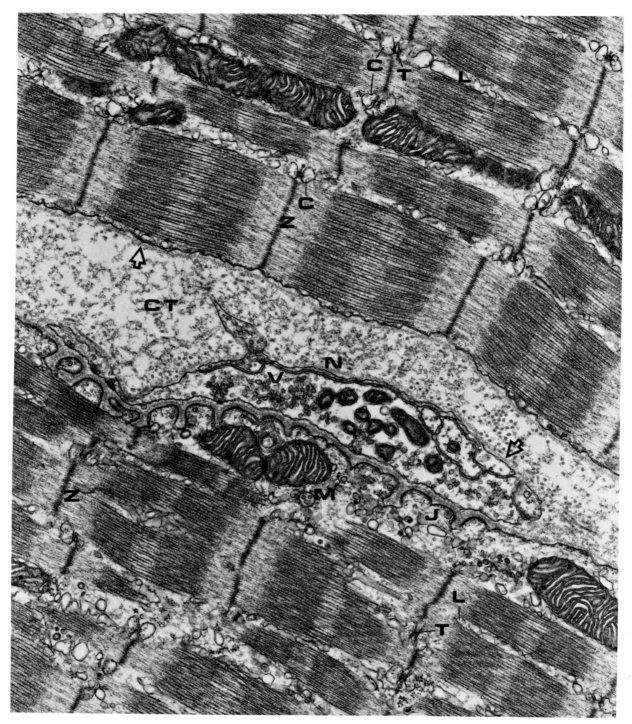

Figure 13.11. An electron micrograph of longitudinal sections through two fibers of amphibian skeletal muscle. The longitudinally oriented *(L)* and terminal cisterns *(C)* of the sarcoplasmic reticulum extend between the myofibrils. The terminal cisterns and transverse tubules *(T)* form triads at the level of the Z line *(Z)*. Mitochondria *(M)* occur in subsarcolemmal and interfibrillar positions. A nerve ending *(N)* forms a neuromuscular complex with the muscle cell. Note the clear (ACH-containing) presynaptic vesicles *(V)* within the neuronal ending and the junctional folds *(J)* of the sarcolemma. The plasmalemma of the muscle cells and axonal terminal are covered by a basal or external lamina *(open arrows)*. The connective tissue *(CT)* between the muscle fibers contains collagen in longitudinal and cross section. ×26,000. (Courtesy D. E. Kelly and included with permission from Copenhaver, W. M., Kelly, D. E. and Wood, R. L.: *Bailey's Textbook of Histology*, Williams & Wilkins, Baltimore, 1978.)

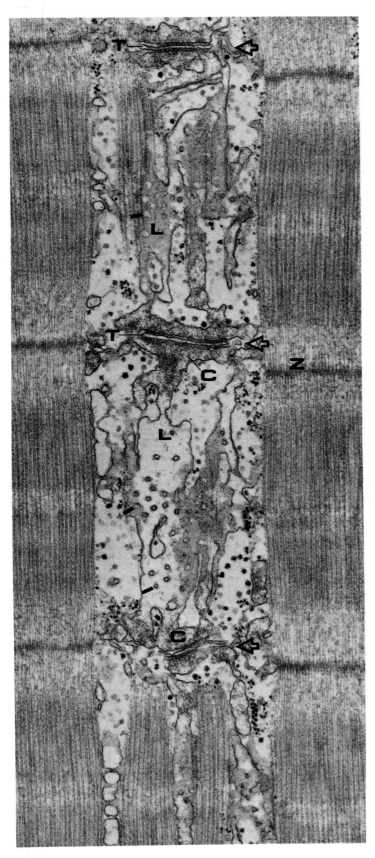

Figure 13.12.   An electron micrograph of a longitudinal section of amphibian skeletal muscle. The triads *(open arrows)* occur at the level of Z lines *(Z)*. The membranes of the longitudinal components *(L)* of the sarcoplasmic reticulum contain numerous perforations *(bars)*. Longitudinal components terminate as dilated cisterns *(C)* in association with transverse tubules *(T)*. Two cisterns and a transverse tubule comprise a triad. Three triads are evident in this section. Dark-staining glycogen granules are scattered throughout the cytoplasm. ×34,000. (Courtesy D. E. Kelly and included with permission from: Copenhaver, W. M., Kelly, D. E. and Wood, R. L.: *Bailey's Textbook of Histology*, Williams & Wilkins, Baltimore, 1978.)

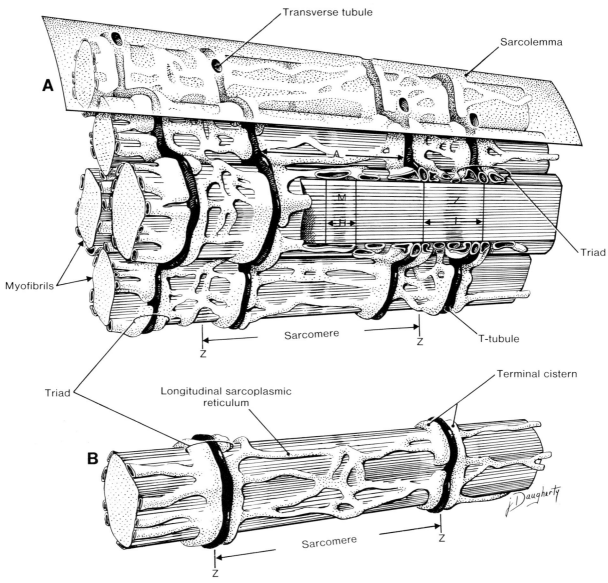

Figure 13.13. A diagrammatic three-dimensional drawing to demonstrate the retaionships of myofibrils, sarcoplasmic reticulum, and T tubules in mammalian skeletal and cardiac muscle. *A*, skeletal muscle; *B*, cardiac muscle. The triads of mammalian skeletal muscle occur at the A/I junctions; thus, two triads characterize each sarcomere. The triads of cardiac muscle and amphibian skeletal muscle occur at the Z lines *(Z)*. The T tubules are invaginations of the sarcolemma that surround the myofibrils at specific locations in association with the terminal cisterns of the sarcoplasmic reticulum. (Redrawn and modified from Peachey.)

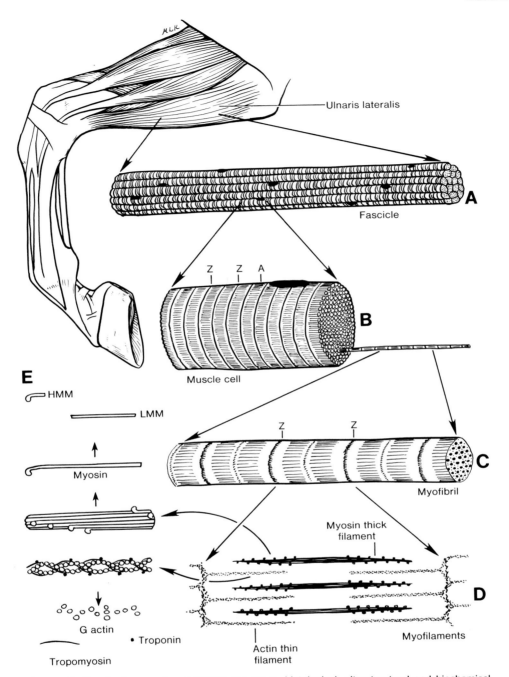

Figure 13.14. A diagram demonstrating the gross, histological, ultrastructural and biochemical relationships of skeletal muscle. The equine thoracic limb demonstrates the gross relationships. Low magnification examination of a muscle fascicle with a light microscope reveals elongated striated cells *(A)*. High magnification light microscopy *(B)* demonstrates Z lines, A bands, and I bands. The examination of myofibrils with the electron microscope (*C* and *D*) reveals the intimate relationships between myofilaments of the sarcomere. Biochemical analyses *(E)* have been used to characterize the thin and thick myofilaments. (Redrawn and modified from Bloom, W. and Fawcett, D. W.: *A Textbook of Histology*, 9th edition, W. B. Saunders, Philadelphia, 1968.)

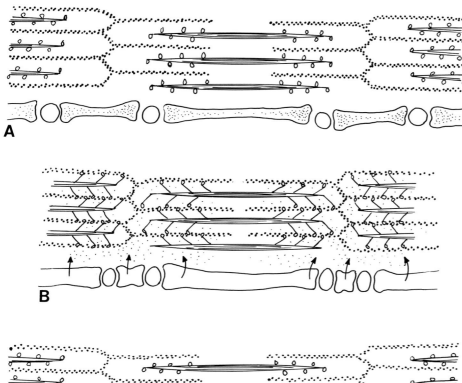

A

B

C

Figure 13.15. Calcium and the contractile mechanism. During relaxation *(A)*, calcium is stored in the sarcoplasmic reticulum. The wave of depolarization moves along the sarcolemma and probably alters the membrane potential of the transverse tubules. The altered membrane potential presumably induces a change in the sarcoplasmic reticulum that permits the movement of calcium into the cytoplasm *(B)*. The inhibition is removed and the globular heads of myosin contact the G actin monomers. The return to the resting state *(C)* is achieved upon return of calcium to the sarcoplasmic reticular profiles.

three types of muscle fibers are identifiable (Fig. 13.18):**type I—slow-twitch, oxidative; type IIa—fast-twitch, oxidative-glycolytic; type IIb—fast-twitch, glycolytic**

Red muscle consists predominantly of type I fibers. These muscles have slow contraction cycles and use aerobic metabolic mechanisms in which glucose and fatty acids are the primary energy sources. White muscle consists of type II fibers. These muscles have fast contraction cycles and use aerobic metabolic mechanisms in which glucose is the primary source of energy. Muscles consist of characteristic mosaic patterns of these fiber types. Specific distribution patterns in specific muscles of different animals and individuals are functional adaptations to diverse behavior.

Type I muscle fibers are small muscle cells that have numerous mitochondria and an abundance of the pigment *myoglobin*. The respiratory pigments (cytochrome system) of the mitochondria and the myoglobin impart the red color. The extensive mitochondria with their numerous cristae occupy interfibrillar and subsarcolemmal positions. Sarcoplasmic reticular profiles, especially in the region of the H band, are more complex than described previously. Also, Z lines are thick. An extensive capillary bed surrounds these muscle fibers. The transport of oxygen from the capillary bed to the cytochrome system of the mitochondria is facilitated by myoglobin, which has a high affinity for oxygen. Prolongation of contraction and relaxation times means that these types of fibers are not fatigued easily. Storage of oxygen by myoglobin may preclude fatigue.

Type II muscle fibers are large muscle cells that have small amounts of myoglobin and minimal mitochondria. Sarcoplasmic reticular profiles are simple and Z lines are thin. The scant amount of myoglobin requires that oxygen is transferred directily from the capillary bed to the few mitochondria. Type IIa fibers are fast contracting and fatigue-resistant; whereas, type IIb fibers are fast contracting and easily fatigued. Lactic acid accumulates readily.

Functional Correlates

The contractile mechanism is dependent upon ATP as a source of energy. The hydrolysis of ATP results in the formation of ADP and inorganic phosphate with the release of energy. Unfortunately, there is an insufficient supply of ATP in a muscle cell to sustain contraction for a long time. Most muscle cells have a storage of ATP that would last less than 1 second. Active and continual contraction requires that ATP be replenished rapidly. This occurs through glycolysis and the tricarboxylic acid cycle. Additionally, muscle fibers have developed a backup and storage system that replenishes ATP rapidly. This system uti-

band, a light-staining H band is apparent in the middle of the A band.

The morphology of the contracted state depends upon the degree of contraction. As muscles contract they become shorter and wider than their resting length and width. Commensurate changes are noted in the sarcomere. The I bands decrease in length and are eventually obliterated when 50% contraction is achieved. The H band changes proportionally with the I band alterations. Although the A band does not change length during normal contraction cycles, an M line may appear as actin filaments slide past the myosin filaments and overlap or interact in the center of the A band. During extremes in contraction, a *contraction zone* may appear adjacent to the Z line. This may represent an overlap of myosin thick filaments at the Z line.

When muscle is stretched, the length of the A band remains constant, while the I band and H band length is increased.

Types of Muscle Fibers

Grossly, skeletal muscle is not a homogeneous mass of muscle fibers. Obvious coloration differences are apparent between species and among individual muscles within the same species. These coloration differences range from a deep red through an intermediate shade to a pale color. The two extremes are termed red and white muscle. The hindlimb, red muscles may be contrasted with the white, pectoral muscles of the domestic fowl. Further studies have correlated specific histochemical and ultrastructural characteristics with different physiological properties of these muscle types.

Based upon metabolic characteristics demonstrable with histochemical techniques,

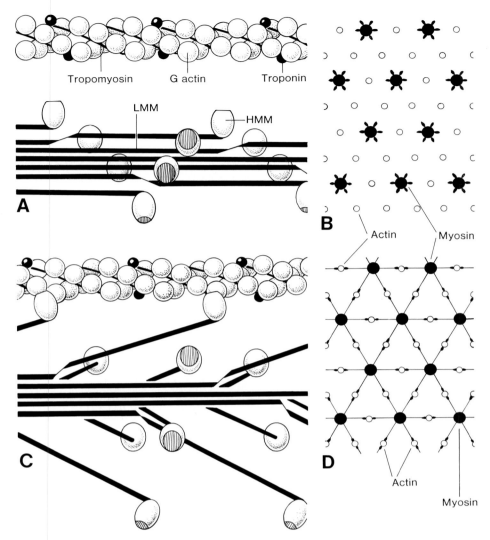

A

B

C

D

Tropomyosin   G actin   Troponin

LMM   HMM

Actin   Myosin

Actin

Myosin

Figure 13.16. A diagram of the relationships between actin and myosin during relaxation and contraction. The globular heads radiate around the myosin thick filament in close association with the actin thin filaments (A). Cross sections (B) through myofilaments reveals that six actin thin filaments surround each myosin, but actin thin filaments are shared by adjacent myosin thick filaments. Upon contraction (C), the globular heads swing laterally and contact G actin monomers. Each actin thin filament is contacted by two globular heads (D). The scales between the longitudinal (A,C) and cross-sectional (B, D) representations are not equal. (Redrawn and modified from Ham, A. W.: *Histology*, 7th edition, J. B. Lippincott, Philadelphia, 1974.)

aerobic conditions. This results in a diminished supply of ATP, an inadequate charging of the creatine and the accumulation of lactic acid. The accumulation of lactate involves an *oxygen debt* that must be satisfied during its metabolism back to pyruvate. Lactate leaks from the cell and causes a localized vasoconstriction that exacerbates the problems. Lactate is carried in the blood to the liver where it is metabolized. The local accumulation of lactate accounts partially for the muscular soreness associated with strenuous exercise. Lactate is converted back to pyruvate within the muscle as the oxygen supply relative to contractile activity is increased.

The energy for muscular contraction is generated by the degradation and metabolism of glycogen stores in the muscle cells. Aerobic respiration is the most efficient energy-generating process and is the source of energy for protracted muscular activity. Such events are dependent upon good glycogen stores and an increased ability for oxygen consumption. The lactic acid system, anaerobic respiration, is the source of energy for short, demanding periods of muscular activity. Because the CP-ATP system is depleted rapidly, these other sources of energy are essential for the types of activities described.

Besides serving as the source of energy for contraction, ATP is required for the movement of calcium from the sarcoplasm into the sarcoplasmic reticulum. Depletion of ATP results in the accumulation of calcium and the inability of the myosin globular heads to release from the G actin. This contraction after the cessation of stimulation may account for *muscle cramps* as well as *rigor mortis*.

A reduction of blood calcium is associated classically with a *hypocalcemic tetany*. Despite the depletion of extracellular calcium, muscle cells do not readily lose their intracellular calcium. Hypocalcemia results in a hyperexcitability of motor nerve fibers and muscle cells that results in the tetanic stimulation and response of the muscle fibers. Hypocalcemic tetany usually occurs as a sequel to acute calcium loss. Canine *eclampsia*, hypocalcemic tetany in the postpartum lactating female, is a classic example. Tetany, however, is not always a sequel to acute calcium loss. *Bovine milk fever, post parturient paresis,* is a hypocalcemic condition characterized by a flaccid paralysis rather than tetany.

Skeletal muscle fibers are adaptive morphologically to the functional demands made upon them. Increased use results in an increased gross muscle size. The increased muscle mass results from the *hypertrophy* of individual muscle fibers. Cytoplasm and the amount of contractile proteins increase. Hypertrophy results from an increased number of myofibrils, not an increase in myofibrillar thickness. A thick-

lizes a *phosphagen, creatine phosphate (CP, phosphocreatine)* that functions to store phosphate bond energy (Fig. 13.19).

During periods of low demand, ATP reacts with *creatine* to form creatine phosphate. The ratio of CP:ATP is approximately 30:1. The ATP for the production of CP is derived from the metabolism of glucose through glycolytic and tricarboxylic acid pathways. The tricarboxylic acid cycle is 19 times more efficient in the production of ATP than is glycolysis.

During periods of exercise, ATP is degraded constantly to ADP, whereas CP constantly rephosphorylates ADP and makes more ATP available for contraction. This phosphorylation is catalyzed by the enzyme *creatine phosphokinase (CPK)*. As long as an adequate oxygen supply is maintained to muscle during exercise, the high ATP yield from aerobic metabolism and the tricarboxylic acid cycle continuously charges the creatine and forms CP. The CP is the most readily available reserve source of ATP.

During strenuous exercise, the oxygen supply is inadequate to drive the tricarboxylic acid cycle. Muscle metabolism then switches to anaerobic respiratory mechanisms. Pyruvic acid is converted to lactic acid instead of being metabolized to carbon dioxide and acetylcoenzyme A as it is under

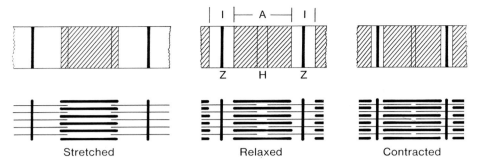

Stretched   Relaxed   Contracted

Figure 13.17. A diagram showing the sarcomeric banding and relationships of the myofilaments during three different physiological conditions. Refer to the text for a complete description of these relationships.

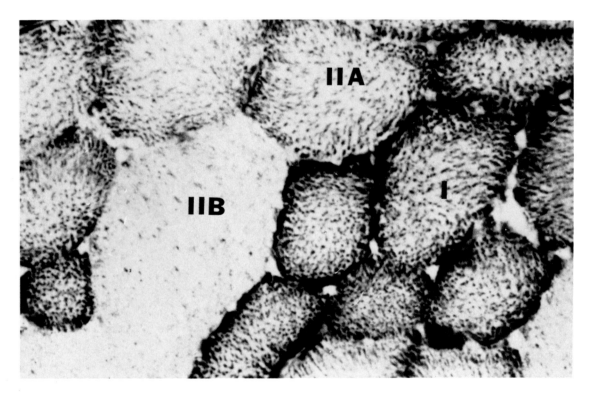

Figure 13.18. Muscle fibers stained histochemically for mitochondrial NAD-reductase. The biopsy sample was obtained from the middle gluteal muscle of a Quarter Horse mare. *I*, slow-twitch, oxidative, fatigue resistant; *IIA*, fast-twitch, oxidative-glycolytic, fatigue resistant; *IIB*, fast-twitch, glycolytic, fatigue easily. ×16 (Courtesy of T. Spurgeon.)

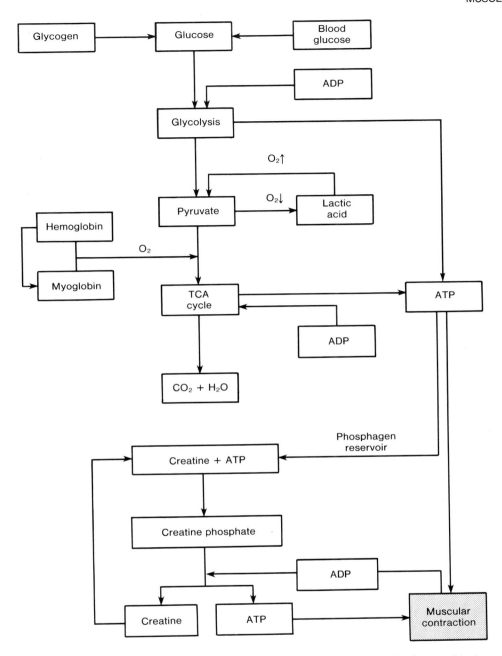

Figure 13.19. Energy sources and muscle contraction. Muscle metabolism is discussed in the text.

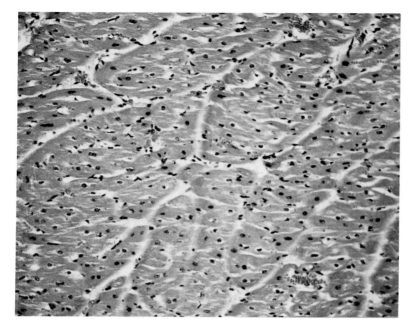

Figure 13.20. Section of cardiac muscle. The branched fibers contain nuclei located in the center of the sarcoplasm. ×40.

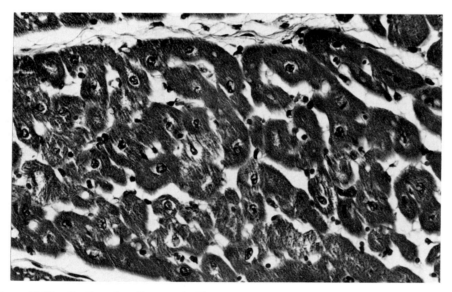

Figure 13.21. Section of cardiac muscle. The central location of the nuclei and perinuclear halos are prominent features of the branched muscle fibers. ×100.

is involuntary. Only those features characteristic of cardiac muscle are presented. If a specific characteristic is omitted, the student is to assume that it is similar to skeletal muscle.

Six morphological features of cardiac muscle are distinctive aids in identification. The cardiac muscle fibers are branched (Plates V.5 and V.6). In any given section of cardiac muscle, longitudinally, transversely, and obliquely sectioned fibers may be observed (Fig. 13.20). The connective tissue surrounding each muscle fiber is prominent in cardiac muscle.

The nucleus of a cardiac muscle cell is centrally located and surrounded by a pale-staining cytoplasmic region—a *perinuclear halo* (Fig. 13.21). The sarcoplasm contains myofilaments that are arranged in a manner described previously. Bundles of myofilaments, however, reflect the branching of the muscle fibers. Moreover, the striations that are readily apparent in skeletal muscle are not as prominent in cardiac muscle. Distinct, transversely oriented, dark-staining bands are scattered throughout the cardiac muscle. These *intercalated discs* are points of end-to-end contact between contiguous muscle fibers. They appear as stepwise striations in the muscle mass (Fig. 13.22).

Ultrastructural Features

The ultrastructural features of cardiac muscle cells are similar to those described for skeletal muscle (Fig. 13.23). Only the significant differences are discussed herein. The *intercalated disks*, as points of contact and adhesion between adjacent cardiac muscle cells, are composed of various types of junctional complexes between terminal Z lines (Fig. 13.24). These complexes include *desmosomes, gap junctions*, and *fasciae adherentes*. Focal areas of dense filamentous materials are the attachment points of actin filaments to the sarcolemma. These regions are the fasciae adherentes (singular, fascia adherens), which are similar to the zonula adherens of epithelial tissues. The fasciae adherentes are irregular and discontinuous regions rather than distinct belt-like zones that characterize zonula adherens. The desmosomes are typical and serve as points of adhesion between cells. The laterally oriented cellular interfaces consist of gap junctions or nexi. Nexi are points of low electrical resistance that couple the cells together electrically. The fasciae adherentes couple the cells together mechanically.

The *sarcoplasmic reticulum* consists of longitudinally oriented and highly anastomotic profiles. Although terminal cisterns are absent, sarcoplasmic reticular profiles make intimate contact with *transverse tubules (T tubules)* as diadic structures. These *diads* generally occur at the level of Z lines. T tubules are larger than their counterparts

ness limit probably exists beyond which functional efficiency is lost. Myofibrils are known to split during the growth process.

Disuse of a muscle or group of muscles results in *atrophy*. Atrophy is a decreased size of individual fibers and a loss of contractile protein. The atrophy of disuse may result from confinement, immobilization associated with fracture repair, or loss of motor nerve input. Because muscular contraction is essential to maintain the integrity of skeletal elements with which they are associated, the muscular atrophy resulting from fracture immobilization also re-

sults in a loss of skeletal mass in the local area. Muscular atrophy is also an important clinical sign of neurological diseases involving the *final common pathway (lower motor neuron, α-motor neuron)*. Neuronal stimulation and exercise are essential for the maintenance of muscular mass.

Cardiac Muscle

Histological Structure

This tissue is similar to skeletal muscle. Both are striated; however, cardiac muscle

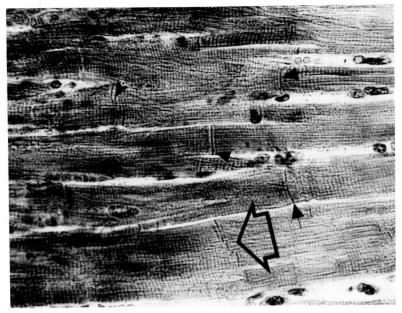

Figure 13.22 Intercalated discs of cardiac muscle. The discs *(solid arrows)*, delimit the end-to-end boundaries of adjacent muscle cells. The intercalated disks may appear as straight boundaries or have a stepwise appearance *(large arrow)*. ×160.

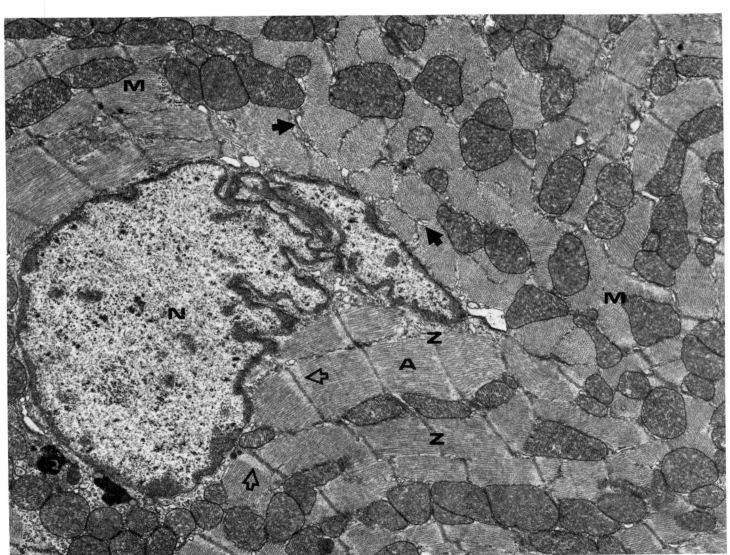

Figure 13.23. An electron micrograph of a cardiac muscle cell. The nucleus *(N)* is surrounded by bundles of myofilaments that are longitudinally and cross-sectioned. Z lines are not registered with each other *(Z)*, and I bands *(open arrows)* are almost obliterated. A bands *(A)* are adjacent to Z lines. Numerous mitochondria *(M)* surround the nucleus and are scattered among the myofibrils. Profiles *(solid arrows)* of the sarcoplasmic reticulum surround the myofibrils. ×11,400.

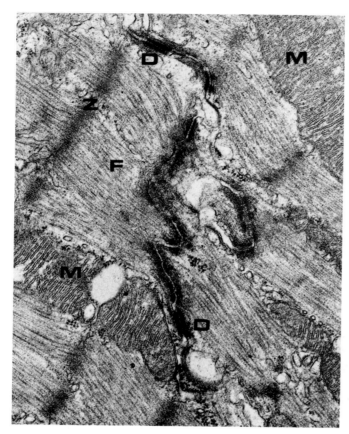

Figure 13.24. An electron micrograph of an intercalated disk. The tortuous path of the disk is apparent. Desmosomes *(D)* are components of the disk. Myofilaments *(F)* extend from Z lines *(Z)* and terminate at the disk. Mitochondria *(M)* are indicated. ×26,000.

in skeletal muscle and contain basal laminar material. Mitochondria occur in greater numbers than in skeletal muscle. Cardiac muscle fibers of the atria contain dense, membrane-bound granules the function of which is yet to be determined. *Atrial granules* do not occur in ventricular muscle cells.

Functional Correlates

The contractile mechanism of cardiac muscle is the same as described for skeletal muscle. The spontaneous and rhythmic contraction of this tissue is an unique functional characteristic, whereas the spread of excitation from one fiber to another is similar to visceral or single unit smooth muscle. The presence of *pacemaker cells* establishes a beat that may be modified by the nerve fibers of the autonomic nervous system.

Cardiac muscle cells have an extensive vascular supply, abundant mitochondria, and large quantities of myoglobin. Hypoxic conditions that lead to anaerobic metabolism cannot support cardiac muscle contraction because of inadequate energy production.

The cardiac muscle cell is capable of hypertrophy, which accounts for its increased size during growth. Hypertrophy is one of the mechanisms by which the heart responds to an increased work load.

Purkinje Fibers

Purkinje fibers are specialized cardiac muscle cells that are modified as impulse-conducting cells (Fig. 13.25). These fibers conduct impulses from the A-V node through the interventricular septum to the ventricles. In cross section the Purkinje fibers are much larger than typical cardiac muscle cells. Also, the Purkinje fibers have an abundant pale-staining, acidophilic sarcoplasm that is rich in glycogen. Myofibrils are few and, when present, are usually located peripherlly. Nuclei are centrally located. In longitudinal section these fibers appear as swollen cardiac muscle cells with scattered myofibrils. These fibers are joined to cardiac muscle cells by intercalated disks.

Repair and Regeneration

Mitotic activity has been noted in smooth muscle cells. This activity appears to be limited and may not be a major factor in repair and regeneration. New smooth muscle cells may be derived from pericapillary mesenchymal cells also. The regenerative powers of smooth muscle are limited; healing occurs primarily through the formation of a connective tissue scar.

The regeneration of damaged skeletal muscle fibers is limited. Healing occurs

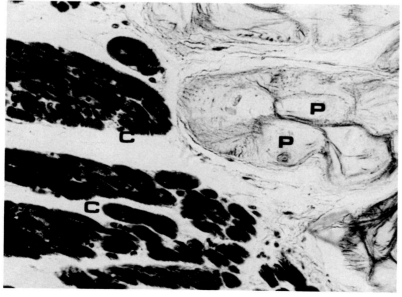

Figure 13.25. Cardiac muscle cells and Purkinje fibers. The Purkinje fibers *(P)* are larger than the cardiac muscle cells *(C)*. ×100 (phosphotungstic acid-hematoxylin (PTAH)).

primarily by scar tissue formation. There are instances, however, during which new skeletal muscle fibers are derived from *myoblasts*. Satellite cells may be myoblasts that have persisted from fetal into adult life. These cells proliferate, fuse, and form typical skeletal muscle cells. The simultaneous formation of scar tissue rarely permits the return to 100% function.

Cardiac muscle cells do not regenerate. Repair is achieved by the formation of scar tissue.

References

Smooth Muscle

Ashton, T. T., Somlyo, A. V. and Somlyo, A. P.: The contractile apparatus of vascular smooth muscle: Intermediate high voltage stereo electron microscopy. J. Mol. Biol. *98:*17, 1975.
Cooke, P.: A filamentous cytoskeleton in vertebrate smooth muscle fibers. J. Cell Biol. *68:*539, 1976.
Kelly, R. E. and Rice, R. V.: Ultrastructural studies on the contractile mechanism of smooth muscle. J. Cell Biol. *42:*683, 1969.
Gabella, G.: Fine structure of smooth muscle. Proc. Trans. Royal Soc. Lond. (Biol) *265:*7, 1973.
Gabella, G. and Blundell, D.: Nexuses between smooth muscle cells of the guinea pig ileum. J. Cell Biol. *82:*239, 1979.
Garamvolgyi, N., Vizi, E. S. and Knoll, J.: The regular occurrence of thick filaments in stretched mammalian smooth muscle. J. Ultrastruct. Res. *34:*135, 1971.
Lane, B. P.: Alterations in cytological detail of intestinal smooth muscle cells in various stages of contraction. J. Cell Biol. *27:*199, 1965.
Small, J. V.: Studies on isolated smooth muscle cells: The contractile apparatus. J. Cell Sci. *24:*327, 1977.
McNutt, N. S. and Weinstein, R. S.: The ultrastructure of the nexus. J. Cell Biol. *47:*666, 1970.
Osvaldo-Decima, L.: Smooth muscle in the ovary of the rat and monkey. J. Ultrastruct. Res. *29:*218, 1970.

Skeletal Muscle

Averill, D. R.: Diseases of the muscle. Vet. Clin. N. A.: *10:*223, 1980.
Braund, K. G., Hoff, E. J. and Richardson, K.: Histochemical identification of fiber types in canine skeletal muscle. Amer. J. Vet. Res. *39:*561, 1978.
Cardinet, G. H., III: Neuromuscular diseases: The diagnosis and classification of muscle diseases in the dog. 4th Kal Kan Symposium, pp 1–10, 1980.
Close, R. I.: Dynamic properties of skeletal muscle. Physiol. Rev. *52:*129, 1972.
Cohen, C.: The protein switch of muscle contraction. Sci. Amer. *233:*36, 1975.
Franzini-Armstrong, C.: The structure of a simple Z line. J. Cell Biol. *58:*630, 1973.
Franzini-Armstrong, C. and Porter, K. R.: The Z disc of skeletal muscle. Z. Zellforsch. *61:*661, 1964.
Granger, B. L. and Lazarides, E.: The existence of an insoluble Z disc scaffold in chicken skeletal muscle. Cell *15:*1253, 1978.
Hanson, J. and Huxley, H. E.: Structural basis of the cross-striations in muscle. Nature *172:*530, 1953.
Huddart, H.: *The Comparative Structure and Function of Muscle.* Pergamon Press, Oxford, 1975.
Huxley, A. F.: Muscular contraction. J. Physiol. (London). *243:*1, 1974.
Huxley, A. F.: The contraction of muscle. Sci. Amer. *199:*67, 1958.
Jones, J. K., Cohen, C., Szent-Gyorgyi, A. G. and Longley, W.: Paramyosin: Molecular length and assembly. Science *163:*1196, 1969.
Knappeis, G. G. and Carlsen, F.: The ultrastructure of the M line in skeletal muscle. J. Cell Biol. *38:*202, 1968.
Peachey, L. D.: The sarcoplasmic reticulum and transverse tubules of the frog's sartorius. J. Cell Biol. *25:*209, 1965.
Shafia, S. A., Gorycki, M., Goldstone, L. and Milhorat, A. T.: The fine structure of fiber types in normal human muscle. Anat. Rec. *156:*283, 1966.
Squire, J. M.: Muscle filament structure and muscle contraction. Ann. Rev. Biophys. Bioeng. *4:*137, 1975.

Cardiac Muscle

Johnson, E. A. and Sommer, J. R.: A strand of cardiac muscle. Its ultrastructure and the electrophysiological implication of its geometry. J. Cell Biol. *33:*103, 1967.
Katz, A. M.: Contractile proteins of the heart. Physiol. Rev. *50:*63, 1970.
Legato, M. J.: Sarcomergenesis in the human myocardium. J. Molec. Cell Cardiol. *1:*425, 1970.
Rhodin, J. A., Missier, P. and Reid, L. C.: The structure of the specialized impulse-conducting system of the steer-heart. Circulation *24:*349, 1961.
Simpson, F. O. and Oertelis, S. J.: Relationship of the sarcoplasmic reticulum to the sarcolemma in sheep cardiac muscle. Nature *189:*758, 1961.
Sommer, J. R. and Waugh, R. A.: The ultrastructure of the mammalian cardiac muscle—with special emphasis on the tubular membrane systems. Am. J. Pathol. *82:*191, 1976.
Spiro, D.: The ultrastructure of heart muscle. Trans. N. Y. Acad. Sci. *24:*879, 1962.

14: Nervous Tissue

General Characteristics

Form and Function. Nervous tissue is distributed throughout the soma and is intimately associated with most tissues. The anatomical unit of nervous tissue is the *neuron*. Neurons are modified for a limited spectrum of comprehensive functions—receive and transmit stimuli. The implementation of these functions is the basis for a complexity of visceral and somatic behavior. Neurons function to receive stimuli from the internal *(interoception)* and external *(exteroception)* environment. Then, they integrate and associate the information. Subsequently, these cells transmit information to the effectors of the body—muscle and glands.

The well-developed cytoplasmic characteristics of *irritability* and *conductivity* suit them uniquely to their tasks. Moreover, their well-developed cellular processes ensure contact with most parts of the body. These processes are the anatomical bases for the transmission of information throughout the soma. Intimate contact between neurons and cellular processes is achieved through functional regions called *synapses*.

Neurons are intimately associated with other cell types called *neuroglia*. **Neurons and neuroglia comprise nervous tissue.** These cells are responsible for the protection, nutrition, and structural integrity of nervous tissue.

Neurons

General Properties

Introduction. Neurons are the genetic, morphological, functional, and trophic units of the nervous system. Although no single description encompasses all neurons, they do have characteristics in common despite the diversity of their three-dimensional morphology. A neuron or *nerve cell* consists of *cell body (cyton, soma)* and a variable number of cellular processes. The cellular processes are the *dendrites* and *axon* (Fig. 14.1). The *perikaryon* is that portion of the cell body surrounding the nucleus.

Development. All of the nervous tissue components, with the possible exception of

microgliocytes, are derivatives of neuroectoderm. Nervous tissue is modified epithelium (Chapter 17).

Classification

The morphological diversity of neurons is manifested in numerous ways (Fig. 14.2). These different morphological features are adaptations to the numerous and diverse functional demands made upon these cells. Neurons may be divided into two general groups—transmission neurons and neurosecretory neurons (Fig. 14.3).

Conducting Neurons. *Transmission (conducting) neurons* comprise the majority of the neuronal types and are those neurons that only secrete neurotransmitters at synapses. Generally, these cells have dendrites, a cell body, and an axon. Various morphological features are used to classify conducting neurons (Fig. 14.4). *Golgi type I* neurons have numerous dendrites and a very long axon. The ventral horn cells of the gray column of the spinal cord (α-motor neurons), the sympathetic and parasympathetic preganglionic neurons, the sympathetic postganglionic neurons and other motor neurons are Golgi type I neurons. *Golgi type II* neurons have numerous dendrites and a short axon. They include interneurons and cells of the cerebral and cerebellar cortex. Golgi type I and II neurons are commonly called *multipolar* neurons, because they have numerous dendritic processes. *Bipolar* neurons have one main dendrite and an axon; the processes are located at opposite poles of the cell body. These cells are confined to regions of special visceral and somatic sensation. *True unipolar* neurons have only an axon and are confined generally in distribution to the developing nervous system. *Pseudounipolar* neurons have an axon and a dendrite that are fused close to the cell body but separate some distance from the cell body. Both processes appear morphologically as axons. These are the typical neurons of the cranial and spinal ganglia. Some neurons such as the amacrine cells of the retina, do not have axons and are referred to as *anaxonic* neurons.

Neurosecretory Neurons. *Neurosecretory neurons* are specialized cells that synthesize *neurosecretory substances*, transport these

products along their axons as Herring bodies and ultimately release these substances into the blood. The intimate relationships of the axonal terminals of these cells to blood vessels are called *neurohemal organs* (Fig. 14.3). Some neurosecretory cells of the hypothalamus secrete *oxytocin* and *antidiuretic hormone* into the capillaries of the neurohypophysis of the pituitary gland. Other neurosecretory cells of the hypothalamus elaborate *releasing factors (releasing hormones)* or *inhibiting factors (inhibiting hormones)* that regulate the secretory activity of the cells of the adenohypophysis of the pituitary gland. (Chapter 25).

Bodian Classification. Classic discussions of the functional relationships of neuronal components invariably include that:

1. the dendrites become stimulated and carry information to the cell body *(afferent)*;
2. the axon then carries information away from the cell body *(efferent)*;
3. this information eventually is transferred to the next element in the series, another neuron or effector organ.

These relationships clearly establish the neuron or chains of neurons as the morphological basis of behavior. (The terms *afferent* and *efferent* are relative terms whose specific meanings are dependent upon naming a site of reference. With the cell body as the reference point, the afferent information is that which flows toward the cell body, whereas efferent information flows away from the cell body. (If neurons A and B were in a chain, the the axonal or efferent informational output from neuron A becomes the afferent informational input to neuron B.)

The relationship of the cell body to these afferent (dendritic) and efferent (axonal) components of neurons is variable. Nevertheless, location of the cell body for specified types of neurons is constant. The specific location of the cell body in relation to the geometric organization is not important when the excitation, conduction, and information transfer functions are considered. According to the *Bodian classification*, the three functionally significant zones are dendritic zone, axonic zone, and

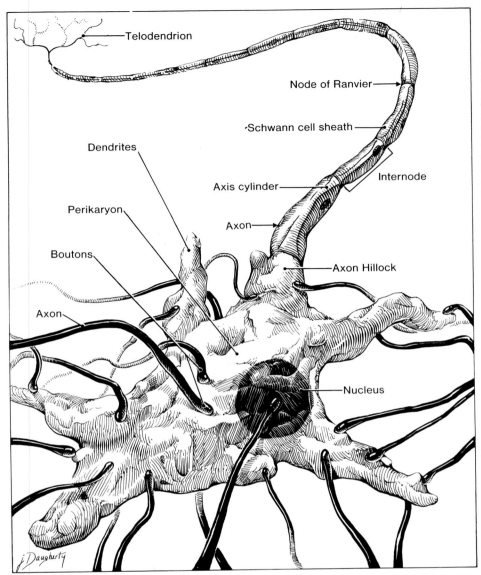

Figure 14.1. Stylized drawing of a neuron. This is an example of a multipolar neuron. The dendrites, cell body, axon, and telodendrion are the conspicuous morphological features. According to the Bodian classification, the dendrites, cell body, and initial segment of the axon comprise the dendritic zone of the neuron. This is the region of the neuron that receives afferent information. The axon carries information away from the dendritic zone. The telodendrion is the site of interaction (point of information transfer) with an effector or another neuron.

philic. The abundant, granular basophilic inclusions are the *Nissl bodies (Nissl substance, tigroid granules)*. They are scattered throughout the perikaryon and the cytoplasm of the dendrites (Fig. 14.7) but are not present in the axon. A clear region, the *axon hillock*, delimits the origin of the axon in the perikaryon (Fig. 14.8). Nissl substance varies in shape, size, and distribution within the neuron. Also, the amount of Nissl substance varies with the functional state of the neuron. Nissl bodies are especially prominent in large neurons such as α-motor neurons. The granules are actually clusters of rough endoplasmic reticulum, free ribosomes, and free polysomes (Fig. 14.9). Neurons renew as much as one-third of their proteins per day. Nissl substance is labile and may dissolve *(chromatolysis)* when the cell body and/or its processes are injured. The dissolution of Nissl substance is accompanied by an increase in smooth endoplasmic reticular profiles, an increased amount of free ribosomes, and polysomes and an increased total cellular RNA content. Although chromatolysis is now considered to be a restorative process, it may still indicate degeneration in some neurons. The restorative aspects of this change are dependent upon the neurons involved, the severity of the injury, and the location of the injury to the cell.

Golgi apparatus functions, however, relate to the formation of lysosomes, the condensation and segregation of cellular products, and the replenishment of the plasmalemma. A neuron is a secretory cell. Most secretory cells have a prominent Golgi apparatus. Secretory vesicles are transported a short distance from the Golgi stack to the apical cell membrane. This region of most secretory cells is specialized for exocytosis. The neuron performs the same activities, but the distances over which secretory vesicles must travel are great. The portion of the neuronal plasma membrane specialized for exocytosis is the presynaptic member or terminal portion of the axon. The presynaptic terminal, then, is homologous to the apical cellular membrane of a typical secretory epithelial cell.

Mitochondria occur in large numbers within the cell body; the organelle is especially prominent in axonal terminals (Fig. 14.9). *Lipofuscin* occurs in nerve cells and may be linked to the high rate of metabolism and organelle turnover that characterize these cells. The lipofuscin pigment is thought to be contained within residual bodies from autophagocytic phenomena. Its presence within these cells is associated with cellular dysfunction. *Neurofilaments* and *neurotubules (microtubules)* are present in the cell body and the cellular processes (Fig. 14.9). Although the plasmalemma is typical morphologically and conforms to the fluid mosaic model, it is not structurally and functionally uniform.

telodendritic zone (Fig. 14.5). The *dendritic zone* is the region of the neuron subjected to excitatory and inhibitory stimulation. It includes the dendrites, cell body, and initial segment of the axon. Impulses impinging upon these surfaces produce graded receptor potentials that propagate passively to the *initial segment (trigger zone)*. This propagation may or may not result in the generation of an action potential. The *axonic zone* includes the initial segment of the axon, axis cylinder and part of the arborizing axonal terminal. It is the all-or-none conducting portion of the neuron. The *telodendritic zone* includes those terminal modifications that permit the trans-

fer of information to the next element in the pathway. Activity in these elements that results from the electrical or chemical activity of the telodendria produces a graded response.

Neuronal Components

Cell Bodies

Structure and Function. The cell body of a neuron varies from 4–135 μm in diameter. A prominent, round, large, vesicular nucleus is usually located centrally. A prominent nucleolus is present also (Fig. 14.6).

The cytoplasm is granular and baso-

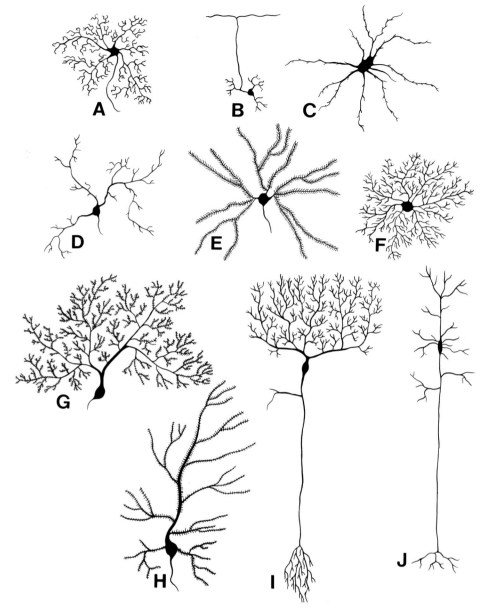

Figure 14.2. A diagram of examples of different neurons that are components of the central nervous system. *A*, neuron of an olivary nucleus; *B*. granule cell of a cerebellar cortex; *C*, neuron from a reticular formation; *D*, large neuron of the spinal nucleus of the trigeminal nerve; *E*, neuron of a basal ganglion; *F*, neuron of a thalamic nucleus; *G*, Purkinje cell of a cerebellar cortex; *H*, pyramidal cell of a cerebral cortex; *I*, Purkinje cell with its long axon and telodendrion; *J*, Pyramidal cell with its long axon and telodendrion. (Redrawn and modified from Truex, R. C. and Carpenter, M. B.: *Human Neuroanatomy.* 5th edition, Williams & Wilkins, Co., Baltimore, 1966.)

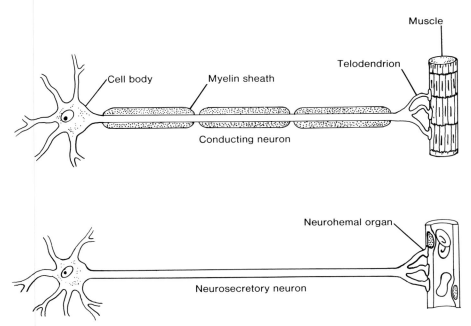

Figure 14.3. A diagram of conducting and neurosecretory neurons. Conducting neurons occur more commonly than neurosecretory neurons. Despite their limited distribution, neurosecretory neurons are important members of the endocrine system.

Dendrites

Structure and Function. The *dendrites* are processes of the cell body that increase surface area. They are like the branches of a tree (Gr.; *dendron*, tree). The dendritic processes are usually shorter than the axon, branch continuously, and gradually taper at the ends (Fig. 14.1). The surface of these processes, as well as that of the cell body, are covered with numerous *spines* or *gemmules* that represent the synaptic connections with *axon terminals* of other nerve cells. The cytoplasmic content of these processes is similar to the cell body. Nissl substance is confined to the proximal portions of the processes, although neurotubules, neurofilaments, and mitochondria are present also. Classically, the dendrites are considered to carry information toward the cell body.

Axons

Structure. The *axon* or *axis cylinder* arises generally from the *axon hillock* region of the perikaryon (Figs. 14.1 and 14.8). This single process has a smooth surface and a uniform diameter. It branches extensively as the *telodendrion* before its termination on an effector. The plasma membrane of the axon is termed the *axolemma*. Although the cell membrane of the axon is typical, it has functional and morphological alterations at various points along its course. The *initial segment* of the axon extends from its point of emergence from the cell body to the point of initiation of myelin. It is the first 50–100 μm of the

axon. Also, the initial segment has a lower threshold of excitation than the dendrites and cell body. Nodes of Ranvier occur along myelinated axons and are foci of discontinuity in the myelin sheath at which points the axons are covered by cytoplasmic processes of the glial cells. The axon may be thicker at nodes of Ranvier. Functionally, the nodes account for *saltatory conduction* of impulses; i.e., the jumping of the wave of depolarization from node to node. Axon terminals are modified in various ways to facilitate information transfer.

Axonal Transport. The cytoplasm of the axon is termed the *axoplasm*. Mitochondria, neurotubules, neurofilaments, and smooth endoplasmic reticular profiles are the conspicuous organelles. Nissl substance does not occur in the axon hillock and axon. Transport problems are manifested in the axon. Materials move constantly away from *(somatofugal)* and to *(somatopetal)* the cell body. Somatofugal movement has been characterized by experimental techniques as *slow axoplasmic flow* and *fast axoplasmic flow*. Most of the materials within the axoplasm moves slowly at rates of 0.5–5.0 mm/day and are believed to involve large molecules utilized in the maintenance, turnover, and repair of the axon. Some materials, however, move very rapidly at rates of 10–200 mm/day. The materials involved in fast axoplasmic flow utilize neurotubules for their transport. These materials are believed to be those involved with the synaptic functions of the axon. Since the cell body is responsive to alterations in its axon, *retrograde (somatopetal) flow* occurs also.

Information Transfer

Focal Sites of Transmission

Electrotonic Transmission

Structure and Function. *Electrotonic transmission* in nervous tissue occurs at specific sites called *ephapses, electrotonic junctions,* or *electrical synapses.* In tissues discussed previously, these sites of electrical transmission between cells (Fig. 13.5) were called *gap junctions (nexi).* The essence of this relationship is the ionic coupling of intimately apposed cellular membranes with minimal intercellular space (Fig. 14.10). Electrical stimulation of cells related in this manner allows the unpolarized spread of excitation by ionic current flow between junctional components. The contributing cell membranes function as a single unit and transmission is achieved rapidly. Ephapses are confined generally to the retina and limited sites within the central nervous system of vertebrates.

Synapses

Structure. *Synapses* are *electrochemical transmission* sites that occur commonly between neurons or neurons and effector cells. The electrical activity of the *presynaptic* nerve cell membrane causes the release of a neurotransmitter substance that traverses the intercellular space and joins to a *receptor site* on the adjacent *postsynaptic* cell membrane. **The union of the neurotransmitter substance with the receptor site results in subsequent events in the adjacent cell that may be excitatory or inhibitory.** The events associated with the release, diffusion, and union of the neurotransmitter substance at the receptor site result in *synaptic delay*.

The following description is applicable to most synapses. Axonal terminations are the *presynaptic* membranous elements, whereas the membranes of adjacent cells are the *postsynaptic* membranous elements. The pre- and postsynaptic membranes are separated by an intercellular space *(synaptic cleft)* that varies in width from 6–20 nm (Fig. 14.11) and contains electron-dense materials and fine filaments. The fine filaments or fibrous materials appear to be attached to the pre- and postsynaptic membranes, projecting from each component like the bristles of a brush. Glycoproteins and glycolipids occur within the cleft. These substances probably are modified materials of the glycocalyx that hold the synaptic members together. Pre- and postsynaptic components can be isolated as discrete units—*synaptosomes*—from disrupted nervous tissue.

This type of morphology typifies a synapse that is described as *directed*. The target area on the postsynaptic member is small but the distance to the target is short. The

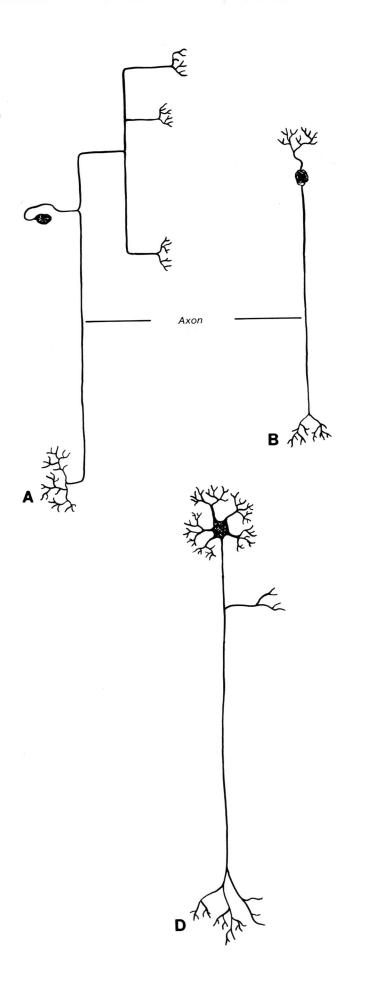

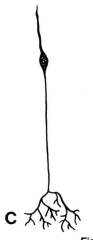

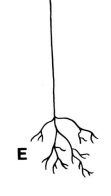

Axon

A

B

C

D

E

Figure 14.4. A diagram of different neurons that are components of the peripheral nervous system. *A*, neuron of a spinal ganglion; *B*, α-motor neuron; *C*, olfactory neuron; *D*, sympathetic ganglion cell; *E*, epithelial receptor and bipolar neuron from the membranous labyrinth of the inner ear. Part of the axon and the telodendrion of the spinal ganglion cell *(A)* occurs within the central nervous system; the remainder of the axon, cell body, and dendritic zone occur within the peripheral nervous system. The α-motor neuronal cell body with associated dendritic zone and part of the axon occurs within the central nervous system; the remainder of the axon and telodendrion occurs within the peripheral nervous system. (Redrawn and modified from Copenhaver, W. M., Kelly, D. E. and Wood, R. L.: *Baileys's Textbook of Histology.* 17th edition, Williams & Wilkins, Baltimore, 1978.)

least directed synapses are those associated with neuroendocrine secretions at neurohemal organs. Adrenergic terminals may be intermediate or *nondirected* in their relationships with effector targets; the localized release of neurotransmitters manifests a widespread influence on effector cells.

Filamentous densities associated with the postsynaptic membrane constitute the *subsynaptic web*. The presynaptic terminal consists of mitochondria, neurofilaments, neurotubules, and *synaptic vesicles*. Cytoplasmic densities may be associated with both the pre- and postsynaptic membranes *(symmetrical synapse)* or either membrane *(asymmetrical synapses)*. Intermediate forms exist also. **Chemical synapses have a distinct morphological presynaptic to postsynaptic polarity that is manifested functionally as a polarized or unidirectional flow of information from the presynaptic membrane to the postsynaptic membrane.**

Appositional Relationships. The presynaptic portion of the axis cylinder expands into bulb-like processes called *end bulbs, end feet, boutons,* or *boutons terminaux* (Fig. 14.12). Enlargements along the course of the axis cylinder are called *boutons en passage.* Boutons en passage occur along the axons of unmyelinated nerves or at nodes of Ranvier of myelinated nerves. Axonal terminals form synapses with various parts of other neurons (Fig. 14.13). The *neuromuscular junction* is a special type of synaptic relationship between neurons and striated muscle. (See Chapter 16.)

Neurochemical Transmission

Presynaptic Components

Neurotransmitters. *Neurotransmitters* are special chemical compounds that link the presynaptic neuron to the postsynaptic neuron or effector organ. Although many compounds have been implicated as being neurotransmitters, only a few qualify on the basis of rigid experimental criteria that must be satisfied. These include *acetycholine, dopamine, norepinephrine, γ-aminobutyric acid, serotonin, histamine, glycine,* and *glutamate.* Despite the diversity of compounds, **a neuron characteristically only uses one neurotransmitter substance to accomplish its functions.**

The presynaptic enlargement contains numerous *synaptic vesicles.* Neurotransmitter substances are contained within or are bound to these vesicles. Upon appropriate presynaptic electrical stimulation, exocytosis occurs. Exocytosis is an indirect consequence of the action potential reaching the axonal terminal. The action potential opens voltage-gated calcium channnels permitting the entry of calcium into the axonal terminal from the surrounding microenvironment. Neurotransmitters are released in discrete, fixed amounts called

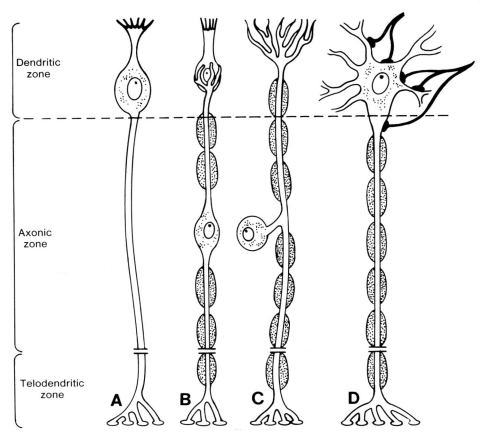

Figure 14.5. A diagram of the zones ascribed to various neurons by the Bodian classification. The position of the cell body varies, but three distinct zones are apparent. The position of the cell body occurs independently of the ability of the neuron to transmit an action potential. The three zones of the classification are indicated. The initial segment, although an anatomical part of the axon, is actually part of the dendritic zone of the cell. *A,* olfactory neuron; *B,* epithelial cell and bipolar neuron of the membranous labyrinth of the inner ear; *C,* dorsal root ganglion cell; *D,* α-motor neuron.

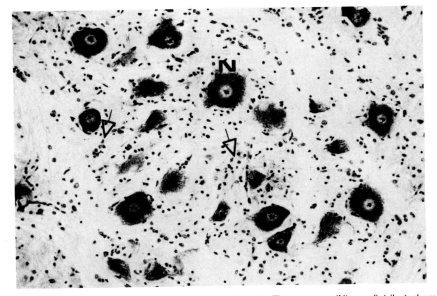

Figure 14.6. Nervous tissue from the brain stem of a pig. The neurons *(N)* are distributed among numerous neuroglial cells *(open arrows).* The cell body at *N* is dark-staining. The round, pale-staining nucleus, with a prominent nucleolus, is located centrally. X40.

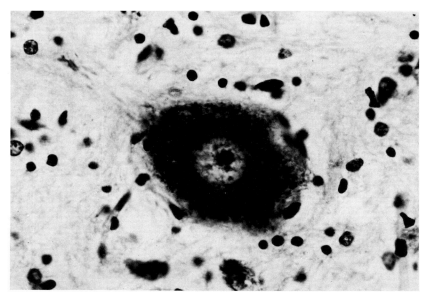

Figure 14.7. Nissl substance of a neuron. The Nissl substance is the dark-staining material within the cytoplasm. The nuclei of cells surrounding the neuron are those of neuroglial cells. Note the size difference between neurons and neuroglial cells. X160.

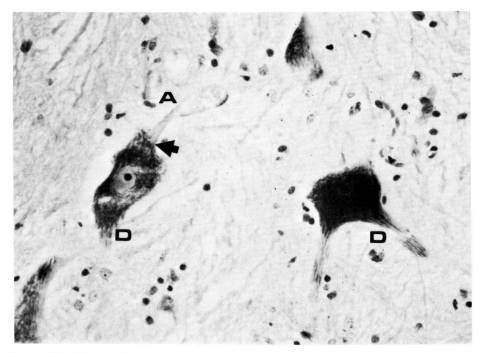

Figure 14.8. Neurons from the brain stem of a dog. The axon hillock *(arrow)*, devoid of Nissl substance, delimits clearly the origin of the axon within the cell body. The initial segment of the axon is an important region for the generation of action potentials. *A,* axon; *D,* dendrites. X100. (Nocht's stain.)

quanta. Each synaptic vesicle, containing several thousand molecules, represents a single quantum. Calcium influx increases the number of quanta released upon stimulation. Calcium may bind to the inside of the presynaptic member at *release* or *active sites* causing a transient binding of vesicles

to the membrane. The vesicles open, release their contents, close and reenter the cytosol.

Two distinct populations of synaptic vesicles are identifiable. *Clear vesicles* occur in those neuronal terminals in which *acetylcholine* is the neurotransmitter. *Dense*

core or *granular vesicles* occur in association with neurons that release *norepinephrine* or other catecholamines.

Cholinergic Terminals. Acetylcholine is synthesized from choline and *acetyl-coenzyme A* (Fig. 14.14). This reaction is catalyzed by *choline acetylase.* The enzyme is active in the neuronal terminal and is a specific marker for cholinergic nerves. Acetylcholine is stored in clear synaptic vesicles in synaptic terminals of cholinergic neruons and is released into the synaptic cleft upon stimulation of the terminal and appropriate entry of calcium. *Acetyl-cholinesterase (true cholinesterase, specific cholinesterase)* occurs in the postsynaptic cell membrane and is responsible for the hydrolysis and subsequent inactivation of this neurotransmitter at cholinergic receptor sites.

Acetylcholine is the neurotransmitter used by the α-motor neurons of the spinal cord and the cranial nerves that innervate skeletal muscle. It is an important neurotransmitter in the autonomic nervous system. Preganglionic sympathetic and parasympathetic neurons are cholinergic; postganglionic parasympathetic neurons are also cholinergic. Acetylcholine is used as a neurotransmitter by various cells of the brain.

Adrenergic Terminals. The synthesis of dopamine, norepinephrine, and epinephrine occurs according to the scheme in Figure 14.15. Some of the synthesis occurs within the dense-core vesicles of *adrenergic neurons.* Phenylalanine or tyrosine enter the metabolic pathway for the synthesis of these *catecholamines.* (Catecholamines are compounds that consist of an o-dihydroxybenzene ring and an akylamine sidechain.) *Tyrosine hydroxylase* is an oxidase that converts tryosine to *L-dihydroxyphenylalanine (L-DOPA).* This is the rate-limiting step in the synthetic process. The L-DOPA is decarboxylated within the cytoplasm to *dopamine.* In noradrenergic nerves, dopamine is converted to *norepinephrine* by *dopamine β-hydoxylase,* an oxidase located within dense-core vesicles. Finally, norepinephrine is converted to *epinephrine* in the adrenal medulla by the activity of *methyl transferase.*

Norepinephrine is the neurotransmitter of the postganglionic nerves of the sympathetic nervous system. Adrenergic nerves are also located within specific foci within the brain stem. Dopaminergic nerves, those that secrete the neurotransmitter dopamine, occur within specific foci in the brain. Sympathetic ganglia also contain *small intensely fluorescent (SIF) cells* that are dopaminergic.

The most important process in terminating the activity of norepinephrine and epinephrine is their reentry into the adrenergic neuronal terminals (Fig.14.16), wherein

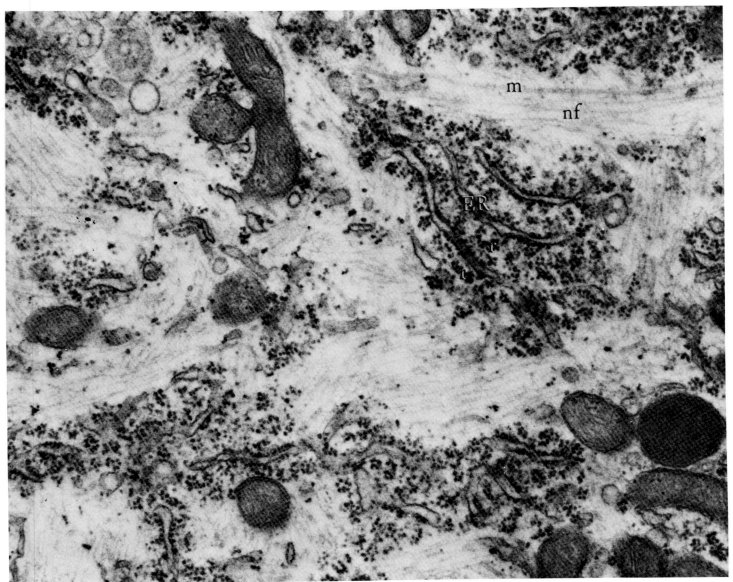

Figure 14.9. An electron micrograph of the cytoplasm of a murine dorsal root ganglion cell. The cytoplasm contains discrete Nissl substance composed of rough endoplasmic reticulum *(ER)* and free ribosomes *(r)* and polysomes. Numerous neurofilaments *(nf)* and microtubules *(m)* are scattered throughout the cytoplasm. X49,000. (Reprinted with permission from Peters, A., Palay, S. L. and Webster, H. F.: *The Fine Structure of the Nervous System: The Neurons and Supporting Cells.* W. B. Saunders, Philadelphia, 1976.)

these substances are oxidized by a mitochondrial enzyme, *monoamine oxidase (MAO)*. The deaminated metabolites enter the blood and are excreted in the urine. The kidney and liver may deactivate norepinephrine and epinephrine also. *Catechol-o-methyl transferase (COMT)* of the kidney, liver, and postsynaptic membrane may assist in the deactivation process by the methylation of these substances. The inactivated metabolites resulting from COMT and MAO activity may be conjugated with glucuronides via the activity of the hepatic enzyme *glucuronyl transferase* and subsequently secreted in the bile.

Postsynaptic Components

Receptors. A *receptor* on or within the postsynaptic membrane is conceived as a molecular structure with which a single neurotransmitter substance reacts. The site may be an enzyme and/or a structural protein component of the membrane. Conformational changes of the receptor protein after its fusion with the neurotransmitter may account for membrane permeability alterations that follow this interaction. The stimulation of a receptor site results in two important postsynaptic events—excitation or inhibition. **Excitation as a result of receptor stimulation is associated with a decreased polarity (hypopolarization) of the postsynaptic membrane.** Chemical gates or channels are associated with the receptor sites. Activation opens these channels and increases the permeability of the membrane to Na^+ and K^+. These events reduce the negativity of the membrane potential due to a net inward flow of positive charges. The alteration in polarity can be measured electrically as an *excitatory postsynaptic potential (EPSP)*. **Inhibition as a result of receptor stimulation is associated with an increased polarity (hyperpolarization) of**

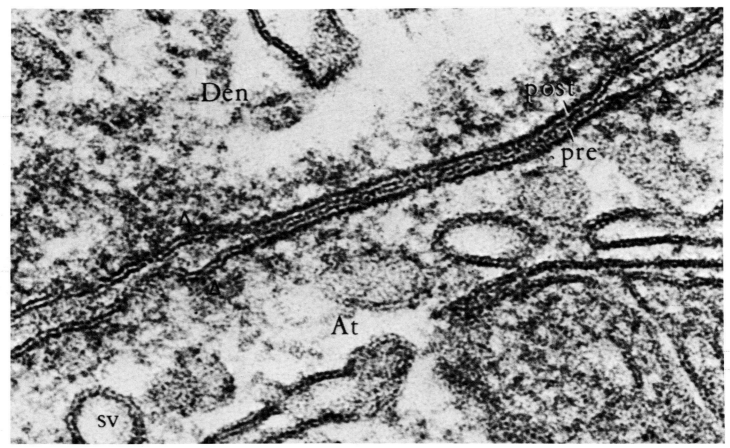

Figure 14.10. An electrical synapse between a mossy fiber *(At)* and a granule cell dendrite *(Den)* within the cerebellum of a viper. Note the intimate juxtaposition of the presynaptic and postsynaptic membranes, that diverge at the margins (△) of the gap junction to form punctate junctions. Synaptic vesicles *(SV)* are present within the mossy fibers also. Although this form of communication between mammalian neurons is not common, this method is important for other cells (epithelia and muscle cells) and some neurons. X305,000. (Reprinted with permission from Peters, A., Palay, S. L. and Webster, H. F.: *The Fine Structure of the Nervous System: The Neurons and Supporting Cells.* W. B. Saunders, Philadelphia, 1976.)

the postsynaptic membrane. This altered polarity is measurable as an *inhibitory postsynaptic potential (IPSP)*. The receptor site functions as a chemical gate in which stimulation results in a flow of chloride ions (in some cases, K$^+$) that increases the negative potential (hyperpolarization) beyond the normal resting potential. **The potential for excitation or inhibition of the postsynaptic membrane resides with the receptor site,** because a given neurotransmitter may elicit excitatory and inhibitory postsynaptic events.

The generation of an EPSP means that the postsynaptic membrane permeability status is more likely to lead to an action potential, whereas the generation of an IPSP means that the permeability status and increased potential is less likely to lead to an action potential. The *spatial* and *temporal summation* of EPSPs and IPSPs generally determine the ultimate response of the postsynaptic element (neurons or effector organs).

Cholinergic Sites. The fusion of acetyl-choline with the receptor sites at a neuro-muscular junction of skeletal muscle results in the influx of sodium ions, the depolarization of the cell membrane above the threshold for action potential generation, and the activation of the cell. In the heart, the fusion of acetycholine with cardiac muscle receptor sites results in an increased potassium permeability, the stabilization of the diastolic membrane potential and the resultant inhibition of the effector organ. The single neurotransmitter, acetycholine, results in two different physiological effects that are the result of different acetylcholine receptors.

Adrenergic Sites. Adrenergic receptor sites are responsive to norepinephrine, the neurotransmitter substance of adrenergic fibers. Also, these adrenergic sites are responsive to the secretion of the adrenal medulla—*epinephrine.* **Norepinephrine manifests local effects, but the effects of epinephrine are manifested throughout the body.** These two substances are classified as *catecholamines.*

On the basis of the differential effects of epinephrine and norepinephrine (and other drugs) upon adrenergic receptor sites, two different receptors are defined. These are α- and β-receptors. Alpha-receptors are stimulated by epinephrine and norepinephrine, whereas β-receptors are affected by epinephrine and to a lesser extent by norepinephrine. Classically, the α-receptors are described as those receptors that mediate acitivation of the postsynaptic element, such as smooth muscle contraction resulting in vasoconstriction. There is one exception—α-receptors are inhibitory to the smooth muscle of the intestines. Alpha-receptors are now subdivided into α_1- and α_2-receptors. Alpha$_1$-receptors are the classical excitatory receptors, except for their effects upon intestinal smooth muscle. The α_2-receptors have been demonstrated on presynaptic components of cholinergic and adrenergic nerves. These receptors inhibit the prejunctional release of acetylcholine and norepinephrine. The placement of α_2-receptors at these prejunctional sites in-

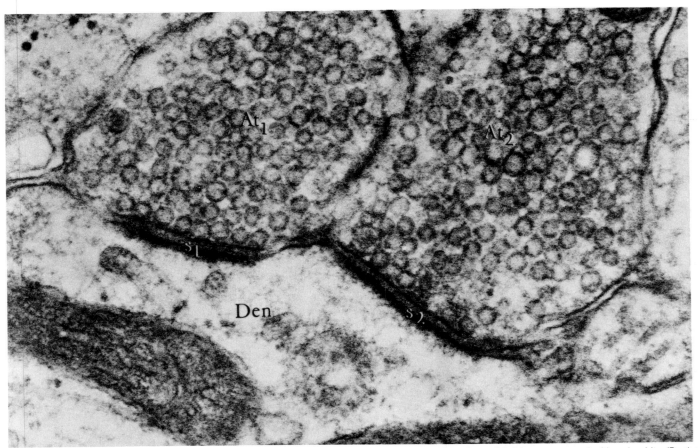

Figure 14.11. Two asymmetrical synapses (S_1 and S_2) of a rat visual cortex. Two axon terminals (At_1 and At_2) have synapsed with a dendrite *(Den)* of a stellate cell. The presynaptic and postsynaptic membranes are separated by a cleft that contains dense intercellular material. The postsynaptic membrane has dense material associated with its cytoplasmic face. Note the numerous vesicles in the axon terminals. X100,000. (Reprinted with permission from Peters, A., Palay, S. L. and Webster, H. F.: *The Fine Structure of the Nervous System: The Neurons and Supporting Cells.* W. B. Saunders, Philadelphia, 1976.)

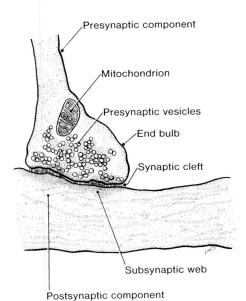

Figure 14.12. Diagram of a synapse. The primary constituents of the synpase are labeled. Synaptic morphology varies.

creases the regulation of neurotransmitter release locally.

Beta-receptors are now divided into two types: β_1- and β_2-receptors. *Beta$_1$-receptors* are stimulatory to the myocardium and inhibit smooth muscle of the intestines. The β_1-receptor stimulation of the heart results in an increased cardiac rate *(positive chronotropy)* and an increased strength of contraction *(positive inotropy)*. *Beta$_2$-receptor* activation is manifested as inhibition of smooth muscle contraction in the bronchioles, vascular beds, and uterus. Beta$_2$-receptors are also located on presynaptic terminals. At these foci, β_2-receptors are stimulatory. Their responsiveness to epinephrine tends to amplify the sympathetic effect achieved by the increased release of norepinephrine from these nondirected synapses.

Current evidence indicates that α- and β-receptors may represent different conformations of a metabolically controlled single molecular entity. Such modulation of receptor structures with its concomitant

functional manifestations would permit the organism to respond to varying physiological and/or pathological conditions. Induced conformational changes may contribute to or result from various disease processes. Additionally, these conformational changes may account for intraspecific and interspecific differences noted upon adrenergic stimulation in domestic animals.

Neuroglia

General Considerations. The development of the central nervous system is characterized by the proliferation of closely juxtaposed cells and the differentiation of these cells into two distinct populations. Both populations, neurons and neuroglia, develop complex geometric patterns. The *neuroglia*, serving as the supportive network or stroma of the nervous system, constitute the "neural glue" that binds neurons together. Besides a supportive function, they also protect, nourish, and perform

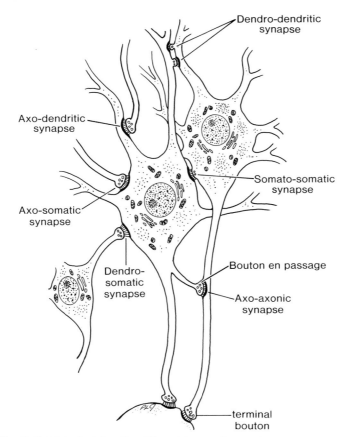

Figure 14.13. A diagram depicting the different types of synaptic patterns. Although all of the synapses are drawn as the asymmetrical type, other patterns exist.

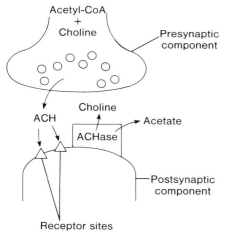

Figure 14.14. A diagram of a cholinergic synapse. After attachment at the receptor sites, acetylcholine *(ACH)* is degraded to acetate and choline by acetylcholinesterase *(ACHase)*. Acetate diffuses into the surrounding tissues, whereas choline is returned to the presynaptic terminal.

other functions vital to the integrity of the neurons.

The neuroglial cells may be subdivided on the basis of their size. The *macroglia* include oligodendrogliocytes, astrocytes, ependyma, amphicytes, Schwann cells, and Müller cells. The *microglia* are the microgliocytes. The neuroglia may be subdivided also on the basis of their association with the central or peripheral nervous systems. The *central glia* includes oligodendrogliocytes, astrocytes, ependyma, Müller cells, and microgliocytes. The *peripheral glia* includes the amphicytes and Schwann cells.

Routine staining techniques are not useful for the demonstration of the cell bodies and cytoplasmic processes of most neuroglial cells (Fig 14.17). The routine identification of the glial elements is based upon nuclear morphology.

Neuropil is a term used to describe the complex, felt-like network in which the nerve cell bodies of the central nervous system are embedded. The neuropil consists of axonal and dendritic processes and neuroglial elements of the gray matter.

Central Glial Elements

Oligodendrogliocytes. *Oligodendrogliocytes* are the most numerous of the neuroglial elements (Fig. 14.18). These cells are characterized by a small, oval or round nucleus that contains a fair amount of heterochromatin. The nucleus, however, may vary from large and pale to small and dark. Generally, this nucleus is smaller and more round than that of the astrocyte. The oligodendrogliocyte contains scant amounts of cytoplasm and few cellular processes. These cells are interdigitated between nerve cell processes and nerve cell bodies. Also, oligodendrogliocytes are intimately associated with the capillaries of the vascular bed. Oligodendrogliocytes, therefore, may be *perineuronal, perivascular,* or *interfascicular.* Perineuronal oligodendrogliocytes may perform some type of nutritional function. In some regions of the feline brain as much as 90% of the surface area of the cell body may be covered by these cells. Oligodendrogliocytes are responsible for myelination of nerve cell processes within the central nervous system.

Astrocytes. *Astrocytes* are the second most frequently encountered neuroglial cells of the central nervous system (Fig. 14.18). Astrocytes or spider cells are divided into two different types, *fibrous* and *protoplasmic.* The latter type has more cytoplasm than the former. The fibrous type is abundant in the white matter and the protoplasmic type is common in the gray matter. Both have a large, round or oval nucleus that is usually pale-staining. Chromatin granules are fine but may be clumped next to the inner nuclear membrane.

Astrocytes are important cells in the structural support of the brain and spinal cord. The processes impart a weave-like texture and supportive framework around the neuronal processes. Astrocytes form the *outer glial limitans.* These cells are responsible for the repair of nervous tissue defects and the formation of central nervous system scars. Astrocytes can become hypertrophic, hyperplastic, and phagocytic. Astrocytes isolate neuronal receptor surfaces by performing an insulating function.

Microgliocytes. *Microgliocytes* are characterized by a scant cytoplasm that contains a small, dark nucleus (Fig. 14.18). The nucleus may be round, indented, or irregularly shaped. The cell body has numerous short processes. These cells may be members of the macrophage system. Microgliocytes seem capable of phagocytosis in response to minor injury. Subsequent to extensive injury, phagocytic cells migrate from blood vessels and accomplish functions ascribed to microgliocytes.

Müller Cells. *Müller cells* are associated with the retina.

Ependyma. *Ependymal cells* line the neural canal (Fig. 14.19). Because of the embryonic origin of the nervous tissue, a tube is formed that is lined with epithelium varying from squamous to columnar. The epithelial lining is retained in the adult

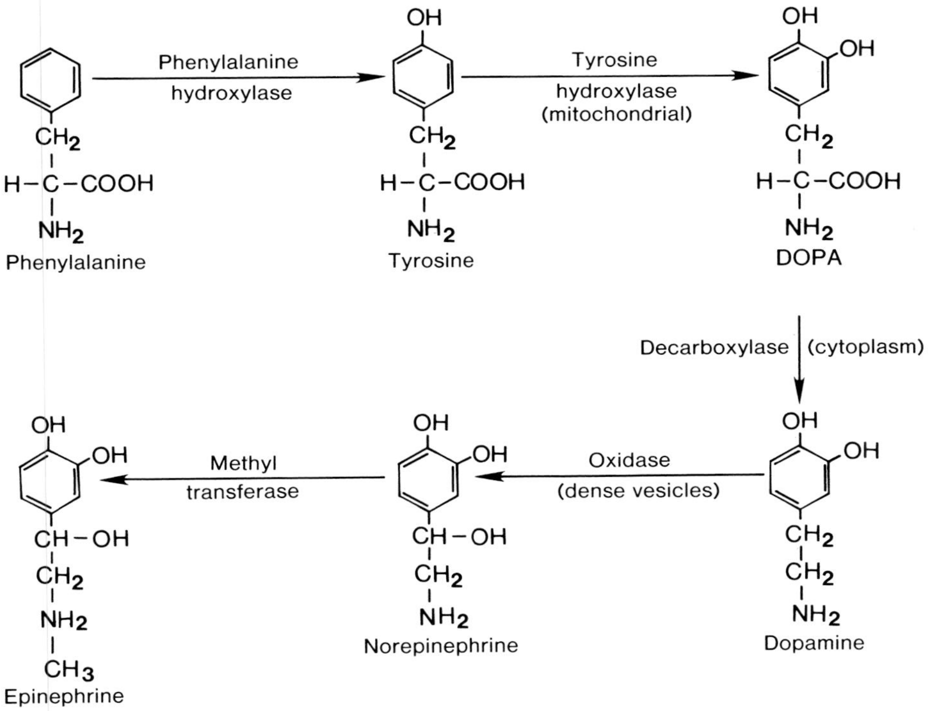

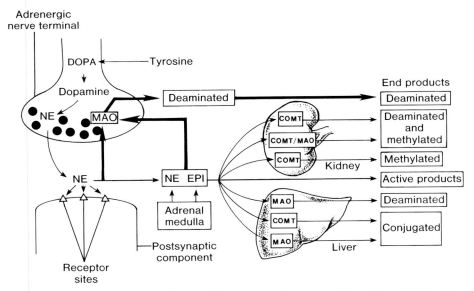

Figure 14.15. The biosynthesis of catecholamines.

Figure 14.16. The secretion and degradation of norepinephrine *(NE)* and epinephrine *(EPI)*. Deaminated, methylated, and conjugated products of epinephrine and norepinephrine are removed from the body by excretion and elimination. The most important inactivation process involves the deamination of the active products by adrenergic nerve terminals.

Ependymal cells contribute to the formation of cerebrospinal fluid. This formative process occurs at scattered sites throughout the ventricular system. The ciliated ependymal cells are responsible for the movement of cerebrospinal fluid within the ventricular system. Nerve endings within the ependymal lining impart a sensory function to this layer of cells. The ependymal cells transport hormones. *Tanycytes* are specific cells of the ependymal lining that occur principally in the walls of the third ventricle. These cells have long, unbranched basal processes extending into the subependymal region. The processes are juxtaposed to subependymal capillaries. Although they seem to serve a structural function, as evidenced by their morphological configuration, they may be involved in transport and/or secretory activities.

The *subependymal organ* or region may be responsible for the replacement of neuroglial cells throughout the life of the organism.

Peripheral Glial Elements

Amphicytes. *Amphicytes (satellite cells, capsule cells)* are neuroglial cells that surround the neurons of ganglia (Fig. 14.21). Amphicytes are probably closely related to oligodendrogliocytes and Schwann cells.

Schwann Cells. *Schwann cells* are associated with nerve cell fibers (Fig. 14.22). They surround these fibers and are responsible for the formation of myelin. These cells, also, are probably closely related to oligodendrogliocytes.

Cellular Investments of Neurons

The neurons of the nervous system are associated intimately with neuroglial cells. Oligodendrogliocytes establish unique relationships with central neurons by virture of myelin sheath formation on nerve cell processes. Schwann cells form similar relationships in the periphery.

Cell Bodies

Ganglion Cell Sheaths. *Ganglion cells* are neurons that are part of the peripheral nervous system. Accumulations of their nerve cell bodies are called *ganglia.* The nerve cell bodies are covered by a layer of cells called *amphicytes* (Fig. 14.21). Amphicytes usually form a continuous covering over sensory ganglion cells; the covering may be incomplete in autonomic (motor) ganglia (Fig. 14.23). Amphicytes terminate at points of Schwann cell initiation. The distinction between amphicytes and Schwann cells may be artificial.

Neuronal Processes

Unmyelinated Nerve Fibers. The Schwann cell is the cellular investment of nerve cell processes. *Unmyelinated fibers*

and is observed as the lining of the central canal of the spinal cord and the four ventricles of the brain (Fig. 14.20). This lining is especially prominent and modified in regions where the *choroid plexuses* are formed. Embryonic ependyma are ciliated cells of a low cuboidal or low columnar configuration. The latter is retained in the adult; islands of cilia may be observed projecting from the brush-like luminal border. These cells have large, pale nuclei with one or more nucleoli. The basal borders, in the adult, reside on a basement membrane and are separated from the nervous tissue. In younger animals, however, the basal modifications are complex and cellular processes may extend through the mantle layer of the developing nervous tissue.

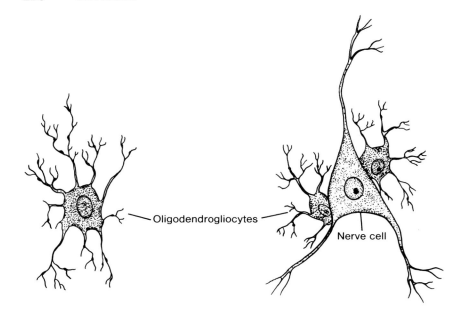

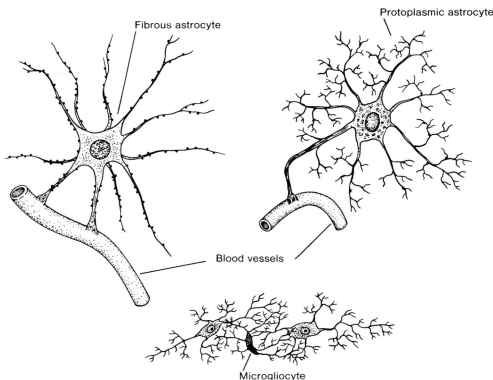

Figure 14.17. A diagram of the morphology of central neuroglial cells as visualized with silver staining techniques. (Redrawn and modified from Copenhaver, W. M., Kelly, D. E. and Wood, R. L.: *Bailey's Textbook of Histology*. 17th edition. Williams & Wilkins Co., Baltimore, 1978.)

Schwann cell can invest many neuronal processes.

Because a single Schwann cell only invests a neuronal process over a limited distance, the neurolemmal sheath is composed of numerous juxtaposed Schwann cells. A basal lamina, located peripheral to the neurolemmal sheath, covers the Schwann cell and separates it from the surrounding connective tissue space (Fig. 14.24). Unmyelinated nerve fibers are small processes with relatively slow impulse conducting speeds.

Myelinated Nerve Fibers. These nerve fibers are the largest and most rapidly conducting fibers in the body. The myelin functions in a manner similar to the insulator on an electrical conductor. The oligodendrogliocytes and the Schwann cells are responsible for the formation of myelin. Although their methods and end products are slightly different, the result is that the nerve fiber is invested with a sheath of myelin.

The *axis cylinder* or neuronal process contains axoplasm and is limited to a cell membrane, the *axolemma* (Fig. 14.22). The space adjacent to the axis cylinder is occupied by the myelin sheath. In routine preparations, however, the removal of lipids seriously alters the appearance of these membranous whorls. All that remains is the nonlipid component of the myelin sheath, *neurokeratin* (Fig. 14.25). Finger-like projections of neurokeratin appear as the spokes of a wheel. The Schwann cells are peripheral to the remnants of the myelin sheath. These cells have a large, vesicular nucleus in which chromatin is clumped peripherally. The cytoplasmic, circumscribing remnants of Schwann cells are referred to as the *neurolemma* or the *sheath of Schwann*.

Breaks in continuity between contiguous Schwann cells are called *nodes of Ranvier* (Fig. 14.26). The nodes appear as constrictions along the nerve fiber at which point the myelin configuration stops, but the processes of the Schwann cell continue to contact the axolemma (Figs. 14.27 and 14.28). Although the myelin sheath stops at the node, the axis cylinder continues through the nodal region uninterruptedly (Fig. 14.29).

The myelin sheath consists of continuous whorls formed by cytoplasmic processes of the neuroglial cell (Figs. 14.24, 14.29 and 14.30). An *inner mesaxon* is formed by juxtaposed cellular processes of the Schwann cell adjacent to the nerve cell processes. An *outer mesaxon* represents the same relationship at the periphery of the myelin. The outer portion of the myelin sheath is covered by the cytoplasm of the neuroglial cell responsible for the myelination. A basal lamina covers the Schwann cell.

(fibers of Remak) are small fibers that are either unmyelinated or are invested only by a trace of myelin. Such fibers are contained within elongated invaginations in the Schwann cell (Fig. 14.24). The fibers, however, are not within the Schwann cell cytoplasm but are covered by the plasma-lemma of the investing cell. Such investments are called *sheaths of Schwann* or *neurolemmal sheaths*. Similarly, Schwann cells are also called *neurolemmal cells*. The juxtaposed plasmalemmal components of the Schwann cell that encircle the axis cylinder are called *mesaxons*. A single

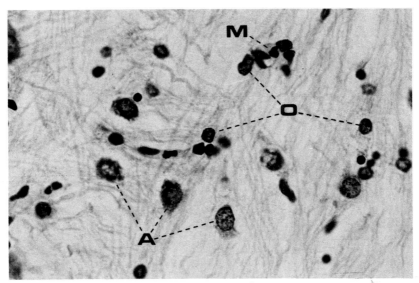

Figure 14.18.   Neurogliocytes from the brain stem of a pig. The oligodendrogliocytes *(O)*, astrocytes *(A)*, and microgliocytes *(M)* are indicated. X160.

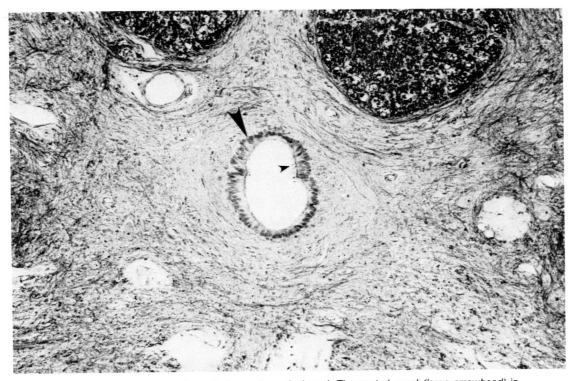

Figure 14.19.   The central canal of a canine spinal cord. The central canal *(large arrowhead)* is lined by columnar cells. Some of the cells are ciliated *(small arrowheads)*. The ependymal lining is intermittently ciliated. X40. (Myelin stain).

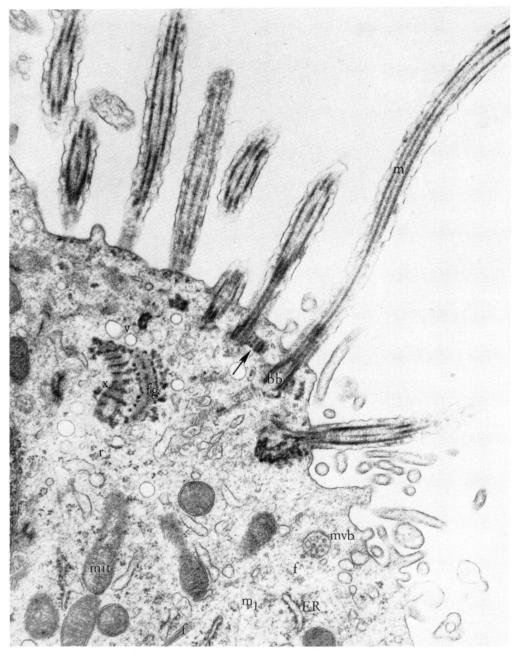

Figure 14.20. An electron micrograph of an ependymal cell from the lining of a murine lateral ventricle. A tuft of cilia contain microtubules *(m)* that originate from a basal body *(bb)*. A basal foot *(arrow)* and ciliary rootlet *(x)* protrude laterally from the basal body. A fibrogranular *(fg)* aggregate is also apparent and may be confused with the ciliary rootlet. Mitochondria *(mit)*, granular endoplasmic reticulum *(ER)*, free ribosomes*(r)*, vesicles *(v)*, microtubules *(m₁)*, filaments *(f)*, and multivesicular bodies *(mvb)* are apparent. (Reprinted with permission from Peters, A., Palay, S. L. and Webster, H. F.: *The Fine Structure of the Nervous System: The Neurons and Supporting Cells.* W. B. Saunders, Philadelphia, 1976.)

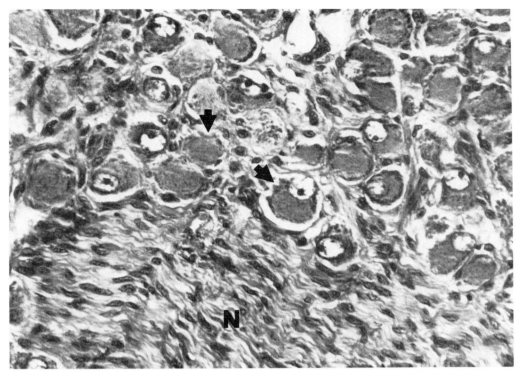

Figure 14.21. Amphicytes and ganglion cells of a dorsal root ganglion of a dog. The amphicytes *(arrows)* surround the ganglion cells. The amphicytes have been separated from the ganglion cells artifactually by processing. N, neuronal processes. X125.

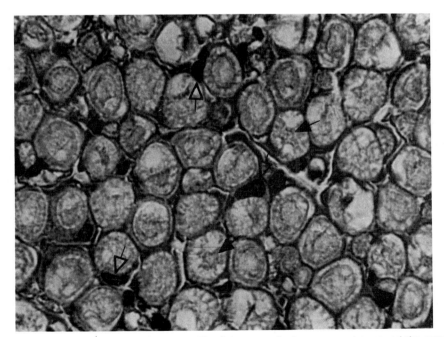

Figure 14.22. A cross section of a nerve. The Schwann cells *(open arrows)* surround the nerve cell processes. The axoplasm *(solid arrows)* is surrounded by the myelin sheath. X160.

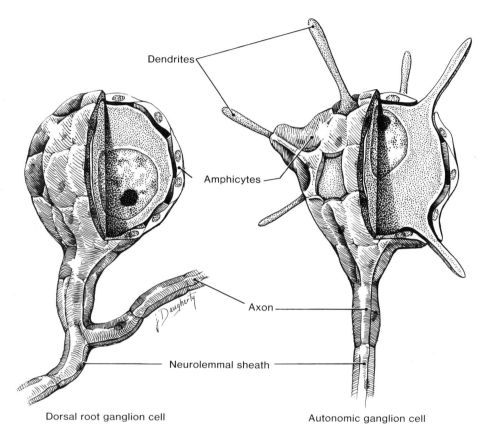

Dendrites

Amphicytes

Axon

Neurolemmal sheath

Dorsal root ganglion cell

Autonomic ganglion cell

Figure 14.23. A diagram of the relationships of amphicytes to different types of ganglion cells. The amphicytes form a complete covering around the ganglion cells of the dorsal root ganglia. The covering may be incomplete in autonomic ganglia. The pseudounipolar neurons of the dorsal roet ganglia only have a single cellular process extending from the cell body. These are sensory cells. The multipolar neurons of the autonomic ganglia have numerous dendrites and a single axon that perforate the amphicytic covering. These ganglion cells are motor neurons.

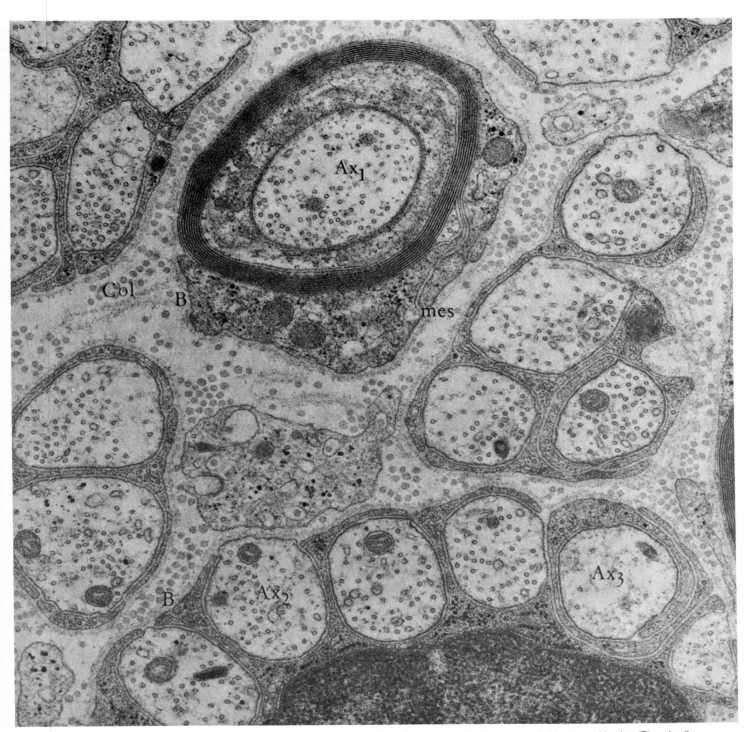

Figure 14.24.   A cross section of the ischiatic nerve of an adult rat. A myelinated nerve fiber *(top)* is surrounded by a basal lamina *(B)* and collagenous fibers *(Col)*. The axon *(Ax₁)* is juxtaposed to the Schwann cell cytoplasm. Note the outer mesaxon *(mes)* and its continuity with the myelin. Other axons are unmyelinated. Note the Schwann cell relationship to *Ax₂*, which is covered incompletely. A finger-like process of the Schwann cell surrounds Ax₃. The collagenous fibers are part of the endoneurium. X48,000. (Reprinted with permission from Peters, A., Palay, S. L. and Webster, H. F.: *The Fine Structure of the Nervous System: The Neurons and Supporting Cells*. W. B. Saunders, Philadelphia, 1976.)

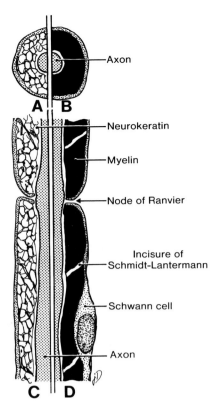

Axon

A | B

Neurokeratin

Myelin

Node of Ranvier

Incisure of
Schmidt-Lantermann

Schwann cell

Axon

C | D

Figure 14.25. A diagram of a sectioned nerve. Sections *C* and *D* are longitudinal sections; *A* and *B*, cross sections. The techniques and stains used to demonstrate the nerve alter appreciably the way it appears in section. The paraffin technique is represented in *A* and *C*. The myelin appears vacuolated, because of protein remnants called neurokeratin. Preservation of the lipids and staining with osmium (*B* and *D*) represents the nerve fiber differently. Compare *A* and *C* with Figures 14.22 and 14.26. Compare *B* and *D* with Figures 14.27 and 14.28. (Redrawn and modified from Bloom, W. and Fawcett, D. W.: *A Textbook of Histology*. 10th edition, W. B. Saunders, Philadelphia, 1975.)

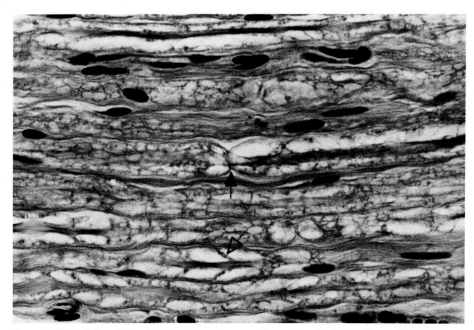

Figure 14.26. A longitudinal section through nerve fibers. A node of Ranvier *(solid arrow)* and a cleft of Schmidt-Lanterman *(open arrows)* are visible. X160.

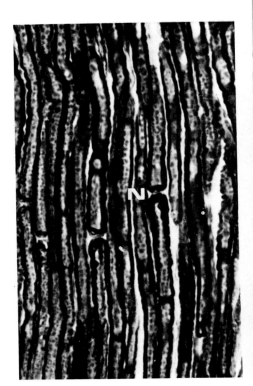

Figure 14.27. A longitudinal section of an ischiatic nerve stained with osmium tetroxide. *N*, node of Ranvier. Compare with Figure 14.26. X100.

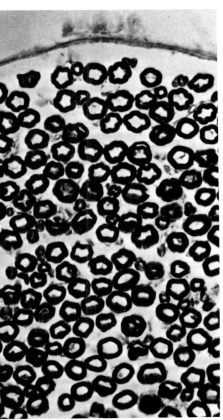

Figure 14.28. A cross section of an ischiatic nerve stained with osmium tetroxide. The axis cylinders are unstained. Compare with Figure 14.24. X100.

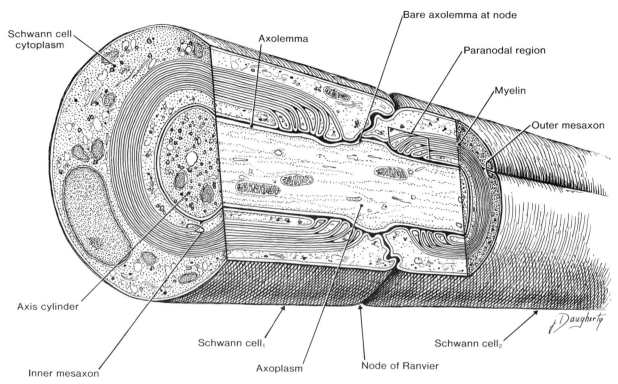

Figure 14.29. A diagrammatic representation of the components of a myelinated nerve cell process. The anatomy depicted typifies the relationships between a Schwann cell and a nerve cell process. The relationships between oligodendrogliocytes and neuronal cell processes are different. (Redrawn and modified from Bloom, W. and Fawcett, D. W.: *A Textbook of Histology*, 10th edition, W. B. Saunders, Philadelphia, 1975.)

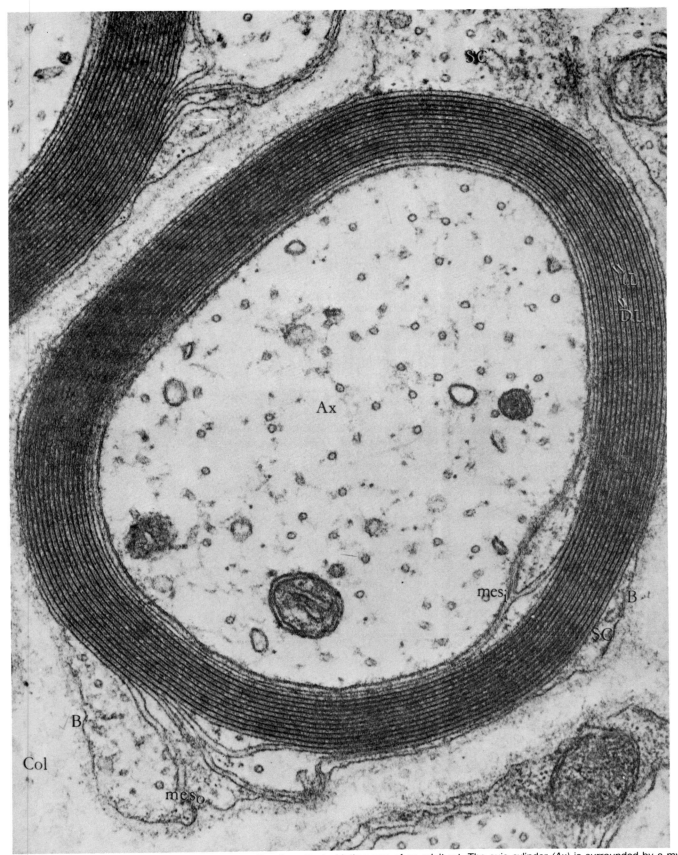

Figure 14.30. A cross section of a myelinated nerve fiber from the ischiatic nerve of an adult rat. The axis cylinder *(Ax)* is surrounded by a myelin sheath composed of spiralled sheets of the Schwann cell plasma membrane. Note the inner mesaxon *(mes$_i$)* and outer mesaxon *(mes$_o$)*. *SC*, Schwann cell; *B*, basal lamina; *Col*, collagenous fibers. Major dense period lines *(DL)* and intraperiod lines *(IL)* are apparent. X100,000. (Reprinted with permission from Peters, A., Palay, S. L. and Webster, H. F.: *The Fine Structure of the Nervous System: The Neurons and Supporting Cells*, 10th edition, W. B. Saunders, Philadelphia, 1976.)

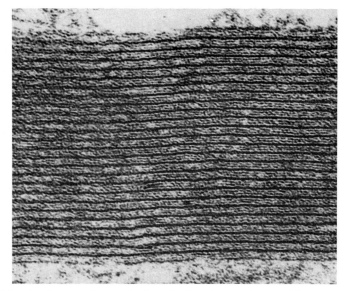

Figure 14.31. An electron micrograph of myelin. The dark, major period lines and light, interperiod lines are visible. X154,000.

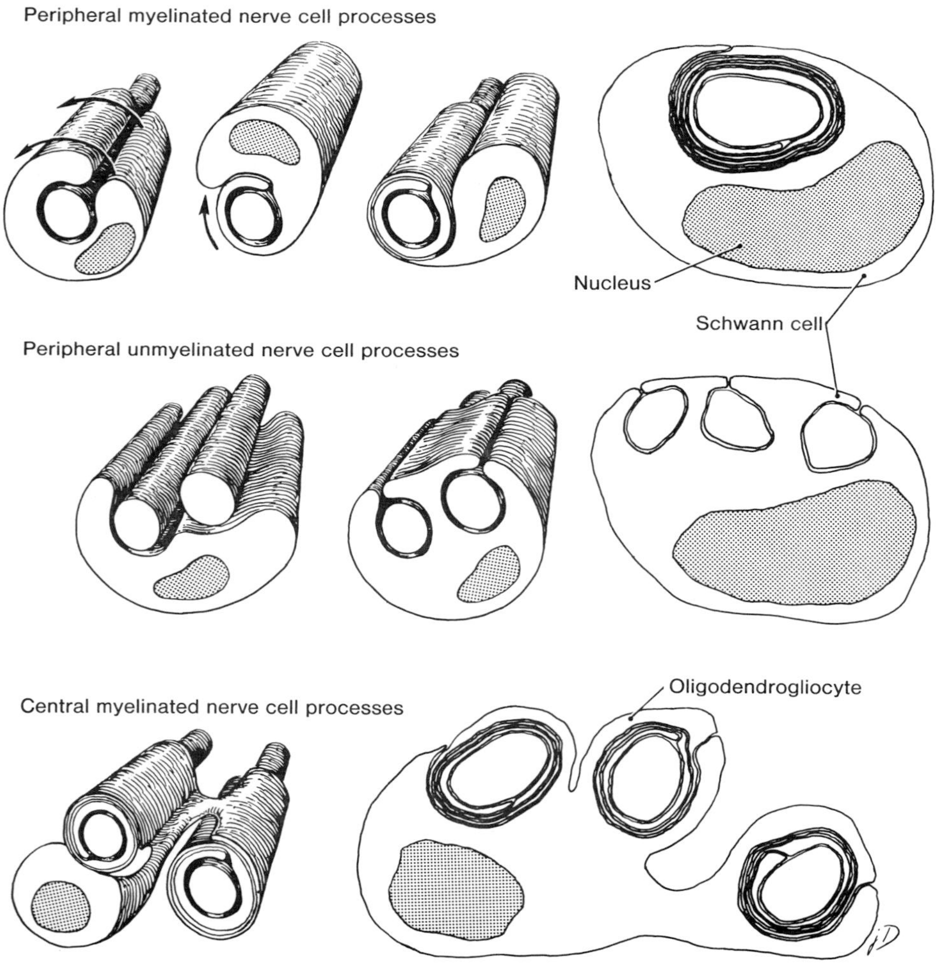

Peripheral myelinated nerve cell processes

Nucleus

Schwann cell

Peripheral unmyelinated nerve cell processes

Central myelinated nerve cell processes

Oligodendrogliocyte

Figure 14.32. A diagrammatic representation of myelination in the central and peripheral nervous systems. The relationship of Schwann cells to unmyelinated nerve fibers is depicted also. See the text for a complete description of the process.

The juxtaposition of successive layers of plasma membrane accounts for myelination. The outer leaflets of contiguous membranes fuse to form *intraperiod lines*, whereas the inner leaflets of adjacent plasma membranes fuse to form the *major dense lines* as the cytoplasm is extruded from the encircling process (Fig. 14.31).

Myelination. *Myelination* of a nerve cell process results from the intimate relationship established between these processes and Schwann cells or oligodendrogliocytes (Fig. 14.32). During *peripheral myelination*, a single neuronal process occupies an invagination along a Schwann cell. A tongue-like projection of the Schwann cell winds around the axis cylinder (Fig. 14.32). As the cytoplasm within this process is lost, the plasma membranes become juxtaposed and fusion of membrane components occurs as descibed previously. The degree of myelination, or thickness of the myelin sheath, is proportional to the number of whorls that occurs during this process (Figs. 14.24 and 14.32). A single Schwann cell is responsible for the internodal myelination of one nerve cell process and one internodal region.

Central and Peripheral Myelin. Although the process of *central myelination* by oligodendrogliocytes is similar to that which occurs peripherally, a few differences exist (Fig. 14.32). Connective tissue elements are not associated intimately with central nervous tissue; adjacent myelinated neuronal processes are not separated by a basal lamina. The repetitive unit of intraperiod and major dense lines is narrower in central myelin than in peripheral myelin. Centrally myelinated neuronal processes do not have much oligodendrogliocytic cytoplasm associated with the myelin sheath. The cell body of the oligodendrogliocytes is not juxtaposed to the myelin sheaths but is connected to them by cellular processes.

Also, one oligodendrogliocyte may myelinate more than one internodal region along the same fiber.

The neuroglial cells maintain the myelin sheath as well as produce myelin after demyelination that accompanies some diseases and injuries (Chapter 17).

References

Cellular Components

Bodian, D: The generalized vertebrate neuron. Science *137*:323, 1962.

Bondareff, W. and Hyden, H.: Submicroscopic structure of single neurons isolated from rabbit lateral vestibular nucleus. J. Ultrastruct. Res. *26*:399, 1964.

Eccles, J. C.: *The Physiology of Nerve Cells.* Johns Hopkins Press, Baltimore, 1957.

Fogelson, M. H., Gonates, N. K., Rorke, L. B. and Spiro, A.: Oligodendroglial lamellar inclusions. Arch. Neurol. *19*:150, 1968.

Glees, P.: *Neuroglia: Morphology and Function.* Charles C Thomas, Springfield, 1955.

Grafstein, B. and Forman, D. S.: Intracellular transport in neurons. Physiol Rev. *60*:1167, 1980.

Hamberger, A., Hansson, H. and Sjostrand, F.: Surface structure of isolated neurons. J. Cell Biol. *47*:319, 1970.

Luse, S. A.: Ultrastructure of reactive and neoplastic astrocytes. Lab. Invest. *7*:401, 1958.

Palay, S. L. and Palade, G. E.: The fine structure of neurons, J. Biophys. Biochem. Cytol. *1*:69, 1955.

Peters, A., Palay, S. and Webster, H. F.: *The Fine Structure of the Nervous System: The Neurons and Supporting Cells.* W. B. Saunders, Philadelphia, 1976.

Quarton, G. C., Melnechuk, T. and Schmitt, F. O.: *The Neurosciences.* Rockefeller University Press, New York, 1967.

Sandborn, E. B.: Electron microscopy of the neuron membrane systems and filaments. Canad. J. Physiol. Pharmacol. *44*:329, 1966.

Schwartz, J. H.: The transport of substances in nerve cells. Sci. Amer. *242*:152, 1980.

Stevens, C. F.: The neuron. Sci. Amer. *241*54, 1979.

Vaughn, J. E.: an electron microscopic analysis of gliogenesis in rat optic nerve. Z. Zellforsch. *94*:293, 1969.

Nerve Cell Processes

Bischoff, A. and Moor, H.: Ultrastructural differences between the myelin sheaths of peripheral nerve fibers and CNS white matter. Z. Zellforsch. *81*:303, 1967.

Cravioto, H.: The role of Schwann cells in the development of human peripheral nerves. J. Ultrastruct. Res. *12*:634, 1965.

Douglas, W. W. and Ritchie, J. M.: Mammalian nonmyelinated nerve fibers. Physiol. Rev. *42*:297, 1962.

Hursh, J. B.: Conduction velocity and diameter of nerve fibers. Am. J. Physiol. *127*:131, 1939.

Napolitano, L. M. and Scallen, T. J.: Observations on the fine structure of peripheral nerve myelin. Anat. Rec. *163*:1, 1969.

Peters, A.: Observations on the fine structure of peripheral nerve myelin. Anat. Rec. *98*:125, 1964.

Uzman, B. G. and Nogueira-Graf, G.: Electron microscope studies of the formation of nodes of Ranvier in mouse sciatic nerves. J. Biophys. Biochem. Cytol. *3*:589, 1957.

Transmission

Akert, K. and Waser, P. G. (eds.): Mechanisms of Synaptic Transmissions. Progr. Brain Res. 31, 1969.

DeRobertis, E. D. P.: *Histophysiology of Synapses and Neurosecretion.* The Macmillan Company. New York, 1964.

Dewey, M. M. and Barr, L.: Intercellular connection between smooth muscle cells: The nexus. Sci. *137*:670, 1962.

Grundfest, H.: Synaptic and ephaptic transmission. *In* Quarton, G. C. et al. (eds.). *The Neurosciences.* pp. 353–372. Rockefeller University Press, New York, 1967.

Gobel. S. and Dubner, R.: Axo-axonic synapses in the main sensory trigeminal nucleus. Experientia *24*:1250, 1968.

Jones, D. G.: The morphology of the contact region of vertebrate synaptosomes. Z. Zellforsch. *95*:263, 1969.

Kandel, F. R.: and Schwartz, J. H.: *Principles of Neuroscience.* Elsivier/North Holland, New York, 1981.

Katz, B.: *Nerve, Muscle and Synapse.* McGraw-Hill, New York, 1966.

Katz, B.: *The Release of Neural Transmitter Substances.* Charles C Thomas, Springfield, 1969.

Kelly, R.B., Deutsch, J.W., Carlson, S.S. and Wagner, J.A.: Biochemistry of neurotransmitter release. Ann. Rev. Neurosci. *2*:399, 1979.

Priedkalns, J. and Oksche, A.: Ultrastructure of synaptic terminals in nucleus infundibularis and nucleus supraopticus of *Passer domesticus.* Z. Zellforsch. *98*:135, 1969.

Takeno, K., Nishio, A. and Yanagiya, I.: Bound acetylcholine in the nerve ending particles. J. Neurochem. *16*:47, 1969.

COLOR PLATES

Plate I: Various Stains of Selected Tissues and Organs

Figure I.1. A section of haired skin. The stratified squamous epithelium stains purple, whereas the dense connective tissue of the dermis stains blue. The hairs are yellow; the associated sebaceous glands are stained red. ×40. (Masson's trichrome).

Figure I.2. A sample of bovine haired skin. The hair follicle in the center of the field is surrounded by yellow-staining dense connective tissue of the dermis. A sebaceous gland is apparent in the upper left portion of the micrograph. ×40. (Hematoxylin-phloxine-safran).

Figure I.3. A dense white fibrous connective tissue, regularly arranged. Collagenous fibers are stained pink. Sections of arterioles, a venule, and nerve fibers are apparent in the upper portion of the micrograph. ×40. (Hematoxylin and Eosin [H and E]. This is one of the most common staining combinations used in histology.)

Figure I.4. A porcine cerebellum. Purkinje cells are the large, pink-staining cells at the interface between the granular (right) and molecular (left) layers of this organ. ×40. (H and E).

Figure I.5. A porcine cerebellum similar to that of Figure I.4. The large, dark-staining cells are Purkinje cells. This staining technique permits the visualization of neuronal processes. ×40. (Silver impregnation).

Figure I.6. A feline ovary. Two vesicular follicles occupy the center of the field. The pink band around the oocyte is the zona pellucida. Primordial follicles are evident along the right margin of the micrograph. ×40. (H and E).

Figure I.7. A feline ovary similar to the section in Figure I.6. The vesicular follicle in the center of the field is more mature and larger than those in the previous micrograph. ×40. (Lendrum's phloxine tartrazine).

Figure I.8. A canine proximal femoral growth plate. This physis was associated with the development of the femoral head. The hyaline cartilage of the growth plate and primary spongiosa stains dark blue. Bone stains pale blue. The bone marrow imparts a high cellularity to the primary spongiosa. ×40. (Alcian blue).

Figure I.9. A ground section of lamellar bone about 75 μm thick. Pale-staining areas are old bone, whereas orange stains newer bone. Red staining areas represent the newest bone. The green band internal and adjacent to the newest bone *(red)* is the osteoid seam. A resorption space is apparent *(upper left)*. ×40. (Tetrachrome stain).

Figure I.10. A tetracycline-labeled, ground bone section of bone from the fracture repair site of an equine third carpal bone. The fluorescent bands indicate new bone depostion at the time of the serial injections of the antibiotic. ×40. (Fluorescent microscopy).

Figure I.11. A section of elastic cartilage. A perichondrium *(yellow)* surrounds the mass of cartilage. ×40. (Pentachrome stain).

Figure I.12. An equine intestinal mucosa. Goblet cells are stained purple. ×40. (Periodic acid-Schiff [PAS]).

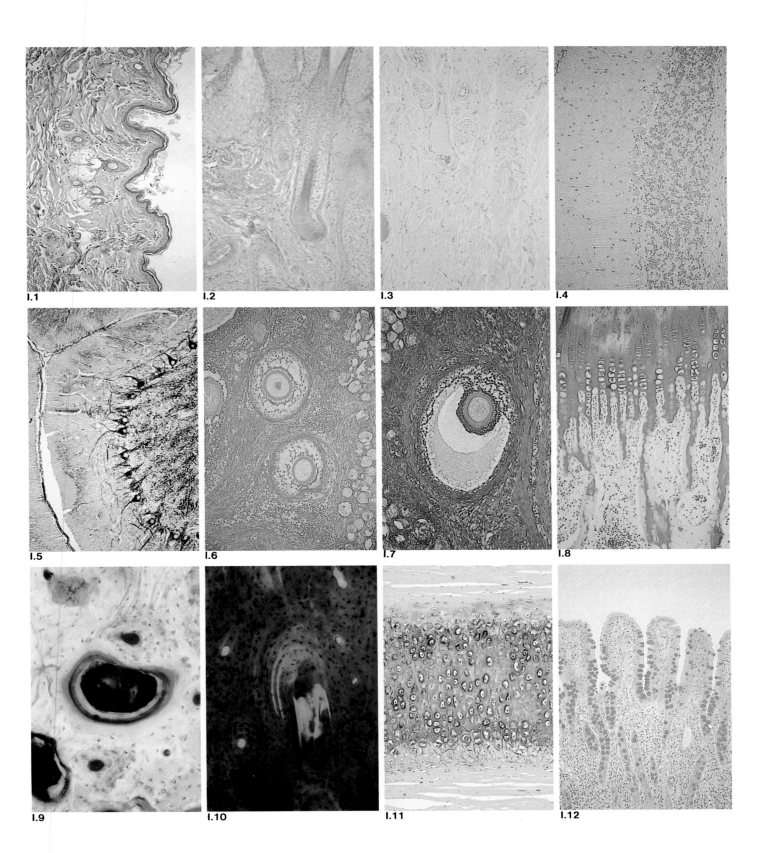

I.1

I.2

I.3

I.4

I.5

I.6

I.7

I.8

I.9

I.10

I.11

I.12

PLATE I

Plate II: Characteristics of Selected Cells

Figure II.1. Leydig cells of a porcine testis. These steroid-producing cells occupy the interstitial space between the seminiferous tubules. The cells are also called interstitial cells. They have an acidophilic, foamy cytoplasm. The foamy appearance results from the leaching of lipid products from the cytoplasm. ×400. (H and E).

Figure II.2. A seminiferous tubule of a porcine testis. A Sertoli cell *(lower center)* has a large triangular nucleus positioned along the basal border of the cell. The cytoplasm is difficult to discern. The identification of the cell is predicated upon nuclear morphology. Sertoli cells form an effective blood-testis barrier. Spermatocytes *(round nuclei) and spermatozoa (elongated nucleus)*. ×400. (H and E).

Figure II.3. Steroid-producing cells of the zona fasciculata of an equine adrenal cortex. The cells have vesicular nuclei. The cytoplasm is foamy and acidophilic. The foamy appearance results from the leaching of lipids during processing. ×400. (H and E).

Figure II.4. An osteoclast from bone. The large cell is multinucleated. The acidophilic, finely granular cytoplasm contains numerous vacuoles. The brush border is apparent at the cell-bone interface. These cells are fusion products of macrophages, or their precursors, that remove bone and cartilage. The osteoclast and the chondroclast are the same cell. Although the names are used interchangeably, the term osteoclast is used more commonly even when the cell is associated with cartilage. ×400. (H and E).

Figure II.5. Osteoblasts from developing bone. The osteoblasts line the surface of a spicule of bone *(center)*. An active cell has a vesicular nucleus and a basophilic cytoplasm. The basophilia is from extensive quantities of rough endoplasmic reticulum. A negative-staining Golgi zone is apparent in one of the cells *(left center)*. The cells assume an epithelioid appearance when active; they appear spindle-shaped when inactive. ×400. (H and E).

Figure II.6. Mesenchymal cells from loose connective tissue. The large prominent nucleus is the prominent feature of this cell. Definitive identification of this cell type is virtually impossible. The slightly basophilic cytoplasm is visible as the perikaryon. Cellular processes are difficult to distinguish from the collagenous fibers that are present also. ×400. (H and E).

Figure II.7. Cells of a bovine abomasum (glandular stomach). The round to oval cells with acidophilic cytoplasm are parietal cells. The cytoplasmic granularity results from numerous mitochondria. The cells secrete hydrochloric acid. The foamy cells in the center of the field are mucus-secreting cells. ×400. (H and E).

Figure II.8. Serous cells associated with the olfactory mucosa. The cuboidal cells have a centrally positioned nucleus surrounded by a finely granular, acidophilic cytoplasm. ×400. (H and E).

Figure II.9. Mucous cells from the glands associated with an equine ureter. The low columnar cells have a foamy cytoplasm and a basally positioned and flattened nucleus. ×400. (H and E).

Figure II.10. A cross section through a pancreatic acinus *(arrow)*. The pancreatic cells have an apical acidophilia and a basal basophilia. The basophilia results from an accumulation of ribosomes and rough endoplasmic reticulum in the basal part of the cell, whereas the apical acidophilia is from zymogen granules. ×400. (Gomori's chrome alum-hematoxylin). (Courtesy of R. A. Kainer).

Figure II.11. Nerve cell and satellite cells in a dorsal root ganglion. The ganglion cell has a large, vesicular nucleus with a prominent nucleolus. Nissl substance is barely evident as a focal cytoplasmic basophilia. A nerve fiber is sectioned longitudinally *(right)*. ×400. (H and E).

Figure II.12. A longitudinal section of skeletal muscle. The striations result from the registration of the myofibrils. A dark A band is separated by a light I band. The I band contains a Z line. The *arrow* indicates connective tissue elements of the endomysium. ×400. (Courtesy of R. A. Kainer).

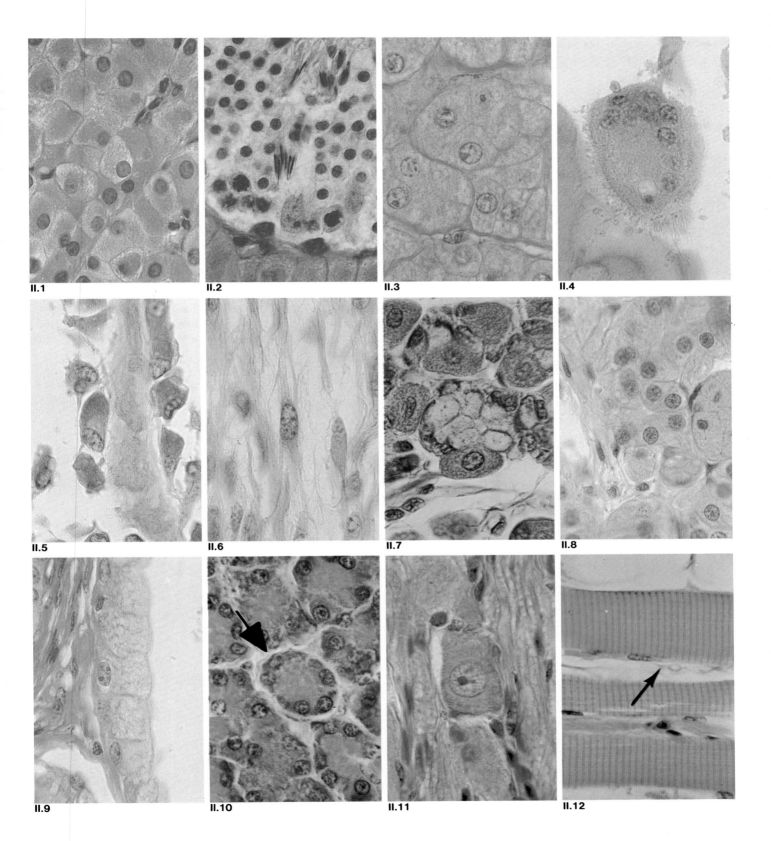

II.1

II.2

II.3

II.4

II.5

II.6

II.7

II.8

II.9

II.10

II.11

II.12

PLATE II

Plate III: Surface and Glandular Epithelia
Lining Epithelia
Figure III.1. Simple cuboidal epithelium of a salivary duct. ×100. (Hematoxylin-phloxine-safran).
Figure III.2. Simple columnar epithelium of a canine stomach, The apical borders of the cells are clear. ×100. (H and E).
Figure III.3. Simple columnar epithelium and goblet cells of a feline jejunum. The pale blue-staining cells are goblet cells. ×100. (Mallory's azan).
Figure III.4. Simple columnar epithelium and goblet cells of an equine intestinal mucosa. The goblet cells and striated border are stained purple. ×100. (PAS).
Figure III.5. Keratinized stratified squamous epithelium of a canine muzzle. The pale-staining material *(top)* is keratin. Note the epidermal pegs and dermal papillae. ×100. (H and E).
Figure III.6. Nonkeratinized stratified squamous epithelium of a canine esophagus. ×100. (Hematoxylin-phloxine-safran).
Figure III.7. Pseudostratified ciliated columnar epithelium with goblet cells from a murine trachea. Bundles of smooth muscle fibers are present in the lamina propria mucosae. ×100. (H and E).

Glandular Epithelia
Figure III.8. Adenomere of an apocrine tubular gland surrounded by dense white fibrous connective tissue. ×100. (Masson's trichrome).
Figure III.9. A section of sebaceous glands within the dermis. These branched alveolar glands are associated with a hair follicle. ×100. (Masson's trichrome).
Figure III.10. Equine pyloric glands. Note the typical mucous cell characteristics. ×100. (H and E).
Figure III.11. Mucous and serous cells within adenomeres of glands associated with a respiratory mucosa. ×100. (H and E).
Figure III.12. Hepatocytes from a procine liver. The epithelial cells are arranged in cords. ×100. (H and E).

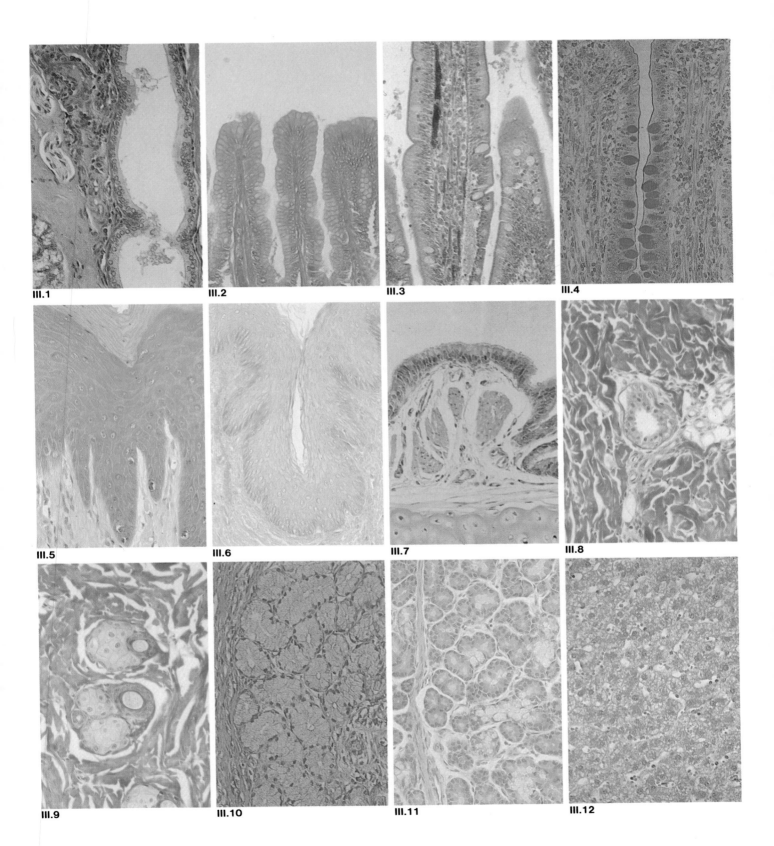

III.1

III.2

III.3

III.4

III.5

III.6

III.7

III.8

III.9

III.10

III.11

III.12

PLATE III

Plate IV: Connective Tissue

Proper Connective Tissue

Figure IV.1. Loose connective tissue. The connective tissue is composed of a loose array of pink-staining collagenous fibers and typical cells of the resident population. A venule *(top left)*, arteriole *(top right)* and a nerve fiber *(lower left)* are evident. ×100. (H and E).

Figure IV.2. Hyperplastic loose connective tissue of the pharyngeal mucosa. Numerous mononuclear cells comprise part of the resident cellular population. These cells perform immunological protective functions in regions exposed to continual antigenic insult. ×100. (H and E).

Figure IV.3. Dense white fibrous connective tissue, irregularly arranged, of a dermis. Pink-staining elastic fibers are scattered among the collagenous fibers. ×100. (Hematoxylin-phloxine and safran).

Figure IV.4. A longitudinal section of a nuchal ligament from a lamb. Elongated nuclei are interspersed between pink-staining, wavy fibers. ×100. (H and E).

Figure IV.5. A longitudinal section of a tendon. The flattened, dense nuclei of fibroblasts are scattered among the pink-staining collagenous fibers. The cytoplasm of the cells is not apparent. ×100. (H and E).

Figure IV.6. A longitudinal section of a tendon. The cells are scattered among the yellow-staining, collagenous fibers. Some loose connective tissue elements and part of a sectioned blood vessel are apparent along the left margin of the micrograph. ×100. (van Gieson).

Supportive Tissue

Figure IV.7. Section of growing hyaline cartilage. Dark-staining nuclei of chondrocytes are apparent within the chondrocytic lacunae. The capsular margins (territorial matrix) stain a dark purple. The interterritorial matrix is light purple. The tissue is surrounded by a perichondrium, the fibrous layer of which blends insensibly with the surrounding connective tissue. ×100. (Hematoxylin and eosin).

Figure IV.8. A section of mature hyaline cartilage. The homogeneous, pink-staining matrix is a conspicuous feature of this tissue. The territorial and interterritorial matrical staining differences are not apparent in this section. The perichondrium occupies the upper portion of the micrograph. ×100. (H and E).

Figure IV.9. Hyaline cartilage associated with a developing bone. The articular cartilage *(top)* and growth plate *(diagonally from right central margin to lower central margin of micrograph)* is hyaline cartilage. The epiphyseal *(upper left)* and metaphyseal *(lower right)* bone stains pink and contains cores of pale-staining calcified cartilage that stains similarly to the hyaline cartilage of the articular surface and growth plate ×100. (H and E).

Figure IV.10. A section of elastic cartilage. The elastic fibers are red and are especially obvious in the young cartilage adjacent to the perichondrium *(bottom)*. ×100. (Pentachrome stain).

Figure IV.11. Fibrocartilage from a canine meniscus. Note the columns of chondrocytes between the collagenous fibers. ×100. (H and E).

Figure IV.12. Osteons within the compact bone of a diaphysis. The limit of the osteon *(lower center)* is the reversal line (cement line). ×100. (Mallory's).

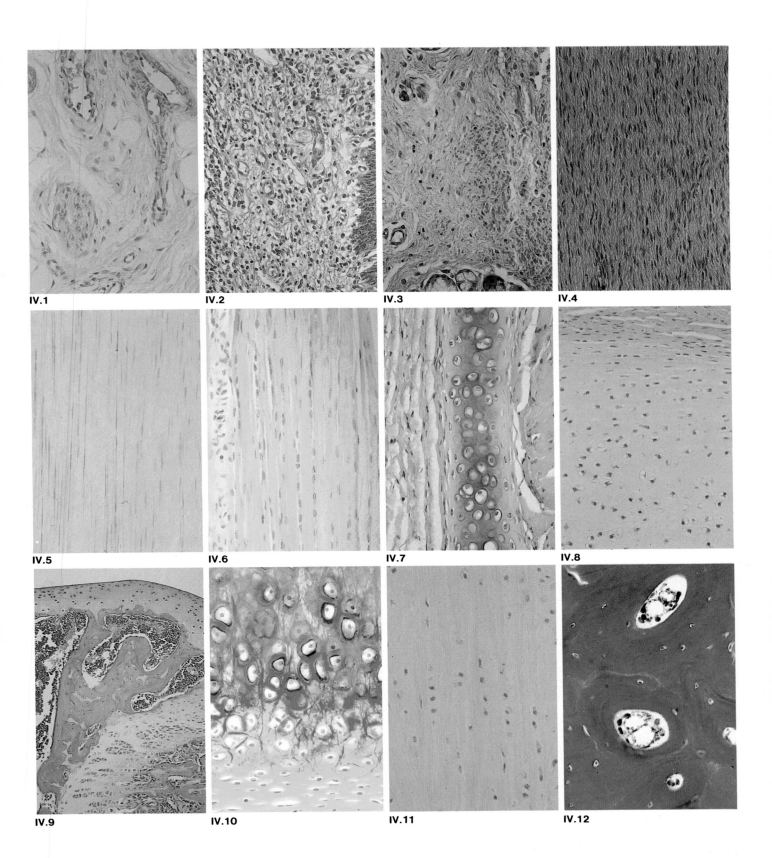

IV.1

IV.2

IV.3

IV.4

IV.5

IV.6

IV.7

IV.8

IV.9

IV.10

IV.11

IV.12

PLATE IV

Plate V: Muscular, Nervous, and Adipose Tissue
Muscular Tissue
Figure V.1. A longitudinal section of a sheet of smooth muscle from the tunica muscularis of an intestine. ×100. (H and E).
Figure V.2. A cross section of bundles of smooth muscle. ×100. (H and E). (Courtesy of R. A. Kainer).
Figure V.3. A longitudinal section of skeletal muscle. ×100. (H and E). (Courtesy of R. A. Kainer).
Figure V.4. A cross section of skeletal muscle. The muscle fibers are grey and the endomysial connective tissue is blue. ×100. (Masson's trichrome).
Figure V.5. A longitudinal section of cardiac muscle. Striations are not as well defined as in skeletal muscle. ×100. (H and E).
Figure V.6. A cross section of cardiac muscle. ×100. (H and E).

Nervous Tissue
Figure V.7. A longitudinal section of a myelinated nerve. ×100. (H and E).
Figure V.8. A longitudinal section of a myelinated nerve. ×100. (Osmium tetroxide).
Figure V.9. A cross section of a fascicle of a myelinated nerve. ×100. (H and E).
Figure V.10. A section of a brain stem of a pig. A large neuron occupies the center of the field. The cytoplasmic blue-staining material is Nissl substance. The small, dark-staining nuclei are those of neuroglial cells. ×100. (Nocht's stain).

Adipose Tissue
Figure V.11. Yellow adipose tissue. ×100. (H and E).
Figure V.12. Brown adipose tissue. ×100. (H and E).

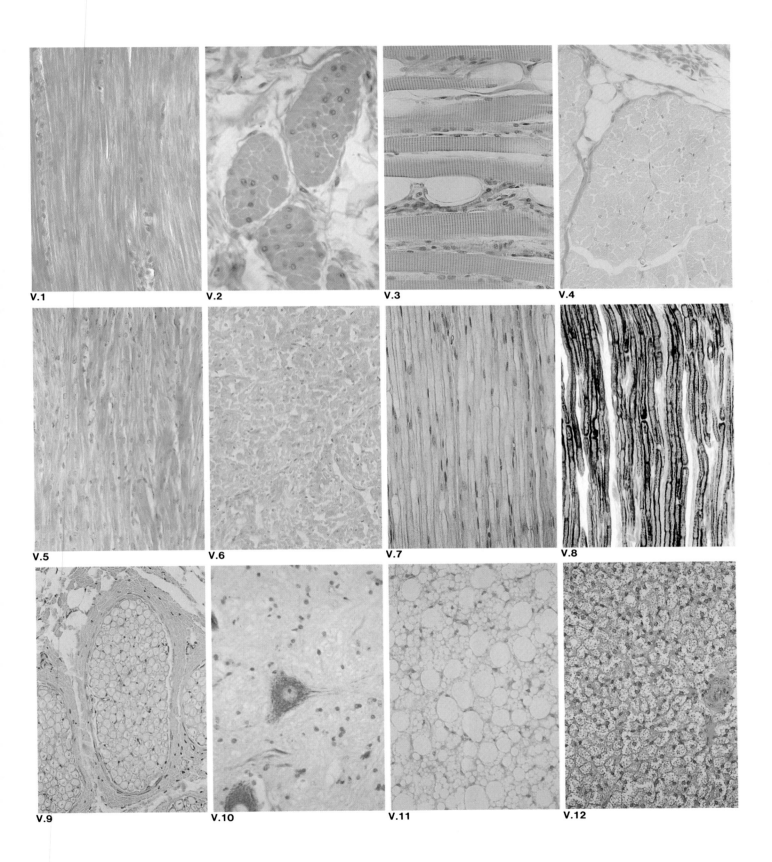

V.1 V.2 V.3 V.4

V.5 V.6 V.7 V.8

V.9 V.10 V.11 V.12

PLATE V

Plate VI: Peripheral Blood Cells
   All of the blood smears were stained with a Romanowsky stain and photographed at 400×.

Neutrophils

Figure VI.1.   Canine peripheral blood smear.
Figure VI.2.   Feline peripheral blood smear.
Figure VI.3.   Equine peripheral blood smear.
Figure VI.4.   Bovine peripheral blood smear.

Lymphocytes

Figure VI.5.   Canine peripheral blood smear.
Figure VI.6.   Feline peripheral blood smear.
Figure VI.7.   Equine peripheral blood smear.
Figure VI.8.   Bovine peripheral blood smear.

Monocytes

Figure VI.9.   Canine peripheral blood smear.
Figure VI.10.   Feline peripheral blood smear.
Figure VI.11.   Equine peripheral blood smear.
Figure VI.12.   Bovine peripheral blood smear.

Eosinophils

Figure VI.13.   Canine peripheral blood smear. (Courtesy of M. A. Thrall).
Figure VI.14.   Feline peripheral blood smear. (Courtesy of M. A. Thrall).
Figure VI.15.   Equine peripheral blood smear. (Courtesy of R. A. Kainer).
Figure VI.16.   Bovine peripheral blood smear. (Courtesy of M. A. Thrall).

Basophils

Figure VI.17.   Canine peripheral blood smear.
Figure VI.18.   Feline peripheral blood smear.
Figure VI.19.   Equine peripheral blood smear.
Figure VI.20.   Bovine peripheral blood smear.

Miscellaneous Blood Cells

Figure VI.21.   Canine lymphocyte. Note the indented nucleus.
Figure VI.22.   A canine rubricyte in a peripheral blood smear.
Figure VI.23.   Toxic neutrophilic bands in a feline peripheral blood smear. Note the Barr body.
Figure VI.24.   Erythrophagocytosis by a blood monocyte.

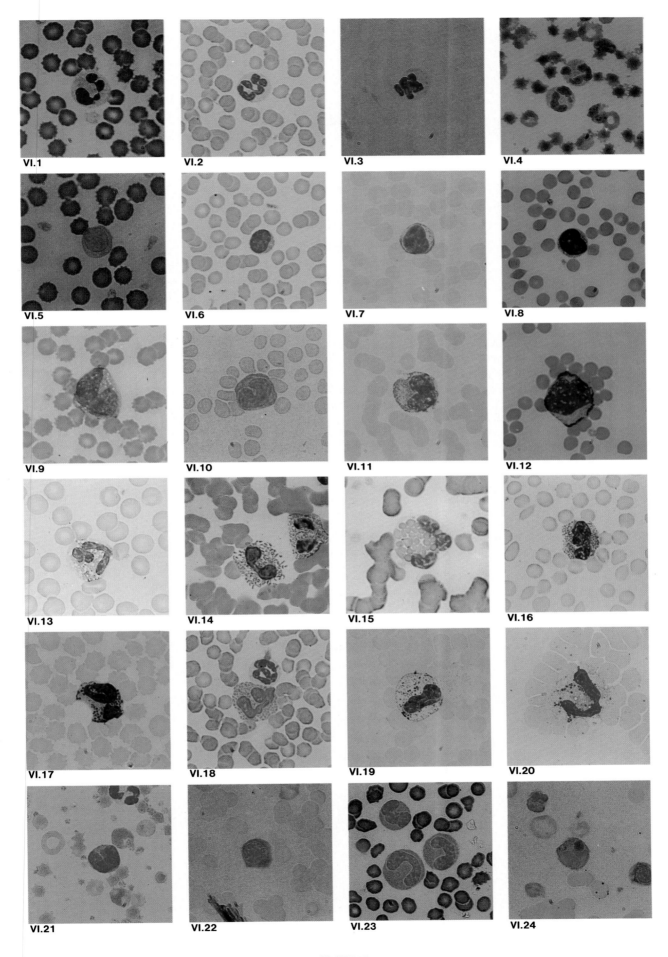

VI.1

VI.2

VI.3

VI.4

VI.5

VI.6

VI.7

VI.8

VI.9

VI.10

VI.11

VI.12

VI.13

VI.14

VI.15

VI.16

VI.17

VI.18

VI.19

VI.20

VI.21

VI.22

VI.23

VI.24

PLATE VI

245

Plate VII: Peripheral Blood and Exfoliative Cytology
    All of the specimens were atained with a Romanowsky stain and photographed at 400×

Miscellaneous Blood Cells

Figure VII.1.   A feline neutrophilic band with toxic granulation.

Figure VII.2.   A bovine lymphocyte with azurophilic granules.

Figure VII.3.   A canine monocyte *(top)*, neutrophilic band cell *(middle)*, and a neutrophil *(bottom)*.

Figure VII.4.   Polychromasia in a canine peripheral blood smear.

Figure VII.5.   Canine peripheral blood cells *Top to bottom* — platelet, monocyte, rubricyte, and metarubricyte.

Exfoliative Cytologic Preparations

Figure VII.6.   A cerebrospinal fluid tap. A macrophage with hemosiderin is apparent in a cerebrospinal fluid sample from a dog with head trauma.

Figure VII.7.   An aspirate of a reactive canine lymph node. Large lymphoblasts *(upper left)*, mature lymphocytes, plasma cells *(center)*, and a Mott cell *(lower right)* are apparent. Note that the spoke-wheel configuration of the plasma cell nucleus, apparent in sectioned materials, is not obvious in smeared samples. A lymphoglandualr body is in the center of the field just below the plasma cell.

Figure VII.8.   An aspirate of a canine popliteal lymph node. Metastatic mast cell tumor cells *(upper left)*, plasmablast *(upper center)*, and a plasma cell *(upper right)* are present. Mast cell granules from ruptured cells are scattered throughout the sample.

Figure VII.9.   Transitional epithelial cells from an impression smear of the urinary bladder of a normal dog.

Figure VII.10.   A tracheal wash from a normal dog. Ciliated columnar cells are present.

Figure VII.11.   A tracheal wash from a dog with chronic bronchitis. Vacuolated macrophages, neutrophils and a reactive lymphocytes are present.

Figure VII.12.   An impression smear of thyroid follicular cells from a normal dog.

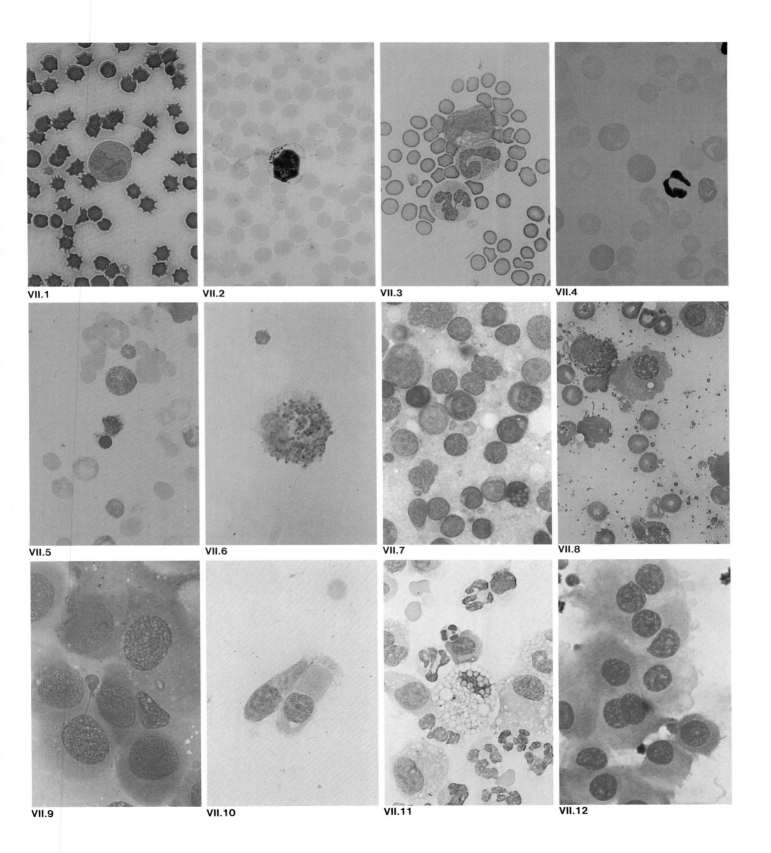

VII.1

VII.2

VII.3

VII.4

VII.5

VII.6

VII.7

VII.8

VII.9

VII.10

VII.11

VII.12

PLATE VII

Plate VIII: Exfoliative Cytology
   All of the specimens were stained with a Romanowsky stain and were photographed at 400×.

Figure VIII.1.   An impression smear of thyroid follicular cells from a normal dog. The cells contain dark blue, cytoplasmic granules.

Figure VIII.2.   An aspirate of a canine salivary gland. The vacuolated cells are secretory cells. Note the contamination of the sample with blood.

Figure VIII.3.   An aspirate of a normal canine prostate gland. Note the size and shape of the normal epithelial cells.

Figure VIII.4.   An aspirate of a canine hyperplastic prostate gland. The cells are more columnar than normal.

Figure VIII.5.   An aspirate of a canine prostate gland with adenocarcinoma. The large, binucleated cell has prominent nucleoli. Note the size difference of this cell. This micrograph is magnified 400× also.

Figure VIII.6.   An aspirate of a canine prostate gland with squamous cell metaplasia. The cells are squamous, have pyknotic nuclei, and abundant cytoplasm.

Figure VIII.7.   A canine vaginal smear during early estrus. Cornified epithelial cells have numerous bacteria on their surfaces. Some erythrocytes are present.

Figure VIII.8.   A canine vaginal smear during diestrus. Intermediate epithelial cells contain neutrophils.

Figure VIII.9.   A smear of fluid obtained by abdominal centesis from a normal horse. A cluster of mesothelial cells, some macrophages and some neutrophils are present.

Figure VIII.10.   A smear of fluid obtained by abdominal centesis from a normal horse. Erythrocytes and a neutrophil with a pyknotic nucleus *(center)* are present.

Figure VIII.11.   A smear of a conjunctival scraping from a normal dog. The epithelial lining cells are typical.

Figure VIII.12.   A smear of a conjunctival scraping from a dog with keratoconjunctivitis sicca. Goblet cells are prominent features of the sample.

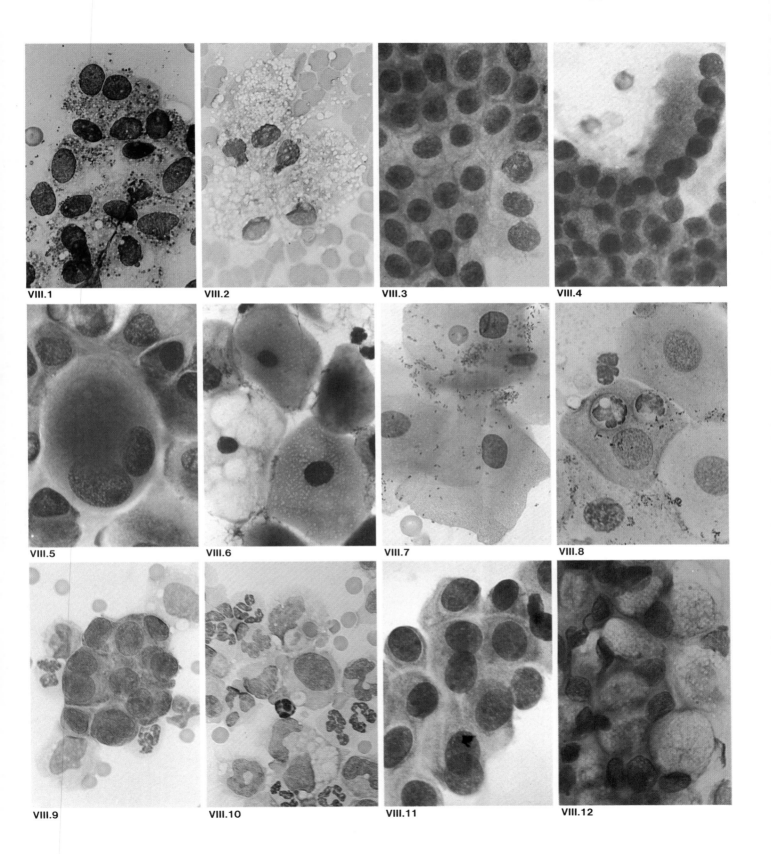

VIII.1 VIII.2 VIII.3 VIII.4

VIII.5 VIII.6 VIII.7 VIII.8

VIII.9 VIII.10 VIII.11 VIII.12

PLATE VIII

SECTION IV:

COMPARATIVE ORGANOLOGY

15: Organization of Organs

Introduction

All of the organs of the body are formed by various combinations of different types and amounts of one or more of the basic tissues. Specific cellular and tissue constituents and unique geometric patterns are distinguishing features of organs.

Parenchyma and Stroma

Understanding the architecture of an organ is fundamental to understanding its function. Although all of the contributing tissues are essential elements, one tissue usually performs the vital functions that characterize the organ. This tissue is the parenchyma. **The distinguishing or specific cell types of a structure constitute the parenchyma and perform the functions by which the organ is characterized.**

Often, the parenchyma is the epithelial constituent. Neurons characterize the functions of the organs of the nervous system. Secretory epithelial cells characterize the function of the glandular stomach. Similarly, the seminiferous tubules of the testis and the secretory and absorptive cells of the small intestine perform the characteristic functions of these organs. The definition does not confine the application of the concept to epithelia. Skeletal muscle fibers are the characteristic cell of the numerous muscles. Also, cardiac muscle cells are the characteristic fibers of the heart.

The parenchyma is bound together by various connective tissues. **The connective tissue of an organ is the stroma.** The stroma transmits the blood vessels, lymphatics, and nerve fibers that are essential for the "nutritional and regulatory support" of the organ.

Tubular Organs

General Form

Most tubular organs consist of four concentric layers that are called *tunics* (Fig. 15.1). From the luminal surface to the periphery, they are: tunica mucosa, tunica submucosa, tunica muscularis, and tunica adventitia (or tunica serosa). All of the tunics may be present, one or more may be reduced or eliminated, or one or more may be modified to meet specific local needs. These variations, in conjunction with other characteristics, permit identification of an organ.

Tunica Mucosa

The tunica mucosa is the innermost or luminal coat and consists of three layers (Fig. 15.2): lamina epithelialis mucosae,

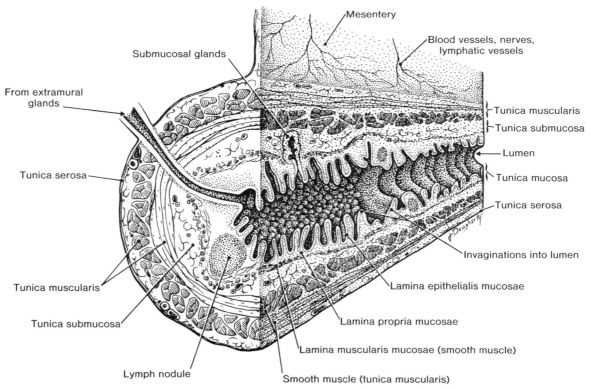

Figure 15.1. A stylized drawing of a tubular visceral organ. Refer to the text for a complete description of the components.

252

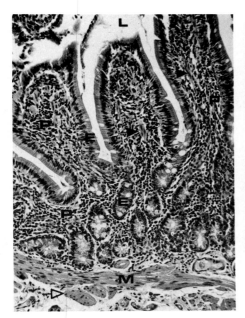

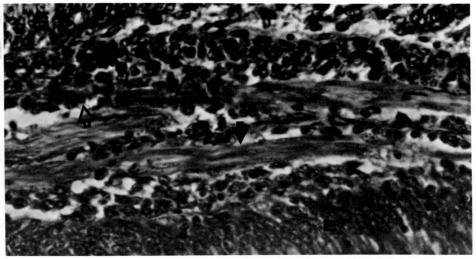

Figure 15.2. Tunica mucosa of an equine duodenum. The lamina epithelialis mucosae *(E)* is adjacent to the lumen *(L)* and invaginates into the lamina propria mucosae *(P)*. The lamina propria mucosae is hyperplastic. The lamina muscularis mucosae *(M)* consists of inner circular and outer longitudinal layers *(open arrow)* of smooth muscle. Extensions of the lamina muscularis mucosae *(solid arrows)* are apparent within the lamina propria mucosae. ×29.

Figure 15.3. Lamina propria mucosae of an equine duodenum. The villus is covered by the lamina epithelialis mucosae *(E)* and contains a core of hyperplastic loose connective tissue *(open arrow)*. Smooth muscle *(solid arrows)* from the lamina muscularis mucosae extends into the lamina propria mucoase. ×125.

lamina propria mucosae, and lamina muscularis mucosae.

The *lamina epithelialis* mucosae is the epithelial layer. This lamina may consist of one or more types of epithelial cells as per the specific function of an organ or portion of an organ. This layer is a consistent lamina of the tunica mucosa. A basement membrane is a constant feature between epithelial cells and the subjacent connective tissue.

The *lamina propria mucosae*, the essential connective tissue that underlies the epithelial layer, is usually areolar and/or reticular connective tissue. Small vessels, nerves and infoldings of the lamina epithelialis mucosae occupy this space. The connective tissue of this space may contain large numbers of protective cells either free or within lymph nodules. Besides a defensive function, this layer is the means by which epithelia are nourished and controlled.

The *lamina muscularis mucosae* consists of one or more layers of smooth muscle cells. Inner circular and an outer longitudinal layers may be apparent. The sheets of the smooth muscle within this lamina are usually continuous; however, the occurrence of this lamina varies. It is the means by which local mobility of organs is achieved. Also, it expresses secretory products from glands that may invaginate into the lamina propria mucosae (Fig. 15.3). It is a sharp line of demarcation between the connective tissue of the lamina propria mucosae and the tunica submucosa.

Tunica Submucosa

The *tunica submucosa* consists of areolar connective tissue that is more coarsely ar-

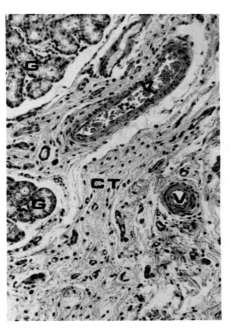

Figure 15.4. Tunica submucosa of an equine duodenum. The areolar connective tissue *(CT)* surrounds vessels *(V)* and glands *(G)* within the tunica submucosa. Nerves and lymphatic vessels are present also. ×34.

ranged than the connective tissue of the lamina propria mucosae (Fig. 15.4). Large blood vessels, nerves, nerve plexuses, and autonomic (intramural) ganglia are present. In some organs, glands may be present also. This tunic permits motility of the tunica mucosa. When a lamina muscularis mucosae is not present, the lamina propria mucosae and the tunica submucosa are referred to collectively as the lamina propria mucosae (*lamina propria-submucosa, tunica submucosa*).

Tunica Muscularis

The *tunica muscularis* is usually well-developed and consists of two layers of muscle (Fig. 15.5). In some organs, however, it may be absent. Although these layers usually consist of smooth muscle, skeletal muscle may be present. The most common arrangement of this tunic is to be subdivided into inner circular and outer longitudinal layers. The inner layer is actually disposed in a tighter helical pattern than the outer, more loosely oriented helix. Vascular and neural plexuses and autonomic ganglion cells usually separate the two layers. This tunic is responsible for the tone of the organ, size of the lumen, and the movement of materials through the hollow organ.

Tunica Adventitia and Tunica Serosa

The *tunica adventitia* is a collection of loose connective tissue over the periphery of an organ. Blood vessels, nerves, ganglia, and adipose tissue may occur within this tunic. This type of outer covering is part of organs that are not intimately associated with the celomic spaces. Also, the tunica

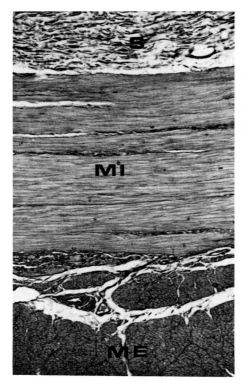

Figure 15.5. Tunica muscularis of a feline stomach. The tunica muscularis is peripheral to the tunica submucosa *(S)*. The tunica muscularis consists of inner *(MI)* and outer *(ME)* layers of smooth muscle. Compare with Figure 13.4. ×40.

serosa is part of organs that are close to the celomic spaces but are not covered by mesothelium.

Organs that are intimately associated with the celomic cavities are surrounded by a layer of mesothelium. In these cases, the most peripheral tunic is referred to as the *tunica serosa* (Fig. 15.6). It consists, therefore, of mesothelium and connective tissue. It is through the tunica adventitia or tunica serosa that the vascular, lymphatic, and nerve supplies gain access to an organ. Further, these tunics are responsible for the suspension of organs either through the union of the tunica adventitia with surrounding connective tissue or by the reflection of mesothelium and associated connective tissue as *mesenteries.*

Surface and Glandular Modifications

Tubular organs use many methods to increase their surface areas (Fig. 15.7). The cellular elements of a flattened tunica mucosa may evaginate into the lumen of the organ and form villous projections (Figs. 15.7*B* and 15.8), rugae (Fig. 15.7*F*), and other effacable and noneffacable folds. The cellular elements of the tunica mucosa may invaginate into the lamina propria mucosae independent of surface projections (Fig. 15.7*F*) or in association with surface projections (Fig. 15.7*C*). This usually results in the thickening of the lamina propria mucosae.

Elements of the lamina muscularis mucosae may interdigitate between these invaginations of the lamina epithelialis mucosae (Figs. 15.7*C, D* and *F*) and extend into the evaginations of the tunica mucosa (Figs. 15.7*C, D* and *F*). Glandular structures that remain within the lamina propria mucosae are called *mucosal glands* (Fig. 15.7*C, D* and *F*). Invaginations of the lamina epitheliallis mucosae may perforate the lamina muscularis mucosae and the adenomeres may occupy the tunica submucosa. Such glandular structures are called *submucosal glands* (Fig. 15.7*D*). In specialized cases, the lamina epithelialis mucosae is continuous with glandular structures positioned remotely from the lumen of the organ (Fig. 15.7*C*). This type of organization typifies the relationship of the liver and pancreas to the gut lumen.

Organization of Solid Organs

Form and Function

The parenchyma and stroma are distinct entities of solid organs, too (Fig. 15.9). Small, parenchymatous units are surrounded by a fine meshwork of areolar or reticular connective tissue in which vessels and nerves are located. Small units of parenchyma may be grouped as larger units and surrounded by a more coarse areolar connective tissue, or the connective tissue of these small groups may be continuous with coarse areolar connective tissue *trabeculae*. In either case, the connective tissue is progressively more dense and is continuous with the dense white fibrous connective tissue of the capsule. This continuity affords structural support and facilitates the entry and/or exit of vessels and nerves.

Membranes as Simple Organs

Mucous Membranes

Mucous membranes include some or all of the components of the tunica mucosa. These membranes consist of a **moistened epithelial lining and an underlying connective tissue** (Fig. 15.10). These membranes are kept moist by secretions from cells within the lamina epithelialis mucosae and/or from glands located within the lamina propria mucosae and/or tunica submucosa. The lamina epithelialis mucosae may consist of stratified squamous, cuboidal, columnar, or pseudostratified columnar epithelium. A mucous membrane consisting of stratified squamous epithelium (keratinized or nonkeratinized) is termed a *cutaneous mucous membrane*. It typically occurs as part of the digestive and reproductive systems (Fig. 15.11). Mucous membranes lined by transitional epithlium occur in the urinary system (Fig. 15.12).

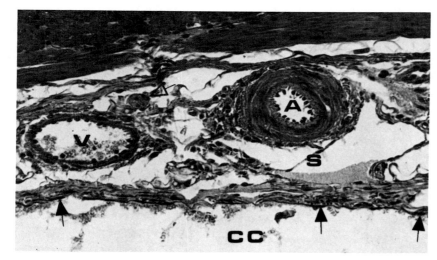

Figure 15.6. Tunica serosa of a feline stomach. The tunica serosa, visceral peritoneum, is the outer covering of the organs associated intimately with the peritoneal cavity. The celomic cavity *(CC)* (peritoneal cavity) is bounded by mesothelial cells *(solid arrows)* that contribute to the visceral and parietal serosal membranes. Subserosal connective tissue *(S)* is areolar. Arteries *(A)*, veins *(V)*, and nerves *(open arrow)* are present. The spaces within the connective tissue are artifacts of sectioning. ×63.

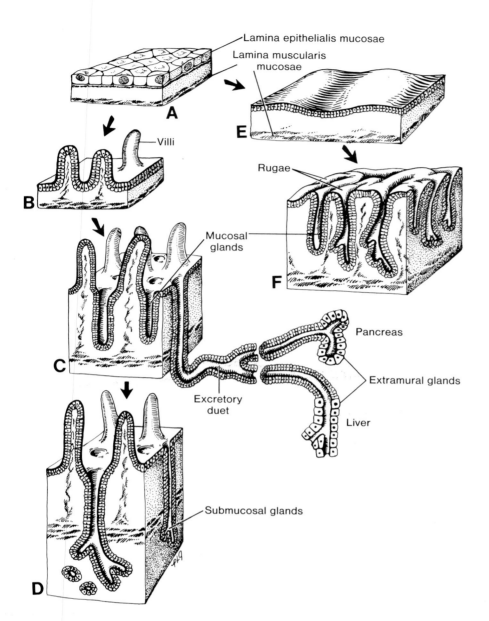

Figure 15.7. A diagram of the devlopment of surface modifications and glands associated with the mural elements of tubular visceral organs. A flat epithelial surface *(A)* is a common feature of many visceral organs. Differential growth of the epithelium may result in an undulating surface *(E)*. Differential growth may become exaggerated, resulting in the formation of mucosal glands that are located within the lamina propria mucosae but are continuous with the lamina epithelialis mucosae *(F)*. Surface alterations of the lamina epithelialis mucosae and underlying lamina propria mucosae may result in the formation of evaginations from the surface called villi *(B)*. Differential growth of the surfaces and underlying connective tissue may result in the formation of complementary invaginations (glands) as mucosal glands between the villi *(C)*. Continued growth of the epithelial lining may result in the formation of ducts and adenomeres of glands that are displaced away from the organs of origin as extramural glands *(C)*. The growth of the lamina epithelialis mucosae through the lamina propria mucosae into the tunica submucosa establishes submucosal glands *(D)*.

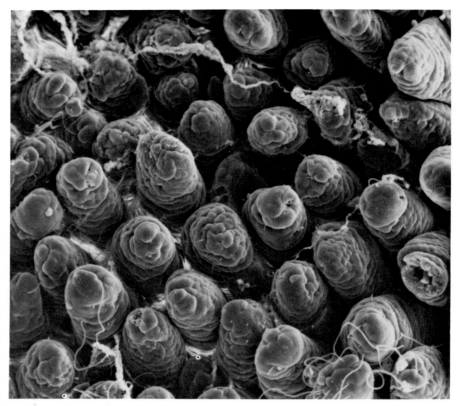

Figure 15.8. A scanning electron micrograph of villi from the jejunum of a mouse. The villi project from the mucosal surface into the lumen of the organ. (Courtesy of D. L. Eisenbrandt.)

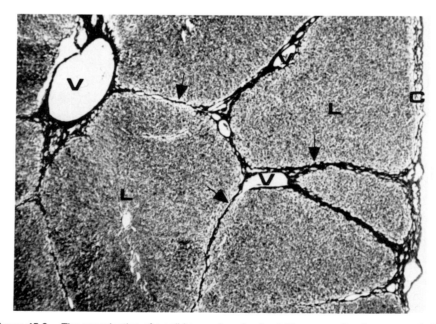

Figure 15.9. The organization of a solid organ (porcine liver). The connective tissue capsule *(C)* is continuous with large connective tissue trabeculae *(arrows)* that subdivide the organ into small anatomic units (lobules). Fine reticular fibers extend a short distance into the lobules *(L)*. Large vessels *(V)* are located within the trabeculae. ×10. (Snook's reticulum.)

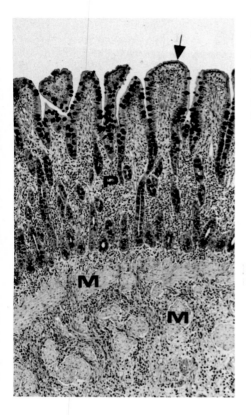

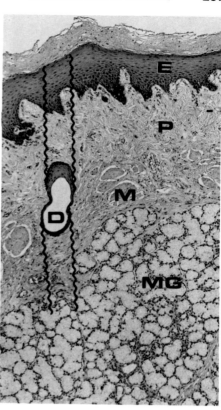

Figure 15.10. A mucous membrane lined by simple columnar epithelium from a canine jejunum. The epithelium *(arrow)* invaginates into the lamina propria mucoase *(P)*. The lamina muscularis mucosae *(M)* consists of smooth muscle oriented into longitudinal and circular configurations. The dark-staining cells of the lamina epithelalis mucosae are goblet cells and other mucous-secreting cells. ×16. (Alcian blue and PAS.)

Figure 15.11. A mucous membrane lined by stratified squamous epithelium from a porcine esophagus. This combination of epithelial tissue, with or without keratinization, and underlying connective tissue is called a cutaneous mucous membrane. The lamina epithelialis mucosae *(E)* is covered by a mucoid secretory product and underlaid by the lamina propria mucoase *(P)*. The lamina muscularis mucosae *(M)* is discontinuous. Mucosal glands *(MG)* are responsible for the moistened surface. The secretory products of these glands reach the surface *(wavy lines)* through the excretory duct *(D)* and its continuations. ×16.

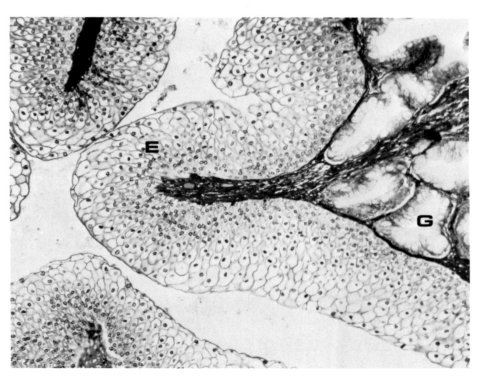

Figure 15.12. A transitional mucous membrane from an equine ureter. Mucous glands *(G)* moisten the surface of the transitional epithelium *(E)*. ×40.

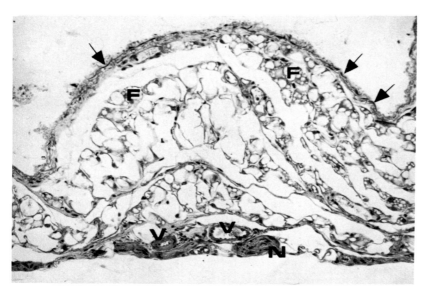

Figure 15.13. A serous membrane (tunica serosa). The mesothelium *(solid arrows)* and its associated areolar connective tissue contains the typical components including adipocytes *(F)*, vessels *(V)* and nerves *(N)*. Compare with Figure 15.6. ×40.

Serous Membranes

Serous membranes consist of a layer of mesothelium and associated connective tissue (Fig. 15.13). They line the celomic spaces and are moistened by the fluids contained within these spaces.

Serosal investments of organs are significant contributors to the repair process of the visceral organs. Fibrin deposition in the submesothelial and subserosal connective tissue decreases leakage after repair by sealing the wound. Excessive and/or rough handling of the peritoneum can cause fibrin deposition in focal regions. The subsequent activity of fibroblasts and the deposition of collagen in such regions are the bases for *adhesions*.

References

Specific references for the subject material of this chapter are included in subsequent chapters that cover the specific organs.

16: Musculoskeletal System

General Characteristics

Form and Function. All of the basic tissues contribute to the formation of this system. Bone gives support as well as serving as points of attachment against which the muscles operate to perform work. Skeletal muscle is the means by which the contractility of the fibers is converted into the work involved in support and locomotion. Dense white fibrous connective tissue in ligaments and tendons provide attachment of bone to bone and muscle to bone. Cartilage facilitates growth as well as serving as the substrate for bone to bone contact (articular surfaces). The proper connective tissues bind various parts of the system together and allow for the passage of blood vessels, lymphatics, and nerves.

Bone as an Organ

Physical Properties of Bone

Density and Composition. The *density* of bone is the basis of many of its mechanical properties. Density is usually reported as the mass/unit volume of fully hydrated, defatted bone. The density of compact bone normally is in the range of 1.9–2.1. Trabecular bone is approximately 15% less dense than compact bone. These figures actually represent the density of the osseous tissue. The methods used compensate for any discontinuities (osteonal canals, communicating canals, interosseous space) in the bone.

The mineral content of bone contributes to bone density. Although the mineral content is usually reported maximally as 69% of the defatted dry weight, variations occur. Newly formed bone, which is incompletely mineralized, is *low density bone*, whereas older bone that may approach complete mineralization is *high density bone*.

The ash content of a bone is the inorganic residue following the incineration of a bone sample. *Ash/unit volume* is generally 69% of the defatted dry weight. Calcium is about 25% and phosphorus is about 12% of the defatted dry weight. Carbonate, sodium, magnesium, chloride, and trace elements are present also.

A reduction in bone mass without a change in ash content is a quantitative change in bone. This quantitative change results from increased remodeling. The skeletal mass is reduced but the quality of the bone is maintained normally in the *quantitative osteopenias—osteoporosis.* **A reduction in ash content with or without a decrease in bone mass indicates a qualitative change in bone.** The *qualitative osteopenias (rickets, osteomalacia)* are manifested as incompletely, inappropriately, or nonmineralized osteoid. Osteoid seams are thickened and/or increased in number.

Bone density Radiographic Density

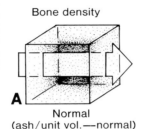
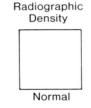
A
Normal
(ash/unit vol.—normal)
Normal

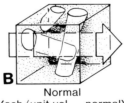
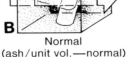

B
Normal
(ash/unit vol.—normal)
Normal
(< sample A)

C
< Normal
(ash/unit vol. < normal
< Normal

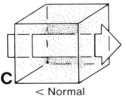
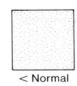
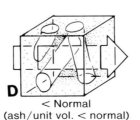
D
< Normal
(ash/unit vol. < normal)
≪ Normal

Bone density is not equivalent to radiographic density. Radiographic density is equivalent to *tissue density.* The radiographic manifestation of tissue density is the sum of all tissue densities present at a particular locus (Fig. 16.1).

Piezoelectricity. Bone has the ability to react to mechanical energy by first converting (transducing) the energy into a useable signal (stimulus). The transducer property of bone is a function of the highly ordered, crystalline nature of hydroxyapatite and the ordered arrangement of collagen. The transduced information is in the form of electrical energy that affects the cells' electrical environment and controls their behavior. Presumably, the generation of an

Figure 16.1. A series of diagrams comparing bone density, ash/unit volume and radiographic density. *A.* A cube of dense cortical bone has a normal density that translates radiographically as a specified amount of radiolucency or radiodensity. The ash/unit volume is normal. *B.* A cube of bone, despite numerous vacuities (osteonal canals, resorption spaces, Volkmann's canals), has a normal bone density and a normal ash/unit volume. These parameters are typical of quantitative bone changes. The same parameters could apply to a cube of bone obtained from trabecular bone in which the cavities represent the interosseous spaces associated with cancellous bone. The bone density of these types of samples would be normal. The radiographic density of sample *B* would be less than that of sample *A.* The radiographic density under these circumstances could represent normalcy or abnormal circumstances, depending upon the amount of bone loss that had occurred. *C.* A cube of bone similar to sample *A* may not contain the proper amount of mineral. Such changes are characteristic of qualitative changes in bone. The bone density and ash/unit volume would be less than normal and distinguishable from the parameters for samples *A* and *B.* The radiographic density of sample *C* would be similar and indistinguishable from the radiographic density of sample *B.* *D.* A cube of bone with decreased mineral (qualitative change) and increased cavities and/or increased interosseous spaces (quantitative change) would have a low bone density and low ash/unit volume. The decreased bone density results from the qualitative change, not the quantitative change. The radiographic density of sample *D* would be much less than normal. Based upon radiographic density only, it is impossible to distinguish between samples *B,* *C* and *D.*

electrical potential results from a separation of charge through the movement of ions. This generation of electrical potential in response to mechanical stimulation is termed *piezoelectricity*. It explains the predictable responsiveness of bone to mechanical loading (Fig. 16.2).

Biomechanical Properties of Bone

Stress and Strain. The magnitude, direction, duration, and rate at which a force *(stress)* is applied to bone influences its responsiveness. The stress may be sufficient to fracture the structure or may alter its three-dimensional relationship to the rest of the skeletal mass. Bone responds to applied stress by developing *strain* within it. The strain is a measure of the deformation that occurs in the structure. If the strain results in an elongation of the structure, then the strain is *tensile*. If the strain results in a shortening of the structure, then it is *compressive*. *Flexure, shearing,* and *torque* are influential stresses, also.

The collagenous fibers of bone impart the tensile strength, whereas the hydroxyapatite crystals impart the compressive strength. **Since the compressive properties of bone are greater than the tensile properties, bone fracture generally occurs in tension.**

Flexure-Drift Relationships. The application of a flexural stress of sufficient magnitude to bone may cause the structure to bend (Fig. 16.3). When this occurs, compressive strain is developed along the concave surface, whereas a tensile strain is developed upon the convex surface. If the flexural force were repeated and/or maintained for a protracted period of time, then the bone would drift through space toward the concave surface (Fig. 16.4). This movement is predicated upon a separation of charge resulting from piezoelectricity. Osteoblastic activity occurs on the compressive or concave surface in association with a negative potential. Osteoclastic activity occurs on the tensile or convex surface in association with a positive potential.

This type of osseous spatial adjustment does occur under various circumstances. The autocorrection of misaligned fracture fragments, the osseous remodeling associated with the sub-luxation and luxation of joints, or any other alteration in normal weight-bearing result from this mechanism. This does not imply that bones with natural curvatures will eventually assume a straightened configuration.

Adaptive bone behavior is dependent upon intermittent deformation and the generation of strain within the organs. High strain rates (vigorous activity) are more potent stimuli for adaptive behavior than less vigorous activity. The amount of periosteal remodeling activity is proportional to the strain generated. Endosteal remodeling activity increases whether the strain increases or decreases.

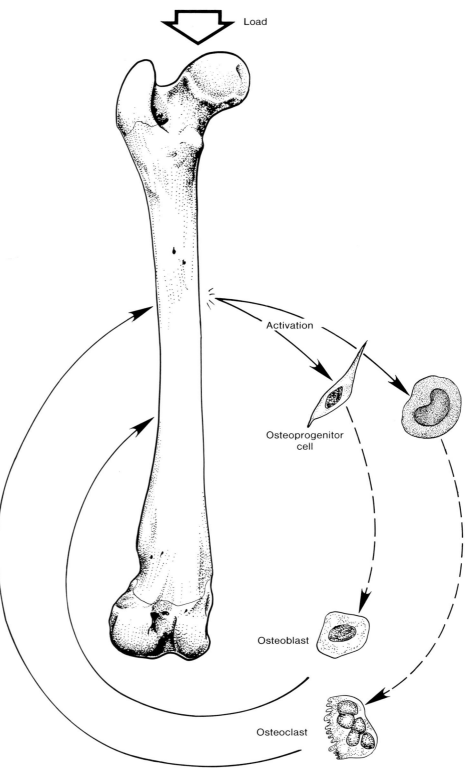

Figure 16.2. A diagram indicating the responsiveness of bone to mechanical stimuli. The loading of a bone, especially manifested if the loading is abnormal, activates osteoprogenitor cells and macrophages within the osseous envelopes. The activation of these cells determines the type of response—formation or resorption—manifested by the organ.

Cartilage and Bone Modeling. Stress influences growth plate orientation, columnation of cells within the plate, and the responsiveness of the growth plate to al-

tered stress patterns. Two types of growth plates or growth cartilage configurations exist in developing bones (Fig. 16.5). One is a *pressure growth plate (compression*

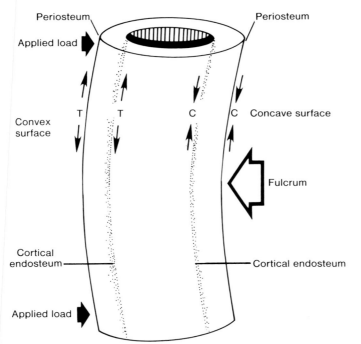

Figure 16.3. A diagram demonstrating the type of strain developed within a loaded living bone. The loading of the bone as indicated induces compressive strain along the concave surface and tensile strain along the convex surface. The tension and compression are greatest along the periosteal surfaces.

growth plate, pressure epiphysis) that is subject generally to compressive forces. The capital femoral growth plate and epiphysis are good examples. The other is a *tension growth plate (tension epiphysis, traction epiphysis)* that is subject generally to tensile forces. The greater trochanter of the femur is a good example of a traction epiphysis.

The application of normal, even and sustained compression upon pressure growth plates results in the even growth of the plate and the proper spatial orientation of the bone. These plates, however, are differentially responsive to compression. Increased compression within the "normal range" accelerates growth of the plate, whereas an increased compression in the "abnormal range" retards growth of the plate. An uneven and sustained loading of a bone surface can result in an altered spatial orientation of the growth plate and associated articular surface.

These principles can be used to correct angular limb deformities (Fig. 16.6). Some foals are born with angular limb deformities of the carpus (and other joints) in which the distal portion of the limb projects laterad (carpus valgus). If the problem is attributable to the distal radial growth plate, then the principles of growth plate response

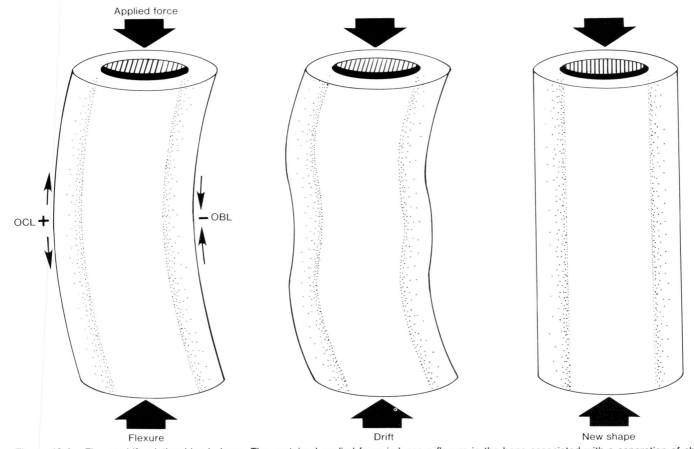

Figure 16.4. Flexure-drift relationships in bone. The sustained applied force induces a flexure in the bone associated with a separation of charge (biopotential). The concave surface, associated with compression, drifts as a result of osteoblastic *(OBL)* activity. The surface under tension, the convex surface, drifts as a result of osteoclastic *(OCL)* activity. The new shape of the bone results from the predictable activity of bone cells under the specified loading conditions. Bones will drift toward the concave surface.

to compression are applicable. A nonexpandable fixation device is bridged across the medial aspect of the distal radial physis and is anchored in the adjacent metaphysis and epiphysis. As the plate continues to grow, it is assumed that nonphysiological compressive forces retard the growth of the plate on that side. The lateral aspect of the plate continues to grow normally and eventually the lateral growth compensates with a resultant correction of the limb. The fixation device is then removed.

Hemicircumferential periosteal elevation is a technique that is used effectively to correct the type of angulation deformities just discussed. In a carpus valgus deformity, an inverted T incision is made over the lateral aspect of the distal radial metaphysis and the periosteum is elevated. This procedure, *alone* or in conjunction with transphyseal fixation, corrects the angular deformity. The mechanism by which this technique accomplishes the correction is not understood. A plausible explanation follows: The longitudinal fibers of the periosteum are anchored in each growth plate at the perichondral ring. The stress on these fibers during growth is manifested as tension within the growth plate. Excision and elevation of the periosteum as described releases the growth plate from the inhibitory effects of tension.

Biological Properties of Bone

Dynamic Properties. The biological behavioral properties of bone are: **endochondral ossification, remodeling, modeling, repair**, and **calcium metabolism**. Modeling and fracture repair are discussed herein.

The long bones move through space in three dimensions as they grow (Fig. 16.7). This growth phenomenon is, of course, the result of integrated cellular and tissue activity. The growth plate is responsible for elongation. The final three-dimensional configuration of the distal and proximal heads results from the activities of the secondary ossification centers. The periosteum is responsible for the thickening or centrifugal growth of the diaphysis, whereas the endosteum is responsible for the thinning of the diaphysis. These two envelopes result in *osseous drift*, the three-dimensional movement of the diaphysis through space. Numerous factors influence the activity at the growth plate and diaphysis. *Modeling* is the response of these activities to varied influencing factors and results in the definitive form of a bone.

The growth plate is an example of a joint between two bones, those of the epiphysis and diaphysis. This type of joint is a *synchondrosis* (Fig. 16.8). Coincident with skeletal maturation, the cartilage of the growth plate is replaced totally by bone. This *synchondrosis* then becomes a *synostosis*. This transition represents the completion of bone elongation. At closure, the balance of activity favors the total replacement of the cartilage with bone.

Vascular, Neural, and Lymphatic Com- **ponents of Bone.** The primary sources of blood supply to a typical long bone are the *nutrient artery, metaphyseal arteries, epi-*

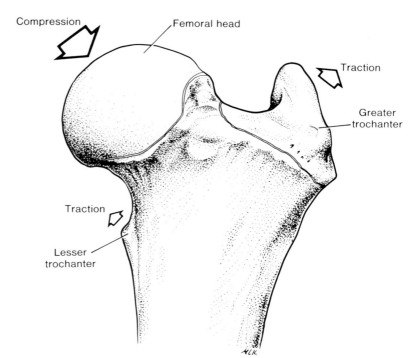

Figure 16.5. A diagram depicting pressure and traction epiphyses of the proximal femur.

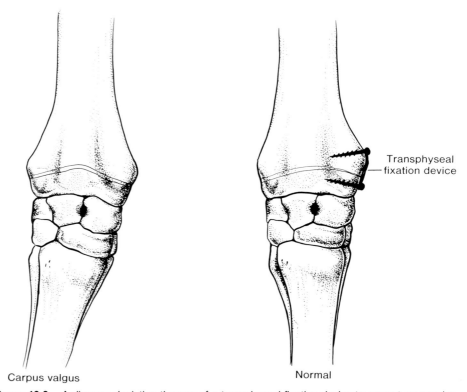

Figure 16.6. A diagram depicting the use of a transphyseal fixation device to correct an angular limb deformity in a foal attributable to an altered growth rate in the distal radial physis. Nonphysiological compression retards the physis after the application of the devise. The lateral side, growing normally, straightens the limb. If the device were not removed after straightening, then a medial deviation would result.

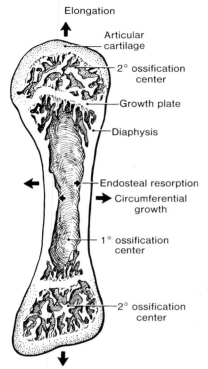

Elongation

Articular cartilage

2° ossification center

Growth plate

Diaphysis

Endosteal resorption

Circumferential growth

1° ossification center

2° ossification center

Figure 16.7. The growth of a long bone. The growth plate is responsible for elongation. The periosteum adds new bone, whereas the cortical endosteum removes bone. These combined activities result in circumferential growth of the diaphysis and enlargement of the marrow cavity.

physeal arteries, periosteal arteries. The relationships of some of these vessels vary slightly but significantly in growing and mature bones (Fig. 16.9).

The *nutrient artery* and vein enter the shaft of the long bone through an oblique canal. Upon entrance into the marrow cavity, proximal and distal divisions branch throughout this cavity. This vessel and its branches are the primary blood supply to the marrow cavity. Some of these branches are incorporated into the cortical endosteum, penetrate the cortex, and become osteonal vessels of at least the inner two-thirds of the cortex. Proximal and distal branches of the nutrient artery eventually anastomose with the metaphyseal arteries.

Metaphyseal arteries and veins gain access to the marrow cavity through numerous small foramina located in the compact bone of the proximal and distal metaphyses. These vessels anastomose with nutrient arterial branches and form capillary loops in association with the osseous replacement that characteries development in the metaphyses. **A dual circulation characterizes the vascular supply to the growth plate. Capillary loops, as branches of anastomotic nutrient and metaphyseal vessels, are one-half of the dual circulatory pattern. The capillary extensions of epiphyseal arteries are the other half.** The metaphyseal capillary loops support the osseous replacement activity of the primary ossifi-

cation center, the epiphyseal capillaries provide nutrition to the growth plate.

Numerous *epiphyseal arteries* and veins enter the epiphyses (secondary ossification centers) through many small foramina in the compact bone. These vessels mimic the supportive role of the anastomotic vessels of the primary ossification center. Additionally, this vascular bed supplies the nutritional needs of the proliferative zone of the growth plate cartilage. Before growth plate closure, the epiphyseal capillary beds are independent of the capillary loops of the primary ossification center. Upon closure of the growth plate, the epiphyseal vessels anastomose with the vessels of the primary ossification center.

The method of entry of epiphyseal vessels into the epiphyses varies with the dispositon of the articular cartilage over the epiphyses (Fig. 16.10). Epiphyseal vessels generally enter the epiphyses through the perichondral ring. In those epiphyses in which there is a discontinuity between the articular cartilage and the growth plate, the epiphyseal arteries perforate the area of discontinuity to gain access to the epiphysis. The first configuration may subject the epiphyseal region to vascular compromise when trauma results in a fractured growth plate.

Periosteal arterioles enter the cortical bone at points of heavy fascial attachments. **Under these circumstances, these vessels are the vascular supply to the outer one-third of the cortex. The outer cortex is supplied by vessels derived from the medullary cavity in regions in which the cortex is overlaid by loosely attached periosteum.** This pattern is generally typical of those bones that develop from endochondral ossification and have more than one ossification center. Minor deviations from this pattern occur in specific bones.

The venous drainage is similar to the afferent blood supply. The metaphysis is drained by numerous *metaphyseal veins.* In regions of the cortex supplied only by the medullary arteries (regions of the cortex beneath loosely attached periosteum), *cortical venous channels* drain the deep cortex and *periosteal venous channels* drain the superficial cortex. Cortical regions beneath heavy fascial attachments are drained similarly. The medullary cavity is also drained directly to the outside by *emissary veins* that perforate the osseous substance, as well as by the *nutrient vein.*

The presence of lymphatic vessels within bone has never been demonstrated satisfactorily; however, lymphatics occur within the periosteum.

Similarly, the innervation of bone remains an enigma. Nerves have been demonstrated within the marrow cavity and within osteonal canals. These poorly myelinated fibers probably are postganglionic vasomotor fibers of the sympathetic nerv-

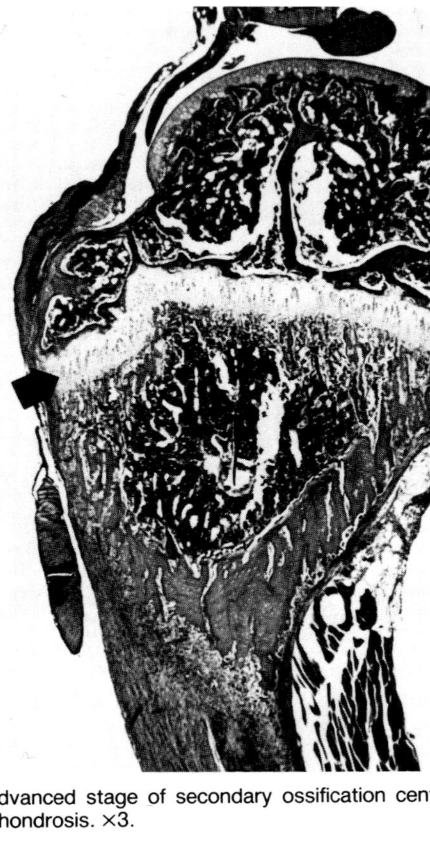

Figure 16.8. Advanced stage of secondary ossification center development. The growth plate *(arrow)* is a synchondrosis. ×3.

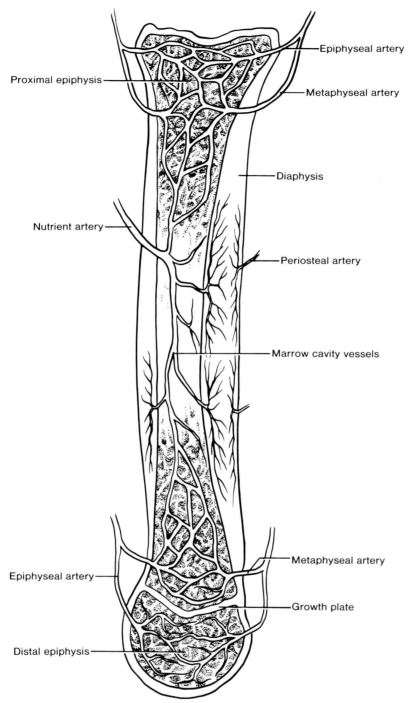

Figure 16.9. Diagram of the typical blood supply to a long bone. Before growth plate closure, the epiphyseal and metaphyseal vasculature is separate. After closure, these vessels anastomose.

ous system. The modality of pain is associated with the nerve endings that occur in the fibrous coverings of bones (periosteum, fibrous joint capsule).

Vascular Relationships—Functional Correlates. The integrity of the blood supply is essential for the maintenance of normal structure and function. Alterations to the venous drainage can have profound effects upon bone.

Muscular activity is an important component of the mechanisms of osseous vascular integrity. The contraction of muscles temporarily occludes venous channels and elevates bone marrow vascular pressure. This pump-like action of muscles is important to vascular drainage and bone structure. Prolonged immobilization of limbs during fracture repair is associated with a reduction in bone mass (quantitative osteo-

penia) proximal and distal to the fracture site.

The removal of the periosteum at points of heavy fascial attachments, either naturally or during surgical intervention, can devitalize the outer one-third of the cortex locally. The revascularization of the region from the medullary vessels should insure that devascularization problems are temporary.

In adult bones, the epiphyseal-metaphyseal-nutrient arterial anastomoses ensure that damage to one of these components has no adverse effects upon bone. Because of the anastomosis of the metaphyseal and nutrient arterial supply, few problems are anticipated when one or the other of these vessels is disrupted during growth. Disruption of the epiphyseal vessels during growth, however, can result in premature closure of the growth plate or epiphyseal *avascular necrosis.*

Fracture Repair

General Features

Influential Factors

Introduction. Fractures are loss of osseous structural integrity. Attendant changes may alter normal function, may cause a loss of function, or may affect changes elsewhere that may be symptomatic of the fracture. Fractures, however, may be accompanied by no apparent loss of normal function. Although various management procedures are utilized to facilitate repair, there are only a few ways that bone as an organ will respond to fracture. Normal repair is achieved by *primary intention* or *secondary intention* mechanisms.

Factors Influencing Repair. Nutritional and metabolic factors influence bone. A well-balanced *diet* is an essential repair component. All of the essential nutrients, some vitamins, and many minerals are necessary for the proper synthesis and maintainence of the organic and inorganic matrix of bone. The *age* of the animal is a contributing factor. Older animals tend to have a lower osteogenic activity than their younger counterparts. Similarly, the presence of intercurrent *disease* processes may alter the process. *Infection,* either naturally induced during the impact stage or introduced iatrogenically during the manipulation of the fracture, has a devastating influence upon repair.

Stability and Vasculature. Three other factors significantly affect the outcome of the fracture repair process: **the stability and immobilization of the fracture site during the repair process; the maintenance of good vascular integrity; the ability to return the fracture fragments to their original relationships (reduction).** These are factors over which the practitioner generally exercises some influence.

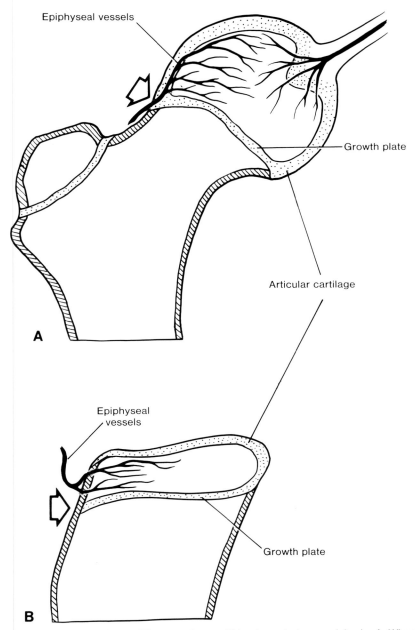

Figure 16.10. A diagram of two different patterns of blood supply to an epiphysis. *A.* When the articular cartilage covers the articular surface entirely and is continuous with the growth plate, the epiphyseal vessels enter the epiphysis by traversing the perichondral ring at the periphery of the physis *(arrow)*. Fractures of the physis or neck can disrupt the vascular supply. *B.* When an epiphysis is covered partially with articular cartilage, the epiphyseal vessels enter the epiphysis at the gap *(arrow)*. These vessels are less apt to be disrupted from growth plate fractures. (Redrawn and modified from Dale, G. G. and Harris, W. J.: Prognosis of epiphyseal separation. J. Bone Joint Surg. *40(B)*:116, 1958).

pliant nature of such skeletons generally leads to greenstick fractures. Optimal mineralization is generally associated with a young adult skeleton.

The amount of cortical or cancellous bone influences the mechanical properties of the organ. The rate at which a load is applied to cortical bone affects its ability to resist the load. Also, cortical bone manifests its strongest properties when loaded parallel to its long axis. The mechanical properties of cancellous bone differ from those of compact bone. As each spicule of the cancellous bone fractures, the total specimen becomes weaker until ultimate failure occurs.

The ability to absorb compressive energy is about twice as large as the ability to absorb tensile energy. Therefore, **bones tend to fail in tension.** Rigid internal fixation is generally applied to the tension band side of a bone for this reason.

Stages of Fracture Repair

The process of fracture repair is a continuum of cellular events that progresses from the insult (impact) through the successful remodeling of the injured site. It is useful to divide the process into distinctive yet interrelated stages based upon the predominant activity apparent. The stages of fracture repair are: *Impact, Induction, Inflammation, Repair,* and *Remodeling.*

Impact Stage. A sufficient amount of energy must be absorbed by the bone to result in failure. The direction, magnitude, and rate of bone loading interact with numerous biological properties to result in diverse fractures. This stage may be characterized by no loss of function or varying degrees of impaired function. Hemorrhage and the natural sequelae to injury may be anticipated. An increased sympathetic discharge may occur. Devitalization of hard and soft tissue results; this may be accompanied by contamination or infection.

Induction Stage. The identification of this stage as a separate and distinct entity is probably articifial, because the events of this stage occur throughout the repair process. Identifying this stage, however, does point to its significance. Cells must be induced to differentiate into various new cellular populations. Vascular changes, tissue hypoxia, and related increases in hydrogen ion concentrations locally are probably stimulatory. Alterations to this stage may lead to delayed union or nonunion.

Inflammatory Stage. This stage, initiated immediately after the insult, results from the disrupted vasculature, the attendant hemorrhage, and resulting hematoma. Hypoxia and acidosis are significant features of the microenvironment. The resultant necrosis is sufficient stimulation for invasion by inflammatory cells. The processes of migration, chemotaxis, recognition, opson-

Osseous Factors. Bone is not a homogeneous, biological, building material. It consists of diverse components, each of which affects directly its biomechanical properties prior to, during, and after the fracture repair.

Intermolecular cross-linking of collagen is the essential feature of the macromolecule that accounts for its tensile properties. Defects in collagen metabolism related to reduced cross-linkage reduce the tensile

properties of bone. Age changes in bone are accompanied by an increased amount of collagenous cross-linkages. Such changes, associated with increased mineralization as well, tend to make older bones more stiff than younger bones. Older bones, therefore, are more brittle than younger bones.

Skeletal mineralization is not homogeneous. Young bones are less mineralized than their older counterparts. The com-

ization and phagocytosis are performed by the invading inflammatory cells.

Inflammation is an essential feature of fracture repair; devitalized tissue is removed and the hematoma is reorganized and removed also. If inflammation does not occur, then repair cannot be achieved. If inflammation is excessive, then repair may be protracted or not accomplished. This typically occurs with infected fracture repair sites *(osteomyelitis)*. Insufficient inflammatory reactions can also protract the repair process.

Reparative Stage. This stage involves activities that progress from induction through inflammation and result in the formation of callus. The events of this stage lead to the restoration of anatomical continuity between the fracture fragments. This stage, too, is an artificial division of events, because repair continues throughout the entire process.

Remodeling. Stimulated bone metabolic units are responsible for the reorganization of the osseous tissue during repair. Complete success results in the fracture site not being identifiable with radiographic or histological techniques.

Types of Repair Mechanisms

Direct and Indirect Bone Formation. Although the fracture repair process can be a complicated event, it is, in its simplest form, a reiteration of events studied previously. Repair mechanisms involve three fundamental biologic activities of bone: *remodeling, intramembranous ossification, and endochondral ossification.* The circumstances associated with the repair process dictate which of these mechanisms, singly or in combination, will mediate the fracture repair process.

Primary intention healing is direct bone formation during the repair process involving remodeling and intramembranous ossification. Second intention healing is indirect bone formation that involves the three mechanisms.

The two examples used to describe primary and secondary intention healing of bone must be considered stereotypical. Many variations of these basic themes exist. Moreover, a single fracture may be characterized by both primary and second intention healing.

Primary Intention Healing

General Characteristics. *Primary intention healing* is characterized by the direct formation of bone without the formation of an extensive, intermediary, cartilaginous, supportive structure *(callus)*. This description is based upon the following assumptions: vascular integrity is good, immobilization is excellent, reduction of the two fragments is excellent and the ends of the fractured fragments are smooth. Rigid fixation, immobilization, and reduction of

the fracture site are achieved by the application of a metallic plate across the fracture site.

Contact Repair

Mechanism. Contact repair is the simplest form of fracture repair that is performed by the body (Fig. 16.11). The general circumstances associated with primary intention healing are operable. **Remodeling is the mechanism responsible for contact repair.**

Soft tissue injury and inflammation occur after the impact. As a result of the fracture, vascular channels within the bone are disrupted. This results in the death of bone cells (osteoprogenitors, osteoblasts, osteocytes) and endothelial cells some distance from the ends of the fracture fragments. Accordingly, the fracture site is bordered by dead bone to the level of the first viable anastomosis with functional vessels. Proliferation of numerous perivascular and endothelial cells occurs within the viable bone adjacent to the dead bone bordering the fracture site. The events that result from the insult are stimulatory to the basic metabolic units (BMUs). The cells of these units and new vessels grow toward the fracture site. Eventually, osteoclasts begin to remove bone from the osteonal canals in the same manner described with remodeling. The cutting cones cross the fracture site and establish the basis for the formation of new osteons. Osteoblasts fill the canals with lamellar bone and establish continuity between the fracture fragments by bridging the small gap with new (secondary) osteons. The situation is analogous to drilling holes (resorption spaces) in a piece of wood and using dowels (secondary osteons) to hold the wood together.

The side of the bone opposite the plate may be the site for the formation of a small periosteal callus. The size and extent of the callus relates to the stability of that portion of the fracture.

Gap Repair

Mechanism. Small spaces (gaps) may remain between the fracture fragments, because rigid fixation may be achieved without perfect reduction of the gap. This may occur when the fragments are fractured irregularly. Then, the space will fill temporarily with woven bone that serves as a spot weld between the fragments. **Intramembranous ossification and remodeling are the processes used to achieve fracture repair under this circumstance.** Canalization and new osteon formation occurs subsequently as described with contact repair. This process may be compared to the union of two pieces of wood with dowels in which irregularities between the pieces of wood must be filled with wood putty. Contact and gap repair commonly occur simultaneously. A comminuted fracture with a

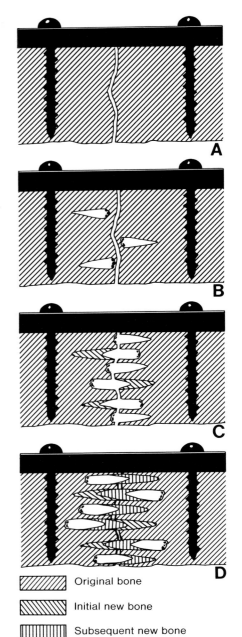

Original bone

Initial new bone

Subsequent new bone

Figure 16.11. Stylized diagrams of the sequence of events of gap type of primary intention healing of bone in which rigid internal fixation was achieved with screws and a bone plate. After the open reduction of the fracture site *(A)*, osteonal remodeling units become activated *(B)*. The remodeling units cross the gap and establish a basis for osteonal bridging of the fracture site *(C)*. The cutting cones form the cavity in which initial new bone formation occurs. The process continues *(D)* until new bone subsequently bridges the gap. Regions in the fracture gap between remodeling units may be "spot welded" with woven bone. The new osteons result in fracture repair having been achieved.

large butterfly fragment, if rigidly immobilized as described previously, will use both mechanisms of primary intention healing.

Second Intention Healing

Introduction. Second intention healing involves the formation of an external supportive structure of cartilage, *callus*, during repair. It is the type of repair expected when casts, pins, and other devices are used. **This repair sequence occurs when vascular integrity may have been compromised, immobilization and stability of the fracture site are not perfect, and reduction has not been achieved perfectly.** For the sake of clarification, the following description assumes that the previously described conditions relating to instability and reduction pertain to a closed, transverse, noncomminuted fracture in which the fracture fragments are smooth and fixation is achieved externally. **Intramembranous ossification, endochondral ossification, and remodeling are the contributing mechanisms through which repair is achieved.** The repair sequence is diagrammed in Figures 16.12–16.17.

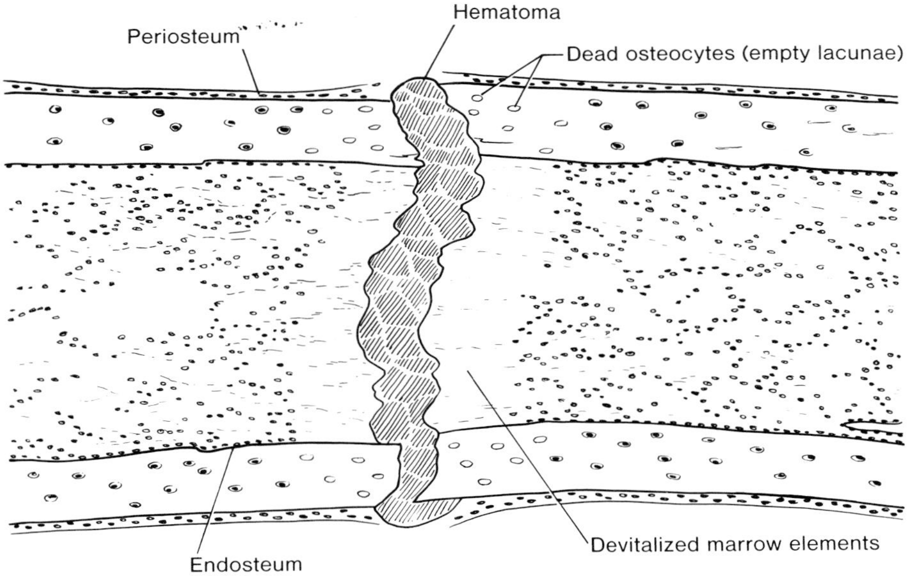

Impact Stage

Consequences of Fracture. The energy absorbed upon impact is responsible for the type and extent of damage manifested. Because of their physical characteristics, bones fracture more readily with rapid loading than with slow loading. The impact accounts for loss of osseous continuity and attendant soft tissue damage usually associated with such phenomena (Fig. 16.12). This results in the devitalization of the tissues by disrupting vascular beds. Clot formation exacerbates the vascular damage of the soft and hard tissues. Periosteal and marrow elements, endosteal components, and bone die back on either side of the fracture to the level of the first functional vascular anastomosis. Bone death is evidenced by the degeneration of osteocytes and empty osteocytic lacunae.

Induction Stage

Initiation and Maintenance. The significance of this stage was discussed previously.

Inflammatory Stage

Onset and Extent. This stage was described previously (Fig. 16.13). Classically, this stage ends when the cardinal signs of inflammation (redness, pain, swelling, and heat) are no longer apparent.

Reparative Stage

Induction Through Callus Formation. This stage involves numerous cellular activities that are initiated with induction, progress through inflammation, and ultimately end with callus formation. As the hematoma is reorganized and invaded by phagocytic and fibroblastic cells, the osseous envelopes are characterized by extensive mitotic activity of osteogenic and entothelial cells (Fig. 16.13). New cells and blood vessels from the endosteum migrate toward

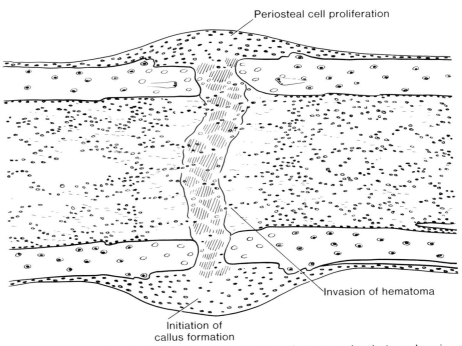

Figure 16.12. Hematoma formation after fracture. Refer to the text for a complete description of the events involved in the fracture repair sequence as represented in Figures 16.12–16.17. (Figures 16.12–16.17 were based upon, modified and expanded from the descriptions by Ham, A. W. and Harris, W. R.: Repair and transplantation of bone. *In*: Bourne, G. H. (ed.): *The Biochemistry and Physiology of Bone*, Vol. III, pp. 337–399, Academic Press, New York, 1971.)

Figure 16.13. Induction of cells from the marrow cavity, periosteum, and endosteum. Invasion of the hematoma has occurred and callus formation is initiated.

the fracture site, invade the hematoma and bridge the gap with a fibrocellular, hyperplastic tissue that eventually forms bone (Fig. 16.13). This tissue is the precursor of the bone that forms within the marrow cavity and within the gap between the fracture fragments. The new osseous tissue (woven bone) derived from the endosteum is called the *internal (endosteal) callus* (Fig. 16.14).

Concomitant with the endosteal events, the cells of the periosteum proliferate and produce a hypercellular mass that differentiates into bone and cartilage. These new cartilaginous and osseous tissues (woven bone) constitute the *external (periosteal) callus* (Fig. 16.14).

Callus Formation. *Callus* is the new tissue that forms around, between, within, and adjacent to the fracture site. The formation of callus actually begins with the formation of the expansive, hyperplastic, and fibrocellular tissue that forms from the osseous envelopes and ends with the deposition of bone across the fracture gap. Many terms are used to describe callus: *internal (endosteal), external (periosteal), bridging, permanent, provisional, temporary, soft and hard callus.* Despite the numerous names for this entity, only one callus forms in association with fracture repair. It changes character as the fibrocellular tissue from which it originates develops into bone, proliferates, and is eventually remodeled.

External Callus. Proliferation of the osteogenic cells of the periosteum occurs initially within an adequate vascular environment. As a result, they produce new periosteal bone along the margin of the fracture some distance removed from the fracture gap. This osteogenic activity culminates in *periosteal new bone formation.* Eventually, this proliferating layer of cells bridges the fracture gap and forms a thickened cellular layer peripheral to the regressing hematoma. It is believed that the osteogenic cells in this region are proliferating faster than their associated periosteal vessels. Accordingly, they differentiate into chondroblasts. Thus, the *external callus* consists of new bone peripherally and cartilage adjacent to the fracture gap. These tissues are covered peripherally by the periosteum (Fig. 16.15). As the cartilaginous mass continues to grow by appositional and interstitial mechanisms, it becomes further separated from its vascular supply. The chondrocytes along the cartilage/bone interface hypertrophy and their associated matrix becomes mineralized. From within outward from this interface, there is a progression from calcified cartilage, hypertrophic chondrocytes, maturing chondrocytes, and proliferating cells. Vascular invasion and osseous replacement are initiated at the cartilage/bone interface. These events continue until the cartilaginous mass is replaced by woven bone. This process is a reiteration of endochondral ossification.

The formation of an external callus under these circumstances of repair indicates that the repair process is progressing normally; in other circumstances the external callus is indicative of complications to repair that may lead to *delayed union* or *nonunion.* **The primary function of the external callus is the stabilization of the fracture site.** The actual repair of the fracture site is achieved via the endosteal callus.

Internal Callus. The *internal (endosteal) callus* is the new tissue that develops from the endosteal envelopes and is responsible for the actual repair of the fracture (Figs. 16.14 and 16.15). These events occur simultaneously with those events described for the periosteum. Proliferating cells from the trabecular and cortical endosteum invade the regressing hematoma. These cells form bone that attaches to the inner surface of the bone on one side of the fracture. The tissue bridges the gap and becomes continuous with bone on the other side of the fracture. There are two significant features of the internal callus. **Bone forms directly without a cartilaginous intermediary.** Also, **the internal callus is the tissue through which actual repair of the fracture is achieved.**

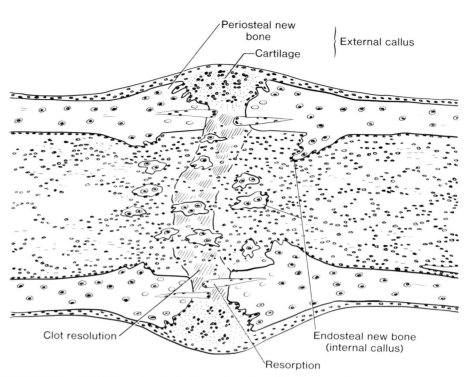

Figure 16.14. Periosteal and endosteal bone formation at the fracture site. Bone formation in the callus is intiated.

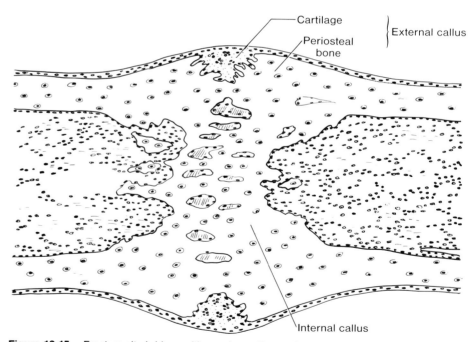

Figure 16.15. Fracture site bridges with new bone. External and internal callus is established.

Remodeling Stage

Resolution. The formation of the internal and external callus results in the deposition of cancellous woven bone. Progressive appositional growth converts this tissue configuration into dense cancellous and compact bone (Fig. 16.15). The new bone that is formed at or adjacent to the fracture site is bonded to dead and live bone. At this point in repair, the marrow cavity may be occluded with bone, the fracture gap is filled with bone and the fracture is surrounded by an expanded sleeve of bone. Osteoclastic activity is responsible for removal of the surplus bone (Fig. 16.16). Simultaneously, remodeling activity, as described with primary intention healing, produces new osteons that traverse the fracture site. Eventually, only the cortical bone of the diaphysis remains (Fig. 16.17).

Circumstances of Repair

"Simply placing feline bones in the same room is enough to bring about repair" is an an expression of the ease with which repair is achieved in this species. While such a statement certainly applies to a cat, similar statements may be made about other species. Some bones, as well as certain regions of specific bones, heal more easily than others. Return of the involved anatomical unit to as near perfect function as possible is the most important consideration.

Reduction. The return of the fracture fragments to the prefracture configuration is termed reduction. Three circumstances are part of the reduction process—distraction, displacement, angulation. *Distraction* implies that the reduction has not been perfect, because a gap remains between the fracture fragments. Perfect reduction of distracted fragments is difficult to achieve clinically. The gap should never exceed one-half the diameter of the distracted fragments. The general prognosis for successful repair decreases as the gap increases. Under circumstances of rigid immobilization, the primary problem is requiring the osseous system to create new bone within the gap. Cancellous bone grafts may have to be used when fragments are distracted markedly. Such grafts provide a temporary scaffold upon which new bone formation occurs. *Displacement* is the improper registration of the fracture fragments in such a way that the cortices and marrow cavity are not perfectly aligned. Small overlaps still permit repair to be achieved. Flexure-drift principles usually apply to the correction of minor displacement problems. Return to normal function, however, can be delayed with improperly registered fragments. *Angulation* between the fracture fragments will not alter the repair process, even if the fragments are at a 45° angle to each other. Repair can be achieved under these circumstances; however, return to clinical function will be virtually impossible. Angulations problems less than 20° repair nor-

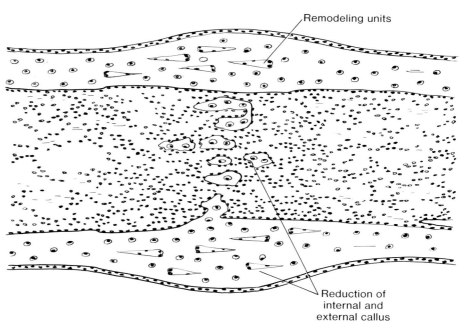

Figure 16.16. Remodeling of internal and external callus. The bone mass is reduced and remodeled.

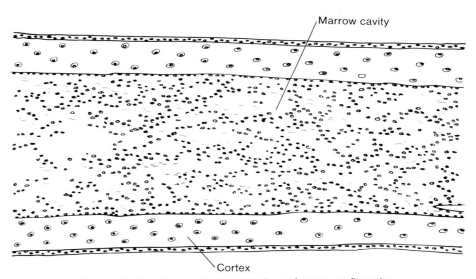

Figure 16.17. Return of the bone to the prefracture configuration.

mally and autocorrect by flexure-drift mechanisms.

Strength of Fractures. The flexural strength of a cylindrical object is defined mathematically. The rectangular moment of inertia, I_o, is a measurement of the resistance of such an object to flexural stresses, accordingly: $I_o = \frac{1}{4} \pi r^4$. Since all values on the right side of the equation, except the radius (r), are constants, the rigidity or resistance of a cylindrical object to flexural stress is a function of the fourth power of the radius. Doubling the radius results in a sixteen-fold increase in flexural strength. Periosteal callus, therefore, increases the flexural strength of a fracture during the repair process.

The area of contact between fracture fragments also has an effect upon the strength of the fracture site. The strength of the fracture site increases as the square of the area ($a = \pi r^2$). Biologically, larger surface areas are associated with larger cellular populations. For this reason, metaphyseal fractures heal faster than diaphyseal fractures.

Articulations

General Characteristics

The means by which two or more bones are joined together are called joints or articulations. These structures are modified morphologically to serve various functions, all of which relate directly or indirectly to weight-bearing, locomotion, and stability.

Composition and Classification. Bones are held together or connected by various connective tissues. Some joints may consist only of a single connective tissue type, whereas others may consist of more than one connective tissue. The following tissues may contribute to the formation of articulations: hyaline cartilage, fibrocartilage, dense white fibrous connective tissue (DWFCT), loose connective tissue, bone, and adipose tissue. The most widely accepted classification scheme is that predicated upon the predominant type of tissue characteristic of the joint: *fibrous, cartilaginous, osseous and synovial joints.*

Fibrous joints are those formed by DWFCT; whereas, cartilaginous joints consist typically of hyaline and/or fibrous cartilage. Osseous joints consist of bone. Synovial joints, however, consist of most or all of the tissues previously mentioned as contributing to articulations.

Functions. The following functions are ascribed generally to joints: *stabilize and unite two or more bones without movement; stabilize and unite two or more bones with some movement; facilitate movement between two or more bones; facilitate the growth of bones; resist the predominant stress manifested at a joint surface.* Joints may subserve one, a combination of, or all of these functions simultaneously.

Types of Articulations

Fibrous, Cartilaginous, and Osseous Joints

Syndesmosis. A *syndesmosis* is the union of bone surfaces by DWFCT. This is typical, as in the skull, when bones develop from separate ossification centers. The edges of the bones mark the limits of the *fontanelles.* The fontanelles contain the connective tissue of the joint, as well as the cells responsible for appositional growth. Progressive closure of the fontanelles results in a *suture.* Because the cells necessary for the continued deposition of bone are present, syndesmoses are commonly replaced by synostoses.

Synchondroses. A *synchondrosis* is the union of two bones by hyaline cartilage (Fig. 16.8). The most common example is the growth plate of the long bones. This joint permits a unidirectinal growth of diaphyseal bone while joining the diaphyseal and epiphyseal bones. Some synchondroses, however, permit a two-dimensional growth of fused bones. The ultimate fate of a synchondrosis is conversion to a synostosis.

Symphyses. The predominant tissue in a *symphysis* is fibrocartilage. DWFCT and hyaline cartilage may be constituents. The ends of the contributing bones are covered by hyaline cartilage. The symphysis pubis

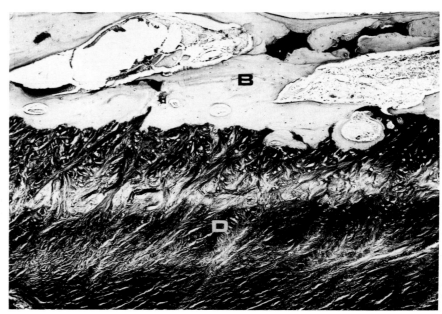

Figure 16.18. A portion of an intervertebral disk from a dog. The bone (B) of a vertebral body is connected to an adjacent vertebral body by an intervertebral disk (D). The fibrocartilage of the anulus fibrosus is apparent as alternating bands of light- and dark-staining materials. ×160. (Periodic acid Schiff [PAS"].

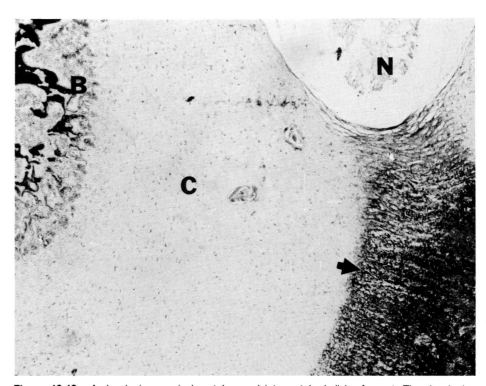

Figure 16.19. A developing cervical vertebra and intervertebral disk of a cat. The developing anulus fibrosus (arrow) consists of fibrocartilage. Remnants of the nucleus pulposus (N) are apparent. The cartilage (C) contributes to the developing vertebral body (B) through endochondral ossification. ×25. (Specimen courtesy of M. J. Burke).

and intervertebral joints are different examples of symphyses (Figs. 16.18 and 16.19).

Synostosis. A *synostosis*, fusion of bones by bone, ensures stability and immobility.

Synovial Joints

Diarthroidal joints (synovial joints, true joints) are the commonest form of bone-to-bone articulation and permit the greatest latitude of motion. These joints are discussed in greater depth than the other joints because of their significance in clinical medicine and surgery.

Origin and Nature. Presumptive bone centers are separated from each other by a mass of mesenchyme. As chondrogenic centers elongate, the bulk of the intervening mesenchyme degenerates, and the remaining mesenchyme forms the contributing components of the synovial joint (Fig. 16.20). The perichondrium of the articular surface degenerates simultaneously. Although the joint space develops as a cavitation process within the mesoderm, mesothelial cells are not developed in association with a synovial joint. Rather, the synovial space is lined by epithelioid cells that are not separated from the surrounding connective tissue by a basal lamina.

The basic components of diarthroses are *articular cartilage* and *articular capsule* (Fig. 16.21). The tissues mentioned previously as components of joints are either involved directly with synovial joints or are closely associated with them.

Histological Structure. The articular surface is composed of hyaline cartilage (Fig. 16.22). The hyaline cartilage in these loci accounts for the bulk of this tissue in the adult (Plate IV.9). The hyaline cartilage, which is devoid of a perichondrium, is divisible into four poorly defined but functionally significant subdivisions (Fig. 16.23): superficial zone, intermediate zone, deep zone, and mineralization zone.

The *superficial (surface) layer* consists of small, flattened chondrocytes, the long axes of which are oriented parallel to the articular surface. An *intermediate (transitional) zone* is characterized by round cells in various stages of maturation. These cells may be arranged in columns that are oriented perpendicular to the articular surface. The *deep zone* characteristically consists of mature and hypertrophic cells. The *mineralization zone* is present at the point of union of the articular cartilage with the underlying compact bone of the epiphysis *(subchondral bone)*. The superficial edge of the mineralization zone is demonstrable histologically by the presence of *tidemarks* (Fig. 16.23). Tidemarks represent the advancing waves of mineralization.

During development, the interstitial growth of the *presumptive articular cartilage* occurs from a mitotic region deep to the surface. (See Epiphyseal Growth, Chapter 10.) These cells divide, move toward the surface and mature (Fig. 16.24). The attainment of the adult configuration marks the end of the effective mitotic activity of articular chondrocytes. Chondrocytic mitoses, however, are evident in degenerative joint disease as *chondrones*. These are cellular nests that represent abortive or ineffective attempts at repair.

The *articular capsule* consists of a *fibrous*

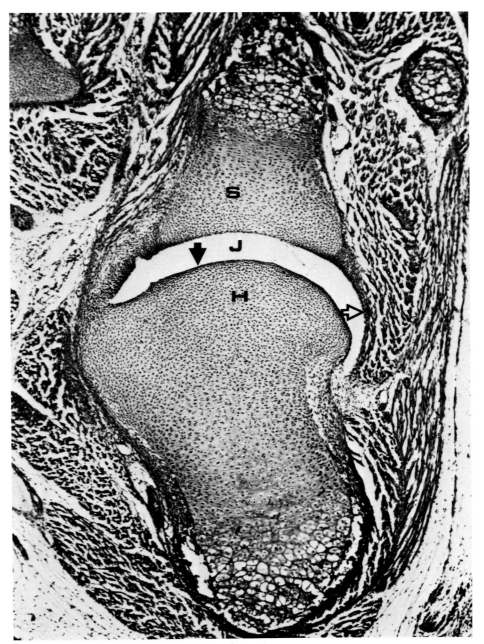

Figure 16.20. Developing scapulo-humeral articulation in a fetal dog. The scapula *(S)* and humerus *(H)* are separated by the joint space *(J)*. The synovial membrane *(open arrow)* has been formed. Note that the articular cartilage *(solid arrow)* is devoid of a perichondrium. ×10.

layer (fibrous capsule) and *synovial membrane* (Figs. 16.21 and 16.22). The fibrous layer consists of DWFCT that contains some elastic fibers. This fibroelastic tissue blends with the proper ligaments of the joint. The fibrous capsule and some ligaments attach circumferentially at a *transition zone* between the fibrous periosteum and the articular cartilage of the contributing bones called the *perichondral ring*. The inner surface of the fibrous capsule is lined by the synovial membrane (Fig. 16.25). The synovial membrane is reflected upon, blends with and is attached to the

nonweight-bearing portion of the articular surface. The membrane forms and delimits the closed space of the joint cavity.

The synovial membrane consists of lining cells and subsynovial connective tissue (Fig. 16.26). The connective tissue blends imperceptibly with the fibrous capsule. The lining (epithelioid) cells are flattened or rounded cells that form a membrane from one to four cells thick. These cells are fibroblasts; no basal lamina lies between them and the associated subsynovial connective tissue. Macrophages are components of this lining also.

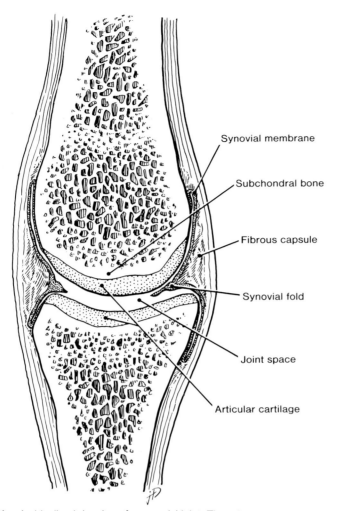

Figure 16.21. An idealized drawing of a synovial joint. The primary components are labeled.

Synovial membrane

Subchondral bone

Fibrous capsule

Synovial fold

Joint space

Articular cartilage

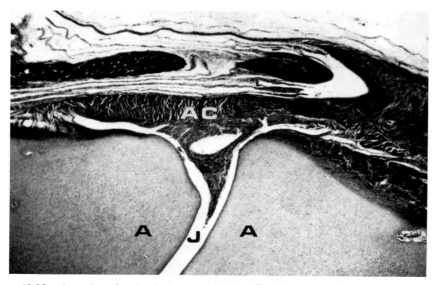

Figure 16.22. A portion of a developing synovial joint. The ligaments and muscles traverse the lateral aspects of the joint in the upper part of the micrograph. The articular capsule *(AC)* surrounds the joint and projects into the joint cavity *(J)*. The articular surfaces *(A)* are composed of hyaline cartilage. ×10.

Prominent infoldings of the synovial membrane into the synovial space are called *synovial folds*, whereas slender projections are called *synovial villi*.

Types of Synovial Membranes. Synovial membranes are classified on the type of tissues with which they are associated. *Fibrous, areolar*, and *adipose* synovial membranes exist. The *fibrous type* is associated with the fibrous capsule, proper ligaments, and tendons that cross the joint. The thin cellular lining of this membrane rests upon the fibroelastic tissue of these components. The *areolar type* of synovial membrane is separated from the fibrous capsule by loose connective tissue, permitting extensive mobility of the synovial membrane. The *adipose synovial membrane* is associated with deposits of adipose tissue that are integral components of some synovial joints.

Perichondral Ring. The *perichondral ring* was described previously as a *transition zone* between the periosteum of the diaphysis and the articular cartilage (Fig. 16.27). This structure is the attachment site of the fibrous capsule and many ligaments of diarthroidal joints. The perichondral ring is a perichondrium. In growing bones, it is positioned as a belt or ring at the peripheral margin of the growth plate. In adult bones, it retains its cartilage-producing potential in its same relative position to the closed growth plate. Stimulation of this region in growing bones is followed by some developmental anomalies characterized by excessive lateral deposition of cartilage and/or bone by endochondral ossification.

If trauma to bones and joints involves tearing the fibrous capsule and/or the ligaments at their points of attachments at the perichondral ring, then cartilage and/or bone formation via endochondral ossification can be expected. These bone spurs are called *periarticular osteophytes*.

Sharpey's fibers are collagenous fibers that anchor fibrous capsules, ligaments and tendons to bone by being incorporated in bone during developmental processes (Fig. 16.33). The relationship is established by bone (or cartilage) growing around the fibrous components of these structures. Periarticular osteophytosis is an attempt by the perichondral ring to re-anchor torn fibers. Unfortunately, this process leads to compromised joint function. Sharpey's fibers also occur in the attachment of tendons to bones.

Synovial Fluid

Characteristics. *Synovial fluid* forms as a transudate from the blood that is altered by the secretory activity of synovial lining cells. Glycosaminoglycans, principally *hyaluronic acid*, are added to the synovial fluid by these cells. The viscosity of syn-

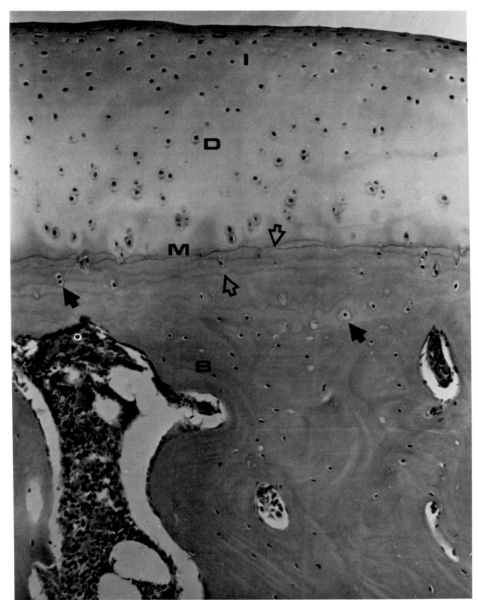

Figure 16.23. Mature articular cartilage and subchondral bone from the head of a feline femur. The superficial (S), intermediate (I), deep (D) and mineralized (M) zones of the articular cartilage are evident. The tidemarks (open arrows) represent the advancing waves of mineralization of cartilage. Pockets of calcified matrix (solid arrows) occur deep to the tidemarks adjacent to subchondral bone (B). Note the relatively smooth interface between subchondral bone and articular cartilage. ×40.

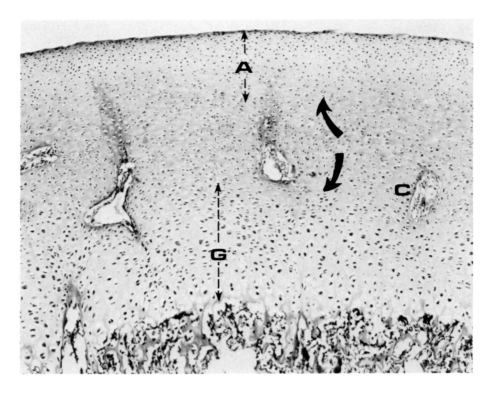

Figure 16.24. A section of a canine growing bone before the formation of a secondary ossification center. Cartilage canals (C) are scattered throughout the chondroepiphysis. Presumptive articular cartilage (A) is not invaded by cartilage canals, The presumptive growth plate is apparent. Cartilage is "fed" into the developing articular surface and growth plate from a mitotic zone in the general region of the bases of the curved arrows. G, presumptive growth plate. ×25.

Figure 16.25. Periarticular relationships in a developing bone. The joint space (J) is outlined by the synovial lining (solid arrow) and the articular cartilage (A). The fibrous capsule (F) is peripheral to the synovial lining cells. The synovial lining cells are reflected on the nonweight-bearing surface of the articular surface (open arrows). The presumptive growth plate (GP) is bounded peripherally by the perichondral ring (P). ×16.

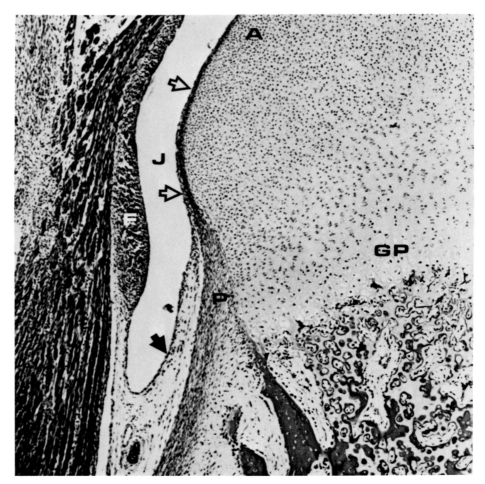

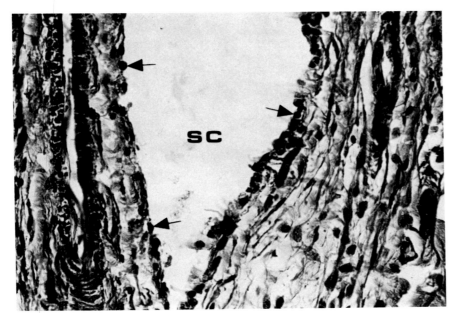

Figure 16.26. Synovial membrane. The synovial cavity (SC) is delimited by a fibrous synovial membrane. Flattened fibroblasts *(arrows)* are the predominant lining cells. ×100.

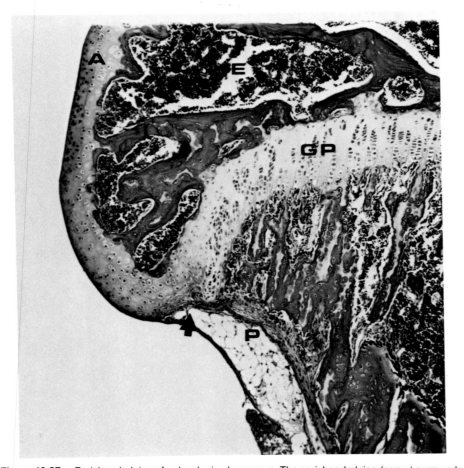

Figure 16.27. Perichondral ring of a developing humerous. The perichondral ring *(arrow)* surrounds the peripheral limits of the growth plate *(GP)* at the transition point between articular cartilage *(A)* and periosteum *(P)*. *E*, epiphyseal ossification center. ×16.

ovial fluid, which derives primarily from the hyaluronic acid, is one of its most conspicuous features. Low molecular weight proteins that are electrophoretically and immunologically identical to plasma proteins are present in this fluid in low concentration. Lysosomal enzymes and proteoglycan degradation products of the lining cells and cartilaginous matrix, respectively, are components of this fluid. The "weeping" of articular cartilage also adds some components to synovial fluid.

The turnover and absorption of synovial fluid is not understood completely. Substances may pass between or through the lining cells to be returned to the vascular bed or accompanying lymphatic vessels in a manner similar to the mechanisms responsible for the turnover of extracellular fluids.

Three functions are ascribed to the synovial fluid: *lubrication of the joint surfaces; nutrition of articular cartilage; protection of joint surfaces.*

Lubrication. *Lubrication* of joint surfaces has been attributed to the high viscosity of the synovial fluid. Because hyaluronic acid is the primary contributor to this viscosity, it has been assumed intuitively that this compound is responsible for reducing friction between joint surfaces. The lubrication of joint surfaces, however, is a complex and dynamic process that cannot be explained simply by the presence of hyaluronic acid.

The precise mechanism by which the articular surfaces and the synovial membrane are lubricated are subject to much controversy. Two mechanisms of mechanical lubrication are applicable to cartilage—fluid film lubrication and boundary lubrication.

Fluid film lubrication occurs when opposing surfaces are separated completely by a lubricating fluid. Four types of fluid film lubrication (hydrodynamic, hydrostatic, elastohydrodynamic and squeeze film) have been implicated in joint surface lubrication. Fluid film lubrication functions when articular surfaces are loaded at various rates.

Boundary lubrication occurs when molecules absorbed at surfaces maintain lubricating properties. A glycoprotein yet to be characterized is believed to be the boundary lubricant of articulations. Boundary lubricants function independently of load and rate of loading.

Mixed lubrication—a combination of fluid film and boundary lubrication—occurs in synovial joints under different circumstances. Three other types of lubrication mechanisms unique to articular cartilage have been identified, although their significance is controversial. *Weeping lubrication* of cartilage is the movement of substances to the surface in response to loading. When the load is removed, the materials move back into the matrix ready for another cycle. *Boosted lubrication* results from the separation of water from the rest of the synovial fluid. Movement of water into the cartilaginous matrix increases the viscosity and lubricating properties of the synovial fluid. *Lipid lubrication* results from the lipid constituents of articular cartilage reducing the coefficient of friction between opposing surfaces.

The lubrication mechanisms involved at articular surfaces are complex and probably involve a combination of mechanisms. The high viscosity of synovial fluid results from the hyaluronic acid content. Intuitively, then, the viscosity and, thus, the hyaluronic acid content must account for the lubricating properties. Hyaluronidase digestion of hyaluronate reduces the viscosity, but the removal of the hyaluronate does not alter the lubricating properties. The glycoprotein mentioned earlier as having been isolated but not characterized is responsible for the lubricating properties of synovial fluid. The reasons for the high viscosity of synovial fluid, since they do not seem to be related to lubrication, remain obscure.

Nutrition and Protection. *Nutrition* of the articular cartilage is an important function of this fluid. There is little evidence to substantiate the metabolic support of articular cartilage from the vascular beds of the subchondral bone. Rather, the weeping of articular cartilage may provide a mechanism that complements diffusion of nutrients and waste products through this avascular tissue. The cells of articular cartilage, all cartilage cells as well, are suited ideally for anaerobic metabolism by containing high concentrations of lactic dehydrogenase.

Protection is manifested in a number of ways. Its lubricating properties protect against mechanical damage. The presence of lysosomal enzymes, as well as phagocytic cells being components of the lining membrane, protects against foreign bodies and microbes. Synovial fluid is a good growth medium for microbiological agents. Additionally, the synovial cells and/or the articular chondrocytes may secrete an activator of the plasminogen system that prevents the formation of clots within synovial fluid or on articular surfaces.

Functional Correlates. The synovial tissues are well vascularized. The large capillaries, many of which are fenestrated, ensure a rapid exchange of tissue fluid. Despite the alteration of tissue fluid by the secretory activity of the lining cells, it is reasonable to consider the joint space as an expanded portion of the connective tissue. The mechanisms governing the exchange of tissue fluid are applicable. Extensive lymphatic capillaries are characteristic of this region also.

The fibrous capsule and associated ligaments are well innervated. Pain and proprioception are the important modalities transmitted by the neuronal processes. Postganglionic fibers of the sympathetic nervous system, as vasomotor nerves, are present also.

The characterization of the synovial fluid is an invaluable aid to diagnosis of various joint abnormalities (Table 16.1).

Joints are evaluated commonly with radiology. The articular cartilage, however, is radiolucent. The radiographic interface between two joint surfaces actually represents the mineralized cartilage and the subchondral bone of each surface. Subchondral bone is an important support component for articular cartilage. Many changes in articular cartilage are accompanied by changes in subchondral bone. Therefore, an evaluation of the subchondral bone is useful in the diagnosis of joint problems.

Repair of Articular Cartilage. The repair of articular cartilage was discussed in depth in Chapter 8. The primary concern after full-thickness damage to an articular surface is the inability of that surface to repair itself appropriately. Abortive attempts at repair usually are followed by degenerative joint disease. *Continuous passive motion* of damaged joints has been a stimulant for full-thickness articular cartilage damage to be repaired by hyaline cartilage. This treatment has been effective in experimental circumstances; it has little direct application to veterinary orthopedics at this point. The insights gained from this approach, however, may be applicable in the future.

Muscle as an Organ

Muscle-Tendon Relationships

Muscle

Organization. The constituents of muscles as organs include: skeletal muscle, loose and dense connective tissues, vessels,

lymphatics, and nerves. Individual muscle fibers are the structural units for gross muscle masses. Grossly, skeletal muscle masses are distinct entities separated from each other by a DWFCT called *fascia*. Fascia may be considered the capsule of the organ and is called *epimysium* by histologists (Fig. 16.28). This outermost covering extends into the muscle mass and forms a covering around individual bundles of muscle fibers, the *perimysium*. Individual fibers of the bundles or *fascicles* are separated from each other by a delicate network of loose connective tissue, the *endomysium*. The connective tissue investments are continuous with the each other. These investments bind these components as a single morphological unit and allow nerves and vessels to reach all of the muscle fibers (Fig. 16.29). Additionally, the investments are continuous with the DWFCT of the tendons of origin and insertion. Lymphatic vessels are present in the epimysial and perimysial connective tissue but are not components of the endomysium.

Myotendinous Junctions. The connective tissue investments of muscles are continuous with the connective tissues to which they are anchored. This continuity is the means by which the mechanical activity of contraction is converted to work. The *muscle-tendon junction* is also the point wherein the actin filaments within the muscle cell are attached to the sarcolemma (Fig. 16.30). The collagen of the tendon is attached to the basal lamina at invagination points along the sarcolemma. The increased length of muscle during growth occurs by the addition of new sarcomeres at this junction.

Tendons

Morphology. A *tendon*, which is composed of DWFCT (regularly arranged), connects muscles to their points of attachment (Fig. 16.30). Whereas the tensile strength of muscle is in the range of 80

Table 16.1.
Synovial Fluid Analysis of Selected Conditions

Parameter	Normal	Trauma	Sepsis
Clarity	Clear	Clear-Bloody	Cloudy
Color	Straw	Straw-Xanthochromic-bloody	Pink-grey-green
Viscosity	High	High	Low
Mucin Clot	Good	Good	Poor
Fibrin Clot	0	0-slight	Minimal-marked*
pH	7.0–7.8	7.0–7.8	Decreased
Total Protein	1.0–1.5	Variable	Increased
RBCs	0	Variable†	+
WBCs	500–3000**	Normal-slight increase	30,000
Cytology	Healthy cells	Healthy cells	Toxic/degenerative
Monocytes	90%	70–80%	10–20%*
Neutrophils	10%	20–30%	80–90%*

* Varies with the type of agent.
† + if acute, 0 if chronic.
** Some species variations: horse-500, dog-3000.

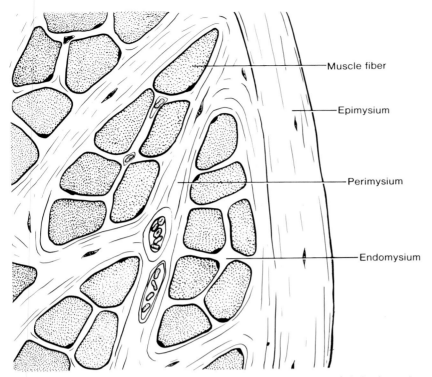

Figure 16.28. A diagram of the connective tissue investments of skeletal muscle.

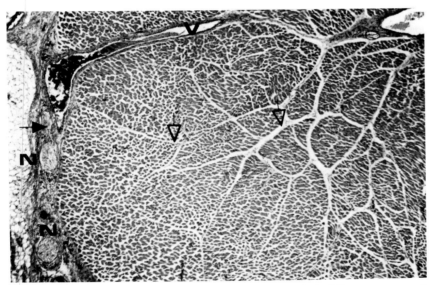

Figure 16.29. A cross section of a skeletal muscle. Groups (fascicles) of fibers are surrounded by the perimysium *(open arrows)*. This connective tissue is continuous with the epimysial *(solid arrows)* and endomysial connective tissues. Nerves *(N)* and vessels *(V)* are visible within the perimysium. ×10.

paths. The tendon sheaths are composed of two layers of flattened cells. The inner layer is intimately associated with the epitendineum and provides a smooth surface for movement. The outer layer is attached to surrounding paratendinous tissues. The intervening space between the two layers is filled with a lubricating fluid similar to synovial fluid. The synovial membranes of joints may establish similar relationships to tendons such that the intervening space between the layers of the sheath is continuous with the joint space. The *mesotendon* is a zone of continuity and contact between the inner and outer layers of the synovial sheath. Blood vessels and nerves enter the tendon through the mesotendon. The relationship between the tendon and the tendon sheath is similar to that established when a cylinder is laid upon a slightly inflated balloon and then pushed into the balloon (Fig. 16.31). The cavity of the balloon is comparable to the lubricating space between the layers of the sheath. To provide proper lubrication, the visceral layer is attached to the epitenon; the entire tendon and visceral layer move within the synovial fluid space as a unit.

Fibrocartilage, often the tissue interface between a tendon and its osseous or cartilaginous attachment (Fig. 16.32), serves to strengthen the point of origin or insertion. The actual attachment of the tendon to the bone or cartilage is achieved by *Sharpey's fibers* (Fig. 16.33). Intrinsic attempts to reattach Sharpey's fibers to bone are characterized by *periosteal new bone growth (exostosis)*.

Intrinsic and Extrinsic Repair. Two functional requirements must be met if repair phenomena are to return tendons to normal function. **The tensile properties of the tendon must be restored and the ability to glide over great distances must be maintained.** Proliferation of fibroblasts and the secretion and polymerization of procollagen are essential for the restoration of tensile properties. Unfortunately, the contribution of fibroblasts from the paratendinous tissues can impair the necessary gliding property. *Extrinsic repair* is an essential component of tendon restoration, but it can lead to *adhesions* (collagenous connections) between the tendon and the surrounding tissues. Although the contribution of paratendinous tissues (fibroblasts and capillaries) is significant, tendons do have the ability to undergo *intrinsic* repair.

Repair Sequence. The sequence of tendon repair occurs in distinct yet interrelated stages: insult (impact), induction, inflammatory, fibroblastic (reparative), and maturation (remodeling). The stages in the process correspond to those described for fracture repair.

The partial or complete severing of a tendon during the *insult stage* not only results in damage to the tendon proper but

pounds per square inch, that of tendons may be 225 times larger. Thus, heavy muscle masses may function effectively through their small tendinous attachments. The ability to perform work is dependent upon tendons moving or gliding great distances through the associated soft tissues.

Tendons consist of bundles of collagenous fibers bound together by perimysial-like connective tissue called *endotenon* (Fig.

16.30). Blood vessels and nerves are also present within tendons. The entire tendon is surrounded by a connective tissue sheath, *epitendineum (epitenon)*, which is similar to the epimysium. Areolar connective tissue, adipose tissue, or synovial sheaths between tendons and their fibrous sheaths are called *paratendon (paratenon)*. Tendons are enclosed within *tendon sheaths (synovial sheaths)* at points of friction along their

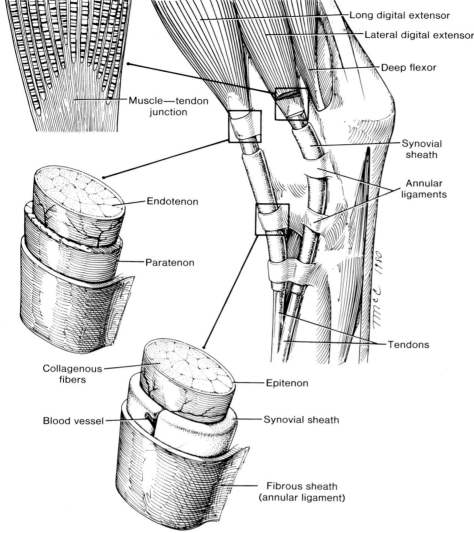

Figure 16.30. An illustration of the superficial muscles and tendons associated with the equine tarsus. The components of these structures are labeled.

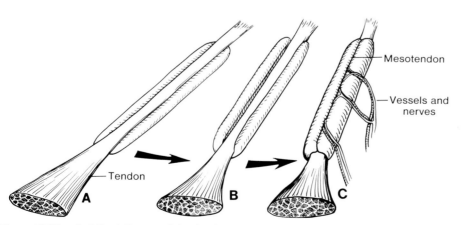

Figure 16.31. A stylized diagram of the development of a tendon sheath around a tendon. *A*, initial tendinous invagination into sheath; *B*, continued invagination and encirclement of tendon; *C*, established relationship.

is accompanied by other soft tissue damage and devitalization. Hemostasis may exacerbate devitalization. Because the blood supply to tendons within synovial sheaths is segmental, the location and extent of the lesion in relation to the blood supply is an important factor in the amount of devitalization. Because the synovial fluid contained within the synovial sheath is also a source of nourishment, its disruption can complicate repair.

The *induction stage*, as described previously for bone, is probably an artificial separation of events occuring throughout the repair process. The stimuli for induction of new cells during tendon repair may be tissue hypoxia. Fibroblasts proliferate rapidly within and adjacent to the tendon and new capillaries rapidly invade the tendon from the paratendinous tissues.

The *inflammatory stage* occurs as a sequel to tissue damage, and the amount of inflammation depends upon the extent of the damage. The cardinal signs of inflammation are apparent throughout this stage. An excessive amount of inflammation can result in an excessive amount of collagen formation *(fibrosis)* at the repair site.

The *fibroblastic stage* is characterized by proliferation of fibroblasts and their secretion of procollagen. The cells of the epitenon and endotenon are responsible for intrinsic repair events. These regions become hyperplastic, and an extensive amount of collagen is deposited randomly within the repair site. The synovial sheath and paratendinous tissues also contribute cells and collagen as the extrinsic aspect of the repair process.

During the *maturation stage*, the collagenous fibers become oriented parallel to the long axis of the tendon, fuse, and interdigitate with other fibers. The tendon eventually separates from the surrounding paratendinous tissues. The degree to which this separation is accomplished determines the extent to which normal function is restored. Collagenous, fibrous adhesions from the tendon to the paratendinous tissues limit functional gliding.

Numerous factors influence successful repair of a tendon. Careful management procedures of these histological events can result in return to near-normal function.

The events responsible for the repair of a torn tendon from its attachments to bone are similar to those described. The important difference is the necessity to reestablish the attachments of Sharpey's fibers.

Muscle-Nerve Relationships

Motor Unit. Large nerve fibers enter the epimysial connective tissue space, branch throughout the perimysium and send fine terminals into the endomysium (Fig. 16.34). High innervation ratios character-

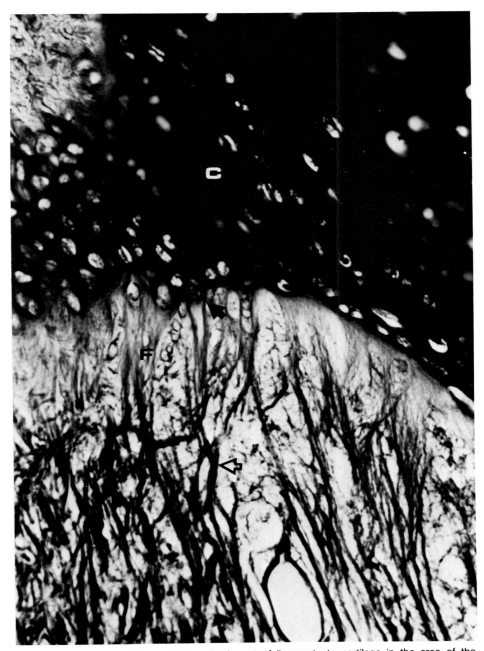

Figure 16.32. Fibrocartilage and the attachment of ligaments to cartilage in the area of the perichondral ring. Collagenous fibers *(open arrow)* continue through the fibrocartilage (F) to become anchored in cartilage *(C)* as Sharpey's fibers *(solid arrow)*. ×100 (Aldehyde fuschin).

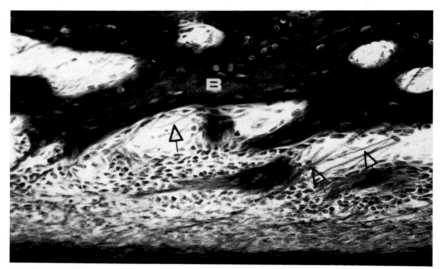

Figure 16.33. Attachment of muscle to bone through dense white fibrous connective tissue. Sharpey's fibers *(arrows)* anchor the connective tissue to the bone *(B)*. ×40.

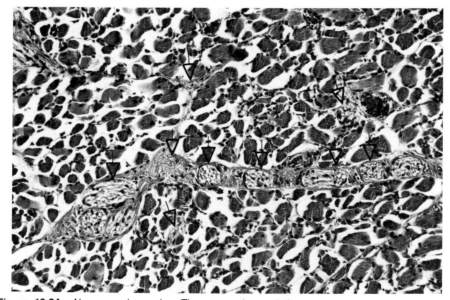

Figure 16.34. Nerves and muscles. The nerves *(arrows)* that are associated with muscle are indicated. Branches from the nerve fibers innervate the adjacent musculature. ×40.

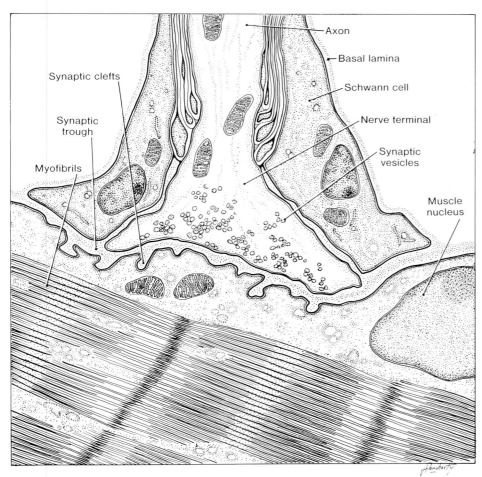

Figure 16.35. A diagram of a myoneural junction. The components have been labeled. Compare with Figure 13.11.

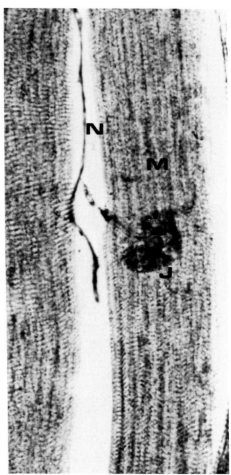

Figure 16.36. Neuromuscular junction. A branch of a nerve fiber *(N)* terminates as a neuromuscular junction *(J)* upon a muscle fiber *(M)*. ×100 (Gold impregnation).

ize the antigravity muscles or coarse movers of the body; whereas, low innervation ratios are characteristic of muscles noted for fine movement. The muscle fibers and the nerve innervating them are called a *motor unit*. **A motor unit includes: the cell body located in the ventral grey column of the spinal cord; the axon as it passes through the white matter of the spinal cord; the continuation of the axon in the ventral root; the axon within the main stem, and the dorsal and ventral branches of the spinal nerve; the myoneural junction; the muscle fibers.** (This concept applies to the equivalent components of the cranial nerves.)

Myoneural Junction. The point of junction between the neuronal terminal and the muscle fiber(s) is called the *motor end-plate* or *myoneural junction* (Figs. 16.35 and 16.36). As the axon of a neuron approaches a muscle fiber, the myelin sheath terminates (Fig. 16.35). The Schwann cell, however, continues and covers the point of contact with the muscle fiber. The terminal arborization of the axon continues into

recesses in the muscle called *synaptic troughs (primary synaptic clefts)*. The *subneural apparatus* consists of modifications to the sarcolemma that include numerous infoldings of the plasmalemma and the basal lamina, the *secondary synaptic clefts* (Fig. 13.11). The axon and plasma membrane are always separated by the intervening basal lamina.

The neuromuscular junction is a highly directed chemical synapse. The telodendria of the axons contain numerous small vesicles and mitochondria. The vesicles, *synaptic vesicles*, contain the neurotransmitter substance, acetylcholine, which is released into the synaptic trough when the nerve is stimulated.

Synaptic vesicles undergoing exocytosis do not fuse with the inner surface of the presynaptic membrane randomly. A series of *dense bars* is attached along the inner surface of the presynaptic membrane opposite the apex of the postsynaptic membranous folds. Synaptic vesicles align themselves along the edges of these bars. This combination of dense bars and aligned syn-

aptic vesicles is called an *active zone*. An active zone is actually the specialized region within synapses at which neurotransmitters are released. Once the neurotransmitter is released, the vesicle is recycled for use by the neuron. (Active zones are features of most neurons. The morphology and frequency of attachment sites vary.)

Acetylcholine binds to receptor sites on the apex of the membranous folds of the subneural apparatus. Neurotransmitter/receptor interaction opens chemically gated Na^+ channels that permit Na^+ to rush into the muscle cell. The rapid influx of sodium causes a rise in the membrane potential of the end-plate. This potential is called the *end-plate potential*. Once the end-plate potential raises the local membrane potential to threshold, an action potential results. Subsequent depolarization spreads from this site as an action potential and activates the muscle cell. The motor end-plate or myoneural junction is a synapse.

Neuromuscular Spindle Apparatus. *Neu-*

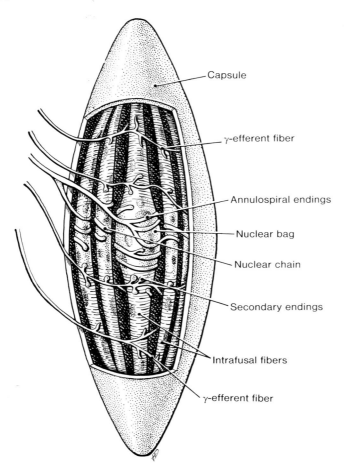

Figure 16.37. An idealized drawing of a spindle apparatus. Refer to the text for a complete description of these components.

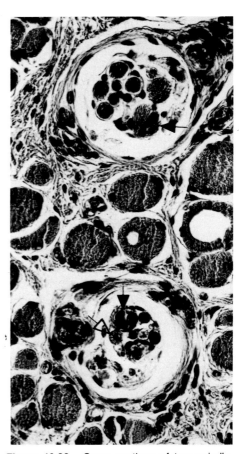

Figure 16.38. Cross sections of two spindle apparatus from the extraocular musculature of an elk. Nuclear bag *(solid arrows)* and nuclear chain *(open arrow)* regions are apparent. Note the connective tissue capsule that separates the small intrafusal fibers from the large extrafusal fibers. ×100.

romuscular spindles are scattered throughout muscles and are responsible for maintaining the tone of a muscle, as well as minimizing the possibility of damage by excessive stretching of muscles. Spindles mediate their activity through a *stretch reflex* that involves two neurons at the level of the spinal cord.

Spindles consist of muscle fibers, nerve endings, and connective tissue (Fig. 16.37). A loose connective tissue capsule separates the smaller, *intrafusal* fibers of the spindle from the ordinary and larger, *extrafusal* fibers of the muscle mass. Intrafusal fibers vary in length from 2 to 10 mm and are approximately 200 μm in diameter. Two types of intrafusal fibers are present, a *nuclear bag fiber* (Fig. 16.38) and a *nuclear chain fiber* (Fig. 16.39). Of the 20 fibers that may form a spindle, the nuclear chain fibers outnumber the nuclear bag fibers by a ratio of two or three to one. Both types of fibers are attached to the capsule at their poles.

Both fibers are typically striated and have distinct *equitorial regions*. The nuclear bag fiber is enlarged in the center, filled with

nuclei and devoid of contractile elements in this region. The smaller and shorter nuclear chain fibers are not expanded in the center, but large nuclei are prominent and contractile elements are missing in this central region.

Numerous afferent and efferent nerve endings are associated with these fibers (Fig. 16.37). Afferent endings associated with the equators of both fibers are called *primary (anulospiral endings)*. When the equators are stretched, the fibers transmit an impulse to the spinal cord resulting in the contraction of extrafusal fibers of the same muscle mass. The same input signal from the primaries causes inhibition of the antagonistic muscle mass. This accounts for the stretch reflex (Fig. 16.40) This type of activity explains the intuitive thought that excitation of a particular muscle mass must be accompanied by the relaxation of its antagonist.

The input from the primaries informs the spinal cord and higher brain centers at a subconscious level about the rate of muscle lengthening or stretching and the actual length of the muscle.

Afferent *secondary endings (flower spray endings)* originate on either side of the equatorial region (Fig. 16.37). Their precise function within the spindle is not understood. They do, however, transmit information about muscle length to the central nervous system at a subconscious level.

Small efferent fibers (*gamma efferents, γ-efferents*) innervate the intrafusal fibers at their respective poles (Fig. 16.37). They establish the degree of stretch on equatorial regions, thereby functioning to raise or lower the threshold of primary ending discharge. This makes the spindle more or less sensitive to stretching. Once the extrafusal fibers contract, the tension or stretching on the equatorial region would relax and cause a collapse of these regions. By γ-efferent discharge, tension on these regions is maintained throughout the entire range of the contraction. This ensures a constant informational input to the spinal cord and higher brain centers about the degree of

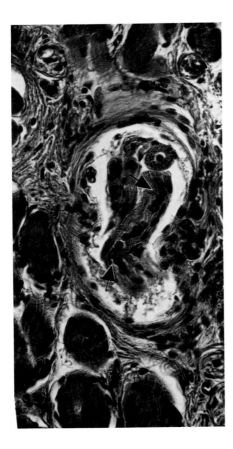

Figure 16.39. An oblique section of a spindle apparatus from the extraocular musculature of an elk. *Arrow*, equitorial regions of nuclear chain fibers. ×100.

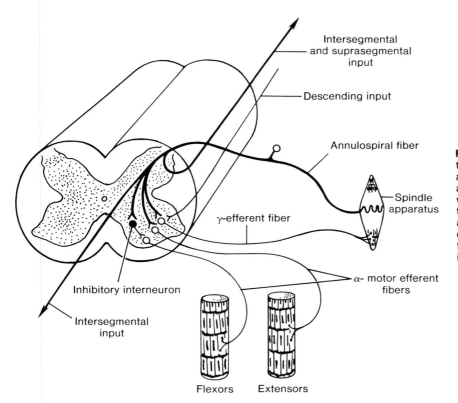

Figure 16.40. A schematic representation of the myotatic reflex. Stimulation of the spindle apparatus by stretching induces the firing of the annulospiral afferent fibers. Collaterals synapse with α-motor neurons in the ventral gray column that cause contraction of the extensors. A synapse with an interneuron inhibits the contraction of the flexors. Collaterals from the annulospiral fibers descend and ascend the spinal cord to intersegmental and suprasegmental levels.

stretch or lack thereof in a particular muscle mass.

Neurotendinous Relationships. *Neurotendinous organs (Golgi tendon organs)* are located in-tendons close to their junction with the muscle mass. The Golgi tendon organs consist of collagenous fibers that are contained within a connective tissue capsule. Numerous cells and afferent terminals are also present. They transmit information concerning the amount of stretch or tension on tendons. This type of information, therefore, also indicates the amount of contraction in a muscle mass. With excessive tension on a tendon, the afferent discharge results in an inhibition to further contraction. Although the informational input is transmitted at a subconscious level throughout the entire range of muscular contraction, ultimately these organs minimize the possibility of tendons being torn from their points of attachment to bone or muscle.

Although the input from spindles and neurotendinous organs is at a subconscious level, conscious input is achieved through other mechanisms. Naked nerve endings (Ruffini-like) are embedded within the connective tissue of joint capsules. Subjected to the compression and tension associated with joint movement, they transmit *kinesthetic* information; i.e., information concerning the relative positions of various parts of the body.

References

Bone as an Organ

Arnold, J. S.: Quantitation of mineral of bone as an organ and tissue in osteoporosis. Clin. Orthop. *17*:167, 1960.

Butler, W.F.: Age changes in alcian blue staining of glycosaminoglycans in sheep articular cartilage. Res. Vet. Sci. *22*:303, 1977.

Cooke, A.F., Dowson, D. and Wright, V.: Lubrication of synovial membrane. Ann. Rheum. Dis. *35*:56, 1976.

Cooper, R. R., Milgram, J. W. and Robinson, R. A.: Morphology of the osteon. An electron microscopic study. J. Bone Joint Surg. *48A*:1239, 1966.

Elliot, H. C.: Studies on articular cartilages. I. Growth mechanisms. Amer. J. Anat. *58*:127, 1936.

Frost, H. M.: *Bone Modeling and Skeletal Modeling Errors.* Charles C Thomas, Springfield, 1973.

Frost, H. M.: New Concepts of bone remodelling and of the nature of osteoporoses. J. Med. Surg. *1*:41, 1961.

Frost, H. M.: *Bone Remodelling Dynamics.* Charles C Thomas, Springfield, 1963.

Frost, H. M.: *The Physiology of Cartilaginous, Fibrous and Bony Tissue.* C. C. Thomas, Springfield, 1972.

Frost, H.M.: A chondral modeling theory. Calc. Tiss. Res. *28*:181, 1979.

Haines, R. W.: The development of joints. J. Anat. *81*:33, 1947.

Hancox, N. M.: *Biology of Bone.* University Press, Cambridge, 1972.

Hirohata, K. and Morimoto, K.: *Ultrastructure of Bone and Joint Diseases.* Grune and Stratton, New York, 1971.

Ketchum, L. D.: Tendon Healing. *In:* Hunt, T. K. (ed.): *Fundamentals of Wound Management in Surgery: Selected Tissues.* 121–153. Chirurgecom, Inc., South Plainfield, New Jersey, 1977.

Kincaid, S.A. and Van Sickle, D.C.: Regional histochemical and thickness variations of adult canine articular cartilage. Amer. J. Vet Res. *42*:209, 1981.

Koch, J. L.: The laws of bone architecture. Amer. J. Anat. *21*:177, 1917.

Radin, E.L., Swann, D.A. and Weisser, P.A.: Separation of a hyaluronate free lubricating fraction from synovial fluid. Nature *228*:337, 1970.

Roy, S.: Ultrastructure of articular cartilage in experimental hemarthrosis. Arch. Path. *86*:69, 1968.

Silberberg, M., Silberberg, R. and Hasler, M.: Fine structure of articular cartilage in mice receiving cortisone acetate. Arch Path. *82*:569, 1966.

Sokoloff, L. and Bland, J. H.: *The Musculoskeletal System.* Williams & Wilkins, Baltimore, 1975.

Urist, M. R. (ed.): Symposium: Articular cartilage in health and disease, Clin. Orthop. *64*:3, 1969.

Wilson, F. C.: *The Musculoskeletal System.* J. B. Lippincott, Philadelphia, 1975.

Fracture Repair

Ham, A.W. and Harris, W.R.: Repair and transplantation of bone. *In:* Bourne, G.H. (ed.): *The Biochemistry and Physiology of Bone.* Vol. III. pp. 337–399. Academic Press, New York, 1971.

Heppenstall, R.B.: Fracture and cartilage repair. *In: Fundamentals of Wound Management in Surgery: Selected Tissues.* pp 1–35, Chirurgecom, Inc., South Plainfield, NJ, 1977.

Peacock, E.E., Jr. and Van Winkle, W., Jr.: *Surgery and Biology of Wound Repair.* W.B. Saunders Co., Philadelphia, 1970.

Perrin, S. Cortical bone healing. Acta Orthop. Scan. *Suppl.* 125, 1969.

Sumner-Smith, G. (ed.): *Bone in Clinical Orthopaedics: A Study in Comparative Osteology.* W. B. Saunders, Philadelphia, 1982. 435p.

Urist, M. R. (ed.): *Fundamental and Clincal Bone Physiology.* J. B. Lippincott Company, Philadelphia, 1980. 416p.

Muscle as an Organ

Bowman, J. P., Jr.: *The Muscle Spindle and Neuronal Control of the Tongue: Implications for Speech.* Charles C Thomas, Springfield, 1971.

Cohen, L. A.: Contributions of tactile musculo-tendinous and joint mechanisms to position sense in human shoulder. J. Neurophysiol. *21*:563, 1958.

Cooper, S: Afferent impulses in the hypoglossal nerve on stretching the cat's tongue. J. Physiol. *126*:32P, 1954.

Lentz, T. L.: Development of the neuromuscular junction. J. Cell Biol. *47*:423, 1970.

Mathews, P. B. C.: Muscle spindles and their motor control. Physiol. Rev. *44*:219, 1964.

Nystrom, B.: Muscle-spindle histochemistry. Science *155*:1424, 1967.

Sokoloff, L. and Bland, J. H.: *The Musculoskeletal System.* Williams & Wilkins, Baltimore, 1975.

Spiro, A. J. and Beilin, R. L.: Histochemical duality of rabbit intrafusal fibers. J. Histochem. Cytochem. *17*:348, 1969.

Wilson, F. C. *The Musculoskeletal System.* J. B. Lippincott, Philadelphia, 1975.

Yelin, H.: A histochemical study of muscle spindles and their relationship to extrafusal fiber types in the rat. Amer. J. Anat. *125*:31, 1969.

17: Nervous System

General Characteristics

Form and Function. The nervous system is a complex group of organs that is formed by the nervous tissue, connective tissue, and vascular components. The complexity is based upon neurons communicating with each other and effector cells. The system perceives stimuli, processes the information, and causes the appropriate response that contributes to its *homeostasis*. The neuron is the anatomical unit of the system and is the basis for the massive intercommunicating, three-dimensional network of cells and cellular processes. The essence of organization is the segregation of neurons into hierarchical levels of responsibility that contribute to the interdependent functions of stimulus perception, information processing, and initiation of appropriate response.

The nervous system is divisible into two anatomical subdivisions, the *central nervous system (CNS)* and *peripheral nervous system (PNS)*. The CNS is comprised of the brain, its extensions, and the spinal cord. The units consist of numerous pools of segregated neurons that are interconnected by the dendritic and axonal processes of its constituent cells. The PNS includes the nerve trunks (cranial and spinal nerves), accumulations of peripherally positioned neuronal cell bodies and neuronal terminals. The PNS receives stimuli and tranduces them into useful information as action potentials and transmits this information to the CNS. The information elicits a segmental or intersegmental response (reflex) and is transmitted to higher (suprasegmental) levels, which are responsible for the integration, association and interpretation of the information. The appropriate response transmitted over neuronal processes forming descending pathways, is carried eventually to the effector organs (glands and muscles) by the nerve trunks of the PNS.

The PNS may be subdivided upon an anatomical basis into the *somatic nervous system* and *autonomic nervous system*. The somatic nervous system includes those neurons that carry information from the external environment to the CNS and back to skeletal muscles. The autonomic nervous system functions similarly. Although the origination of informational input varies, the subsequent evocation of a response involves the internal or visceral organs.

The conducting neuronal components of the CNS and PNS function in such a manner as to allow the organism to respond immediately and usually for a short period of time to alterations in the external and internal environment. The neurosecretory neuronal components, because of their influence on the endocrine system, permit gradual and longer term responses to environmental alterations than their conducting counterparts.

Anatomical Considerations

Development. The basic form of the vertebrate CNS is a dorsal, hollow, tubular structure derived from a thickened plate of *neuroectoderm* (Fig. 17.1). This *neural plate* is a longitudinal thickening dorsal to the notochord during the presomite stage of development. The neural plate invaginates to form the *neural groove*, the lateral margins of which grow centrally and fuse along the longitudinal axis to form the *neural tube*. As these two layers of ectoderm separate from each other, a longitudinally oriented mass of cells segregates as the *neural crest cells*.

The rostral end of the neural tube is associated with an extensive accumulation of developing nerve cells and is characterized by the development of vesicles that are destined to differentiate into various components of the brain (Fig. 17.2). This process of *cephalization* is identifiable early in development by the appearance of three vesicles: prosencephalon, mesencephalon, rhombencephalon (Fig. 17.3). The *prosencephalon* divides into two vesicles, the *telencephalon* and *diencephalon*. The telencephalic vesicles grow extensively; they completely cover the rostral portions of the vesicles as the *cerebral hemispheres*. The *diencephalon* differentiates into the thalamus and its various subdivisions (*epithalamus, thalamus, metathalamus, subthalamus* and *hypothalamus*) and is associated directly with the developing eye *(optic vesicle)*. Throughout this development the rostral portion of the neural tube becomes tortuous, but the integrity of the lumen of the neural tube is maintained. The lumen associated with telencephalic development becomes the two *lateral ventricles*, whereas the lumen associated with diencephalic growth and development becomes the "donut-shaped" *third ventricle*. The third ventricle maintains its communication with the lateral ventricles through two laterally positioned foramina *(foramina of Monro, interventricular foramina)*. The *mesencephalon* does not subdivide into other vesicles but gives rise directly to the midbrain. The constricted portion of the lumen of the neural tube in the midbrain is called the *mesencephalic aqueduct*. It is the connection between the third ventricle rostrally and the *fourth ventricle* caudally. The fourth ventricle develops in association with the rhombencephalon. The *rhombencephalon* subdivides into the metencephalic and myelencephalic vesicles. The *metencephalon* gives rise to the cerebellum dorsally and the pons ventrally. The *myelencephalon* becomes the medulla oblongata. The medulla oblongata ends at the foramen magnum; the spinal cord continues caudally. The continued growth and development of the brain is contingent upon the continued differentiation of the five vesicles of the neural tube (Fig. 17.3).

Cellular Differentiation, Development, and Orientation. The rapid growth and development of the neural tube (especially the rostral portion) results from the marked proliferative activity of the neuroepithelial cells that form it. The neuroepithelium segregates into three distinct populations of cells: neural crest cell, neuroblasts, and glioblasts. *Neural crest cells* separate from the neural tube and differentiate into numerous cell types scattered throughout the soma, some of which maintain their relationship with the nervous system (Fig. 17.4). Neuroblasts differentiate into the neurons of the CNS, whereas the *glioblasts (spongioblasts)* differentiate into the central neuroglial cells (Fig. 17.4).

Although the extent of the proliferative activity varies in different parts of the neural tube, the pattern of cellular differentiation, organization, and orientation is maintained throughout the wall of this structure (Fig. 17.5). The innermost zone, which lines the lumen of the tube, is termed

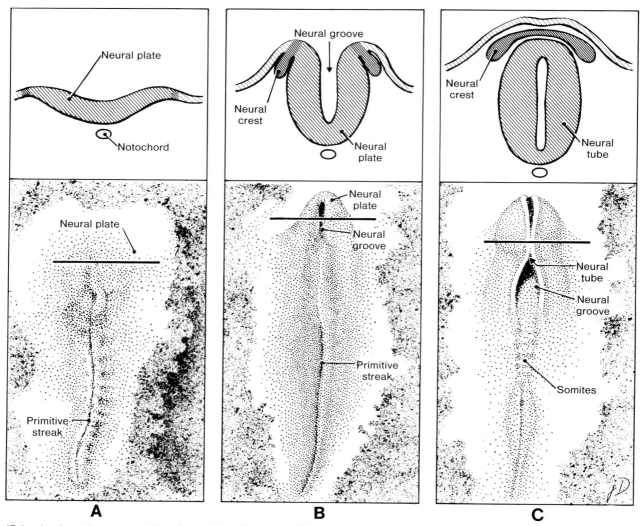

Figure 17.1. A schematic representation of neural tube development. *Upper*, cross sections; *lower*, dorsal views. *A.* The ectoderm thickens as the neural plate during the presomite stage of development. *B.* The neural plate continues to thicken and forms an invagination, the neural groove. *C.* The neural groove closes as a neural tube and neural crest cells are differentiated.

the *germinal* or *matrix layer*. It consists of actively dividing neuroepithelial cells. As these cells divide, their daughter cells migrate peripherally and form a centrally positioned *mantle layer*. The neuroblasts of this layer may send processes rostrad and/or caudad to form the outermost *marginal layer*. Or, the processes may perforate the neural tube to become motor fibers of the PNS. Glioblasts differentiate into neuroglial cells and assume their characteristic relationships to neurons in the three layers. Upon the culmination of CNS development, the three layers of the developing neural tube will have become the white matter (marginal layer), the grey matter (mantle layer) and the ependymal layer (germinal or matrix layer). The additional proliferation of neuroepithelial cells within the specific vesicles of the developing brain accounts for additional neuronal pools associated with these adult structures.

A longitudinal groove, the *sulcus limitans*, is present in the wall of the neural tube from the mesencephalon caudad. A plane coincident with the sulcus limitans divides the neural tube into two distinct anatomic and functional regions (Fig. 17.6). The mantle layer of the dorsal plate, *alar plate*, is associated functionally with sensory input into the CNS, whereas the mantle layer of the ventral plate, *basal plate*, is associated functionally with motor output from the CNS. Within the spinal cord, these two plates assume the relationships described (Fig. 17.7). Within the brain stem the relative positions of these two plates is maintained; however, the altered growth pattern in this region of the neural tube accounts for the lateral positioning of the alar plate and medial position of the basal plate (Fig. 17.7). The relative positioning of the neurons and neuronal pools that form these plates or columns is main-

tained in the neural tube from the mesencephalon caudally into the spinal cord.

Physiological Considerations

Functional Organization

The PNS was described previously as consisting of nerve trunks, ganglion cells, and neuronal terminals. The brief discussion of the development of the CNS indicated that the motor fibers exiting the CNS to innervate various effector organs originate from the motor plate. Functionally and anatomically, these neurons contribute to the PNS. Similarly, the ingrowth of neuronal processes from cranial and spinal ganglion cells from the periphery contributes to both the PNS and CNS. Numerous neuronal processes (axons), originating from various afferent neuronal terminals (dendritic zones) throughout the body are components of these systems. The classifi-

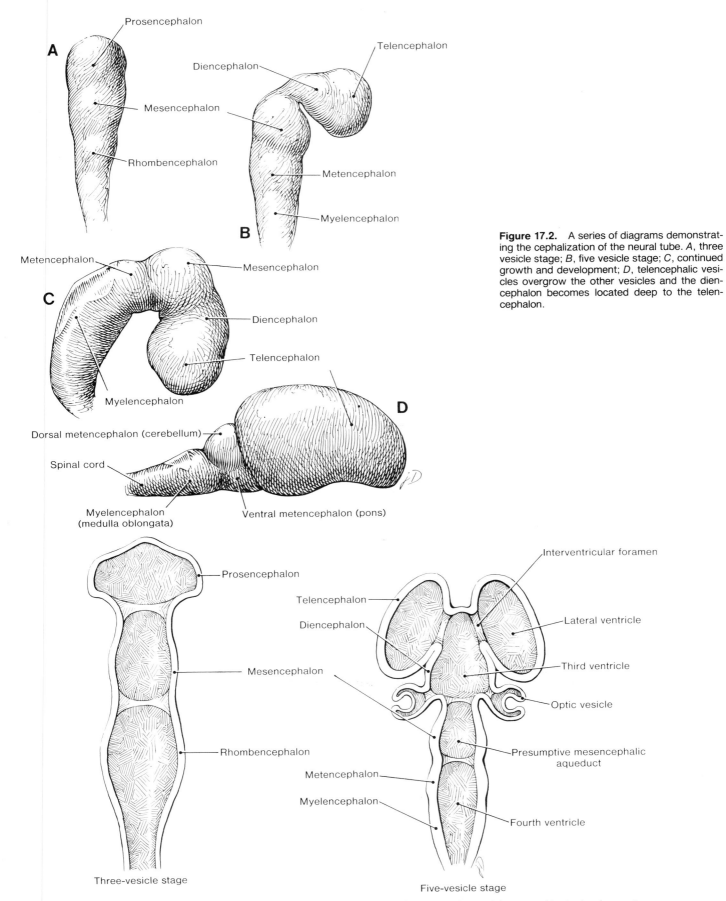

Figure 17.2. A series of diagrams demonstrating the cephalization of the neural tube. *A*, three vesicle stage; *B*, five vesicle stage; *C*, continued growth and development; *D*, telencephalic vesicles overgrow the other vesicles and the diencephalon becomes located deep to the telencephalon.

Figure 17.3. Diagrams of frontal sections through the three-vesicle and five-vesicle stage of brain development.

287

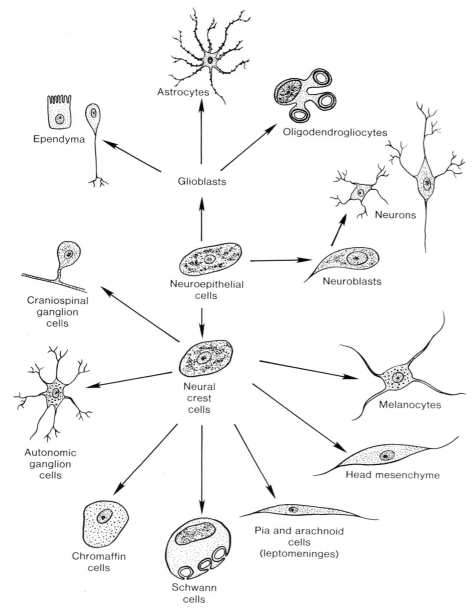

Figure 17.4. A diagram of the cellular intermediates and derivatives of neuroepithelial cells.

cation of the nervous system on a purely anatomical basis de-emphasizes the contribution these systems make to each other. Functionally, the neurons and their processes may be considered from different perspectives:

1. the location of the dendritic zone;
2. the location of the axon telodendria;
3. the type of information transmitted by the nerve fibers.

These criteria provide a basis for a functional classification scheme. Although the classification scheme is neither perfect nor complete, it does simplify the approach by grouping functionally similar neurons together (Table 17.1).

Efferent Systems. Information carried over nerve trunks is either going to or exiting from the CNS. The *motor* or *efferent fibers* innervate the effectors of the body. Their dendritic zones and cell bodies are located in the spinal cord and brain stem grey matter (basal plate). Their axonal processes form the cranial nerves, spinal nerves and splanchnic nerves. Those neurons whose axon telodendria are distributed generally throughout the body to the skeletal muscle mass comprise the *general somatic efferent (GSE) system*. The neurons that form this system are called the *lower motor neurons* or *final common pathway*.

Those neurons whose axon telodendria are distributed generally throughout the body to cardiac muscle, smooth muscle and glands comprise the *general visceral efferent (GVE) system*. This system is the efferent limb of the autonomic nervous system. **The GVE system is a two-neuron system.** (See Autonomic Nervous System, this chapter.)

Because of the unique embryological origin of certain skeletal muscle masses within the branchial arches, the nerve fibers that innervate them are given a special designation. Furthermore, these skeletal muscle fibers are associated with visceral functions. Accordingly, the neurons that innervate these unique skeletal muscle cells constitute the *special visceral efferent (SVE) system*.

Afferent System. The *sensory* or *afferent fibers* arise from dendritic zones scattered throughout the body. These fibers carry information to the brain and spinal cord and contribute to the alar plate region. The nerve cell bodies, dendritic zones, and part of their axons comprise the PNS. These fibers contribute to the cranial nerves, spinal nerves, and splanchnic nerves. Their telodendria, however, are located in the CNS.

Those neurons the dendritic zones of which are scattered throughout the body generally and are responsive to external stimulation by pain, touch, and temperature form the *general somatic afferent (GSA) system*. General proprioception (GP) is that system of neurons the dendritic zones of which are located in muscles, tendons, and joint capsules. They respond to changes in tension and length and add valuable conscious and unconscious information about body position and the relative position of body parts to each other. The GSA system is considered by some authors to include the GP system. All cranial nerves with GSE and SVE fibers probably transmit this type of information.

Certain organs are modified uniquely as sensory receptors that transmit information about the relationship of the organism to the external environment. The dendritic zones of the neurons that are integral components of the eye and ear, constitute the *special somatic afferent (SSA) system*. Vestibular functions of the ear comprise *special proprioception (SP)* and are considered to be part of the SSA system by some authors.

Those neurons the dendritic zones of which are located in the walls of the visceral organs constitute the *general visceral afferent (GVA) system*. The receptors respond to mechanical and chemical alterations within and/or associated with these organs.

Some organs are modified uniquely for the perception of *special visceral afferent* information—olfactory and gustatory sensations.

Reflex Arc

Introduction. Although the nervous system has the ability to initiate activity seem-

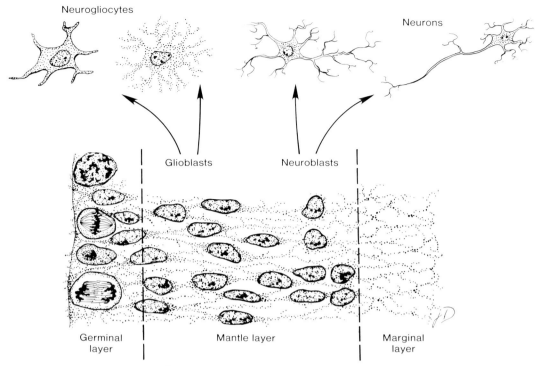

Figure 17.5. A diagram of a cross section through the developing neural tube. The zones of the neural tube and the derivatives of the component cells are indicated.

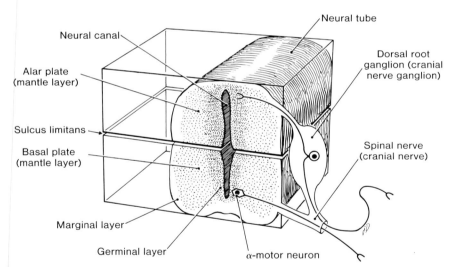

Figure 17.6. A diagram of the relationships of the alar and basal plates in the developing neural tube.

ingly independent from extraneous stimulation, the functional significance of the system is apparent when an activity is initiated in response to some sort of stimulus. Any given activity (movement of a limb, secretion of glands, increased heart rate, pupillary constriction) in response to a stimulus requires that afferent pathways are linked to efferent pathways. The involuntary activity that results from this linkage is called a *reflex*. The afferent and efferent limbs, as well as the interneurons that may

contribute, form the *reflex arc*. The reflex, generally, is a short-term, stereotypic response to a stimulus that serves the immediate needs of the organism.

Reflexes are not uniform involuntary events that occur in response to stimuli. Anatomically, they may vary from *monosynaptic* (involving only two neurons) to *polysynaptic* (involving more than two neurons). They may involve a simple knee jerk in response to increased patellar tendon tension (patellar reflex), increased cardiac

rate in response to decreased blood pressure (arterial pressoreceptor reflex), or a decreased cardiac rate in response to deep visceral pain during surgery (vago-vagal reflex). **Reflex motor activity does not occur as an event that is isolated from the rest of the nervous system. Reflexes, invariably, involve segmental, intersegmental, and suprasegmental contributions.**

Monosynaptic and Polysynaptic Reflexes. The simplest arrangement of neurons in a reflex arc is the *monosynaptic reflex* or *stretch reflex* (Fig. 17.8). A pseudounipolar nerve cell with its cell body located in the *dorsal root ganglion* has an axonal process extending from a stretch receptor that receives general proprioceptive information. The axon is a component of the *spinal nerve* and *dorsal root* and extends into the *dorsal grey column* of the spinal cord. Its axon telodendrion synapses with the dendritic zone of nerve cells located in the *ventral grey column*. Upon sufficient stimulation, the excitatory postsynaptic potentials (EPSP) result in an action potential in these *α-motor neurons (lower motor neurons, final common pathways)*. The axons of the neurons exit the spinal column, form the *ventral root*, and continue to the periphery in the *spinal nerve*. The telodendria of the GSE fibers innervate the skeletal muscle that is responsive to the proprioceptive stimulation.

Inhibition is achieved by the interposition of another neuron in the circuit, an *interneuron*. Stimulation of the interneuron

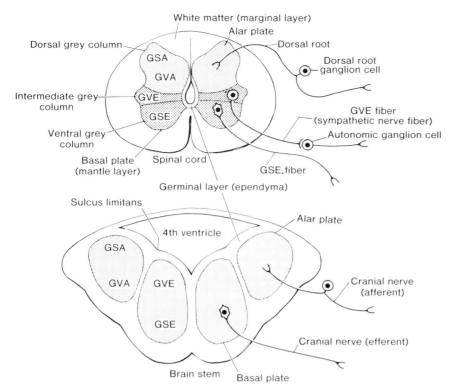

Figure 17.7. Diagrams depicting the relationships of the alar and basal plates in the spinal cord and brain stem. Refer to the text for an explanation of the functional classification of components.

Table 17.1.
Functional Organization of the Cranial and Spinal Nerves

System	Information Carried	Location of Telodendritic and Dendritic Zones	Nerves Involved*
EFFERENT			
GSE	Contraction	Skeletal muscle	III, IV, VI, XII, all spinal nerves
GVE	Contraction, secretion	Smooth and cardiac muscle and glands	III, VII, IX, X, XI, all spinal nerves
SVE	Contraction	Branchial arch skeletal muscle	V, VII, IX, X, XI
AFFERENT			
GSA	Pain, touch, temperature, general proprioception	Somatopleure derivatives	V, VII, IX, X, all spinal nerves
SSA	Optic, auditory, vestibular	Retina, membranous labyrinth	II, VIII
GVA	Mechanical, chemical	Splanchnopleure derivatives	VII, IX, X
SVA	Taste, smell	Tongue, olfactory mucosa	VII, IX, X, I

* Roman numerals refer to cranial nerves.

results in the generation of IPSPs in the α-motor neuron of the antagonistic muscle mass. The α-motor neuron becomes hyperpolarized and the antagonistic muscle mass relaxes. At the same time branches from the proprioceptive fibers ascend the spinal cord to transmit GSA information to higher brain centers (cerebrum, cerebellum). Suprasegmental transmission is complemented by branches from the fibers ascending and descending to other spinal cord segments (intersegmental). The reflex is a complex interaction between segmental, intersegmental, and suprasegmental neurons.

A *multisynaptic (polysynaptic) reflex* involves more than two neurons in the reflex arc (Fig. 17.8). The *withdrawal reflex* is an example of a multisynaptic reflex pathway. The application of excessive pressure to the interdigital region of the forelimb of a dog results in the withdrawal (flexion) of the forelimb. The GSA information is transmitted as described previously; however, an additional neuron is added to the circuit. The excitation of the α-motor neurons that innervate the flexors must be complemented by the inhibition of the extensors as described previously. Segmental, intersegmental, and suprasegmental relationships described previously also pertain to the reflex. The withdrawal and myotatic reflexes demonstrate the principle of *reciprocal innervation*. Excitation of the flexors requires the inhibition of the extensors. The converse is true also.

Cranial Nerve Reflex Patterns. The pattern of multisynaptic reflex activity also occurs with the cranial nerves and visceral nerves. The reflex activity associated with cranial nerves follows the same basic pattern described previously; however, such activity may involve more than one cranial nerve. One cranial nerve may serve as the afferent limb and another may serve as the efferent limb. Naturally, they are connected by interneurons. Although the spatial arrangement of cranial nerve reflexes is different from the spinal nerve reflexes, they are logical if the relationships between the alar plate (sensory plate) and basal plate (motor plate) are kept in mind. A V-VII reflex arc is an example of this type of relationship. Noxious stimulation to the head (cornea, palpebra, muzzle) is transmitted as GSA information to the sensory region (alar plate) of the trigeminal nerve (V). An interneuron connects this sensory region to the motor nucleus (basal plate) of cranial nerve VII (facial nerve). The SVE fibers of the cranial nerve VII innervate the skeletal muscles responsible for the response (squint, blink, menace).

Peripheral Organizational Components

Ganglia

Sensory Ganglia

Accumulations of nerve cell bodies outside the CNS are called *ganglia*. Corresponding accumulations within the CNS are called *nuclei*. Two types of ganglia are distinguished, *craniospinal ganglia (sensory)* and *autonomic ganglia (motor)*. The craniospinal ganglia include the *dorsal root ganglia* of the spinal nerves and the *cranial ganglia* of the cranial nerves. The autonomic ganglia include the *paravertebral* and *prevertebral ganglia* of the sympathetic nervous system. The parasympathetic ganglia are called *terminal ganglia*. They may be close to, upon, or within the wall of various organs. Those within the wall of organs are *intramural ganglia*.

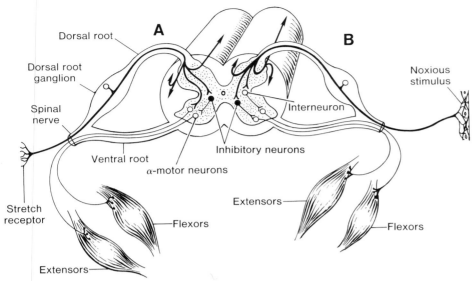

Figure 17.8. A diagram of a stretch reflex *(A)* and a withdrawl reflex *(B)*. The stretch reflex is monosynaptic; the axon telodendrion of the afferent neuron synapses with the α-motor neuron to the extensors. The withdrawl reflex is multisynaptic; the axon telodendrion of the afferent fiber synapses with an interneuron. The interneuron synapses with the α-motor neuron to the flexors.

Ganglia, although variable in size, are usually surrounded by a connective tissue capsule the fine collagenous and reticular fibers of which are scattered throughout the organ. Blood vessels, axons, dendrites, peripheral neuroglia, and nerve cell bodies are enmeshed within the supportive framework. Amphicytes are intimately associated with the nerve cell bodies.

Craniospinal Ganglia. Ganglion cells are features of all afferent neuronal fibers to the CNS. The ganglion cells of spinal nerves are located in *dorsal root ganglia*. Ganglion cells are components of all sensory nerves. This probably includes all cranial nerves. (Even the cranial nerves described as exclusively motor probably have general proprioceptive fibers.) The ganglion cells of the optic nerve are located in the retina. The ganglion cells for the remaining cranial nerves (I, V, VII-XI) are patterned after the dorsal root ganglia. (The ganglion cells of cranial nerve VIII, however, are bipolar neurons.)

The *dorsal root ganglia* are representative of craniospinal ganglia (Fig. 17.9). These globular structures are encapsulated (Plate II.11). Their size is variable. Each neuron is surrounded by amphicytes (Fig. 17.10). These flattened or cuboidal cells are in such intimate contact with the perikarya that indentations in the nerve cell bodies are often apparent. The amphicytes are continuous with the neurolemmal sheath of the axon. Axons comprise the remainder of the organ.

Motor Ganglia

Sympathetic and Parasympathetic Ganglia. The *sympathetic ganglia* and the multipolar neurons that comprise them are smaller than dorsal root ganglia and their constituent cells. Nerve fibers are scattered diffusely throughout these ganglia. *Parasympathetic ganglia* are similar to sympathetic ganglia. Those located within the organs *(intramural ganglia)*, however, are not as structured as those described previously (Fig. 17.11). Parasympathetic ganglia consist of a few multipolar nerve cell bodies and neuronal processes. In most instances, these perikarya are devoid of amphicytes; however, fibroblasts may replace the satellite cells. These ganglia, too, are motor ganglia.

Neuronal Processes

Nerve Trunks

The organization of peripheral neuronal processes into nerve trunks of varying size follows the basic pattern described for the organization of solid organs. The organization of nerve trunks is detailed in Figure 17.12.

Spinal Nerves. The nerve trunks or nerves are aggregations of axons (Bodian classification) connecting the brain, brain stem, and spinal cord to the peripherally positioned dendritic zones or axon telodendria of neurons. The *spinal nerves*, formed by the dorsal and ventral roots contain afferent and efferent fibers (Table 17.1). All spinal nerves contain GSA, GSE, and GVE components. The *viseral nerves*, which supply the visceral organs of the thoracic, abdominal, and pelvic cavities, are similar to the spinal nerves. They consist of GVA and GVE components.

Cranial Nerves. The cranial nerves are organized in different patterns. Dorsal and ventral roots are not apparent. The cranial nerves consist of nerve trunks that may be sensory only (I, II, VIII), motor only (III, IV, VI, XII), or sensory and motor (V, VII, IX, X, XI). The mixed (sensory and motor) cranial nerves are similar to the spinal nerves. The sensory cranial nerves deviate slightly from the basic pattern. The olfactory, optic, and vestibulocochlear nerves consist of axons of ganglion cells located in the olfactory bulbs, ganglionic layers of the retina, and vestibular and spiral ganglia, respectively. The cranial nerves that are motor only may be considered similar to the ventral roots and efferent components.

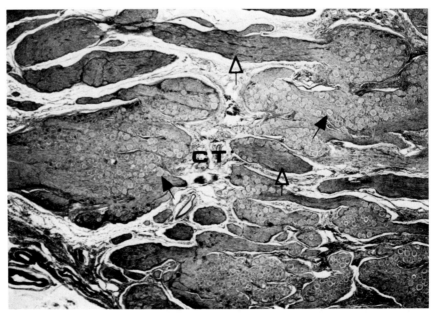

Figure 17.9. A section of a dorsal root ganglion. The organ consists of nerve cell bodies *(solid arrows)*, nerve cell processes *(open arrows)*, and connective tissue *(CT)*. ×4.

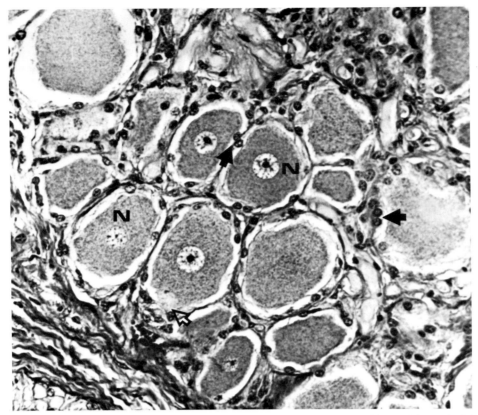

Figure 17.10. Cells of a dorsal root gangion. The neurons *(N)* are surrounded by amphicytes *(solid arrows)*. Note the axon hillock of one neuron *(open arrow)*. Compare with Figure 14.21. ×63. (Iron hematoxylin).

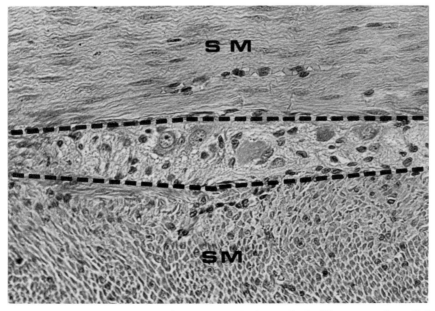

Figure 17.11. An intramural ganglion from a myenteric plexus. *Dashed lines*, approximate limits of the ganglion. The ganglion is interdigitated between two masses of smooth muscle *(SM)* of the tunica muscularis. ×100.

of the spinal and visceral nerves. The cell bodies of these nerves are contained within specific nuclei of the motor column (basal plate) of the brain stem.

Histological Organization

Epineurium. Nerve trunks consist of bundles *(fascicles)* of neuronal fibers in-

vested with connective tissue (Fig. 17.12). The outermost covering of nerves is the *epineurium* (Plates V.7, V.9 and Figs. 17.12 and 17.13). The epineurium, considered the capsule of these organs, consists of dense white fibrous connective tissue (DWFCT), irregularly arranged. The outermost covering of a single fascicle is epineurium. When numerous fascicles are joined together, as is the usual case, epineurium not only covers the entire nerve but individual fascicles are bound by epineural connective tissue.

Perineurium. The *perineurium* is the connective tissue investment of individual nerve fascicles (Figs. 17.13–17.15). The perineurium may consist of 1 to 10 layers of cells. As fascicles divide and become smaller, the perineurium becomes thinner. Ultimately, a single neuronal process is covered by a single layer of perineural cells. Capsules of afferent terminals (Pacinian and Meissner's corpuscles, muscle spindles) may be formed by perineural cells; whereas, naked neuronal processes emerge from their single perineural cellular investment at their terminations.

Perineural cells form alternating layers of cells between layers of collagenous and reticular fibers. The perineural cells may be continuous with or derived from the leptomeninges. Although referred to variously as fibroblasts throughout the literature, these cells are surrounded by basal laminae. If they are fibroblasts, then they are unique. Also, the margins of these cells dovetail and interlock with each other. At points of intimate contact, tight junctions are apparent. They may reasonably be considered epithelioid on the basis of these characteristics.

Endoneurium. The *endoneurium* is the connective tissue that extends from the surface of Schwann cells to the inner layer of perineural cells. It is the connective tissue space whose limits are defined by the basal laminae of the innermost perineural cells, Schwann cells, and endothelial cells (Figs. 17.15 and 17.16). Numerous collagenous fibers are scattered throughout this space. Fibroblasts may comprise between 5 and 25% of the nuclear profiles observed in section. (Coincidentally, these fibroblasts do not have a basal lamina associated with them.) The endoneurium also contains numerous capillaries. As capillaries enter the endoneurium from the perineurium, they carry extensions of the perineural cells with them.

Functional Correlates. These investments provide support for these peripherally positioned, delicate structures. The sheaths contribute to the elasticity that precludes their tearing during normal ranges of motion.

The perineurium and endoneurium contribute to the maintenance of a constant environment for neuronal processes. The perineuronal and endothelial cells of the

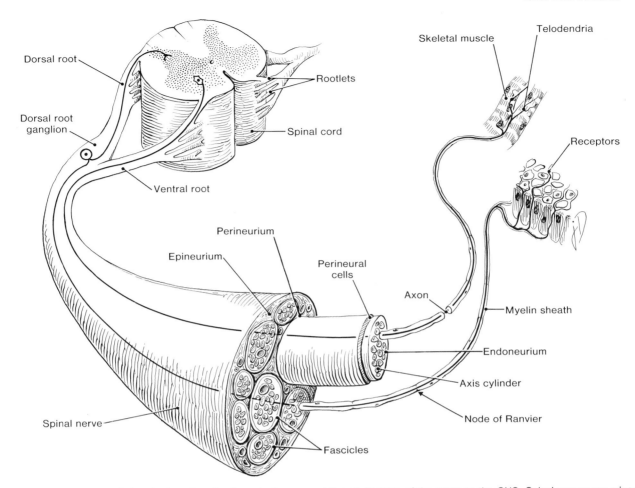

Figure 17.12. A diagram depicting the investments of a spinal nerve and the relationship of the nerve to the CNS. Spinal nerves are mixed nerves; their axons carry sensory and motor information.

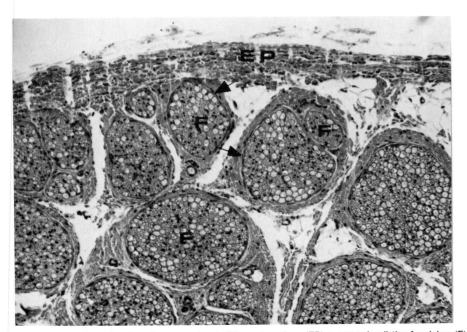

Figure 17.13. Organization of a nerve trunk. The epineurium *(EP)* surrounds all the fascicles *(F)*. Individual fascicles are surrounded by the perineurium. *Solid arrows* indicate the perineural cell sheath that surrounds individual fascicles deep to the perineurium. (Compare with Fig. 17.16.) The endoneurium surrounds individual nerve cell processes. ×40.

endoneurial capillaries form an incomplete *blood-nerve barrier* that prevents certain substances gaining entry to the endoneurium. Breaks exist at three sites: the terminations of neuronal processes where the perineurium ends; the entry points of blood vessels into the endoneurium at the end of the perineural cells; points at which collagenous fibers perforate the perineurium.

Afferent Terminals

Classification. The afferent nerve terminals (dendritic zones) are transducers that convert various types of modalities (pain, touch, warmth, pressure, etc.) into a form usable by the nervous system. Receptors have been classified in numerous ways: source of the stimuli and location of the receptors; types of modalities transduced by the receptors; form of the stimuli required to stimulate the receptors; the structure of the receptors. Two anatomical subdivisions are used to classify receptors: *free and diffuse, encapsulated.*

Free and Diffuse Endings. The *free and diffuse nerve endings* are the most ubiquitous. Although they are most numerous in the epidermis, they also occur in mucous

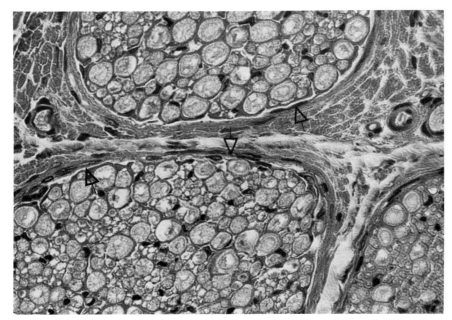

Figure 17.14. A section of a nerve and its investments. Layers of perineural cells *(arrows)* surround individual fascicles deep to the perineurium. ×160.

and serous membranes, muscles, joints, and the connective tissue of the viscera. The extensively arborized fibers may be myelinated or unmyelinated and may terminate as flattened or bulb-like endings scattered among epithelial or connective tissue cells (Fig. 17.17). They are usually considered touch receptors.

Merkel's disks are modified free nerve endings that are associated with deep epidermal cells. The terminal branches are flattened or disk-like and in contact with these modified cells. They generally occur in hairless skin. These receptors are associated with tactile stimulation that is pain associated.

Encapsulated Endings. The *encapsulated receptors* vary from slight to heavy encapsulation. These include: Meissner's corpuscles, Krause's endbulbs, Golgi-Mazzoni corpuscles, genital corpuscles, Vater-Pacinian corpuscles, Herbst corpuscles, Ruffini corpuscles, neuromuscular spindles, and Golgi tendon organs (Fig. 17.17).

Meissner's corpuscles are one of the most ubiquitous encapsulated receptors of hairless skin (Fig. 17.18). They occur in the dermal papillae of the soles and palms. The corpuscles are about 100 μm long and approximately 25 μm wide. They are slightly encapsulated and contain the terminals of one or more nerves arranged in a helical order around a mass of cells similarly arranged. The overall form is that of an imbricated fir cone. These corpuscles are receptors for tactile discrimination. Merkel's disks may be rudimentary forms of this corpuscle.

Krause's endbulbs are slightly encapsulated, spherical receptors that are located in the skin and associated mucous mem-

branes (especially the conjunctiva). In one type, the neuronal terminal enters the granular mass within the capsule and terminates at the opposite pole in a slightly expanded ending. In a second type, the nerve enters the granular mass within the capsule, undergoes arborization, and terminates in expanded endings. This corpuscle is a cold receptor.

Golgi-Mazzoni corpuscles are similar to Meissner's corpuscles. They are, however, smaller and more thickly encapsulated than Meissner's corpuscles. They are believed to be pressure receptors that occur in the connective tissue of hairless skin and associated mucous membranes. They also occur in the dermis of the glans penis, the digital pads of carnivores, and the connective tissue associated with the hoof.

Genital corpuscles are similar to, as well as larger and more encapsulated than, Golgi-Mazzoni corpuscles. Genital corpuscles may also be lobulated. The number of neuronal processes entering the capsule varies from one to ten. They arborize and form a spiral, interlacing network of naked neuronal terminals. These corpuscles, occurring in the clitoris and glans penis, are considered pressure receptors.

The *Vater-Pacinian corpuscles* are the largest encapsulated nerve endings (Fig. 17.19). They may be 3 to 4 mm long. A single axon enters the corpuscle and terminates in a bulbous enlargement surrounded by a mass of granular material. Concentric layers of epithelial cells (perhaps perineural cells), connective tissue cells, and capillaries impart an onion-like appearance (Fig. 17.20). The corpuscles are pressure receptors and are extremely ubiquitous. They occur in the deep connective

tissue, mesenteries, and serous membranes, as well as in the connective tissue of visceral organs, muscle, and that associated with tendons and ligaments.

Herbst corpuscles are smaller versions of Pacinian corpuscles that function as pressure receptors in the tongues and beaks of birds.

Ruffini corpuscles are composed of an arborization of neuronal processes interlacing throughout a granular mass enclosed by a connective tissue capsule. These corpuscles are believed to be heat receptors, but Ruffini-like receptors are associated with kinesthetic sensations.

Efferent Terminals

Neuromusclar spindles and *Golgi tendon organs* were described previously.

Some question relating to the specificity of given afferent terminals for a specific modality exist. The distinctness of some corpuscles is also questioned. Meissner's corpuscles, Merkel's disks, Golgi-Mazzoni corpuscles, Krause's end-bulbs and genital corpuscles are closely related. Similarly, Pacinian and Herbst corpuscles may be closely related. Evidence also exists that receptors continuously break down and reorganize throughout life.

Central Organizational Components

Meninges

The CNS is well protected by its placement within the bones of the skull and spinal column. Additional protection is afforded by the association of dense and loose connective tissue with the CNS (Fig. 17.21). These tissues are disposed as three fibrous membranes totally enclosing the system: dura mater, arachnoidea, and pia mater. The dura mater is also called the pachymeninx; the arachnoid and pia mater are called the leptomeninges. These membranes are intimately associated with *cerebrospinal fluid (CSF)* and the vascular supply of the CNS.

Pachymeninx

Dura Mater. The *dura mater* is a tough DWFCT covering of the brain and spinal cord that consists of collagen, some elastic fibers and blood vessels (Fig. 17.22). In association with the brain, it consists of two layers. The outer layer is the fibrous periosteum of the inner surface of the cranial bones. This layer contains a number of blood vessels associated with the cranial bones. An inner, poorly vascularized layer (meningeal layer) blends insensibly with the outer or periosteal layer. These layers become distinct in specific regions of the brain where they separate and form the *dural sinuses*. These sinuses are responsible for the collection of cerebrospinal fluid and its return to the vascular system. The dura

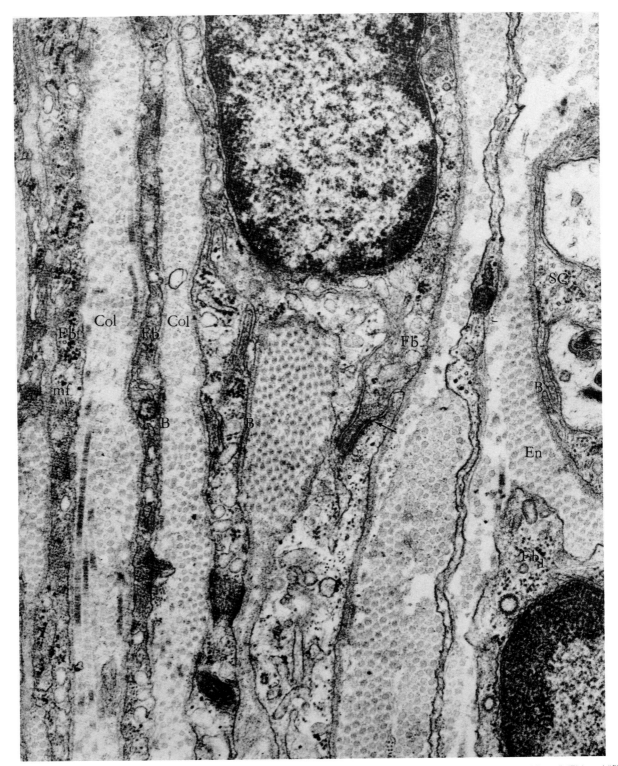

Figure 17.15. A transmission electron micrograph of the perineurium and endoneurium of a murine ischiatic nerve. "Fibroblasts" *(Fb)* and "fibroblastic processes" *(Fb)* alternate with layers of collagen *(Col)* within the perineurium. Note, however, that these "fibroblasts" are surrounded by a basal lamina *(B)*. Microfilaments among other typical organelles are visible within these cells. A Schwann cell *(SC)* within the endoneurium is covered by a basal lamina *(B)*, whereas an endoneural *(En)* fibroblast *(Fb₁)* is not surrounded by a basal lamina. Junctional complexes *(arrow)* also characterize the attachments of adjacent "fibroblastic cells" within a given cellular lamina. (Reprinted with permission from Peters, A., Palay., S. L. and Webster, H. F.: *The Fine Structure of the Nervous System: The Neurons and Supporting Cells*. W. B. Saunders, Co., Philadelphia, 1976.)

is separated from the arachnoid membrane by a potential *subdural space.*

The dura mater of the spinal cord is a single layer (meningeal dura) and is separated from the periosteum that lines the vertebrae by an extensive space called the *epidural space* (Fig. 17.23). This space is filled with loose connective tissue, adipose tissue, and extensive veins and venous si-

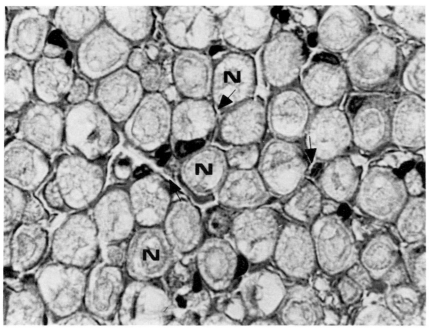

Figure 17.16. A section of a nerve and its investments. Individual nerve cell processes *(N)* are surrounded by the endoneurium *(arrows)*. Note the axis cylinders and neurokeratin of the altered myelin sheaths. ×320.

nuses. The epidural space is used for the administration of some anesthetics *(epidural anesthesia)*.

Leptomeninges

Arachnoidea. The *arachnoidea* consists of a distinct membrane and numerous fibrous trabeculae on its inner surface (Fig. 17.24). Both are composed of fine collagenous and elastic fibers. The extensive network of trabeculae that extends to the pia mater forms the supportive framework for the *subarachnoid space.* This space is occupied by cerebrospinal fluid. Blood vessels, also, are scattered on the floor of this space in the pia mater. Protrusions of com-

ponent tissues from the subarachnoid space extend through the inner layer of the dura mater and form *arachnoid villi (arachnoid granulations)* that project into the sinuses of the dura. Through this association, cerebrospinal fluid from the subarachnoid space is returned to the blood vascular system.

Pia Mater. The *pia mater* is the most intimate protective membrane of the brain and spinal cord (Figs. 17.22 and 17.24). It extends into the numerous depressions and fissures that characterize the CNS. This membrane is composed of very fine collagenous and elastic fibers, as well as small vessels. It is covered by a continuous membrane of flattened, fibroblastic cells. Blood vessels entering the depths of the nervous tissue are accompanied by connective tissue of the pia mater.

Cerebrospinal Fluid

Choroid Plexus

Histological Organization. The embryonic, tubular nature of the CNS is extensively modified during development. The simple tube of the embryo is converted to large ventricles and a canal in the brain that is continuous with a central canal in the spinal cord. The ependymal lining of this modified tube is retained in the adult. In specific areas (roof and walls of the ventricles), the ependyma is closely associated with the vascular pia mater. Usually, the pia mater is separated from the ependyma by numerous neurons and neuroglia elements. Juxtaposition of pia mater and

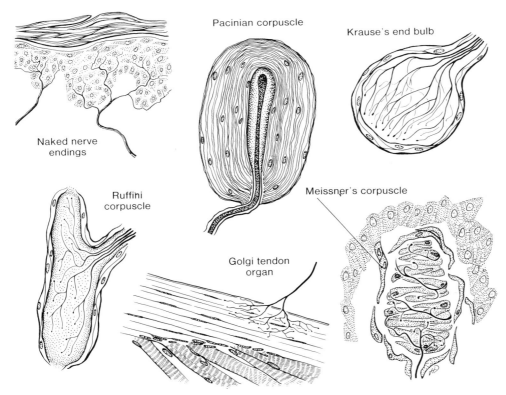

Figure 17.17. Diagrams of various types of receptors.

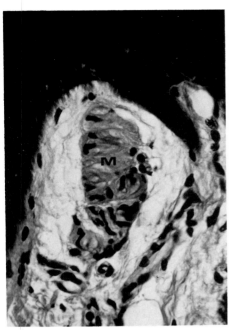

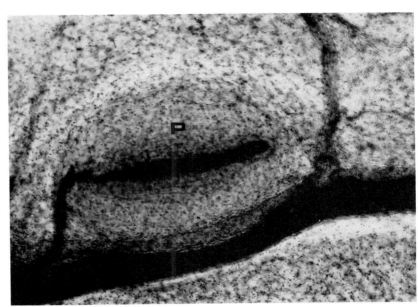

Figure 17.19. A whole mount preparation of a Vater-Pacinian corpuscle (P) from a mesentery. ×16.

Figure 17.18. A section of the skin. A Meissner's corpuscle (M) is apparent in the dermis. ×117.

ependyma occurs in regions in which interdigitated neurons and neuroglia do not develop.

The intimate juxtaposition of the pia mater (with its blood vessels and connective tissue) and ependyma forms the choroid plexus (Fig. 17.25). The choroid plexus consists of three distinct yet interrelated components: ependyma, tela choroidea, and choroid plexus (Fig. 17.26). The *ependyma* is a thin layer of epithelial cells, *lamina epithelialis*, that lines the ventricular space and is associated intimately with the peripherally positioned pia mater (Fig. 17.27). The cuboidal or columnar cells of this lamina have well-developed brush borders and are joined along their lateral margins by tight junctions that serve as an effective seal between the ventricular and extracellular fluid space of the pia mater (Fig. 17.28). The thin, web-like connective tissue of the pia mater is termed the *tela choroidea*. The vascular plexus *(choroid plexus)* is contained within the delicate connective tissue. These elements project into the ventricular system as extensive folds (villi).

Dynamic Relationships

General Features. The CSF is a clear, colorless fluid that fills the ventricular system and the central canal of the spinal cord. The CSF also occupies the subarachnoid space in association with the brain and spinal cord. The fluid is in continuity with both these spaces through two laterally positioned foramina in the roof of the fourth ventricle, the *foramina of Luschka*. The

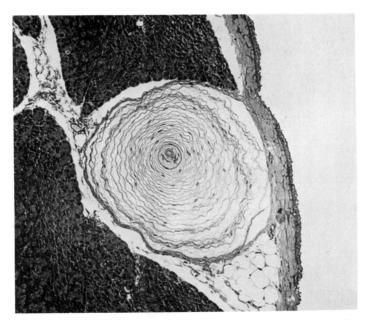

Figure 17.20. A cross section of a Vater-Pacinian corpuscle in the connective tissue associated with a feline pancreas. The concentric layers of components impart an onion-like appearance. ×25.

CSF is not confined to these spaces. Rather, it penetrates into and permeates all of the tissue of the CNS. The fluid serves as an hydraulic protective and supportive medium as well as a medium for the nutrition of neural tissue of the CNS.

As much as 40% of CSF may be produced at sites other than the choroid plexus—the general ependymal lining cells of the ventricular system, leptomeningeal coverings and blood vessels of the brain and spinal cord.

Formation of Cerebrospinal Fluid. CSF is produced as an *ultrafiltrate* or *dialysate*

of the blood and by *active secretion* by the ependymal cells. The principles of tissue fluid formation apply generally to CSF formation. Although CSF formation normally continues at a constant rate, its production rate is independent of blood hydrostatic pressure but is influenced by vascular colloid osmotic pressure. The selective permeability and active secretion of ependymal cells account for significant differences between CSF and tissue fluid. The CSF contains less calcium, potassium, glucose, and protein and more magnesium, sodium, and chloride than tissue fluid.

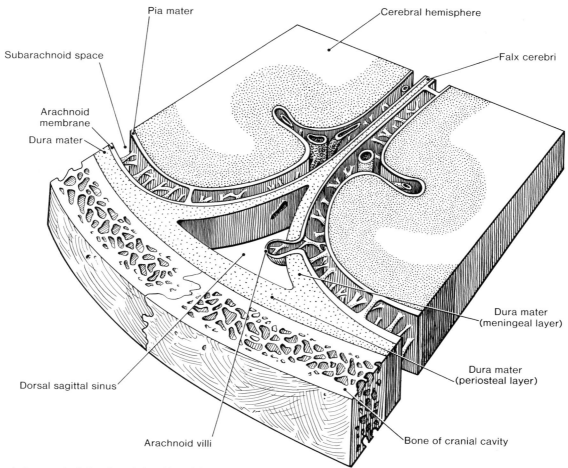

Figure 17.21. A diagram depicting the relationships of the cranial meninges in cross section. The separation of the two layers of the dura mater in the region depicted forms the dorsal sagittal sinus and the falx cerebri.

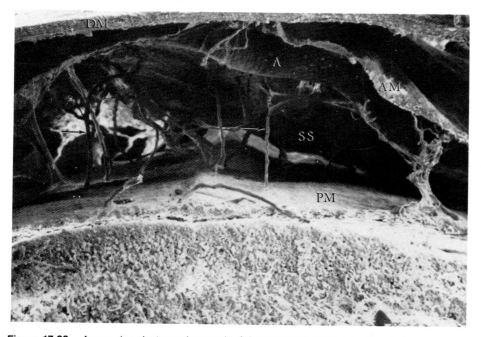

Figure 17.22. A scanning electron micrograph of the meninges of the spinal cord of a young dog. *DM*, dura mater; *A*, arachnoidea; *SS*, subarachnoid space; *PM*, pia mater: *arrows*, arachnoid trabeculations. (Reprinted with permission from Peters, A., Palay, S. L. and Webster, H. F.: *The Fine Structure of the Nervous System: The Neurons and Supporting Cells.* W. B. Saunders, Co., Philadelphia, 1976.

Circulation of Cerebrospinal Fluid. The bulk of CSF is produced by the plexuses of the lateral ventricles. The fluid flows into the third ventricle through the lateral ventricular foramina, and additional fluid is added by the choroid plexus of the third ventricle. The fluid continues its flow caudad through the cerebral aqueduct into the fourth ventricle where more CSF is added by the choroid plexus of the fourth ventricle. Although some fluid continues caudad into the central canal of the spinal cord, this flow pattern is not dynamic. CSF gains access to the subarachnoid space via the foramina of Luschka. Once within this space, the CSF bathes and covers all aspects of the brain and spinal cord. The fluid is returned to the vasculature by passing through the *arachnoid villi (granulations)*, which project into the *dural venous sinuses*. The arachnoid villi appear to function as pressure-dependent, unidirectional flow valves. Whereas the formation of CSF seems to be independent of vascular hydrostatic pressure, the return of CSF to the dural sinuses is dependent upon CSF/blood pressure gradients. Excessive pressure in the dural sinuses can collapse the villi and shut down the return of CSF.

Functions of Cerebrospinal Fluid. CSF

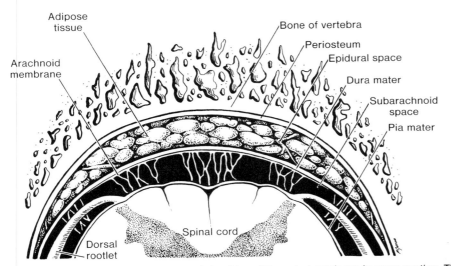

Figure 17.23. A diagram depicting the relationships of the spinal meninges in cross section. The dura mater of the spinal cord is separated from the periosteum by the epidural space.

Labels on figure: Adipose tissue; Arachnoid membrane; Bone of vertebra; Periosteum; Epidural space; Dura mater; Subarachnoid space; Pia mater; Dorsal rootlet; Spinal cord.

helps to maintain a constant extracellular microenvironment. The fluid seeps into the nervous tissue bathing all cells. The CSF is in dynamic equilibrium with the extracellular fluid. The specific gravity of CSF serves the important function of hydrostatic cushioning of the CNS. The weight of the brain in CSF is reduced to about one-third its weight in air.

The free movement of CSF into the extracellular fluid environment means that this fluid serves as the transport medium for the ingress and egress of various substances. Since lymphatic channels are not associated with the organs of the CNS, the CSF may be considered to perform this function. Various substances can reach the brain through the CSF. Finally, receptors in the fourth ventricle are responsive to hydrogen ion concentrations in CSF. The fluid, therefore, contributes to respiratory function.

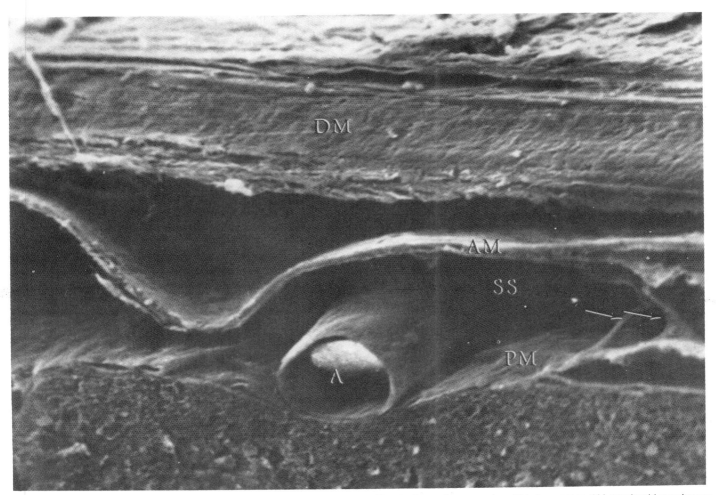

Figure 17.24. A scanning electron micrograph of the meninges of the cerebral hemisphere of a young dog. *DM*, dura mater; *AM*, arachnoid membrane; *SS*, subarachnoid space; *A*, arachnoidea; *PM*, pia mater; *SS*, subarachnoid space; *arrows*, subarachnoid trabeculations. A subdural space—an artifact of preparation— is apparent. (Reprinted with permission from Peters, A., Palay, S. L. and Webster, H. F.: *The Fine Structure of the Nervous System: The Neurons and Supporting Cells.* W. B. Saunders Co., 1976.)

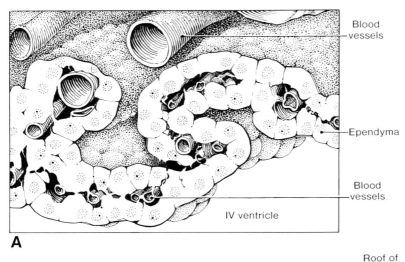

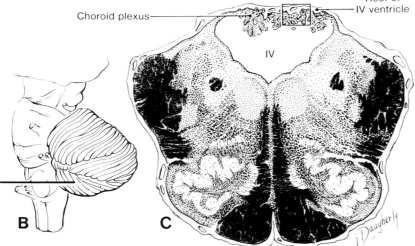

Figure 17.25. A composite drawing depicting the choroid plexus and its relationship to the fourth ventricle. *A*, an artist's interpretation of a scanning electron micrograph of the choroid plexus; *B*, the relationship of the choroid plexus to the fourth ventricle in cross section; *C*, the level from which the section was drawn.

Brain-Associated Barriers

Blood-Cerebrospinal Fluid Barrier

Structure and Function. The unique composition of CSF results from the high degree of regulation imposed upon its formation. The anatomical interface between blood and CSF consists of various components from without inward: diaphragmmed, fenestrated capillary endothelium, basal lamina, delicate connective tissue, basal lamina, and ependymal cells. These constituents form the *blood-CSF barrier* (Fig. 17.29). A minimal barrier is formed by the intimate juxtaposition of the endothelial cells and the ependymal cells and a fusion of their basal laminae. Perforations in the capillary endothelial cells imply a nonrestrictive movement of tissue fluid into the tela choroidea; therefore, the ependyma probably perform the significant barrier functions.

The free movement of CSF into the nervous tissue and the dynamic equilibrium of CSF and extracellular fluid are essential for the maintenance of the proper microenvironment for neuronal function. The movement of materials between these spaces is selective. The selectivity or barrier functions are not the exclusive domains of the interfacing anatomic components. Transport relates to specific structural and functional properties of endothelial and ependymal cells and the properties of the materials being transported.

Blood-Brain Barrier

Current Concepts. The blood vessels located within the subarachnoid space are bathed by CSF and are separated from the neural tissue by the pia mater (Fig. 17.29). As large blood vessels penetrate the substance of the neural tissue, they are sepa-

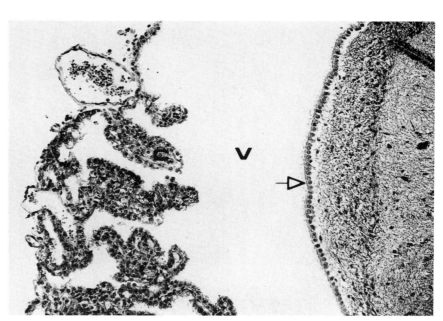

Figure 17.26. A section of a choroid plexus from a fourth ventricle. The choroid plexus *(C)* is suspended from the roof of the fourth ventricle *(V)*. Ependymal cells are integral components of the choroid plexus. The ependymal cells *(arrow)* also cover the nervous tissue of the brain stem adjacent to the fourth ventricle. ×40.

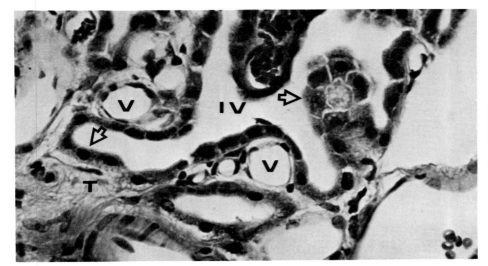

Figure 17.27. Components of the choroid plexus of the fourth ventricle *(IV)*. The ependymal cells *(arrows)* are associated intimately with the vessels *(V)* of the choroid plexus. Connective tissue components of the tela choroidea *(T)* are evident. ×125.

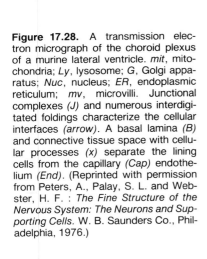

Figure 17.28. A transmission electron micrograph of the choroid plexus of a murine lateral ventricle. *mit*, mitochondria; *Ly*, lysosome; *G*, Golgi apparatus; *Nuc*, nucleus; *ER*, endoplasmic reticulum; *mv*, microvilli. Junctional complexes *(J)* and numerous interdigitated foldings characterize the cellular interfaces *(arrow)*. A basal lamina *(B)* and connective tissue space with cellular processes *(x)* separate the lining cells from the capillary *(Cap)* endothelium *(End)*. (Reprinted with permission from Peters, A., Palay, S. L. and Webster, H. F. : *The Fine Structure of the Nervous System: The Neurons and Supporting Cells*. W. B. Saunders Co., Philadelphia, 1976.)

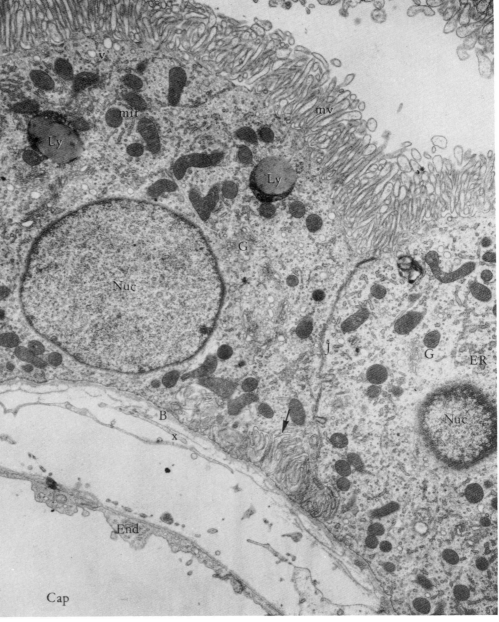

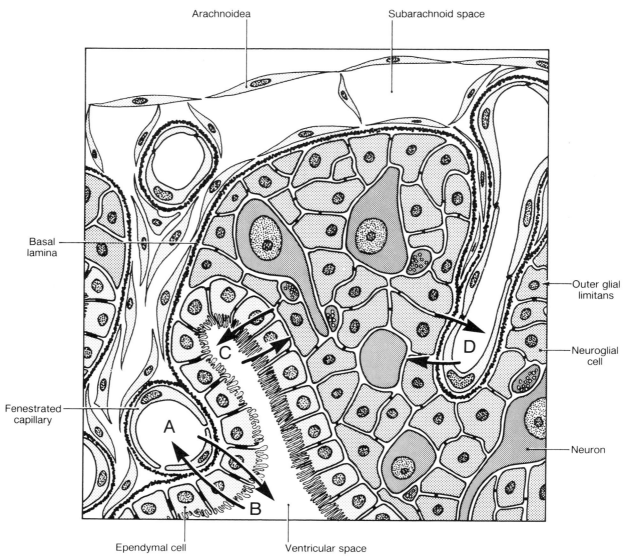

Arachnoidea   Subarachnoid space

Basal lamina

Fenestrated capillary

A

B

C

D

Outer glial limitans

Neuroglial cell

Neuron

Ependymal cell   Ventricular space

Figure 17.29. An artist's conception of the blood-CSF and blood-brain barriers. *A.* Tissue fluid forms by ultrafiltration of the plasma. *B.* Ependymal cells modify the ultrafiltrate as cerebrospinal fluid. *C.* CSF enters the substance of the nervous tissue, freely bathing the neurons and neuroglia. *D.* Endothelial cells serve as the blood-brain barrier. Fluid and dissolved substances enter the nervous tissue, bathing the neurons and neuroglia.

rated from the pia mater by a pericapillary space. This perivascular *space of Virchow-Robin* becomes progressively smaller and eventually is obliterated when the capillaries become juxtaposed to the neuroglial cells (astrocytes) that form the *outer glial limitans*. Juxtaposition of neuroglial cells between capillary beds and neurons provides the anatomical basis for a blood-neuron interface. This interface has been called the blood-brain barrier. The astrocytes forming this barrier have foot-like processes that are associated intimately with the basal lamina of the endothelial cells. Astrocytes *were* considered the cells through which materials passed between the capillary bed and neurons. Current evidence, as discussed previously, has established clearly that the neurons and neuroglia are bathed continuously by the CSF (Fig. 17.29). Moreover, some materials move readily

from the capillary bed between neuroglial cells and gain access to the neurons. **The blood-brain barrier is formed by the endothelial cells of the brain capillaries.**

The reasons governing the selective behavior of these capillary endothelial cells is not clear. Tight junctions, glial foot processes, specialized transport systems within endothelial cells (carrier-mediated transport) and the specific properties of the substances being transported impart barrier functions to these endothelial cells. The capillary endothelium of the brain should be considered a secretory lining epithelium.

Specific Organs

Spinal Cord

The spinal cord varies in configuration at the cervical, thoracic, lumbar, and sacral

levels. The following pattern, however, is similar at all levels of the cord.

The cord is generally round to oval and is surrounded by the pachymeninx (inner layer) and the leptomeninges (Fig. 17.30). The bulk of the cord is divided into two distinct regions, grey matter and white matter. The *grey matter* is arranged in a pattern often described as an H or butterfly. The grey matter consists of nerve cell bodies, unmyelinated fibers, some myelinated fibers, protoplasmic astrocytes, oligodendrogliocytes, microgliocytes, and some blood vessels with fine perivascular connective tissue fibers. Although neurons are aggregated or scattered throughout the grey matter, they are especially distinct in the *ventral columns*. These large multipolar neurons (α-motor neurons) give rise to axons carrying information to effector organs of the body. Neurons of medium size are

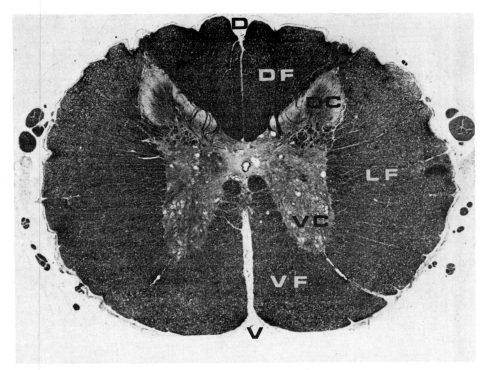

Figure 17.30. A typical section through the cervical region of the spinal cord. The dorsal *(DC)* and ventral *(VC)* columns are prominent grey matter components. The dorsal *(DF)*, lateral *(LF)* and ventral *(VF)* funiculi comprise the white matter of the spinal cord. *D*, dorsal; *V*, ventral. ×4. (Myelin stain).

those derived from the myelencephalon, metencephalon, mesencephalon, and diencephalon. Various nuclei and tracts are distributed in a specific manner throughout the brain stem (Plate V.10 and Fig. 17.3). The general pattern of nerve cell body and tract distribution for the cranial nerves rostral to the myelencephalon follows the general relationships described for the alar and basal plates. Additional nuclei occur within the region, and numerous ascending and descending tracts occur.

Cerebellum. The cerebellum is also divided into grey and white matter (Fig. 17.32). The white matter is covered by a thin layer of grey matter. Three distinct zones of grey matter are apparent: *outer molecular layer, central layer of Purkinje cells* and *deep granular layer.* The granular layer is contiguous to the white matter (Plates I.4 and I.5).

The outer molecular layer consists of some small neurons and numerous unmyelinated fibers. The Purkinje cells of the central layer are large, pyramidal cells that are very prominent (Figs. 17.33 and 17.34). **(Do not confuse Purkinje cells with Purkinje fibers!)** The neurons of the granular layer are small and tightly packed within this region. The details of the connections among these cells, as well as connections with *mossy* and *climbing fibers,* are available in texts of neuroanatomy.

located in the *lateral columns* of the thracolumbar segments. These neurons give rise to axons that connect with autonomic ganglia. Small neurons characterize the *dorsal columns.* Their axons project up and down the spinal cord. The spinal canal (lined by ependyma) is contained within the *central intermediate substance* or *grey commissue.*

The *white matter* is composed of myelinated and unmyelinated fibers, scattered neuroglial elements and blood vessels. A *dorsal funiculus* occupies the region between the dorsal columns; a *lateral funiculus* is between two adjacent dorsal and ventral columns; and a *ventral funiculus* is between the two ventral columns.

The diameter of the spinal cord is not uniform from the cervical to sacral regions. Because most of the thoracic limb is innervated by the cervical segments of the spinal cord, there is a corresponding enlargement at this level. The *cervical (brachial) enlargement* or *intumescence* occurs between the levels C_6-T_1. A similar enlargement, the *lumbar intumescence,* occurs in the caudal aspect of the spinal cord in relation to the pelvic limb between segments L_4-S_2. The enlargements result from greater quantities of white and grey matter in these portions of the spinal cord than in other segments.

The white matter of the spinal cord is divisible into specific regions characterized by ascending and descending fiber tracts. Species differences exist in the distribution,

size, and relative positions of these tracts within the spinal cord.

Brain Stem

The brain stem is a complex structure that is continuous with the spinal cord caudally and higher brain centers rostrally. The structures that form the brain stem are

Cerebrum

The diverse and complex functions of the cerebrum are reflected in its cytoarchitecture. Although six layers of cells have been described, the degree of development of each layer varies with the section of cerebral cortex being studied (Fig. 17.35). The grey (outer) region of the cerebral cor-

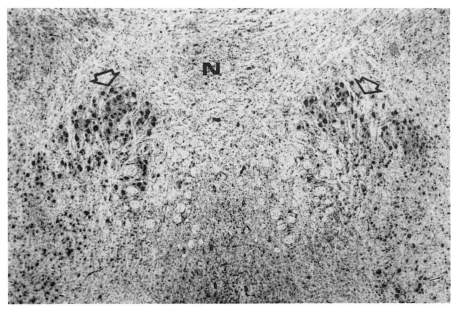

Figure 17.31. A frontal section through the brain stem of a pig. The nerve cell bodies of two prominent nuclei *(arrows)* are apparent within the rest of the nervous tissue *(N)* of the organ. ×4.

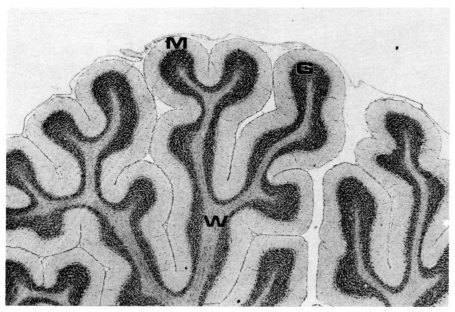

Figure 17.32. A section through a cerebellum. The molecular layer *(M)* and the granular layer *(G)* are peripheral to the white matter *(W)*. ×4.

tex consists generally of the following cellular regions: *molecular layer, outer granular layer, pyramidal cell layer, inner granular layer, ganglion* or *inner pyramidal cell layer,* and *polymorphic cell layer.*

Throughout these regions are neuroglial elements, myelinated and unmyelinated nerve fibers and vessels. The student is referred to a text of neuroanatomy for further discussion of the cerebral cortex.

Autonomic Nervous System

Organization

System Characteristics

Introduction. The regulation of a constant and optimal internal environment (*homeostasis* or *homeokinesis*) is the function of the autonomic nervous system (ANS). It is complemented in its activity by the endocrine system. Together, these systems function to provide the fine control of the numerous parameters that permit the normal expression of cellular activities.

The regulatory effects of the ANS are manifested via its influence on four types of effector systems: (1) smooth muscle (e.g., intestines, urinary bladder, blood vessels); (2) cardiac muscle; (3) exocrine glands (salivary, sweat, mucous); (4) some endocrine glands (adrenal medulla); The ubiquitous distribution of smooth muscle and exocrine glands exemplifies the broad influence of this system upon the body. The effects of cardiac function manifest broad influences. The primary hormone of the adrenal medulla (epinephrine) has broad effects.

Components—Central and Peripheral. Often, the ANS is presented as an efferent

(motor) system that links the CNS to the aforementioned effectors. The efferent portion of this system may be the most obvious, but the autonomic regulation of visceral function requires more than efferent pathways. The ANS consists of: *sensors, afferent pathways, central integration centers, control centers, efferent pathways and effectors.* Together, these function in the maintenance of the internal environment. The system consists of centrally and peripherally located components (Fig. 17.36). The receptors (sensors) for the ANS are located throughout the viscera.

Afferent Input. The common modalities monitored by the receptors are: stretch, distention, pressure and chemical changes.

Impulses from these receptors course over nerves toward the central nervous system. The fibers, carrying generalized sensory information from the viscera, are referred to as GVA fibers. Upon entry into the spinal cord, a reflex pathway is established through an *internuncial neuron (interneuron).* The afferent information also ascends to higher centers (suprasegmental). This may be at the conscious level (e.g., visceral pain) or the unconscious level. The impulses, directly or indirectly, reach the *hypothalamus,* the integration center of the autonomic nervous system. The hypothalamus, then, influences metabolic centers in the midbrain, pons, and medulla. Efferent fibers originate in these centers, as well as the spinal cord, and innervate visceral effectors via specific cranial nerves, spinal nerves, and splanchnic nerves. These fibers, carrying general motor impulses to the visceral effectors, are referred to as GVE fibers.

Because the ANS is involved in the regulation of visceral functions, the fibers of the GVA and GVE systems are essential constituents. The sensory input to the ANS, however, is not restricted to that transmitted by GVA fibers. All sensory systems (GVA, SVA, SSA, and GSA) supply input to the ANS.

Reflex Arc—Basis of Regulation. The ANS is a system designed to function spontaneously or indepedently of volition. The *reflex arc* is central to such an organizational scheme. The higher centers, specifically the hypothalamus, serve to modulate the response. Through the integrative functions of the hypothalamus, the effectors of

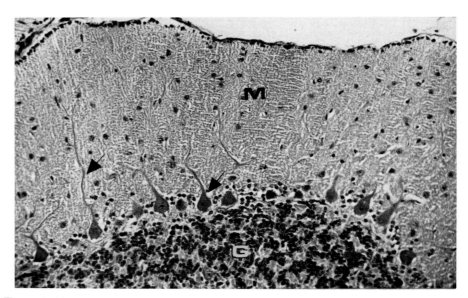

Figure 17.33. Purkinje cells of a cerebellum. The Purkinje cells *(arrows)* occur at the interface between the molecular *(M)* and granular *(G)* layers. ×4.

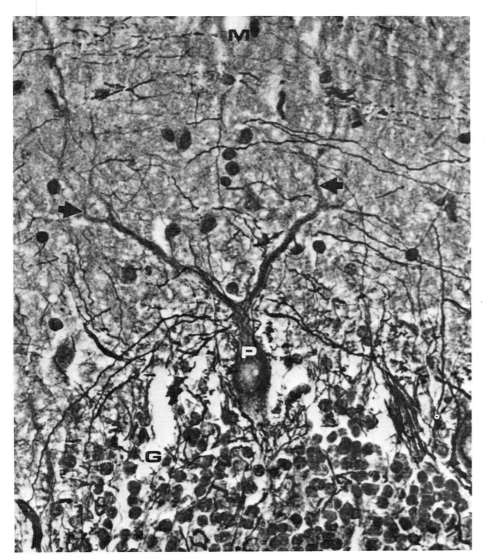

Figure 17.34. A Purkinje cell of a cerebellum. The Purkinje cell *(P)* has dendritic processes *(arrows)* extending into the molecular layer. The axon of the cell extends through the granular layer *(G)* and synapses with neurons in the cerebellar nuclei. ×100 (Silver stain).

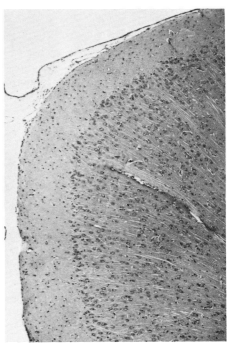

Figure 17.35. A section through a cerebrum. The occurrence and distribution of layers of the grey matter differ in various regions of the cerebrum. ×10.

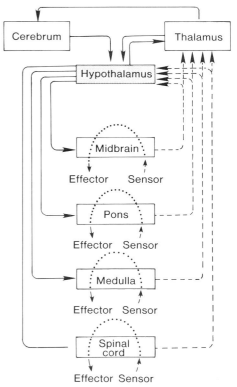

Figure 17.36. A schematic diagram of the components of the autonomic nervous system. *Solid lines,* efferent pathways; *dashed lines,* afferent pathways; *dotted lines,* reflex pathways through the midbrain, pons, medulla oblongata, and spinal cord.

the ANS manifest a basic level of normal activity *(tone)* that may be modified by afferent input and efferent output.

In a polysynaptic somatic reflex (Fig. 17.37: (1) GSA fibers reach the *dorsal root* from the spinal nerve and enter the *dorsal grey column.* (2) a synapse occurs with an *interneuron.* (3) the interneuron synapses with a neuron in the *ventral grey column (α-motor neuron, lower motor neuron, final common pathway).* (4) GSE fibers enter the *ventral root* and *spinal nerve* and subsequently reach the skeletal muscle effector.

In the typical autonomic reflex: (1) GVA fibers reach the *dorsal root* and enter the *dorsal grey column.* (2) a synapse occurs with a neuron *(pregnaglionic neuron)* located in the *intermediate grey column.* (3) this axon courses out of the spinal cord and synapses with a second neuron *(postganglionic neuron)* that is located in a motor ganglion. (4) the GVE impulses are transmitted over postganglionic fibers (axons) to the visceral effectors.

Some authors refer to the neuron in the intermediate grey column as the interneuron, whereas others refer to it as the lower motor neuron. It is the author's opinion that **it is consistent with the terminology applied to a somatic reflex to consider the first neuron (preganglionic) as the interneuron and the second neuron (postganglionic) as the lower motor neuron.** The cell bodies of the second neurons (postganglionic) may be located in *vertebral (paravertebral), prevertebral (collateral)* or *terminal (peripheral) ganglia.* The unmyelinated axons of postganglionic neurons terminate on visceral effectors. **The autonomic reflex, then, always consists of least three neurons: an afferent neuron, a preganglionic neuron, a postganglion neuron.**

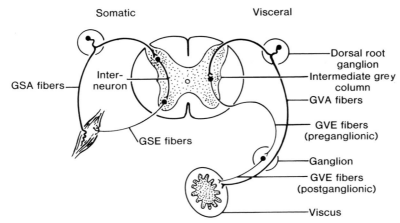

Figure 17.37. A diagrammatic comparison between a somatic and visceral reflex. Note the additional neuron located in a ganglion in the visceral reflex.

Sympathetic and Parasympathetic Divisions

General Features. The ANS is divided into two subdivisions: *sympathetic* and *parasympathetic nervous systems*. Part of the rationale for these subdivisions is predicated upon the anatomical location of the first neuron (preganglionic neuron). These neurons are located in three regions of the central nervous system—*brain stem, thoracolumbar spinal cord* and *sacral spinal cord* (Fig. 17.38).

In the sympathetic nervous system, the cell bodies of the preganglionic neurons are located in the intermediate grey column of the *thoracolumbar spinal cord*. These neurons extend from approximately the first thoracic to the fifth lumbar segment of the spinal cord. This portion of the ANS is also called the *thoracolumbar system*. In the parasympathetic nervous system, the cell bodies of the preganglionic neurons are located in the *brain stem* in *nuclei of cranial nerves III, VII, IX, X*, and *XI* and in *sacral segments of the spinal cord*. This outflow pattern is the basis for referring to this system as the *craniosacral system*.

The Sympathetic Nervous System

Origin and Distribution. Numerous patterns characterize the distribution of pre- and postganglionic sympathetic nerve fibers. Notably, the postganglionic fibers are long. The synapses between the pre- and postganglionic neurons occur some distance away from the effectors innervated. **Synapses within the paravertebral ganglia occur for fibers being distributed to the periphery generally. Synapses within pre-vertebral ganglia are for fibers being distributed to the deep visceral organs.**

Specific nerves may be identified after a careful dissection of the sympathetic nervous system. The nerves and associated prevertebral ganglia form extensive plexuses that are intimately associated with major arteries.

Generally, preganglionic fibers originating cranial to T_5 are distributed cranially, whereas those nerves originating caudal to T_5 are distributed caudally. The extent of the ganglionated sympathetic trunk is actually greater than the site of origin of preganglionic fibers. The trunk extends from the cranial cervical region to the cranial caudal region. In the cervical region, the sympathetic trunk is enclosed within a common sheath with the vagus nerve, forming the *vagosympathetic trunk*.

The Parasympathetic Nervous System

Origin and Distribution. The spatial relationships between GVA fibers and the GVE fibers of the sacral portion of the parasympathetic nervous system follow the basic pattern discussed previously. Afferent information reaches the spinal cord via the pelvic and splanchnic nerves. The cell bodies for the fibers, as described previously, are located in the dorsal root ganglia. These neurons synapse with the preganglionic neurons located in the intermediate horn. Preganglionic fibers are than distributed to the viscera via the pelvic nerve and plexus. Their terminal ganglia are the sites for synapses with the postganglionic neurons. These synapses, generally, occur within the walls of the organs innervated. Accord-

ingly, they are referred to as intramural ganglia. The postganglionic fibers are very short.

Afferent information at the level of the sacral cord also ascends the spinal cord to higher brain centers. Also, afferent information may be carried via the splanchnic nerves to the vagus nerve and then to higher centers.

The reflex pattern for the cranial portion of the parasympathetic nervous system is organized in a manner slightly different than described previously for the autonomic spinal reflexes. These organizational differences are related to the different embryological events characteristic of spinal cord and brain stem development.

The parasympathetic nuclei of cranial nerves III, VII, IX, X and XI are homologous to the intermediate grey columns of the spinal cord (thoracic, lumbar, and sacral segments). These nuclear regions are the sites of origin of the preganglionic fibers of these parasympathetic nerves. Synapses with postganglionic neurons occur in terminal ganglia that are located close to or within the organs innervated.

Afferent information may enter the brain stem in a variety of ways and from various sources. The cell bodies of afferent fibers are located in specific sensory ganglia that are homologous to the dorsal root ganglia of the spinal cord. (One exception to this is the use of SSA information.) Upon entry into the brain stem these afferent fibers project rostrad and caudad in the *solitary tract*. These fibers terminate on interneurons of the *nucleus of the solitary tract*, the fibers of which synapse (directly or indirectly) with the preganglionic neurons of cranial nerves VII, IX, X, and XI. Despite the altered organizational patterns, all of the components necessary for an autonomic reflex are present.

Functional Correlates

Dual Innervation. Most of the visceral organs of the body have a dual innervation. The functional influence of the sympathetic and parasympathetic innervation upon these organs has been described classically as antagonistic. One system, in fact, may enhance and/or accelerate visceral functions, whereas the other may inhibit and/or decelerate visceral functions. They manifest a synergistic effect upon visceral function to achieve a desired end—homeostasis.

There are notable exceptions to the previous generalities. Both divisions seem to

Figure 17.38. An idealized drawing of the autonomic nervous system. The diagram is simplified for clarity. Not all the permutations possible are shown. Moreover, fusion of nerves into each other is not typical of the antomy but is used to reduce the number of lines on the drawing. The sympathetic innervation of the integument (arrector pili muscles, vessels, glands) is only indicated for one segment to the *left* to reduce the complexity of the drawing. The innervation of other visceral organs is shown to the *right*. The specific pathways of the sympathetic innervation to the cervical organs via the vertebral nerve is not indicated. Sympathetic nerves are red, parasympathetic nerves are blue. Preganglionic fibers are *solid*, postganglionic fibers are *dashed*.

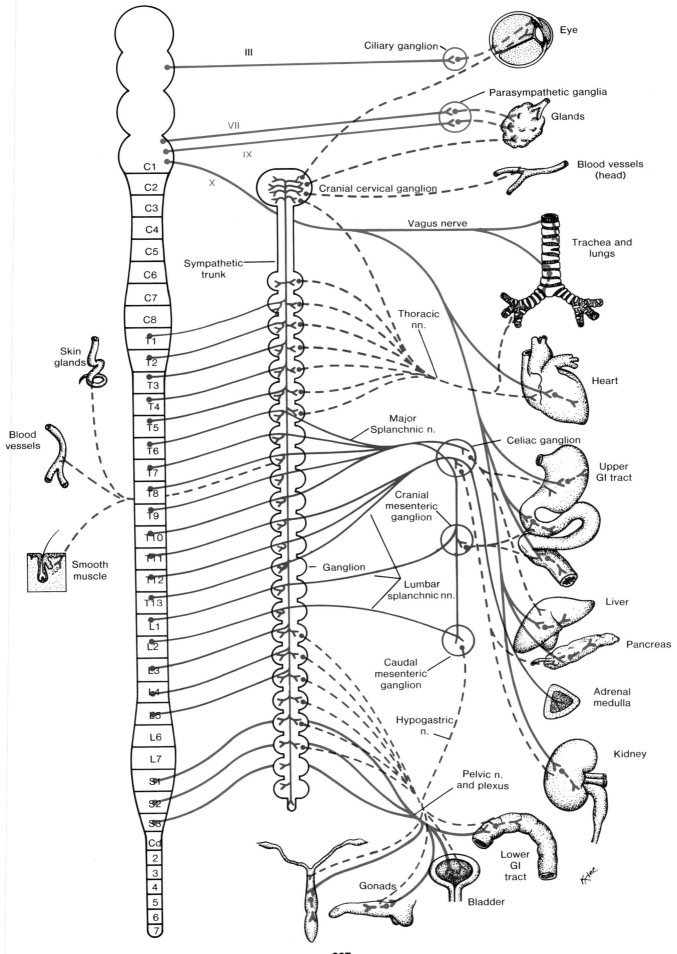

III

VII

IX

X

C1
C2
C3
C4
C5
C6
C7
C8
T1
T2
T3
T4
T5
T6
T7
T8
T9
T10
T11
T12
T13
L1
L2
L3
L4
L5
L6
L7
S1
S2
S3
Cd
2
3
4
5
6
7

Ciliary ganglion

Eye

Parasympathetic ganglia

Glands

Blood vessels (head)

Cranial cervical ganglion

Vagus nerve

Sympathetic trunk

Trachea and lungs

Thoracic nn.

Heart

Skin glands

Major Splanchnic n.

Celiac ganglion

Upper GI tract

Cranial mesenteric ganglion

Blood vessels

Ganglion

Lumbar splanchnic nn.

Liver

Smooth muscle

Pancreas

Caudal mesenteric ganglion

Adrenal medulla

Hypogastric n.

Kidney

Pelvic n. and plexus

Gonads

Lower GI tract

Bladder

307

stimulate salivary and pancreatic secretion. Moreover, not all organs have a dual innervation. The adrenal medulla, spleen, pilomotor muscles, sweat glands, and probably all of the blood vessels of the body are innervated exclusively by the sympathetic division. The parasympathetic division provides the exclusive innervation for the ciliary and pupillary sphincter muscles, whereas the sympathetic division innervates the pupillary dilator.

Comparison of Systems. For those organs that are innervated exclusively by the sympathetic nervous system, tone variations are still possible. Normally, most vessels are constricted partially by the basal level of activity of this system. An increased level of activity constricts the vessels *(vasoconstriction)*, whereas a decreased level of activity permits dilation of the vessels *(vasodilation)*.

The preganglionic fibers of the autonomic nervous system are myelinated and relatively slow-conducting B fibers. Each preganglionic fiber potentially may diverge to numerous postganglionic neurons that give rise to mostly unmyelinated C fibers. By comparison to the somatic system, the autonomic output is diffuse and slow.

The two systems manifest differences in the degree of response. These differences may be explained, in part, on the basis of the different *innervation ratios* in the two systems. The relatively short preganglionic fibers of the sympathetic nervous system synapse with numerous neurons some distance from the organs innervated, permitting a diffuse response over the long postganglionic fibers to the organs innervated. This innervation ratio of preganglionic axons to ganglion cells may be one to twenty or more. The relatively long preganglionic fibers of the parasympathetic nervous system synapse with numerous neurons close to or within the organs innervated, permitting a more discrete and limited response than its sympathetic counterpart. In some organs, the innervation ratio seems to be one to one; however, estimates of the ratio of preganglionic vagal fibers to ganglion cells of the submucosal plexus are as high as 1:8000. The distinction between the two systems based upon discreteness of response does not apply to all sites.

The innervation ratios, alone, do not distinguish the two systems. Postganglionic synapses with effector cells are described as *intermediate forms* of *directed synapses*. Local effects of adrenergic neurotransmitters, or the degree of nondirectedness, may exceed the the local effects of acetylcholine upon its effectors.

Synaptic Relationships

Transmitters

Specific Substances. Transmission at the synapses between the pre- and postgan-glionic neurons and between the postganglionic neuron and effector organs is chemically mediated. *Neurotransmitters* act upon receptors to affect postganglionic neurons and/or effector organs. The principal neurotransmitters of the ANS are *acetylcholine (ACH)* and *norepinephrine* (Fig. 17.39).

Pre- and Postganglionic Fibers. Sympathetic and parasympathetic preganglionic fibers release ACH. These fibers are called *cholinergic* fibers. The parasympathetic postganglionic fibers are *cholinergic* fibers. The neurotransmitter secreted by sympathetic postganglionic fibers is *norepinephrine*; they are *adrenergic* fibers.

Cholinergic Receptor Sites

General Features. These types of receptors are discussed in Chapter 14; additional information is required now as to relate their function to the ANS. Drugs that mimic ACH are termed *cholinergic drugs*. ACH receptor sites are termed *cholinergic receptors*. Although ACH is released by preganglionic sympathetic and parasympathetic nerves and postganglionic parasympathetic nerves, the properties of the preganglionic and postganglionic receptor sites are different. These two sites manifest a differential responsiveness to two plant alkaloids, muscarine and nicotine.

Muscarinic Sites. *Muscarine*, a mycotic alkaloid, has little effect upon autonomic ganglion cells; however, it does mimic the stimulatory effect of ACH upon effector organs innervated by postganglionic parasympathetic nerves. These specific ACH-receptor sites are termed *muscarinic receptors* (Fig.17.39). Drugs that act in the same manner as muscarine are termed *muscarinic drugs*.

Certain drugs have the ability to block the effects of ACH at its receptor sites, preganglionic or postganglionic. These types of drugs are called *anticholinergic drugs*. Anticholinergic drugs that specifically block the receptor sites of postganglionic parasympathetic nerves are termed *antimuscarinic drugs*. Atropine, glycopyrrolate, and scopolamine are examples of antimuscarinic drugs.

Muscarinic receptors are present as prejunctional receptors on adrenergic terminals. Stimulation of these receptors inhibits the release of norepinephrine; thus, local inhibitory control of adrenergic terminals tends to amplify the parasympathetic influence on effector organs.

Nicotinic Sites. *Nicotine*, a plant alkaloid, mimics the effect of ACH on autonomic ganglion cells and on the receptors of the motor end-plates of skeletal muscle. Nicotine in small amounts stimulates these receptor sites. In large doses, nicotine blocks autonomic ganglion cell transmission and the stimulation of skeletal muscle. These receptor sites are referred to as *nicotine receptors* and the drugs that manifest these effects are called *nicotinic drugs* (Fig. 17.39). Neuromuscular junctions are considered slightly different nicotinic receptor sites.

Response to Stimulation. The uniqueness of the receptor sites at the postganglionic parasympathetic synapses is important clinically. The selective blockage of muscarinic sites can be achieved by the judicious use of antimuscarinic drugs.

Although all cholinergic receptors respond to ACH, not all of these receptors result in the activation of effector organs. Activation of specific receptor sites can manifest excitatory or inhibitory effects upon the effector organ by the generation of EPSPs or IPSPs. (See Chapter 14, Neurochemical Transmission.) Cholinergic stimulation of the heart results in a de-

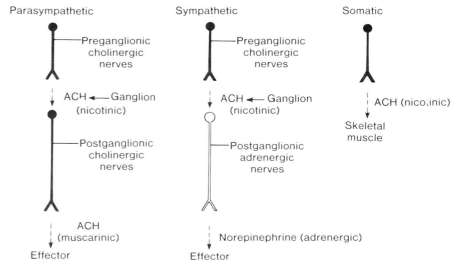

Figure 17.39. A diagram of cholinergic and adrenergic nerves. Refer to the text for a complete description of these relationships.

creased heart rate; similar stimulation of the pupillary sphincter muscle and smooth muscle of the gastrointestinal tract results in smooth muscle contraction. Generally, the muscular sphincters of the alimentary canal relax or decrease tone upon cholinergic stimulation.

Adrenergic Receptors

Classification of Receptor Sites. The differential effects of catecholamines (norepinephrine, epinephrine, and isoproterenol) upon effector cells was the basis for identifying two subdivisions of adrenergic receptors. These were named α- and β-receptors. Norepinephrine is a strong α-stimulator but a weak β-stimulator. Epinephrine is a strong α- and β-stimulator, whereas isoproterenol is a strong β-stimulator but a weak α-stimulator. Since the original descriptions of these major subdivisions, other drugs have been used to identify subpopulations of these receptors—α_1-, α_2-, β_1-, β_2-receptor sites (Chapter 14).

α**-Adrenergic Sites.** The classic stimulatory effects of α-receptor stimulation is attributed to α_1-adrenergic receptors. Stimulation of these receptors results in vasoconstriction, pupillary dilation and pilomotor smooth muscle contraction. Stimulation of these receptors in the wall of the intestine, however, results in inhibition (decreased smooth muscle tone).

The effects of α_2-stimulation at postjunctional sites (on the effector cells) have not been clarified completely. These receptors have been identified on some vascular smooth muscle; they stimulate these muscle fibers. Alpha$_2$-receptors have been identified on prejunctional adrenergic and cholinergic terminals. Prejunctional α_2-receptors on adrenergic terminals inhibit the release of neurotransmitter substance and function as the mediators of a local negative feedback mechanism. Prejunctional α_2-receptors on cholinergic terminals function similarly; they inhibit the release of ACH. The prejunctional effect upon cholinergic terminals would tend to amplify the local adrenergic effect by decreasing local parasympathetic tone.

Alpha-adrenergic receptors mediate metabolic effects also. Alpha$_1$-receptors mediate hepatic glycogenolysis, whereas α_2-receptors inhibit lipolysis in adipocytes. Additionally, stimulation of α_2-receptors on platelets causes their aggregation. The mechanisms by which α-receptors mediate their effects are not understood completely. The receptors may use calcium and cyclic adenosine monophosphate.

β**-Adrenergic Sites.** The β_2 receptors, generally, result in inhibition of smooth muscle. This includes smooth muscle inhibition in blood vessels, intestines. bronchioles, uterus, and splenic capsule. The secretions of some glands are inhibited by stimulation of constituent β_2-receptors. Prejunctional β_2-receptors are located on adrenergic terminals. In these loci, the β_2-receptors are stimulatory to the adrenergic terminals in response to epinephrine stimulation. This type of responsiveness tends to amplify the local effects of sympathetic discharge.

The β_1-receptor is an exception to the postjunctional inhibitory role of β receptors. Beta$_1$-receptor stimulation is excitatory to the heart muscle and has a positive chronotropic and positive inotropic effect upon the cardiac muscle mass. The effects of β-receptor stimulation are mediated through cyclic adenosine monophosophate (cAMP).

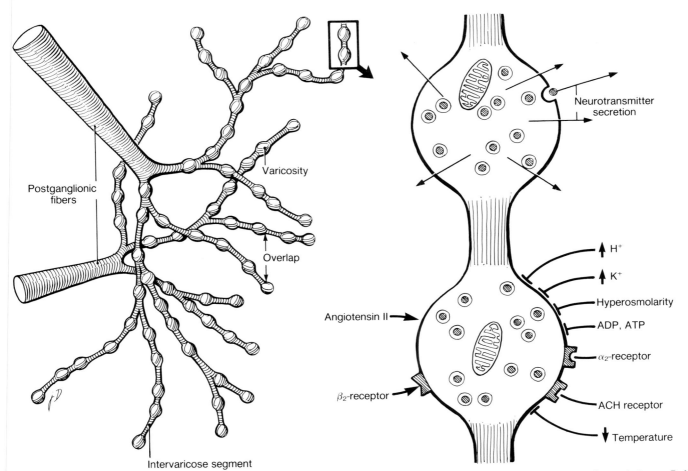

Labels: Postganglionic fibers · Varicosity · Overlap · Intervaricose segment · Neurotransmitter secretion · H$^+$ · K$^+$ · Hyperosmolarity · ADP, ATP · α_2-receptor · ACH receptor · Temperature · Angiotensin II · β_2-receptor

Figure 17.40. Diagrams illustrating adrenergic varicosities and the varied local factors that influence the release of neurotransmitter substance. Refer to the text for a complete description of these influences.

Distribution of α- and β-Receptors. Many organs contain either α- or β-receptors and react accordingly; some organs contain both α- and β-receptors. The vessels of the dermis, mucosa, kidney, and other visceral organs have more α- than β-receptors; the vessels of the heart and skeletal muscle have more β- than α-receptors. In the smooth muscle of the gut wall, the α- and β-receptors are both inhibitory.

Adrenergic Varicosities. The postganglionic neurons of the sympathetic nervous system are excellent examples of intermediate forms of nondirected synapses. The axonal terminals arborize extensively, and the branches have numerous beads or varicosities along the tract (Fig. 17.40). The varicose axonal terminals of adjacent neurons overlap extensively. The overlap helps to account for the diffuse effects of sympathetic discharge.

Each varicosity represents a presynaptic member from which norepinephrine is released. The synaptic clefts associated with these varicosities are wide; norepinephrine spreads some distance to influence effector cells.

Numerous local factors modulate the activity of adrenergic varicosities associated with vascular smooth muscle (Fig. 17.40). Such modulation may reduce or amplify the output of adrenergic terminals and have the effect of isolating the local neuroeffector activity from the rest of the system. Metabolic factors that inhibit neurotransmitter release include: acidosis, increased K^+ concentrations, hyperosmolality, adenosine and adenine nucleotides. These local factors are associated with increased muscular activity. Local modulation, in this instance, inhibits norepinephrine release, the vascular tone decreases and vasodilation is achieved.

Alpha$_2$-receptors and muscarinic receptors on the varicosities inhibit the release of norepinephrine. These substrates, then, tend to self-regulate or amplify the desired local effect, respectively. Histamine, a strong vasodilator, also has a inhibitory effect upon these varicosities.

Cutaneous blood vessels and their associated adrenergic varicosities are subject to modulation by reduced temperatures. Reduced temperatures increase the effector site affinity for the neurotransmitter and decrease the uptake of norepinephrine into the varicosity. Despite the neurotransmitter release in this circumstance, the desired vasoconstriction and heat conservation is achieved.

The stimulation of prejunctional β$_2$-receptors by epinephrine augments the sympathetic tone locally by increasing norepinephrine release from noradrenergic varicosities.

Adrenal Medulla

Relationship to the Autonomic Nervous System. A discussion of the relationship of the adrenal medulla to the ANS is useful for several reasons: (1) it has a unique innervation pattern; (2) it demonstrates the link between the nervous and endocrine systems; (3) it is a useful model in understanding the relationships, distribution, and effects of various receptors, and (4) it is important for an understanding of stress and "fight or flight" reactions.

The adrenal medulla is a unique organ that is innervated by *preganglionic sympathetic nerves*. The anatomical basis for this is simple. The cells of the adrenal medulla (as well as others such as dorsal root ganglion cells, autonomic ganglion cells and extra-adrenal medullary tissue) are derived from neural crest ectoderm. The chromaffin cells of the adrenal medulla, therefore, are *postganglionic neurons*. These cells secrete epinephrine and norepinephrine (≅ 85:15).

Functions. The adrenal medulla is an important but nonessential component of the sympathetic nervous system. It is the means by which generalized sympathetic overflow manages to affect all cells of the body (Fig. 17.41). Adrenal medullary secretions, primarily epinephrine, affect the following processes:

1. facilitate adrenergic transmission
2. increase heart rate(β_1)
3. increase cardiac contraction strength (β_1)
4. increase glycogenolysis (diabetogenic)
5. release free fatty acids from adipose tissue.

These effects ready the animal body for stress such as that accompanying violent muscular activity, hypotension, hypoxia, fear, anger, anxiety. Simultaneously, blood is shunted from the vessels of the skin (α-receptors) and viscera (α>β) to the vessels of skeletal muscle (β>α). This reactivity or sudden surge of adrenal medullary activity is described as the "fight or flight reaction." Rather, it is better described as preparing

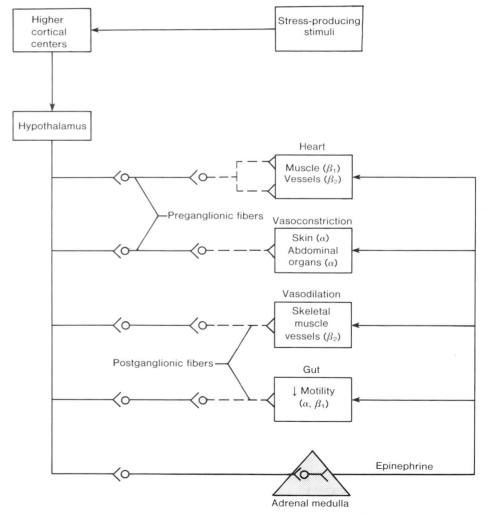

Figure 17.41. A diagram of the relationship of the adrenal medulla to the sympathetic nervous system. The innervated organs react to neural stimulation as indicated. The release of epinephrine complements the neural stimulation.

the animal for stressful circumstances that threaten its physical well-being and/or homeostasis. The examining room is a good place to observe the effects of the adrenal medulla.

As the rest of the sympathetic nervous system, the adrenal medulla is not essential for life, as long as emergencies are minimized. In fact, demonstration of the deficiencies of complete sympathectomy is difficult if nonstressful conditions are maintained.

Pharmacological Considerations

Introduction. The autonomic drugs are those that act primarily on the ANS and include those chemicals that mimic *(agonists)*, intensify or block *(antagonists)* the effects of the neurotransmitters of the sympathetic and parasympathetic divisions of the ANS. Autonomic drugs may manifest their mimetic effects by several mechanisms. Some drugs *(congeners)* are sufficiently similar to the neurotransmitter that they are able to *combine with the receptor site* and elicit the effector response. The similarity between epinephrine, norepinephrine, and dopamine is apparent in Figure 14.15. Some drugs may *cause the release of the neurotransmitter* from the axon telodendria. Other drugs *inhibit the enzyme activity* responsible for the degradation of the neurotransmitter, causing it to accumulate and prolong the effector response.

The blocking effect of certain autonomic drugs can be achieved in several ways. Certain compounds are sufficiently similar to the neurotransmitters that they bind with receptor sites and *competitively inhibit* the normal neurotransmitter-receptor site reaction. Others prevent the release or synthesis of the neurotransmitter substances.

Drugs that act in the manner described are classified into four general categories: parasympathomimetic, parasympatholytic, sympathomimetic, sympatholytic.

Parasympathetic System

Parasympathomimetics. Parasympathomimetic drugs mimic the effects of parasympathetic neuronal stimulation of the effector organs. Drugs in this category are also called *cholinergic* drugs. They are effective at sites in which ACH is the chemical mediator. Some cholinergic drugs are choline esters that act directly on the postganglionic neurons and the effector organs. They are resistant to hydrolysis by cholinesterase and manifest relatively fewer sympathomimetic actions than the cholinergic alkaloid nicotine. The *cholinomimetics* are effective at ganglionic synapses (parasympathetic and sympathetic), parasympathetic postganglionic neuroeffector junctions, and neuromuscular junctions of skeletal muscle.

Choline esters that are functional para-

sympathomimetic drugs are acetylcholine, methacholine, carbachol, and bethanechol (Fig. 17.42). Although acetylcholine is the stereotypic cholinergic drug, the others are sufficiently similar to it to manifest parasympathomimetic effects. These effects may be muscarinic or nicotinic. Muscarinic and nicotinic effects are manifested by acetylcholine and carbachol; the latter is dose-dependent. Methacholine and bethanechol are muscarinic drugs; the CH_3 group on the β-carbon effectively eliminates nicotinic effects. Carbachol is a strong muscarinic used for the stimulation of the gastrointestinal and urinary tract.

Other cholinergic drugs are inhibitors of acetylcholinesterase (ACHase). They bind with the ACHase and reduce the hydrolysis and subsequent inactivation of ACH. Some ACHase inhibitors are physostigmine, neostigmine, and organophosphates. Physostigmine is a topical agent used in the treatment of glaucoma. Neostigmine is an effective symptomatic treatment for myasthenia gravis. Organophosphates are used as insecticides and their potential effect

upon the body after accidental ingestion should be recognized. The cholinergic effects of the plant alkaloids, muscarine and nicotine, were discussed previously.

Parasympatholytics. Drugs that block the effects of the parasympathetic nerves are termed *parasympatholytics* or *anticholinergics*. The drugs in this category actually block muscarinic receptors as *antimuscarinic drugs*. (Some effector organs, sweat glands, and some blood vessels in skeletal muscle have muscarinic receptors but are innervated by sympathetic postganglionic cholinergic nerves. Some smooth muscle cells have cholinergic receptors but lack cholinergic innervation.)

Atropine is the typical antimuscarinic drug. The antimuscarinic effects of atropine and similar compounds (scopolamine, glycopyrrolate) are manifested through a competitive inhibition of ACH. Atropine competes with ACH for receptor sites and the effectiveness of this antimuscarinic drug is dependent upon the concentration of ACH and atropine at these sites. The effects of an antimuscarinic drug are ex-

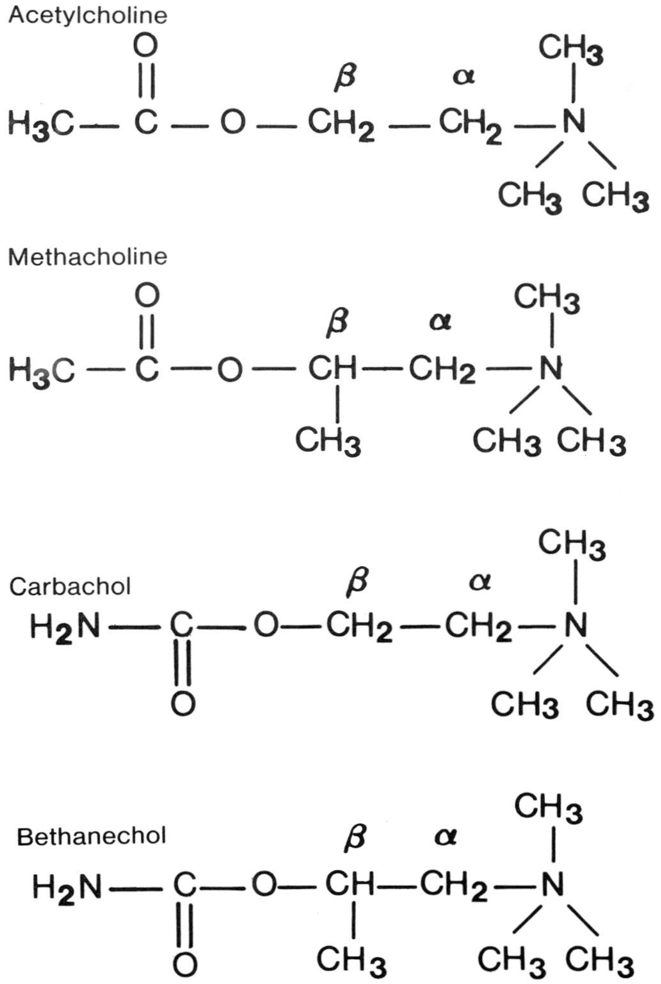

Figure 17.42. The chemical nature of four cholinergic drugs. Note their similarities and subtle differences.

pressed generally as sympathetic effects. This points out the significance of a balanced parasympathetic and sympathetic input to establish the tone of an organ.

Sympathetic System

Sympathomimetics. The catecholamines and other compounds comprise a complex group of drugs that may partially or completely mimic the effects of sympathetic postganglionic neuronal discharge. These drugs are called *sympathomimetics* or *adrenergics.*

The α- and β-*stimulators* include epinephrine and ephedrine. Epinephrine is used effectively in anaphylaxis and cardiac arrest, whereas ephedrine, a noncatecholamine, is a strong vasopressive agent that has good decongestant effects.

Dopamine activates β_1-receptors of the heart. At high dosages, this drug is a vasoconstrictor, activating α_1-receptors. Specific dopaminergic receptor sites are present in autonomic ganglia. This drug has a dilatory effect upon renal and splanchnic arteries.

An effective, noncatecholamine β_1- and β_2-*stimulator* is isoproterenol. This drug is a more potent β-agonist than epinephrine and norepinephrine. It has instantaneous positive inotropic and chronotropic effects upon the heart and causes vasodilation and bronchodilation.

Selective β_2-*stimulators* were developed primarily for the treatment of bronchial asthma. Salbutamol is an effective β_2-stimulant; it is a bronchodilator that has minimal cardiac side-effects.

Sympatholytics. Sympatholytic drugs are also called *antiadrenergics.* All of these drugs generally function as competitive inhibitors of norepinephrine and epinephrine. The α-adrenergic blocking agents include phentolamine, phenoxybenzamine and the ergot alkaloids. Propanolol is the prototype and effective β-adrenergic blocking agent.

Neuronal Response to Injury

Introduction. The high degree of neuronal specialization is accompanied by the loss of mitotic potential. Among the numerous complexities that relate to neuronal functions, and is yet to be explained, is the dynamic interaction that occurs among neurons and between neurons and their effector organs. The death of a neuron results in the irreplaceable loss of that cell and its processes. Neurons or neuronal pools that lose their innervation are subject to *transneuronal (trans-synaptic) reactions.* Transneuronal reactions also affect the neurons that "innervate" the damaged neurons. So, presynaptic and postsynaptic neurons may be affected. These reactions may range from subtle to degenerative.

Neuroglial cells, especially astrocytes, fill in the space that had been occupied by the neuron or neuronal pools. Neuron/effector organ relationships function in a similar manner. The denervation of a skeletal muscle mass results in its atrophy, which is reversed upon reinnervation. The disrup-

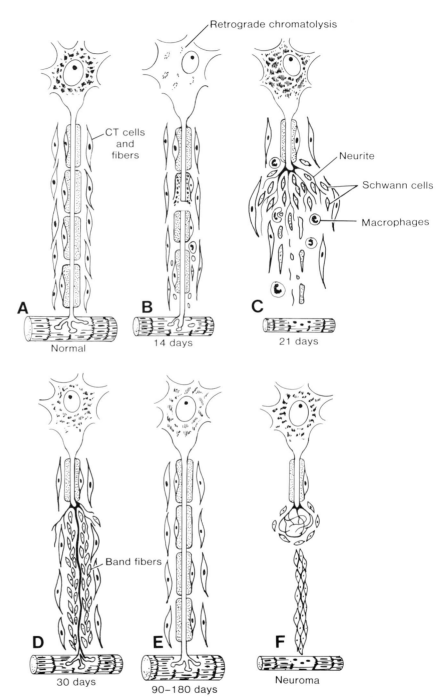

Figure 17.43. A series of diagrams depicting the degeneration and regeneration of a nerve fiber. *A*, normal neuromuscular relationships. The muscle size is considered normal for subsequent comparisons. *B*, primary neural degeneration. The myelin sheath is degenerating and the muscle is undergoing neurogenic atrophy. *C*, reactivity to neural degeneration. Schwann cells have become reactive and macrophages have invaded the region. Neurites have begun to grow from the proximal stump of the axon. Distal degeneration is almost complete, and muscular atrophy is progressing. *D*, band fiber formation. Schwann cells establish themselves as band fibers to guide the predominant neurite. *E*, re-establishment of innervation. The relationships have returned to normal. *F*, neuroma formation. A whorled arrangement of growing neurites, Schwann cells, and connective tissue establish the neuroma. (Redrawn, modified and combined from Junqueira, L. C.: *Basic Histology.* Lange, Los Altos, 1975 and Quarton, G. C., Melnechuk, T and Schmitt, F. O. (eds.): *The Neurosciences.* Rockefeller University Press, New York, 1967.)

tion of an axonal process results in the degeneration of the myelin sheath. Similarly, the loss of myelin sheaths from disease processes affects the functional integrity of axis cylinders. (The axons are unable to transmit action potentials.) The exact trophic relationships and influences between and among these components has not been clarified, but they have an *obligatory symbiotic relationship (obligatory symbiosis)*.

Neuronal processes damaged within the PNS result in degenerative and regenerative alterations of the cellular process and may involve the nerve cell body. Neurons within the CNS react similarly to damage; however, the time frame for regeneration is slower than their peripheral counterparts. The changes in neurons in response to injury are referred to as *primary* and *secondary degeneration*.

Response to Injury. The transection of a nerve results in damage proximal and distal to the site of injury (Fig. 17.43). Proximally, the *primary degeneration*, which may include disintegration of the myelin sheath and loss of part of the axis cylinder, extends over a few internodal segments (Fig. 17.43B). The nature of the injury dictates the degree of proximal involvement. The proximal portion of the axon, maintaining its continuity with the nerve cell body, soon begins to undergo regeneration and new branches of the axon *(neurites)* radiate from the stump (Fig. 17.43C).

After the separation of the distal segment from the nerve cell body, the axonal terminal undergoes degeneration first, *terminal degeneration*. Subsequent degeneration of the myelin sheath and axis cylinder occurs. This process, *secondary* or *Wallerian degeneration*, is characterized by progressive degenerative changes in the distal segment. The axis cylinder, separated from the trophic influence of the nerve cell body, assumes a beaded appearance, breaks up into irregular fragments and eventually disintegrates. The myelin sheath undergoes similar alterations in association with the fragmented axis cylinder. All of these changes occur within the limits of the endoneurium. The peripherally positioned connective tissue fibers form a cylindrical envelope around the reacting nerve fiber.

Macrophages invade the *zone of trauma* and assist with the removal of debris. Schwann cells enlarge and proliferate. Reactive Schwann cells are responsible for removing cellular detritus and myelin fragments from the regions away from the zone of trauma. Schwann cell proliferation results in the formation of *band fibers (cellular tubes, protoplasmic bands)* along the length of the disintegrated distal segment (Fig. 17.43D). Band fibers are important as a guiding tubular framework for the neurites of the proximal segment into the distal fragment and eventually to the neuron or effector organ. When a neurite establishes contact with the pathway supplied by the band fibers, the remaining neurites degenerate (Fig. 17.43E).

The changes that occur in the axis cylinder are accompanied by alterations of the cell body. *Retrograde chromatolysis* occurs within the cell body very rapidly (Fig. 17.43B). Eventually the nerve fiber is restored to its original relationship and regeneration will have been achieved (Fig. 17.43E). The transection of a nerve may result in the opening of a large gap between the proximal and distal segments or the distal segment may be missing, as would result from an amputation. In either case, the neurites and associated cells may form a large, painful nodule called a *neuroma* (Fig. 17.43F). Neuroma formation is not a problem in the dog but is a significant problem in the horse. Neuromas can be significant complications of digital neurectomies that may be used as salvage operations for navicular disease. The folding and suturing of the epineurium over the transected proximal fragment *(epineurial capping)* significantly decreases the occurrence of these neuromas in the horse.

The regeneration of nerve fibers within the CNS occurs at a much slower rate than within the PNS. The absence of band fiber formation from oligodendrogliocytes may account for the slow progression of repair. Peripheral regeneration may occur at a rate of 2–4 mm/day, whereas complete disintegration and phagocytosis of severed distal segments within the CNS may take six months. Importantly, functional regeneration within the CNS probably does not occur.

References

General

Chrisman, C.L. (ed.): Symposium on advances in veterinary neurology. Vet Clin. North Amer, *10*:1, 1980.

DeLahunta, A.: *Veterinary Neuroanatomy and Clinical Neurology*. 2nd edition. W.B. Saunders. Philadelphia, 1983.

Ettinger, S.J. (ed.): *Textbook of Veterinary Internal Medicine: Diseases of the Dog and Cat*. Vol. I. W.B. Saunders, Phildadelphia, 1975.

Hoerlein, B.F.: *Canine Neurology: Diagnosis and Treatment*. 3rd ed. W.B. Saunders, Philadelphia, 1978.

Kandel. E.R. and Schwartz, J.H.: *Principles of Neural Science*. Elsevier/North Holland, New York. 1981.

Quarton, G.C., Melnechuk, T. and Schmitt, F.O (editors): *The Neurosciences*. Rockefeller University Press, New York, 1967.

Peripheral Nervous System

Bradley, W.G.: *Disorders of Peripheral Nerves*. Blackwell, Oxford, 1974.

Cauna, N.: Structure of digital touch corpuscles. Acta Anat *32*:1, 1958.

Cauna, N. and Mannan, G.: The structure of human digital pacinian corpuscles (corpuscula lamellosa) and its functional significance. J. Anat. *92*:1, 1958.

Dyck, P.J., Thomas, P.K., Lambert, E.H. and Bunge, R.: *Peripheral Neuropathy*. Vol I. 2nd edition, W. B. Saunders, New York, 1984.

Fernand, V.S.V and Young, J.Z.: The sizes of the nerve fibers of muscle nerves. Proc. Roy. Soc. (Biol.). *139*:38, 1951.

Gamble, H.J. and Eames, R.A.: An electron microscpe study of the connective tissue of human peripheral nerve. J. Anat. *98*:655, 1964.

Griffiths, I.R., Duncan, I.D. and Lawson, D.D.: Avulsion of the brachial plexus. 2. Clinical aspects. J. Small Anim. Prac. *15*:177, 1974.

Grillo, M.A.: Electron microscopy of sympathetic tissues. Pharmacol. Rev. *18*:387, 1966.

Hess, A.: The fine structure of young and old spinal gangia. Anat. Rec. *123*:399, 1955.

Heuser, J.E., Reese, T.S., Dennis, M.J., Jan. Y., Jan, L. and Evans, L.: Synaptic vesicle exocytosis captured by quick freezing and correlated with quantal transmitter release. J. Cell Bio. *81*:275, 1979.

Jones, L.M. et al.: *Veterinary Pharmacology and Therapeutics*. Iowa State University Press, 4th edition, 1977.

Kunos, G.: Adrenoreceptors. *In*: George, R. et al. (eds.): *Annual Review of Pharmacology and Toxicology*. Vol. 18. Annual Reviews, Inc., Palo Alto, 1978.

Kuntz, A.: *The Autonomic Nervous System*. Lea and Febiger, Philadelphia, 1953.

Meyers, F.H.: *Review of Medical Pharmacology*. 5th edition, Lange, Los Altos, 1976.

Ortiz-Picon, J.M.: The neuroglia of the sensory ganglia. Anat. Rec. *121*:513, 1955.

Schanthaveerappa, T.R. and Bourne, G.H.: The "perineural epithelium," a metabolically active, continuous protoplasmic cell barrier surrounding peripheral nerve fsciculi. J. Anat. *96*:527, 1963.

Sheperd, J.T. and Vanhoutte, P.M.: Local modulation of adrenergic neurotransmission. Circulation *64*:655, 1981.

Spencer, P.J. and Schaumberg, H.H.: The pathology of dying back polyneuropathies. Prog. Neuropathol. *3*:253, 1977.

Central Nervous System

Bradbury, M.: *The Concept of a Blood-Brain Barrier*. Wiley & Sons, New York, 1979.

Barringer, J. R.: A simplified procedure for spinal fluid cytology. Arch. Neurol. *22*:305, 1970.

Elliott, H.C.: Studies on the motor cells of the spinal cord. Amer. J. Anat. *70*:95, 1942.

Globus, E.G. and Scheibel, A.B.: Pattern and field in cortical structure. J. Comp. Neurol. *131*:155, 1967.

Hartley. W.J.: Lower motor neuron disease in dogs. Acta Neurolpathol. *2*:334, 1963.

Herndon, R.M.: The fine structure of the Purkinje cell. J. Cell Biol. *18*:167, 1963.

Maxwell, D.S. and Pease, D.C.: Electron microscopy of the choroid plexus. Anat. Rec. *124*:331, 1956.

Palmer, A.C.: Pathogenesis and pathology of the cerebellovestibular syndrome. J. Small An. Pract. *11*:167, 1970.

Weed, L.H.: Meninges and cerebrospinal fluid. J. Anat. *72*:181, 1938.

Wright, J.A.: Evaluation of cerebrospinal fluid in the dog. Vet. Rec. *103*:48, 1978.

Yeo, J.D.: A review of experimental research in spinal cord injury. Paraplegia. *14*:1, 1976.

18: Cardiovascular System

General Characteristics

Form and Function. The cardiovascular system consists of components to pump, transport, and distribute required elements to the cells and tissues of the soma (Fig. 18.1).

The histological aspects of vessel construction cannot be separated from the hemodynamic role they fulfill. The arterial side of the system carries a low volume of blood under high pressure at a high velocity. The capillary system carries a large volume of blood under appreciably diminished pressures and velocities. The venous system transports a high volume of blood at low pressures and velocities.

Mural Organization

Organizational Scheme. Although various patterns in mural morphology are observed to accommodate the pressure-volume relationships, the basic scheme consists of *tunica intima, tunica media,* and *tunica adventitia* (Figs. 18.2 and 18.3).

The *tunica intima* consists of three distinct subdivisions: *endothelium, subendothelial coat,* and *internal elastic membrane* (Figs. 18.2–18.4). The endothelium is typical squamous cells that line the lumen of the organ. This cellular layer is a common and consistent feature of all blood vessels and the heart. Typically, the nucleus is prominent and may bulge into the lumen, whereas the marginal cytoplasm is difficult to discern with the light microscope. The cells reside upon a basement membrane that separates the endothelium from the peripheral fibroelastic connective tissue and fibroblasts of the *subendothelial coat.* For the most part, these elements are oriented longitudinally (parallel to the long axis of the vessel). Smooth muscle fibers may be present, as well as cells that normally occupy connective tissue spaces. The *internal elastic membrane* is a condensation of elastic fibers that separates the tunica intima from the tunica media.

The *tunica media* consists of a mixture of smooth muscle cells, collagenous fibers, elastic fibers, and fibroblasts (Figs. 18.2, 18.3, and 18.5). The smooth muscle cells are arranged in a circular pattern around the lumen. They are in intimate association with collagenous and elastic fibers. *Nervi* and *vasa vasorum,* the nerve and blood supplies of the vessels, may be observed within this tunic of large vessels.

At the junction between the tunica media and tunica adventitia, an *external elastic membrane* may be present. It, too, is a condensation of elastic fibers. This membrane demarcates the media from the adventitia. The *tunica adventitia* is formed of this membrane and dense fibroelastic connective tissue (Figs. 18.2, 18.3, and 18.5). Generally, it is difficult to distinguish the end of the adventitia and the beginning of the surrounding connective tissue. Nervi and vasa vasorum ramify in the tunica adventitia.

Not all vessels contain all of the aforementioned elements; nor, if present, are all of them represented equally in all vessels.

The endothelium, however, is the constant feature of all vascular components.

Exchange System

Capillaries. *Capillaries* are the means by which metabolites gain access to and waste products leave the connective tissue space. Capillaries are simple endothelial-lined tubes with a diameter of 7–9 μm. Due to this size limitation, they are able to accommodate a single red blood cell at a time. Peripherally, this tube is covered by a basement membrane (Fig. 18.6).

In section with light microscopy, a thin rim of acidophilic cytoplasm delimits the extent of the capillary (Fig. 18.7). The dark nucleus of the endothelial cell occurs along the margin of the lumen and may bulge into the lumen. Capillaries are accompanied along their entire length by connective

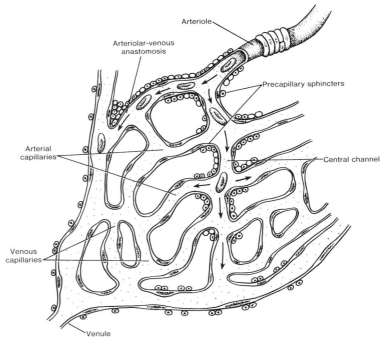

Figure 18.1. A diagram illustrating the relationships of capillaries to arterioles and venules. The central channel, surrounded by smooth muscle, has been named the metarteriole. Contraction of the smooth muscle shunts blood through the capillary bed. (Redrawn and modified from Copenhaver, W. M., Kelly, D. E. and Wood, R. L.: *Bailey's Textbook of Histology.* Williams & Wilkins, Baltimore, 1978.)

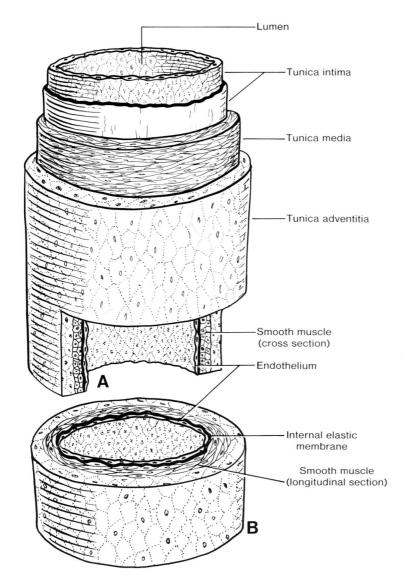

Lumen

Tunica intima

Tunica media

Tunica adventitia

Smooth muscle (cross section)

Endothelium

A

Internal elastic membrane

Smooth muscle (longitudinal section)

B

Figure 18.2. A diagram of the mural organization of an artery. When sectioned longitudinally *(A)*, the smooth muscle of the tunica media is cross sectioned. When the vessel is cut in cross section *(B)*, the smooth muscle is cut in longitudinal section.

from other sinusoids because of the association of endothelial cells with macrophages (Fig. 18.10). These phagocytic cells are intimately associated with endothelial cells.

Venous sinuses are larger than sinusoids, the basal lamina is discontinuous, and the lining cells are not phagocytic.

Various cells assume intimate relationships with the endothelial cells of capillaries. They are called *pericapillary cells (perivascular cells, adventitial cells)* and include *histiocytes, fibroblasts, mesenchymal cells, mast cells,* and *Rouget cells.* Rouget cells are smooth muscle cells intimately associated with the capillary endothelium. These cells are probably the smooth muscle cells of *metarterioles* and *precapillary sphincters* (Fig. 18.1).

High Pressure System

Arterioles. There is a gradual transition from capillaries to arterioles. A *metarteriole* is a branch of an arteriole that has a discontinuous layer of smooth muscle fibers surrounding it (Fig. 18.1). These vessels function as sphincters and control the amount of blood flowing through the *central* or *thoroughfare channel* that courses through the capillary bed and joins the venous side of the circulation. *Precapillary sphincters* are capillaries with a single layer of smooth muscle fibers that control blood flow through the metarterioles into the capillary bed proper. Contraction of these vessels completely stops flow in the specific capillary bed. A capillary bed bypass may be achieved by arteriolar-venular anastomoses (Fig. 18.1).

Arterioles have a diameter less than 100 μm (Fig. 18.11). The smallest arterioles consist of a tunica intima devoid of a subendothelial coat. The only recognizable elements are the endothelium and thin internal elastic membrane, the latter of which appears as a bright scalloped line (Fig. 8.12). The tunica media consists of one to three layers of smooth muscle among which are scattered some fine collagenous fibers and elastic fibers. An external elastic membrane is not present and the loose connective tissue of the tunica adventitia blends insensibly with the surrounding connective tissue.

It is not unusual to observe a scalloped endothelial layer, the individual cells of which appear to protrude into the lumen (Fig. 18.13). It is probably due to excessive contraction of the vessel at the time of fixation.

Small and Medium-Sized Arteries. There is no sharp line of distinction between arterioles and small arteries. The small and medium-sized arteries are also termed *muscular* or *distributing arteries* (Fig. 18.3). The tunica intima is typical. An external elastic membrane is often well-defined, and the tunica adventitia is typical.

tissue cells, thin collagenous fibers, and reticular fibers. Among the many cells closely associated with them, fixed macrophages, mesenchymal cells, and Rouget cells are especially prominent.

All capillaries are similar with the light microscope. Ultrastructural studies, however, demonstrate that five types of capillaries exist: continuous capillaries, fenestrated capillaries, sinusoidal capillaries, sinusoids, and venous sinuses.

Continuous capillaries have no interruptions or pores in the endothelial cells (Fig. 18.8). This type occurs typically in muscle, lungs and, nervous system.

Fenestrated (perforated) capillaries have pores scattered throughout the walls of the endothelium (Fig. 18.9). These pores may be covered by a diaphragm that is thinner than the cell membrane. These capillaries

occur in the endocrine glands, intestines, and kidneys, loci at which fluid transport is a significant function. Continuous and fenestrated capillaries have a complete basal lamina.

Sinusoidal capillaries are larger and more irregularly shaped than continuous and fenestrated capillaries. A basal lamina is not a prominent feature of these vessels. The lining (endothelial) cells of the sinusoidal capillaries are not phagocytic and macrophages are not associated with the cells. These capillaries characterize the endocrine organs and the aortic and carotid bodies.

Sinusoids are larger than sinusoidal capillaries. The basal lamina of sinusoids is not a prominent feature and is commonly absent. These vessels occur in the bone marrow and liver. The hepatic sinusoids differ

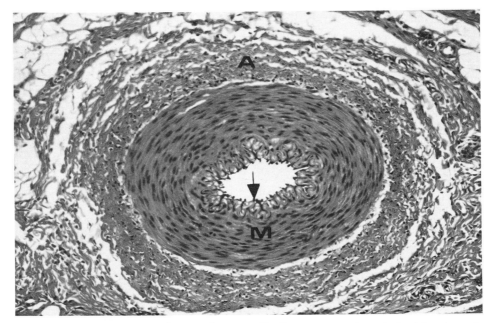

Figure 18.3.   Mural elements of a muscular artery. The three components are tunica intima *(arrow)*, tunica media *(M)*, and tunica adventitia. X40.

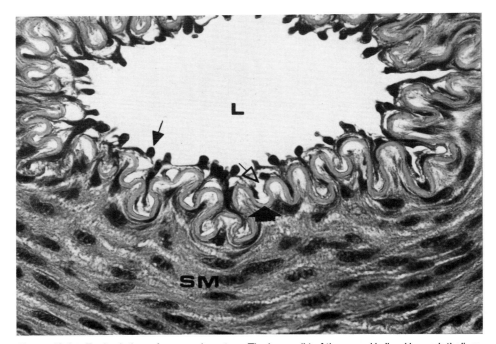

Figure 18.4.   Tunica intima of a muscular artery. The lumen *(L)* of the vessel is lined by endothelium *(solid arrow)*, the cells of which protrude into the lumen. The protrusion results from agonal contractions of the tunica media during sample acquisition. The accentuation of the subendothelial space *(open arrow)* is an artifact of preparation. The internal elastic membrane *(large solid arrow)* is adjacent to the smooth muscle *(SM)* of the tunica media. X160.

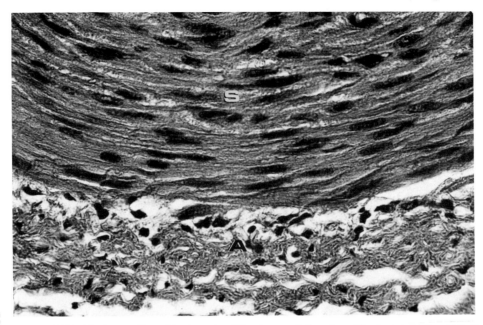

Figure 18.5. Tunica media and tunica adventitia of a muscular artery. The tunica media contains smooth muscle cells *(S)*, whereas the tunica adventitia *(A)* consists of fibroelastic connective tissue. X160.

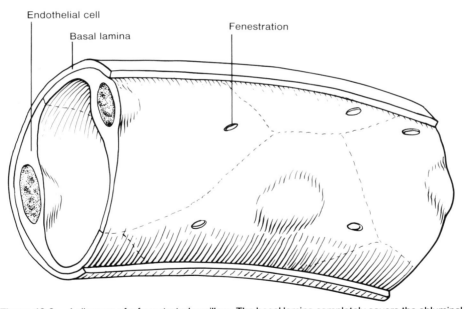

Figure 18.6. A diagram of a fenestrated capillary. The basal lamina completely covers the abluminal surface of the endothelium.

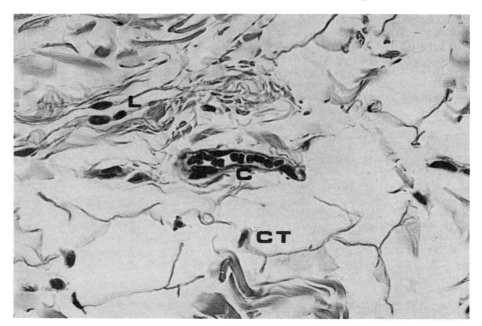

Figure 18.7. Capillaries in loose connective tissue. The connective tissue *(CT)* contains a blood capillary *(C)* and a lymphatic capillary *(L)*. X160.

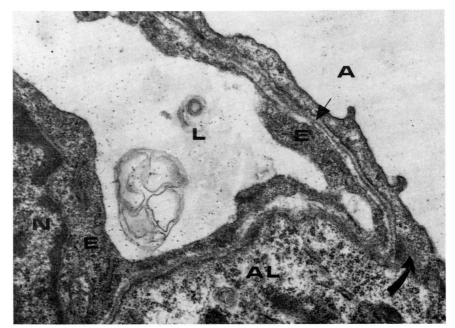

Figure 18.8. An electron micrograph of a continuous capillary from a bovine lung. The alveolus *(A)* is defined by the perikaryon of the alveolar lining cell *(AL)* and the attenuated cellular process of the lining cells *(curved arrow)*. The lumen of the capillary *(L)* is delimited by the endothelial cells *(E)* and its nucleus *(N)*. The basal lamina *(small arrow)* is complete and the endothelial lining is continuous. X20,000.

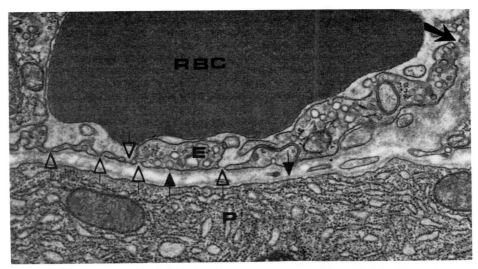

Figure 18.9. An electron micrograph of a fenestrated capillary. The endothelium *(E)* of the capillary is separated from a pancreatic acinar cell *(P)* by two basal laminae *(small solid arrows)*. The capillary contains an erythrocyte *(RBC)*. Numerous fenestrations *(open arrows)* are covered by diaphragms, whereas one fenestration *(large solid arrow)* is not. X25,000.

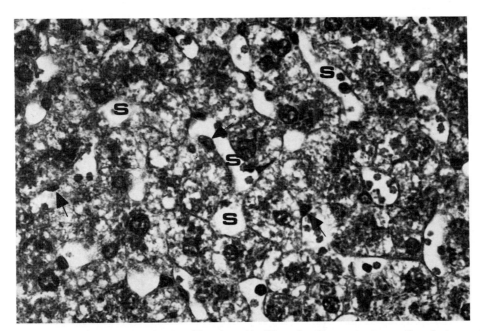

Figure 18.10. Sinusoids of a liver. The sinusoids *(S)* are lined by some phagocytic cells *(arrows)*. X160.

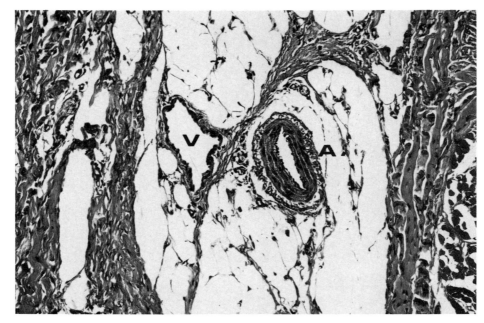

Figure 18.11. An arteriole and companion venule. The arteriole *(A)* has three layers of smooth muscle in the tunica media. The companion venule *(V)* does not contain smooth muscle. X40.

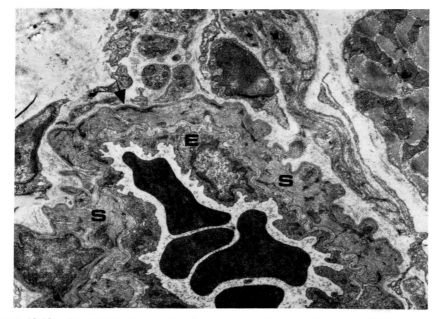

Figure 18.12. An electron micrograph of an arteriole. The smooth muscle *(S)* surrounds the endothelial cell *(E)*. A basal lamina *(arrow)* ia apparent at the peripheral border of the smooth muscle cell. X14,000. (Micrograph courtesy of G. P. Epling).

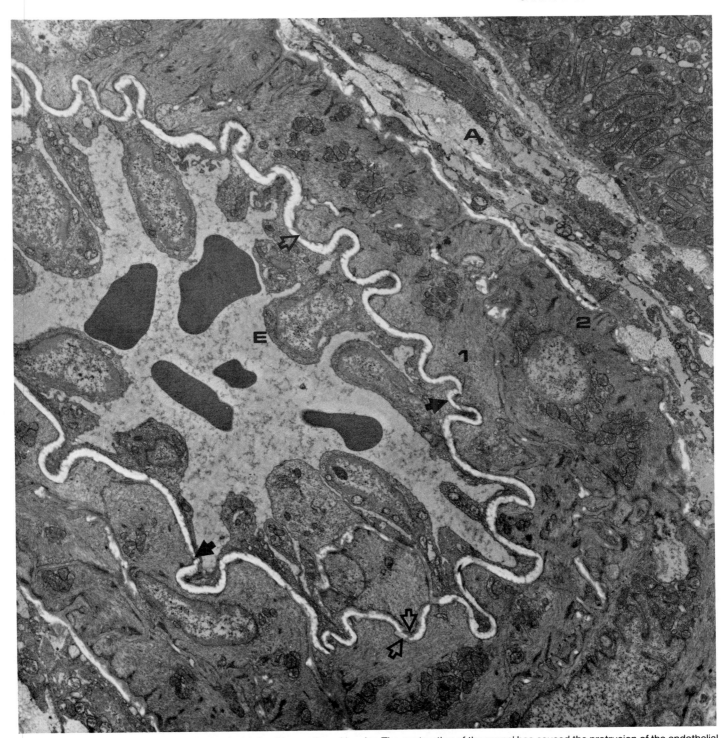

Figure 18.13.   An electron micrograph of an arteriole with a scalloped border. The contraction of the vessel has caused the protrusion of the endothelial perikaryons into the lumen of the vessel *(E)*. The internal elastic membrane is folded for the same reason *(solid arrows)*. Two smooth muscle cells *(1,2)* comprise the tunica media. Portions of the basal lamina are apparent on the luminal and abluminal surfaces of the internal elastic membrane *(open arrows)*. Elastic fibers, collagen, and fibroblasts are apparent in the adventitial connective tissue.

Elastic Arteries. The *elastic arteries* are the largest arteries (Fig. 18.14). Compared to their luminal volume, they have a rather thin wall.

All the elements of the tuncia intima are present. The endothelial layer consists of polygonal cells rather than the expected flattened cells. The subendothelial layer consists of collagenous fibers, elastic fibers, fibroblasts, and smooth muscle cells in a loose connective tissue. An internal elastic membrane is present; however, it is not always distinct because the tunica media consists of large quantities of elastic fibers that are oriented in such a manner as to be interpreted as repeating elastic membranes. Between the coarse elastic fibers are fine collagenous fibers, fine elastic fibers, fibroblasts, and smooth muscle cells. A distinct external elastic membrane is not present. The connective tissue of the tunica adventitia is thin and blends insensibly with the surrounding connective tissue.

Low Pressure System

Venules. *Venous capillaries* attain large diameters (up to 20 times those of capillar-

ies) and gradually become associated with other mural elements. In distinction to arterial capillaries, venous capillaries usually become associated with connective tissue first and later develop smooth muscle within their walls.

Venules consist of a simple endothelial tube surrounded by a loose connective tissue (Fig. 18.11). Smooth muscle cell investment occurs as the venules become small veins. The tunica adventitia of these vessels is thick compared to the tunica media.

Small and Medium-Sized Veins. These vessels are lined by a thin tunica intima that consists of polygonal endothelial cells and a very small subendothelial connective tissue layer (Fig. 18.15). The tunica media is thin and consists of circularly oriented muscle cells, collagenous fibers, and fine elastic fibers. The tunica adventitia is well-developed and forms the bulk of the wall.

Many of these veins are equipped with *valves* (Fig. 18.16). These are invaginations of the tunica intima into the lumen of the vessel. Valves are lined by flattened endothelial cells and contain a core of subendothelial connective tissue (Fig. 18.17).

These intimal modifications are especially prominent in vessels located below the heart.

Large Veins. The tunica intima is thicker than observed in smaller veins and an internal elastic membrane may be present. The tunica media consists primarily of collagenous and elastic fibers, whereas the smooth muscle component is reduced or even absent. The tunica adventitia is well-developed and is the thickest part of the wall. Scattered bundles of smooth muscle may be present within this coat and oriented parallel to the long axis of the vessel. Valves are absent in the venae cavae and the hepatic portal vein.

High and Low Pressure Systems Compared

Generally, the mural elements of a vein of a given size, when compared with the companion artery, are less distinct. The following distinguishing characteristics are usually apparent in sections:

1. **Blood rarely occurs in sectioned arteries, but it is typically present in veins.**

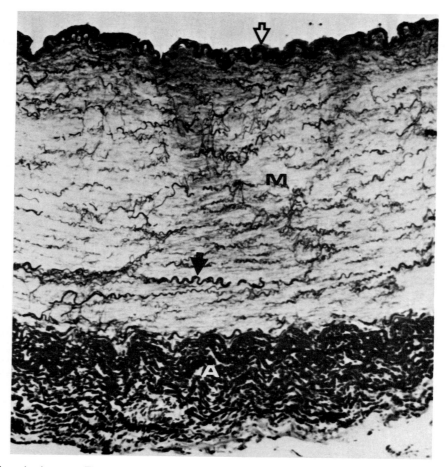

Figure 18.14. A section of an elastic artery. The section of aorta is stained for elastic fibers. The tunica intima contains a well-defined internal elastic membrane *(open arrow)*. The tunica media *(M)* consists of smooth muscle *(not stained)* and elastic fibers *(solid arrow)*. The tunica adventitia (A) has numerous elastic fibers also. X25. (Orcein stain).

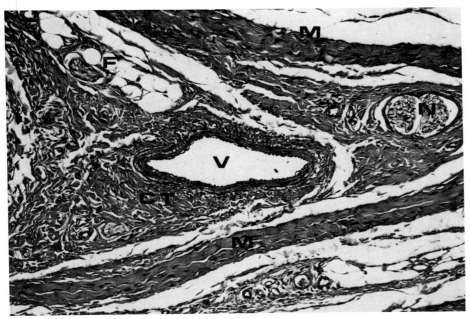

Figure 18.15. A section of a small vein. The small vein *(V)* is surrounded by connective tissue *(CT)*. Adipocytes *(F)*, nerves *(N)*, and skeletal muscle are present also. X40.

2. The tunica media is well-developed in arteries, whereas the tunica adventitia is well-developed in veins.
3. Luminal diameters are greater than mural thicknesses in veins, whereas luminal diameters of arteries are smaller than mural thicknesses.
4. During agonal changes, veins are subject to irregular contractions, whereas arteries contract more regularly.
5. Internal elastic membranes may be present in arterioles, but these membranes are usually confined to large veins.
6. The tunica adventitia of veins is usually the thickest coat of the wall.

Heart

Mural Organization

The heart is a thick-walled, highly muscularized tube that propels the blood through the body. The mural elements of the heart are organized in a manner similar to the peripheral vessels. The heart consists of three coats: an inner coat or *endodocardium*, a middle coat or *myocardium* and an outer coat or *epicardium* (Fig. 18.18).

Endocardium. The endocardium, the cardiac counterpart of the tunica intima, consists of *endothelium* and a *subendothelial coat*. A *subendocardial coat* is deep to these components (Fig. 18.19). The endothelium consists of polygonal cells that reside on a basement membrane. This lining is continuous with the endothelial lining of the peripheral vessels. The *subendothelial coat* of fine collagenous and elastic fibers is continuous with a deeper or more peripheral *subendocardial coat* of loose connective tissue. The latter contains collagenous and elastic fibers, adipose cells, smooth muscle fibers, blood vessels, and nerves. Besides attaching the endocardium to the myocardium, this coat also contains the impulse-conducting system of the heart (Purkinje fibers) in the ventricles.

Myocardium. The *myocardium* is comparable to the tunica media (Fig. 18.20). It consists, primarily, of cardiac muscle. Connective tissue fibers, nerves and blood vessels are also present (Chapter 13).

Epicardium. The *epicardium* is actually a serous membrane—the *visceral pericardium* of gross anatomy (Fig. 18.21). The mesothelial lining resides upon a thin layer of loose connective tissue. It is continuous with a loose connective tissue layer that contains variable deposits of adipose tissue, blood vessels and nerves—the *subepicardial coat*.

Cardiac Skeleton. The cardiac muscle and valves are supported by a skeleton of dense white fibrous connective tissue (DWFCT). Some components of this skeleton may also be cartilaginous or osseous. The following elements form the cardiac skeleton: (1) four fibrous rings (anuli fi-

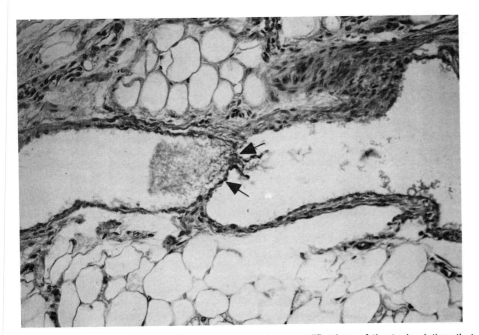

Figure 18.16. A valve in a vein. The cusps *(arrows)* are modifications of the tunica intima that prevent the reversal of blood flow. X50.

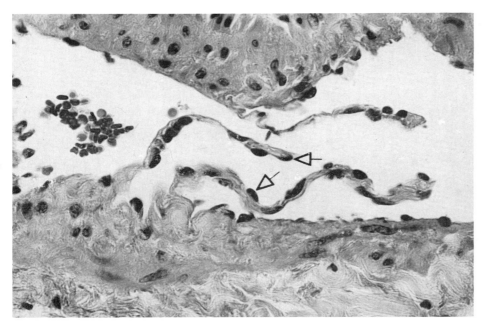

Figure 18.17. Components of a valve. The cusps are composed of endothelial cells *(arrows)* that surround a core of subendothelial connective tissue. X160.

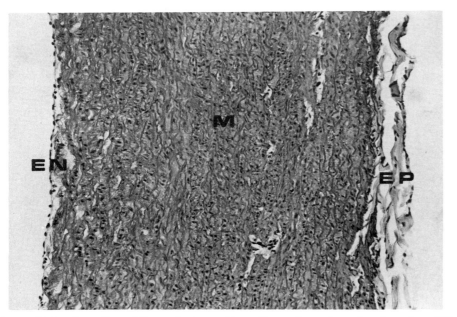

Figure 18.18. A section of the wall of an atrium. The wall consists of endocardium *(EN),* myocardium *(M)* and epicardium *(EP).* The epicardium is also called the tunica serosa and visceral pericardium. X40.

brosi), (2) a fibrous triangle (trigonum fibrosum), (3) a fibrous and membranous septum (septum membranaceum).

The *anuli fibrosi* are DWFCT rings that surround the *semilunar valves* of the pulmonary artery and aorta and the two atrioventricular valves. These rings are continuous, directly or indirectly, with the *trigonum fibrosum*. This is a mass of DWFCT between the atrioventricular canals. Similarly, it is continuous with the DWFCT of the interventricular septum—the *septum*

membranaceum. These skeletal elements serve as points of attachment for the cardiac muscle mass.

Cartilage and/or bone may occur in the fibrous rings. In the ox, especially, ossification of the fibrous ring of the aortic semilunar valve results in the formation of an *os cordis*.

Cardiac Valves. The cardiac valves are invaginations of the endocardium into the lumen of the heart (Fig. 18.22). The connective tissue of the anuli fibrosi is contin-

uous as a supportive core in the valves between the two layers of endocardium. The connective tissue of the atrioventricular valves is continuous with the collagenous fibers of the tendinous cords *(chordae tendineae)*, which are attached to the ventricular surfaces of the valves. Naturally, a thin layer of endocardium is reflected over these tendinous cords and is continuous with the endocardium of the papillary muscles. Elastic fibers are more numerous on the side of the valve facing the back pressure.

The semilunar valves are similar to the atrioventricular valves. A dense nodule of collagen or cartilage may be present on the edge of the three cusps. Each nodule is called a *nodule of Arantius.*

Cardiac Conduction System. The myocardial muscle mass is modified uniquely for contractile and conducting functions. Despite the ability of cardiac muscle cells to generate and conduct impulses throughout the myocardial mass, a specialized impulse-generating and impulse-conducting system has been developed that ensures the proper origination of impulses and the subsequent proper sequencing of atrial and ventricular contractions. The generating and conducting system consists of the sinoatrial (SA) node, atrioventricular (AV) node and the atrioventricular bundle (Fig. 18.23). Purkinje fibers are the histological components of this system (Fig. 18.24).

The *SA node* is positioned within the wall of the right atrium at the point of confluence with the major vessels that enter the right atrium. The SA node contains Purkinje fibers that are described as *pacemaker cells.* The wave of depolarization spreads radially throughout the atrial myocardial mass and is eventually conducted to the *AV node.*

This ill-defined mass of Purkinje fibers and connective tissue converges as the *atrioventricular bundle (bundle of His)* close to the ventricles. The atrioventricular bundle courses craniad and ventrad through the trigonum fibrosum and extends into the septum membranaceum dividing into the *right* and *left bundle branches.*

The impulse originating and conducting system affords a number of advantages to the myocardial mass. The cells of the SA node, because of their relatively more rapid rate of depolarization and repolarization, assume a pacemaker function that normally precludes *ectopic foci* from assuming that role. The initial spread of excitation over the atrial musculature permits the contraction of this musculature to fill the ventricles. The AV nodal delay facilitates maximal ventricular filling before the initiation of contraction. The atrioventricular bundles speed the impulses toward the apex and permit the wave of contraction to proceed from the apex back to the base of the heart. This sequence of contraction repre-

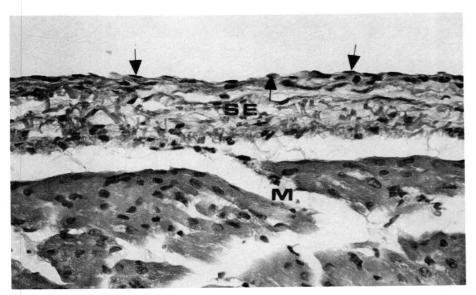

Figure 18.19. A section of atrial endocardium. The endothelium *(arrows)* is underlaid by subendothelial connective tissue *(SE)* that is adjacent to the myocardium *(M)*. X100.

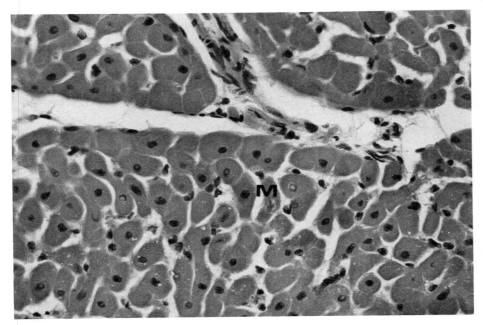

Figure 18.20. A section of ventricular myocardium. Most of the cardiac muscle cells have been cut in cross section. The myocardium consists of cardiac muscle cells separated by a well-vascularized endomysium. X100.

sents an efficient means of ejecting blood from the ventricles into the pulmonary and aortic circulations.

Cardiac Blood Vessels, Lymphatic Vessels, and Nerves. The heart is richly vascularized through its coronary arteries. These vessels originate from the aortic arch immediately distal to the aortic valve. The extensive capillary network throughout the myocardial mass is an obvious feature of its histology. Lymphatic vessels are present in the three coats of the heart. Numerous nerve fibers from the autonomic nervous system innervate the myocardial mass, nodes, and smooth muscle of the coronary vessels.

Cardiac Activity

Regulatory Mechanisms

Introduction. Regulation of the cardiovascular system is subject to the influence of numerous factors—myogenic, neurogenic, humoral, chemical, metabolic, barometric, and volumetric influences. Cardiovascular regulation is the sum of the regulation of the peripheral circulation and the heart.

The essence of cardiovascular regulation is to ensure an adequate amount of blood to the tissues of the body, *tissue perfusion* (Fig. 18.25). Proper tissue perfusion is dependent upon an adequate volume of blood being presented to the capillaries under appropriate pressure.

Types of Influences. The *myogenic* influence upon the heart stems from the automaticity of the pacemaker cells. *Neurogenic* influences from the sympathetic or parasympathetic nerves can increase or decrease the rate of depolarization of the cells of the SA node. Epinephrine from the adrenal medulla exerts an *hormonal influence* upon the α- and β-receptors of the cardiovascular system. A *chemical influence* is exerted by special receptors that are sensitive to P_{CO_2}, P_{O_2}, and pH. *Barometric* or blood pressure changes influence neurogenic cardiac regulation. The heart is capable also of ejecting a given stroke volume against an increased aortic pressure *(homeometric autoregulation)*. *Volumetric influences* are manifested as an integral part of regulation, because the heart tends to eject whatever is returned to it. This stroke volume-diastolic filling relationship constitutes *Starling's law of the heart* and is dependent upon changes in myocardial fiber length *(heterometric autoregulation)*. *Pain* may have a stimulatory or inhibitory effect upon cardiac activity. Added to the above are numerous local autoregulatory factors that affect tissue perfusion. These include the kinins, lactate, histamine, carbon dioxide, and oxygen.

Specialized Chemoreceptors

The *carotid bodies* and *aortic bodies* are specialized chemoreceptors that exert a significant influence upon the cardiovascular and respiratory systems through their responsiveness to blood levels or partial pressure (P) of carbon dioxide (P_{CO_2}) and oxygen (P_{O_2}).

Carotid Bodies. The *carotid bodies* are small nodules of cells that are positioned in association with the common carotid arteries. These receptors are highly vascularized structures that consist of parenchymal cells enclosed by a capsule of connective tissue. The epithelioid cells are divisible into two distinct groups. *Type I cells (glomus cells)* are large, contain a round nucleus, and are usually clumped together in small groups. Numerous nerve fibers ramify throughout the carotid bodies and terminate on Type I cells. The glomus cells are surrounded by *Type II cells (sustentacular cells)*. The precise mechanism by which Type I cells function has not been determined.

Glomus cells have ultrastructural features of sensory and effector (secretory) cells; their innervation appears to be both afferent and efferent. During periods of normal P_{O_2} and P_{CO_2}, Type I cells appar-

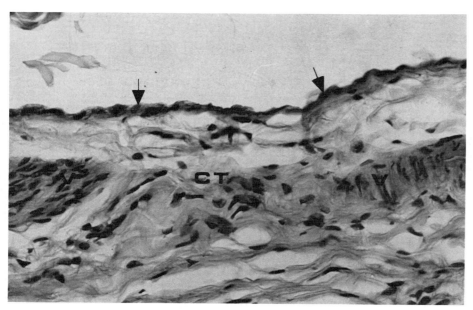

Figure 18.21. A section of atrial epicardium. The mesothelial lining *(arrows)* resides upon a layer of connective tissue *(CT)*. The smooth muscle is part of vessels *(V)* that have been sectioned obliquely. X100.

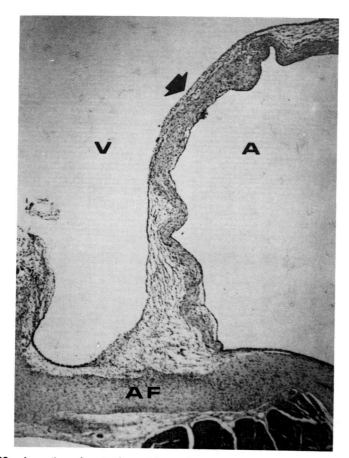

Figure 18.22. A section of part of an atrioventricular valve. The valve *(arrow)* separates the ventricle *(V)* from the atrium *(A)*. The connective tissue of the fibrous ring *(AF)* is continuous with the connective tissue core of the valve. The valve is covered by endothelium. X10.

ently secrete dopamine, and the afferent terminals (dendritic zones) associated with them discharge spontaneously. This discharge has a negative feedback control on centers located within the brain stem. During periods of low P_{O_2} and elevated P_{CO_2}, the spontaneous discharge of afferent terminals decreases, resulting in a release of central inhibition, and efferent terminals become active. The carotid bodies are innervated by general visceral afferent and general visceral efferent fibers from the glossopharyngeal nerve.

Aortic Bodies. The *aortic bodies* are structures similar to the carotid bodies. Although these structures have not been studied as extensively as the carotid bodies, they probably function in a similar manner. The bodies are innervated by fibers from the vagus nerve.

Specialized Baroreceptors

Carotid and Aortic Sinuses. The *carotid sinus* and *aortic sinus* are specialized receptor regions responsive to alterations in blood pressure. The carotid sinus is a dilation of the internal carotid artery as it originates from the common carotid artery. The tunica media of the carotid sinus has fewer smooth muscle fibers and more elastic and collagenous fibers than adjacent portions of the artery. Numerous afferent terminals from the glossopharyngeal nerve ramify in the tunica adventitia of this structure. The vagus nerve innervates the aortic sinus. These receptors cause a stimulation of central control centers resulting in a reflex bradycardia, dilation of splanchnic vessels, and a fall in systemic blood pressure.

Neuroregulation

Central Components and Afferent Input. The regulatory influence of the hypothalamus upon the cardiovascular system is mediated through various autonomic nerve centers—vasomotor centers, motor nuclei of cranial nerves, and the lateral grey columns of the throacic and lumbar spinal cord. The control of this sytem by the hypothalamus is manifested as a basic level of normal activity or *tone* that is altered in response to varied types of afferent input.

The *vasopressor region* and *cardiac stimulator center*, as well as the *vasodepressor region*, are large, diffuse regions within the medullary reticular formation. The *cardiac inhibitory center* or *dorsal motor nucleus of the vagus nerve* is a discrete nucleus within this region.

Physiological Correlates. The dual innervation of the myocardium provides an effective and precise means for the regulation of cardiac activity. This activity is determined by the balance exerted between the inhibitory cholinergic nerves of the vagus and the stimulatory adrenergic fibers of sympathetic nerves.

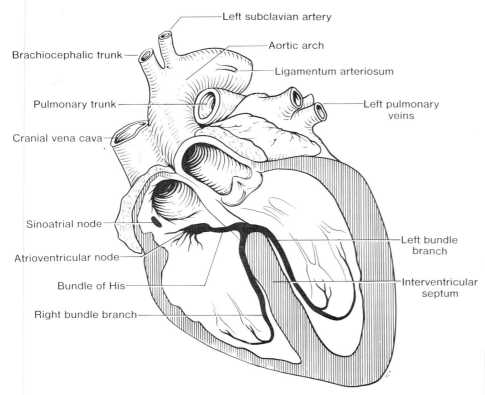

Figure 18.23. A cut away diagram of a canine heart. The conduction system and the major components of the heart are indicated.

The stimulation of the heart by the sympathetic nerves results in a *positive chronotropy* (increased heart rate), a *positive inotropy* (increased strength of contraction and a *positive dromotropy* (increased velocity of conduction. An increased vagal tone results in negative chronotropy, negative inotropy and negative dromotropy.

The heart rate of a resting animal is primarily under the inhibitory influence of the vagus nerve that exerts a braking effect upon the resting heart rate. Bilateral vagotomy or the use of antimuscarinic drugs result in tachycardia. Massive vagal stimulation or the use of muscarinic drugs can reduce the heart rate (bradycardia) to the point of sinus arrest. Sympathectomy or the use of β_1-blocking agents result in bradycardia, whereas sympathetic stimulation or the administration of β-stimulators results in tachycardyia. The chronotropic effects upon the heart are mediated through an alteration of the depolarization rate of nodal tissue. A change in the slope of the prepotential determines the rapidity of nodal firing.

The inotropic effect of these nerves upon the heart is not equivalent. Although the sympathetic nerves exert a marked positive inotropy upon the venticular myocardium, the negative inotropic effect of the vagus nerve is not equivalent. The mechanism by which these nerves exert their inotropic effects is not clear. The positive inotropy exerted through β_1-receptor activity is me-

diated through cyclic adenosine monophosphate (cAMP). Many xanthines, which decrease the breakdown of cAMP by the inhibition of phosphodiesterase activity, are positive inotropes also. The cardiac glycosides and other antiarrhythmic drugs are believed to exert their positive inotropy upon the myocardium by the inhibition of Na^+-Ka^+-dependent adenosine triphosphatase. The increased intercellular Na^+ followed by an influx of Ca^{++} causes an enhanced excitation-contraction coupling.

The dromotropic effect is manifested as an alteration in atrial and ventricular conduction speeds, as well as an alteration to nodal delay. The dromotropic effect complements the chronotropic effect. These factors plus the inotropic effect determine cardiac performance or *cardiac output*. **The cardiac output is the heart rate multiplied by the stroke volume.**

The adrenergic receptors located in the smooth muscle of the coronary vessels are β_2-receptors. The heart is required to do more work under sympathetic stimulation. Coronary vessel dilation via these receptors ensures an ample blood supply to the myocardium commensurate with the increased work demands imposed upon it.

Autonomic Reflex Activity

Arterial Pressoreceptor Reflex. Arterial baroreceptors are located throughout the body as integral components of the mural elements of these vessels. They are respon-

sive to alterations in the stretch of blood vessels that accompanies alterations in blood pressure.

An increased blood pressure stretches the wall of the vessel and results in an increased rate of discharge (Fig 18.26). This information reaches the vasomotor centers and stimulates the vasodepressor region while blocking the vasopressor region. This effectively decreases the sympathetic tone to the cardiovasular system. Concomitantly, these afferents reach the cardiac inhibitory center (dorsal motor nucleus of the vagus nerve); the vagal tone to the heart is increased. Thus, an increased blood pressure reflexively results in a decreased cardiac output and peripheral vasodilation. This combination effectively lowers the blood pressure. A decreased blood pressure has the reverse effect upon the cardiovascular system (Fig. 18.26).

The specific arterial pressoreceptor reflex involving the carotid sinus is called the *carotid sinus reflex, baroreceptor reflex*, and *depressor reflex*. It is an important negative

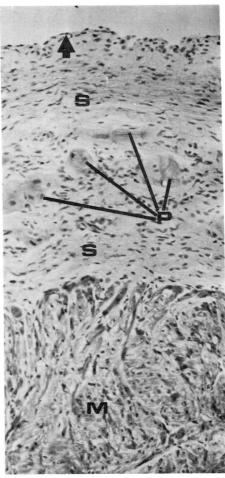

Figure 18.24. Subendocardial Purkinje fibers of a porcine heart. *Arrow*, endothelium; *S*, subendothelium; *P*, Purkinje fibers; *M*, myocardium. The Purkinje fibers are part of the bundle branches of the ventricles. X40.

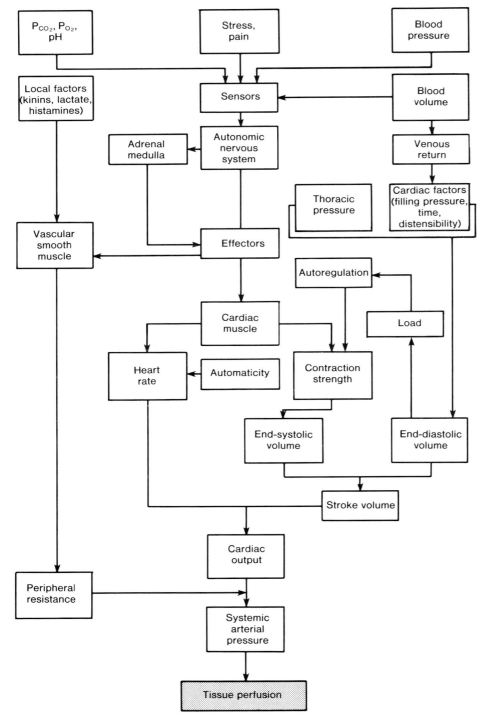

Figure 18.25. A flow chart demonstrating the various influences upon the cardiovascular system that affect tissue perfusion.

basis. The mechanism of action was discussed previously. Note that an increased discharge, as in the baroreceptor reflex, results in a release of central inhibition. The primary effects, however, are mediated through the respiratory centers. Minimal cardiac effects are noted, because peripheral hypoxia depresses cardiac activity; a central hypoxia stimulates cardiac activity. Chemoreceptors help to coordinate pulmonary and cardiac activity to ensure proper ventilation/perfusion ratios.

It is possible that blood flow to the brain could be impaired without stimulation of the carotid or aortic receptors. Under these circumstances the medullary receptors are important monitors of P_{CO_2} and pH. Cerebral ischemia, then, would result in increased activity in the cardiovascular and respiratory systems.

Pain. Most of the sensory modalities are involved in the reflex activity associated with cardiovascular regulation. Pain manifests diverse influences upon the system. Generally, a painful stimulus results in a rise in blood pressure through an increased activity of the vasopressor centers. Vasoconstriction and increased cardiac output account for a rise in blood pressure.

Severe cutaneous pain and deep visceral pain usually have the opposite effect—bradycardia and decreased blood pressure. A vagovagal reflex involving the visceral organs occurs under a variety of circumstances but may be especially significant during abdominal surgery.

Hormonal Influence

Adrenomedullary and Antidiuretic Hormone Influence. The effects of the adrenal medullary secretions are discussed with the autonomic nervous system (Chapter 17).

Antidiuretic hormone (ADH) is released from the nerve fibers of the neurohypophysis at neurohemal organs. Volume receptor stimulation in the left atrium influences the release of ADH. This hormone is also released after hemorrhage. Beside the advantage of water retention, ADH may have a direct pressor effect upon the blood vessels. This effect may be significant in the long term adjustments of blood volume after minor blood loss.

Lymphatic Vessels

Capillaries and Larger Vessels. Lymph capillaries are very similar to continuous blood capillaries and are most difficult to distinguish from one another in section (Fig. 18.7). Three features generally may be used to make the distinction. Lymph capillaries are partially or completely devoid of a basement membrane. Their abluminal surfaces may have microvilli that anchor the vessels in the connective tissue space. Also, they are generally devoid of formed elements; however, agranulocytes may be encountered.

feedback loop that is significant in cardiovascular homeostasis. Generally, stimulation of baroreceptors inhibits the cardiovascular system. One notable exception to this generality exists. When the heart is operating under the influence of increased vagal tone, stretching of the right atrium results in an increased heart rate *(Bainbridge reflex)*.

Chemoreceptor Reflexes. These reflexes utilize the carotid and aortic bodies. Medullary receptors on the floor of the fourth ventricle near the obex are involved also. The receptors for chemical reflexes are sensitive to P_{O_2}, P_{CO_2} and pH.

The carotid body, as an example, consists of a glomus of cells that is one of the most vascularized organs of the body. It receives approximately 200 times more blood than the rest of the body on a ml/min/gram

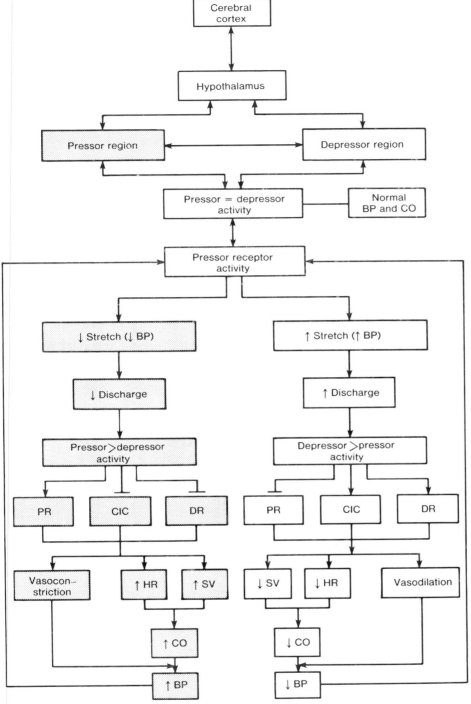

Figure 18.26. A flow chart showing the effects of the arterial pressoreceptor reflex upon blood pressure. *PR*, pressor region; *CIC*, cardiac inhibitory center (dorsal motor nucleus of the vagus nerve); *DR*, depressor region; *SV*, stroke volume; *HR*, heart rate; *CO*, cardiac output; *BP*, blood pressure. *Arrows* indicate the direction of flow or simulation; *bars* indicate inhibition. An increased discharge rate inhibits the *PR* but stimulates the *CIC* and *DR*; a decreased blood pressure results. The reverse occurs when a decreased blood causes a decreased receptor discharge.

The larger vessels are not well-organized. Although the three mural regions may be present, they are not well-defined. Generally, the lymphatics vessels have thinner walls than the veins of a corresponding size. Valves occur in lymph vessels of a smaller size than the corresponding appearance of valves in veins.

References

Vasculature

Abramson, D.I.: *Circulation in the Extrmities.* Academic Press, New York, 1976.

Ahmed, M.M.: The fine structure of endothelium in coronary arterioles. Acta Anat. *69:*327, 1968.

Bennet, H. S., Luft, J.H. and Hampton, J.C.: Morphological classification of vertebrate blood capillaries. Amer. J. Physiol. *196:*381, 1959.

Bruns, R.R. and Palade, G.E.: Studies on blood capillaries. I. General organization of blood capillaries in muscle. J. Cell Biol. *37:*244, 1968.

Cliff, W.J.: *Blood Vessels.* Cambridge University Press, Oxford, 1976.

Fernando, N.V.P.and Movat, H.Z.: The capillaries. Exp. Molec. Pathol. *3:*87, 1964.

Hayes, J. R.: Histological changes in constricted arteries and arterioles. J. Anat. *101:*343, 1967.

Keech, M.K.: Electron microscope study of the normal rat aorta. J. Biphys. Biochem. Cytol. *7:*533, 1960.

Leak, L.V. and Burke, J.F.: Fine structure of the lymphatic capillary and the adjoining connective tissue area. Amer. J. Anat. *118:*785, 1966.

Rhodin, J.A.G.: Fine structure of vascular walls in mammals with special reference to smooth muscle component. Physiol. Rev. *42:*447, 1962.

Wood, J.E.: *The Veins: Normal and Abnormal Function.* Little, Brown, Boston, 1965.

Heart

Bolton, G.R.: *Handbook of Canine Electrocardiography.* W.B. Saunders, Philadelphia, 1975.

Eckner, F.A.O., Brown, B.W., Overll, E. and Glagov, S.: Alterations of the gross dimensions of the heart and its structures by formalin fixation: Aquantitative study. Virchow Arch. Path. Anat. *346:*318, 1969.

Ettinger, S.J. and Suter, P.F.: *Canine Cardiology.* W.B. Saunders, Philadelphia, 1970.

Ghidoni, J.J., Liotta, D. and Thomas, H.: Massive subendocardial damage and accompanying prolonged ventricular fibrillation. Amer. J. Path. *56:*15, 1969.

Hogan, P.M. and Davis, L.D.: Evidence for specialized fibers in the canine right atrium. Crc. Res. *23:*387, 1968.

James, T.N. and Sherf, L.: Ultrastructure of myocardial cells. Amer. J. Cardiol.*22:*389, 1968.

James, T.N., Sherf, L. and Urthaler, F.: Fine structure of the bundle branches. Br. Heart J. *36:*1, 1974.

Langer, G.A. and Brady, A.J.: *The Mammalian Myocardium.* John Wiley & Sons, New York, 1974.

Merkin, R.J.: Position and orientation of heart valves. Amer. J. Anat. *125:*375, 1969.

Mitomo, Y., Nakao, K. and Angrist, A.: The fine structure of the heart valves of the chicken. Amer. J. Anat. *125:*147, 1969.

Muir, A.R.: Observations on the fine structure of the Purkinje fibers in the ventricles of the sheep's heart. J. Anat. *91:*251, 1957.

Nabors, C.E. and Ball. C.R.: Spontaneous calcification in hearts of DBA mice. Anat. Rec. *164:*153, 1969.

Rhodin, J.A.G., Delmissier, P. and Reid, L.C.: The structure of the specialized conducting system of the steer heart. Circulation. *24:*349, 1961.

Regulation

Aars, H.: The baroreflex in arterial hypertension. Scand. J. Clin. Lab. Invest. *35:*97, 1975.

Armour, J. A. and Randall, W.C.: Functional anatomy of canine cardiac nerves. Acta Anat. *91:*510, 1975.

Denn, M.J. and Stone, H.L.: Autonomic innervation of the dog coronary arteries. J. Appl. Physiol. *41:*30, 1976.

Feigl, E.O.: Sympathetic control of coronary circulation. Circ. Res. *20:*262, 1967.

Feigl, E.O.: Carotid sinus reflex control of coronary blood flow. Circ. Res. *23:*223, 1968.

Feigl, E.O.: Parasympathetic control of coronary blood flow in dogs. Circ. Res. *25:*509, 1969.

Granger, H.S. and Guyton, A.C.: Autoregulation of the total systemic circulation following destruction of the central nervous system in the dog. Circ. Res. *25:*379, 1969.

Gross, D.: Pain and autonomic nervous system. Adv. Neurol. *4:*93, 1974.

Osborne, M.P. and Butler, P.J.: New theory for receptor mechanism of carotid body chemorecptors. Nature *254:*701, 1975.

19: Lymphatic System and Immunity

General Characteristics

Form and Function. The lymphatic and vascular systems form a functional unit, the *hemic-lymphatic system*, that is a *secondary defense system*. The *primary defense system* is the skin and the mucous membranes. The defensive aspects of the lymphatic system are manifested by:

1. Production of defensive cells.
2. Transport of materials via the lymphatic vessels.
3. Filtration of lymph and blood.
4. Phagocytosis.
5. Production of immunoglobulins.

The filtration function is complemented by phagocytosis. The phagocytic function is achieved by aggregation of phagocytic cells as the *macrophage system*.

Classification of Lymphatic Tissues. The tissues and organs of the lymphatic system may be grouped into morphological subdivisions:

1. Diffuse, unencapsulated lymphatic tissues (subepithelial lymphatic tissue associated with somatic orifices and tracts of the respiratory, digestive, and urogenital systems).
2. Dense, unencapsulated lymphatic tissue (subepithelial accumulations of lymphatic tissue associated with the respiratory, digestive, and urogenital tracts).
3. Dense, encapsulated tissues scattered throughout the body (lymph nodes, spleen, hemal nodes, hemolymph nodes, thymus, bursa of Fabricius).

Diffuse Lymphatic Tissue

Generalized Distribution of Lymphoid Cells. Lymphoid cells occur within any locus of the body. The connective tissue of the lamina propria mucosae is replete with these defensive cells. They may occur with sufficient frequency to impart a hypercellular nature to this connective tissue (Fig. 19.1). In those organs that are subjected continually to insult from foreign materials (respiratory, digestive, and urogenital systems), these cells become part of the resident population of the connective tissue.

They are an effective second line of defense in these loci.

Dense Lymphatic Tissue

Solitary Lymph Nodules. Lymph nodules are scattered throughout the body. Solitary nodules, as spheres of lymphoid cells and supportive stroma, occur within the connective tissue of the digestive, respiratory, and urogenital tracts (Fig. 19.2). The lymphocytes from the outer corona migrate into the surrounding lamina propria mucosae or tunica submucosa. The connective tissue surrounding these nodules is drained by lymphatic vessels. Some of these nodules may be encapsulated.

Avian Lymphatic Tissue. Many avian species, with the exception of swamp, shore and sea birds, do not have lymph nodes.

Solitary accumulations of lymphatic tissue as nodules characterize the walls of the digestive tract, serous membranes, and skin (Fig. 19.3).

Aggregated Lymph Nodules. Accumulations of large and even confluent lymph nodules occur throughout the soma (Fig. 19.4). Often, aggregated lymph nodules are referred to as tonsils, in which case Peyer's patches of the intestinal wall may be considered "intestinal tonsils."

Tonsils. Tonsils are formed of solitary or aggregated nodules and diffuse lymphatic tissue as part of the pharyngeal mucosa (Fig. 19.5). The unencapsulated nodules have large germinal centers with dense cortices. Extensive infiltration of lymphocytes into the surrounding pharyngeal mucosa is usually evident.

Although all tonsils are similar, two dis-

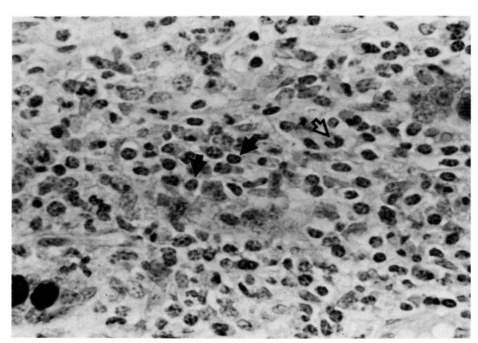

Figure 19.1. A section of lamina propria mucosae associated with the gastrointestinal tract. The tissue is hyperplastic. Numerous plasma cells *(solid arrows)*, macrophages *(open arrow)*, and other mononucleated cells are present. ×160.

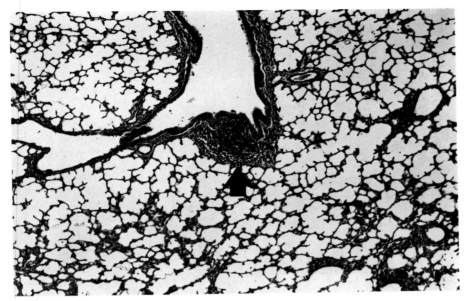

Figure 19.2. A solitary lymph nodule in a lung. The lymph nodule *(arrow)* is associated closely with a bronchiole. ×16.

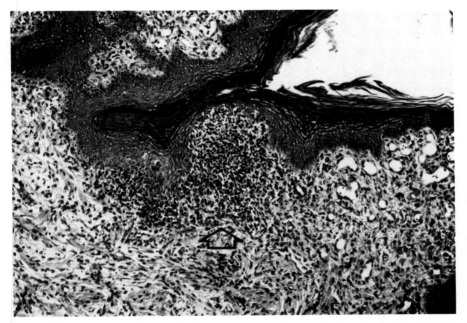

Figure 19.3. Lymphatic tissue in the dermal connective tissue of the comb of a bird. The dermis contains a lymphatic nodule *(arrow)* and loose lymphatic tissue.

tinguishable groups are defined on the basis of tonsillar tissue relationships with the surface epithelium—*tonsils with crypts* and *tonsils without crypts.* The *crypt* is a blind and sometimes branched invagination of the surface epithelium. A crypt and the associated lymphatic tissue is referred to as a *tonsillar follicle* (Fig. 19.6). A group of follicles constitutes a tonsil of this type. A *tonsil without crypts* is formed by a single lamina of lymphatic tissue that may secondarily protrude into the lumen or be slightly folded to increase surface area (Fig.

19.5). The invaginations of the tunica mucosa are significant, because they serve as foci of infection and corresponding inflammatory processes.

The morphological features and specific sites of tonsillar tissue vary among domestic species:

1. Tonsils with crypts (follicular tonsils): palatine tonsils in man, horse, ruminant, swine; lingual tonsils in man, horse, ruminant, swine; tubual tonsils in swine; paraepiglottic tonsils in sheep, goat, swine.

2. Tonsils without crypts: palatine tonsils in

carnivores; pharyngeal tonsils in all domestic animals except carnivores; tubal tonsils in ruminants.

Tonsils do not possess afferent lymphatic channels. Efferent lymphatic channels drain the aggregated nodules.

Lymphatic Organs

Lymph Node

Histological Structure. These organs are dense, encapsulated components of the system that occur constantly in specific regions called lymphocenters. Lymph nodes are usually bean-shaped and vary in size from about 1 mm to several centimeters. The nodes, sometimes called glands, consist of a *capsule, stroma, cortex, medulla, nodules, and hilus* (Fig. 19.7).

The capsule consists of dense white fibrous connective tissue (DWFCT) that is continuous with trabeculae of the same tissue. The fine stromal elements of the organ are reticular fibers (Fig 19.8).

The *cortex* consists of nodules, trabeculae, fine stromal elements, and lymph sinuses (Fig. 19.9). This region contains primarily B lymphocytes and their progeny, macrophages and dendritic cells. Dendritic cells of lymph nodes are comparable to Langerhans cells of the skin. Dendritic cells are stellate cells whose interlacing web of cellular processes traps antigens effectively. The *medulla* consists of cellular aggregates, a cellular and fine fibrous stroma and sinuses. The medulla is arranged as aggregates of cells in cords *(medullary cords)* that are separated by connective tissue and

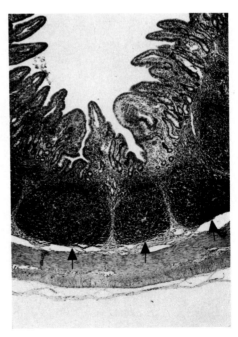

Figure 19.4. Peyer's patches in the wall of an ileum. The patches *(arrows)* are aggregates of lymphatic nodules. ×8.

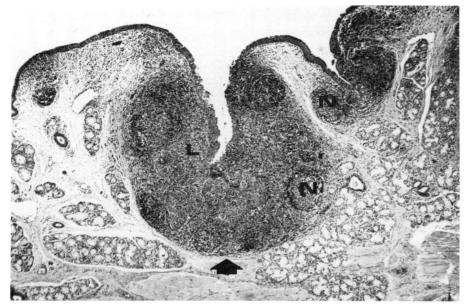

Figure 19.5. A tonsil without crypts. The tonsil *(arrow)* is composed of nodular *(N)* and loose *(L)* lymphatic tissue. The tunica mucosa is folded slightly. Extensive infiltration of lymphocytes into the lamina propria mucosae and lamina epithelialis mucosae is evident. Because of the infiltration, the epithelial lining is not readily apparent *(center)*. ×10.

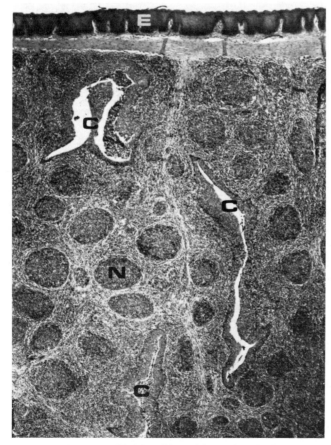

Figure 19.6. A tonsil with crypts. Nodular *(N)* and loose lymphatic tissues are the primary components. The lamina epithelialis mucosae *(E)* is folded extensively and forms deep crypts *(C)* or invaginations. ×10.

lymph sinuses (Fig. 19.10). The hilus is a connective tissue space that contains efferent lymphatic vessels.

Cellular Populations. Lymphocytic populations are organized into nodules within the lymph node. *Primary nodules (follicles)* are devoid of germinal centers. *Secondary nodules* are characterized by germinal centers. Medullary cords are sometimes called *tertiary follicles*. An immunologically competent, responsive, and active nodule *(secondary nodule)* consists of a *germinal center* and outer *corona* (Fig. 19.11). The germinal center contains various mature and immature cells. *Dendritic cells* form a cellular reticulum. Mature lymphocytes and lymphoblasts are predominant cell types, although plasma cells, dendritic cells, and macrophages are present also. The lymphoblasts and their progeny of lymphocytes are B cells. Some T cells occur at the interface between the germinal center and the corona. These centers are paler than the peripheral corona because of the presence of pale-staining and fewer cells. As lymphocytes are produced, they migrate peripherally to form the corona or *cortex of the nodule*.

The region subjacent to the lymph nodules of the cortex, *paracortical* or *subcortical zone*, is occupied primarily by T lymphocytes.

Medullary cords contain accumulations of plasma cells and their progenitors, some B lymphocytes and macrophages. In ideal preparations, these regions are clearly delimited by large medullary sinusoids.

Lymph Circulation. *Afferent vessels* enter at the capsule and empty into a prominent *subcapsular (marginal) sinus*. Percolation of lymph continues through the *cortical sinuses* and nodules into the *medullary sinuses*. The latter are confluent with *efferent lymphatic vessels* at the hilus. Flow through a lymph node is unidirectional—capsule to hilus.

Blood Vessels and Nerves. Arteries enter the lymph node at the hilus and are distributed through trabeculae. The venous drainage is typical; however, the *postcapillary venules* of the paracortical region are lined by thickened endothelial cells. These vessels are involved in *recirculation* of lymphocytes from the blood.

Nerves also enter the hilus. Most of these are probably vasomotor nerves. Some nerves, which are independent of the vasculature, occur within the trabeculae, capsule, and medullary cords.

Species Differences. The porcine lymph node has the reverse pattern of that observed in other species (Fig. 19.12). Lymphatic nodules are located in the central or medullary regions of the organ, whereas the medullary cords and related aggregates of cells are located at the peripheral or cortical region. Flow of lymph, similarly, is the reverse of other domestic species; i.e., it

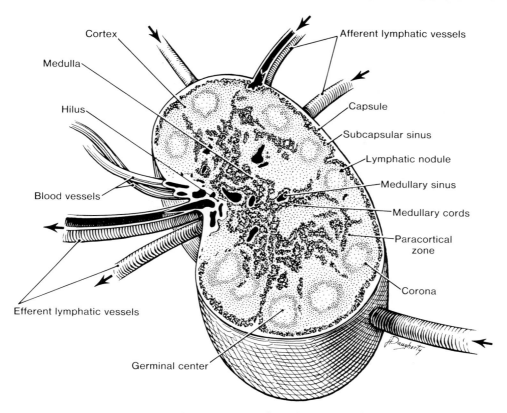

Figure 19.7.   A diagram of a typical lymph node.

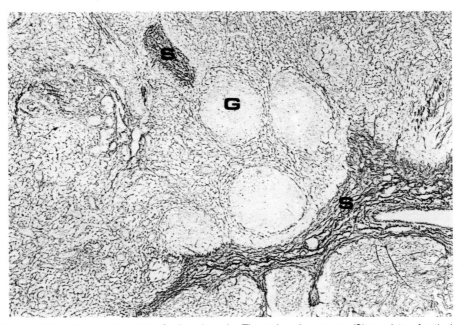

Figure 19.8.   Stromal elements of a lymph node. The trabecular stroma *(S)* consists of reticular and collagenous fibers, whereas other interstitial regions of the lymph node are composed of reticular fibers exclusively. The germinal centers of the lymphatic nodules *(G)* contain a paucity of fibrous elements. ×16. (Snook's reticular stain.)

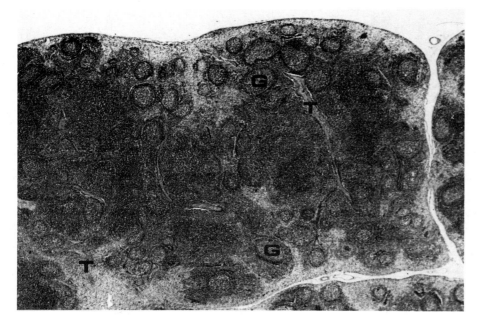

Figure 19.9. A section of a an equine lymph node. The cortex consists of nodules with germinal centers *(G)*, trabeculae *(T)* and sinuses. ×4.

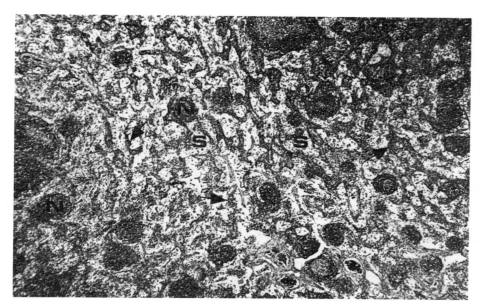

Figure 19.10. The medulla of a canine lymph node. Nodules *(N)* are apparent at the periphery of the medulla. Medullary cords *(arrows)* and sinuses *(S)* are the primary constituents of the medulla. ×10.

enters at the hilus and emerges at the capsular area.

Important variations in lymph nodes occur in many species. In the horse, a fusion of cortical nodules is common. The ox possesses very large germinal centers. The age and physiological state of the organism alter lymph node morphology.

Functional Correlates. Lymph nodes *produce lymphocytes, filter lymph, phagocytose foreign materials*, and *produce antibodies*. Extensive mitotic activity within

the germinal centers of lymph nodules is responsible for B lymphocyte production.

The walls of lymphatic capillaries are readily permeable to foreign materials (macromolecules, particulate matter, microbial agents) and connective tissue cells (Fig. 19.13). The obvious result of this property is the ability of these vessels to transport various materials and cells to the lymph nodes wherein filtration and phagocytosis can occur. The permeability of the endothelial lining of the lymphatic chan-

nels within the lymph node facilitates these basic protective functions. The free movement of particulate matter, microbial agents and cells from the lymphatic channels to the lymph node with subsequent access to blood vessels and efferent lymphatic vessels also facilitates the spread of infectious agents and the metastasis of cancer cells.

The synthesis of antibodies is an important function of the B cell population in lymph nodes. Antigens that reach the lymph nodes are subjected to phagocytosis by macrophages of the medullary cords. These cells migrate to the cortex to interact with antigen-sensitive progenitor B cells of the germinal centers. Macrophages secrete a helper substance called *interleukin 1* that activates *T helper cells*. These cells secrete helper substances that enhance the stimulation of B lymphocytes into plasma cells. Stimulated cells that do not become identifiable plasma cells and are indistinguishable from the progenitor B cells are retained as *memory cells*. Dendritic cells of the cortex are effective antigen trappers after initial antigenic stimulation. Their activity enhances the secondary immune response. T cells respond to antigenic stimulation similarly—requiring the helper substances of macrophages and T helper cells. The mitotic and differentiation response produces large populations of: *cytotoxic effector cells (killer cells), memory cells, and lymphokine-producing cells.*

Hemal Nodes and Hemolymph Nodes

Histological Structure. The sinuses of *hemal nodes* are filled with blood rather than lymph (Fig. 19.14). Also, lymph vessels are not demonstrable. The capsule and trabeculae contain smooth muscle fibers. The organs, described as miniature spleens, look much like typical lymph nodes. Hemal nodes occur in ruminants in retroperitoneal postions along the vertebral column and in association with some of the visceral organs. They also occur in the jugular furrow.

Hemolymph nodes, as believed by some, may be hemorrhagic lymph nodes. Evidence exists, however, that they are normal and distinct entities. These organs receive blood and lymph that intermix in the sinuses. They may represent an intermediate form of lymphatic organ between the two aforementioned types. Hemolymph nodes occur in the perirenal region of the sheep and goat and have been observed in the lumbar region of the ox. Because of the significance of lymph nodes in diagnostic histopathology, awareness of these structures is essential. These, otherwise, may be mistaken for hemorrhagic lymph nodes.

Spleen

Histological Structure. The spleen is the largest mass of lymphatic tissue (Fig.

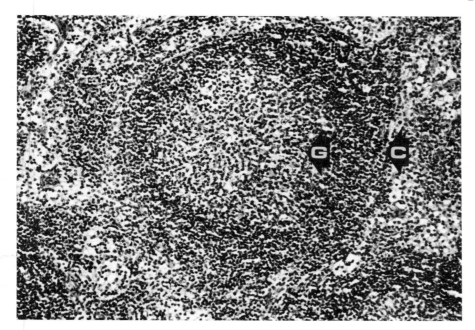

Figure 19.11. A lymphatic nodule from a lymph node of an immunologically competent animal. The nodule consists of a central germinal center *(G)* and an outer corona *(C)*. ×40.

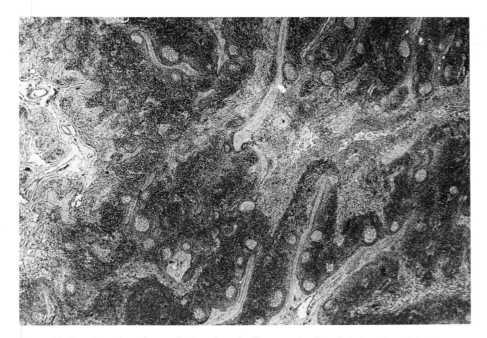

Figure 19.12. A section of a porcine lymph node. The organization of the lymph node is the reverse of that which occurs in other mammals. ×10.

19.15). This large organ has multiple functions: *blood cell formation, hemoglobulin and iron metabolism, red blood cell destruction, blood filtration, blood storage, phagocytosis, and immune response.*

The associated connective tissue of its serous membrane blends with the DWFCT of its capsule. Trabeculae of DWFCT extend into the parenchyma and subdivide it into smaller compartments (Fig. 19.16). Smooth muscle fibers and elastic fibers are present in the capsule and trabeculae of this organ (Fig. 19.17). Reticular fibers are the primary stromal elements. The arrangement of the capsular and trabecular smooth muscle is species variable. Large volume changes are accommodated, and smooth muscle facilitates discharge of blood from the organ.

The spleen is a mixture of phagocytic sinuses, reticular fiber stroma, and a cellular parenchyma. A distinct cortex or me-

dulla are not apparent. The parenchyma consists of nodules scattered among a cellular parenchyma—*white pulp* and *red pulp.* Lymph nodules *(splenic corpuscles)* and *periarterial lymphatic sheaths (PALS)* comprise the white pulp (Fig. 19.18). An arteriole, sometimes called the *central artery*, occupies a central or paracentral position within nodules. This vessel is sometimes called the *nodular arteriole* (Fig. 19.15). It is not observed in all sections because the plane of section may parallel its course. The presence of nodules is dependent upon the same factors that influence germinal center development or regression in lymph nodes.

White and Red Pulp. The *white pulp* consists of dense lymphatic tissue that is associated intimately with branches of the trabecular arteries. Nodular enlargements, *splenic corpuscles*, are randomly distributed along the course of the arteries of the white pulp and are intercalated with the periarterial lymphatic sheaths (Figs. 19.19 and 19.20). The composition, nature, and distribution of cellular components within a splenic corpuscle are similar to those of a lymphatic nodule; however, each germinal center of a splenic nodule is surrounded by a *mantle layer (mantle zone)*, which is continuous with the periarterial sheath. The peripheral limits of the white pulp are interfaced with the red pulp by a *marginal zone*, which consists of sinuses, a sheath of dendritic cells, macrophages, and a layer of lymphatic cells. The periarterial lymphatic sheath and marginal zone are thymic-dependent regions that are occupied by T cells; the splenic corpuscle produces B cells.

The regions between the splenic corpuscles and trabeculae are the regions of the *red pulp*, so named because of the extensive vascularity. The red pulp consists of splenic sinuses and splenic cords (Fig. 19.21). The splenic sinuses are discontinuous and are lined by phagocytic cells. These sinuses open into the splenic cords. The cords are composed of granulocytes, granulocyte progenitors, reticular cells, and phagocytic cells. In some species smooth muscle fibers also occur. The sinuses and cords are an integral filtration and phagocytic unit with many fixed and wandering macrophages. These phagocytic cells, of course, are responsible for the removal of cellular detritus, damaged erythrocytes, and foreign substances from the blood. A yellow-brown pigment, *hemosiderin* (a breakdown product of hemoglobin), is usually present in the phagocytic cells of the sinuses and cords.

The three-dimensional relationships of splenic components are illustrated in Figure 19.22.

Splenic Circulation. An understanding of the circulatory pattern through the spleen is essential for a general comprehension of its function (Fig. 19.23). *Splenic arteries*

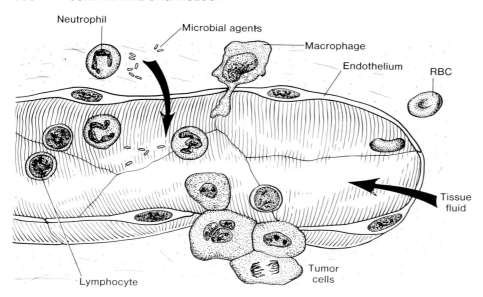

Figure 19.13. A diagram of the initial portion—lymphatic capillary—of lymphatic channels. White blood cells, some RBCs, proteins, particulate matter, parasites, microbial agents, and certain tumor cells gain access readily to the lymphatic vessels. Whereas such access serves as a method of involving the lymph nodes in the defense of the organism by transporting foreign materials, infectious agents may spread to other parts of the body via the lymphatic system. Also, some tumors metastasize (spread) through the lymphatic system.

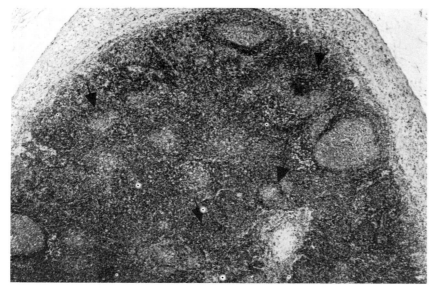

Figure 19.14. A bovine hemal node. The organ is similar to a lymph node. Sinuses (arrows), however, are engorged with blood. ×10.

enter at the hilus and divide into *trabecular arteries.* Upon entering the splenic parenchyma, lymphocytes accumulate in the adventitia of the vessels. This sheath of lymphocytes is continuous with splenic nodules. The vessel is then referred to as the *nodular arteriole.* Branches from this vessel supply capillaries in the white pulp and marginal region of the white pulp. The capillaries empty into the *red pulp sinuses* or into *pulp veins.* The nodular arteriole emerges from the white pulp and divides into several smaller branches, *penicillar ar-* terioles. Penicillar arterioles are divisible into *red pulp arterioles, sheathed arterioles,* and *terminal arterial capillaries.* Sheathed arterioles have thickened walls *(sheath of Schweigger-Seidel)* composed of concentric laminae of reticular cells and reticular fibers (Fig. 19.24). The continuation of blood from terminal arterial capillaries is a subject of controversy. Blood from terminal arterial capillaries may open directly into venous sinuses *(closed theory).* This presumably occurs in man, rat, and dog. The terminal arterial capillaries may open

into the reticulum of the red pulp and filter into the venous sinuses *(open theory).* This is supposedly characteristic of the mouse, cat, horse, ox, and swine. Some authors claim that both methods are utilized, whereas others claim that the circulation may change between both extremes.

Species Differences. Three types of spleens have been described: *defensive, intermediate, and storage* types. The first type has few trabeculae and muscle fibers but abundant lymphatic tissue (lagomorphs, man). The storage type has many trabeculae and smooth muscle fibers. It is relatively large and has less white pulp than the other form (horse, dog, cat). Intermediate forms are typical of ruminants and swine. Red blood corpuscular destruction is typical of all spleens; it is well demonstrated in horses and swine.

Lymph Vessels and Innervation. The spleen does not receive afferent lymph vessels from other portions of the body. Lymphocytes filter through the spleen from the blood. Only efferent lymphatic vessels occur in the white pulp; the predominant efferent channels occur in the trabeculae, capsule, and hilus of the organ.

Some myelinated neuronal processes occur in the spleen: these are probably sensory nerves. The predominant nerves are postganglionic sympathetic fibers that are distributed to the smooth muscle of vessels (vasomotor), capsular smooth muscle, trabeculae, and pulp regions.

Physiological Correlates. The spleen is not essential for life. After splenectomy, other organs—especially the bone marrow—assume some of its functions.

Splenic filtration removes foreign particles, microbial agents, and old or degenerating blood cells from the circulation. Filtration and removal of blood-borne materials is achieved by splenic architecture and the macrophage system components, respectively. Sluggish blood flow through splenic cords and marginal zones enhances phagocytosis by the perivascular macrophages of splenic cords. Although the lungs, liver, and bone marrow contribute to this cleansing function, the spleen has the greatest capacity for it. The ability of the spleen to separate blood cells from plasma complements the cleansing function. The sympathetic stimulation of splenic veins increases pressure within the spleen and forces plasma into the lymphatic channels. Additionally, this separation results in a concentration of red blood cells (RBCs) within splenic cords.

The storage function of some spleens is enhanced by the separation phenomenon. The spleens of horses and carnivores may have a reservoir capacity for RBCs that approximates one-third of the circulating blood volume. Sympathetic discharge and the release of adrenomedullary secretions in response to stress (physical examination,

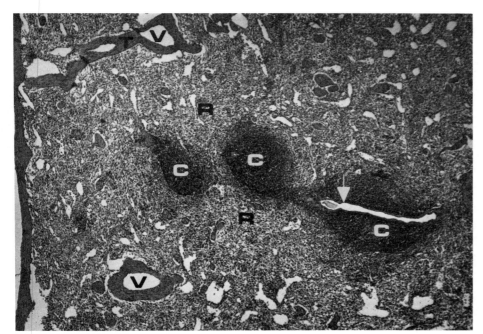

Figure 19.15. General organization of the spleen. Trabeculae *(T)* invaginate into the parenchyma from the capsule. Trabeculae contain arteries and veins *(V)*. The parenchyma consists of splenic corpuscles *(C)*. Nodular arterioles *(arrow)* occur within the splenic corpuscles. The corpuscles are surrounded by red pulp *(R)*. ×10.

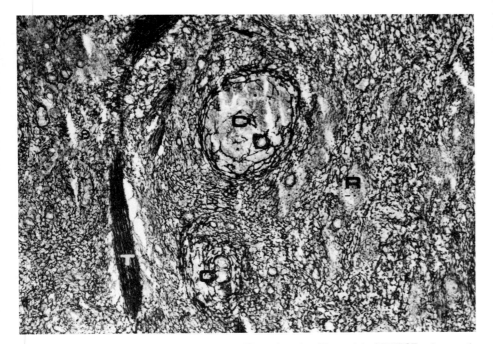

Figure 19.16. Stromal elements of the spleen. The trabeculae *(T)* consist of DWFCT, whereas the remaining stromal elements are reticular fibers. Splenic corpuscles *(C)* are delineated by the red pulp *(R)*. The germinal centers of the splenic corpuscles contain a paucity of stromal elements. ×40. (Snook's reticular stain.)

an enlarged spleen may be associated with a thrombocytopenia.

The sluggish flow of blood through the spleen facilitates the removal of aged or damaged erythrocytes by this organ. Cells that are incapable of surface deformation as they move through the spleen, such as the spherocytes of autoimmune hemolytic anemia, are subject to erythrophagocytosis. Similarly, the spleen is capable of removing particulate matter (HJ bodies, Heinz bodies) and parasites from the surface of erythrocytes.

The spleen functions as a hematopoietic organ during fetal and neonatal life. It is not a significant contributor to this function in the adult; however, the hematopoietic potential is retained throughout adulthood. The spleen may function as a storage depot for immature erythrocytes during which time they mature.

The spleen functions in cell-mediated immunity and humoral antibody responsiveness by virtue of its B and T lymphocyte populations.

Thymus

Embryonic Origin. The thymus is derived from the third and fourth pharyngeal pouches in accompaniment with the parathyroid derivative of the same pouches. The thymic anlagen, eventually separated from the parathyroid derivatives, occupy part of the cranial mediastinum, thoracic inlet, and ventral cervical region.

Most endodermally derived structures (liver, pancreas and other glands) assume a solid organ configuration in which the epithelial component becomes the obvious parenchyma. The densely packed mass of thymic epithelial cells becomes more loosely arranged as a cellular reticulum coincident with vascularization. Subsequent invasion by lymphocyte progenitors from the bone marrow converts the gland into a *lymphoepithelial organ* in which the predominant feature is the presence of *thymocytes*. These lymphocytes are the parenchyma of the organ. As the gland continues to grow, the epithelial cells—*epithelial-reticular cells*—become stellate cells that are attached to each other by desmosomes. Some of these cells form continuous sheets that become the peripheral limits of a system of labyrinths occupied by thymocytes and stellate-shaped epithelial-reticular cells. The deep portion of the gland *(medulla)* has fewer thymocytes than the outer portion of the gland *(cortex)*. The lobules of the gland, containing cortical and medullary components, form as a consequence of vacular invasion during development.

Histological Structure. Both lobes of the organ are covered by a capsule of loose connective tissue from which septa of similar tissue arise and subdivide the organ into lobules (Fig. 19.25). These septa extend to the corticomedullary junction. The

venipuncture) can cause splenic capsular contraction. Contraction of the spleen results in the discharge of a concentrated mass of erythrocytes into the circulation with a corresponding increase in the packed cell volume. Similarly, some drugs (anesthetics, tranquilizers) may cause a splenic

engorgement that is manifested as a decreased packed cell volume.

The storage function of the spleen is extended to platelets also. The spleen may store as much as one-third of the total number of circulating platelets. Splenectomy may cause a thrombocytosis, whereas

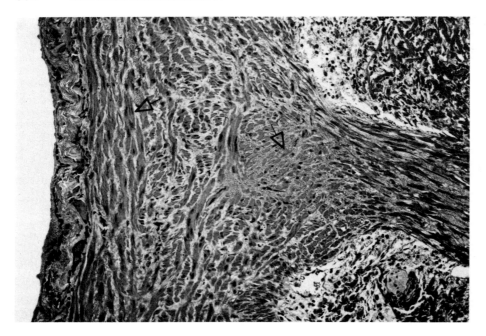

Figure 19.17. Smooth muscle of the capsule and trabeculae of a cervine spleen. The smooth muscle *(arrows)* is a prominent splenic feature. ×40.

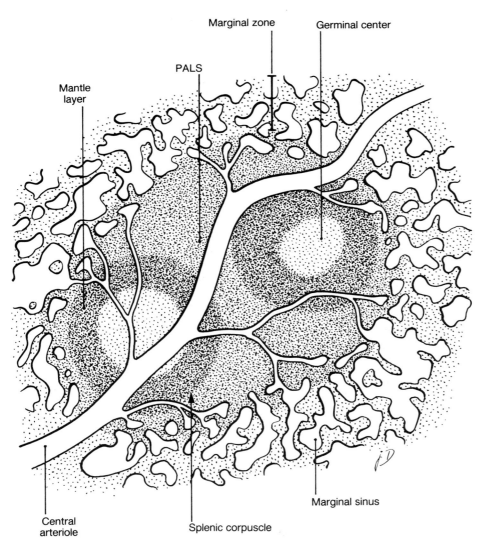

Figure 19.18. A diagram illustrating the components of the white pulp. PALS—periarterial lymphatic sheaths.

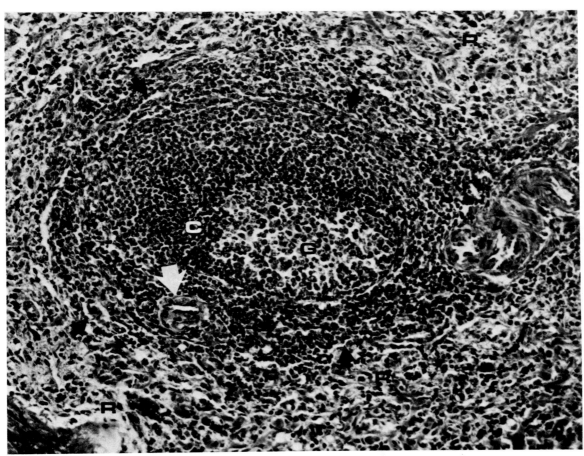

Figure 19.19. Splenic corpuscle and red pulp of a canine spleen. A germinal center *(G)*, corona *(C)* or mantle layer and paracentral arteriole *(white arrow)* are apparent. The marginal zone *(black arrow)* separates the nodule from the red pulp *(R)*. ×40.

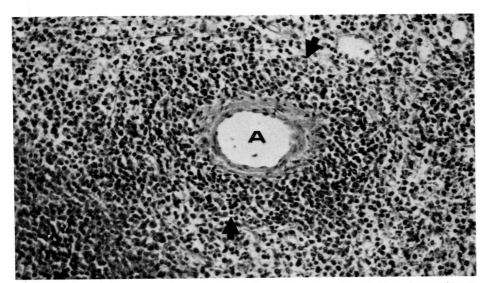

Figure 19.20. A periarteriolar sheath of lymphatic tissue. A condensation of white pulp constituents *(arrows)* surrounds an arteriole *(A)*. T lymphocytes occur within this locus. ×40.

incomplete septation results in the lobules being continuous with each other. Reticular connective tissue forms the bulk of the perivascualr stroma.

Epithelial-reticular cells assume two different configurations that are integral to the structure and function of this organ. The periphery of the organ is lined by a complete sheet of these cells (Fig. 19.26). Similarly, complete sheets of these cells en-

sheath the vessels associated with the thymus. These sheets of cells form the periphery of the labyrinths discussed previously. Epithelial-reticular cells also assume stellate configurations within the labyrinths forming a cellular reticulum (Fig. 19.26). Cellular processes of adjacent cells, both within the labyrinths as well as at their surfaces, are attached to each other by desmosomes. So, epithelial-reticular cells delimit the labyrinths as well as form a supportive *cytoreticulum*.

The organ consists of a distinct *cortex* and *medulla* (Fig. 19.25). The cortex and medulla consist of dense accumulations of small lymphocytes *(thymocytes)* that obliterate the cytoreticulum formed by the epithelial-reticular cells (Fig. 19.27). The thymocytes of the medulla are not as densely packed as the cortex; therefore, the medulla appears lighter than the cortex. The definitive feature of the organ, however, is the presence of *thymic corpuscles (Hassall's corpuscles)*, which occur in the medulla (Fig. 19.28). These acidophilic bodies vary in diameter from 20 μm to more than 100 μm. They are concentric whorls of epithelial-reticular cells in various stages of degeneration. The hyaline-appearing cells can

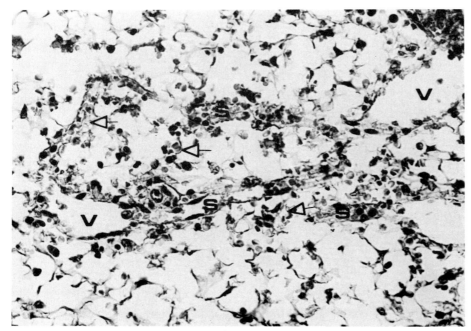

Figure 19.21. Red pulp of a canine spleen that was flushed with physiologic saline during acquisition. Most of the free cells within the red pulp have been removed. Splenic cords *(arrows)*, splenic sinusoids *(S)*, and venous sinuses *(V)* are evident. ×100.

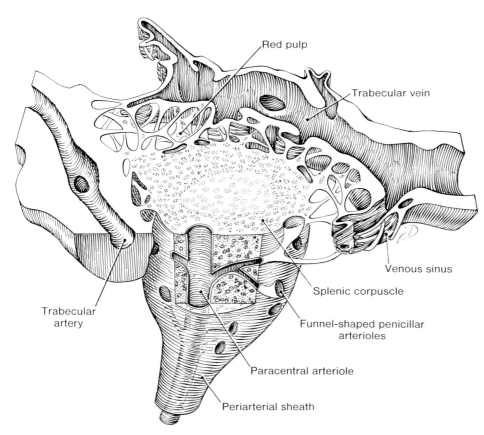

Figure 19.22. A three-dimensional drawing of a portion of the spleen.

tion. The peripherally located cells of the corpuscles are continuous with the cellular stroma. Their exact thymic function is unknown.

Blood Vessels and the Blood-Thymic Barrier. The arteries to the thymus ramify in the interlobular connective tissue and enter the substance of the organ at the corticomedullary junction of the lobules (Fig. 19.29). Arterial capillaries penetrate and traverse the cortex to the periphery of the cortical parenchyma. Although some of these vessels are confluent with thymic venules within the capsule, most of them reverse their direction, forming arcades within the cortex and drain into venules of the corticomedullary junction and medulla. The capillaries of the cortex are impermeable to macromolecules.

Arteriolar branches from the corticomedullary vessels extend into the medulla, branch into capillaries, and return as medullary veins to the corticomedullary junction. Postcapillary venules are permeable to macromolecules and lymphocytes.

The *blood-thymic barrier* consists of epithelial-reticular cellular investments of the vascular beds within the thymic parenchyma (Figs. 19.26 and 19.29). Actually, the selective permeability characteristics of the cortical region limit the applicability of the term barrier to the cortical relationships. The medullary vessels are sufficiently permeable to macromolecules and lymphocytes that the postcapillary venules of the medulla and corticomedullary junction function in a manner similar to those vessels described with lymph nodes. Accordingly, these postcapillary venules do not contribute to a blood-thymic barrier. The identical structural features of the epithelial-reticular cellular relationships throughout the gland do not match their differential barrier functions.

Lymphatic Vessels and Innervation. Afferent lymphatic vessels are not associated with the thymus. Efferent lymphatic vessels occur as components of the connective tissue peripheral to the lobules.

Although some nerve fibers may occur freely within the parenchyma of the thymus, most of the nerve fibers of the gland, which are derived from the vagus and sympahtetic nerves, are distributed to mural elements of the blood vessels.

Physiological Correlates. The thymus is the primary lymphatic organ of mammals. Lymphocytes (thymocytes), which differentiate in the thymus, leave the organ and populate secondary lymphatic organs (lymph nodes, spleen, tonsils, bone marrow, and other aggregates of lymphatic nodules scattered throughout the body) with T cells. The movement of thymocytes through postcapillary venules to secondary lymphatic organs, *peripheralization*, is a significant aspect of cell-mediated immunity.

undergo keratinization and even mineralization. High concentrations of immunoglobulin A (IgA) are present within the

corpuscles of the ox. Pyknosis and karyolysis are common. The corpuscles are often observed in advanced stages of involu-

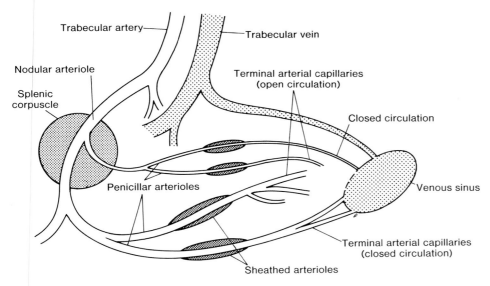

Figure 19.23. A schematic drawing of open and closed splenic circulation.

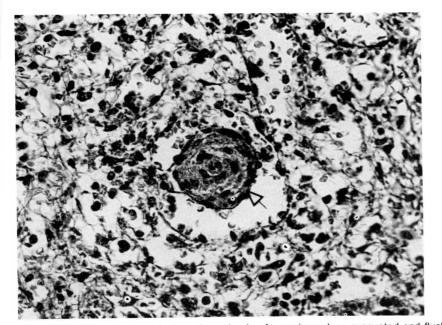

Figure 19.24. A sheathed arteriole from the red pulp of a canine spleen evacuated and flushed with physiological saline during aquisition. The sheathed arteriole *(arrow)* is surrounded by concentric whorls of reticular cells and fibers. ×100.

A gradual and continued involution of the thymus is accelerated after puberty and is characterized by a decrease in organ weight, a loss of cortical lymphocytes, infiltration by adipose cells, and an increase in thymic corpuscles. Eventually, the infiltration of adipose cells completely replaces the organ.

The significant role of the thymus in immunity is demonstrated aptly by neonatal thymectomy in some species. This causes an impaired delayed hypersensitivity. The ability to produce an antibody-mediated response is impaired also, since antibody production requires assistance from T cells.

Thymosin and *thymopoietin I* and *II* are hormones produced by the thymus that influence the development of progenitor cells into T cells.

Bursa of Fabricius

This structure is characteristic of birds (Fig. 19.30). It is a blind sac that opens on the dorsal wall of the proctodeum. It is often referred to as the "*cloacal tonsil*" or "*cloacal thymus.*" The wall of the organ is extensively folded and covered by a simple columnar or pseudostratified columnar epithelium. Lymphatic nodules are located between the folds of the epithelium. Germinal centers are present.

Immunity

Organisms of different species and individuals within a species, except for identical twins, possess a unique chemical identity. Although individuals within a species consist of similar chemical constituents, their specific macromolecular composition is different. Moreover, various mechanisms have been developed by the body to protect it from foreign materials introduced exogenously. **The essence of these mechanisms is to maintain the chemical uniqueness by excluding all foreign materials.**

Nonspecific Immunity

Protective Factors. *Nonspecific responses or mechanisms* are integral components of the organism's resistance to exogenous macromolecules and various agents of disease. The innate genetic compositon of some organisms precludes the successful invasion of a potential host by certain types of disease agents. *Similarly, specific anatomical, physiological and biochemical factors afford nonspecific protection.* The skin, mucociliary apparatus, lacrimation, urination, defecation, and pH are part of nonspecific mechanisms. Neutrophilic phagocytosis, lysosomal and β-lysin secretion, and the properdin system are part of nonspecific protection also.

Specific Immunity

General Features. The *specific immune response* is an adaptive, protective mechanism that permits the body to recognize and respond to specific foreign materials. The foreign materials that are capable of eliciting a specific immune response have a unique surface configuration *(antigenic determinant)* and are called *antigens.* Macrophages, lymphocytes, and plasma cells are responsive to antigenic stimulation. The responsiveness is manifested as *humoral antibody* or *cell-mediated immune responses.*

Humoral Antibody Response. The humoral antibody response is a function of the B lymphocytes. Macrophages and T helper cells assist with the response by secreting *helper substances (interleukins)* that are necessary for the resulting cellular transformation. Upon initial exposure to an antigen, the B lymphocyte is stimulated, becomes transformed into a blast cell, proliferates, and produces a population of sensitized B lymphocytes and plasma cells *(clonal expansion).* This population includes effector cells producing *antibodies (immunoglobulins)* and *memory cells.* Memory cells are inactive but are capable of responding to the antigen (Ag) at some future time. The initial response to an Ag, resulting in the production of antibodies (Ab), is called the *primary response.* A measurable Ab titer to the specific Ag can be determined after a variable but relatively long period of time *(latent period).* The

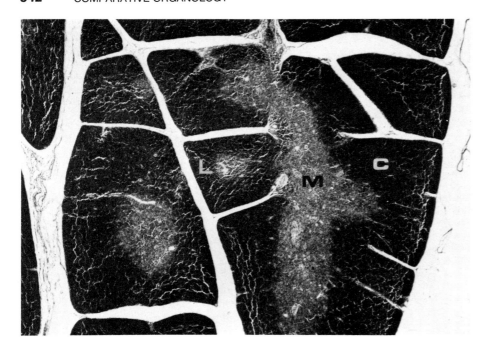

Figure 19.25. A section of a canine thymus gland. The loose connective tissue capsule covers the organ and divides it into distinct lobules *(L)*. The light-staining medulla *(M)* is surrounded by a dark-staining cortex. The thymus may be considered one large nodule; individual nodules do not occur within the organ. ×10.

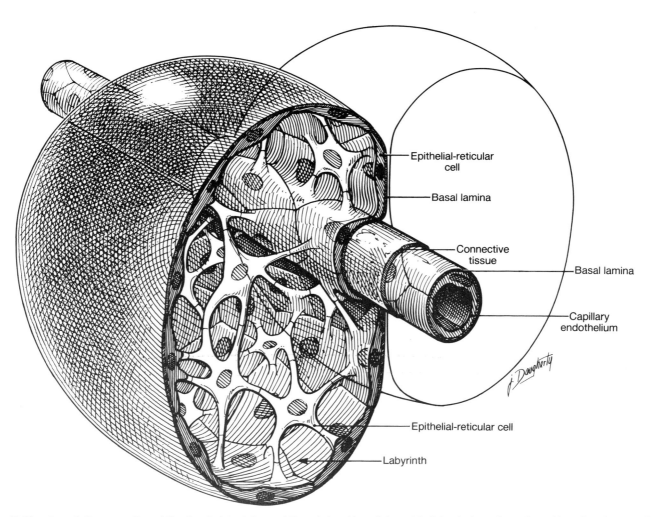

Figure 19.26. An artist's conception of the thymic labyrinths and the relationships of the epithelial-reticular cells to them. Note that the vasculature and connective tissue are separated from the labyrinthine spaces by epithelial-reticular cells. The labyrinths are filled with thymocytes.

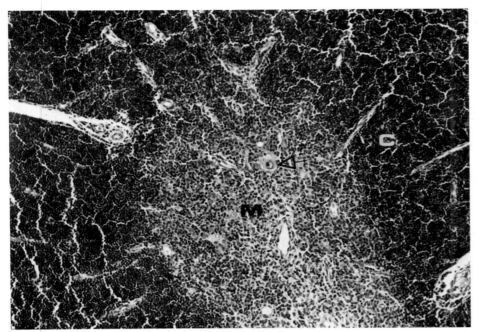

Figure 19.27. The cortex and medulla of a canine thymus gland. The cortex *(C)* contains more dense aggregations of thymocytes than does the medulla *(M)*. A characteristic thymic corpuscle *(arrow)* is present. ×40.

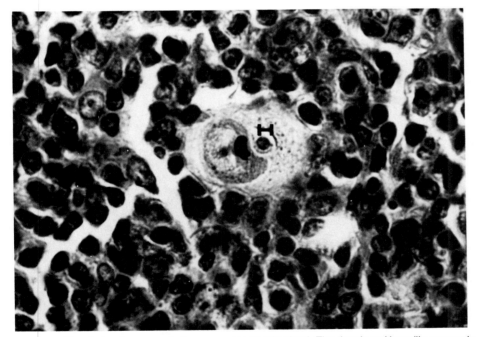

Figure 19.28. A thymic corpuscle from a canine thymic gland. The thymic or Hassall's corpuscle *(H)* is a morphological feature of the medullary portion of the gland. ×320.

subsequent exposure of the body to the same Ag can activate memory cells that were sensitized previously. This second exposure results in a more rapid and greater Ab-producing reaction than in the primary response and is termed the *secondary* or *anamnestic response.*

An *immunoglobulin* is a Y-shaped molecule whose Ag reaction sites are located at the ends of the arms of the Y (Fig. 19.31). A small chain is attached parallel to each of the arms. *Light* and *heavy chain* components result from appropriate chemical treatment. The Fc fragment is the portion of the immunoglobulin that is responsible for its various biological properties—activation of complement, binding to cells, and opsonization.

Abs bind to specific Ags and facilitate their removal from the body. This binding may:

1. Result in the precipitation of the Ab-Ag complex with subsequent phagocytosis.
2. Inhibit the uptake of certain antigens (viral) by cells.
3. Induce the lysis of microbial agents by the activation of complement.
4. Facilitate the phagocytosis of various agents by macrophages (opsonization).

Antibodies (immunoglobulins, Ig) are plasma proteins that occur in the globulin fraction. Several classes of immunoglobulins have been identified: *immunoglobulin G (IgG), immunoglobulin M (IgM), IgA, immunoglobulin E (IgE)*, and *immunoglobulin D (IgD).*

IgG comprises about 80% of all immunoglobulins. Because it is small, it leaves the vascular bed readily. This immunoglobulin is the major Ab produced in response to infections and immunizations. It is the predominant immunoglobulin of the anamnestic response. Although it is an effective *opsonin, agglutinin*, and *precipitin* of Ags, it is not an efficient activator of complement. The half-life of IgG is species variable (dog—7 to 8 days; ox—23 days).

IgM comprises about 10% of the immunoglobulins. It is a large pentameric compound whose protective functions are probably confined to the vascular system. Although IgM is the predominant Ig of the primary response, it is also produced anamnestically. The level of IgM in the secondary response does not exceed the level of the primary response. This Ab functions similarly to IgG, but IgM is an efficient activator of complement. IgM is the first antibody response in the fetus. IgM has less specificity than IgG.

IgA comprises about 10% of the immunoglobulins. It is the major immunoglobulin in external secretions wherein it affords primary antibody protection for the mucous membranes of the respiratory, gastrointestinal, and genitourinary systems and eye. This immunoglobulin may assume polymeric forms. The dimeric form of IgA passes through intestinal epithelial cells, salivary gland cells, and hepatocytes. During the passage, a *secretory* or *transport piece* of protein is added to the dimeric structure, forming *secretory IgA*. The secretory piece increases the resistance of secretory IgA to proteolysis. Secretory IgA may prevent the adherence of microbial agents to epithelial surfaces. Protection of mucosal surfaces by IgA may be broad spectrum and is not characterized by an anamnestic response.

Although IgE comprises less than 1% of the total immunoglobulins, it possesses some unique characteristics that are integral components of the Type I hypersensitivity reactions. IgD is a lymphocyte surface

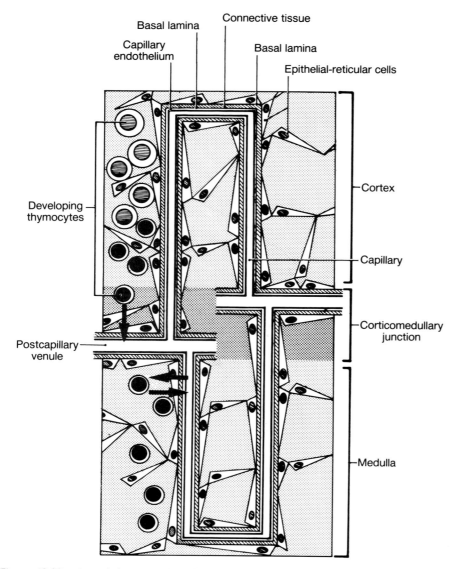

Figure 19.29. An artist's conception of the organization of the thymic-blood barrier. Epithelial-reticular cells separate the labyrinths from the blood vessels. (Compare with Fig. 19.26.) The cortical barrier is functional, whereas the medullary barrier is not. Cells move freely between the vascular spaces of the postcapillary venules and the labyrinthine spaces at the corticomedullary junction.

Ab that occurs in laboratory animals, man, and chickens. This immunoglobulin has not been demonstrated in other domestic mammals.

Cell-Mediated Immune Response. The T cells are the population of lymphocytes that are responsible for cell-mediated immunity (CMI). The T cells are programmed to recognize and respond to specific Ags also. The combination of Ag with T-cell surface receptors results in mitosis and differentiation. The interleukins secreted from macrophages and T-helper cells help to regulate the activation process. The binding of Ag to T-cell receptors initiates a blastoid transformation resulting in expansion of specific lymphocytic populations. The resulting T-cell population includes memory, effector,

and secretory cells. The activities of the effector cells are varied, but the response to Ag stimulation does not include their synthesis and secretion of humoral Abs.

Some activated or sensitized T cells become *cytotoxic lymphocytes (T-killer cells)*. Upon intimate contact with the foreign cells that activated them, T lymphocytes cause lysis of them immediately. The mechanism probably involves a T cell-induced alteration of plasma membrane permeability.

The T lymphocytes also secrete soluble, non-Ag specific, short-lived proteins called *lymphokines*. Lymphokines, among their other activities, affect the functions of B lymphocytes and macrophages.

The T cells also secrete complex protein-

aceous conglomerates called *helper substances* that are essential for an optimal T- and B-cell responsiveness. The precise mechanism for this macrophage/T cell interaction with B cells and other T cells is unknown. Helper substances may attach to macrophages so as to fix Ags to macrophage surfaces in a manner that permits recognition and response by the B cells. Alternatively, the helper substances may bind to the T or B cells in such a way as to permit their responsiveness to Ags presented by macrophages.

Whereas some T cells serve as helper cells, others serve as suppressor cells. The *T-suppressor cells* limit the T- and B-cell responsiveness. The secretion of soluble *suppressor factors* may be the influential mechanism. These factors decrease B-cell recognition of Ags, interfere with T-helper cell interactions with B cells, or limit the responsiveness of B cells to Ag stimulation. Suppressor T cells may be involved in the *tolerance phenomenon*, the inability to respond to Ag stimulation. Tolerance to self-antigens is an essential T-suppressor cell function.

Cellular Interactions in Immunity. The myelolymphoid organs and the macrophage system are essential components of normal immune responsiveness. Lymphocytes and macrophages cooperate in clearing foreign materials.

The precise mechanisms of cellular cooperation in the production of humoral antibodies has not been determined; various theories have been proposed to explain B-cell, T-cell and macrophage interactions in this process. Macrophages play a central role in the immune response. They trap and process Ags and facilitate T- and B-cell interaction. Whereas Ag trapping and processing is probably a nonspecific recognition activity of macrophages and dendritic cells, the subsequent cellular interactions lead to a specific Ab response.

The strategic positioning of macrophages and dendritic cells throughout the body and their positioning within lymph nodes ensures that these cells are exposed to foreign materials. Ag processing and cellular interactions may occur in peripherally positioned diffuse and nodular lymphatic tissues. Macrophage-processed and/or free Ags reach the lymph nodes by the vascular and/or lymphatic channels that enter these organs. The architecture of the lymph nodes (as well as other lymphoid organs) ensures that Ags trapped by macrophages and dendritic cells will contact the cells responsible for specific immune responses.

Although the neutrophil performs phagocytic functions that protect the organism, these cells are not involved in Ag processing. **Their entry into tissue spaces and their subsequent phagocytic activity culminates in their death and lysis within the tissue spaces.**

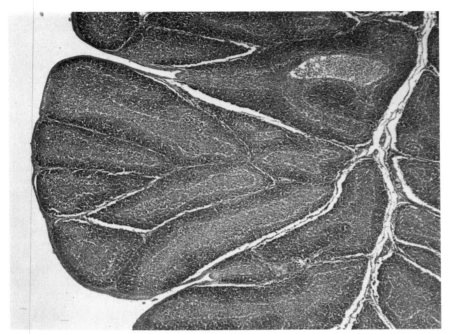

Figure 19.30. A section of the avian bursa of Fabricius. Lymphatic nodules are aggregated in such a way as to impart architectural characteristics that appear similar to the thymus. ×10.

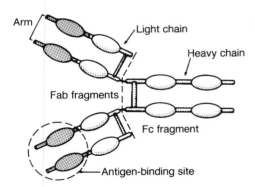

Figure 19.31. A diagram of a typical immunoglobulin. A light chain is attached to each arm. A heavy chain includes an arm and one-half of the tailpiece. Two Fab fragments and an Fc fragment result from hydrolysis along the dashed line (hinge region). The Fab fragments contain the Ag-binding sites. The Fc fragment is responsible for the biological properties of the molecule.

Hypersensitivity Reactions

Type I Hypersensitivity

The *Type I hypersensitivities (allergies, anaphylaxis)* may be generalized or localized reactions of mast cells and basophils to certain Ags mediated by IgE. Because of its cellular binding activity, it is called a *cytotrophic antibody*. The interaction of Ag, IgE, and the reactive cells involves the release of pharmacologically active substances, the most significant of which is *histamine*. Although the Type I reaction serves protective functions through its induction of an acute inflammatory response

and the elimination of Ag substances, it has deleterious side effects that can be life-threatening.

Although certain Ags may induce IgE production, not all individuals can produce this immunoglobulin. The production of IgE in response to Ag stimulation *(atopy)* is determined genetically.

Upon initial exposure to the exciting Ag, the B cell population reacts by secreting IgE. Mast cells and basophils, which have specific receptors for the Fc portions of this immunoglobulin, bind IgE. After re-exposure to the same Ag, the Ag binds with the Ag-binding fragments of IgE. This Ab-Ag reaction causes degranulation and/or lysis of these cells with the subsequent release of various active substances.

The substances released include: histamine, serotonin, eosinophilic chemotactic factors of anaphylaxis (ECF-A), platelet-activating factor (PAF), prostaglandins, leukotrienes (LT), bradykinin.

Histamine, the most important of these substances, is an amine that results from the decarboxylation of histidine. Many of the stereotypical tissue responses relate directly to the activity of this compound. The primary effects of histamine are directed to smooth muscle and glands. Most blood vessels dilate and increase their permeability in response to stimulation by histamine. Increased permeability is responsible for the characteristic wheal and flare of this reaction. The vascular smooth muscle of some organs, however, contracts in response to histamine. The nonvascular smooth muscle constituents of the lungs,

stomach, intestines, uterus, and urinary bladder contract in response to histamine stimulation. Excessive pulmonary mucous secretion, salivation, and lacrimation are typical exocrine responses to histamine release.

Histamine exerts its influence upon target cells through *histamine receptors* located on surface membranes. Based upon the activities of histamine antagonists—those drugs that compete with or block histamine from binding to these receptors—two types of receptors have been identified—H_1 and H_2 receptors. Membrane permeability alterations to calcium and/or release of calcium from intracellular, sequestered stores results from stimulation of these receptors. The cause and effect relationship of histamine stimulation and increased cyclic adenosine monophosphate (cAMP) needs clarification.

Serotonin is a metabolite of tryptophan. Mast cells of laboratory rodents and large ruminants contain this substance. The effects manifested by serotonin are directed to cardiac and smooth muscle fibers. Vasoconstriction and increased cardiac activity are typical effects. Increased vascular permeability in response to serotonin occurs in laboratory rodents.

ECF-As are small polypeptides that are released from mast cells upon stimulation. They attract eosinophils to sites of mast cell stimulation and degranulation. They are also responsible for the withdrawl of eosinophils from the reactive region.

PAF is a phospholipid that induces aggregation of platelets and causes them to release their contents. This promotes serotonin release and prostaglandin synthesis.

A family of compounds called *eicosanoids* is derived from a 20-carbon compound with double bonds. This parent compound is arachidonic acid. The family includes: prostaglandins, thromboxanes, prostacyclin, and leukotrienes (Chapter 24).

Five types of LTs have been identified and designated LTA, LTB, LTC, LTD, and LTE. Smooth muscle contraction and increased vascular permeability occur as a result of LTC_4 and LTD_4 activity, the compounds that heretofore had been described as the *slow-reacting substances of anaphylaxis*. The LTs are responsible for a slow onset but sustained smooth muscular contraction. LTB is a neutrophilic and eosinophilic chemotactic factor. *Prostaglandin $F_{2\alpha}$* promotes vascular and nonvascular smooth muscle contraction. Other prostaglandins *(PGE)* and *prostacyclin (PGI$_2$)* inhibit vascular and nonvascular smooth muscle contraction. The effects manifested by prostaglandins and prostacyclins locally are dependent upon the types and quantities of substances released from specific tissues. *Thromboxanes* function in a manner similar to $PGF_{2\alpha}$.

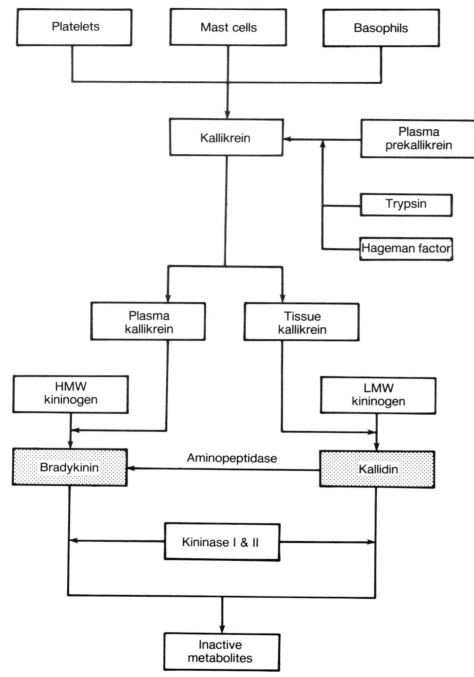

Figure 19.32. A diagram depicting the kallikrein-kinin system. This system is a contributory component of the Type I hypersensitivity reaction.

Kinins are vasodilator peptides that are activated from *kininogens* by the enzymatic action of *kallikreins (kininogenases)*. Kinins also increase vascular permeability. Tissue kallikreins are derived from activated platelets; they may also be activated from the plasma (Fig. 19.32). Plasma kallikreins are produced by the liver. Kallikreins are *serine proteases*—enzymes with serine at their active site.

Two types of kininogens occur in the plasma. A *low-molecular-weight kininogen (LMW kininogen)* diffuses into the connec-tive tissue space and becomes the substrate for tissue kallikrein. A *high-molecular-weight kininogen (HMW kininogen)* re-mains in the plasma and is the essential substrate for plasma kallikrein. The *kalli-krein-kinin system* is an active part of va-soregulatory mechanisms and a contribu-tory component of Type I hypersensitivity.

Eosinophils are integral components and modulators of type I hypersensitivity reac-tions. They release enzymes (histaminase, arylsulfatase, phospholipase D) that neu-tralize the active substances secreted by mast cells. *Histaminase* degrades hista-mine, whereas *arylsulfatase* inactivates the LTs. Additionally, *phospholipase D* deac-tivates platelet activating factor. Moreover, eosinophils secrete *PGE*, which are inhibi-tors of histamine secretion and stimulators of vasodilation.

Additional regulation of this process is directed toward the neuroregulation of the mast cell. Neuroregulation of mast cell de-granulation is achieved through their com-plement of α- and β-adrenergic receptors. Alpha stimulation enhances degranulation, whereas β-adrenergic stimulation depresses mast cell degranulation. Both effects are mediated through cAMP.

The clinical manifestations of Type I hypersensitivities vary. Cutaneous reactiv-ity is manifested by swelling and erythema (wheal and flare) associated with insect bites. Generalized atopic reactivity *(ana-phylactic shock)* may be manifested as car-diopulmonary distress and/or gastrointes-tinal upset. The type of response is species-specific, since various organs *(shock organs)* of domestic species and man have a differ-ential responsiveness to the biological activ-ity of the active substances. Numerous Ags *(allergens)* are capable of inducing localized and/or generalized Type I reactions.

Type II Hypersensitivity

General Mechanisms. *Type II hypersen-sitivity* is also called *cytotoxic* or *cytolytic reactivity*. These types of reactions involve immunoglobulins (IgG, IgM), comple-ment, neutrophils, macrophages, and tissue Ags.

Cytotoxic reactions are characterized by the reaction of circulating Abs (IgG, IgM) with Ags that are attached to cell surfaces or Ags that have become intimate compo-nents of cell surfaces. The binding of im-munoglobulins with these Ags activates the complement system. The subsequent bind-ing of complement at the site of Ag-Ab reaction results in the lysis of the surface-modified cell. Alternatively, the Ag-Ab re-action at the cell surface permits the adher-ence of phagocytic cells (neutrophils and macrophages) to the cell surface. Cell lysis and phagocytosis result. These processes are enhanced when complement is bound to the Ag-Ab complex. Additionally, the release of hydrolases by the phagocytic cells causes surrounding tissue damage.

Reactions to incompatible transfusions, neonatal isoerythrolysis, RH factor incom-patabilities in man (erythroblastosis fetalis), autoimmune hemolytic anemia, immune thrombocytopenia and certain other im-mune-mediated disease processes are char-acterized by Type II hypersensitivity reac-tions.

Type III Hypersensitivity

The *type III hypersensitivity* response is also called the *toxic complex reaction*. Ags result in the formation of immune complexes that activate the complement system. The initiation of the complement cascade results in the release of factors that cause platelet aggregation, mast cell degranulation, and the accumulation of neutrophils. Extensive tissue damage, inflammation, and necrosis result.

Type III reactions are characterized by two responses to Ags. The *Arthus reaction* is the result of the localized accumulation of immune complexes. The generalized circulation of immune complexes initiates the second type III response, *serum sickness.* Type III reactions may be manifested when excessive amounts of Ag-Ab complexes are formed.

The Arthus reaction may be initiated when an Ag to which the organism is able to respond is introduced into the subcutis, as might occur after a vaccination booster injection. The Ag within the connective tissue reacts with IgG. Some controversy exists relating to the function of IgE in this reaction. The immune complexes of IgE and Ag may cause the release of vasoactive amines from mast cells. The resultant increase in vascular permeability may permit the leakage of IgG from the vascular bed and may facilitate the formation of Ag and IgG immune complexes. Importantly, the immune complex involving IgG fixes complement. Various products of the complement cascade, C3a, C5a, C3b, and C567, initiate helpful and damaging sequelae. The release of C567 attracts neutrophils to the local area, whereas the release of C3b facilitates the adherence of neutrophils to the immune complexes. The opsonizing influence of C3b results in phagocytosis and clearance of the immune complexes. *Anaphylatoxins* (C3a, C5a) cause mast cell degranulation and the release of vasoactive substances. The release of hydrolases (collagenases, elastases, proteases) by the neutrophils causes the localized damage that characterizes the Arthus reaction. Vascular wall damage exacerbates the localized response by attracting more neutrophils that release more hydrolases. Damaged endothelial cells also release kallikreins and aid in the generation of kinins. The resultant hemorrhage leads to clot formation and necrosis of the tissues that have been deprived of their vascular supply *(ischemic necrosis).* The complement cascade induction of platelet aggregation also exacerbates the tissue necrosis. The severe localized inflammatory response of the Arthus reaction may be observed in dogs either infected or vaccinated with live adenovirus type I (infectious canine hepatitis virus) and is manifested as "blue eye." Hypersensitivity pneumonitis is a Type III response to actinomycetes spores. Staphylococcal hypersensitivity dermitis is also an example of a Type III reaction. Arthus reactions, however, can occur in any localized focus of Ag-Ab accumulation.

Serum sickness involves similar initiating mechanisms as those described for the Arthus reaction. A portion of the complexes that are insoluble are cleared by macrophages. The soluble complexes circulate throughout the vascular system and eventually deposit themselves on vascular endothelial cells. Their deposition initiates those events attributable to various complement factors described for the Arthus reaction. Severe damage to the kidney (glomerulonephritis) can result when these complexes are deposited within the glomerus. Although the precise mechanism of kidney damage is not understood, it occurs without the involvement of neutrophils. Mesangial, endothelial, and epithelial cell proliferation, as well as basement membrane alterations cause excessive protein loss in the urine. Arteritis and arthritis are also sequelae of serum sickness.

Type IV Hypersensitivity

Type IV hypersensitivity is also called *delayed hypersensitivity* and *CMI.* The delayed hypersensitivity reaction does not require immunoglobulins and occurs initially over a period of 8–12 days. Cytotoxic lymphocytes, lymphokines, and macrophages are contributing components. The infiltration of mononuclear cells into regions of antigen concentration is the characteristic histological feature. The rejection of foreign skin grafts, the response to intradermal injections of tuberculin, the skin reactivity to certain contact agents, and the response to certain arthropods are examples of Type IV hypersensitivity reactions.

Autoimmunity

The essence of immune mechanisms is the ability to recognize those substances that are "self" and those that are foreign. The inability to recognize self results in the formation of autoantibodies and the destruction of somatic tissues. Various mechanisms are proposed to explain this self-destructive phenomenon. Autoantibodies may be produced against body components that normally are not "seen" by the lymphocytes following damage that results in exposure to the surveillence cells. New Ags may be developed within the body as a result of viral influence and/or the incorporation of foreign materials with normal body components. These and other mechanisms may be responsible for activation of the immune processes against "self." Autoimmunity is manifested as Type I-IV hypersensitivity reactions. Systemic lupus erythematosis, autoimmune thyroiditis, myasthenia gravis, and rheumatoid arthritis are examples of autoimmune or *immune-mediated diseases.*

References

Adams, D.O.: The granulomatous inflammatory response: A review. Am. J. Pathol. *84:*164, 1976.

Breaven, M. A.: Histamine. N. Engl. J. Med. *294:*30, 1976.

Burnet, F. M.: The thymus gland. Sci. Amer. *207:*50., 1962.

Clark, S.L., Jr.: The reticulum of lymph nodes in mice studied with the electron microscope. Amer. J. Anat. *110:*217, 1962.

Cohn, Z.A.: The structure and function of monocytes and macrophages. Adv. Immunol. *9:*163, 1968.

Edwards, V.D. and Simon, G.T.: Ultrastructural aspects of red cell destruction in the normal rat spleen. J. Ultrastruct. Res. *33:*187, 1970.

Fujisaki, S.: The fine structure of Hassall's corpuscles and reticular cells in the mouse thymus. Acta Med. Biol. *14:*107, 1966.

Hayes, T.G.: The marginal zone and marginal sinus in the spleen of the gerbil. A light and electron microscopic study. J. Morphol. *141:*205, 1973.

Hoshino, T., Takeda, M., Abe, K. and Ito, T.: Early development of thymic lymphocytes in mice studied by light and electron microscopy. Anat. Rec. *164:*47, 1969.

Jaroslow, B.N.: Genesis of Hassall's corpuscles. Nature. *215:*408, 1967.

Kay, A.B.: The role of the eosinophil. J. Allergy Clin. Immunol. *64:*90, 1979.

Levin, P.M.: The development of the tonsil of the domestic pig. Anat. Rec. *45:*189, 1930.

Metz, S.A.: Anti-inflammatory agents as inhibitors of prostaglandin synthesis in man. Med. Clin. N. A. *65:*713, 1981.

Meyer, A.: Hemal nodes in bovines and goats. Amer. J. Anat. *21:*359, 1917.

Moe, R.E.: Electron microscopic appearance of the parenchyma of lymph nodes. Amer. J. Anat. *114:*341, 1964.

Movat, H.Z.: and Fernando, N.V.P.: The fine structure of the lymphoid tissue during antibody formation. Exp. Molec. Pathol. *4:*155, 1965.

Murray, R.G., Murray, A. and Pizzo, A.: The fine structure of thymocytes of young rats. Anat. Rec. *151:*17, 1965.

Payne, F. and Breneman, W.R.: Lymphoid areas in endocrine glands in the fowl. Poult. Sci. *31:*155, 1952.

Peck, H.M. and Hoerr, N.L.: The intermediary circulation in the red pulp of the mouse spleen. Anat. Rec. *109:*447, 1951.

Raviola, E. and Karnovsky, M.J.: Evidence for a blood-thymus barrier using electron-opaque tracers. J. Exp. Med. *136:*466, 1972.

Regoli, D. and Barabe, J.: Pharmacology of bradykinin and related kinins. Pharmacol. Rev. *32:*81, 1980.

Renston, R.H., Jones, A.L., Christiansen, W.D., Hradek, G.T. and Underdown, B.J.: Evidence for a vesicular transport mechanism in hepatocytes for biliary secretions of immunoglobulin A. Science. *298:*1276, 1980.

Roberts, D.K. and Latta, J.S.: Electron microscopic studies on the red pulp of the mouse spleen. Anat. Rec. *148:*81, 1964.

Samuelsson, B. and Hammarstrom, S.: Nomenclature of the leukotrienes. Prostaglandins *19:*645, 1980.

Schachter, M.: Kallikreins (kininogenases): A group of serine proteases with bioregulatory actions. Pharmacol. Rev. *31:*1, 1980.

Song, S.H. and Groom, A.C.: A scanning electron microscope study of the splenic red pulp in relation to the sequestration of immature red cells. J. Morphol. *149:*437, 1974.

Tehver, J. and Grahame, I.: Capsule and trabeculae of spleens of domestic animals. J. Anat. *65:*473, 1931.

Theofilopoulos, A.N. and Dixon, F.J.: The biology and detection of immune complexes. Adv. Immunol. *28:*89, 1979.

Tizard, I.R.: *An Introduction to Veterinary Immunology.* 2nd edition. W.B. Saunders, Philadelphia, 1982.

Unanue, E.R.: The regulatory role of macrophages in antigenic stimulation. Adv. Immunol. *15:*95, 1972.

Weiss, L.: *The Cells and Tissues of the Immune System: Structure, Functions, Interactions.* Prentice-Hall, Englewood Cliffs, 1972.

Yamori, T. and Mori, Y.: Electron microscopic observation of reticuloendothelial system. Tohoku J. Exp.Med. *81:*330, 1964.

20: Integumentary System

General Characteristics

Form and Function. The integumentary system consists of the basic tissues discussed previously. The outermost layer of the skin, *epidermis*, is stratified squamous epithelium (Figs. 20.1, and 5.8–5.12). The epidermis is divisible into distinct layers; the number of layers varies with different regions of the body (Plate I.1). The *dermis* or *corium* underlies the epidermis and varies from loose connective tissue to dense white fibrous connective tissue (DWFCT) (Fig. 20.2). The *hypodermis* or *subcutis* consists of loose connective tissue that connects the dermis to underlying periosteum, perichondrium, or deep fascia. The nature of the hypodermis (superficial fascia) varies with the location of the body. Some regions contain high quantities of adipose cells (footpads), whereas others have few adipose cells (scrotum, eyelids, ears). The dermis and hypodermis contain numerous blood vessels, nerves, and lymphatic vessels.

Many structures are derivatives of the skin: hair, nails, claws, feathers, horns, antlers, combs, wattles, sweat glands, sebaceous glands, mammary glands, and hooves. The skin and its diversified structures perform numerous and varied functions.

The skin is an effective two-way *barrier* between the internal and external environment. The skin prevents water loss *(desiccation)* and the movement of electrolytes and macromolecules into the external environment. Also, it minimizes the ingress of physical, chemical, and microbial agents. The secretory products of tubular glands (in some animals), the hair coat, and cutaneous blood supply are mediators of *temperature regulation*.

The cutaneous vascular supply also contributes to alterations in *blood pressure*. The skin glands contribute to the diverse *secretory functions* of this organ (sebum, sweat). Milk is a secretory product of the mammary gland, a discrete organ of this system. In some species, the skin glands contribute an *excretory function*. The skin is involved in *calcium homeostasis* by virture of the ultraviolet light conversion of 7-dehydrocholecalciferol to cholecalciferol within the sebaceous glands; however, the ultraviolet component of solar radiation is capable of damaging living tissues. The pigmentation of the skin *protects against ultraviolet radiational (actinic) damage*. The elasticity and strength of the skin provide for *motion* and *external form*; highly cornified structures provide for *locomotion*. *General behavioral patterns, sexual behavioral displays*, and *mechanical protection* are afforded by this system, also. The skin is an extensive *sensory organ*. General somatic afferent modalities, including pain, pressure and temperature, as well as special somatic afferent information from the eyes and ears, function to integrate the organism within its surrounding external environment.

Clinically, the skin is an important organ. Besides being the largest organ of the body, it may reflect a variety of external and internal disease processes (ectoparasitism, immune-mediated disease, endoparasitism, endocrine disorders, nutritional problems).

Mammalian Integument

Typical Skin

Development. The epidermis develops from ectoderm, whereas the dermis and hypodermis are derivatives of the mesoderm. Initially, the epidermis is composed of a layer of simple cuboidal epithelial cells.

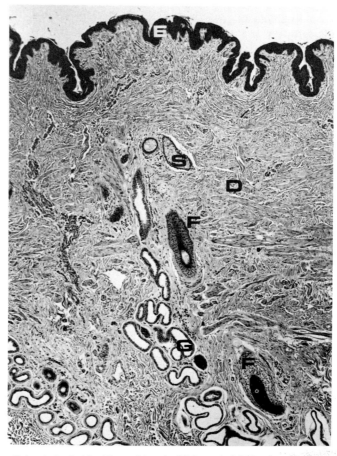

Figure 20.1. Ovine haired skin. The epidermis *(E)* is underlaid by an extensive dermis *(D)* that contains hair follicles *(F)*, sebaceous glands *(S)* and tubular glands *(G)*. ×10.

348

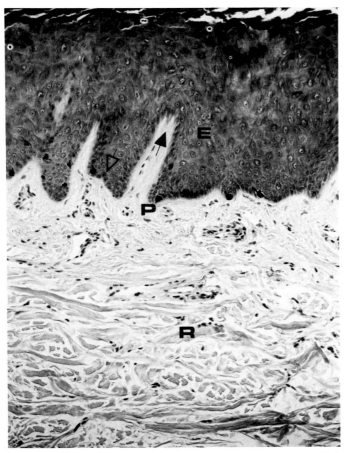

Figure 20.2. Papillary and reticular zones of the dermis. The papillary zone *(P)* is immediately adjacent to the epidermis *(E)* and is continuous with the reticular zone *(R)*. Dermal papillae *(solid arrow)* and epidermal pegs *(open arrow)* are well developed. ×40.

Cellular proliferation results in the stratification of cells that typifies the epidermis. Basal cell layer proliferation adds progressively to the thickness of this outer covering. Additionally, basal cell proliferation and invagination into the underlying dermis and hypodermis account for the formation of hairs, feathers, and glands, the cells of which are continuous with the cellular layers of the epidermis.

The dermis and hypodermis develop from typical mesenchyme. Progressive proliferation and differentiation of mesenchymal cells result in the establishment of resident cellular populations that typify loose and dense connective tissues.

Organization of the Skin

Epidermis. The *epidermis* is composed of distinct layers that comprise the outer layer of the body (Figs. 20.1 and 5.8). The relative amounts of these layers vary from region to region. The most basal layer is termed the *stratum basale* (Fig. 5.9). The cells of this zone vary from cuboidal to columnar. A *stratum spinosum* or *para-*

basal layer is located peripheral to the basal layer (Fig. 5.10). The stratum spinosum varies in thickness and is characterized by *apparent* intercellular bridges. The cells gradually change from polyhedral to squamous. Pigment, when present, extends into this zone as far as the transition into the next region of the epidermis. The stratum spinosum varies in thickness, being thick in hairless regions and thin in heavily haired regions.

The *stratum granulosum* consists of flattened rhomboidal or squamous cells that possess *keratohyalin granules* (Fig. 5.11). These basophilic and histidine-rich granules contained within membranes form the interfibrillar substance of soft keratin. These granules are not consistent features of all keratinized regions; they are present at sites in which soft keratin is formed. The term *intermediate layer* is applicable to this zone.

The *stratum lucidum* consists of several layers of homogeneous, translucent, squamous cells that are only slightly stainable. Keratohyalin granules are no longer visible, but a substance called eleiden is present.

This zone is especially prominent and limited to very thick epidermal regions of the body, such as the footpads of carnivores, epidermis of the nose (planum nasale, planum nasolabiale, planum rostrale), perioplic epidermis, and teat.

The superficial *stratum corneum* consists of several to many layers of anucleated, squamous, cornified (keratinized) cells (Fig. 5.12). A fibrous protein, keratin, is abundant. In noncornified regions, the term *superficial layer* is used. Dead cells are sloughed from the peripheral portion of this zone.

The surface covering of the integument, *keratin*, is the transformation product of basal cell differentiation. Once differentiation of these cells occurs, their progeny are considered classic examples of fixed postmitotic cells. This process needs a copious supply of stem cells.

Cells undergoing keratinization become enucleated, flattened cells filled with a secretory product—keratin. Keratin is actually a mixture of low sulfur content proteins (microfibrils) that are embedded within an amorphous matrix rich in high sulfur content protein. Autophagocytosis increases with the accumulation of keratin, resulting in the digestion of all cellular organelles. The cell membranes of contiguous cells are still connected by desmosomes, despite the intracellular alterations.

Soft keratin characterizes the majority of the epidermis and those cutaneous mucous membranes that are keratinized. *Hard keratin* is typical of the skin appendages—feathers, parts of hair, hooves and others. Keratohyalin granules are evident during the formation of soft keratin. Desquamation of *keratinocytes* is a continual feature of the process. *Hard keratin* has high quantities of cystine and numerous disulfide bonds. This induces great strength and stability to the substance. Keratohyalin granules are not apparent during the formation of hard keratin. Also, desquamation is not a feature of the process.

Dermis. The *dermis* or *corium* is separated from the epidermis by a typical basement membrane. Two zones are described in the dermis, a *papillary* and a *reticular* zone (Fig. 20.2). They are, however, similar and blend insensibly with each other. The papillary (superficial) zone conforms generally to the contours of the stratum basale. The thickness of the areolar connective tissue of the papillary region varies with the species. The papillary zone generally contains those epidermal structures that invaginate into the dermis from the epidermis. The deep (reticular) zone is DWFCT. The name of this zone refers to the arrangement of collagenous fibers into a network or reticulum.

Dermal papillae are finger-like projections that extend into the epidermis from the dermis (Fig. 20.2). Corresponding *epi-*

dermal pegs are also evident as complementary configurations associated with dermal papillae. Confluent epidermal pegs form epidermal ridges. This is the means by which the epidermis and dermis become highly interdigitated. The dermal papillae increase surface contact with the epidermis. This type of junctional interface is typical in regions subjected to mechanical loading—footpads of carnivores and equine hooves. Heavily haired skin is usually not papillated. Dermal papillae also contain numerous vessels and various special receptor terminals of neurons. Lymphatic tissue, glands, and smooth muscle also occur in the dermis.

The skin (epidermis and dermis) resides upon a *hypodermis* or subcutaneous layer of areolar connective tissue. The hypodermis attaches the skin to deep structures and permits integumentary motility over these structures. When the hypodermis is infiltrated by numerous adipose cells, the layer is called the *panniculus adiposus*. The hypodermis blends into the underlying dense connective tissue of the deep fascia, periosteum, or perichondrium. Infiltration of adipose tissue is typical in the digital pads of carnivores and the digital cushion of the equine foot. They function in mechanical cushioning. Alternating compression and decompression of the equine digital cushion is essential for venous return from the foot.

Vascular, Neural, and Lymphatic Components. The blood supply to typical haired skin is extensive and is organized into three vascular plexuses: *superficial* or *subpapillary plexus, middle* or *cutaneous plexus,* and *deep* or *subcutaneous plexus. Simple cutaneous arteries* emerge from the fascial planes between muscle masses to supply the deep plexus primarily. *Mixed cutaneous arteries* supply the muscle mass and eventually terminate in the deep plexus secondarily. Branches from the subcutaneous plexus form the cutaneous plexus. The cutaneous plexus is associated intimately with those structures that have invaginated into the dermis (hairs, glands). Branches from the cutaneous plexus form the subpapillary plexus. The veins of these plexuses are satellites of the arteries.

Regional and interspecific variations from this pattern exist. Haired skin is devoid generally of extensive capillary loops into dermal papillae, whereas glabrous skin has extensive capillary loops into the papillary zone.

The nerves to the skin are a mixture of motor and sensory nerve fibers. General visceral efferent fibers of the sympathetic nervous system innervate the smooth muscle of the walls of blood vessels, the arrector pili muscles and the myoepithelial cells associated with tubular glands. The majority of the nerves to the epidermis and dermis are general somatic afferent fibers. **The skin is a vast and important sensory organ.** Various sensory modalities (touch, pain, temperature, itch) are received by afferent neuronal terminals. Sensory nerve endings occur in the hypodermis, dermis, and epidermis.

Branches of cutaneous nerves innervate the hair follicles and form a *hair follicle network.* Sensory nerve endings wrap around the hair follicles and form a significant tactile receptor in mammalian haired skin. This relationship is especially well-developed in sinus or tactile hairs. The sensory nerves of the dermis, *dermal network,* is more extensive in glabrous skin than haired skin.

Blind-ended lymphatic capillaries located within dermal papillae continue into a network of lymphatic vessels in the papillary region.

Specialized Skin Regions

The mammalian integument is not uniform throughout its distribution. Some portions of the skin are haired, whereas others are glabrous. A thick epidermis may characterize some portions of the body; a thin epidermis, others. Similarly, the dermis may assume various thicknesses throughout its distribution. The dermis is the thickest part of the skin. Regional skin variations relating to amount and type of pelage, distribution and type of glands, and skin thickness are functional adaptations that ideally suit the organism to its external environment.

Digital pads. The *footpads* or *digital pads* of carnivores are highly cornified, thickened, highly pigmented, and hairless portions of the skin. The digital pads resist abrasion and are effective shock absorbers. The epidermis of the digital pads, which is the thickest epidermis of the carnivore skin, consists of all layers described previously, including a stratum lucidum. The stratum corneum is a predominant feature; the surface is smooth in the cat and papillated in the dog. Prominent dermal papillae interdigitate with epidermal pegs. The hypodermis consists of adipose tissue and proper connective tissue, the *digital cushion.* Coiled, tubular sweat glands (merocrine glands) are present in the dermis and hypodermis.

Scrotum. The skin of the scrotum is usually the thinnest skin of the body. The stratum corneum is not well-developed and the dermis is not extensive. Apocrine tubular and sebaceous glands are present, but species variations exist. Hair follicles are not abundant and the hairs that are present are short and fine. Smooth muscle fibers of the tunica dartos are interspersed with collagenous and elastic fibers within the dermis. The *tunica dartos* is responsible for the relative position of the testes to the body wall. This is an effective mechanism for regulating scrotal temperature; sperm production is a temperature-dependent phenomenon.

Nose. Integumentary modifications characterize the external nose of varied domestic species. The *planum nasale* of carnivores is composed of a thickened and highly cornified epidermis devoid of sebaceous and tubular glands. The *planum nasolabiale* of the ox and the *planum nasale* of small ruminants (sheep and goat) are devoid of hairs but contain tubular merocrine glands that moisten the surface. The epidermis is thickened and highly cornified. The highly cornified *planum rostrale* of the pig contains many tubular merocrine glands and is covered sparsely by fine hairs. Fine hairs and sebaceous glands are characteristic of the thin skin around the nostrils of the horse.

External Auditory Meatus. The *external auditory meatus* or *external ear canal* connects the external auditory opening with the tympanic membrane. The canal is lined by skin. Small hair follicles, sebaceous glands and modified, apocrine, tubular glands are present. The modified, apocrine, tubular glands are the *ceruminous glands* of the external auditory meatus. The dermis of this canal blends with the perichondrium and periosteum of the supportive cartilage and bone. The external auditory meatus is moistened by the ceruminous secretions. Despite being moistened, this structure is **not** a mucous membrane. **The external auditory meatus is lined by skin.** This structure is subject to many of the typical disease problems associated with the integument. *Otitis externa* is a common problem of companion animals, especially those with droopy ears.

Mucocutaneous Junctions. *Mucocutaneous junctions* are points of transition between typical skin and *cutaneous mucous membranes.* Mucocutaneous junctions occur at all body orifices.

Hairs

Development. Hair follicles form as invaginations of the presumptive epidermis into the underlying dermis. The onset of development is marked by an epidermal thickening that becomes a prominent cellular cord. The solid cord of invaginating epidermis undergoes canalization forming a space for the future hair. The remaining, invaginated epidermis is continuous with the *external root sheath.* This sheath becomes continuous as the *germinal matrix* at the base of the developing follicle. The germinal matrix forms the hair and internal root sheath. Although the epidermal ingrowth is described as invagination into the dermis, a basal lamina separates epidermal and dermal structures.

Follicular Organization. These modified structures occur variably within the system and serve various functions: *insulation, protection,* and *sensory reception* (Plate I.2).

The drawing in Figure 20.3 is a typical hair in the anagen stage of its growth cycle.

A connective tissue sheath from the dermis is oriented circumferentially around the *hair follicle* (Fig. 20.4). A basement membrane *(glassy membrane)* separates the connective tissue from follicular epithelium. The *external root sheath* continues with the *stratum basale, stratum spinosum,* and *stratum granulosum* (Fig. 20.5). An *internal root sheath* is subdivided into three regions: peripheral *Henle's layer,* intermediate *Huxleys' layer* and inner *cuticle of the root sheath* (Fig. 20.8). *Henle's layer* consists of a single layer of flattened cells. *Huxley's layer* consists of several layers of cells that contain *trichohyalin* granules, keratohyalin granules of hair. Henle's, Huxley's, and the cuticular layers of the internal root sheath are not continuous with the surface. These layers do not extend beyond the opening of sebaceous glands into the follicle. The *cuticle of the root sheath* is a single layer of cornified cells that abuts the cuticle of the hair. These cells interdigitate with the cornified cells of the cuticle of the hair.

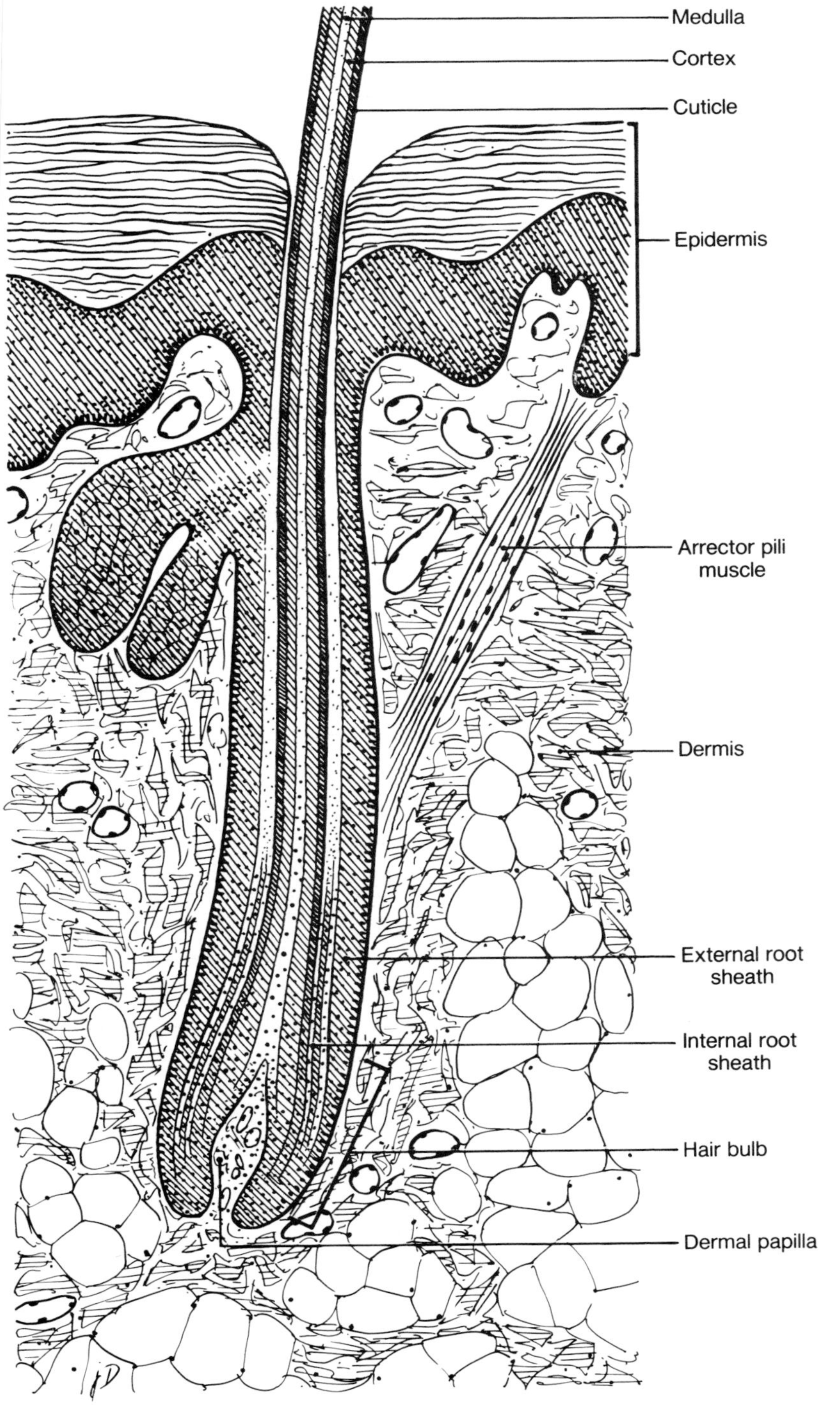

The hair consists of three regions: a *cuticle,* a *cortex,* and a *medulla* (Figs. 20.5 and 20.6). The *cuticle* is a single layer of enucleated, cornified cells that interdigitate with the cuticle of the root sheath. The *cortex* forms the bulk of the hair shaft. It consists of several layers of flattened, cornified cells that contain hard keratin. Pigment may be present and numerous air spaces characterize the intercellular spaces. The *medulla* may be absent in some hairs. When present, it consists of cornified, cuboidal cells that are separated by air spaces (Fig. 20.6). The cuticular, cortical, and medullary characteristics are so specific that identification to species is possible with careful examination.

The hair follicle terminates in a cone-shaped epidermal peg *(hair bulb)* that defines the limits of the *dermal papilla* (Fig. 20.7). While dermal papillae may provide some vascularization, most nutrients are supplied by a cicumscribing follicular vascular bed. Dermal papilla may induce growth and regulate differentiation within the germinal matrix. Hair growth is achieved in a simple fashion. The epidermal cells at the apex of the papilla give rise to medullary cells. The epidermal cells lateral to the apex give rise to cortical cells and cuticular cells. The cells at the depths of the epidermal pegs five rise to the inner root sheath, whereas more laterally located cells give rise to the outer root sheath.

A sheath of smooth muscle, the *arrector pili muscle,* attaches to the connective tissue associated with the hair follicle and the connective tissue of the papillary region associated with the skin proper (Fig. 20.8). Its contraction not only erects the hair but may help to express the sebaceous glands that are located between the mass of muscle and the hair follicle.

Species Differences. Hairs typically occur in groups *(hair beds)* of three primary follicles and variable numbers of secondary follicles. These groupings may not always be apparent in adults or at the surface. In dogs, hair beds contain follicles that may open separately or through a common opening at the surface. Compound follicles (clusters) consist usually of one *principal* or *guard hair* and three to nine *auxiliary (secondary)* or *wool hairs* (Fig. 20.9). A guard hair is approximately 150 μm in diameter and has a cuticle, cortex, and medulla. The wool hairs are approximately 70 μm in diameter and are devoid of a medulla. Clustering of hairs may be as exaggerated as in

Figure 20.3. A diagram of a typical hair follicle.

Labels on figure:
- Medulla
- Cortex
- Cuticle
- Epidermis
- Arrector pili muscle
- Dermis
- External root sheath
- Internal root sheath
- Hair bulb
- Dermal papilla

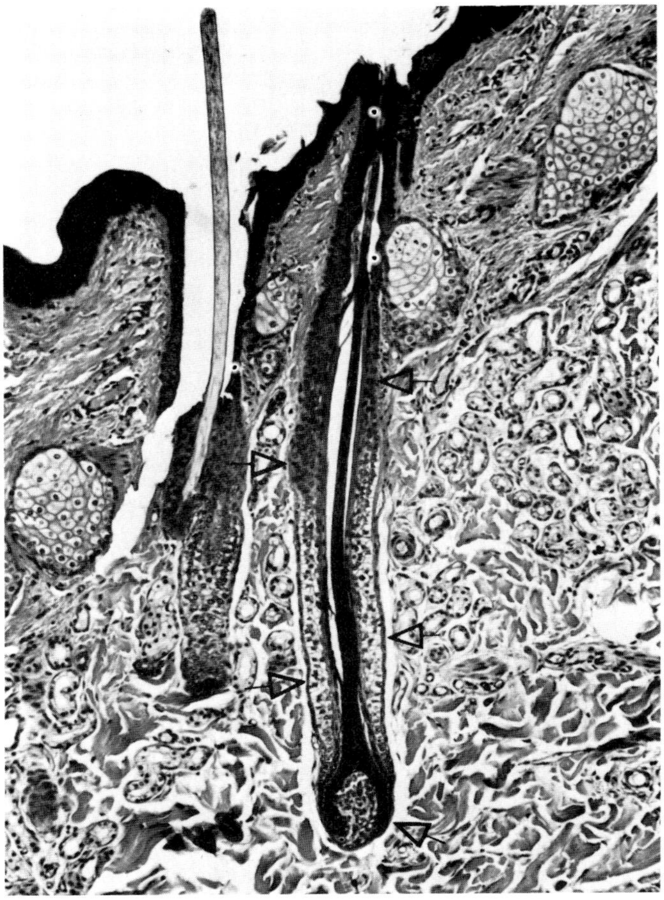

Figure 20.4. Hair follicle. The margins of the follicle *(arrows)* have been separated partially from the surrounding connective tissue. Note the continuity of the cellular components of the follicle with the surface cells. The intimate association of the dermal papilla to the hair bulb is apparent at the *lowest arrow*. ×25.

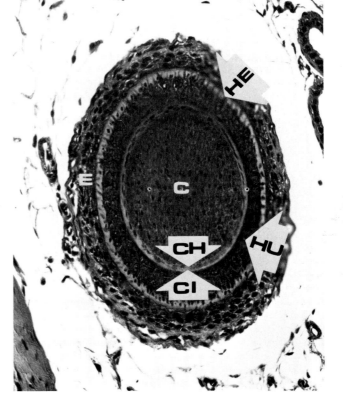

Figure 20.5. A cross-sectioned hair follicle. The external root sheath *(E)* surrounds the hair and is separated from the connective tissue by a glassy membrane (not apparent). The internal root sheath consists of Henle's layer *(HE)*, Huxley's layer *(HU)* and an inner cuticular layer *(CI)*. The hair consists of a cuticular layer *(CH)* and cortex *(C)*. A medulla is not present. ×63.

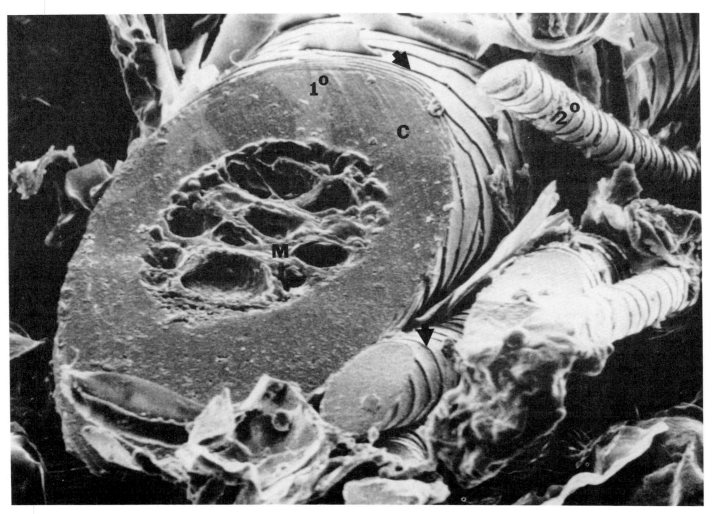

Figure 20.6.   A scanning electron micrograph of hairs from the saddle region of a beagle. Cross sections of the main (1°) and secondary (2°) hair shafts are apparent. The main shaft has a cortex *(C)* and a honeycomb-like medulla *(M)*. A medulla is not present in the secondary hairs. The cortices of the primary and secondary hair shafts are protected by organized layers of cuticular cells *(arrows)* that overlap each other in a telescoping pattern. (Courtesy of F. Al-Bagdadi.)

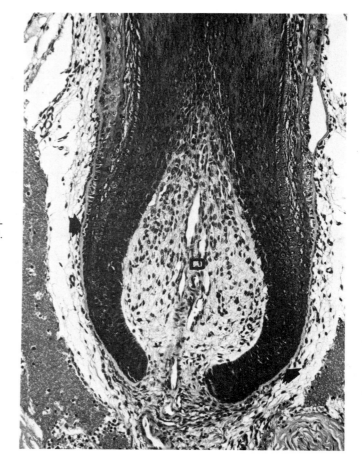

Figure 20.7. Hair bulb and dermal papilla. The cone-shaped hair bulb surrounds the dermal papilla *(D)*. The glassy membrane *(arrows)* is apparent. ×40.

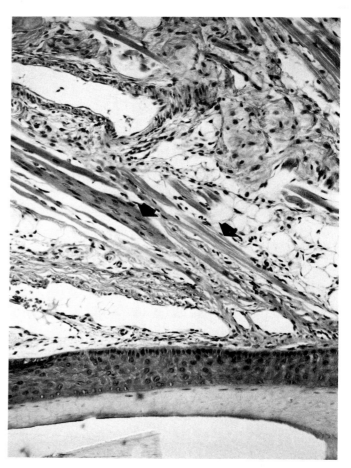

Figure 20.8. Arrector pili muscle. The muscle *(arrows)* attaches to the hair follicle and papillary region of the dermis.

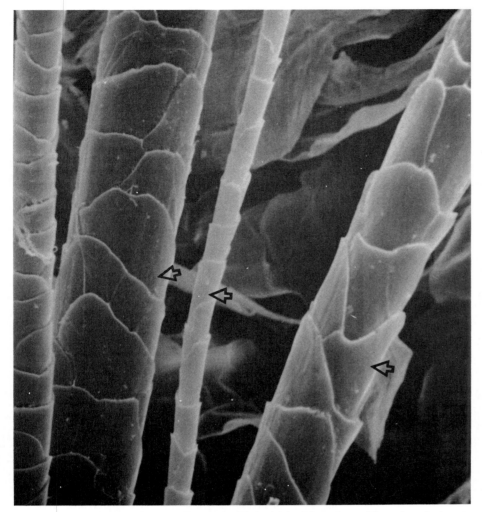

Figure 20.9. A scanning electron micrograph of hair obtained from the saddle region of a beagle. Four hair shafts of different diameters are covered by cuticular cells *(arrows)*. The cuticular cells have different shapes. Hair shafts of different sizes form the typical compound hairs of this species. (Courtesy of F. Al-Bagdadi.)

the chinchilla in which as many as 75 hairs may comprise a cluster with a single surface opening. The single guard hair is approximately 15 μm in diameter whereas the numerous wool hairs are maximally 11 μm in diameter.

Hair Cycle. The normal growth and shedding of hairs occur in cycles that are influenced by the photoperiod. A complete hair cycle consists of three stages—anagen, catagen, and telogen (Fig. 20.10). *Anagen* is the period within the cycle during which time hair growth is accomplished. *Catagen* is the transitory stage that occurs before the resting period, *telogen*.

The hair is produced by the mitotic activity of the constituent cells of the hair bulb during anagen. The continual apposition of new cells to the shaft of the hair results in its elongation. During catagen the hair bulb becomes a solid, keratinized mass of cells, whereas the distal follicle becomes thin. The club-shaped bulb that is formed is fused to the hair-shaft and migrates to the level of the sebaceous glands. These hairs, devoid of an association with distinct papillae, are called *club hairs*. A secondary germ develops deep to the club hair. This morphological configuration marks telogen and may be maintained for weeks or months. During early anagen, the secondary germ grows deeper, forming a new hair bulb in association with a dermal papilla. Continued mitosis throughout anagen results in the elongation of the shaft. The new growth eventually displaces the club hair, which is shed, and the cycle continues again.

Knowledge about the growth and shedding of hairs in domestic animals is incomplete. Many laboratory rodents shed their hairs in *synchronized waves* that are initiated ventrally and progress laterad and dorsad. Carnivores and man, however, have an *asynchronized mossaic pattern* of hair growth and shedding in which each follicle has its own intrinsic rhythm. Hair cycles are also influenced by the photoperiod.

Many disease conditions are characterized by a lusterless or dull hair coat in which the cuticular cells are not flattened against the cortex; thus, light is not reflected normally. The anagen stage of hair growth may be shortened in various disease states. Accordingly, many hairs in telogen may be shed synchronously.

Sensory Hairs. These structures are called *tactile hairs* or *sinus hairs* (Fig. 20.11). Although the distribution of this type of hair is rather specific, the structure of the hair and follicle is similar to normal hairs. The connective tissue sheath adjacent to the glassy membrane is thickened and separated by connective tissue trabeculae from a peripherally located connective tissue sheath. The intertrabecular spaces are filled with venous blood contained within the venous sinuses. Free nerve endings and Merkel's disks are associated with the epidermal cells and connective tissue fibers.

Special Skin Cells

Melanocytes and Langerhans' Cells. The presence of melanin-bearing cells in the skin and mucous membranes (conjunctival sac, buccal cavity) imparts characteristic pigmentation (Fig. 20.12). Melanin also protects the organism from harmful ultraviolet radiation. Ultraviolet solar radiation may contribute to the increased incidence of ocular squamous cell carcinoma in cattle in the Rocky Mountain West. Despite their protective function, melanoblasts and melanocytes are responsible for the formation of a highly malignant tumor, malignant melanoma.

Langerhans' cells are round cells with a clear cytoplasm when processed by routine staining techniques with hematoxylin and eosin (H and E). They occur in the peripheral portion of the stratum spinosum. Special staining techniques (gold chloride) have demonstrated these cells to have a stellate or dendritic shape. Langerhans' cells share some morphological and histochemical characteristics with melanocytes and were once considered to be effete melanocytes. Experimental evidence, however, has demonstrated the presence of Langerhans' cells in skin grafts devoid of neural crest ectodermal elements. Moreover, Langerhans' cells appear to be distributed more constantly throughout the skin than melanocytes, the latter being subject to regional differences. Langerhans' cells also are capable of phagocytosis.

Current evidence indicates that Langerhans' cells are derivatives of the bone marrow. The cells possess surface receptors for the Fc segment of immunoglobulin G (IgG) and C3, receptor sites similar to those that

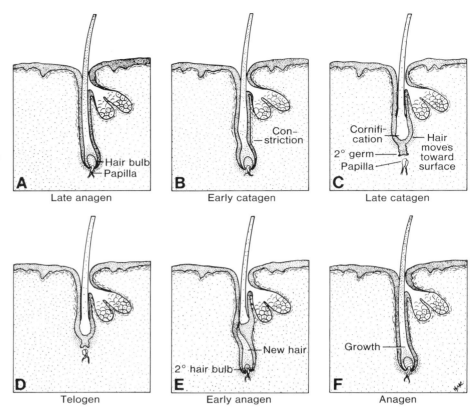

Figure 20.10. A diagram of the sequence of events in a typical hair cycle. *A*, hair growth begins to slow down; *B*, club hair starts to form at constriction in follicle; *C*, club hair cornifies and secondary germ forms. Club hair moves toward the surface. *D*, resting stage; *E*, secondary germ forms a new (secondary) hair bulb and club hair is pushed from the follicle as new hair growth progresses; *F*, new hair growth continues and the cycle is completed.

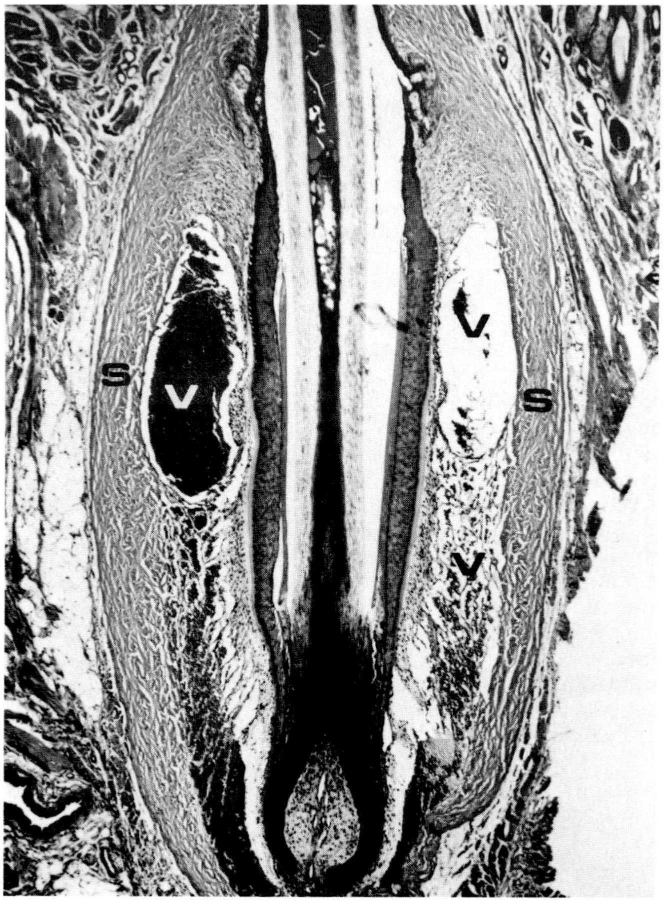

Figure 20.11. Sinus hair from a cat. The sinus hair is surrounded by a well-developed connective tissue sheath *(S)* that contains venous sinuses *(V)*. ×10.

Melanin granules

Cells of stratum spinosum

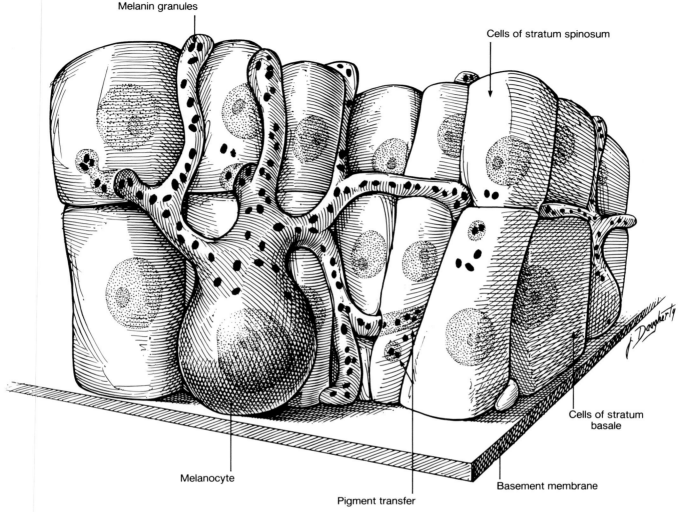

Melanocyte

Pigment transfer

Cells of stratum basale

Basement membrane

Figure 20.12.   An artist's conception of the relationship of melanocytes to cells of the epidermis.

characterize the surfaces of macrophages. These receptors permit the binding of antibodies without disabling the antigenic property of antigen binding. The Langerhans' cells belong to a group of relatively nonphagocytic macrophages that assist with the "processing" of antigen. Specifically, these cells are similar to the *dendritic cells* of lymph nodes. The extensive cytoplasmic processes form a web that is capable of antigen trapping. The trapped antigen is a potent stimulant for antigen-sensitive cells. Langerhans' cells may facilitate or assist the T lymphocyte in graft rejection responses.

Glands of the Mammalian Skin

Sebaceous and Tubular Glands

The glands of the skin are generally those that are associated with hairs. These are the *sebaceous glands* and the *tubular skin glands.* The former typically deposit their excretory product into the follicle; some may empty independently on the skin surface. The tubular skin glands occur in close association with follicles or open independently on the surface.

Sebaceous Glands. Sebaceous glands in association with hairs are evaginations of the epithelial lining of the root canal in the form of simple, branched alveolar glands (Figs. 5.27 and 5.32). They vary in size from 0.2–2.0 mm. The *peripheral cell layer* of squamous or cuboidal cells resides on a basement membrane. These are the stem cells of the gland. The holocrine nature of sebaceous glands requires a copious supply of cells. The lumen of the alveolus is filled with polyhedral cells. The cells are forced to the center of the gland during which time they accumulate lipids and undergo degeneration. Numerous examples of pyknosis and karyolysis are usually present. The accumulated lipids (fatty acids, cholesterol) and entire cell constitute the secretory product, *sebum* (Fig. 20.13).

The basal cells of the alveolus are con-

nected to the root canal by a short, wide, excretory duct that is lined by a stratified squamous epithelium. Contraction of the arrector pili muscle may express the glands. The secretory product enters the follicle and then spreads over the surface of the skin.

The functions of sebaceous glands are varied: sebum diminishes the possible entry of microorganisms into the skin; the secretory product diminishes water loss; it contains precursors to vitamin D; sebum keeps the hairs and outer skin surface soft and pliable.

Some areas of the skin are devoid of sebaceous glands: foot pads, hooves, claws, horns, and others.

Tubular Skin Glands. The tubular glands of the skin are simple, coiled, tubular structures. They are extensively developed in the horse and man and are absent in the bird. There are two general types: *merocrine (eccrine)* and *apocrine.*

The adenomere consists of a low cuboidal epithelium in the merocrine glands, whereas the epithelial lining of the adenomere of apocrine glands is a low columnar type. Blebs on the luminal surface are indicative of the apocrine secretory mechanism. The adenomeres of both types of glands are arranged as a *glomus* (a tuft or ball). The glomus may connect to the surface directly. Usually, the apocrine glands open into the neck of the root canal above the opening of the sebaceous gland by a loosely coiled or straight excretory duct. The duct consists of a single or double layer of cuboidal cells. Myoepithelial cells are associated with the adenomeres.

Although the merocrine tubular glands are the primary sweat glands of man, they open independently of hair follicles They are restricted to the footpads of carnivores (Fig. 20.14), the frog of ungulates, porcine carpus, and nasolabial region of ruminanats and swine. In man, sweat glands are usually confined to the mammary, axillary, pubic, and perineal regions. The apocrine tubular gland is the predominant sweat gland in domestic animals (Figs. 20.1, 5.24, 5.25, and 5.31). These glands are distributed generally throughout the skin. The canid has extensive tubular glands over the entire body, but apparently they are minimally functional as sweat glands. The equine apocrine tubular glands are active and produce an obvious secretion during physical exertion.

Sweat glands serve as a cooling mechanism for the body, as well as an excretory organ. The secretory product is mostly water (serous) and slightly alkaline. In the horse, however, it is strongly alkaline and contains albuminoids, serum globulins, and some urea.

Special Skin Glands

Glands of the Perianal Region

These glands may be divided into three types according to their association with the rectum and anus: *anal glands, glands of the anal sac,* and the *circumanal* or *perianal glands.*

Anal Glands. *Anal glands,* present in dogs, cats, and pigs, are modified tubuloalveolar sweat glands that occupy the submucosa of the columnar and intermediate zones of the anal canal and open into the anus (Fig. 20.15). Anal glands of carnivores secrete lipid materials, whereas those of pigs secrete mucoid substances (Fig. 20.16). Nodular and diffuse lymphatic tissue and venous erectile tissue may be present.

Anal Sacs. The *anal sacs* or *perianal sinuses* are paired, lateral cutaneous diverticula of the anus that are lined by a keratinized stratified squamous epithelium. Each sac has mural glands that open into it (Fig. 20.17). A typical lamina propria is underlaid by a dense fibroelastic connective

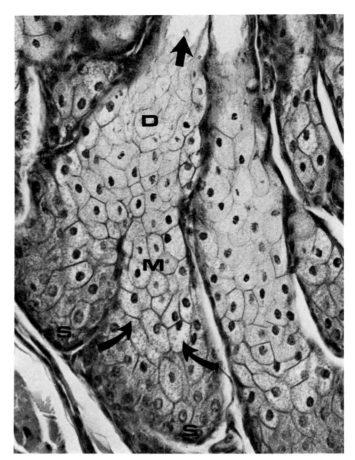

Figure 20.13. Secretory sequence in a sebaceous gland. The stem cells *(S)* migrate from the periphery *(curved arrows)*, mature *(M)*, disintegrate *(D)* and are propelled to the excretory duct *(straight arrow)*. ×100.

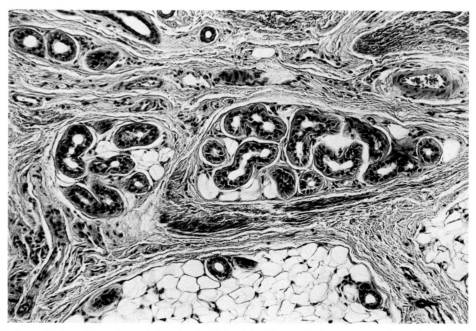

Figure 20.14. Merocrine tubular glands of the feline footpad. These are not the typical tubular glands of domestic animals. ×40.

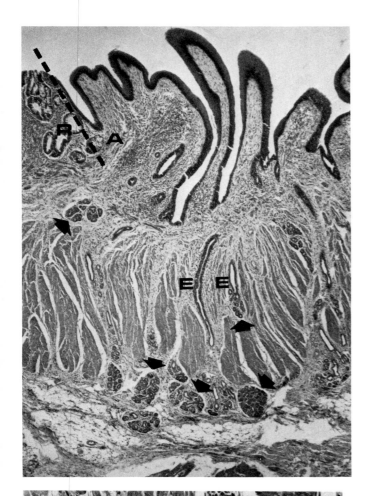

Figure 20.15. Porcine anal glands. The anal glands *(arrows)* are located in the submucosa of the columnar and intermediate zones of the anal canal. *A*, anus; *R*, rectum; *dashed line*, anorectal junction. The excretory ducts *(E)* of these glands open into the anus. ×10.

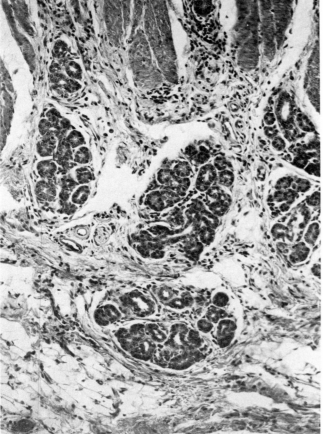

Figure 20.16. Adenomeres of porcine anal glands. These tubuloalveolar glands of the pig secrete mucoid substances. ×40.

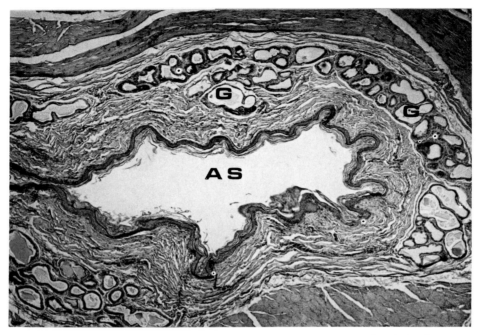

Figure 20.17. Canine perianal sinus. The anal sacs are paired cutaneous diverticula of the anus that contain numerous apocrine tubular glands *(G)* in their walls. *AS*, one of the anal sacs. ×10.

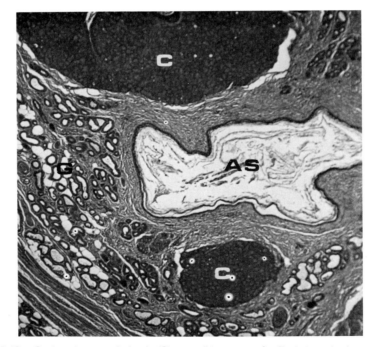

Figure 20.18. Canine circumanal glands *(C)* are solid masses of cells that are in close association with the anal sacs *(AS)*. *G*, apocrine tubular glands. ×10.

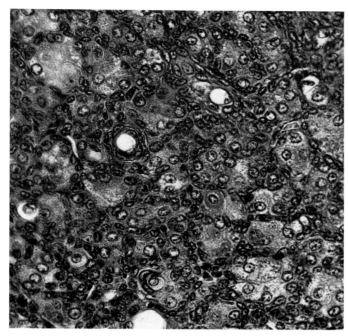

Figure 20.19. Parenchyma of the circumanal glands. The parenchyma consists of a solid mass of polygonal cells that are acidophilic. Although ducts are present in this section, the ducts are not patent as they leave the gland. ×100.

tissue. Much smooth and skeletal muscle is present in the connective tissue.

The anal sac is present in carnivores and many rodents. In the dog, the glands of the anal sac are apocrine tubular; in the cat, apocrine tubular glands and sebaceous glands are present. In both species, both types of glands open into the excretory duct or neck of the anal sac.

The excretory products of the glands of the anal sac, sloughed cells and excrement, may occlude the opening of the sacs to the anus. The anals sacs may have to be expressed periodically in dogs.

Glands of the Circumanal Region. The *glands of the circumanal region* include: *sebaceous glands* and *circumanal glands* (Fig. 20.18). The former are typical and may not be associated with hairs.

The circumanal glands of the dog are nonpatent masses of parenchymal cells that have often been described as *hepatocyte-like* (Fig. 20.19). The cells have a finely granular, acidophilic cytoplasm and pale nuclei. Numerous proteinaceous granules are present. The cells may be polygonal or tall columnar.

Nonpatent ducts from the circumanal glands have been reported to connect with the sebaceous glands of the region. It is concluded, therefore, that these glands are nonsecretory, abortive sebaceous glands. Many of the glands, however, are located some distance from sebaceous endpieces. Circumanal glands are predisposed to neoplasia.

Mammary Gland

General Features. The following description generally applies to all species but is especially applicable to the cow. The organ is a compound, tubuloalveolar gland that is believed to be a modified sweat gland (Fig. 20.20). Lipids of the gland are secreted by the apocrine method, whereas proteins and carbohydrates are secreted by the merocrine method.

The mammary gland consists of *teats* and *udder*. The udder consists of a capsule, interstitial connective tissue, secretory epithelium, and a system of excretory ducts. Actively lactating glands have much parenchyma and little connective tissue, whereas the reverse is true of nonlactating glands.

For a cow to produce 40 lb of milk per day, approximately 8 tons of blood must pass through the udder. This same amount of milk is produced, secreted, suspended, and subsequently removed from the udder in a short milking period from a sac of tissue that weighs approximately 50 lb. These relationships necessitate extensive secretory tissue, blood supply, and supportive connective tissues.

Lactating Gland. The secretory components include the alveolar epithelial lining cells and those of the initial portion of the *intralobular ducts (secretory tubules)* (Figs. 20.20 and 20.21). The active cells assume a columnar configuration with their apical borders protruding into the lumina (Fig.

20.22). Typical apical blebs are indicative of the apocrine secretory method. The accumulation of fat droplets is manifested by the foamy appearance of the cells. These small droplets may become confluent and form a single large droplet. The lateral cell borders usually are indistinct. The nucleus may be basally displaced or may be positioned apically during the secretory process. It may even be discharged into the lumen and become part of the secretory product.

Sloughed secretory cells, macrophages, and leukocytes may comprise part of the secretory product throughout lactation (Fig. 20.23). Macrophages and leukocytes, however, are especially prominent during early lactation when they comprise part of the *colostrum*. Colostrum functions as a laxative, but most importantly in some species it imparts a passive immunity to the nursing offspring until they achieve immunological competency.

Inactive secretory cells assume a low profile that may result from a diminished or terminated secretory phase or from mechanical distortion due to the accumulation of the secretory product in the lumen. Not all the cells of a given secretory unit or all the secretory tubules and alveoli are active at any given moment.

One or two *alveoli* drain into a single *secretory tubule*. This tubule or *intralobular duct* is lined by cuboidal epithelium: however, the initial secretory portion is lined by columnar epithelium. Intralobular ducts drain into a *lobular duct* lined by a nonsecretory cuboidal or columnar epithelium. The lobular duct, as the primary excretory duct for a lobule, drains into a *lobar duct*. The lobar duct is formed by the confluence of numerous lobular ducts. The lobar duct, which is the primary excretory duct for a lobe, is lined by a bistratified columnar epithelium. Ducts may expand to store milk. Numerous lobar ducts drain into the *gland sinus (gland cistern, lactiferous sinus)*, which is lined by a bistratified epithelium also. This is a common chamber at the base of each quarter of the udder. The volume of this cistern is variable. A slight constriction or *anulus* separates the *gland sinus* from the *teat sinus (teat cistern)*; the latter is lined by a bistratified columnar epithelium. Because the teat sinus and gland sinus are not always separated by an anulus, they are called collectively the *lactiferous sinus*. The teat sinus is continuous with the skin via the *streak canal (papillary duct, teat canal)*. The internal orifice of this canal is marked by an abrupt change to stratified squamous epithelium (keratinized). The epithelium and connective tissue of this region is organized into longitudinal folds called the *rosette of Furstenburg*. The epithelium of the teat canal continues through the external orifice and is continuous with the epidermal covering of the teat.

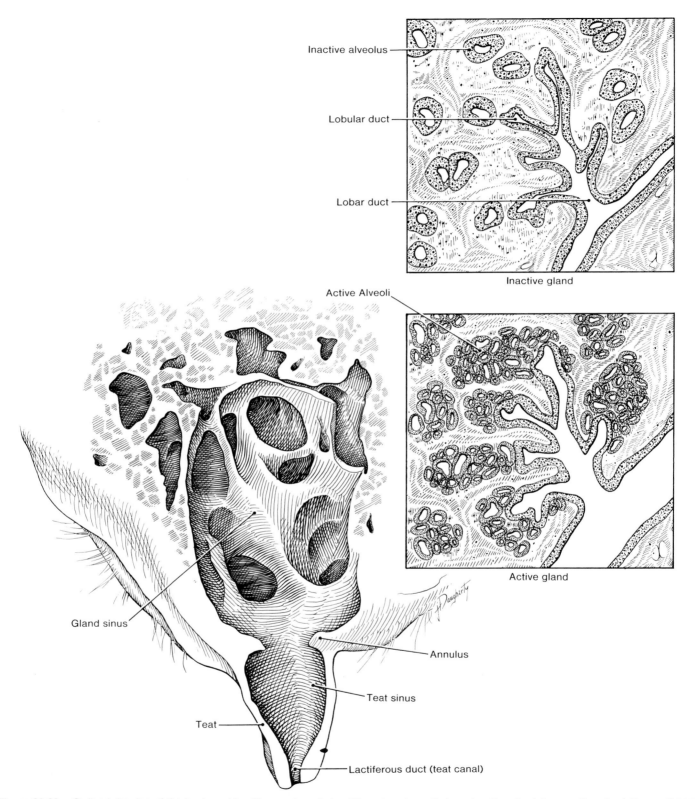

Inactive alveolus

Lobular duct

Lobar duct

Inactive gland

Active Alveoli

Active gland

Gland sinus

Annulus

Teat sinus

Teat

Lactiferous duct (teat canal)

Figure 20.20. Stylized drawing of the bovine udder. The number of alveoli is reduced greatly in an inactive gland. In an active gland, the number of alveoli increase at the expense of interstitial connective tissue.

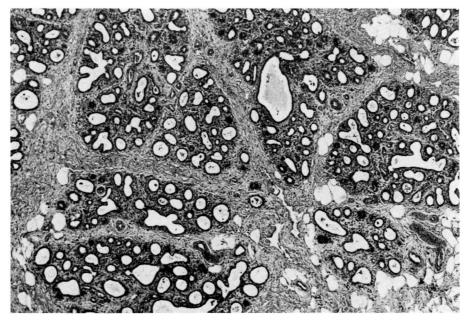

Figure 20.21. Lactating bovine mammary gland. The parenchyma of the organ is predominant. Compare with Figures 20.21 and 20.25. ×16.

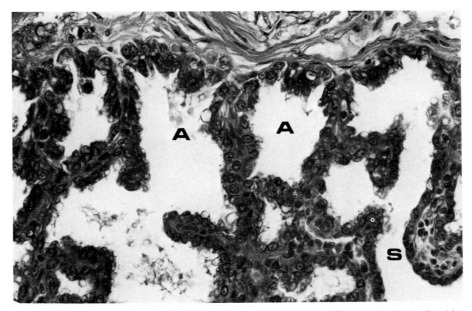

Figure 20.22. Adenomeres of a lactating bovine mammary gland. The alveoli *(A)* are lined by a columnar epithelium that has blebs along its apical surface. The secretory tubules *(S)* are lined by a cuboidal epithelium. ×100.

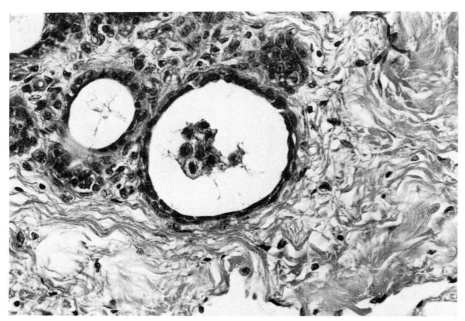

Figure 20.23. Cells within an alveolus. The cells may be sloughed epithelial cells or migratory cells from the connective tissue. ×100.

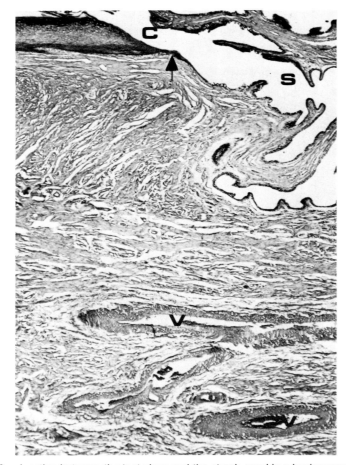

Figure 20.24. Junction between the teat sinus and the streak canal in a bovine mammary gland. The junction *(arrow)* between the teat sinus *(S)* and the internal orifice of the streak canal *(C)* is marked by a transition from bistratified columnar to stratified squamous epithelium. Vessels *(V)* are oriented longitudinally in this region. ×10.

The connective tissue of the gland varies with its position within the organ. Sparse areolar or reticular intralobular connective tissue is well vascularized. Numerous myoepithelial cells are present in association with adenomeres. Interlobular (intralobar) and interlobar connective tissue is areolar. Bundles of smooth muscle and elastic fibers are present around large ducts.

The capsule is a fibroelastic connective tissue especially rich in elastic fibers that divides the organ into four quarters. The external lamina of the capsule is DWFCT and comprises the *lateral suspensory ligament*. The *medial suspensory ligament* is especially rich in elastic fibers.

The epithelium and associated connective tissue of the teat sinus and teat canal are in close association and are continuous with the dermis (corium) and epidermal covering of the teat. The bistratified columnar epithelium is underlaid by a dermis that is rich in elastic fibers. Strands of smooth muscle fibers are apparent in the connective tissue. In the region of the internal orifice of the streak canal, they are disposed as a sphincter. At the junction between the teat and gland sinuses, this muscle also forms a sphincter. Extensive longitudinal blood vessels, thick-walled veins, and lymphatic vessels are associated with smooth muscle, especially in the regions of the sphincters (Fig. 20.24). The connective tissue peripheral to the smooth muscular fibers is the corium. It is typical but is especially rich in elastic fibers. The epidermal covering of the teat in the cow is hairless and nonglandular.

Nonlactating Gland. The parenchyma is greatly reduced and replaced by areolar connective tissue (Figs. 20.20 and 20.25). Extensive lymphocytic infiltration into the connective tissue and parenchyma is typical. Extensive adipose tissue may be present. The predominant loss of parenchyma is associated with the alveoli and secretory tubules. During mammary gland development, the alveoli are believed to be derived from the residual duct system.

During advanced stages of milk production, a gradual involution of the udder occurs that eventually leads to a morphology associated with inactivity. Throughout lactation, but especially apparent in advanced stages, *corpora amylacea* are common (Fig. 20.26). These are concretions of casein (milk protein) and cellular detritus.

Species Differences. There are numerous gross and subgross anatomical differences among the mammary glands of domestic species. Although there are some histological differences, they are academic. The number of teats, gland cisterns, and teat canals per teat vary. The number of teat canals per teat in various species is: ruminants, one; sow, two to three; mare, two to four; queen, four to seven; bitch, 8–20; woman, 15–24.

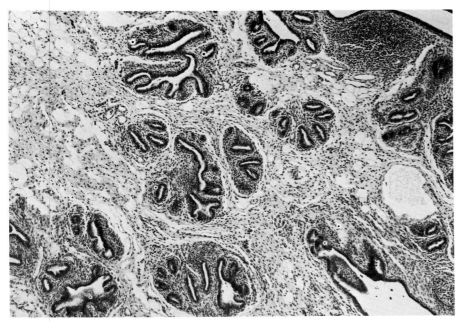

Figure 20.25. A nonlactating bovine mammary gland. The parenchyma is reduced, whereas the amount of connective tissue is increased. Compare with Figures 20.20 and 20.21. ×16.

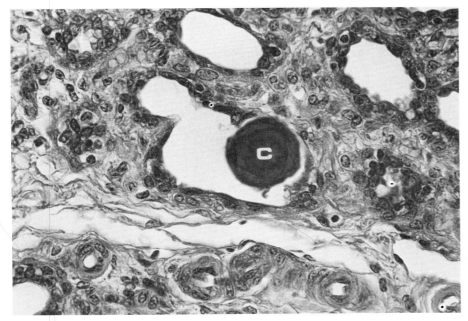

Figure 20.26. Amylaceous corpuscle in an alveolus of the bovine mammary gland. The corpuscle (C) is a concretion of milk protein and cellular debris. ×100.

Miscellaneous Glands

Numerous other glandular structures are localized to specific regions in different domestic species. Although these special skin glands do not possess unique histological structural features, they do have interesting and/or unique gross relationships to other structures. These specialized glands, however, are not hair associated.

Special Sebaceous Glands. The *infraorbital glands* of sheep form a continuous lining around the infraorbital sinus (Fig. 5.32). The sinus, located rostral and medial to the eye, is lined by thin skin, numerous sebaceous glands and a few apocrine tubular glands peripherally. The *submental organ* of cats is located within the intermandibular space and consists of accumulations of sebaceous glands. The *supracaudal glands* or *tail glands* of dogs and cats are located along the dorsal aspect of the tail. The tail glands of the cat extend along the entire length of the dorsum of the tail;

excessive secretions of these glands impart a waxy appearance to the tail known as "stud tail." In the dog, the tail glands are confined to a small, raised, oval and well-circumscribed region at the base of the tail from which single coarse hairs eminate. The *preputial glands* of the stallion are prominent and active sebaceous glands that elaborate sebum *(smegma)*. The *scent glands* or *horn glands* of the goat are modified sebaceous glands associated with hairs that are located along the caudomedial aspect of the horn base. Their secretory product, which includes caproic acid, imparts the typical odor to male goats.

Special Tubular Glands. The *mental organ* of pigs is an accumulation of apocrine tubular glands in the intermandibular space. Porcine *carpal glands*, aggregations of merocrine tubular glands, are located on the medial aspect of the carpus.

Special Glands—Tubular and Sebaceous. The *interdigital glands* of sheep are located in the interdigital sinus and consist of a mixture of sebaceous and apocrine tubular glands. The lining of the ovine inguinal sinus contains inguinal glands that are constituted similarly.

Hooves and Claws

Equine Foot

Structure of the Hoof

General Features. The hoof is the epidermis and its cornified derivatives. The foot, however, includes the hoof, dermis, and the structures contained therein (Fig. 20.27). Unique geometric relationships exist between the epidermis and related dermis or corium. This is manifested in two distinct ways. In some regions, the dermis is papillated; i.e., typical but pronounced dermal papillae and corresponding epidermal pegs are present. In other regions, the epidermal pegs are confluent as epidermal ridges. As a result, the interdigitated epidermal and dermal regions are *laminar*.

Most parts of the hoof are formed of cornified material that is arranged in a tubular manner. Some regions—those between the tubules—are nontubular. One region is laminar. The hoof, therefore, is composed of *tubular, intertubular* and *laminar horn* (hard keratin).

The histological regions of the hoof are: *periople, coronet, laminae, bars, sole,* and *frog* (Fig. 20.28).

The perioplic, coronary, and laminar epidermises comprise the *wall* of the hoof (Fig. 20.29). In older horses, the coronary and laminar epidermises are the primary constituents of the wall.

Perioplic Epidermis. The *perioplic epidermis* is also called the *stratum externum* or *stratum tectorium* (Fig. 20.30). It is composed of soft, thin, white, shiny and cornified material that extends over the wall and

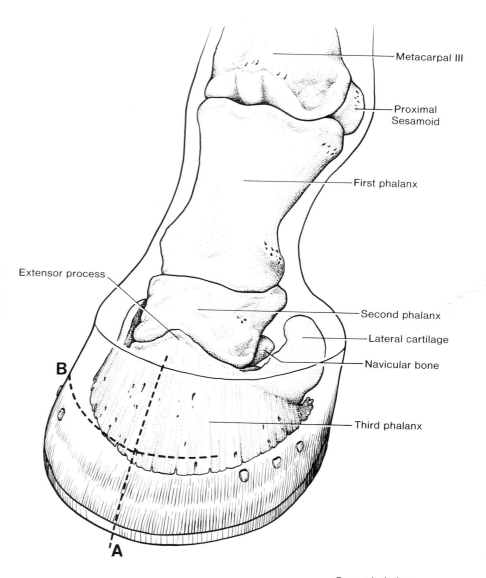

Figure 20.27. A simplified drawing of the equine foot. The *line* at *A* ("perpendicular" to the ground surface) represents the plane of section in Figures 20.28, 20.30, 20.31, 20.33, and 20.34. The *line* at *B* (parallel to the ground surface) represents the plane of section for Figures 20.29, 20.32, and 20.35.

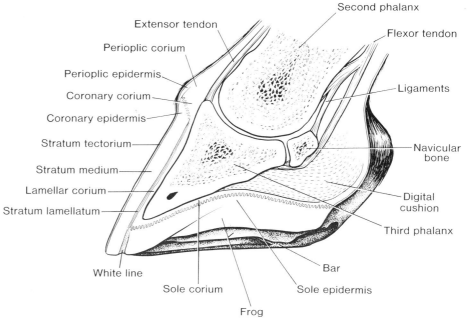

Figure 20.28. A longitudinal section through an equine foot.

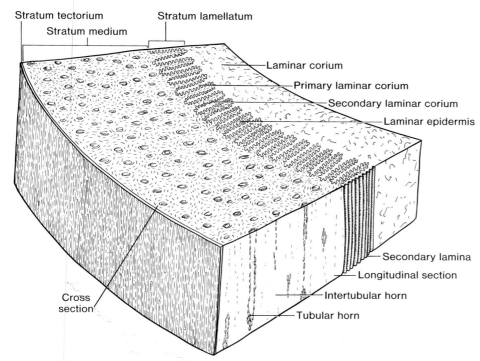

Stratum tectorium

Stratum medium

Stratum lamellatum

Laminar corium

Primary laminar corium

Secondary laminar corium

Laminar epidermis

Secondary lamina

Longitudinal section

Intertubular horn

Tubular horn

Cross section

Figure 20.29. A cross section and longitudinal section through the wall of the equine hoof.

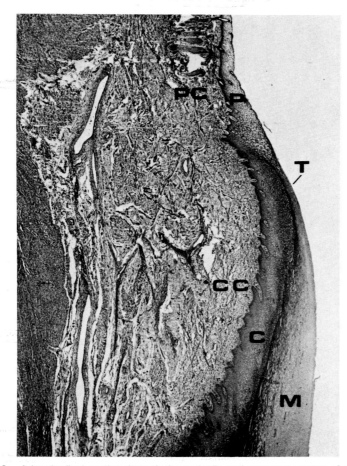

Figure 20.30. A longitudinal section through the perioplic and cornonary region of a fetal equine foot. *PC*, perioplic corium; *P*, periople or perioplic epidermis; *T*, stratum tectorium; *CC*, coronary corium; *C*, coronary epidermis; *M*, stratum medium. ×4.

bulbs. The perioplic epidermis, the means by which the hoof is directly attached to the epidermis of the typical skin, may be absent over the wall in older animals. This wall component is probably the means by which water loss from the young hooves is diminished. The highly vascularized *perioplic corium* is papillated; papillae are oriented "perpendicular" to the ground surface. This orientation results in a downward growth of the perioplic epidermis. **The perioplic corium is typical connective tissue. It supports and nourishes the perioplic epidermis.**

Coronary Epidermis. The *coronary epidermis*, underlaid by the *coronary corium*, is also called the *stratum medium* (Fig. 20.31). Because this portion of the wall is typically hard keratin, this region of the hoof is devoid of a stratum granulosum and a stratum lucidum. The keratin is disposed as prominent tubular and intertubular horn, which forms the bulk of the hoof wall (Fig. 20.32). The tubular horn is elaborated in a manner that may be compared to the growth of hairs (Fig. 20.33). The spaces between the tubular horn are filled with intertubular horn. The tubules of horn arise from the germinal epithelium that covers the lateral and distal portions of the dermal papillae. The intertubular horn is elaborated from the germinal epithelium in the depths of the epidermal pegs. The papillae of this region are elongated and "perpendicular" to the ground surface. This orientation results in the cornified cells forming tubes that are oriented similarly to the ground surface. Again, **the coronary epidermis is underlaid by typical dermis, the coronary corium, that nourishes and supports the epidermis.**

Laminar Epidermis. The *epidermis of the laminar region (stratum lamellatum)* is composed of nontubular horn that is elaborated at a slow pace "perpendicular" to the stratum medium (Fig. 20.34). The stratum lamellatum fuses with the stratum medium and holds the wall proper to the underlying dermal structures. The orientation and configuration of the epidermal "pegs" and dermal "papillae" are altered in this region. The dermal "papillae" and corresponding epidermal pegs are converted to elongated ridges that are oriented "perpendicular" to the ground surface. *Primary* and *secondary laminae* characterize this region (Fig. 20.35). Secondary laminae are oriented at an acute angle to the primary laminae. Primary epidermal laminae are composed of keratinized material. Collectively, these laminae are called the *insensitive laminae* (Fig. 20.36). The remaining secondary laminae with associated naked nerve endings, germinal epithelium, and dermal structures are called the *sensitive laminae*. The laminae of the epidermis (stratum lamellatum) interdigitate with corresponding projections of the *laminar*

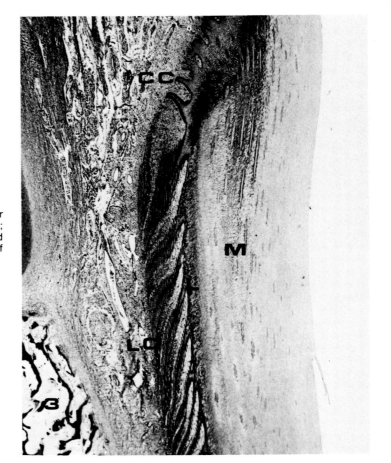

Figure 20.31. Longitudinal section through the coronary and laminar region of a fetal equine foot. *CC*, coronary corium; *C*, coronary epidermis; *M*, Stratum medium; *L*, laminar epidermis; *LC*; laminar corium; *3*, third phalanx. The slight obliquity of the section permits the visualization of individual laminae. ×40.

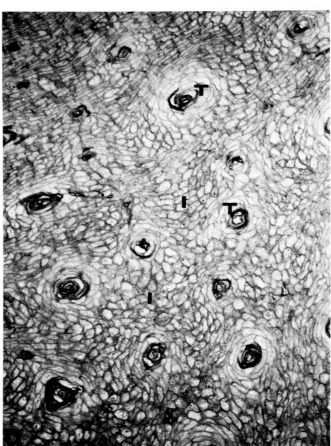

Figure 20.32. Organization of the stratum medium of the equine hoof. The stratum medium is composed of tubular *(T)* and intertubular horn *(I)*. ×40.

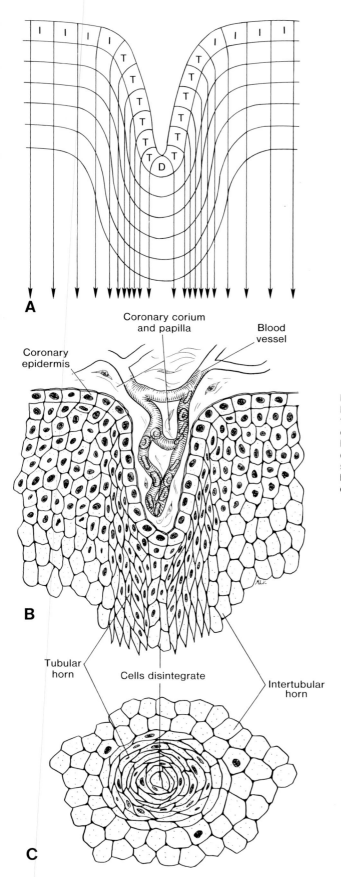

Coronary corium and papilla

Blood vessel

Coronary epidermis

A

B

Tubular horn

Cells disintegrate

Intertubular horn

C

Figure 20.33.   Scheme depicting the elaboration of tubular and intertubular horn by the cornonary epidermis. *A.* This scheme represents a longitudinal section through the coronary region. Cells indicated with a *T* line the shoulders of an epidermal peg. These cells give rise to tubular horn. The cells indicated with an *I* line the apex of an epidermal peg. These cells give rise to intertubular horn. The cells at *D* disintegrate eventually. *B.* This is the cellular representation of the scheme depicted in *A. C.* A cross section through the tubular and intertubular horn or the stratum medium. Drawings *A, B,* and *C* are in register with each other.

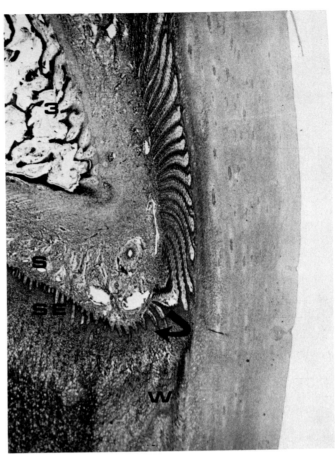

Figure 20.34. Longitudinal section through the laminar and sole region of a fetal equine foot. The corium and epidermis of the laminar region is continuous *(curved arrow)* with the sole corium *(S)* and sole epidermis *(SE)*. The point of transition or reflection of the epidermis is continued to the ground surface as the white line *(W)*. *3*, third phalanx. The change of orientation of keratinized material partially accounts for the appearance of the white line. Primarily, the white line is visible because the degree of keratinization or hardness of horn material is different in the stratum medium, white line, and sole epidermis. The slight obliquity of the section permits visualization of individual laminae. ×4.

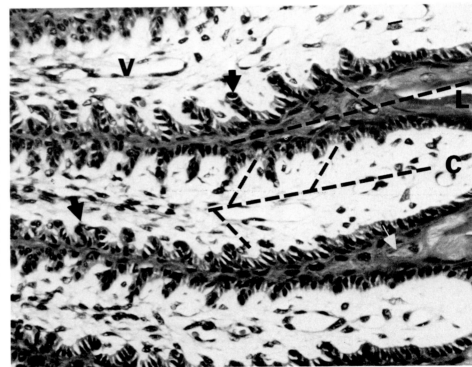

Figure 20.35. A cross section of a fetal equine foot. The laminar epidermis *(L)* and laminar corium *(C)* are evident. The primary and secondary epidermal laminae are indicated with a *dashed line*. The corresponding laminae of the corium are indicated similarly. Secondary epidermal laminae consist of cells *(solid arrows)* that comprise the stratum basale. The primary epidermal laminae consist of a few cells *(white arrow)* undergoing rapid keratinization. Their dermal constituents are typical. *V*, blood vessel. Classically, the epidermal laminae are considered to be the insensitive laminae, whereas the dermal laminae are considered to be the sensitive laminae. Because naked nerve endings probably occur within the secondary epidermal laminae, the sensitive laminae probably also include the secondary epidermal laminae. ×100.

corium. The insensitive laminae continue to the ground surface as the laminae of the wall. The junction between the laminae of the wall and *epidermis of the sole* is called the *white line* (Fig. 20.34).

The epidermis and corium of the laminar region are oriented "perpendicular" to the ground surface. At the white line, these structures reflect around the corner of the wall and become parallel to the ground surface. This point of reflection results in the fusion of horn material that is oriented differently. Thus, the white line is formed. The white line is an important landmark for shoeing horses. **Stratum lamellatum is epidermis. This portion of the hoof wall is nourished and supported by DWFCT, laminar corium.**

Epidermis of the Bars, Sole, and Frog. The *epidermis of the bars, sole,* and *frog* is similar to the papillated regions described previously. The papillae, however, are not as elongated as those described previously and the horn material is softer than that which composes the wall.

Corium of the Foot

Corium and Digital Cushion. The corium of the foot is a continuation of the skin. The corium of the foot, however, does contain numerous elastic fibers. In the region of the coronary corium, an extensive venous plexus is present. In most instances, the corium of the foot is intimately associated with the fibrous periosteum of the enclosed osseous structures. These relationships aid not only in shock absorption but also in attaching the hoof to the deeper structures of the foot. The corium of the frog contains modified sweat glands (merocrine tubular glands) that invaginate into the dermis from the epidermis of the frog.

A *digital cushion* occupies the space between the bones and tendons of the foot and the ground surface of the hoof. This fibroelastic connective tissue is an effective shock absorber. Compressive forces transmitted through the digital cushion to the lateral cartilages of the third phalanx are essential features of the venous return mechanism. Inactivity associated with transport results in edema (stocking) of the distal limb.

Ruminant and Porcine Claws

General Features. Although there are many gross differences between these structures and the equine hoof, there are only a few significant histological differences (Fig. 20.36). The claws of these species consist of: *wall, sole,* and well-developed *bulbs.* The laminar epidermis consists of primary laminae only (Fig. 20.37). These occur with a greater frequency than in the horse. The orientation of the papillae of the sole is more craniad than in the horse. Usually, more zones of the epidermis are apparent.

Claws of Carnivores

General Features. The claws of carnivores consist of a wall and sole (Fig. 20.38). The coronary epidermis and associated corium comprise the majority of the wall and consist of long dermal papillae and corresponding epidermal pegs. Laminar epidermis and associated corium are restricted to the dorsolateral aspects of the wall. The sole corium consists of thick papillae.

Integumentary Appendages

Horns of the Ox. The horn of the ox consists of three basic components: *os cornua, corium,* and *epidermis.* The *os cornua* or *frontal process* is an outgrowth of the frontal bone. The cornual process is covered by typical integumentary corium that is papillated. The associated epidermis gives rise to tubular and intertubular horn. At the base of the horn the epidermis gives

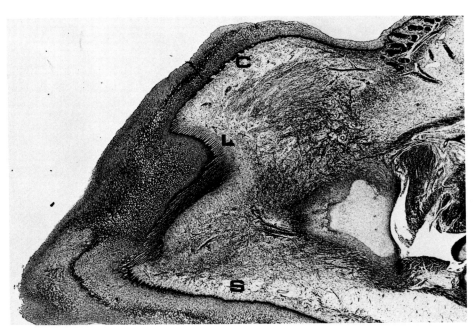

Figure 20.36. Longitudinal section through an ovine fetal claw. The coronary *(C)*, laminar *(L)* and sole *(S)* epidermis and corium are indicated. ×4.

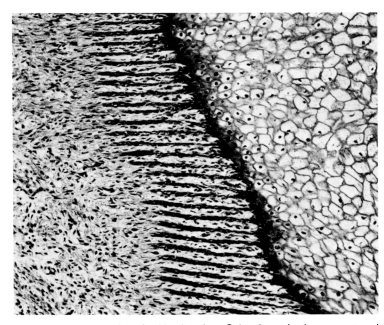

Figure 20.37. Laminae of the fetal bovine claw. Only primary laminae are present. ×40.

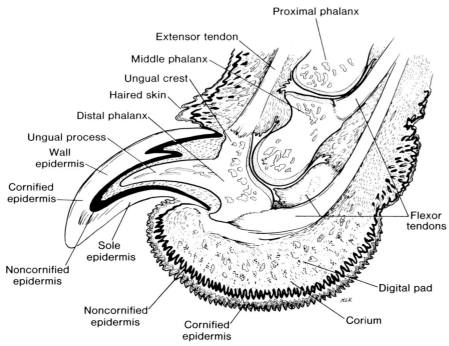

Figure 20.38. A stylized drawing of a sagittal section through the canine foot.

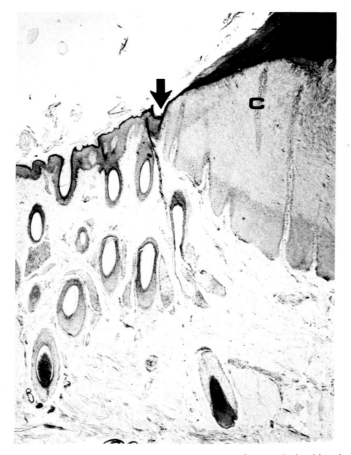

Figure 20.39. Equine chestnut. The point of transition *(arrow)* from typical epidermis to chestnut *(C)* is marked by an increased epidermal thickness and increased keratinization. ×10.

rise to soft horn, the *epikeras*, which is similar to the perioplic epidermis of the hoof. Cellular proliferation of the basal cells of the epidermis is slow and the horn continues to elongate at a very slow pace.

Antlers of Cervids. The antlers of deer and associated species consist of bone and, during certain times of the year, skin (velvet). These structures undergo cyclic growth, maturation, and shedding that is associated with seasonal breeding habits. The bone develops by a modified endochondral ossification. During growth, the developing cartilage is located at the end of each *tine*. It mineralizes and osseous replacement occurs. Eventually, as in the growth plate, the osseous replacement occurs at a faster rate than cartilage differentiation and "closure" occurs. At that point, the core of the antler is bone that is continuous with the *pedicle* of the frontal bone. Throughout development, the developing bone is covered by the integument, *velvet*. Upon maturation, the velvet becomes necrotic and is removed by rubbing. The bony protuberance remains as the mature antler. An abscission zone develops at the base of the antler and it is dropped. Subsequently, the entire process begins again.

Some species grow as much as 25 lb of bone during the 3-month active growing period at a rate of up to 1 cm per day. No mammalian growth process compares with it. Although antlers are usually confined to males, the female caribou and reindeer are antlered.

Miscellaneous Appendages. The horn of the pronghorn is very similar to the horn of the ox; however, the cornified material is shed annually. The frontal process of the giraffe is similar to the antler; however, the frontal process and associated integument are not shed. The horn of the rhinoceros consists of matted hair.

Dewclaws, Chestnut, and Ergot. *Dewclaws* of ruminants, swine, and dogs represent vestigial digits covered by horn material and associated dermis similar to the horn material characteristic of the species. A bony core may or may not be present (limb and species variable). *Chestnut* and *ergots* are regions of the equine epidermis that are highly keratinized and consist of tubular and nontubular horn (Fig. 20.39). They are devoid of hairs and glands. Some authorities consider these to be vestiges of some of the digits.

Repair of the Skin

Introduction. The numerous and varied functions of the skin depend upon the maintenance of morphological integrity. Microbial agents may enter the body through injuries that disrupt integumentary continuity, whereas excessive fluid and protein loss may occur through large foci denuded of their epidermal coverings.

The skin is subject to various types of wounds or disruption in anatomical integrity—abrasions, contusions, lacerations, punctures, and incisions. Three types of healing processes have been described for wounds in which tissues underlying the epidermis are exposed to the external environment—open wounds. *First intention healing* occurs when a clean incisional wound is closed immediately. *Second intention healing* is spontaneous healing without any or minimal surgical intervention. *Third intention healing* is spontaneous healing followed by wound closure.

Skin repair is a dynamic complex of cellular activity that is initiated with injury and continues through the reorganization of the tissues of the injury site. Skin repair represents a continuum of integrated cellular activity that may be divided into stages: *insult (wounding), induction, inflammatory, proliferative,* and *maturation stages.*

The events involved in skin repair—requiring epidermal, dermal, and hypodermal contributions—are similar in most integumentary repair processes. The methods by which the injured sites are handled dictate alterations in the process. Minor abrasions to the epidermis without damage to the underlying dermis generally repair themselves through the mitotic activity of the stratum basale of the epidermis. Although first intention healing may occur faster than second intention healing, all stages of the repair process are integral components of these methods. Excisional wounds in which excessive amounts of tissue are lost are characterized by a marked proliferation of fibrous connective tissue *(granulation tissue).*

For simplicity, a incisional wound undergoing second intention healing is described subsequently. The sequence of events is illustrated in Figures 20.40–20.44.

Insult (Wounding) Stage. Disruption of the integrity of the skin results in hemorrhage, local cell death, and contamination with microorganisms (Fig. 20.40). Hemostatic mechanisms account for clotting of the extravasated blood in the wound gap and plugging of severed vessels. The clot minimizes further fluid loss and forms a seal over the injured region. Deprived of their normal vascular supply, the tissues at the sites of injury undergo desiccation.

Induction Stage. Identification of this stage as a distinct entity may be artificial; however, induction of new cells continuing throughout repair is essential. The precise stimuli for an integrated repair process have not been identified. Initially, the resultant localized tissue hypoxia may induce essential neovascularization (Fig. 20.41). Fibroblasts may respond to local lactic acid accumulations resulting from the activity of macrophages, but collagen synthesis can not occur until essential metabolites are supplied by the vasculature.

Inflammatory Stage. The inflammatory stage begins immediately after the injury (Fig. 20.41). Although vasoconstriction is the immediate localized response to injury, capillary contraction is followed by capillary dilation with an accompanying increase in vascular permeability. The release of vasoactive substances from endothelial cells, mast cells, and platelets—histamine, serotonin, bradykinin, prostaglandin E_2—initiates the localized vascular response. Chemotactic factors released at the injury site attract neutrophils and fibroblasts. Bradykinin and prostaglandin E_2 may also function to attract these cells to the wound.

Neutrophils are the predominant cells at the injury site for the first 3 days after injury. They are effective phagocytes that function to control microbial contamination and remove cellular debris. Macrophages, mast cells, eosinophils, lymphocytes, and plasma cells are also attracted to the injury site.

The duration of the inflammatory stage is dependent upon various factors: the amount of contamination, the extent of the tissue damage, and the presence of infection. A clean wound, one in which no microbial agents are present, may be characterized by a peak inflammatory response in 3–4 days. Progression of repair is accompanied by a gradual and steady diminution of inflammatory cells.

Proliferative Stage. The proliferative stage, involving the mitotic activity of epidermal cells, endothelial cells, and fibroblasts, extends 10–14 days postinjury (Fig. 20.42). Cells of the stratum basale along the margins of the wound migrate across the defect. Similar cells from cut hair follicles within the defect may migrate to cover the wound. Migration is a random process

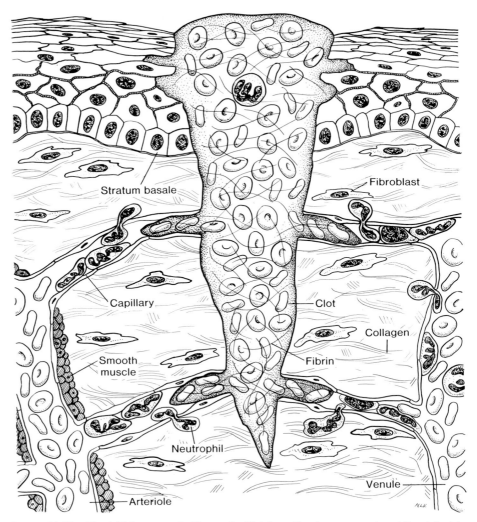

Figure 20.40. The initial events of skin repair. Clot formation has occurred and the defect has been filled. Capillaries have been plugged. Hemostasis has been achieved. The labels on this figure also apply to Figures 20.40–20.44.

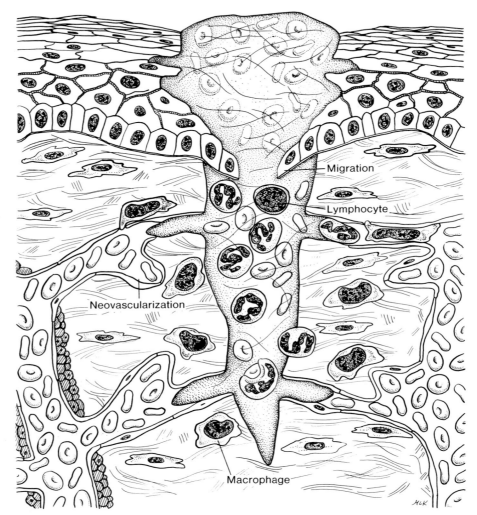

Figure 20.41. Induction and initiation of inflammation. Inflammatory cells have invaded the wound site. Neovascularization and epidermal cells migration have been initiated.

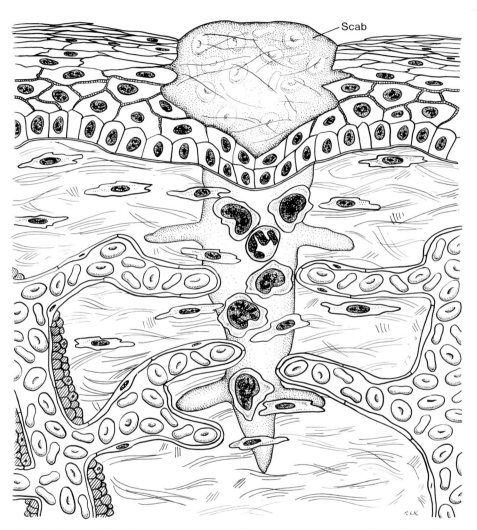
Scab

Figure 20.42. Proliferative stage of wound repair. Inflammation has subsided and the epidermal cells have migrated over the wound site beneath the scab. Neovascularization continues and fibroblasts invade the clot with the new blood vessels.

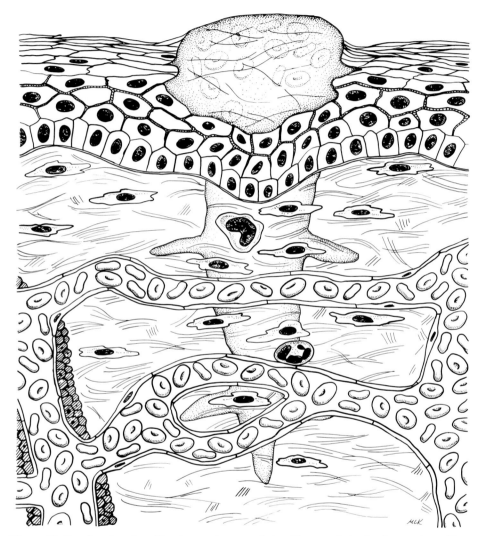

Figure 20.43. Continued proliferation at the wound site. Neovascularization is complete. Fibro-blasts continue to proliferate and produce matrix materials.

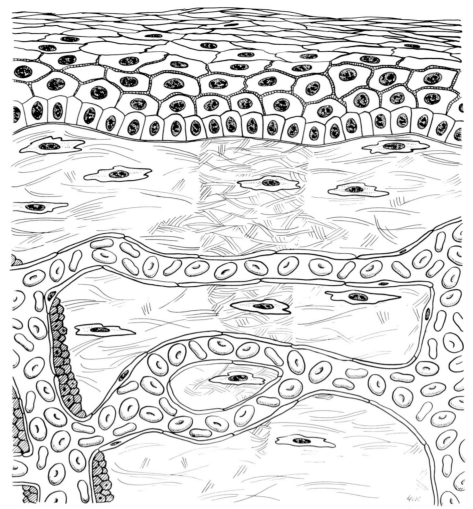

Figure 20.44.   Completion of wound repair. Continued remodeling of the wound site will increase wound strength and result in the removal of excess collagen.

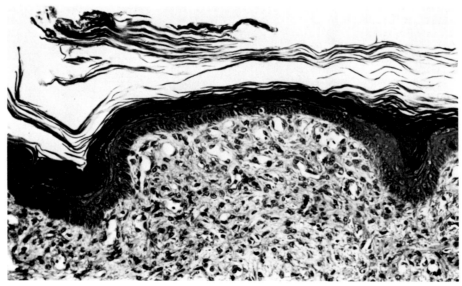

Figure 20.45.   Avian skin. The epidermis has a reduced number of layers. ×63.

that is initiated within the first 24 hours after the injury but is not visible until keratinization occurs. The epidermis adjacent to the wound site subsequently proliferates to replace the migrating cells. The migrating cells, retaining their mitotic potential, proliferate and begin to replace the epidermis. The result of this migratory and proliferative activity is the reestablishment of an epidermal barrier. The barrier overlies the connective tissue of the dermis but is beneath the scab. The scab sloughs in about 7 days.

Endothelial cell proliferation from the ends of severed vessels initiates the reestablishment of vascularity (Fig. 20.43). Fusion of these cells from arterial and venous capillaries completes the neovascularization. Perivascular fibroblasts proliferate and synthesize matrical materials in response to the improved microenvironement. Fibroblasts, moving along fibrin strands that serve as temporary scaffolds, advance with the advancing vascular beds. Some fibroblasts develop the ability to move along matrix materials by contractile mechanisms. These fibroblasts, which contain contractile myofilaments, are termed *myofibroblasts*. The fibroblastic cells dominate the wound site as inflammation diminishes.

The connective tissue at the wound site contains numerous fibroblasts and is well vascularized. White blood cells are numerous also; however, the wound is devoid of nervous tissue. This newly generated tissue, *granulation tissue*, is the mediator of connective tissue repair and is responsible for *wound contraction*—the movement of full thickness skin toward the center of a defect. Wound contraction is an active process that is probably dependent upon the myofibroblast. The myofilaments of myofibroblasts are integral components of this process. Although mesenchymal cell differentiation accounts for the population of fibroblastic cells of granulation tissue, the determinants for the differentiation of myofibroblasts and fibroblasts is unknown. Granulation tissue, typically, contains both populations of cells.

Maturation Stage. The gradual reduction of fibroblasts and a corresponding decrease in capillaries within the wound are the histological features of the maturation stage (Fig. 20.44). The maturation stage is characterized by a balanced synthesis and degradation of connective tissue components. Collagenous fibers typically align themselves along stress lines within the wound. A gradual and continual increase in wound strength can be anticipated. While wound strength may approach 25% of preinjury strength by three weeks postinjury, some wounds may continue to improve wound strength for two years. Innervation of the wound site eventually reoccurs. Nerve regeneration was described previously.

Avian Integument

Epidermis and Dermis. The epidermis of avian skin is thin, loose and dry (Fig. 20.45). Although much thinner than the mammalian counterpart, four strata are defined: *stratum basale, stratum spinosum (stratum intermedium), stratum transitivum*, and *stratum corneum*. The stratum transitivum is probably the avian counterpart to the mammalian stratum granulosum. The dermis and subcutis have been subdivided into as many as eight different strata. The dermis becomes more dense in the depths of the corium and abuts on a very extensive subcutis. Lymphoid tissue is extensive in the corium and subcutis. The corium and epidermis are devoid of glands.

Feathers extend from the epidermis into the corium and assume a configuration similar to hairs. Although they are both epidermal structures, they probably have a different phylogenetic origin.

Feathers. Feathers are of epidermal origin and develop within a follicle. The base of the follicle, however, is not continuous over the dermal papilla. Thus, the core of the feather contains remnants of vascular connective tissue (feather *pulp*).

The principal parts of the feather are the *quill (calamus)* and the *vane (vexillum)* (Fig. 20.46). The quill is contained within the follicle and contains two foramina (*proximal umbilicus* and *distal umbilicus*). As the quill grows, the dermal papilla retracts leaving behind the desiccated central *pulp*. The rachis is the continuation of the quill above the skin surface. The *vane* is the collective term for all of the barbs. The barbs project laterally from the rachis in an oblique and parallel manner. The barbs possess *proximal* and *distal barbules* that are oriented at right angles to the barbs and parallel to the rachis. The distal barbules have hooklets that engage the indentations of the proximal barbules. This relationship

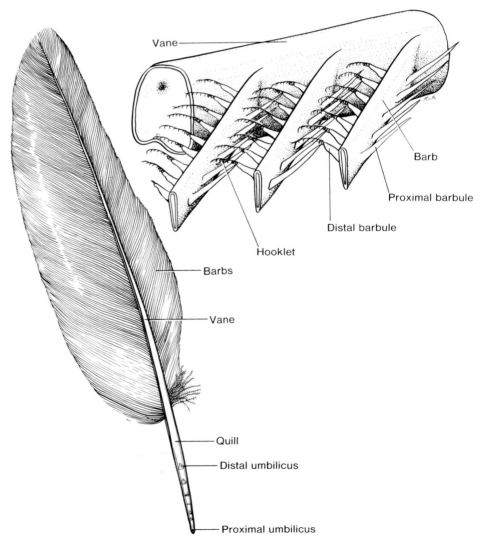

Vane

Barb

Proximal barbule

Distal barbule

Hooklet

Barbs

Vane

Quill

Distal umbilicus

Proximal umbilicus

Figure 20.46.   A drawing of the main components of a flight feather.

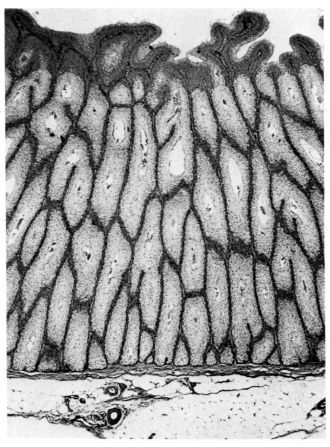

Figure 20.47.   The avian uropygial gland. Numerous sebaceous adenomeres are grouped to form this gland. ×10.

nective tissue, and fat. In some birds (turkey), erectile tissue may be present within these structures.

References

Abercrombie, M., Flint, M. H. and James, D. W.: collagen formation and wound contraction during repair of small excised wounds in the skin of rats. J. Embryol. Exp. Morphol. *2*:264, 1954.

Adam, W. S., Calhoun, M. L., Smith, E. M. and Stinson, A. W.: *Microscopic Anatomy of the Dog: A Photographic Atlas.* Charles C Thomas, Springfield, 1970.

Baker, B. B.: Epidermal cell renewal in the dog. Diss. Abst. Int. *32B*:5526, 1972.

Baker, K. P.: Hair growth and replacement in the cat. Brit. Vet. J. *130*:327, 1974.

Chase, H. B.: Growth of the hair. Physiol. Rev. *34*:113, 1954.

Creed, R. F. S.: The histology of the mammalian skin with special reference to the dog and cat. Vet Rec. *70*:736, 1958.

David, L. T.: Histology of the skin of the Mexican hairless swine *(Sus scrofa).* Amer. J. Anat. *50*:283, 1932.

Findlay, J. D. and Yang, S. H.: The sweat glands of Ayrshire cattle. J. Agric. Sci. *40*:126, 1950.

Godall, A. M. and Yang, S. H.: Myoepithelial cells in bovine sweat glands. J. Agric. Sci. *42*:159, 1952.

Hausman, L. A.: Structural characteristics of the hair of mammals. Amer. Natur. *44*:496, 1930.

Hibbs, R. G.: The fine structure of human exocrine sweat glands. Amer. J. Anat. *103*:201, 1958.

Hunt, T. K. and Van Winkle, W., Jr.: *Fundamentals of Wound Management in Surgery—Wound Healing: Normal Repair.* Chirirgecom, Inc., South Plainfield, NJ 1976.

Katz, S. I., Tamaki, K. and Sachs, D. H.: Epidermal Langerhans cells are derived from cells originating in bone marrow. Nature. *282*:324, 1979.

Lucas, A.M. and Stettenheim, P. R.: *Avian Anatomy: Integument* Parts I and II, U. S. Government Printing Office, 1972.

Maibach, H. I. and Rovee, D. T. (eds.): *Epidermal Wound Healing.* Year Book Medical Publishers, Chicago. 1972.

Moffat, G. H.: The growth of hair follicles and its relation to the adjacent dermal structues. J. Anat. *102*:527, 1968.

Montagna, W.: *The Structure and Function of the Skin.* 9th ed. Academic Press, New York, 1962.

Muller, G. H. (ed.): Symposium on the skin and internal disease. Vet. Clin. North Amer. *9*:1, 1979.

Muller, G. H. and Kirk, R. W.: *Small Animal Dermatology.* W. B. Saunders, Philadelphia, 1976.

Munger, B. L.: The cytology of apocrine sweat glands. I. Cat and monkey. Z. Zellforsch. *67*:373, 1965.

Nielsen, S. W.: Glands of the canine skin. Amer. J. Vet. Res. *14*:448, 1953.

Stump, J. E.: Anatomy of the normal equine foot, including microscopic features of the laminar region. J. Amer. Vet. Med. Assoc. *151*:1588, 1967.

Toker, C.: Observations on the ultrastructure of a mammary ductule. J. Ultrastruct. Res. *21*:9, 1967.

Webb, A. J. and Calhoun, M. L.: The microscopic anatomy of the skin of mongrel dogs. Amer. J. Vet. Res. *15*:274, 1954.

Webber, A. F., Kitchell, R. L. and Sautter, J. H.: Mammary gland studies. I. The identity and characterization of the smallest lobule unit in the udder of the dairy cow. Amer. J. Vet. Res. *16*:255, 1955.

establishes a relatively nonporous and flexible sheet that sheds water and facilitates flight.

Down feathers have a small and thin rachis. The barbs are devoid of barbules. Thus, these feathers are loose and fluffy; they serve as good insulation.

Filoplumes are feathers with a hair-like structure. They are scattered over the body but are especially predominant structures on the head and neck.

Uropygial Gland. The uropygial gland is also called the *oil* or *preen gland* It is the only cutaneous gland that occurs in birds (Fig. 20.47); it is well developed in aquatic species and consists of numerous sebaceous adenomeres opening into a common duct or sinus that empties on the surface on a common papilla. The papilla contains smooth muscle fibers that extend around the excretory duct. The heavily encapsulated, bilobed duct is situated above the last sacral vertebra.

Specialized Structures. There are numerous other epidermal modifications in birds: scales, toe pads, claws, beaks, wattles, spurs, and combs. Claws, spurs, and beaks are similar to the mammalian claw, whereas toe pads may be compared to the pads of carnivores. Scales are comparable to those of reptiles and occur on the legs of all birds as well as on the wings of penguins. Wattles and combs are diverticuli of the skin that contain extensive vasculature, mucous con-

21: Digestive System I— Alimentary Canal

The digestive system is divided into two sections for ease of presentation. The modified tubular and tubular components of the digestive tract (buccal cavity to anus) constitute this chapter. The extramural glands (salivary glands, liver, pancreas) and gallbladder comprise Chapter 22.

General Characteristics

Structure and Function. The digestive system consists of the alimentary canal and accessory structures such as the lips, tongue, teeth, and extramural glands. The *alimentary canal (tract)* is a tubular or modified tubular structure extending from mouth to anus. The alimentary tract is divided conveniently into a number of organs on the basis of structure and anatomical location. The epithelial lining of most of the canal is derived from endoderm; however, the rostral and caudal epithelium is from stomodeal and proctodeal ectoderm, respectively.

Muscularized lips and a tongue aid in *prehension*, whereas teeth permit *mastication*. *Deglutition* (swallowing) results from the muscular activity of the buccal cavity and pharynx. The muscularized esophagus propels the bolus into the stomach wherein *mechanical* and *chemical digestion* is initiated. The remainder of the tube continues digestion and *absorption*. The tube *propels* the luminal contents toward the anus, culminating in the *elimination* of digested residue. Some of the less obvious essential functions are the *synthesis and secretion of enzymes, secretion of digestive juices, vitamin production, plasma protein synthesis and secretion, detoxification of harmful substances* and *elaboration of essential body metabolites.*

The solid, fluid, and semifluid luminal contents of the digestive system are outside the body. Materials do not enter or leave the body through this system until they cross the epithelial barrier of the digestive tract. The selective absorption of materials vital to the organism is a function of the lining cells of this system.

Oral Structures

Buccal Cavity Proper

General Characteristics. The buccal cavity does not have a typical tubular configuration, but its mural organization conforms to the basic pattern. Generally, the buccal cavity may be described as an exten-

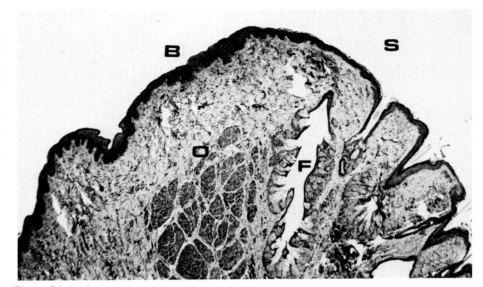

Figure 21.1. A section through a feline lip. The buccal surface *(B)* is a mucous membrane. The skin *(S)* is typical and contains hair follicles *(F)* and associated sebaceous glands. The orbicularis oris muscle *(O)* is in the center of the structure. ×10.

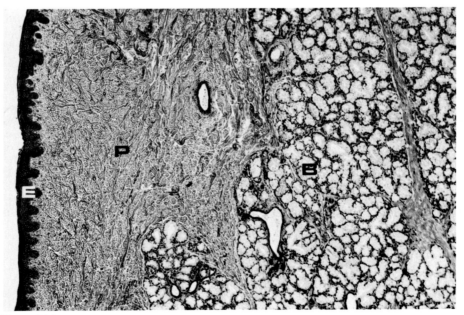

Figure 21.2. A section through a feline cheek. The lamina epithelialis mucosae *(E)* is underlaid by a typical lamina propria mucosae *(P)*. Numerous mucus-secreting buccal glands *(B)* are present. ×16.

sion of the skin that has been modified as a *cutaneous mucous membrane.*

Histological Structure. The lamina epithelialis mucosae is stratified squamous epithelium with varying degrees of cornification. Large epithelial papillae projecting from the surface epithelium assist in the prehension and mastication of food (ruminants). The lamina propria mucosae blends insensibly with the tunica submucosa. Usually, the lamina propria mucosae

is devoid of glands; it possesses only the excretory ducts of submucosal glands that are generally referred to as buccal glands. These are either mucous, serous, or mixed glands. The submucosal tunic or lamina propria mucosae blends with and rests upon the fascia associated with the underlying skeletal muscle. If skeletal muscle is replaced by bone, then the lamina propria mucosae or tunica submucosa is continuous with the periosteum.

Lip

The *lips* are a fold of fibroelastic tissue that marks the entrance to the digestive system. A *mucocutaneous junction* occurs on this structure. At the point of transition, the thin epidermis becomes the thickened cutaneous mucous membrane (Fig. 21.1). The lip is keratinized in species whose diets contain much roughage (ruminants, horse). It is nonkeratinized in the pig and carnivores. The degree or absence of keratinization is diet-dependent.

The core of the lip is composed of fibroelastic connective tissue and skeletal muscle. On the integumentary side of the lip, the dermis and hypodermis are typical. On the labial side, the lamina propria mucosae and tunica submucosa are typical although not distinct from one another. Submucosal glands *(labial glands)* are present. They are mucous in small ruminants and carnivores and mixed in other species. These glands are branched, tubuloalveolar types. They are serous glands in the bovine nasal planum. The tunica muscularis is skeletal muscle (orbicularis oris).

Cheek

The lamina epithelialis mucosae, lamina propria mucosae, and tunica submucosa of the cheek are similar to the structure of the lip (Fig. 21.2). Serous or mucous *buccal glands* occupy the submucosal connective tissue space.

Hard and Soft Palates

The *hard palate* is composed of a keratinized stratified squamous epithelium that

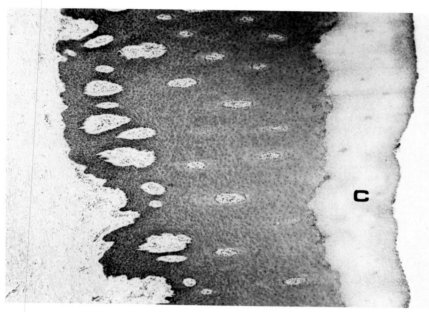

Figure 21.3.   A section of bovine dental pad. This structure replaces the upper incisors of ruminants. The pad has a thickened lamina epithelialis mucosae that is highly cornified *(C)*. ×10.

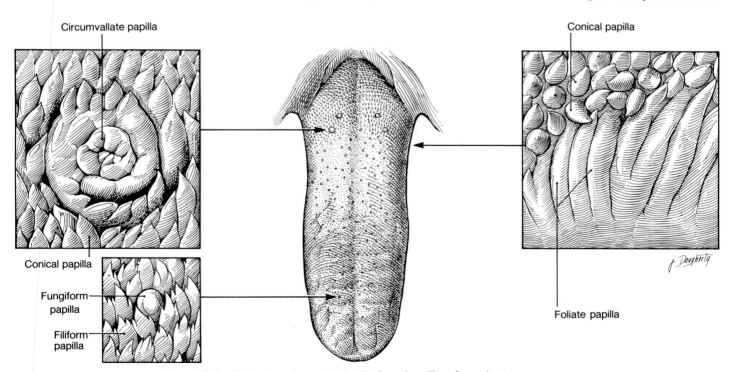

Figure 21.4.   Illustrations demonstrating the lingual papillae of a canine tongue.

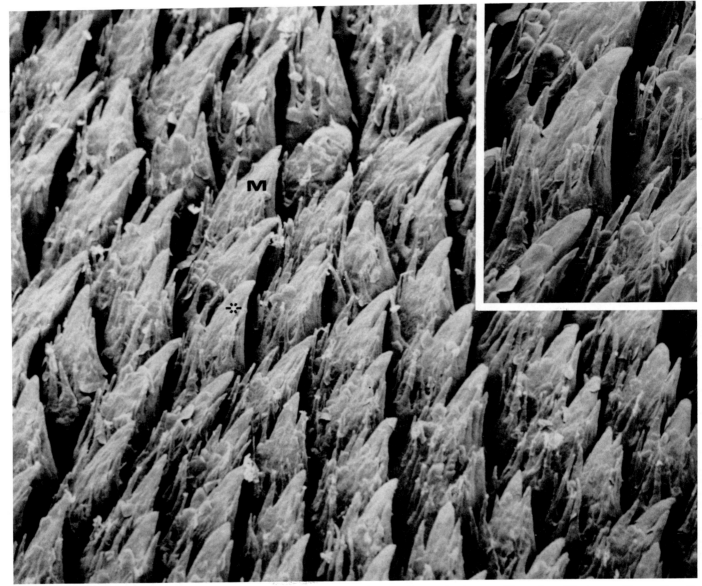

Figure 21.5.   Scanning electron micrographs of the tongue of a foxhound. Filiform papillae predominate on this portion of the tongue. The configuration is a main papilla *(M)* surrounded by four to eight secondary papillae. The papillae project caudally and are highly cornified. Inset: The papillae at the asterisk-like symbol is enlarged. The surrounding secondary papillae are apparent. (Negatives courtesy of F. Al-Bagdadi.)

is especially thick and highly keratinized in the *dental pad* of ruminants (Fig. 21.3). The lamina propria-submucosa is typical and is continuous with the fibrous periosteum of the bony roof of the buccal cavity. Adipose tissue and an extensive vascular bed are present. The caudal region of the hard palate of most species has numerous branched tubuloalveolar glands that may be mucous or mixed. The *soft palate* is a fibrous and muscular caudal extension of the hard palate. On its dorsal aspect (nasopharynx), it is covered by a pseudostratified ciliated columnar epithelium *(respiratory epithelium)*, whereas its ventral side is covered by a typical cutaneous mucous membrane. The connective tissue core may contain glands similar to those in the hard

palate. Lymphatic nodules are encountered frequently. The palatine tonsil of the pig is entirely within the soft palate.

Tongue

Histological Structure. The tongue is a cranial projection from the ventral floor of the buccal cavity that is covered by a cutaneous mucous membrane with a core of skeletal muscle.

The lamina epithelialis mucosae is variously keratinized. Numerous epidermal pegs and dermal papillae are apparent. Extensive invaginations of the dermal papillae into the epithelium result in evaginations of the mucous membrane as *lingual papillae* (Fig. 21.4). In horses and ruminants, the caudodorsal aspect of the tongue has a

thickened mucous membrane that gives rigidity to this structure. The lamina propria mucosae and tunica submucosa are typical and blend with the epimysium of the intrinsic and extrinsic lingual musculature.

The *lyssa* is characteristic of carnivores. It consists of dense white fibrous connective tissue (DWFCT), some adipose tissue, skeletal muscle, and occasionally some cartilage. In the pig, it consists primarily of adipose tissue and some connective tissue. It is not well-developed in horses and ruminants.

Lingual Papillae. *Lingual papillae* are generally confined to the dorsal aspect of the tongue. These differ in size, form, number, distribution, and function. Also, they are species-variable.

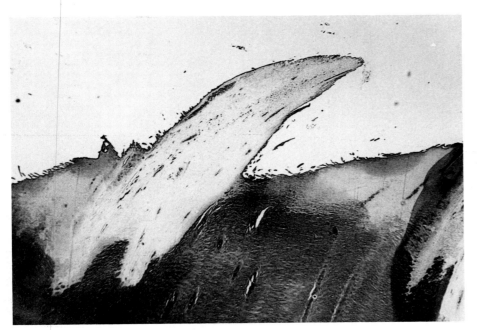

Figure 21.6. A section of typical lingual papilla from a feline tongue. This papilla is entirely an epithelial structure. ×10.

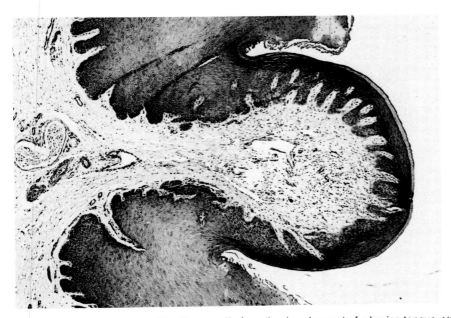

Figure 21.7. A section of typical lentiform papilla from the dorsal aspect of a bovine tongue. ×16.

Filiform papillae are numerous and well-developed in cats and ruminants wherein they serve mechanical functions (Figs. 21.5 and 21.6). The keratinized papillae are shaped like rose thorns with their curvature directed caudad. The core of lamina propria mucosae is typical.

Lenticular or *conical papillae* also serve mechanical functions (Fig. 21.7). The papillae have the form of a biconvex lens. They are especially prominent on the dorsum of the caudal one-third of the tongue.

Fungiform papillae are mushroom-shaped papillae that serve mechanical and gustatory functions (Fig. 21.8). These papillae are not as keratinized as the previous types. The primary papillation of the lamina propria mucosae is typical and secondary papillations may be present.

Foliate papillae are leaf-shaped structures separated from each other by an invagination of the mucous membrane (Fig. 21.9). These papillae have taste buds. The epithelium of these papillae is nonkeratinized. Finger-like (secondary) projections from the lamina propria mucosae are pres-

ent. Branched, tubuloalveolar, serous glands (*von Ebner's glands*) of the lamina propria-submucosa open into the base of an epithelial furrow.

Circumvallate (vallate) papillae are the largest and least encountered papillae (Fig. 21.10). These papillae are not elevated above the lamina epithelialis mucosae; they are surrounded by a deep furrow. Numerous taste buds are located in their lateral walls. The lamina propria mucosae is typical. Branched, tubuloalveolar, serous glands (von Ebner's glands) open into the base of the furrow and cleanse this region of foodstuffs.

Taste Buds. The *taste buds* of the tongue are intraepithelial structures located in the walls of foliate, fungiform, and circumvallate papillae (Figs. 21.11 and 21.12). Taste buds are ovoid masses of cells that extend from the basement membrane and open through a small canal, *taste pore*, at the surface of the epithelium. Microvillous projections of constituent cells extend into the taste pore as "taste hairs."

Three cell types have been described within the taste bud in light microscopic preparations of these structures (Fig. 21.13): *supporting (sustentacular) cells*, *gustatory cells (taste receptor)*, and *basal cells*. Supportive (dark) and gustatory (light) cells, although described as columnar cells, appear spindle-shaped. Gustatory cells have a dense cytoplasm and a vesicular nucleus. Sustentacular cells have a vacuolated cytoplasm and a dense nucleus. A basal cell, apparent in well-fixed specimens, is small and is located along the lateral and basal borders of the taste bud.

Electron microscopic studies indicate four cell types in taste buds—basal, dark, intermediate, and light cells. The basal cell is the stem cell for all of the other cell types. The dark cell differentiates from a basal cell into a light cell. Dark and light cells are receptor cells. The role of the intermediate cell needs further clarification. Cell death and turnover within this structure are rapid. New cells may differentiate from the basal cells every 10 hours, whereas the average life-span of the differentiated cells is approximately 250 hours. The maintenance of functional integrity is dependent upon new cells establishing contact with intraepithelial sensory nerve endings. Humoral substances elaborated by the nerves maintain this functional integrity.

Nerve endings within the taste buds *(intragemmal fibers)* terminate on sensory cells. The basic gustatory modalities of sour taste, sweet taste, salt taste, and water taste have been described in the dog. The distribution of the modalities on the tongue have been mapped and have been associated with various types of lingual papillae.

Teeth

General Characteristics. Although mam-

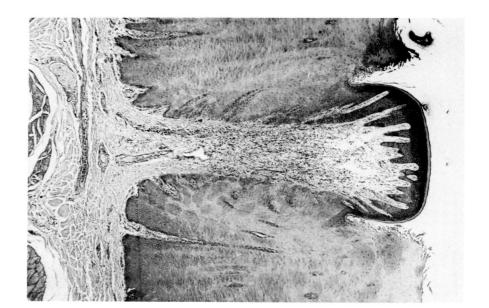

Figure 21.8. A section of typical fungiform papilla from a canine tongue. This structure may be gustatory. ×10.

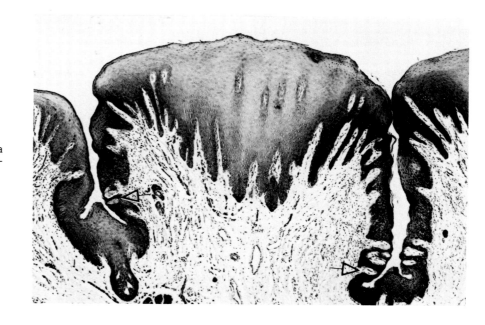

Figure 21.9. A section of typical foliate papilla from a canine tongue. These papillae are gustatory. *Arrows*, taste buds. ×16.

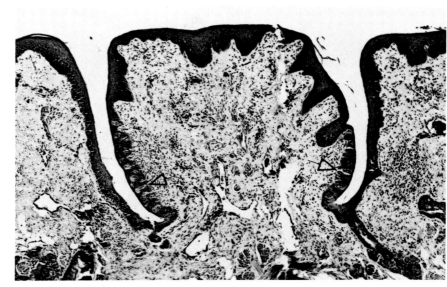

Figure 21.10. A section of typical circumvallate papilla of the canine tongue. Taste buds *(arrows)* are present. ×16.

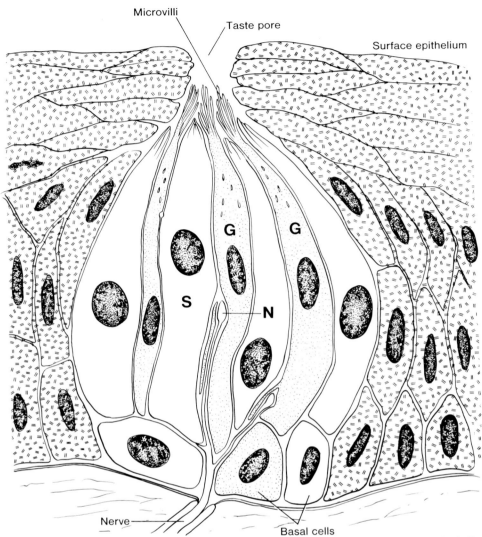

Figure 21.11. An idealized drawing of the electron microscopic appearance of a taste bud. *G*, gustatory cells; *S*, sustentacular cells; *N*, nerve ending.

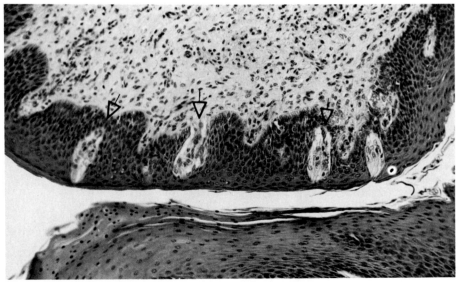

Figure 21.12. Taste buds associated with a circumvallate papilla of a canine tongue. The taste buds *(arrows)* are intraepithelial structures. ×40.

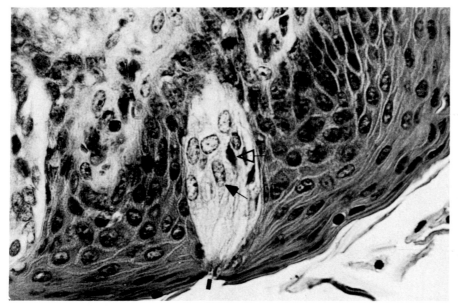

Figure 21.13. The cells of taste buds. Sustentacular cells *(open arrow)* and gustatory cells *(solid arrow)* are spindle-shaped cells. The taste pore *(bar)* opens on the epithelial surface. ×160.

malian teeth differ in gross and subgross appearance, they consist of the same components: *enamel, dentin, cementum,* and *pulp.* Teeth are either simple or complex. *Brachydont (simple)* teeth do not continue to grow at the completion of eruption (Fig. 21.14). Further, these teeth are divisible into a definitive *crown, neck,* and *root.* The *hypsodont (complex)* teeth of ruminants, rodents, and the horse are constantly erupting structures (Fig. 21.15). These teeth do not possess a definitive crown, neck, and root. Rather, they are considered to be composed of root only. The hypsodont teeth include the cheek teeth of ruminants, all of the teeth of the horse, the incisorform teeth of rodents, and the canine teeth of the pig.

Development

Dental Lamina to Cap Stage. The development of teeth requires contributions from the epithelium and the underlying connective tissue (Fig. 21.16). An epithelial ridge, *dental lamina,* develops in the *dental arch* of each jaw and grows into the underlying mesenchymal region. Epithelial proliferation along the lateral border of the lamina further extends this structure into the mesenchyme. From this lateral extension, the *enamel organs* of the *deciduous teeth (milk teeth)* arise. At a later period, medial or lingual outgrowths of the dental lamina give rise to enamel organs of the *permanent teeth.* Proliferation of the invading epithelium as a solid mass of cells continues to the *cap stage* accompanied by a mesenchymal condensation at the base of the cap (Fig. 21.17).

Enamel Organ. By complementary growth of the epithelium and associated mesenchymal tissue of the *dental papilla,* the *bell stage* is achieved (Fig. 21.18). The epithelium is now the *enamel organ* and is divisible into distinct regions: *inner enamel epithelium, stellate reticulum,* and *outer enamel epithelium* (Fig. 21.19). The *inner enamel epithelium* consists of columnar cells, *ameloblasts,* that are separated from the dental papilla by a basement membrane. The epithelium is continuous with the *outer enamel epithelium* at the lower edges (rim) of the bell. The outer epithelium is composed of small, flattened cells. The center of the enamel organ is composed of the *stellate reticulum.* The stellate cells, previously tightly packed, are separated by extensive intercellular spaces. The region of contact between the stellate reticulum and the inner enamel epithelium is occupied by cuboidal cells, the *stratum intermedium* (Fig. 21.19). As development of the tooth progresses, the stellate reticulum *(enamel pulp)* atrophies and the outer enamel epithelium collapses upon the inner enamel epithelium.

The dental papilla is entrapped within the confines of the enamel organ. A thin layer of columnar cells differentiates from the mesenchyme along the inner surface of the basement membrane, the *odontoblasts.* The remainder of the papilla becomes the pulp of the tooth. It consists of blood vessels, nerves, and loose connective tissue.

Dental Sac. A condensed mass of con-

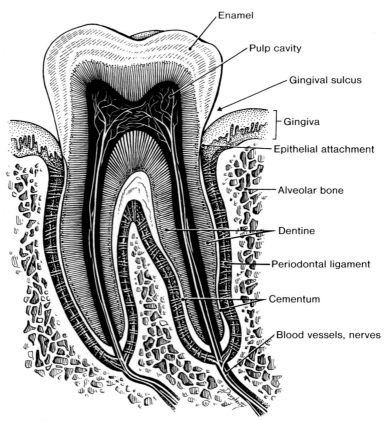

Figure 21.14. A diagram of a brachydont, molariform tooth.

- Enamel
- Pulp cavity
- Gingival sulcus
- Gingiva
- Epithelial attachment
- Alveolar bone
- Dentine
- Periodontal ligament
- Cementum
- Blood vessels, nerves

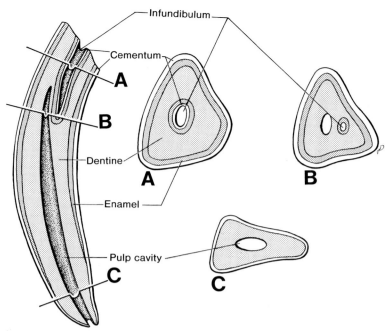

Figure 21.15. Idealized drawings of sections of a hypsodont, incisorform tooth of a horse. The entire peripheral surface is covered by cementum.

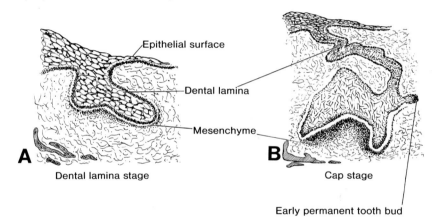

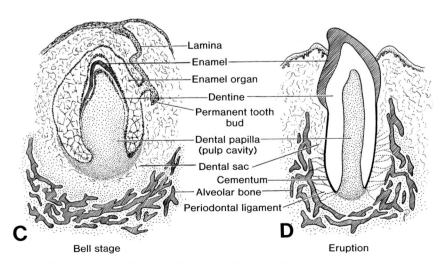

Figure 21.16. A series of diagrams of early development of a deciduous branchydont tooth. *A*. The surface epithelium proliferates and invaginates into the underlying mesenchyme as the dental lamina. *B*. The attached epithelial mass begins to cavitate adjacent to the mesenchymal condensation. *C*. The enamel organ forms during the bell stage. Enamel and dentin have begun to form. *D*. Eruption has occurred. Dentin and cementum are added continually until complete eruption is achieved.

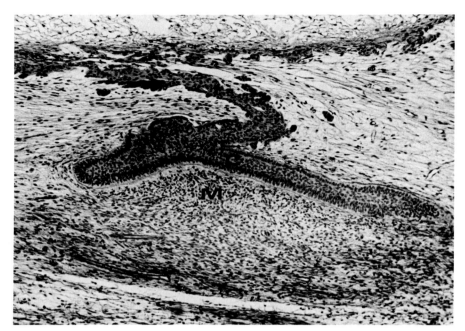

Figure 21.17. Cap stage of a secondary tooth bud. The enamel organ is still a condensed mass of epithelial cells *(C)* associated with mesenchyme *(M)*. The mesenchymal condensation indicated is destined to become dental pulp. ×25.

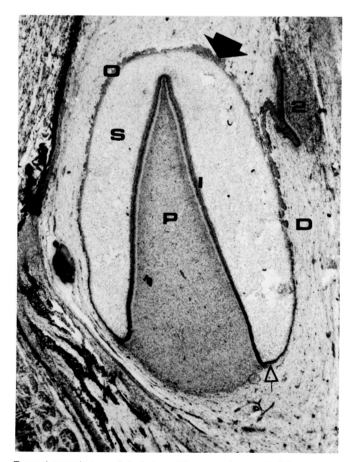

Figure 21.18. Enamel organ in an early bell stage. The enamel organ *(solid arrow)* has a permanent tooth bud attached to it *(2)*. The enamel organ consists of an outer enamel epithelium *(O)* that is continuous with the inner enamel epithelium *(I)* at the rim of the organ *(open arrow)*. The stellate reticulum *(S)* is between the inner and outer epithelial layers. The enamel organ surrounds a mesenchymal condensation, the dental papilla *(P)*. *D*, dental sac. ×6.

nective tissue, *dental sac*, circumscribes the enamel organ and the dental papilla. The dental sac: gives rise to the *alveolar bone* and periosteum surrounding the root; forms a layer of *cementum* peripheral to the dentine of the root; forms a network of anchoring collagenous fibers that connect the cementum of the root to the alveolar bone, the *periodontal membrane*.

Crown and Root Formation. Deposition of enamel is achieved by the secretory activity of ameloblasts. This appositional process proceeds from the apex of the papilla toward the gingiva and rim of the bell. The process is initiated after the deposition of secretory products from the odontoblasts. The odontoblasts secrete their products in such a way that predentine and dentine are deposited at the apex of the papilla, laterally toward the rim, and in a direction opposite to enamel deposition. This process, also, is appositional. Ameloblasts and odontoblastic activity results in the formation of the *crown* of the tooth. The cells secrete their products and retreat away from the matrix; the ameloblasts retreat outwardly and the ondontoblasts, inwardly.

At the point of continuity between the inner and outer enamel epithelium (the future *neck* region of the tooth), a fold of epithelium develops and grows downwardly as the *epithelial root sheath (sheath of Hertwig)*. Dentin continues to develop in this region. Instead of enamel, however, the mesenchyme interdigitates itself between the odontoblasts and the root sheath and cementum develops. The root, therefore, consists of cementum and dentin. The transition from crown to root is the *neck* of the tooth.

Eruption. As the aforementioned processes are occurring, the dental sac gives rise to the alveolar bone and other structures. The downward growth of the root exerts pressure against the stationary alveolar bone. This pressure is translated into upward movement or *eruption*. During eruption, the crown of the tooth breaks through the enamel organ and gingiva. Ameloblastic activity ceases at eruption. The continued deposition of the root during eruption, however, results in the definitive positions of the tooth being achieved.

The subsequent development of the enamel organ of permanent teeth progresses through the same sequence outlined previously. As permanent tooth buds develop, their growth exerts pressure against the roots and associated structures of the deciduous teeth. This pressure results in resorption of the roots of the deciduous teeth and associated alveolar bone. The loss of the deciduous teeth is followed closely by replacement with permanent teeth.

Cellular and Matrical Components

Ameloblasts and Enamel. *Ameloblasts*

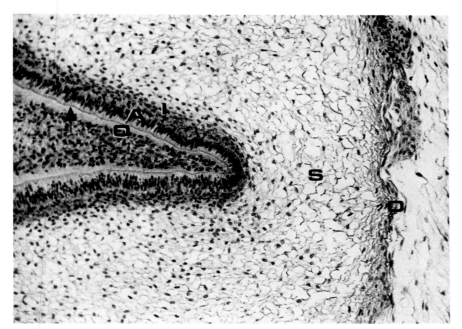

Figure 21.19. Components of the enamel organ. The outer enamel epithelium *(O-right)* is adjacent to the stellate reticulum (S). A layer of cuboidal cells, stratum intermedium *(I)*, underlies the inner enamel epithelium, which is composed of ameloblasts *(A)*. The ameloblasts are separated from the ondotoblasts *(O-left)* of the dental papilla by a basement membrane *(arrow)*. ×40.

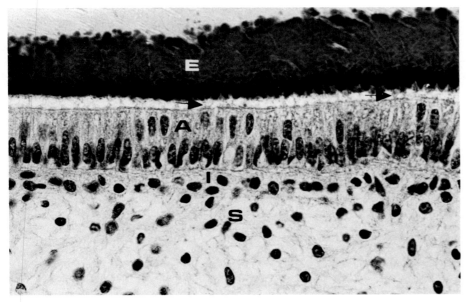

Figure 21.20. Layer of ameloblasts. The ameloblasts *(A)* are associated intimately with the stratum intermedium *(I)* the cells of which are continuous with the stellate reticulum *(S)*. Enamel *(E)* has been deposited and Tome's processes *(arrows)* are apparent. ×160.

are columnar cells that appear hexagonal in cross section (Fig. 21.20). These polarized cells have an elongated, basally positioned nucleus. The basal part of the cell is rich in mitochondria. The apical portion of the cell is rich in granular endoplasmic reticulum and Golgi apparatus. At the apex of the cell, *Tome's processes* (prismatic extensions of ameloblastic apical cytoplasm) are apparent. Material for enamel formation is secreted through these processes in the form of slightly mineralized rods. During the secretory processes, the ameloblasts retreat outwardly before the advancing front of their secretory products. The result is an acellular enamel composed of rods and inter-rod material. The basic structural unit of enamel is the *enamel rod*. Each enamel rod, as evident in demineralized sections viewed with the electron microscope, consists of glycoproteinaceous tubular subunits. Each Tome's process forms the rods; the base of the process forms the *inter-rod* matrix. Mineralization is progressive and is initiated in the enamel rods. The mineral content of rod and inter-rod matrices is identical; however, the orientation of tubular subunits and crystalline materials differ. During development, the most mineralized enamel matrix occurs at the dentino-enamel junction. The least mineralized occurs at the retreating front of ameloblasts.

Enamel consists of approximately 95–97% inorganic material in the form of apatite crystal. It is the hardest substance in the body. Since the ameloblasts eventually disintegrate, enamel is incapable of repair.

Odontoblasts and Dentin. *Odontoblasts* are not tightly packed together (Fig. 21.21). These columnar cells are also polarized. The predominant organelles are the apically disposed granular endoplasmic reticulum and a large supranuclear Golgi apparatus. The initial secretory product of the odontoblasts is *predentin*. It is deposited initially at the dentino-enamel junction and contains *odontoblastic processes (Tome's fibers, dentinal fibers)*. As predentin is secreted, the odontoblasts retreat before the advancing front, but their processes remain and are contained within *dentinal tubules*. Subsequent mineralization of predentin results in *dentin*. This method of secretion is similar to the relationship between osteoid seam and mineralizing bone. Dentin contains about 69% inorganic substances.

Unlike ameloblasts, odontoblasts do not disintegrate upon the completion of their secretory activity. Rather, they are viable and potentially functional cells throughout the life of a tooth.

Cementoblasts and Cementum. *Cementoblasts* are differentiated from the dental sac and give rise to *acellular cementum* and *cellular cementum*. This material with its contained *cementocytes* is very similar to woven or immature bone. Sharpey's fibers become embedded in cementum by an appositional growth of cementum around the collagenous fibers. This process is similar to the means by which the collagen of tendons is incorporated in and attached to bone.

Dental Pulp. *Dental pulp* is the connective tissue from the dental papilla that lines the pulp cavity. The dental pulp contains numerous vessels and nerves within a loose connective tissue framework. These structures enter or exit the pulp cavity through the apical foramen in each root. *Secondary dentin* formation continues throughout the life of the tooth gradually reducing the size of the pulp cavity.

Associated Structures

Periodontal Membrane. The *periodontal*

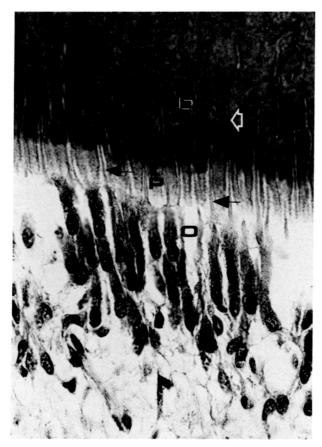

Figure 21.21. Layer of odontoblasts. The odontoblasts *(O)* have apical processes, dentinal fibers *(solid arrows)*, that extend into dentinal tubules *(open arrow)*. Predentin *(P)* is secreted and then mineralized as dentin *(D)*. ×160.

membrane (ligament) consists of coarsely bundled collagenous fibers and fibroblasts. These fibers are embedded in the cementum and associated alveolar bone as Sharpey's fibers. They anchor the tooth in the *alveolus (socket)* and are ruptured during tooth extraction. The teeth are suspended within the alveolus by virtue of the collagenous fibers of this structure.

Epithelial Attachment. The eruption of the teeth through the gingiva creates a break in this cutaneous mucous membrane. The continuity of the barrier is maintained, however, through the attachment of the gingival epithelium to the neck of the tooth. The *gingival crevice* or *gingival sulcus* is the depression between the tooth and gingiva above the point of epithelial attachment (Fig. 21.14). The gingival sulcus and epithelial attachment are especially significant in periodontal disease. *Tartar* or *calculus* commonly accumulates on the tooth in the gingival sulcus. Breaks in the epithelial attachment provide an entry portal for microbial agents and debris into the vital tissues of the periodontal ligament, resulting in periodontitis.

Types of Dentition

Brachydont Dentition. The *crown* of the tooth is covered by enamel and is visible above the *gingiva* (Fig. 21.14). The crown is composed of enamel and dentin. The dentin is visible on the surface in worn teeth from which the enamel has been removed by constant abrasion. The *neck* of the tooth is the point of transition between the crown and the root. It is the point of *epithelial attachment* to the cementum. The root is composed of dentin and cementum in apposition to one another. The periodontal membrane serves as the suspension mechanism between the alveolar bone and cementum of the root. The dental pulp is a loose connective tissue rich in vascular supply and nerves. It is bounded by the dentin of the crown and root (or roots).

Hypsodont Dentition. Constantly erupting teeth differ from the brachydont teeth (Fig. 21.15). This difference is based upon some alterations in the developmental sequence. In brachydont teeth, the enamel organ is intact until the time of eruption. In hypsodont teeth, the enamel organ ruptures before eruption. This brings the connective tissue of the dental sac into close association with the newly formed enamel. As a result, cementum is deposited on the enamel. Also, the resulting morphology of

the mature hyposodont tooth, especially the *infundibular recess*, requires that the enamel organ is more complex in surface morphology than that of simple teeth.

In brachydont teeth, the eruption of the crown is accompanied by the disintegration of the ameloblasts. In hypsodont teeth, ameloblasts do not disintegrate. They continue their activity for an extended period beyond eruption. Although hypsodont teeth are described as root teeth without a definitive crown, neck, and root, this is not entirely true. A typical root (cementum and dentin) is confined to the lower portion of the tooth (Fig. 21.15).

Pharynx

Histology. The *oropharynx* is the extension of the buccal cavity that connects with the esophagus. The lamina epithelialis mucosae is stratified squamous epithelium. Varying degrees of keratinization are species variable. The lamina propria mucosae is typical and contains tonsils, individual lymph nodules, and scattered leukocytes. Numerous papillae are obvious and resemble dermal papillae of the skin. Although a typical lamina mucularis mucosae is not present, a layer of elastic fibers delimits this space from the tunica submucosa. The latter is typical and contains branched, tubuloalveolar, mucous glands. The tunica muscularis is composed of striated muscle that is not oriented in any particular manner. The tunica adventitia is typical and blends with the accompanying deep fascia.

Esophagus

This structure is a muscular tube that is modified for the voluntary and involuntary movement of foodstuffs to and from the stomach.

Mucosa. The lamina epithelialis mucosae is stratified squamous epithelium. Varying degrees of cornification may be apparent; it is apparent in species that ingest hard, dry foodstuffs.

The lamina propria mucosae is typical and may contain numerous lymph nodules and scattered lymphatic tissue (man and pig). These are especially prominent at the esophageal-gastric junction.

The lamina muscularis mucosae is typical but of variable occurrence (Fig. 21.22). This muscular layer is continuous with the elastic fiber layer of the pharynx. It is thick and complete in man. In horses, ruminants, and cats, it consists of scattered muscle bundles that may fuse in the aboral portion of the esophagus. In the dog and pig, it is absent in the cervical portion but may become complete near the stomach (Fig. 21.23).

Submucosa. The tunica submucosa is typical and contains numerous branched, tubuloalveolar, mucous glands. These glands are present the entire length of the

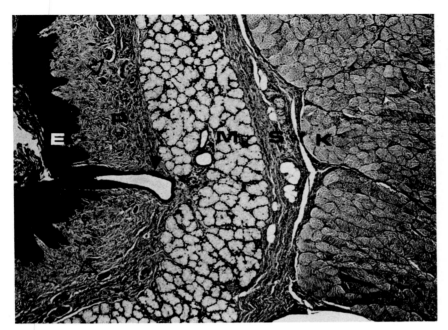

Figure 21.22. Porcine esophagus (lower cervical region). The lamina epithelialis mucosae *(E)* is supported by a lamina propria mucosae *(P)*. The lamina muscularis mucosae consists of scattered bundles of smooth muscle *(open arrows)*. Mucous glands *(M)* are continuous with the epithelial lining via excretory ducts *(solid arrow)*. A tunica submucosa *(S)* is adjacent to the skeletal muscle *(K)* of the tunica muscularis. ×12.

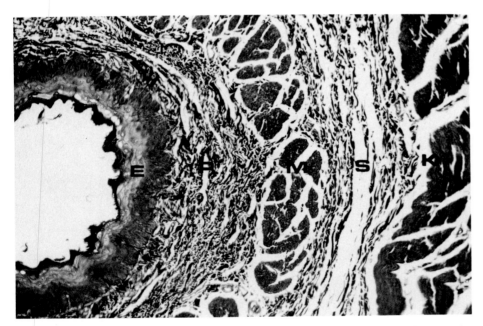

Figure 21.23. Canine esophagus (thoracic region). The lamina epithelialis mucosae *(E)* and lamina propria mucosae *(P)* are typical. The lamina muscularis mucosae *(M)* is extensive. *S*, tunica submucosa; *K*, skeletal muscle of tunica muscularis. ×40.

canine esophagus; in pigs they are present in the cervical portion but sparse in the thoracic portion; in ruminants, horses, and cats they are present in the cervical portion.

The tunica mucosa and tunica submucosa have longitudinal folds that permit expansion of the esophagus.

Muscularis. The tunica muscularis consists of striated muscle, smooth muscle, or a mixture of both. The inner and outer lamina may be distinct in the aboral portion. In ruminants and dogs, the tunic is entirely striated (Fig. 21.24); in pigs, the cervical portion consists of striated muscle,

the thoracic portion is mixed and the caudal portion consists of smooth muscle; in horses and cats, it consists of striated muscle to the middle portion and then consists of smooth muscle.

Serosa/Adventitia. The tunica adventitia or tunica serosa is typical.

Histophysiology. The esophagus has properties that relate to the distribution and type of muscle that comprises the tunica muscularis. The ease of vomition and/or regurgitation in ruminants and the dog is linked to the distribution of skeletal muscle throughout the course of the esophagus. Although emesis and regurgitation are abnormal physiological events in the dog, regurgitation is a normal physiological event in the digestive sequences of ruminants. The pig and cat are capable of vomiting in response to sufficient irritation occuring within the pharynx and stomach. Despite the distribution of skeletal muscle within the cranial two-thirds of the esophagus of the horse, vomition is rare in this species.

The pharyngoesophageal and gastroesophageal junctions serve as physiological sphincters that are capable of maintaining intraesophageal luminal pressure higher than intragastric pressure. The "caudal esophageal sphincter" of the horse has sufficient tone that it remains closed during gastric dilation to the point of gastric rupture without vomiting occurring.

During deglutition, food is propelled into the pharynx by the caudal movement of the tongue. Coordinated voluntary and involuntary muscular activities permit the food to pass through the "pharyngoesophageal sphincter" and into the esophagus. The distention of the cranial esophagus initiates a wave of peristalsis that moves the bolus aborad. Relaxation of the "gastroesophageal sphincter" permits food to enter the stomach.

General visceral afferent and efferent fibers innervate esophageal smooth muscle and glands. Because most domestic species have either all skeletal muscle or a preponderance of skeletal muscle in the tunica muscularis of the esophagus, the innervation of these muscle fibers probably originates as special visceral efferent fibers.

Esophageal dysfunction can result from a number of causes in the dog (foreign body, stricture, perforation). Regurgitation of foodstuffs, not vomition, is the pathognomonic sign of obstructive esophageal disease. Often, surgical intervention is considered in such cases. Unfortunately, the healing potential of the esophagus is less than optimum and leakage into the surrounding regions is common. Poor tissue strength coupled with a minimal amount of adventitial or serosal connective tissue complicates the healing process. A marginal segmental blood supply and the constant movement of thoracic organs (heart, lungs) compounds the healing process. The serosal tunics of visceral organs are effective

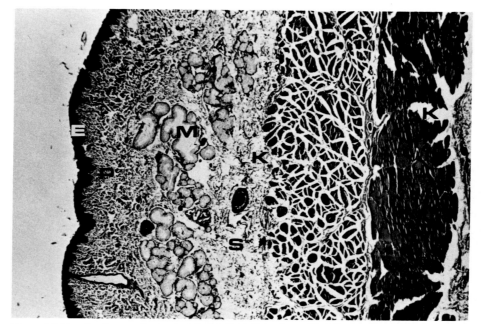

Figure 21.24. Canine esophagus (cervical region). *E*, lamina epithelialis mucosae; *P*, lamina propria mucosae; *M*, mucous glands; *S*, tunica submucosa; *K*, skeletal muscle of tunica muscularis. A lamina muscularis mucosae is not present. ×10.

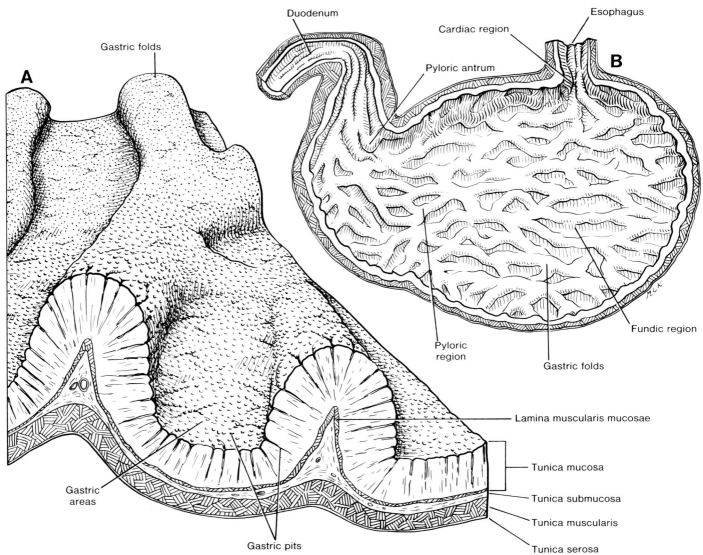

Figure 21.25. A drawing of a longitudinal section of a canine stomach *(B)*. A portion of the wall is enlarged *(A)*.

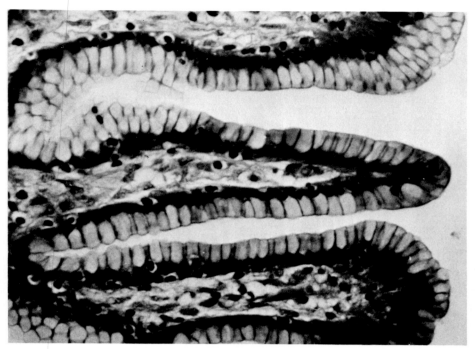

Figure 21.26. Lining cells of an equine stomach. Note the clear zone in the apical portion of the cells. ×160.

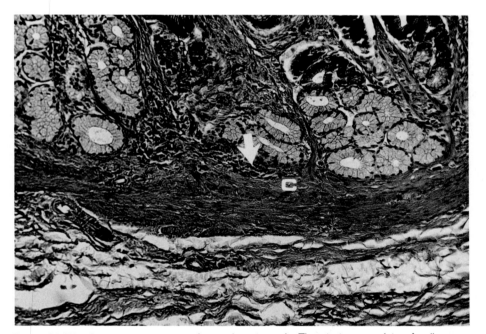

Figure 21.27. Stratum compactum of a canine stomach. The stratum consists of collagenous fibers *(C)*. Note the hypercellularity of the lamina propria mucosae *(arrow)*. ×40.

sealants. The cervical esophagus, however, is devoid of a tunica serosa, and the thoracic esophagus is not associated intimately with a tunica serosa.

Glandular Stomach

Structure

General Characteristics. The *glandular stomach* is modified as an enlarged tube that assumes a sac-like configuration when filled with food. Foodstuffs delayed within the stomach are subjected to the enzymatic and hydrolytic action of gastric juice. The muscular wall of the organ induces the mechanical mixing and breakdown of the foodstuffs. Peristaltic waves of contraction propel the mixed and partially digested foodstuffs *(chyme)* to the duodenum.

Mucosa. The mucosa and part of the submucosa have tortuous folds, *plicae gastricae (gastric folds)* oriented parallel to the long axis of the organ (Fig. 21.25). The prominence of these folds, although not completely effacable, varies inversely with the degree of gastric distention. The epithelial surface is divided into smaller irregular units called *gastric areas (areae gastricae)* by numerous small grooves. The gastric areas are marked with numerous small depressions, *gastic pits (foveolae gastricae)*, into the bottom of which the gastric glands open. The depth of the gastric pits varies with specific regions of the stomach.

The lamina epithelialis mucosae of the stomach, including the gastric pits, is simple columnar epithelium. The lining cells are mucus-secreting. Because mucinogen is not preserved by routine histological preparations, the entire apical portion of the gastric lining cells has a clear zone (Fig. 21.26). The size and the shape of the clear zone varies but is a prominent cellular feature. The shape of the nucleus varies from oval to spheroidal. The shape of gastric lining cells, as well as the chemical composition of its mucinogen, differs from the mucous cells of gastric glands and typical goblet cells. The lining cells become more cuboidal at the openings of the gastric glands. The gastric lining cells are devoid of a striated border; however, some microvilli are present.

The lamina propria mucosae is typical. The connective tissue space usually has numerous lymphocytes, macrophages, and plasma cells that impart a distinct hypercellularity. Scattered lymphatic follicles may be present.

The actual thickness of the lamina propria mucosae varies with the region of the stomach. Gastric glands, which are continuous with the gastric lining cells, penetrate variable distances into the lamina propria mucosae. Although the lamina propria mucosae may be thick, the actual connective tissue constituents are scant, because they are interdigitated between the numerous gastric glands.

The lamina propria mucosae may contain a distinct *stratum compactum* at the junction of the lamina propria mucosae and the lamina muscularis mucosae (Fig. 21.27). This stratum consists of a DWFCT. This stratum, especially well-developed in carnivores, may protect the stomach from perforation by sharp objects.

A lamina muscularis mucosae is present, but its arrangement is variable. Two to four muscle layers may comprise this lamina. The smooth muscle fibers are oriented longitudinally and circularly. Thin strands of smooth muscle extend into the lamina propria mucosae between the glands.

Submucosa. The tunica submucosa is typical. Neuronal fibers and ganglion cell cytons form the *submucosal plexus (Meissner's plexus).*

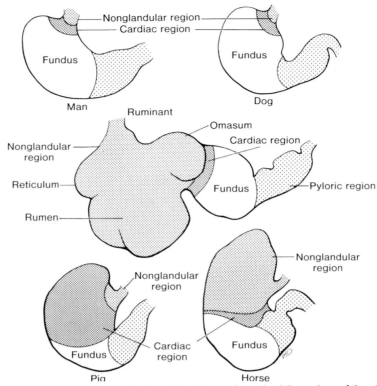

Figure 21.28. A diagram of the distribution of glandular and nonglandular regions of the stomachs of selected animals. The regions indicated are glandular regions. The organs are not drawn to scale.

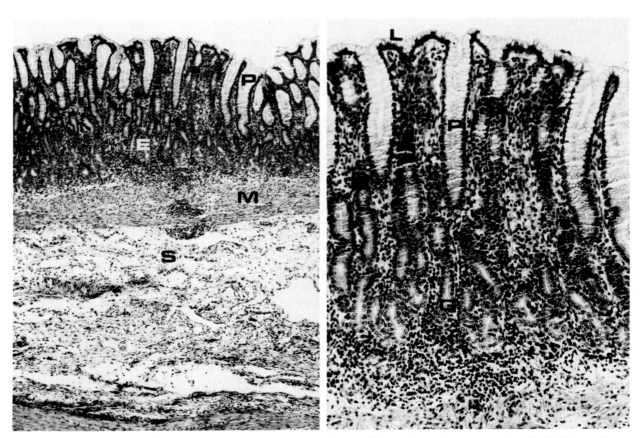

Figure 21.29. Cardiac region of a canine stomach. A simple columnar epithelium (E) lines the surface and gastric pits (P). The lamina muscularis mucosae (M) and tunica submucosa (S) are typical. ×16.

Figure 21.30. Cardiac glands of a canine stomach. The lamina epithelialis mucosae is composed of a simple epithelium that lines the lumen (L), gastric pits (P), and cardiac glands (G). ×40.

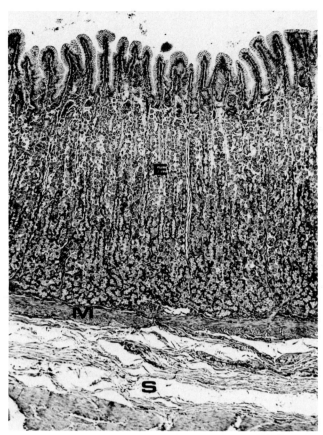

Figure 21.31. Fundic region of a canine stomach. The lamina epithelialis mucosae *(E)* is highly folded. The tunica mucosa is very thick. The lamina muscularis mucosae *(M)* and tunica submucosa *(S)* are typical. ×16.

Muscularis. The tunica muscularis mucosae is typical. Constituent neurons and neuronal processes form the *myenteric plexus (Auerbach's plexus)* between the inner and outer laminae of smooth muscle (Fig. 17.11).

Serosa. The tunica serosa is typical.

Glandular Regions

Regional differences in the tunica mucosa of the stomach permit the histological identification of four distinct gastric regions: esophageal region, cardiac gland region, fundic gland region, and pyloric gland region (Fig. 21.28).

Esophageal Region. The esophageal region of the stomach is the nonglandular portion of the stomach that is lined by stratified squamous epithelium. Keratinization may be present but is dependent upon species and diet.

Cardiac Gland Region. The cardiac gland region is not developed equally in all species (Fig. 21.29). The beginning of the cardiac gland region is marked by a transition from stratified squamous to columnar epithelium.

The *cardiac glands* are branched, tubular, coiled glands (Fig. 21.30). The neck is that portion of the structure nearest the opening of the gastric pit. The body is the remainder of the adenomere. The neck and upper portion of the body are lined by mucus-secreting, cuboidal cells. The remaining cells of the gland are columnar, mucus-secreting cells. Some *parietal cells* may be present in the canine cardiac gland region, whereas some *chief cells* may be present in porcine cardiac glands.

Argentaffin cells (enterochromaffin cells) are small, pyramidal cells with a clear cytoplasm that are located between glandular lining cells and the basement membrane. Special silver staining techniques demonstrate these cells and their numerous silver-containing granules that are located in an abluminal or infranuclear position. Electron microscopic and immunocytological techniques have been used to demonstrate as many as ten different cell types that correspond to argentaffin cells.

The argentaffin cells do not secrete materials into the lumen of the organ. Rather, their products are secreted into the lamina propria mucosae and are distributed by the blood vessels. These cells are hormone-secreting, *gastrointestinal endocrine cells (enteroendocrine cells)*. Secretions of these cells include: *serotonin, histamine, somatostatin, gastrin, endorphins,* and *enteroglucagon.* The secretory and muscular activities of the gastrointestinal organs, including the pancreas and gallbladder, are controlled to a considerable extent by the release of these hormones in response to the changing properties and constituents of luminal contents.

Fundic Gland Region. The *fundic gland region* is similar to the cardiac region (Fig. 21.28). The glands of the fundic region, *fundic glands* or *gastric glands proper,* are branched, tubular glands that are longer than but less frequently branched than their cardiac region counterparts (Fig. 21.31). The length of the fundic glands thickens the lamina propria mucosae (Figs. 21.29 and 21.31). The amount of connective tissue within the lamina propria mucosae is reduced greatly because the glands are packed tightly (Fig. 21.32).

A fundic gland is divisible into four regions: *base, body, neck,* and *isthmus.* The isthmus or opening of the gland is continuous with the constricted neck. The body or main tubular portion of the gland continues from the neck and terminates as a slightly dilated and bent adenomere, the base.

Three cell types are distinguishable readily in routine preparations of fundic glands: *chief cells (zymogen cells), parietal cells,* and *mucous neck cells.* A fourth cell type, the *enteroendocrine cells,* may be seen occasionally or may be demonstrated with special techniques. A fifth cell type, *transitional cell,* is described occasionally in the isthmus. Transitional cells are cuboidal cells that may be responsible for the replacement of lining and glandular epithelial cells.

Mucous neck cells line the neck of the gland and are interspersed among parietal cells. Mucous neck cells are cuboidal or low columnar cells with a pale-staining cytoplasm (Fig. 21.33). The mucoid product of these cells differs from that of the surface lining cells but is similar to the mucoid secretion of the cardiac and pyloric glands. The mucus of the neck cells is less viscous than that of the surface lining cells and contains acidic glycosaminoglycans. The secretory product of the mucous neck cells may protect the fundic gland from the proteolytic and hydrolytic activity of the proteases and hydrochloric acid. Mucous neck cells may be capable of differentiating into surface lining and/or glandular lining cells.

Chief cells (zymogen cells) are the predominant cells of the fundic glands (Fig. 21.34). They are pyramidal-shaped cells with a basally positioned round nucleus. Apically positioned secretory granules *(zymogen granules)* are present in fasted animals; however, the cells are labile to fixation and the secretory granules may be leached from the cell, imparting an apical foamy appearance (Fig. 21.35). The basal portion of the chief cells contains numerous rough endoplasmic reticular profiles

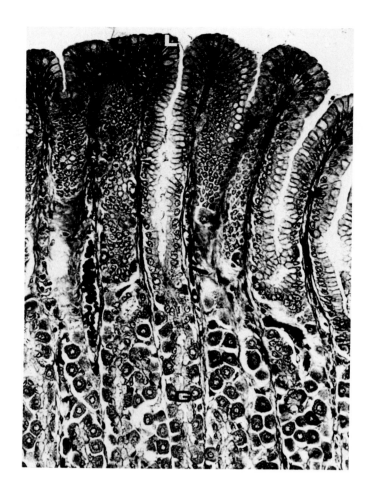

Figure 21.32. Gastric pits and fundic glands of the canine stomach. The lining epithelium *(L)* is columnar, extends into the gastric pits and is continuous with the lining cells of the fundic glands *(G)*. Note the reduced amount of connective tissue between the fundic glands, as evidenced by the intimate juxtaposition of adenomeres. ×63.

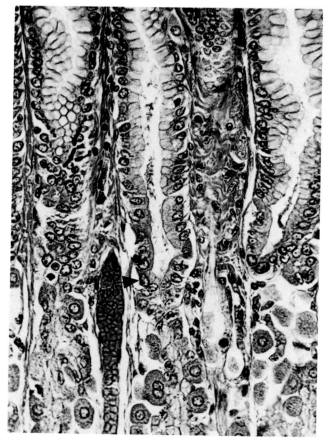

Figure 21.33. Mucous neck cells of the fundic glands of a canine stomach. The neck of the gland is constricted *(arrow)* and is lined by mucous neck cells *(arrow)*. The secretory product of these cells is mucoid; however, the mucoid product differs from that of surface lining cells. ×100.

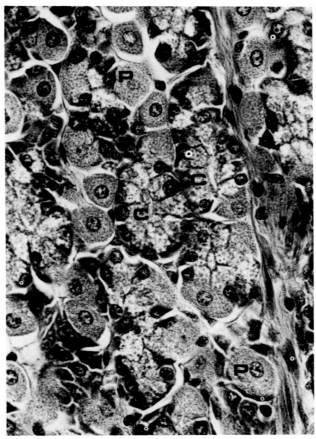

Figure 21.34. Chief cells and parietal cells of the fundic glands of a canine stomach. The chief cells *(C)* have granules along their apical borders. The parietal cells *(P)* are granular and acidophilic. ×160.

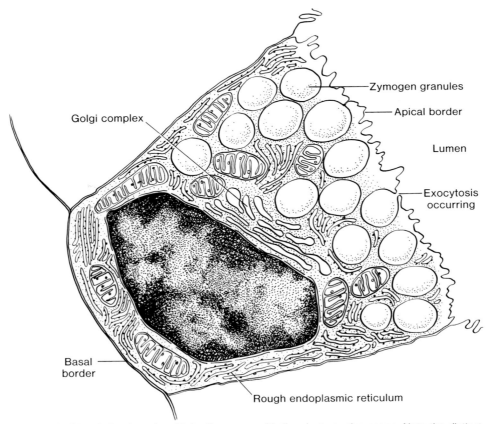

Figure 21.35. A drawing of a chief cell as seen with the electron microscope. Note the distinct cellular polarity.

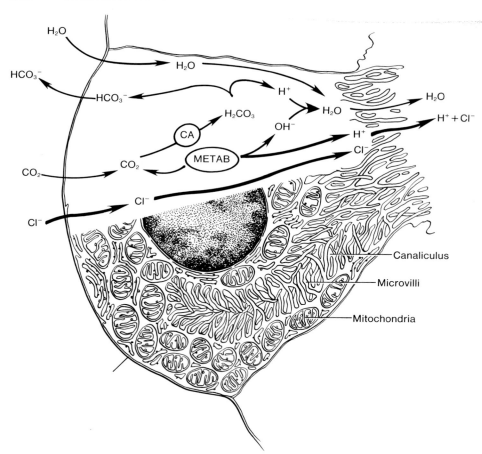

Figure 21.36. A drawing of a parietal cell as seen with the electron microscope. The upper portion of the cell demonstrates the metabolic pathways involved in the synthesis and secretion of hydrochloric acid. Carbon dioxide (CO_2) diffuses into the cell as well as being one of the products of metabolism *(METAB)*. Carbon dioxide is hydrated to carbonic acid (H_2CO_3) under the influence of carbonic anhydrase (CA). Carbonic acid dissociates into hydrogen ion (H^+) and bicarbonate (HCO_3^-). Bicarbonate diffuses into the interstitium. Chloride ion diffuses into the cell, is coupled with H^+ and is transported actively into the lumen of the gland as hydrochloric acid. (See Gastric Acid Secretion.)

and free ribosomes that impart a distinct basophilia. The chief cells are responsible for the synthesis and secretion of gastric enzymes—pepsin, rennin, and gastric lipase.

Parietal cells (oxyntic cells) are distinguished easily from the other cells of the fundic glands because of their bright-staining, acidophilic cytoplasm (Fig. 21.34). They are large cells scattered throughout the gland from neck to base. Their spheroidal or pyramidal configuration with a round nucleus is a distinctive feature (Plate II.7). Parietal cells are "wedged" between the chief cells. Although their basal borders are in contact with the basement membrane, not all of the cells reach the luminal surface directly. Numerous canaliculi extend from the apical plasmalemma as invaginations into the cytoplasm proper (Fig. 21.36). The canaliculi appear to be occluded by numerous microvilli projecting into these spaces. Apical microvilli also

extend between the chief cells and reach the luminal surface. Parietal cells elaborate hydrochloric acid. Also, they may secrete *intrinsic factor*, a substance necessary for the absorption of vitamin B_{12} *(extrinsic factor)* in man. Carnivores probably do not require intrinsic factor for the absorption of vitamin B_{12}.

Pyloric Gland Region. The histological organization of the *pyloric gland region* is similar to the cardiac gland region (Fig. 21.37). The gastric pits are deeper than in other regions of the stomach, but the pyloric glands are similar to the cardiac glands (Fig. 21.38). The pyloric glands are short, simple, or branched tubular glands. The predominant cell is the mucus-secreting cell.

The remaining mural elements are typical; however, a well-developed inner circular lamina of the tunica muscularis is a striking feature of this area. It forms the *pyloric sphincter* at the *gastroduodenal junction* (Fig. 21.39).

Histophysiology

Gastric Motility. The musculature of the stomach is contracting continually. When emptied, mild peristaltic contractile waves begin and increase in intensity over a period of hours. When food enters the canine stomach, an initial period of relaxation is followed by slow waves of contraction *(gastric slow wave)*. These originate from the longitudinal musculature along the rostral portion of the greater curvature. Food is moved toward the pylorus by these propulsive waves of contraction. Subsequently, peristaltic waves originating in the antrum, *antral peristalsis*, propel liquid contents into the duodenum while preventing solid masses of foodstuffs from gaining access to the small intestine. Gastric slow waves are the pacemakers for antral peristalsis. Chyme is gradually and continually squirted into the duodenum. The antrum, pylorus, and cranial duodenum probably function as a contractile unit. Regurgitation of chyme from the duodenum back into the stomach does not occur normally, because the contraction of the pylorus persists longer than that of the cranial duodenum.

Gastric emptying is achieved when antral contractions overcome the resistance of the pyloric sphincter. The rate at which the stomach empties is influenced by the type of food in the diet. Duodenal distention with chyme, increased acidity, and the products of proteolysis activate a neural reflex that decreases gastric motility, the *enterogastric reflex*. Gastric inhibitory peptide and *vasoactive intestinal peptide*, factors that have been isolated from the intestinal mucous, have an inhibitory effect upon gastric motility and secretion. The neural and humoral regulatory mediators permit the small intestine to achieve a more complete digestion of the substances present.

Secretory Activity. *Gastric juice* is the combined secretory product of the lining and glandular epithelial cells of the stomach. Normal gastric juice consists of various organic and inorganic components: Na^+, K^+, Mg^{++}, H^+, Cl^-, $HPO_4^=$, $SO_4^=$, pepsin, rennin (in young animals), lipase, mucus, and water. The function of the mucus is to protect the mucosa from being irritated or digested. The pH of gastric juice, approximately 1.0, is sufficiently strong to damage the mucosa were it not for the mucous coating.

Gastric secretion is controlled and influenced by several mechanisms and is divided conveniently into three phases: *cephalic, gastric, and intestinal.*

The *cephalic phase* represents the reflex activation of the stomach (motility and secretion) in response to the thought, sight, smell, or taste of food. Activity in the brain stimulates the dorsal motor nucleus of the

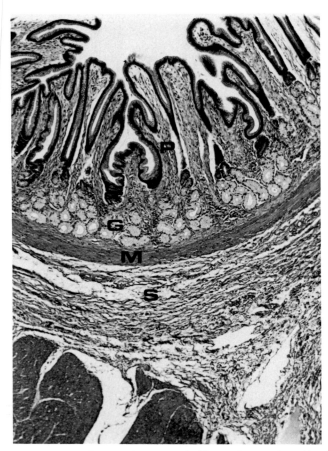

Figure 21.37. Pyloric region of the canine stomach. The surface and gastric pits are typical. Because the tunica mucosa is not as highly folded as in other regions of the stomach, the lamina propria mucosae *(P)* is more visible. Pyloric glands *(G)* are present. The lamina muscularis mucosae *(M)* and tunica submucosa are typical *(S)*. ×16.

vagus nerve. Vagal stimulation also mediates *gastrin* release from enteroendocrine cells within the pyloric antrum. The gastric juice secreted during the cephalic phase has a high concentration of hydrogen ion and is rich in pepsin.

The *gastric phase* of gastric secretion begins when food enters the stomach and continues until gastric emptying is accomplished. The vagus nerve and gastrin are the influencing factors during this phase. The presence of food in the stomach and the distention of this organ are influential. Antral distention also causes the release of gastrin. Similarly, various chemicals present in the partially digested food (meat extracts, amino acids, ethyl alcohol) also stimulate the release of gastrin. Gastrin release in response to local mechanical and chemical factors is mediated through an intrinsic reflex. Intrinsic stimulation of the stomach seems to be the more important mechanism. Histamine is also a potent stimulator of gastric secretion.

The main effect of gastrin upon the stomach is the stimulation of chief and parietal cells. Hydrochloric acid inhibits gastrin secretion.

The *intestinal phase* of gastric secretion has a positive and negative effect upon gastric acitivity. As chyme enters the intestine its constituents function as *secretagogues*; i.e., compounds capable of causing secretion. The secretagogues cause the release of gastrin from the intestinal mucosa *(enteric gastrin)*. Food in the small intestine stimulates the *enterogastric reflex*, an inhibitory reflex to the stomach. Gastric motility, therefore, is decreased when the small intestine is full of chyme. Various secretagogues stimulate the release of *secretin* and *cholecystokinin* from the duodenal mucosa. These hormones antagonize the effects of gastrin upon the stomach. Additionally, *gastric inhibitory peptide* inhibits gastric secretion.

The events of the intestinal phase are predominately inhibitory upon the stomach. They ensure a more complete digestion of the chyme and combine to retard the delivery of chyme to a small intestine that is full.

Gastric Acid Secretion. Hydrochloric acid secretion by parietal cells requires an expenditure of energy, because the acid is moved against a concentration gradient.

The concentration of hydrogen ions in gastric juice is approximately 3 million times greater than that in plasma. The energy for this process is derived from oxidative metabolism within the parietal cell (Fig. 21.36).

The precise origin of the hydrogen ion has not been settled; however, it may be derived from the ionization of water or the cytochrome system. For each hydrogen ion that is secreted, an hydroxyl ion remains. For the pH to remain constant within the cell, the hydroxyl ion must be neutralized. This is achieved by the *carbonic anhydrase* system. Carbon dioxide, which is formed within the cell as a result of normal metabolic processes or diffuses into the cell from the connective tissue, is hydrated to carbonic acid by carbonic anhydrase. The dissociation of carbonic acid into hydrogen and bicarbonate ions provides the buffer for the excess hydroxyl ions. The hydrogen ions react with the hydroxyl ions to form water, while the bicarbonate ions diffuse into the connective tissue.

The movement of ions in and out of parietal cells occurs in an orderly and predictable manner. Chloride ions diffuse from the blood into the parietal cell. An available hydrogen ion is coupled with a chloride ion and actively transported across the cell membrane into the gastric lumen. This active transport mechanism requires energy derived from oxidative phosphorylation and is linked to the uptake of a sodium ion from the gastric lumen. Sodium is pumped actively across the basal cell membrane in exchange for a potassium ion. The potassium ion then diffuses passively out of the cell with the bicarbonate ion that was formed by the dissociation of carbonic acid. The passive and active movement of ions associated with hydrochloric acid secretion occurs in such a manner as to maintain cellular electrical balance.

The bicarbonate ion that leaves the parietal cell enters the general circulation; blood leaving the gastric circulation may be alkaline. The elevated secretion of hydrogen ions associated with a meal is sufficiently high to cause a bicarbonate production that can raise systemic blood pH and alkalize the urine. This mechanism is a reasonable explanation for the *postprandial alkaline tide.*

The secretion of hydrochloric acid is influenced by the vagus nerve and gastrin. Additionally, *histamine* is a potent stimulator of hydrochloric acid secretion. The high histamine content of the gastric mucosa has led to the belief that histamine may be requisite for gastric acid secretion. Two types of histamine receptors, H_1- and H_2-receptors, have been identified. Antihistaminic drugs that are used commonly for the prophylactic treatment of allergies

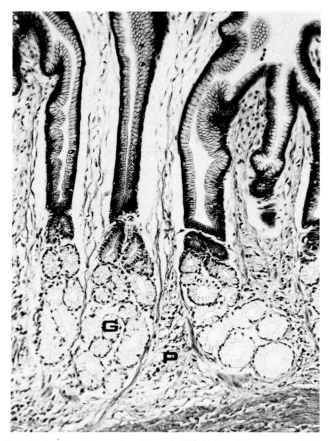

Figure 21.38. Pyloric glands of the canine stomach. The lining of the gastric pit is continuous with the lining of the pyloric glands (G). The lamina propria mucosae (P) is extensive and typical. ×40.

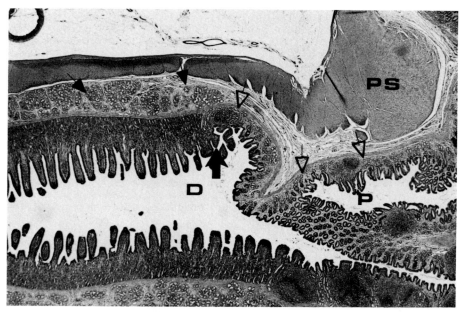

Figure 21.39. Gastroduodenal junction (canine digestive tract). The pyloric region of the stomach (P) is continuous with the duodenum (D). The tunica muscularis is modified as the pyloric sphincter (PS). The pyloric glands *(open arrows)* are similar to the submucosal glands of the duodenum *(small solid arrows)*. The latter may be the intestinal continuation of the former. *Large solid arrow*, actual point of mural reorganization. ×4.

block the H_1-receptor sites. The H_2-receptor sites, the type that occurs on parietal cells, are not blocked by H_1-blocking agents; specific H_2-blocking agents (cimetidine) are required to inhibit gastric acid secretion. Separate yet functionally integrated cholinergic, gastrin, and H_2-receptors may interact to modulate the activity of the parietal cells.

Excessive activity of parietal cells with a predisposing or concomitant alteration in the protective mucous coat can lead to an erosion of the gastric mucosa, a *gastric (peptic) ulcer.* The constant hydrochloric acid secretion of human parietal cells may augment the potential for problems; the dog, although still susceptible to gastric ulceration, secretes hydrochloric acid when stimulated by food. Peptic ulcers in dogs with mast cell tumors are not an uncommon occurrence.

Renewal, Replacement, and Repair. Gastric lining cells may be replaced every three days, whereas glandular cells are replaced every 5–7 days. Mitotic activity is limited to the lining cells in the depths of the gastric pits. As lining cells are exfoliated from the surface, they are replaced by the luminal migration of cells from the zone of mitosis. Similarly, undifferentiated cells in the isthmus migrate toward the base of the gland to replace constituent cells. The chief and parietal cells are replaced slowly.

After a wound in the stomach, the margins of the discontinuity are characterized by epithelial cells that appear to be undifferentiated mucus-secreting cells. These cells divide and migrate over the defect similar to that described for the epidermis. Once the lamina propria mucosae has been covered, the lamina epithelialis mucosae invaginates to form new gastric pits and glands. All of the epithelium is mitotically active during this stage of healing. Eventually, typical surface lining cells are differentiated and mucous neck cells are identifiable within the glands. Chief cells and parietal cells appear to differentiate from mucous neck cells. The remainder of the mural elements repair themselves as described previously. The healing properties of the stomach are excellent.

Compound Stomach

General Characteristics. The ruminant stomach consists of four parts: *rumen, reticulum, omasum,* and *abomasum* (Fig. 21.28). The *forestomach*, consisting of the first three chambers, is derived from the esophageal region of the stomach and is lined by an aglandular stratified squamous epithelium. The forestomach functions to break down ingesta through mechanical and chemical activity. The rumen serves as a large fermentation vat in which microorganisms (bacteria and protozoa) break

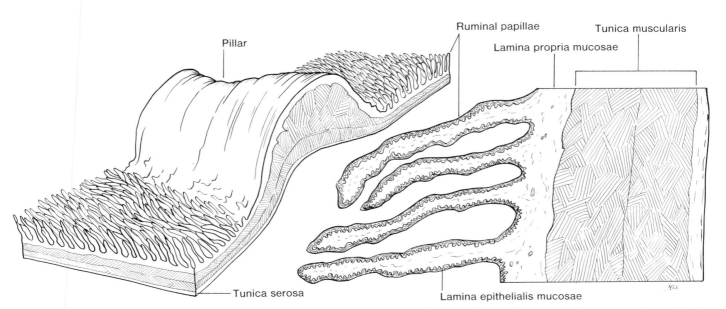

Figure 21.40. A three-dimensional and cross-sectional drawing of the wall of a rumen. The core of connective tissue is all that is contained within the papillae.

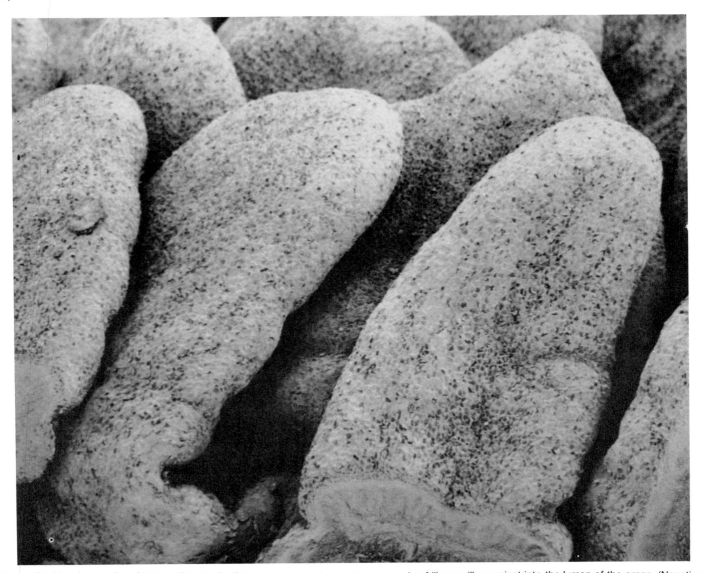

Figure 21.41. A scanning electron micrograph of the ventral sac of a caprine rumen. Leaf-like papillae project into the lumen of the organ. (Negative courtesy of F. Al-Bagdadi.)

down the ingested foodstuffs and produce *volatile fatty acids* (VFAs). VFAs are absorbed across the lamina epithelialis mucosae into the blood vessels of the lamina propria mucosae. The mechanical action of the reticulum and omasum converts fermented ingesta into a mass of fine particulate matter. Absorption of metabolites occurs across the epithelium of the forestomach. The ingesta is then moved into the abomasum wherein enzymatic digestion of the foodstuffs is accomplished.

Rumen. The rumen is also referred to as the *paunch*. The characteristic feature of this chamber is the conical papillae that project into the lumen from the cutaneous mucous membrane (Figs. 21.40 and 21.41). These papillae may be 1.5 cm long and contain a core of highly vascularized connective tissue composed of fine collagenous and elastic fibers.

The lamina epithelialis mucosae is stratified squamous epithelium that is cornified and of variable thickness (Fig. 21.42). The layers of this epithelium are not well-defined. The cells of the stratum corneum are usually swollen or vesiculated. They are typically flattened on the papillary apex.

The lamina propria mucosae is typical and blends insensibly with the tunica submucosa. A condensation of connective tissue fibers in the deep region of the lamina propria-submucosa extends into the papillae. The region may be similar to the stratum compactum; it is sometimes mistaken for a lamina muscularis mucosae. The combined lamina propria-submucosa is generally devoid of lymphatic nodules and is aglandular.

The tunica muscularis is typical. The *pillars* of the rumen are extensive folds of the entire wall that contain a core of muscle

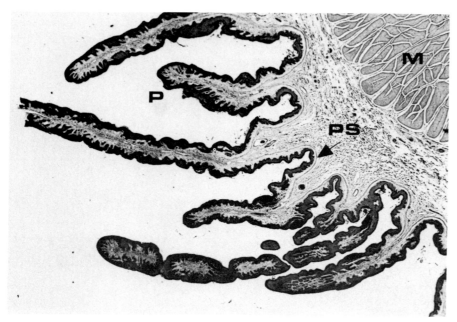

Figure 21.42. A section of a bovine rumen. Conical papillae *(P)* project from the luminal surface of the organ. A lamina muscularis mucosae is not present. The lamina propria-submucosa *(PS)* is typical and adjacent to the tunica muscularis *(M)*. A condensation of connective tissue fibers *(arrow)* should not be mistaken for the lamina muscularis mucosae. ×4.

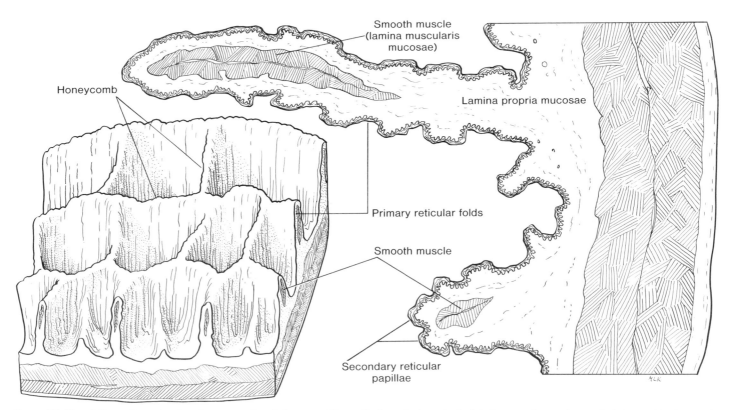

Figure 21.43. A three-dimensional and cross-sectional diagram of the wall of a reticulum. An isolated mass of smooth muscle is located in the tip of the reticular fold.

from the tunica muscularis. The tunica muscularis and tunica serosa are typical.

Reticulum. The reticulum is also called the *honeycomb.* The morphology of the reticulum is similar to that of the rumen. Only those features that distinguish it from the rumen are presented.

The mucous membrane has numerous, anastomotic *primary folds* that are oriented, upon surface view, as a reticulum or honeycomb (Fig. 21.43). From these vertically projecting folds are numerous *secondary* and *tertiary papillae.* Within the lamina propria mucosae of the tips of the primary or *reticular folds* is an isolated mass of smooth muscle of the lamina muscularis mucosae (Fig. 21.44). This mass extends throughout the length of the folds and is continuous with the lamina muscularis mucosae of the esophagus. The course of the smooth muscle, therefore, is oriented parallel to, but above, the plane of the surface lining. The lamina muscularis mucosae is confined to the aforementioned region in this chamber.

The lamina propria-submucosa, tunica muscularis, and tunica serosa are typical.

The functions of this chamber are similar to the functions of the rumen.

Omasum. The terms *many plies* and *book* are also applied to the omasum (Fig. 21.45).

The keratinized cutaneous mucous membrane has numerous, foliate *primary folds (laminae)* as well as smaller papillae. The laminae are covered with short, cornified papillae (Fig. 21.46). The lamina muscularis mucosae is continuous and forms a double layer of smooth muscle that follows the contour of the laminae as well as that of the unraised surface lining. The inner layer of the tunica muscularis is interdigitated between the smooth muscle of the lamina muscularis mucosae within the primary folds. At the apex of the laminae,

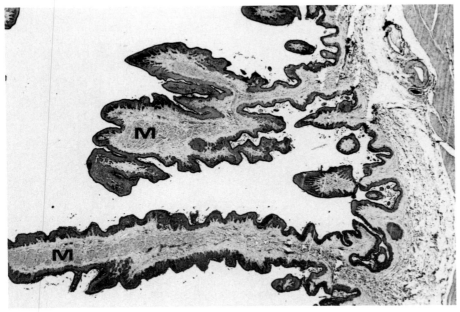

Figure 21.44.   A section of a bovine reticulum. The reticulum consists of primary reticular folds from which numerous secondary and tertiary papillae project laterally. The lamina muscularis mucosae *(M)* is present, but it is confined to the tips of the reticular folds. ×4.

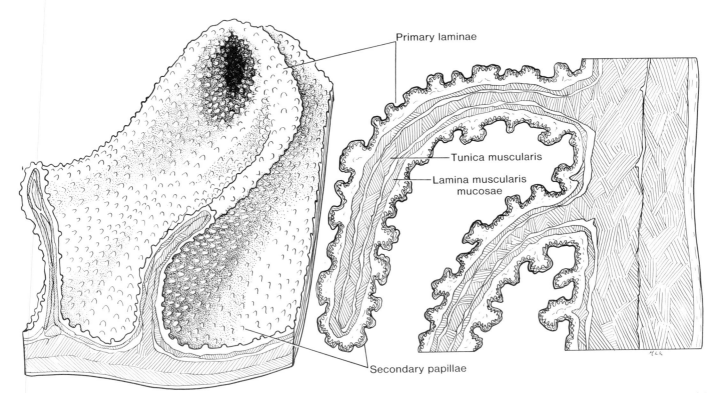

Primary laminae

Tunica muscularis

Lamina muscularis mucosae

Secondary papillae

Figure 21.45.   A three-dimensional and cross-sectional drawing of the wall of an omasum. Note that the core of the laminae contains elements of the lamina muscularis mucosae and tunica muscularis.

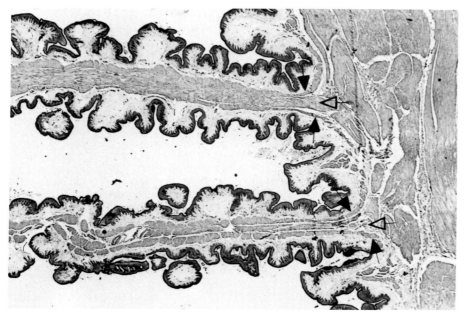

Figure 21.46. A section of bovine omasum. The omasum has numerous laminae from which smaller papillae project. Three layers of smooth muscle occur in the laminae. The two peripheral layers are those of the lamina muscularis mucosae *(solid arrows)*. The central layer is continuous with the smooth muscle of the tunica muscularis *(open arrows)*. ×4.

the smooth muscle masses fuse into a thickened muscular mass. The lamina propria mucosae, tunica submucosa, tunica muscularis, and tunica serosa are typical. At the apices of the laminae, however, a mucous connective tissue is present.

Abomasum. The abomasum is the glandular portion of the ruminant stomach. The description of the glandular stomach applies to this organ.

Histophysiology of Ruminant Digestion

Development. The rumen, reticulum, and omasum comprise approximately 89% of the total weight of the adult bovine stomach. Whereas the four chambers of the compound stomach are evident within the embryo at approximately 60 days of gestation, the relative proportions of these chambers are not the same as in the adult. The abomasum is the predominant chamber and may comprise as much as 56% of the total organ weight at birth. The adult proportions are achieved gradually and are attained eventually at approximately six months of age. The speed with which the adult proportions and chamber capacities are achieved is dependent upon the nature of the diet. An increase in dietary roughage accelerates the development, whereas maintenance on milk or similarly constituted diets retards the development. Similarly, the development and growth of ruminal papillae are dependent upon roughage in the diet.

Motility of the forestomach is essential to accomplish three primary functions:

mixing, regurgitation, and eructation. As a functional unit, the forestomach may be considered to consist of two chambers—rumen-reticulum and omasum. The neuronal regulation of their movements is achieved through medullary control centers.

The *mixing contractions* of the rumen-reticulum are divided into two distinct groups—A-wave and B-wave. Ingesta is propelled caudad by the A-wave contractions. B-wave contractions occur as forward-moving waves of contractions.

Regurgitation contractions, although involuntary, may be regulated and suppressed by the activity of conscious centers. Reverse peristalsis propels the ingesta to the buccal cavity where it is remasticated and eventually reswallowed. Regurgitation permits more thorough processing of the ingesta.

Eructation contractions permit the expulsion of gas from the rumen. The gas passes into the lungs from the pharynx; it is expired during normal exhalation. As much as 50 liters of gas/hour can be produced in the bovine rumen during fermentation processes. Eructation is essential to prevent the accumulation of the gases. Abnormally large accumulation of gas *(bloat)* within the rumen can result in death.

Digestive Activities. The relationship between the ruminant and the population of microbes (bacteria, protozoa) in the fermentation vat (rumen, reticulum) is dependent upon their mutual cooperation *(synergism)*. The ruminant supplies the ideal anaerobic environment (temperature, pH) and food supply, whereas the microbes

degrade plant materials (cellulose), produce VFAs, synthesize microbial proteins, and produce B vitamins. The ruminal microbes continually move into the aboral components of the digestive system wherein they are digested. The microbes, then, including both the bacterial and protozoal components, are sources of nutrients directly. The anaerobic fermentation produces carbon dioxide, water, methane, lactic acid, acetic acid, butyric acid, and propionic acid.

The *VFAs—acetic, butyric* and *propionic acids*—contribute approximately 70% of the ruminant's daily energy needs. Although most of the absorption of VFAs occurs through the ruminal papillae, some of the acids are absorbed by the reticulum and omasum. The amount and type of VFAs absorbed varies with the type of diet. The fate of the individual VFAs differs also. *Acetic acid*, which accounts for about 60% of the absorbed VFAs, is the primary source of acetyl coenzyme A for the synthesis of lipids. Additionally, acetic acid is metabolized by adipose tissue, muscular tissue, and the mammary gland. *Propionic acid*, comprising about 25% of the absorbed VFAs, is the most important source for the production of glucose *(gluconeogenesis)* within the liver. Because only minimal quantities of glucose are available to the ruminant from digestion, propionic acid is essential. *Butyric acid*, which comprises about 15% of the absorbed VFAs, is converted to β-hydroxybutyric acid, a *ketone body*, in the lamina epithelialis mucosae of the rumen. β-hydroxybutyric acid is metabolized in the liver. Ketone bodies *(acetoacetic acid* and *β-hydroxybutric acid)* are oxidized in skeletal muscle also. Acetone is produced from the decarboxylation of acetoacetic acid and isopropanol from the decarboxylation of the β-hydroxybutyric acid.

Although ruminants have essential amino acid requirements, they need not be supplied in the diet. The microbial flora are capable of metabolizing plant proteins to amino acids and subsequently synthesizing microbial proteins. Similarly, the microbes are capable of converting *nonprotein nitrogen* sources to amino acids of microbial proteins. *Urea*, a common nonprotein nitrogen source, gains access to the rumen through salivary secretions, absorption through the ruminal mucosa from the blood, and dietary supplementation.

The microbial flora also produce all of the B vitamins required by the organism. As long as cobalt is supplied in the diet, it is virtually impossible to induce a vitamin B complex dietary deficiency.

Despite the stratified squamous epithelium that lines the forestomach, extensive absorption of nutrients probably occurs in all of the chambers. VFAs, lactic acid, ammonia, inorganic ions, and water are absorbed through the ruminal lamina epithelialis mucosae. The absorption of materials from the omasum probably occurs also. Materials moving slowly through the interlaminar spaces of the omasum are probably subject to greater absorption than those that move through the chamber rapidly. VFAs are probably absorbed by the abomasum also.

Small Intestine

Structure

General Characteristics. The small intestine has numerous modifications to increase the absorptive and secretory surface: *length, plicae, villi* and *microvilli*. Although there are distinctive features of the various regions of the intestine, these regions share many features in common.

An abrupt change in the character of the mucous membrane occurs at the gastroduodenal junction. Gastric folds are replaced by finger-like projections *(villi)* of the mucous membrane (Fig. 5.26). Permanent folds *(plicae circulares)* are present and have villi projecting from them. These folds also contain portions of the tunica submucosa. The openings to *intestinal crypts* occur at the base of the villi.

Mucosa. The lamina epithelialis mucosae consists of three types of cells: *lining cells, goblet cells, and enterochromaffin cells.*

The *lining cells* are typical columnar epithelial cells. The apical border has numerous microvilli arranged in an orderly array *(striated border)*. The finely granular, acidophilic cytoplasm contains the basally displaced, elongated nucleus. These cells are actively engaged in the absorptive process.

The *goblet cells* are typical (Plate I.12). They tend to increase in frequency toward the rectum. Their secretory product protects the lining. In the lower intestine, the mucoid layer facilitates the movement of the luminal contents toward the anus.

Enteroendocrine cells are typical and have been described with the stomach.

Intestinal crypts open at the base of the villi as simple, branched, tubular invaginations. The epithelium consists of *columnar lining cells, goblet cells, argentaffin cells* and *Paneth cells.*

Paneth cells are specialized pyramidal cells of the intestine (Fig. 21.47) with supranuclear acidophilic granules and basally displaced nuclei. The basal portion of the cell is basophilic. Paneth cells are present in ruminants, equids, and man but are absent in the other domestic species. Although the Paneth cells have many of the characteristics of protein or enzyme-secreting cells that suggest a digestive function, no evidence supports this supposition. The bacteriocidal enzymes (lysozyme) that are present within the cells intimate a phagocytic function.

The lamina propria mucosae is usually

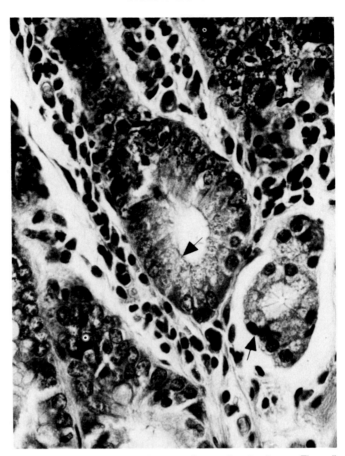

Figure 21.47. Paneth cells of the intestinal crypts of an equine duodenum. The cells are pyramidal-shaped entities *(arrows)* with apical granules. ×160.

described as areolar; however, the accumulation of reticular fibers, granulocytes, and agranulocytes has prompted some to classify it as a *reticuloareolar connective tissue*. Intestinal crypts and lymph nodules are also present. The crypts may occupy the bulk of this layer. The frequency of lymph nodules, however, increases caudally and may occupy the lamina propria mucosae as well as the tunica submucosa, as in the case of *Peyer's patches*. Besides the aforementioned components, numerous lymphatic vessels *(lacteals)* are present and extend with the connective tissue into the core of the villi. A stratum compactum is present in carnivores. The lamina muscularis mucosae is typical. Strands of smooth muscle and connective tissue fibers are interdigitated between the crypts into the cores of the villi.

Submucosa. The tunica submucosa is typical. Submucosal glands are simple, branched, tubuloacinar glands that open into crypts (Fig. 21.48). They may be mucous (ruminants, dog), mixed (cats), or serous (horses, pigs). These glands are called *intestinal submucosal glands (Brunner's glands, duodenal glands)*. In carnivores, man and small ruminants, they are con-

fined to the initial or middle portion of the duodenum. In horses, pigs and large ruminants, they extend into the jejunum. These glands may be the aboral continuations of pyloric glands that have been displaced to the submucosa.

Muscularis. The tunica muscularis with Auerbach's plexus is present and typical. The contraction of this smooth muscle is responsible for peristalsis.

Serosa. The tunica serosa is typical.

Regions of the Small Intestine

Duodenum. The tunica mucosa is highly folded with villi and plicae circulares (Fig. 21.49). Intestinal crypts are prominent. Intestinal submucosal glands may be present. Lymphatic nodules may be present, but they are sparse. The villi, although subject to some variations, tend to be regularly shaped, blunt, and wide.

Jejunum. This region of the small intestine is similar to the duodenum (Fig. 21.50). Intestinal submucosal glands are confined to the initial portion of the jejunum in some species. The villi are thinner, smaller, and fewer in number than in the duodenum (Fig. 21.51). Mucosal-submucosal lymph nodules are present, espe-

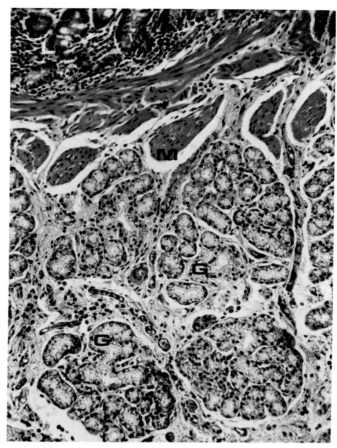

Figure 21.48. Submucosal glands of an equine duodenum. The submucosal glands *(G)* are located peripheral to the tunica mucosa. The glands, however, are continuous with the intestinal crypts.

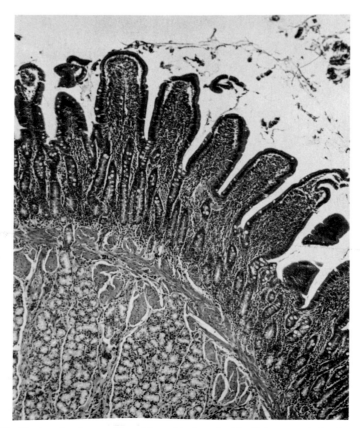

Figure 21.49. Equine duodenum. The villi are blunt and wide. Submucosal glands are present. ×16.

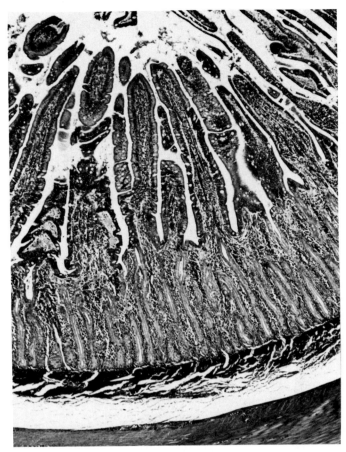

Figure 21.50. Jejunum of a bushbaby. The villi are long and slender. ×16.

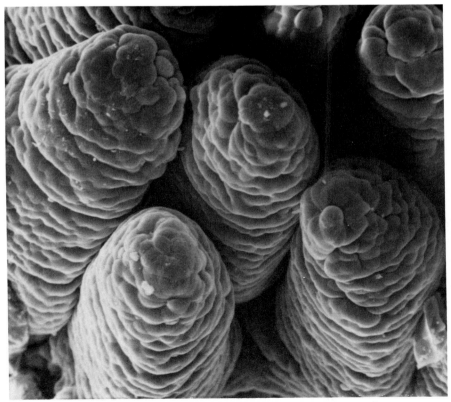

Figure 21.51. A scanning electron micrograph of the villi from the jejunum of a young mouse. Compare with Figure 15.8. (Negative courtesy of D. L. Eisenbrandt.)

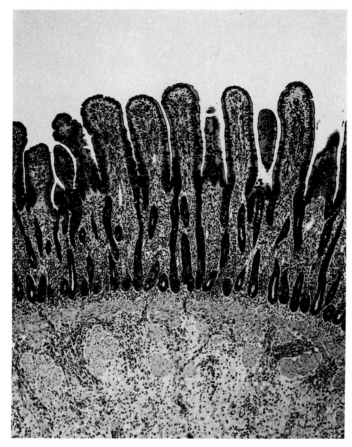

Figure 21.52. A section of an equine ileum. The villi are club-shaped. ×16. (Alcian blue-periodic acid-Schiff.)

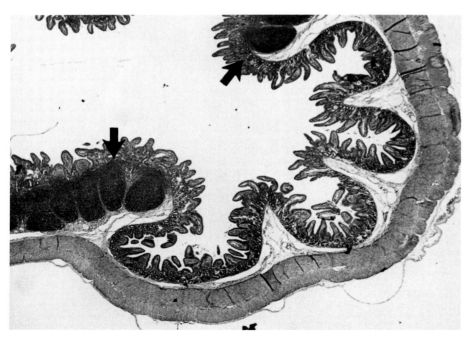

Figure 21.53. A section of a porcine ileum. Peyer's patches *(arrows)* are located in the antimesenteric portion of the ileum. The patches may be sufficiently large to obliterate the villi. ×4.

cially in pigs. The remaining mural elements are typical (Plates III.3 and III.4).

Ileum. This region is similar to the jejunum (Fig. 21.52). Goblet cells are a prominent feature. Lymphatic tissue (Peyer's patches) occurs frequently in the mucosa-submucosa (Fig. 21.53). These lymphatic nodules may become sufficiently prominent to fill or obliterate the villi. In such instances, the mucous membrane is flattened and interrupted by crypts. Because these regions look similar to tonsils and their associated crypts, they are referred to as *lymph craters*. They are especially prominent in swine.

The villi of this region are club-shaped. Plicae are not present; they are most prominent in the jejunum and diminish in size orad and aborad.

Histophysiology of the Small Intestine

Motility. Intestinal motility functions:

1. To mix the chyme to insure that digestive enzymes contact the partially digested foodstuffs.
2. To move the chyme in order that it contacts all absorptive surfaces.
3. To propel the chyme through the intestine.

Segmenting contractions are ring-like contractions that occur in the lamina interna of the tunica muscularis. Denervation does not affect these contractions. Segmenting contractions are not propulsive; they function to mix the contents to facilitate digestion and absorption. *Peristalsis* propels the contents of the lumen aborally. Peristaltsis involves segmental shortening of the longitudinal layer followed by ring-like contractions of the circular layer. Although peristaltic contractions occur independently of extrinsic innervation, the intrinsic nerve supply (submucosal and myenteric plexuses) must be intact.

Contractions of the smooth muscle respond to increased stretch of the intestinal wall *(myenteric reflex)*. Normally, peristalsis occurs slowly enough to permit absorption of materials. Rapidly propagated muscular contractions *(peristaltic rushes)* may traverse the entire intestine. The decreased transport time that results may cause a diarrhea, malabsorption, or maldigestion.

The extrinsic nerve supply influences the strength and frequency of intrinsic intestinal activity. Vagal stimulation augments intestinal smooth muscle activity, whereas sympathetic stimulation decreases or completely inhibits it. Sensory stimulation of various regions may result in inhibition of the intestine. Intestinal motility may cease when any part of the intestine is distended *(intestino-intestinal inhibitory reflex)*. Similarly, trauma, peritonitis, obstruction, and surgery can result in the inhibition of the intestine. Stimulation of the intestine occurs when food enters the stomach or when chyme enters the intestine *(gastrointestinal excitatory reflex).* Gastrin and cholecystokinin stimulate intestinal motility, whereas secretin inhibits it.

Digestion and Absorption. Goblet cells, lining cells of intestinal submucosal glands, and lining cells of intestinal crypts of the oral portion of the small intestine are responsible for the secretion of large quantities of intestinal juice. Intestinal juice contains: water, electrolytes, mucins, secretory immunoglobulin A, and enzymes. Many of the enzymes, intracellular in origin, become components of intestinal juice after the disintegration of cells that have been shed into the lumen of the organ. Localized mechanical and chemical stimulants are effective means of increasing intestinal secretion. Neuronal and humoral stimulation occurs also. Secretin and cholecystokinin stimulate intestinal submucosal glands. A substance contained within an extract of canine small intestine, *enterocrinin,* may stimulate the secretion of intestinal juice.

The complete digestion of foodstuffs and their subsequent absorption into the body are essential functions of the small intestine. Many enzymes, including those from disintegrated cells of the lamina epithelialis mucosae and those from the pancreas, become components of the luminal contents and contribute to digestive processes. Some enzymes *(sucrase, lactase, maltase* and *aminopeptidase)* however, are not secreted into the intestinal lumen; they remain integral components of the plasma membrane of the striated border of intestinal lining cells and are necessary for the complete digestion of nutrients before absorption.

Monosaccharides result from the enzymatic degradation of polysaccharides. The absorption of monosaccharides is by *facilitated diffusion.* Proteins and peptides are digested by gastic enzymes, pancreatic enzymes, and hydrochloric acid. *Aminopeptidases* split amino acids from peptides attached to the striated border. Amino acids and sodium are absorbed by the cell in a manner similar to that described for monosaccharides.

Ordinarily, proteins must be digested before absorption of them is possible. One unique exception to this generalization exists. Some animals, ruminants and horses, confer *passive immunity* upon their young exclusively through the immunoglobulins present in *colostrum.* Carnivores utilize *placental* and *colostral transfer* to confer passive immunity upon their young. The transfer of maternal immunity through the colostrum is dependent upon the intact absorption of *immunoglobulins* by intestinal absorptive cells. Although the mechanism of absorption is not well understood, immunoglobulins are probably subject to endocytosis and may be protected from cellular digestive processes by binding to a receptor molecule within the cell. Finally,

the immunoglobulins are transported through the cells and released into the general circulation. The ability to absorb immunoglobulins diminishes rapidly in the neonatal animal.

Lipids comprise a large group of compounds that include *triglycerides, fat-soluble vitamins (vitamins A, D, E, K), cholesterol,* and *phospholipids.*

The initial digestion of dietary *neutral fats (triglycerides)* is the *emulsification* of large fat droplets with bile salts. Progressive emulsification produces small fat droplets that are then subject to the enzymatic activity of pancreatic lipase. *Pancreatic and enteric lipases* from intestinal lining cells selectively hydrolyze the triglycerides into monoglycerides, free fatty acids, and glycerol. Aggregates of monoglycerides, fatty acids and bile salts form *micelles.* The bile salts function to "transport" the constituents of the micelles to cellular surfaces. The constituents are absorbed by simple diffusion; the bile salts are released from micelles into the lumen to transport more molecules. Monoglycerides and fatty acids diffuse through the plasma membrane, enter the smooth endoplasmic reticulum and are reconstituted into triglycerides. Small vesicles containing triglycerides are pinched off from the smooth endoplasmic reticulum and migrate directly or through the Golgi apparatus to the lateral cell margins at the level of the nucleus. The vesicles fuse with the lateral plasma membrane and the droplets enter the intercellular space. The droplets of triglycerides *(chylomicrons)* migrate to the center of the villi. The chylomicrons enter the lacteals and are carried to the vascular system via the abdominal and thoracic lymph channels. Fatty acids comprised of more than 16 carbons are transported to the blood via the lymph channels, whereas those with less than 16 carbon atoms enter the portal circulation directly.

The entire small intestine is responsible for the absorption of other nutrients—water, bile salts, sodium, hydrogen ion, bicarbonate ion, calcium, phosphate, chloride, sulfate, and iron. The duodenum, however, does not absorb bile salts, vitamin B_{12} or hydrogen ion, whereas the ileum does not absorb sulfates.

Renewal, Replacement, and Repair. The lining cells of the crypts are less differentiated than the lining cells of the villi. The striated border is better developed and the microvilli are longer toward the apex of the villi than at the base of the crypts. Moreover, numerous mitotic figures are present deep in the crypts. These facts, coupled with the evidence obtained from labeled thymidine studies, demonstrate that the lining cells of the villi arise from cells deep in the crypts. Stem cells within the crypts divide, differentiate and migrate toward the tips of the villi; they are then shed into the

intestinal lumen. Lining cells (absorptive cells) of the villi, goblet cells and Paneth cells differentiate from primitive stem cells. Only the Paneth cells do not migrate onto the villi. Most of the intestinal epithelial cells are replaced about every 3 days. The repair of the small intestine is similar to that described for the stomach.

Large Intestine

Structure

General Characteristics. The large intestine is the caudal extension of the alimentary canal. It begins at the ileocecal junction and terminates at the anus. The classical anatomical divisions include the cecum, colon, rectum, and anus. Significant gross modifications characterize the cecum and colon among domestic species. Despite the numerous gross anatomical modifications of the large intestine, specific regions of the organ are difficult to identify based upon histological characteristics.

The organization of the mural elements of the large intestine conforms to the pattern described for the small intestine. Specific features occur in all regions of the large intestine that distinguish it from the small intestine; villi are absent; intestinal crypts, which are elongated and straight, open to the surface at the luminal margin; goblet cells are a conspicuous feature of the lamina epithelialis mucosae, although Paneth cells are absent; the plicae circulares of the small intestine are replaced by longitudinally oriented folds; diffuse lymphatic tissue and lymph nodules are conspicuous histological features.

Regions of the Large Intestine

Cecum. The *cecum* is an intestinal modification in herbivores with a simple stomach (horse, rabbit, guinea pig). The histological features described for the large intestine generally are applicable to the cecum (Fig. 21.54). Lymph nodules may be prominent at the opening of the cecum (ruminants, swine, dogs) or may be distributed more toward the distal part of the organ (horses, cats). The outer layers of the tunica muscularis of pigs and horses have thickened, flat, longitudinally oriented bands of smooth muscle and elastic fibers *(taeniae ceci).*

Colon. The diameter of the colon is greater than that of the small intestine. The mucus membrane of the colon is smooth and conforms to the general description of the large intestine (Fig. 21.55). The other tunics conform to the general pattern, except for modifications of the tunica muscularis. The outer layer of the tunica muscularis is thickened into flat, longitudinally oriented bands of smooth muscle and elastic fibers, *taeniae coli,* in pigs, horses, and man. A thin layer of longitudinally oriented

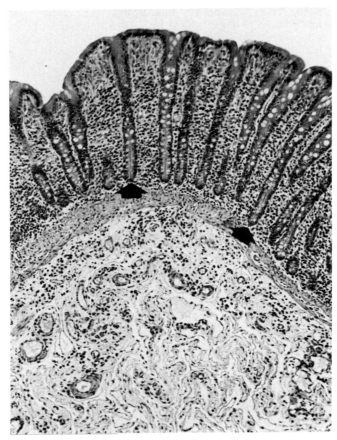

Figure 21.54. Equine cecum. Villi are absent and intestinal crypts *(arrows)* open at the surface. ×16.

smooth muscle occurs between the thickenings.

Rectum. This portion of the gut is similar to other portions of the large intestine. Taeniae coli are absent, but the tunica muscularis is thicker in this region than in the colon. The lining and glandular epithelium contains many goblet cells. Also, a tunica adventitia replaces the tunica serosa. The tunica mucosa has longitudinally oriented folds in which there is a core of erectile tissue within the lamina propria mucosae. The remaining mural elements are typical.

Anus. This region of the gut, a mucocutaneous junction, is marked by a transition from columnar epithelium to stratified squamous epithelium at the *rectoanal junction* (Fig. 21.56). The lamina epithelialis mucosae is similar to the lining of the buccal cavity. At the level of the rectoanal junction, the lamina muscularis mucosae and the outer layer of the tunica muscularis end. The inner layer of the tunica muscularis continues and terminates as the internal anal sphincter. A tunica adventitia is present and blends insensibly with the surrounding connective tissue. In certain species, anal glands, anal sacs, and circumanal glands are associated with the anus (Chapter 20).

Histophysiology of the Large Intestine

Motility and Secretion. The motility of the colon functions in a manner similar to the small intestine. Muscular contractions facilitate the mixing of ingesta and its propulsion to the anus. *Slow wave contractions*, which originate in the intermediate region of the colon, spread toward the cecum or distal colon and account for antiperistaltic and peristaltic movements of the ingesta. *Segmenting contractions* ensure the mixing of ingesta also. *Mass contractile movements*, originating from the distal segment of the colon, can evacuate the colon or propel the feces toward the anal opening over a long distance.

Colonic movements in the proximal segment of the organ can occur independently of extrinsic nerve supply. Distention of the colon is sufficient to initiate its intrinsic contraction. The entry of food into the stomach or duodenum causes a reflex contraction of the colon (*gastrocolic reflex* and *duodenocolic reflex*). The distal segment of the colon, rectum, and anus are more dependent upon extrinsic innervation than the proximal segment.

Mucus, as the primary secretion of the large intestine, lubricates and facilitates the passage of feces as well as protecting the mucosa from mechanical and chemical injury. Acids produced by colonic bacteria are potentially irritating to the mucosa and are neutralized by the alkaline pH of colonic secretions. Upon appropriate stimulation, the large intestine is capable of secreting high volumes of water and electrolyes.

Synthesis, Absorption, and Fermentation. Synthesis of various nutrients occurs to varying degrees in the large intestine of most animals and is attributed to the colonic microflora. The synthesis of vitamins B and K is especially significant. The vitamins may be absorbed by the mucosa or may be eliminated in the feces. In the latter case, *coprophagy* is a behavioral pattern that supplements daily vitamin requirements. The synthesis of many compounds is an important aspect of large intestinal digestion in nonruminant herbivores.

The large intestine absorbs water, sodium, chloride, and vitamins, while secreting potassium and bicarbonate. In man, the small intestine absorbs 20 times more water daily than the large intestine.

The large intestine is a fermentation organ in nonruminant herbivores (horses, rabbits, rodents). Cellulose digestion and the subsequent absorption of its digestive products occur in the cecum and colon of the horse and related animals. Volatile fatty acids, produced from the anaerobic metabolism of cellulose by cecal and colonic microflora, are absorbed by the large intestine. Microbial protein production and subsequent utilization by the host organism are similar to that described previously.

Renewal, Replacement, and Repair. The renewal and replacement of large intestinal lining cells is similar to that described for the small intestine. Whereas dietary intake contributes to the mass of fecal material that is formed and eventually eliminated, dietary intake is not requisite for the elimination of formed feces. The passage of formed feces occurs during starvation. The exfoliated cells of the intestinal tract contribute to this fecal volume.

The repair of the large intestine is accomplished in a manner similar to that described for the small intestine. Numerous factors, however, diminish the healing potential. The large intestine is filled with foreign material (feces) and has a high bacterial count. The blood supply, although adequate for normal functioning, is not sufficient to ensure maximal healing. Leakage from the large intestine is a common sequel to repair. That portion of the large intestine that is in the pelvic cavity is devoid of a serosal covering.

Intestinal Fluids. The absorptive load to which the gastrointestinal tract is exposed daily far exceeds just those substances that result from digestive processes. Water and electrolytes comprise a major component

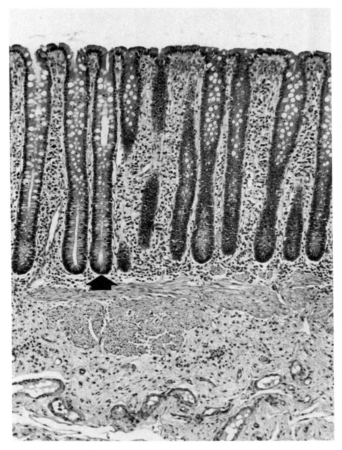

Figure 21.55.   Equine colon. Villi are absent and intestinal crypts *(arrow)* open at the surface. Compare with Figure 21.54. ×16.

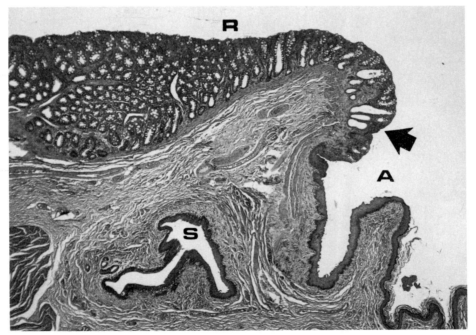

Figure 21.56.   Rectoanal junction (feline digestive tract). The columnar epithelium of the rectum *(R)* changes to the stratified squamous epithelium of the anus *(A)* at the rectoanal junction *(arrow)*. An anal sac (S) is apparent in this region. ×10.

of the absorptive load. Oral fluids, approximately 20–30 ml/lb/day in the normal dog, comprise only a fraction of the water load presented to the intestines. They include major contributions from the salivary glands, gastric mucosa, liver, pancreas, and intestinal mucosa. The normal balance requires that absorption exceeds secretion. The less differentiated cells of the intestinal crypts, as well as goblet cells of the villi, provide most of the intestinal secretory activity. Absorption is accomplished by the differentiated and older cells that line the villi. Although large intestinal absorptive activity is critical for homeostasis, approximately 80% of the absorption of the fluid load is achieved in the small intestine, especially in the midjejunum. Disruptions in absorptive/secretory balance can cause diarrhea.

Avian Digestive System

Specific Components

Buccal Cavity. The buccal cavity and associated structures are different from those observed in mammals generally. A cornified beak is appended to the upper and lower jaw bones. The tongue is narrow, pointed, and contains a bone *(entoglossal bone)*. The cranial portion of the bone is continued by hyaline cartilage. The stratified squamous epithelium of the tongue, which is cornified variously, is continuous with the mucous membrane of the buccal cavity.

Teeth are not present; however, rudimentary tooth buds are present in some birds.

Definitive salivary glands are not present. Instead, the mucosa-submucosa of the buccal cavity has many simple, branched, tubular mucous glands (Fig. 21.57). These glands are lined with large mucous cells.

Esophagus and Crop. The laminia epithelialis mucosae of these two structures is a highly cornified stratified squamous epithelium (Fig. 21.58). The lamina propria mucosae consists of areolar connective tissue with diffuse lymphatic tissue and some lymph nodules. The accumulation of lymphatic tissue is especially prominent caudal to the crop. The mucous membrane is arranged in longitudinal folds. The lamina muscularis mucosae consists of an undulating mass of longitudinally oriented smooth muscle. Simple, branched, tubuloalveolar mucous glands are present in the esophagus. The tunica submucosa, tunica muscularis, tunica adventitia, and tunica serosa are typical.

The *ingluvies* or *crop* is an esophageal diverticulum. The lamina epithelialis mucosae is thicker than that of the esophagus. Simple, branched, tubuloalveolar mucous glands are present in anseriform birds, but the glands are absent in galliform and columbiform birds. In columbiform birds, the

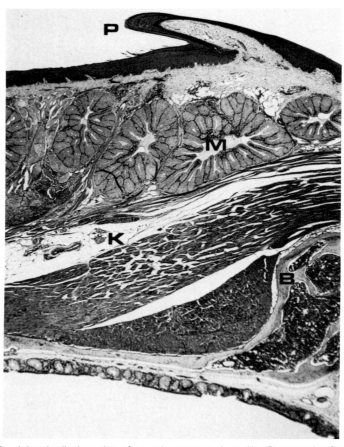

Figure 21.57. A longitudinal section of an avian tongue. A papilla *(P)* protrudes from the dorsal surface. The mass of the tongue consists of mucous glands *(M)*, skeletal muscle *(K)* and bone *(B)*. ×10.

superficial cells of the lamina epithelialis mucosae undergo a fatty change to a substance called *crop milk*. The enlargement of the esophagus serves to moisten foodstuffs through its mucoid secretion as well as to macerate the food through the muscular contractions of its tunica muscularis. The remaining tunics of the wall are similar to the esophagus.

Proventriculus. This structure is the glandular stomach of avian species (Fig. 21.59). Its mural organization conforms generally to the pattern that typifies most digestive organs. Its glands, however, are different from those encountered in mammalian species.

The tunica mucosa is folded extensively into flattened ridges separated by grooves or sulci. *Mucosal glands* or *rugosal glands* (simple, branched, tubular glands) open into the base of the sulci. Elevations in tunica mucosa (papillae) contain the opening of the excretory duct of *submucosal glands* or *subrugosal glands* (Fig. 21.59). The lamina epithelialis mucosae consists primarily of columnar cells. These cells extend into the sulci. The lamina epithelialis mucoase continues into the mucosal glands as a cuboidal epithelium. The lamina propria mucosae is typical and contains numerous accumulations of diffuse and nodular lymphatic tissue. The lamina muscularis mucosae consists of an interrupted band of longitudinally oriented fibers, strands of which are interdigitated between the mucosal glands.

The tunica submucosa is typical but is seemingly displaced by the large and numerous *submucosal glands* (Fig. 21.59). These glands are compound, branched, tubular glands. The adenomeres radiate 360° around a central excretory duct lined by a tall columnar epithelium that may be simple or pseudostratified. The radially oriented glands are lined by secretory cells that may be cuboidal or pyramidal (Fig. 21.60). The apical portions of the secretory cells are not joined together; thus, a serrated appearance is imparted to the lining. These cells have a granular and acidophilic cytoplasm with a centrally or paracentrally positioned nucleus. This is the only cell type in the gland. Because avian gastric juice is similar to the mammalian counterpart, it is assumed that this cell must secrete both enzymatic and acidic secretory products.

The tunica muscularis is modified slightly; inner longitudinal, middle circular,

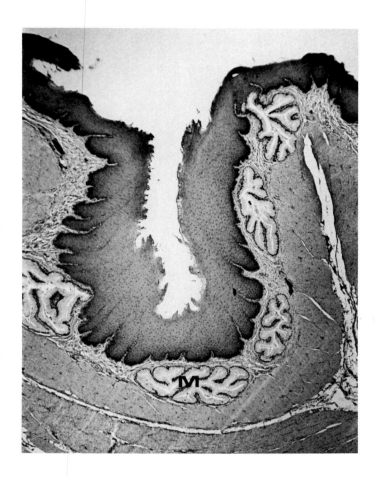

Figure 21.58. Avian esophagus. The lamina epithelialis mucosae is stratified squamous epithelium. *M*, mucous glands. ×10.

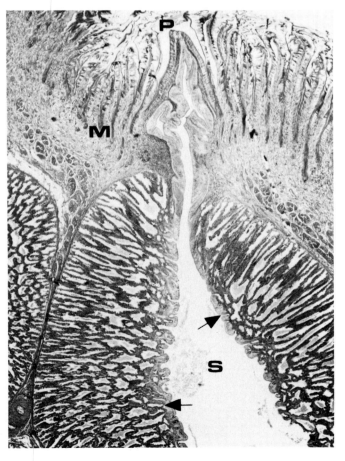

Figure 21.59. Avian proventriculus. Mucosal glands *(M)* are formed by grooves or rugae on the surface of the organ. These are called rugosal glands. Submucosal glands *(S)* or subrugosal glands consist of adenomeres *(arrows)* that radiate from a central excretory duct. The subrugosal glands open on papillae *(P)* at the surface. ×4.

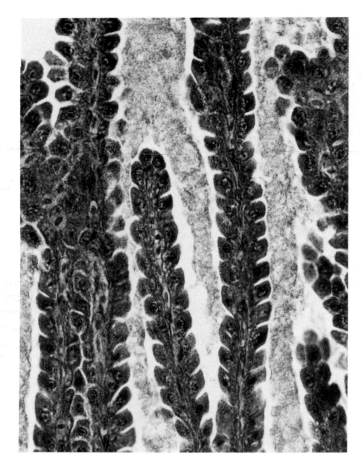

Figure 21.60. Secretory cells of the subrugosal glands (proventriculus). The acidophilic cells are not joined at their apical surface, imparting a serrated appearance to the lining. ×160.

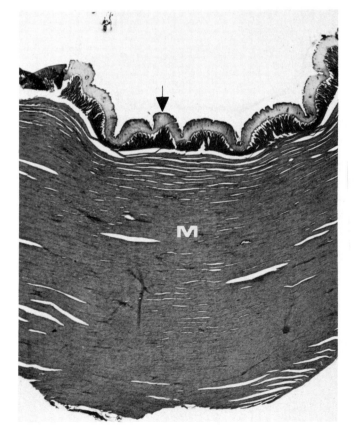

Figure 21.61. Avian ventriculus. The lining *(arrow)* is cornified material secreted by the mucosal glands. The tunica muscularis *(M)* is very thick. ×4.

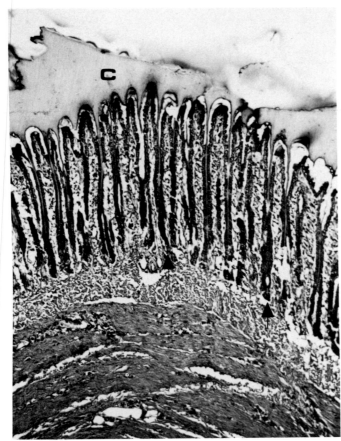

Figure 21.62. Mucosal glands and lining of the avian ventriculus. The cornified material *(C)* is the secretory product of the mucosal glands *(arrows)*. ×40.

and outer longitudinal layers are present. The tunica serosa is typical.

Ventriculus. This portion of the digestive system *(gizzard, muscular stomach)* is connected to the proventriculus by a narrow isthmus that is devoid of submucosal glands. The luminal surface is lined by a cornified secretory product that is produced by the mucosal glands (Fig. 21.61). The surface lining of the tunica mucosa consists of low columnar cells with round and basally positioned nuclei. The surface cells continue into the glands and are replaced by goblet-like cells. The mucosal glands are straight, tubular glands (Fig. 21.62). The lamina propria-submucosa is typical.

A tunica muscularis is present, but it is not typical. It consists of smooth muscle and DWFCT. The lateral border of the gizzard consists of regularly arranged DWFCT. The smooth muscle arises from this connective tissue and spreads throughout the tunic. The tunica serosa is thin.

Lower Digestive Tract. The *small intestine* is not divisible histologically into distinct regions. Except for the following exceptions, the small intestine is similar to that of mammals.

The lamina propria and tunica submucosa contain large quantities of diffuse and nodular lymphatic tissue. These may become aggregated in the caudal portion in a manner similar to Peyer's patches. A third layer of smooth muscle may comprise the inner portion of the tunica muscularis.

The *caeca* are two blind sacs appended to the junction of the small and large intestines. Villi are present at the orifice but diminish and are lost at the end of the organ. The lamina propria mucosae and tunica submucosa contain numerous diffuse and aggregated lymphatic tissue. The accumulation of nodules at the caecal orifices is called a *caecal tonsil*. The junction of this organ to the other portions of the intestine is circumscribed by a sphincter from the inner circular mass of the tunica muscularis. Water absorption occurs in the caeca and some believe that cellulose digestion occurs also.

The *rectum* has short, thick villi and an increased number of goblet cells. Except for these differences, this region is similar to the small intestine.

The *cloaca* is the common orifice for the digestive, excretory, and reproductive organs. The cloaca, which is divisible into a coprodaeum, urodaeum, and proctodaeum, is lined by simple columnar epithelium. The tunica mucosa is folded extensively and accounts for the compartmentalization of this structure. Lymphatic tissue is present in the associated connective tissue. The bursa of Fabricius is an evagination of the proctodaeum.

The tunica mucosa of the *anus* is highly folded and lined by keratinized stratified squamous epithelium. A lamina muscularis mucosae is not present and striated muscle of the tunica muscularis forms the anal sphincter.

References

Buccal Cavity

Anderes, R. L.: Canine tooth structure, development, blood and nerve supply. North Amer. Vet. *16:*37, 1935.

Elwood, W. K. and Bernstein, M. H.: The ultrastructure of the enamel organ related to enamel formation. Amer. J. Anat. *122:*73, 1968.

Garlick, N. L.: The teeth of the ox in clinical diagnosis. I. Developmental anatomy. Amer. J. Vet. Res. *15:*226, 1954.

Hand, A. R.: The fine structure of Von Ebner's gland of the rat. J. Cell Biol. *44:*340, 1970.

Kallenbach, E.: Fine structure of rat incisor enamel organ during alte pigmentation and regression stages. J. Ultrastruct. Res. *30:*38, 1970.

Lester, K. S. and Boyde, A: Scanning electron microscopy of developing roots of molar teeth of the laboratory rat. J. Ultrastruct. Res. *33:*80, 1970.

Murray, R. G., Murray, A. and Fujimoto, S.: Fine structure of gustatory cells in rabbit taste buds. J. Ultrastruct. Res. *27:*444, 1969.

Swenson, M. J. (ed.): *Duke's Physiology of Domestic Animals.* 9th edition, Comstock, Ithaca, 1977.

Weinrab, M. M. and Sharaw, Y.: Tooth development in sheep. Amer. J. Vet. Res. *25:*891, 1964.

Weinstock, M.: Gap junctions in the odontoblasts of the rat incisor teeth. Anat. Rec. *199:*270A, 1981

Tubular Organs

Adkins, R. B., Ende, N. and Gobbel, W. G.: A correlation of parietal cell activity with ultrastructural alterations. Surgery *62:*1059, 1967.

Bonfanti, C.: Duodenal glands in the horse. Rev. Med. Vet. *4.*95, 1952.

Brobeck, J. R. (ed.): *Best and Taylor's Physiological Basis of Medical Practice.* 10th edition, Williams & Wilkins, Baltimore, 1979.

Brunser, O. and Luft, J. H.: Fine structure of the apex of absorptive cells from rat small intestine. J. Ultrastruct. Res. *31:*291, 1970.

Cardell, R. R., Badenhausen, S. and Porter, K. R.: Intestinal triglyceride absorption in the rat. An electron microscopical study. J. Cell Biol. *34:*123, 1967.

Demke, D. D.: A brief histology of the intestine of the turkey poult. Amer. J. Vet. Res. *15:*447, 1952.

Deveney, C. W. and Dunphy, J. E.: Wound healing in the gastrointestinal tract. *In: Fundamentals of Wound Management in Surgery: Selected Tissues.* pp. 61–95. Chirurgecom, Inc., South Plainfield, NJ 1977.

Elias, H.: Comparison of duodenal glands in domestic animals. Amer. J. Vet. Res. *8:*311, 1947.

Freeman, B. M. (ed.): *Physiology and Biochemistry of the Fomestic Fowl.* Academic Press, New York, 1983.

Hampton. J. C.: An electron microscopic study of mouse colon. Dis. Colon Rectum *3:*423, 1960.

Johnson, R. R. and young. B. A.: Undifferentiated cells in the gastric mucosa. J. Anat. *101:*617, 1967.

Leeson, C. R. and Leeson, T. S.: The fine structue of Brunner's glands in the rabbit. Anat. Rec. *159:*409, 1967.

Moon, H. W.: Mechanisms in the pathogenesis of diarrhea: A Review. J. Am. Vet. Med. Assoc. *172*:443, 1978.

O'Brien, T. R., Biery, D. N., Park, R. D. and Bartels, J. E.: *Radiographic Diagnosis of Abdominal Disorders in the Dog and Cat: Radiographic Interpretation, Clinical Signs, Pathophysiology.* W. B. Saunders, Philadelphia, 1978.

Rubin, W.: Enzyme cytochemistry of gastric parietal cells at a fine structure level. J. Cell Biol. *42*:332, 1969.

Sturkie, P.D.: *Avian Physiology.* 3rd edition. Springer-Verlag, New York, 1976.

Titkemeyer, C. W. and Calhoun, M. L.: A comparative study of the structure of the small intestine of domestic animals. Amer. J. Vet. Res. *16*:152, 1955.

Trier, J. S.: Structure of the mucosa of the small intestine as it relates to intestinal function. Fed. Proc. *26*:1391, 1967.

Watson, A. G.: Structure of the canine esophagus, N. Z. Vet. J. *21*:195, 1973.

22: Digestive System II— Extramural Organs

Salivary Glands

General Features. The salivary glands are evaginations from buccal epithelium into the associated lamina propria-submucosa. Although the adenomeres of the salivary glands are located at various distances from the buccal lining, all of their excretory ducts open onto the buccal epithelium. Predicated upon their size, location, and proximity to the buccal cavity, the salivary glands are classified as major or minor glands. The *major salivary glands*—parotid, mandibular, sublingual, zygomatic, and molar glands—are large structures located generally some distance from the buccal cavity; consequently, their excretory ducts may be long. The *minor salivary glands*—labial, lingual, buccal, and palatine glands—are small structures that are approximated closely to the buccal cavity.

The major salivary glands conform generally to the basic pattern described for compound, tubuloalveolar glands (Chapter 5). Structures unique to these salivary glands are *alveoli, intercalated ducts* and *striated ducts*. The striated duct, also called the *secretory tubule*, is the intralobular duct of these glands. **The secretory pathway of the major salivary glands is alveolus—intercalated duct—intralobular duct (secretory tubules)—lobular duct—intralobar duct—lobar duct—excretory duct.**

The adenomeres of the major salivary glands may consist of mucous and serous cells that are distributed variously (Fig. 22.1). Some adenomeres may be mucous, some serous, and others may be mixed (Figs. 22.2, 22.5 and 22.6). The distribution of serous and mucous cells in mixed salivary glands is variable also. Some adenomeres are serous or mucous exclusively. Others consist of single cells or groups of cells of one type intermingled with predominant cells of the other type. Additionally, *serous demilunes* may cap mucous endpieces. *Myoepithelial cells* are juxtaposed intimately to the alveolar secretory cells.

The *intercalated ducts* are small tubules lined by a low cuboidal epithelium (Fig. 22.3). They are nonsecretory ducts that connect alveoli to striated ducts. The *striated ducts* are lined by a columnar epithelium. The naming of these ducts is based upon the infranuclear striations that result from dense accumulations of mitochondria and numerous infoldings of the basal plasmalemma of the lining cells (Fig. 22.4). Striated ducts do not occur in salivary glands that are exclusively mucus-secreting. In the absence of striated ducts, the intralobular duct is lined by simple columnar epithelium.

Bistratified cuboidal or bistratified columnar epithelia may be present at points of transition between intralobular and lobular ducts (Figs. 5.14 and 5.15). Larger ducts (intralobar ducts, lobar ducts) may be lined by pseudostratified columnar epithelium. Eventually, stratified squamous epithelium replaces the other lining tissues. It becomes the characteristic lining of the excretory duct. This lining is continuous with the lining epithelium of the buccal cavity.

The epithelium of the salivary glands (lining and secretory cells) is separated from the surrounding connective tissue by a basement membrane. The intralobular connective tissue consists of reticular or areolar connective tissue. The latter blends with the dense white fibrous connective tissue (DWFCT) of the capsule.

The organization of minor salivary glands, although not as extensive, is similar to that which characterizes the major salivary glands.

Parotid Salivary Gland. This gland is

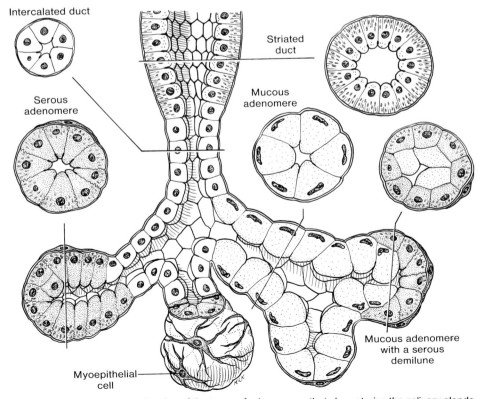

Figure 22.1. An idealized drawing of the types of adenomeres that characterize the salivary glands.

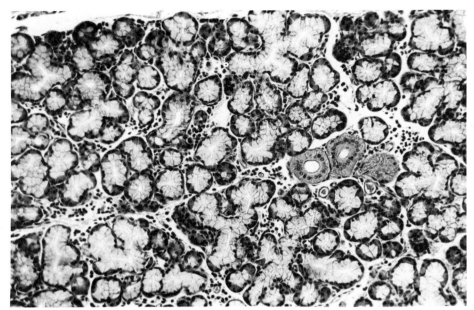

Figure 22.2. An equine sublingual salivary gland. This is a mixed salivary gland. Note the mucous adenomeres and serous demilunes. ×40.

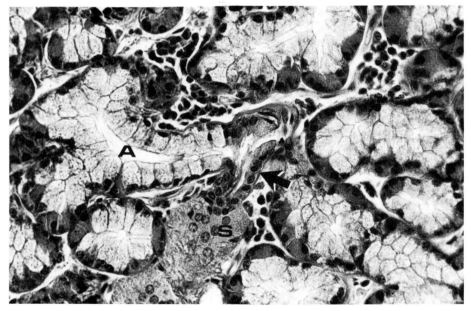

Figure 22.3. Alveolus, intercalated duct and striated duct of an equine mixed salivary gland. The alveolus *(A)* is lined by mucous cells and serous demilunes. The intercalated duct *(arrow)* connects alveoli to striated ducts *(S)*. ×100.

usually a serous gland in all domestic animals, man, and rodents, a few mucous cells or adenomeres may be present in carnivores (Fig. 22.5). Also, it may be a mixed gland in young puppies and lambs.

Mandibular Salivary Gland. This gland is a mucous gland in dogs and cats (Fig. 22.6); serous in rodents; mixed in the horses, man, and ruminants. The distribution of serous and mucous cells in mixed mandibular salivary glands is variable.

Sublingual Salivary Gland. These glands are predominately mucous in ruminants, swine, and rodents; mixed in small carnivores, man, and horses (Fig. 22.7).

Unique Salivary Glands of Carnivores. The *zygomatic salivary gland* of small carnivores is located deep to the zygomatic process of the maxillary bone above the palate and beneath the orbit. Although predominately a mucous gland, some serous demilunes are present. The *molar salivary*

gland of felids is located near the commissure of the lips. The molar glands are similar to the zygomatic glands.

Miscellaneous Salivary Glands. The minor salivary glands comprise a group of small glands that are scattered throughout the buccal cavity. They are located within the lamina propria-submucosa in close proximity to the lamina epithelialis mucosae. Minor salivary glands include the labial, lingual, buccal, and palatine glands. The minor salivary glands are best described as diminutive forms of those major glands described previously. Minor salivary glands are mucous, serous, or mixed.

The *labial glands* are mucous in small ruminants, dogs, and cats; serous in large ruminants, swine, and horses; mixed in man. The *lingual glands* of large ruminants and horses are mixed, whereas those of carnivores and sheep are mucous. *Von Ebner's glands* are specialized lingual glands that secrete a serous product in association with large gustatory lingual papillae. *Dorsal buccal glands* are mucous in large ruminants, carnivores and horses; *ventral buccal glands* of these animals are serous. The buccal glands of man and swine are mixed. Palatine glands are mixed also.

Functional Correlates. *Saliva*, the mixed secretory product of all of the salivary glands, has numerous functions. It moistens the cutaneous mucous membrane and foodstuffs; lubricates and facilitates mastication, deglutition, and phonation; aids in the adjustment of upper digestive tract pH; aids in the dissolution and tasting of foodstuffs; initiates a limited amount of carbohydrate digestion. The pig, however, seems to be the only domestic animal that has a significant amount of salivary amylase to be of any consequence. The salt content of saliva may help regulate electrolytes. Lactoperoxidase and immunoglobulin A (IgA) serve protective functions as a salivary antimicrobial system.

Saliva consists of proteins, glycoproteins, electrolytes, and water. It is a dilute aqueous fluid that is not an ultrafiltrate of blood, because the concentrations of hydrogen ions, chloride ions, potassium ions, sodium ions, proteins, and glucose differ from those within blood. The production of saliva requires energy.

Salivation is under the reflex control of medullary salivary centers of the autonomic nervous system. Afferent impulses originate in sensory receptors in the buccal cavity, pharynx, stomach, and nasal cavity. The presence, odor, taste, and mastication of foodstuffs are stimulatory to the sensory receptors. Parasympathetic components of cranial nerves VII, IX, and X are the motor fibers to the salivary glands. Sympathetic nerves innervate these glands also. **Both components of the autonomic nervous system excite salivary secretion.** Parasympathetic stimulation, the dominant excitatory

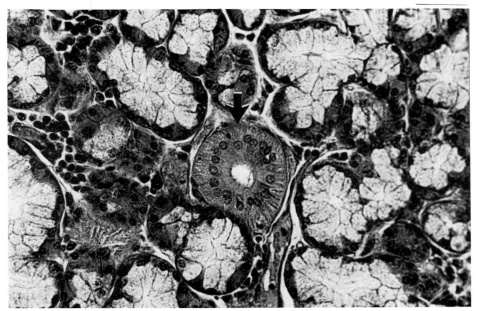

Figure 22.4. Striated duct of an equine mixed salivary gland. The striated duct *(arrow)* is lined by simple columnar epithelium with basal striations. ×100.

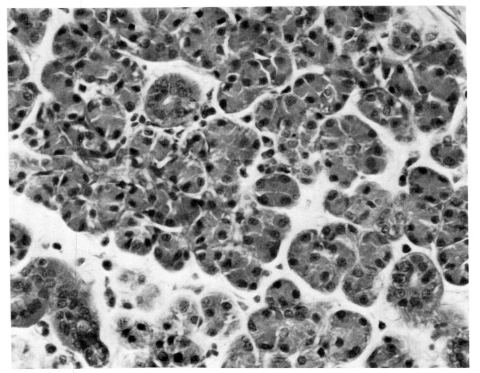

Figure 22.5. A canine parotid salivary gland. The adenomeres are composed of serous cells. ×40.

suggestion of food can cause a *conditioned reflex flow* of saliva in dogs and swine. An *unconditioned refex flow* of saliva occurs in response to the presence of food in the mouth. Ungulates only possess an unconditioned reflex secretion of saliva.

The ion content of saliva is dependent upon the type and rate of salivation. The epithelial lining cells of the striated ducts influence the ionic and water content of the secretion. The basal surface of striated duct epithelium is a large surface area for the rapid transport of fluids and ions. The juxtaposition of energy-producing mitochondria affords a readily available energy source. The basal morphology, with plasmalemmal infoldings and associated mitochondria, resembles other epithelial cells that are involved in the rapid movement of fluid and ions (Fig. 5.51).

The juxta-alveolar connective tissue of the salivary glands contains numerous plasma cells and small lymphocytes, as well as the usual contingent of resident cells. IgA produced by plasma cells in these loci is transported through the alveolar lining cells during which time the secretory piece is added. Secretory IgA, which is resistant to proteolysis, protects the mucous membranes of the buccal cavity from pathogenic microorganisms.

Liver

General Characteristics. The liver, as the single largest gland of the body, accounts for 2–5% of the body weight of the organism. The ratio of liver weight to body weight is usually a constant. The liver is actually a compound, tubular gland with diverse metabolic functions.

The numerous and varied functions of the liver are accomplished by two cell types—the *hepatocyte* and the *von Kupffer cell*. The hepatocyte retains a high mitotic potential while performing diversified and specialized functions. Hepatic functions related directly to the hepatocytes include the following:

1. Synthesis—sugars, plasma proteins, clotting factors, lipids, urea, ketone bodies
2. Secretion—bile salts, bile acids
3. Excretion—bile pigments
4. Storage—lipids, vitamins, glycogen
5. Biotransformation—toxic substances, drugs, hormones
6. Metabolism—lipids, proteins, carbohydrates

Although hematopoiesis is a function during fetal development, the potential for blood cell production is retained in the adult.

The von Kupffer cell, a member of the macrophage system, lines portions of the hepatic sinusoids and is associated intimately with the hepatocyte. The function of the cell accounts for the phagocytic activity of the liver.

stimulus, results in a voluminous, dilute, watery saliva. Sympathetic stimulation brings about a diminished, viscous, mucous saliva. Antimuscarinic drugs effectively curtail salivation.

The amount of saliva secreted by an animal varies with the species. During a 24-hour period, man may produce 1–2 liters; sheep, 1–4 liters; cattle, 90–190 liters; horses, 38 liters. The type of diet influences the amount and nature of the salivation. In the dog, a fresh meat diet stimulates the secretion of a viscous saliva, whereas a dry food preparation elicits a voluminous, watery saliva. The flow of saliva may be influenced by psychic stimulation. The sight or

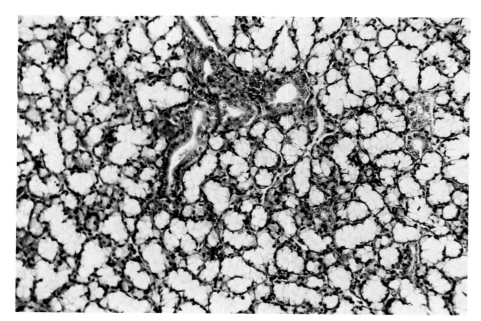

Figure 22.6. Canine mandibular salivary gland. This is a mucous gland. ×40.

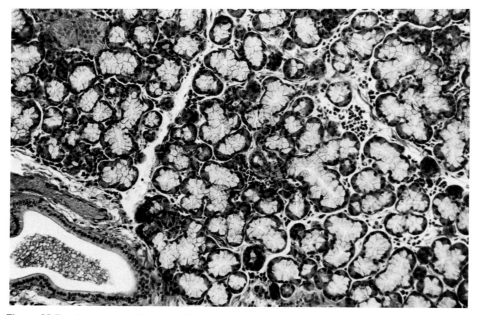

Figure 22.7. An equine sublingual salivary gland. This is a mixed salivary gland. Note the excretory duct in the lower left portion of the micrograph. ×40.

Development. The liver, although removed from the mainstream of the alimentary canal, opens to the gastrointestinal tract. The hepatic parenchyma and ducts are derived embryologically from the endoderm of the gut lining. The extrahepatic bile duct system develops as a duodenal diverticulum. The hepatocytes develop from endodermal cells that secondarily invade the mesenchyme into which the diverticulum advanced. The dual endodermal development accounts for the unique morphological configuration of the liver parenchyma. The plates or laminae of hepatocytes, interdigitated with mesenchymally derived sinusoids, are continuous with the extrahepatic bile ducts that open into the duodenum. Intrahepatic bile ducts develop secondarily from hepatocytes and eventually fuse with the extrahepatic biliary system. If the liver were to develop as a simple diverticulum from the gut, then the relationships would be similar to those described for the exocrine glands.

Histological Organization

Connective Tissue. The fibrous capsule *(capsule of Glisson)*, which consists of DWFCT rich in elastic fibers, underlies a serous membrane *(capsula serosa)*. The capsular connective tissue is continuous with the interstitial connective tissue. The interstitial (interlobular) connective tissue, although scant in most species, is prominent in those interlobular regions called *portal areas* and consists of loose connective tissue. The lobules of the porcine liver, however, are invested completely by loose connective tissue in such a manner that distinct lobules are evident grossly and histologically (Fig. 22.8). Intralobular connective tissue is scant in all species; it is a reticular connective tissue confined to parts of the space of Disse.

Hepatic Lobules. Hepatic lobules, whether distinctly or indistinctly outlined by interlobular connective tissue, comprise the morphological units of the liver. These prismatic, polygonal masses of tissue are comprised of *plates* or *laminae* of hepatocytes interdigitated between anastomotic hepatic sinusoids (Fig. 22.9). The plates of cells and sinusoids appear to radiate from a centrally positioned vessel, the *central vein* (Fig. 22.10). The concept of the hepatic lobule is based upon two simple relationships: the structural organizational pattern and the pattern of blood flow from the periphery through the sinusoids to the central vein.

Hepatocytes. *Hepatocytes* are polyhedral cells, the boundaries of which are usually distinct (Fig. 22.11). The vesicular nucleus contains prominent nucleoli. The centrally positioned nucleus is surrounded by an acidophilic cytoplasm that contains basophilic material (Plate III.12). Binucleate cells may be observed. The histological appearance of the hepatocytes depends upon the physiological state of the organism at the time of sampling. Fasted animals have small, turbid, and indistinctly outlined hepatocytes. After a feeding, the hepatocytes enlarge, become distinctly outlined and are filled with numerous glycogen and lipid inclusions, causing a foamy or honeycombed appearance.

The ultrastructural features of the hepatocyte confirm its functional multiplicity (Fig. 22.12). Numerous mitochondria are scattered throughout the cell, their shape and distribution being dependent upon the functional activity of the cell. An extensive network of clustered rough endoplasmic reticulum and free ribosomes corresponds to the basophilia of light microscopy. The smooth endoplasmic reticulum extends throughout the cytoplasm and is continuous with rough endoplasmic reticular profiles. Lysosomes, peroxisomes, lipid droplets, and glycogen are present also. A prominent Golgi apparatus assumes a juxtanu-

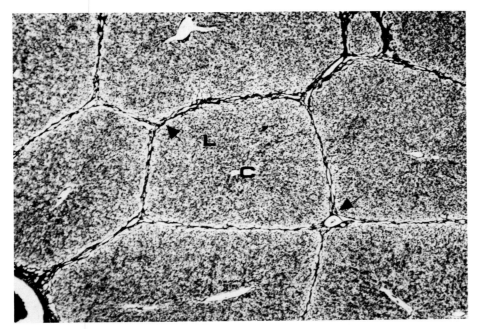

Figure 22.8. A section of a porcine liver. The lobules *(L)* are well defined by the interlobular connective tissue *(arrows)*. A central vein *(C)* is located in the center of each lobule. ×10 (reticular stain).

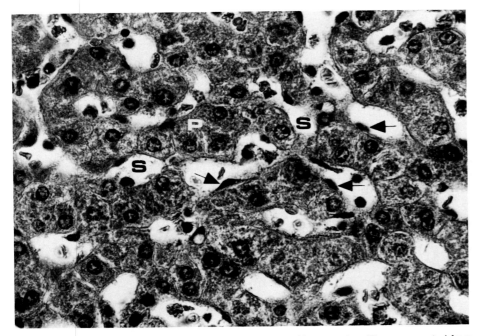

Figure 22.9. Plates and sinusoids of the liver. The plates of hepatocytes *(P)* are separated from each other by sinusoids *(S)* that are lined by von Kupffer cells *(arrows)* and endothelial cells. ×160.

motic network that separates the hepatic plates from each other (Fig. 22.9). All hepatocytes have at least one surface juxtaposed to a sinusoid.

The wide lumen of the sinusoid is lined by two distinct cells. The predominant cell is the typical endothelial cell; the other cell is a member of the macrophage system— *von Kupffer cell*. The Kupffer cells usually reside upon the endothelial cells; however, the phagocytic cells may extend across the sinusoidal lumen or even form part of the wall of the sinusoid.

The hepatic sinusoids, which are generally devoid of a basal lamina and have numerous cellular gaps between the littoral cells, permit the free movement of materials between the plasma and hepatocytes. Despite the juxtaposition of the sinusoids to the hepatocytes, they are separated by a *perisinusoidal space (space of Disse)* that varies in width. Some cells, reticular fibers, and hepatocytic microvilli occupy the perisinusoidal space (Figs. 22.12 and 22.14).

Biliary System and Portal Triads. The *biliary system* of the liver consists of *bile canaliculi, intrahepatic ducts*, and *extrahepatic ducts* for the conduction of bile from the hepatocytes to the duodenum (Fig. 22.15). The system of secretory cells and conducting tubules comprises the exocrine glandular components of the liver. The bile canaliculi are the smallest components of the biliary system and are formed between adjacent hepatocytes (Figs. 22.13 and 22.14). When compared to other exocrine glands, the bile canaliculi and hepatocytes that form them may be considered to be the secretory intralobular ducts of the liver. Bile canaliculi become confluent with small *interlobular bile ducts* located at the periphery of the lobule through small ductules lined by cuboidal epithelium. The small ductules *(ducts of Hering, cholangioles, terminal ductules)* are lined by small, pale-staining cells that may be modified hepatocytes. Interlobular ducts ramify throughout the interlobular connective tissue and anastomose with other interlobular ducts to form larger interlobular bile ducts. The interlobular bile ducts ramify throughout the connective tissue in association with branches of the hepatic artery and hepatic portal vein, forming a *portal triad*.

The bile ducts, located between adjacent lobules, are lined by a low simple cuboidal epithelium surrounded by areolar connective tissue. Larger interlobular bile ducts are lined by a simple columnar epithelium. The areolar connective tissue surrounding larger bile ducts contains smooth muscle and elastic fibers. The interlobular bile ducts become confluent and form progressively larger *intrahepatic ducts*. The latter become the extrahepatic ducts, consisting of *hepatic ducts, cystic duct* from the gallbladder, and *common bile duct (ductus cho-*

clear position. The hepatocytic plasma membrane adjacent to the sinusoids have numerous, short, irregular microvilli. The cell membranes of contiguous hepatocytes have desmosomes and gap junctions. Adjacent plasma membranes of cells comprising the plates have indentations in them that are in registration with each other. Small microvilli project into the indenta-

tions. The small indentations, ramifying between adjacent cells as a system of *bile canaliculi* (Fig. 22.13), are just visible with the light microscope.

Hepatic Sinusoids. The *hepatic sinusoids* are the intralobular vascular supply. Blood from interlobular vessels is transported through the sinusoids to the central veins. The sinusoids comprise a vastly anasto-

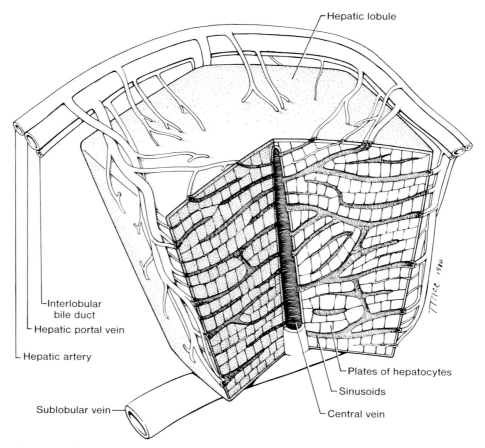

Figure 22.10. A three-dimensional drawing of an hepatic lobule. The hepatic lobule, whether or not distinctly outlined by connective tissue, conforms to this general shape.

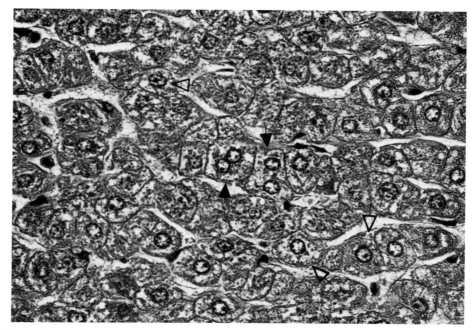

Figure 22.11. Parenchyma of the liver. The hepatocytes may be uninucleated *(open arrows)* or binucleated *(solid arrows)*. ×160.

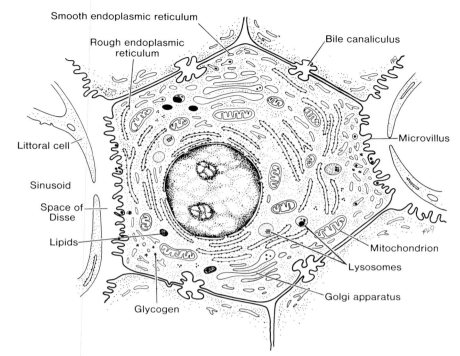

Figure 22.12. A drawing of an electron micrograph of an hepatocyte, adjacent cells, spaces of Disse, and sinusoids.

ledochus), which transport bile to the duodenum.

The epithelium of the duct system blends into and is actually an extension of the lamina epithelialis mucosae of the duodenum. The bile canaliculi located deep in the liver are actually spaces "outside the body."

A *portal triad,* consisting of interlobular branches of a bile duct, hepatic artery, and hepatic portal vein, are especially obvious in regions between three or more lobules in which there is an accumulation of interlobular connective tissue, a *portal canal,* or *portal area.* The portal canal contains a portal triad, nerves, and small lymphatic vessels, as well as interlobular connective tissue (Fig. 22.16). The branch of the hepatic portal vein is usually the most prominent structure, whereas the lymphatics are usually collapsed and inconspicuous. The portal area with its conspicuous portal triad is an important landmark in the organization of the liver and the study of the normal and abnormal livers.

Vascular, Lymphatic, and Neural Relationships. The functional uniqueness of the liver is reflected in its unique dual vascular supply. The *nutritional* arterial vasculature is supplied by the *hepatic artery,* whereas the *functional* venous vasculature is supplied by the *hepatic portal vein* (Fig. 22.10).

The hepatic artery divides into branches that supply the individual lobes of the liver. The lobar branches subdivide into smaller interlobular branches that ramify throughout the interlobular connective tissue space as components of the portal triads. The arterial blood is delivered to the lobules via the hepatic sinusoids. The hepatic arterial blood supply accounts for approximately one-fifth of the vascular supply to the liver.

The hepatic portal vein, originating from capillaries within the small intestines and spleen, supplies approximately four-fifths of the vascular supply to the liver. The hepatic portal vein enters the porta of the liver and divides into lobar and interlobular branches. The ramification of branches of the hepatic portal vein is similar to that of the branches of the hepatic artery. Venous blood of the hepatic portal venules is delivered to the hepatic sinusoids via inlet venules where it is mixed with the arterial blood of the hepatic arterioles (Fig. 22.18).

Venous drainage is accomplished by a convergent sinusoidal drainage toward the *central vein.* The central vein, oriented perpendicular to the long axis of the lobule, drains into *sublobular veins.* The larger *hepatic veins* form from the confluence of sublobular venous drainage.

The dual blood supply to the liver accomplishes two interrelated functions. The hepatic artery, laden with metabolites and rich in oxygen, supports the metabolic requirements of the organ. The hepatic portal vein, although laden with substances derived from intestinal absorption, is deficient in oxygen. The substances within the portal system, including metabolites and toxic materials, are delivered to the von Kupffer cells and hepatocytes for metabolic processing. The venous/arterial mixture (80%:20%) imposes potential restrictions upon hepatocytic function. Any compromise of the arterial blood supply may deprive the hepatocytes in a centrolobular position of required amounts of oxygen, resulting in their death.

The lymph vessels form an extensive network within the interlobular connective tissue and within the connective tissue of the capsule. Lymphatic vessels, however, do not occur within the lobules, despite the observation that more lymph exits the liver than from any other organ of the body. The space of Disse, although not a typical lymphatic channel, has been implicated as the region in which the voluminous amount of lymph forms. Lymph formed within the perisinusoidal space probably flows retrograde to the normograde flow within the sinusoids and is picked up by the interlobular lymph vessels.

The nerve supply of the liver consists predominantly of nonmyelinated fibers of the sympathetic division of the autonomic nervous system. Although most of the nerve fibers are vasomotor, some innervate the bile ducts, but none of the nerves penetrates the lobules.

Liver Units

The histological organization of the liver may be considered from three perspectives—morphological, secretory, and vascular. **The morphological or anatomical unit is the hepatic lobule; the secretory or functional unit is the portal lobule; the vascular unit, the hepatic acinus.**

Hepatic Lobule. The *hepatic lobule* was described previously.

Portal Lobule. The *portal lobule,* as the secretory or functional unit, is based upon the exocrine function of the organ (Fig. 22.18). All of the bile canaliculi drain into interlobular bile ducts. A single, large interlobular bile duct, located within a portal area, eventually drains the exocrine secretions from adjacent hepatic lobules. The interlobular bile duct within the portal area than becomes the central focus of the portal lobule.

Hepatic Acinus. The *hepatic acinus,* as the vascular unit of the liver, represents the organization of the liver from the perspective of the vascular supply to the hepatic lobules (Fig. 22.18). Branches of the hepatic portal vein and hepatic artery radiate from the portal area and extend between hepatic lobules. The end branches of these vessels open into the hepatic sinusoids. Because the axis of the hepatic acinus is perpendicular to the axis of the portal area, the sinusoids and parenchyma of two adjacent hepatic lobules as well as the interlobular blood vessels comprise the acinus. (The interlobular bile ducts follow the same pattern, but the vascular supply is the primary focus of this perspective.) Three zones (*pe-*

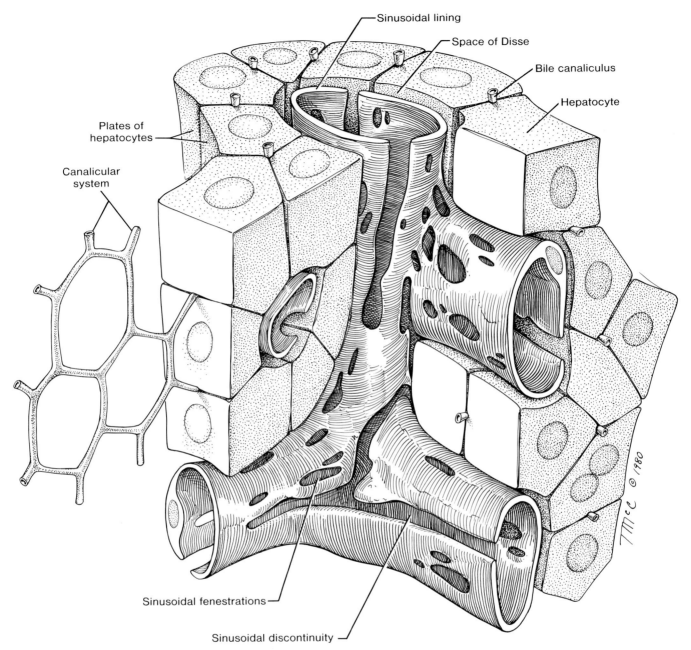

Figure 22.13. A three-dimensional stylized drawing of the relationships between hepatocytes, sinusoids, and bile canaliculi. The canaliculi are represented as tubules for illustrative purposes.

ripheral, intermediate, and *centrolobular*) are identifiable on the basis of their proximity to the interlobular vessels. The perspective afforded by consideration of the organization in terms of the vascular supply is significant in pathology. Certain disease processes of the liver are manifested in a zonular pattern related to the end branches of interlobular vessels.

Histophysiology of the Liver

Synthesis. Besides synthesizing many of the substances necessary for the functional and structural integrity of the component cells, the hepatocytes synthesize many substances for export to other parts of the body—albumin, fibrinogen, α- and β-globulins, lipoproteins, and cholesterol. Glycogen is synthesized from glucose *(glycogenesis)* and stored in the hepatocytes. The release of glucose from glycogen stores *(glycogenolysis)* within hepatocytes occurs upon somatic demand. Similarly, lipids stored in the liver are released in times of somatic need. Numerous vitamins (A, D, K, B-complex) are stored in the liver. Although protein synthesis and secretion comprise major functions of hepatocytes, proteins do not seem to be stored in the liver; they are secreted into the blood as they are synthesized.

Excretion—Biliary Secretions. The liver synthesizes and stores many products that eventually are secreted into the blood and biliary system. The excretory functions of the liver, however, relate to the synthesis and secretion of substances that enter the bile. The secretion of bile comprises the exocrine function of the liver. The primary

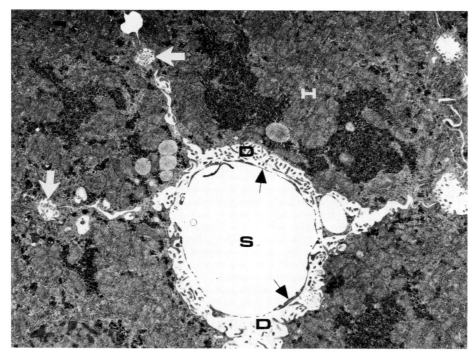

Figure 22.14. An electron micrograph of a liver. The hepatocytes *(H)* form the bulk of the organ. Portions of contiguous borders form bile canaliculi *(white arrows)*. The sinusoids *(S)* are lined by von Kupffer cells and endothelial cells *(black arrows)*. The space of Disse *(D)* separates the sinusoid from the hepatocytes. The cell processes within the space are microvillous projections of hepatocytes. ×6000. (Courtesy of W. Todd.)

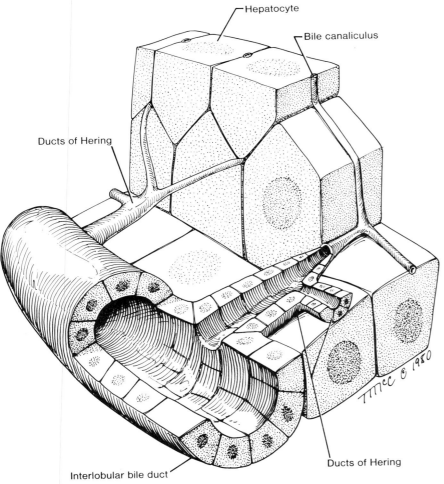

Fig. 22.15. A three-dimensional stylized drawing of the canalicular system and its relationship to intrahepatic bile ducts. The ducts of Hering are modified hepatocytes. The bile canalicular space is outside of the body. Again, the bile canaliculi are represented as tubules for illustrative purposes.

Hepatocyte

Bile canaliculus

Ducts of Hering

Ducts of Hering

Interlobular bile duct

425

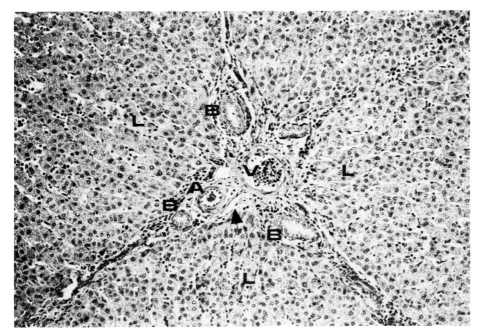

Figure 22.16. Portal area of the liver. This region is located between lobules *(L)*. The region contains branches of the bile duct *(B)*, hepatic portal vein *(V)* and hepatic artery *(A)*. Lymphatic vessels *(arrow)* are present also. ×40.

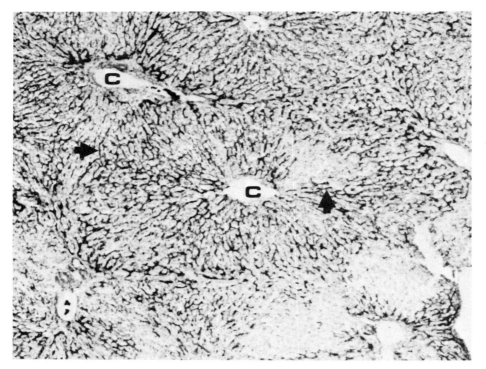

Figure 22.17. A section of galline liver. The bird had been injected with india ink antimortem. The phagocytic cells of the sinusoids have trapped some of the india ink. The sinusoids *(arrows)* are outlined. *C*, central vein. ×16.

Bilirubin, a bile pigment derived from the metabolism of hemoglobin, is conjugated to a glucuronide by *glucuronyl transferase* within the hepatocytes (Fig. 12.8). Although bilirubin constitutes the pigmentary portion of the exocrine secretions of hepatocytes, the conjugation of bilirubin to glucuronic acid is an important detoxifying function of liver cells.

Cholesterol, fats, phospholipids, electrolytes, and other organic compounds are components of bile. Selective reabsorption of some components of bile and their subsequent resecretion by the liver are achieved through the *enterohepatic circulation*.

Biotransformation. Many biologically active and/or toxic compounds are produced by (hormones, metabolites), injected into (drugs), or absorbed by (toxins) the body. Many of these compounds are acted upon by the liver to alter their toxicity, to reduce their acitivity and to eliminate them. These processes, often considered to be detoxification, do not always result in the detoxification of selected substances. As a result of certain types of hepatic activity, some drugs become more toxic to the body after their metabolism. *Biotransformation* better describes the activity of the liver in terms of the alteration and elimination of numerous and varied chemical compounds.

The biotransformation of many chemical compounds occurs within the smooth endoplasmic reticulum, mitochondria, and cytosol of the hepatocytes. Biotransformative reactions may be subdivided into two broad categories—synthetic and nonsynthetic reactions. *Synthetic reactions* or *conjugation reactions* involve the coupling of substances to several endogenous reactive compounds—glucuronide, acetic acid, sulfate, or amino acids. Conjugation reactions occur within the cytosol also. Conjugation of compounds with acetic acid involves several *N-acetyltransferases* and *acetyl coenzyme A*. Nonsynthetic reactions involve the cytosol, smooth endoplasmic reticulum, and mitochondria. Nonsynthetic mechanisms include oxidative, reductive, and hydrolytic reactions.

Although the conjugation reaction is an effective means of detoxifying many substances, not all biotransformations result in detoxification. Ethylene glycol is subject to biotransformation by *alcohol dehydrogenase*. The product of this oxidation reaction, *oxalic acid*, chelates calcium. The complex becomes toxic to the kidneys. The essence of biotransformation reactions is to increase water solubility and polarity. As a result, compounds become less lipid-soluble and are unable to penetrate cell membranes. Accordingly, inactivation and elimination of the compounds are achieved. The phagocytic function of the von Kupffer cell complements the biotransformation activity of the hepatocyte.

constituents of bile are the *bile salts*—sodium and potassium salts of *glycocholic* and *taurocholic acid. Cholic acid*, formed from cholesterol, is conjugated to glycine or taurine to form the bile salts. The bile salts function to emulsify fats in the small intestine, form water-soluble complexes with lipids *(micelles)* in the small intestine to facilitate lipid absorption and activate intestinal lipases.

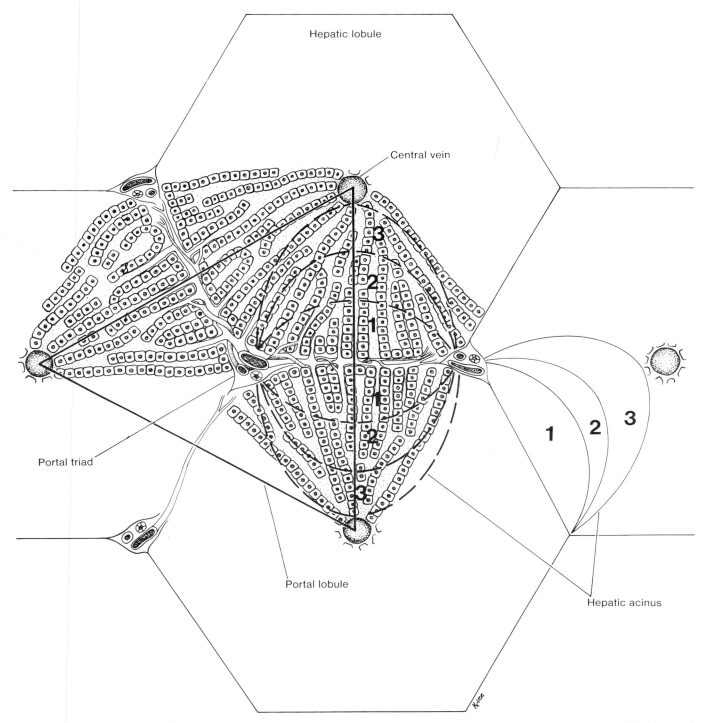

Figure 22.18. Diagram of the organization of the liver. The organization of the liver may be considered from its structure (hepatic lobule), exocrine activity (portal lobule), and vascular supply (hepatic acinus). The hepatic lobule is the histological structure in which the central vein is the central landmark. The portal lobule (outlined as a triangular area) has the interlobular bile duct within the portal area as the centralized landmark. The hepatic acinus represents zones of contiguous lobules that are supplied by the same interlobular vessels. The zone closest to the interlobular region *(1)* has the best blood supply, whereas the zone closest to the central vein *(3)* has the poorest blood supply.

General Metabolism. The liver is involved in all aspects of carbohydrate, protein, and fat metabolism. *Gluconeogenesis,* the synthesis of glucose from *glucogenic amino acids,* citric acid cycle intermediates, and lactic acid, is a significant aspect of carbohydrate metabolism in hepatocytes.

Most of the β-oxidation of fat occurs in hepatocytes. *Ketone body formation* also occurs in the liver.

Protein metabolism includes diverse reactions. *Deamination* and the production of keto acids is important in lipid *(ketogenic amino acids)* and carbohydrate (glucogenic amino acids) synthesis. Ketogenic amino

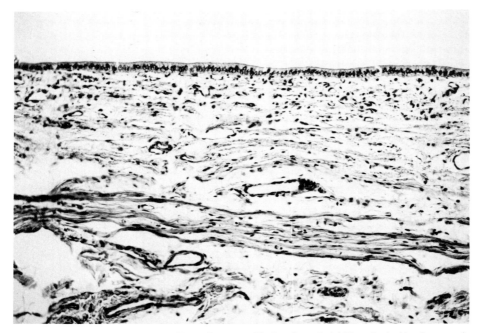

Figure 22.19. Bovine gallbladder. The columnar epithelium is underlaid by a typical lamina propria-submucosa. ×40.

acids yield acetyl coenzyme A when metabolized and can form ketone bodies (acetoacetate), whereas glucogenic amino acids yield glucose precursors. The liver is able to synthesize nonessential amino acids, and the liver and other tissues are able to convert one amino acid to another through *transaminase* reactions. *Alanine aminotransferase (ALT)*, formerly known as serum glutamine pyruvate transaminase (SGPT), is a liver-specific transaminase in carnivores that is used to determine liver function. The enzyme leaks from damaged hepatocytes, and elevation of ALT may be detected in the serum. The formation of urea within hepatocytes is the means by which the body excretes nitrogenous waste prducts. Urea also contributes to the countercurrent mechanism of the kidney; therefore, it is influential in the concentrating of urine.

Although the liver assumes a passive role in vitamin storage, hepatocytic function and bile secretion are essential for the absorption of fat-soluble vitamins (A, D, E, K) from the intestinal tract. The liver also assumes an active role in the metabolism of vitamin D.

Regeneration. The mitotic potential of hepatocytes is retained throughout the life of the organism. Surgical extirpation of part of the liver is followed by a rapid restoration of its original mass. Similarly, liver mass is restored in a short period of time after experimental surgical extirpation of three-fourths of the rat liver; complete restoration of the organ is achieved in 30 days. Mitotic activity and cellular hypertrophy account for the restored mass.

Although acute damage from toxic substances may be followed by complete organ recovery, chronic exposure usually results in altered organ function, decreased organ size, and an increase in intrahepatic fibrous connective tissue *(cirrhosis)*.

Gallbladder

General Characteristics. The *gallbladder (cholecyst)* functions as a storage organ for bile. It also concentrates the secretory product of the liver by absorbing water from its lumen. It is a diverticulum of the common bile duct.

The lamina epithelialis mucosae is composed of simple columnar epithelium (Fig. 22.19). The lamina propria-submucosa consists of areolar connective tissue. The tunica muscularis consists of smooth muscle that is not oriented in any particular manner. The tunica serosa is typical. The tunica mucosa is so extensively folded in the dog and cat that the invaginations are often misinterpreted as simple glands *(Rokitansky-Aschoff sinuses)*. Glands occur in the bile ducts and gallbladder of certain species, notable the ox.

The *hepatic, cystic,* and *common bile ducts* are structurally similar to the gallbladder. The mural smooth muscle is disposed as circular and longitudinal layers.

Functional Correlates. The gallbladder functions to store, concentrate, acidify, and deliver the bile to the duodenum upon demand. Bile is prevented from entering the duodenum by the *sphincter of Oddi*, a smooth muscular modification surrounding the common bile duct as it passes through the duodenal wall. The sphincter remains closed during fasting and forces bile from the hepatic ducts and common bile duct into the cystic duct and gallbladder. When food enters the mouth, the tone of the sphincter decreases. *Cholecystokinin* is released from intestinal cells by stimulation from fatty acids, acid, protein digestive products, and calcium in the duodenum. Relaxation of the sphincter of Oddi and contraction of the smooth muscle of the gallbladder and associated ducts result from

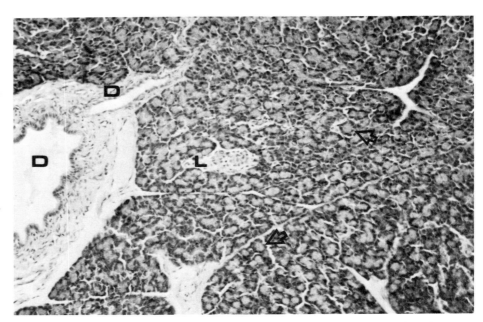

Figure 22.20. A section of canine pancreas. The bulk of the gland consists of exocrine adenomeres *(arrows)* and a duct system *(D)*. *L*, pancreatic islets. ×40.

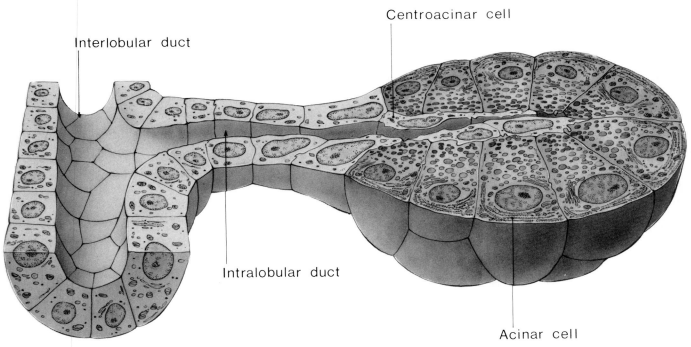

Figure 22.21. An illustration of a pancreatic adenomere and associated ducts. (Copied from a color illustration courtesy of R. A. Kainer.)

cholecystokinin secretion. Substances that cause the gallbladder to contract are called *cholagogues*. The smooth muscle of the gallbladder and ducts is innervated by both divisions of the autonomic nervous system.

Exocrine Pancreas

General Characteristics. The pancreas is a compound, tubuloalveolar gland that is a diverticulum of the epithelium of the gut (Fig. 22.20). It is an exocrine and an endocrine organ. The exocrine portion of the organ is very similar to the morphology described for the salivary glands (Fig. 22.21). The main differences in this organ are its special glandular epithelium, the absence of striated ducts, the absence of basket cells, and the presence of endocrine tissue.

The cells of the glandular epithelium are conical or pyramidal (Fig. 22.22). Although these cells resemble typical serous cells, the pancreatic glandular cells differ in the basal regions. This region possesses radial striations and is basophilic (Plate II.10). This is due to the basal accumulation of numerous mitochondria and rough endoplasmic reticulum. The nucleus is usually in a parabasal position. A supranuclear pale-staining region (Golgi zone) may be apparent. The acidophilic luminal region is granular and may possess zymogen granules (Fig. 22.23). Their presence or absence is related to the physiological state of the organism. Granules accumulate during fasting and are extruded during digestion.

The adenomere opens into a small *intercalated duct* that is lined by a squamous or

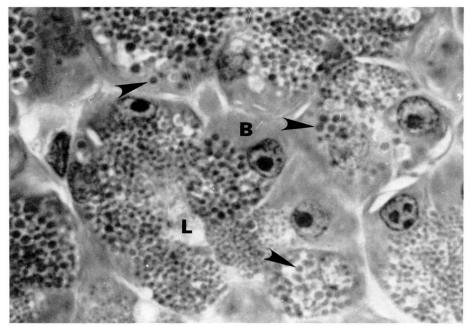

Figure 22.22. Adenomeres of a canine pancreas. This 2-μm, plastic-embedded section has excellent detail. Compare with Figure 22.21. Zymogen granules *(arrowheads)* are preserved well. The basophilia *(B)* of the basal portion of the cell is obvious. *L*, lumen of acinus. ×160. (Glycol methacrylate-embedded section.)

cuboidal epithelium (Fig. 22.21). Rather than the ductular epithelium beginning at the termination of the acinar cells, a variable amount of overlap exists. As such, the lining cells of this duct reside, initially, upon the secretory cells of the acinus. The cells that line this surface are referred to as *centroacinar cells*. These cells do not seem

to impair the secretory process, but their significance is not understood.

As the duct system becomes confluent, a change from cuboidal to columnar epithelium occurs. The epithelium of the larger ducts may contain goblet cells as well as simple, branched, tubuloaveolar, mucous glands.

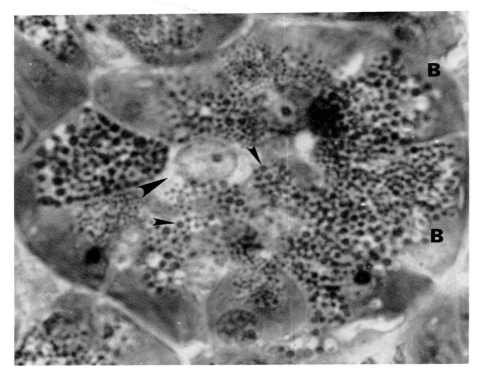

Figure 22.23. An adenomere from a canine pancreas. This, too, is a 2-μm, plastic section. The cellular detail is excellent. Note the centroacinar cell *(large arrowhead)*. *B*, basal basophilia. *small arrowheads*, zymogen granules. ×250. (Glycol methacrylate-embedded section.)

alkalinity of pancreatic juice. Sodium bicarbonate neutralizes the acidity of the fluids entering the duodenum.

The regulation of pancreatic exocrine secretion is mediated by neural and hormonal mechanisms. Parasympathetic stimulation via the vagus nerve causes the secretion of small amounts of pancreatic juice that is rich in enzymes. The mechanisms involved in the cephalic phase of gastric digestion may stimulate pancreatic secretion also.

The presence of acid in the duodenum causes the release of *secretin* from the intestinal mucosa. Secretin influences the intralobular ducts and causes the release of a thin, watery, bicarbonate-rich, and enzyme-poor pancreatic secretion. The neutralization of the acidity reduces secretin release and then reduces pancreatic activity. The release of cholecystokinin from intestinal cells causes the flow of an enzyme-rich pancreatic juice. The hormonal activation of pancreatic activity is the primary mechanism of regulation.

References

Bailey, C. B. and Balch, C. C.: Saliva secretion and its relation to feeding in cattle. Brit. J. Nutr. *15:*371, 1961.

Burkel, W. E. and Low, F. N.: The fine structue of rat liver sinusoids, space of Disse and associated tissue space. Amer. J. Anat. *118:*769, 1966.

Caro, L. G. and Palade, G. E.: Protein sythesis, storage, and discharge in the pancreatic exocrine cell. An autoradiographic study. J. Cell Biol. *20:*473, 1964.

Elkholm, R. and Edlund, Y.: Ultrastructure of the human exocrine pancreas. J. Ultrastruct Res. *2:*453, 1959.

Elias, H. and Sherrick, J. C.: *Morphology of the Liver.* Academic Press, New York, 1969.

Hall, R. L.: Laboratory evaluation of liver disease. Vet. Clin. North Amer. *15:*3, 1985.

Loud, A. V.: A quantitative stereological description of the ultrastructure of normal rat liver parenchymal cells. J. Cell Biol. *37:*27, 1968.

Rappaport, A. M.: The structural and functional unit in the human liver (liver acinus). Anat. Rec. *130:*673, 1958.

Shackleford, J. M. and Wilborn, W. H.: Ultrastructure of bovine parotid glands. J. Morph. *127:*453, 1969.

Swenson, M. J. (ed.): *Duke's Physiology of Domestic Animals.* 9th edition, Comstock, Ithaca, 1977.

Trotter, N. L.: A fine structure of lipid in mouse liver regenerating after partial hepatectomy. J. Cell Biol. *21:*233, 1964.

Wood, R. L.: Evidence of species differences in the ultrastructure of the hepatic sinusoid. Z. Zellforsch. *58:*678, 1963.

Yamada, E.: The fine structure of the gallbladder epithelium of the mouse. J. Biophys. Biochem. Cytol. *1:*444, 1955.

The DWFCT of the capsule subdivides the gland through the formation of connective tissue septa. The finest connective tissue is that which is associated with the adenomeres and smaller ducts, becoming progressively coarse and continuing with septal connective tissue.

Functional Correlates. *Pancreatic juice* is an alkaline fluid (pH = 8.0) that contains numerous enzymes essential in digestion. The enzymes include *trypsin, chymotrypsin, carboxypeptidase A and B, elastase, ribonuclease, deoxyribonuclease, phospholipase, esterase, collagenase,* and *amylase.* The proteolytic and lipolytic enzymes are secreted as enzyme precursors to prevent digestion of the cells in which they are synthesized. *Trypsinogen,* the inactive form of trypsin, is activated by the proteolytic enzyme *enterkinase* released from the intestinal mucosa. Once activated, trypsin can activate other trypsinogen molecules as well as *chymotrypsinogen,* the inactive form of chymotrypsin. Trypsin also activates *prophospholipase A* into the activated form, *phospholipase A.*

The release of activated enzymes into pancreatic tissue, as occurs in pancreatitis, can have devastating effects upon the organism. Phospholipase A splits a fatty acid from lecithin, forming *lysolecithin.* Lysolecithin causes damage to cellular membranes. The activation of other pancreatic enzymes can digest cellular components, destroy the pancreas, and damage other visceral organs after leakage into the peritoneal cavity. Serum elevations of lipase and amylase are suggestive of pancreatic disease.

Numerous electrolytes (Na^+, K^+, Ca^{++}, Mg^{++}, Cl^-, $SO_4^=$, $HPO_4^=$, and HCO_3^-) are components of pancreatic juice; however, the major salt secreted by the pancreas is sodium bicarbonate, which produces the

23: Urinary System

Kidney

General Features

Functional Considerations. The kidney and associated urinary passages *filter* blood, *remove* waste products, *recover* useful metabolites, *store* fluid waste, and eventually *transport* the waste products to the exterior. Because the kidney *regulates* fluid volume, acid/base balance, and electrolyte composition, the organ is central in creating and maintaining an internal environment in which the constituent cells can thrive. Additionally, the kidney functions as an endocrine organ through its secretion of *renin, renal erythropoietic factor (erythrogen),* and active metabolites of vitamin D.

Organization. The kidney is composed of a *cortex* and a *medulla* (Fig. 23.1). The separation into two distinct regions at the *corticomedullary junction* implies that the regions consist of different components. Actually, elements of both regions occur in each other, but a quantitative difference of components occurs in the two distinct regions.

The kidney is a compound, tubular gland composed of *uriniferous tubules* (Fig. 23.1). In some species, only one lobe exists, whereas in others the lobation may persist or secondarily fuse. A lobe consists of medullary and cortical components. The medullary portion is a *pyramid,* the broad base of which is in contact with the cortex. One or more pyramids may join to form a *papilla,* the rounded, apical portion or the pyramid(s) that project(s) into a minor calyx. The tip of the papilla is fenestrated *(area cribrosa);* the perforations correspond to the openings of the uriniferous tubules into the calyces or renal pelvis.

Among the domestic species, swine and large ruminants described as *multipyramidal* or *multilobar* kidneys (Fig. 23.1). A papilla projects into a *minor calyx;* the calyces are continuous with the ureter. *Unipyramidal* or *unilobar* kidneys are characteristic of carnivores, small ruminants, and horses. The kidney has one lobe (cat) or one lobe that fuses from several lobes developmentally. A single, broad-based papilla forms the *renal crest.* The renal crest is associated intimately with the expanded portion of the ureter, the *renal pelvis* (Fig. 23.1).

Tubular Components. The uriniferous tubule consists of a *nephron* and a *collecting duct system* (Fig. 23.2). The kidneys of a medium-sized dog may contain as many as 800,000 nephrons. The nephron is that portion of the uriniferous tubule that produces the urine and consists of a *capsule of Bowman, proximal convoluted tubule, loop of Henle,* and a *distal convoluted tubule.* A tuft of arterial capillaries, the *glomerulus,* and *Bowman's capsule* comprise a *renal corpuscle.* The collecting duct system, which collects, concentrates, and transports the urine, consists of *arched collecting tubules, straight collecting tubules,* and *papillary ducts (ducts of Bellini).*

Two distinct regions are visible in histological sections of the renal cortex. The cortex proper or *cortical labyrinth* is separated by *medullary rays* (Fig. 23.3). The labyrinth contains renal corpuscles, proximal and distal convoluted tubules, and arched collecting ducts. A medullary ray consists of the descending and ascending limbs of Henle's loop and straight collecting tubules. Similarly, the medulla is divisible into an *outer* and *inner zone.* The outer zone, that region juxtaposed to the cortex, contains the loops of Henle of short nephrons and straight collecting tubules. The inner zone contains Henle's loops of long nephrons, straight collecting tubules, and papillary ducts.

Development. Renal development progresses through stages in which three different renal systems evolve. The *pronephros* is the first and most simple renal system. The regression of the pronephros is followed by the developemt of a more sophisticated system, the *mesonephros.* The *metanephros* or definitive kidney develops subsequently. The metanephros originates from two embryonic anlagen—the metanephric blastema and the metanephric duct. The *metanephric blastema,* a derivative of mesoderm, gives rise to the nephron. The metanephric duct, a diverticulum of the mesonephric duct, gives rise to the collecting

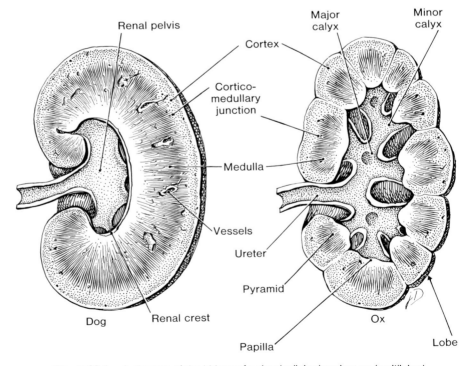

Figure 23.1. A diagram of the kidney of a dog (unilobar) and an ox (multilobar).

431

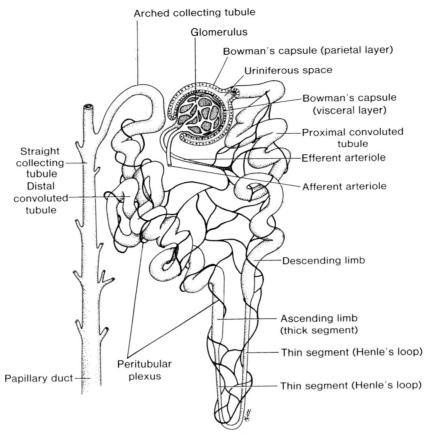

Figure 23.2. An idealized drawing of a nephron and collecting tubules.

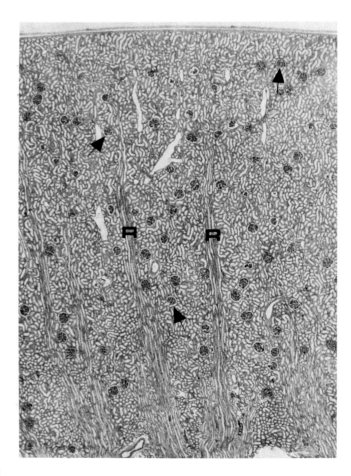

Figure 23.3. Cortex of a canine kidney. Numerous glomeruli *(arrows)* are scattered throughout the cortex among profiles of tubules. The medullary rays *(R)* are prominent. ×4.

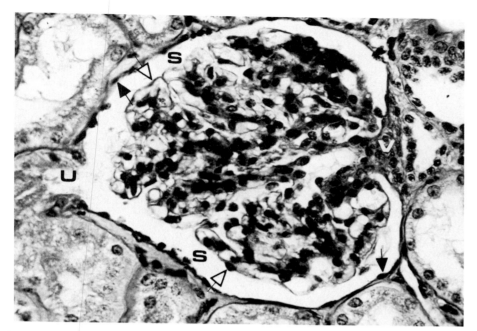

Figure 23.4. A renal corpuscle from a canine kidney. The renal corpuscle consists of a Bowman's capsule and a glomerulus. Bowman's capsule consists of a parietal layer *(solid arrows)* and a visceral layer *(open arrows)* of cells separated by the uriniferous space *(S)*. Vessels enter and leave the glomeroulus at the vascular pole *(V)*. The parietal layer of Bowman's capsule is continuous with the proximal convoluted tubule at the uriniferous pole *(U)*. ×100.

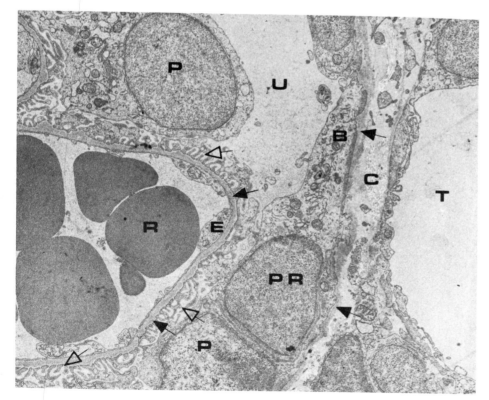

Figure 23.5. An electron micrograph of a portion of a glomerulus. Numerous podocytes *(P)* are in close association with a capillary laden with erythrocytes *(R)*. The podocytic processes *(open arrows)* are adjacent to the well-developed basal lamina *(solid arrows)*. One podocyte *(PR)* is reflected as the parietal layer of Bowman's capsule *(B)*. The parietal layer is bounded by a basal lamina *(solid arrows)* and connective tissue *(C)*. A portion of a uriniferous tubule *(T)* is adjacent to the renal corpusle. *E,* endothelium. ×6000.

duct system, renal pelvis, minor and major calyces, and ureter. *Urogenital sinus* development from the divided ventral portion of the cloaca accounts for the development of the trigone of the bladder and urethra. The body and apex of the bladder develop from the initial part of the allantoic stalk. The differentiation of the urinary system is linked intimately to the organogenesis of the genital system. In the male, the *mesonephric duct (Wolffian duct)* is "discarded" from the urinary system and utilized as the definitive genital tract (ductus deferens and epididymis). In the female, new ducts (*paramesonephric* or *Müllerian ducts*) develop in close association with the mesonephric ducts and form the uterine tubes, uterus, and vagina.

Connective Tissue and Serosa. The kidney is covered by a loosely adherent capsule of dense white fibrous connective tissue (DWFCT). Loose connective tissue attaches the capsule to the parenchyma. Smooth muscle may be present in the inner portion of the capsule. The capsular connective tissue is continuous with the adventitial coat of the ureter or renal pelvis at the hilus of the organ.

The connective tissue stroma associated with the renal parenchyma is scant. Reticular connective tissue forms a delicate meshwork around and between the uriniferous tubules. The adventitial tunics of blood vessels, lymphatic vessels, and nerves also form part of the renal interstitium.

Nephron

Renal Corpuscle

Corpuscular Organization. The *renal corpuscle* is composed of a *tuft* or *glomerulus* of capillaries and *Bowman's capsule*, the expanded end of the nephron (Fig. 23.4). The glomerulus connects the afferent arteriole to the efferent arteriole. Bowman's capsule consists of a *visceral* and *parietal lining* of squamous epithelium or modified squamous cells. The glomerular capillaries are interdigitated with the visceral lining.

Visceral Lining Cells—Podocytes. Because the lining of Bowman's capsule is simple squamous epithelium, it is difficult to distinguish the visceral lining from the capillary endothelium. This endothelial lining is fenestrated and covered by a complete basement membrane (Fig. 23.5). The body of the lining cells is not in direct contact with the basal lamina (Figs. 23.6 and 23.7). Rather, cell bodies are elevated from but contact the basal lamina by cytoplasmic processes (Fig. 23.6). Large cytoplasmic *foot processes*, called *primary* or *major processes*, extend from the perikaryon of the visceral lining cells approximately parallel to the long axis of the capillary bed (Fig. 23.7). *Minor processes (secondary processes)* radiate from the primary

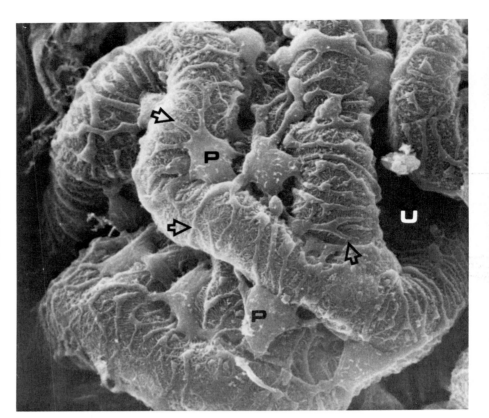

Figure 23.6. A scanning electron micrograph of a freeze-fractured renal corpuscle of a canine kidney. Podocytes *(P)* have large or primary foot processes *(open arrows)* that are associated with the capillaries. Smaller foot processes (secondary foot processes) radiate from the primary foot processes and are separated by filtration slits. *U*, uriniferous space. ×2000. (Negative courtesy of D. L. Eisenbrandt.)

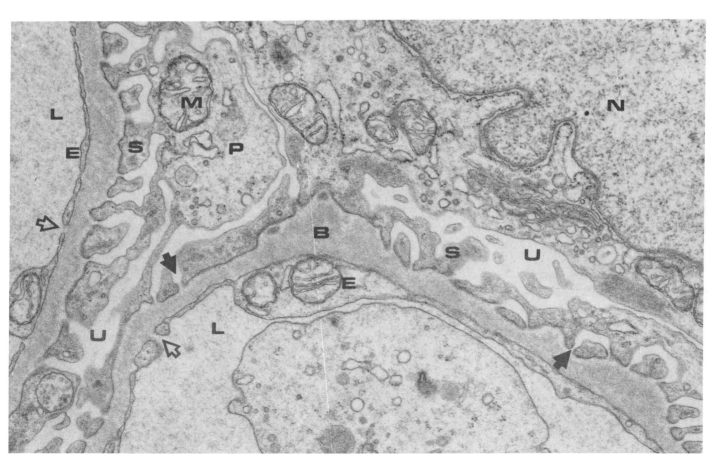

Figure 23.7. An electron micrograph of a podocyte and its processes. Primary foot processes *(P)* have secondary foot processes *(S)* radiating from them. Filtration slits *(solid arrows)* and capillary (E) fenestrations *(open arrows)* are apparent. *B*, basal lamina; *N*, nucleus of podocyte; *M*, mitochondrion; *L*, capillary lumina; *U*, uriniferous space. ×23,000.

processes and minor processes terminate in orderly arranged feet that reside upon a basal lamina. The secondary foot processes interdigitate with each other and are separated from adjacent secondary processes by *filtration slits* (Fig. 23.8). A thin membrane (*filtration membrane* or *slit diaphragm*) extends across the filtration slits. Cells with foot processes (visceral lining cells) are called *podocytes* (foot cells). The podocytes are aligned along the periphery of the capillaries; their foot processes contribute to the filtration barrier (Fig. 23.9).

Basal Lamina and the Filtration Barrier. The *basal lamina* of the kidney is interdigitated between the podocytic foot processes and the endothelial cells of the glomerulus (Figs. 23.5, 23.7–23.9, and 23.17). This basal lamina is two to three times thicker than most basal laminae. Three zones are apparent in this basal lamina. A central, electron-dense zone is the *lamina densa*. This zone is about 100 nm thick and is characterized by granular and fibrillar materials. A *lamina rara externa*, against which podocytic processes abut, is more electron-lucent than the lamina densa. Fibrillar materials are apparent in the lamina rara externa. This portion of the basal lamina is about 100 nm, too. The *lamina rara interna* is between the lamina densa and the endothelial cells. Its morphological characteristics and dimensions are similar to the lamina rara externa.

The *filtration barrier* is a complex of three morphological features: endothelial fenestrations, basal lamina, and slit diaphragms. Endothelial fenestrations, without diaphragms, permit the passage of most materials from the vascular bed, except cells. Molecules in the range of a 6-nm diameter can pass through the basal lamina; molecules with a diameter of about 9 nm cannot pass through the slit diaphragms. Normal glomerular blood flow, size, and the number and types of charges on the molecules are contributory factors in filtration.

Basal laminar materials include type IV collagen. These materials seem to be formed continually by the podocytes in a laminar fashion. Such appositional growth of the basal lamina would result in its becoming thicker throughout life. Since it does not thicken throughout life normally, new materials are added externally and old materials are removed internally. The mesangial cells may phagocytize the old components of the basal lamina.

Mesangial Cells. *Mesangial* or *intercapillary cells* are stellate cells located between the capillary loops of the glomerulus. The mesangial cells are mesenchymally derived cells that are similar to pericytic cells occuring elsewhere in the body associated with capillaries. The cells are enveloped by the basal lamina. Although their precise function has not been defined, they are

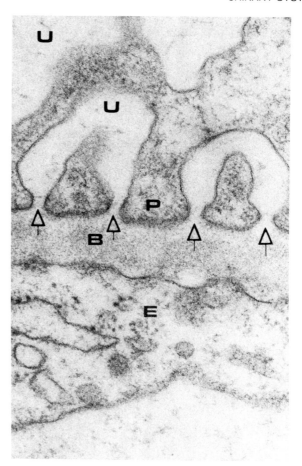

Figure 23.8. An electron micrograph of podocytic processes. Large foot processes have small pedicels *(P)* radiating from them. The pedicles contact the basal lamina *(B)*. Filtration slits *(open arrows)* separate adjacent pedicels. Filtration membranes are apparent *(left and right open arrows)*. *E*, endothelium; *U*, uriniferous space. ×77,000.

phagocytic cells that may remove particulate matter from the renal corpuscle. This phagocytic activity may include the removal of old elements of the basal lamina, as well as general cellular debris.

The mesangial cells also serve a supportive role. The podocytes and their associated basal lamina do not contact every surface of the capillaries. Rather, the basal lamina and foot processes surround groups of capillary tufts. The intervening space is occupied by mesangial cells (Fig. 23.10).

Parietal Lining Cells. The parietal layer of Bowman's capsule consists of typical squamous cells. Generally, only their perikarya and nuclei are evident (Fig. 5.49). A prominent basement membrane is apparent between them and the periglomerular connective tissue when periodic acid-Schiff (PAS) staining is used (Fig. 5.48). The basement membrane completely separates the parietal cells from the surrounding elements. The squamous cells of the parietal layer are continuous with the lining cells of the proximal convoluted tubule.

Vascular and Urinary Poles. Two distinct regions of the renal corpuscle are ap-

parent in ideal sections: a *vascular pole* and a *urinary pole* (Fig. 23.4). The vascular pole is the region of entry and exit of the arterioles and the region in which the *juxtaglomerular apparatus* is located. The urinary pole is the point of continuity between Bowman's capsule and the proximal convoluted tubule. At this point, the squamous epithelium of the parietal layer is continuous with the cuboidal epithelium of the proximal convoluted tubule.

Tubular Components

Proximal Convoluted Tubule. The *proximal convoluted tubule* is the longest, widest, and most developed segment of the nephron (Fig. 23.11). The proximal tubule has been described as consisting of a convoluted portion (*pars convoluta*) and a straight portion (*pars recta*). Now, the straight portion (*tubulis rectus proximalis*) is considered to be part of the loop of the nephron. The function of the proximal convoluted tubule is extremely important, and it is the segment that is easily affected by disease processes and toxic substances. It is lined by cuboidal cells with a well-

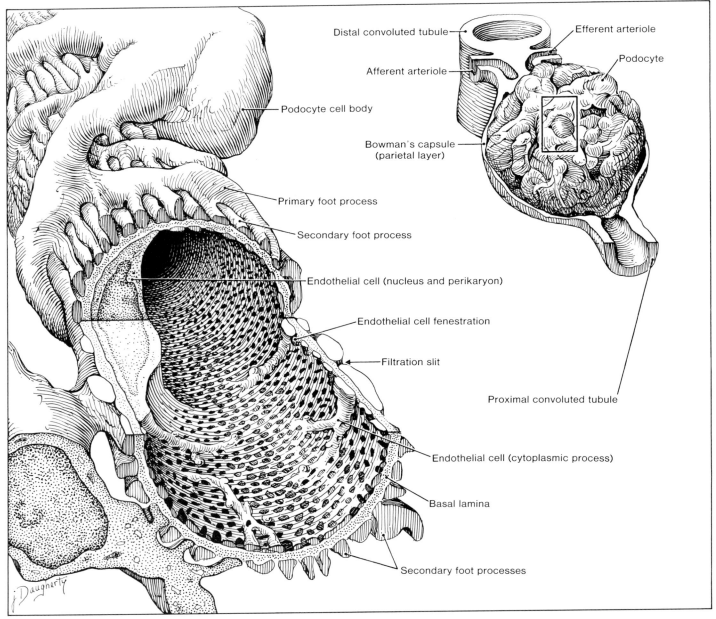

Distal convoluted tubule

Afferent arteriole

Podocyte cell body

Efferent arteriole

Podocyte

Bowman's capsule
(parietal layer)

Primary foot process

Secondary foot process

Endothelial cell (nucleus and perikaryon)

Endothelial cell fenestration

Filtration slit

Proximal convoluted tubule

Endothelial cell (cytoplasmic process)

Basal lamina

Secondary foot processes

j Daugherty

23.9. A diagram of the renal corpuscle and podocytes as visualized with the scanning electron microscope.

developed brush border. With routine staining, the eosinophilic and granular cytoplasm does not contrast markedly with the brush border. A marked difference, however, is noted with PAS staining. The glycocalyx on the microvilli is PAS-positive. The basal surface resides upon a PAS-positive basement membrane. The basal portion of these cells is highly folded and contains numerous mitochondria. The mitochondria contribute to basal striations that may be apparent. Because the lateral borders of cells are highly interdigitated, they are not readily observed in light microscopic sections. The lateral margins of these cells are joined by a shallow belt of tight junctions and a deeper belt of inter-

mediate junctions. The nuclei of these cells are spherical, small, and located in a basal or parabasal position. Varying physiological states contribute to an altered morphology of this segment. Generally, the luminal size is small and the tubule is composed of cells with prominent brush borders.

Loop of Henle. The proximal convoluted tubule continues into the *loop of Henle.* The length of this segment of the nephron varies. Its length is indicative of the ability of the organism to conserve water. The loop of Henle consists of three portions: the *straight portion of the proximal tubule (tubulus rectus proximalis, descending limb),* a *descending* and *ascending thin segment,* and a *straight portion of the distal tubule*

(tubulus rectus distalis, ascending limb). There are some variations in the loop of Henle. Those nephrons in a juxtamedullary positon have long *intermediate segments* (thin segments) the apices of which are deep in the medulla and may extend into the apices of the medullary papillae. Peripherally positioned nephrons (subcapsular) have short loops of Henle that extend a short distance into the medullary region. The transition from the cuboidal epithelium of the descending limb to the squamous epithelium of the *descending thin segment* is abrupt. Because there are numerous blood and lymphatic capillaries in this region of the medulla, the microscopist must look carefully to distinguish the thin

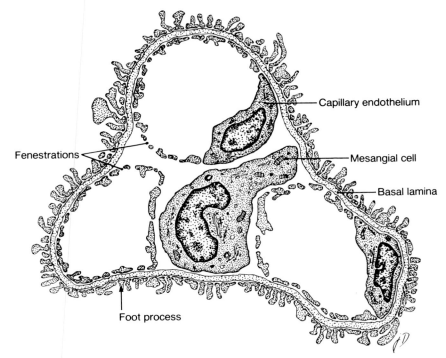

Figure 23.10. A diagram illustrating the relationship of mesangial cells to capillary endothelium and foot processes of podocytes. The basal lamina does not surround each capillary completely. Mesangial cells comprise the core of the capillary tuft that is devoid of a basal lamina.

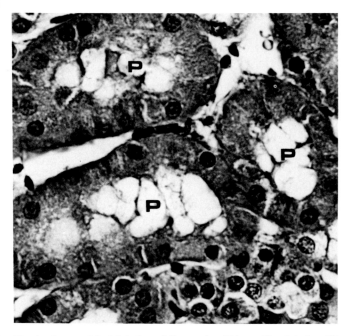

Figure 23.11. Proximal convoluted tubules of the canine kidney. The tubules *(P)* are lined by cuboidal cells. The brush border is not defined clearly. ×160. (See Fig. 5.51.)

part of the wall of this tubule at this point is called the *macula densa*. The tubule continues from its juxtacorpuscular position as the *distal convoluted tubule* (Fig. 23.13).

Distal Convoluted Tubule. Distal convoluted tubules are short and are not encountered as frequently in sections as their proximal counterparts. Although distal convoluted tubules are not as large as proximal convoluted tubules, their luminal diameter to mural thickness ratios are greater than the proximal convoluted tubules. More cells line these tubules, and their lateral borders are better defined than the cells of their proximal counterparts. The cells of distal convoluted tubules are less acidophilic than cells of the proximal tubules. The nuclei of these cells are central to parabasal in position.

Collecting Duct System

The collecting duct system is derived from the metanephric duct. This duct system is continuous with the ureter through the renal pelvis. The collecting duct system may be subdivided into different types of tubules: straight collecting ducts, connecting tubules, arched collecting tubules, and papillary ducts.

The organization of the kidney may be compared to a gland. The nephron represents the adenomere. The connecting tubules and arched collecting ducts may be considered intralobular ducts. The straight collecting ducts are comparable to interlobular ducts, whereas the papillary ducts may be compared to lobar ducts.

Straight collecting ducts occupy the medullary rays within the cortex and medulla. These tubules extend from the cortex through the medulla to join with other straight collecting ducts to form large *papillary ducts*.

Distal convoluted tubules join collecting ducts in two ways. Superficially positioned nephrons empty directly into cortical collecting ducts via *connecting tubules*. Midcortical and juxtamedullary nephrons join straight collecting ducts via *arched collecting tubules*. Connecting tubules of several nephrons join to form these arched tubules. The arched tubules from these nephrons course toward the capsule, turn, descend within medullary rays and join the straight collecting ducts.

The collecting duct system throughout most of its course is lined by cuboidal epithelium. The epithelium of the connecting tubules, arched collecting tubules, and straight collecting ducts consist of cuboidal, pale-staining cells with large, round, dark nuclei. Their lateral cellular margins are distinct. These light or principal cells predominate, but dark cells are observed occasionally. Dark (intercalated) cells have more mitochondria and polyribosomes than light cells. Small folds *(microplicae)*—

segments from other tubules lined by simple squamous epithelium. Usually, the thin segments have larger lumina and more nuclei that protude into the lumina than the capillaries. The morphology of the actual *loop* (Fig. 23.12) and *ascending thin segment* is similar to the descending thin segment. The transition to the cuboidal epithelium of the *ascending limb* is also abrupt. The straight portion ascends to the region of the vascular pole of the renal corpuscle. This portion of the nephron is positioned between the afferent and efferent arterioles. A condensation of cells in

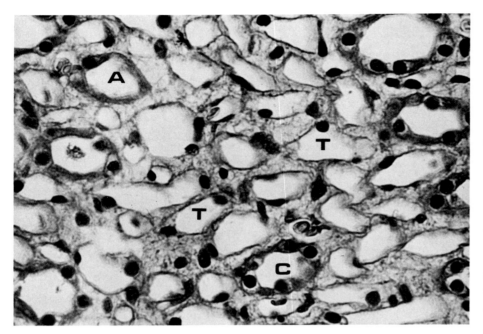

Figure 23.12. Medulla of a canine kidney. Thin segments of Henle's loop *(T)*, ascending limbs *(A)* and collecting ducts *(C)* are indicated. ×160.

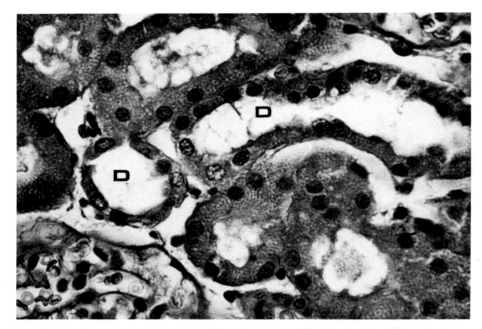

Figure 23.13. Distal convoluted tubules of a canine kidney. The distal tubules *(D)* are lined by a cuboidal epithelium. ×160.

evident with electron microscopy—may characterize their apical surface. The number of dark cells increases as the straight collecting duct continues into the medulla. Also, the epithelial height increases within the medullary collecting ducts (Fig. 23.14).

Straight collecting ducts fuse within the inner zone of the medulla to form papillary ducts. Papillary ductal epithelium is col-

umnar (Fig. 23.15). As the ducts open into the renal pelvis or minor calyses, the *area cribrosa* is formed at the apex of the pyramid or along the renal creast. The ductal epithelium is reflected as the transitional epithelial lining of the intrarenal continuation of the ureter. In ungulates, the transitional epithelium may extend into the papillary ducts for a short distance.

Stromal Elements

Vasculature, Lymphatics, and Nerves. The blood supply for the kidney is the *renal artery* (Fig. 23.16). Upon entering the hilus of the organ the renal artery divides into smaller *interlobar arteries*. The interlobar arteries, coursing parallel to the long axes of the pyramids, turn parallel to the long axis of the kidney at the corticomedullary junction. From this point, they are continued as the *arcuate* or *arciform arteries*.

The blood supply to the cortex is achieved through ascending or perpendicular branches of the arcuate artery, the *interlobular arteries*. The interlobular arteries course through the cortical labyrinth giving rise to numerous short lateral branches, the *afferent arterioles*. The afferent arterioles may be considered *intralobular arterioles*. The afferent arterioles enter the vascular pole of Bowman's capsule and divide into large capillary branches, the *glomerulus*. The capillaries of the glomerulus form a loop and reunite as the *efferent arteriole* that exits Bowman's capsule at the vascular pole (Figs. 23.2, and 23.10). **(N.B.: The capillary bed of the glomerulus is within the arterial circulation.)** The efferent arteriole then divides into a capillary bed that forms a *peritubular plexus* around uriniferous tubules of the cortex.

The medullary blood supply is derived from efferent arterioles originating from renal corpuscles close to the medulla. Vessels extending from these efferent arterioles descend into the medulla along straight paths and are called *false straight arterioles (arteriolae rectae spuriae)*. Vessels originating from the arcuate arteries to supply the medulla are called *true straight arterioles (arteriolae rectae verae)*. Capillary branches of these arterioles enmesh and surround the medullary uriniferous tubules to form a *peritubular plexus*. The arterioles *(arteriolae rectae)*, capillaries, and venules *(venae rectae)* comprise the *vasa recta*.

The interlobular arteries continue to the surface and terminate as a capsular plexus. The venous drainage of the kidney is accomplished through companion vessels to the aforementioned arteries and their branches.

A superficial set of lymph vessels drains the capsular region, whereas a deeper set of vessels, distributed in a manner similar to the blood vessels, drains the renal interstitium.

Many unmyelinated nerves are sympathetic vasomotor fibers, but nerves are not demonstrable within the renal corpuscle. Some branches of the nerves are associated intimately with the tubular epithelial cells; however, these nerves do not enter the epithelial lining. General visceral afferent fibers originate in the capsule, pelvis or calyses, and perivascular region. The precise distribution of parasympathetic fibers to

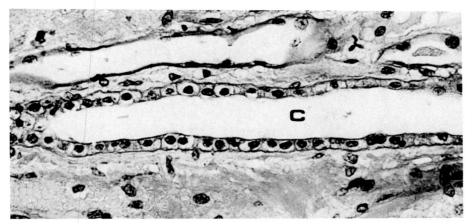

Figure 23.14. Collecting duct from an equine kidney. The collecting duct *(C)* is lined by cuboidal epithelium. The cytoplasm is clear and the lateral cell margins are distinct. ×160.

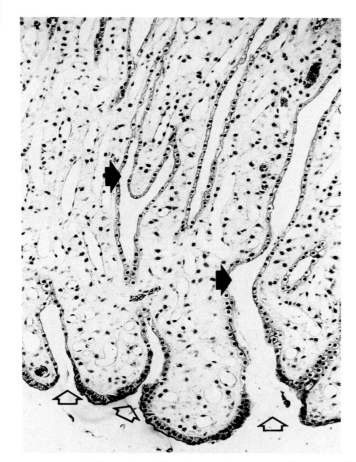

Figure 23.15. Area cribrosa of a feline kidney. The collecting ducts are confluent as papillary ducts *(solid arrows)*. These ducts open into the renal pelvis *(open arrows)* and form an area cribrosa. ×40.

and within the kidney has not been determined. Renal transplants demonstrate aptly that the kidney is able to function without extrinsic nerve supply.

Juxtaglomerular Complex

Histological Components. The *juxtaglomerular complex* or *apparatus* consists of four components: afferent arteriole, efferent arteriole, macula densa, and extraglomerular mesangium (Fig. 23.17). The smooth muscle of the afferent arteriole is modified as myoepithelial cells. These cells are the *juxtaglomerular cells* that contain secretory granules in various stages of synthesis and storage. Although *granular juxtaglomerular cells* predominate, some *agranular jux-*

taglomerular cells contribute to the myoepithelioid cuff. One pole of the juxtaglomerular cells contacts the basal lamina of afferent arterial endothelial cells, whereas the other pole contacts the basal lamina of the macula densa cells in the distal convoluted tubule. *Extraglomerular mesangial cells* are situated between the afferent and efferent arterioles adjacent to the glomerulus. These cells are continuous with intraglomerular mesangium. The precise function of the extraglomerular mesangium *(polkissen cells, lacis cells, polar cushion)* is not understood. The *macula densa* is part of the distal convoluted tubule. The macula densa consists of tall epithelial cells that are thinner than cells in other portions of the distal convoluted tubule. As a result, the region appears as a dense spot (Fig. 23.18). Because of its strategic location in the distal convoluted tubule and its juxtaposition to the juxtaglomerular cells, it is tempting to assign a sensory function to the macula densa. The precise functional relationships of the components of the juxtaglomerular complex, however, have not been determined.

Functional Correlates. Granular juxtaglomerular cells secrete the proteolytic enzyme *renin*. Renin converts *angiotensinogen*, a plasma protein in the α_2-globulin fraction, to *angiotensin I*. Activation of angiotensin I to *angiotensin II* occurs primarily in the lungs through the activity of a *converting enzyme*. Angiotensin II is the most potent arterial constrictor substance known. Also, it reduces vascular volume through constriction of veins. Its pressor activity increases venous return to the heart, thereby increasing cardiac output and blood pressure. The *renin-angiotensin axis* also affects blood volume directly by stimulating the kidneys to retain Na^+ and water. Angiotensin II is also a trophic hormone for the adrenal cortex. This hormone causes the release of aldosterone from the zona glomerulosa of the adrenal cortex. Aldosterone causes increased sodium and water retention by the kidney resulting in an expanded extracellular fluid volume.

The regulation of renin secretion is probably governed by a combination of different mechanisms. Intrarenal baroreceptors, perhaps the juxtaglomerular cells, are sensitive to afferent arteriolar pressure. The release of renin is inversely proportional to this pressure. The macula densa may be a chemoreceptor responsive to sodium levels being transported across the distal convoluted tubule; however, the precise stimuli have not been determined. Similarly, renin release may be inversely proportional to the rate of sodium transport. The sympathetic nervous system exerts two effects upon arterial blood pressure. The direct effect is manifested upon vascular smooth muscle through the appropriate adrenergic receptors. Also, circulating catecholamines

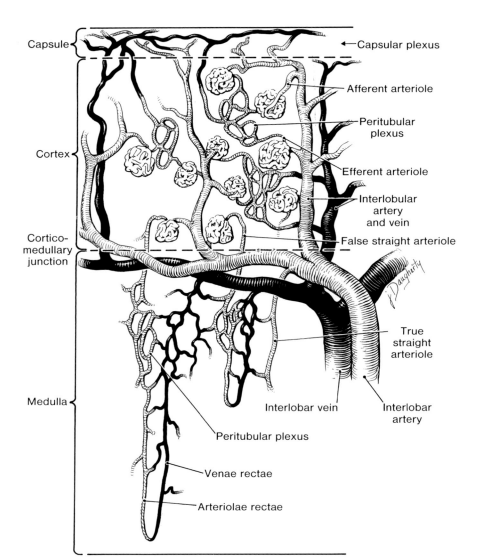

Capsule

Capsular plexus

Afferent arteriole

Peritubular plexus

Cortex

Efferent arteriole

Interlobular artery and vein

Cortico-medullary junction

False straight arteriole

Figure 23.16. A diagram depicting the vascular supply of the kidney.

True straight arteriole

Medulla

Interlobar vein

Interlobar artery

Peritubular plexus

Venae rectae

Arteriolae rectae

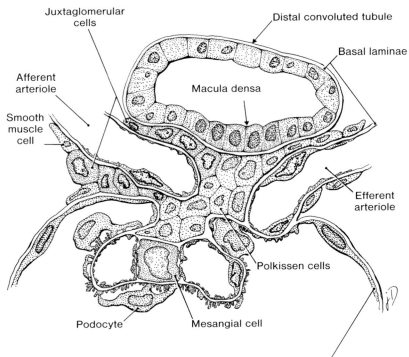

Juxtaglomerular cells

Distal convoluted tubule

Basal laminae

Afferent arteriole

Macula densa

Smooth muscle cell

Figure 23.17. A diagram of the juxtaglomerular apparatus.

Efferent arteriole

Polkissen cells

Podocyte

Mesangial cell

Parietal layer of Bowman's capsule

440

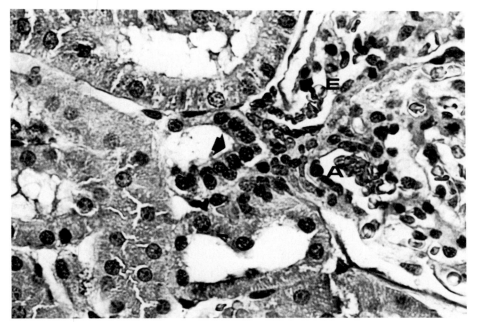

Figure 23.18. Macula densa of a canine kidney. The macula densa *(arrow)* marks the beginning of the distal convoluted tubule. The macula densa is positioned at the vascular pole in close association with the afferent *(A)* and efferent *(E)* arterioles. The cells between the afferent arteriole, efferent arteriole, and macula densa are polkissen cells. ×160.

stimulate the release of renin by direct activiation of β-adrenergic receptors on juxtaglomerular cells. Antidiuretic hormone and angiotensin II inhibit the release of renin. Juxtaglomerular cells also secrete erythrogenin in response to hypoxia and respiratory alkalosis.

Histophysiology of the Kidney

The maintenance of an optimal enviromnment is the primary function of the kidney. The maintenance is predicated upon conserving essential metabolites—ions, sugars, amino acids, water—and secreting metabolic waste products. The proper maintenance of fluid balance is an essential renal function. Three renal mechanisms are used to accomplish these functions—glomerular filtration, tubular reabsorption, and tubular secretion. The essence of renal function is the filtration of all filterable substances and the reabsorption of those that are essential. These mechanisms are complemented by tubular secretion of selected substances.

The kidney is also an essential endocrine organ. Its secretion of erythropoietin affects red blood cell production. Renin is secreted by the juxtaglomerular apparatus. This substance is essential for the endocrine influence on blood pressure and fluid volume. The renal epithelium is involved in calcium metabolism.

Glomerular Filtration. The blood flow to the kidneys represents approximately 20–25% of the cardiac output. Renal blood flow, equivalent to about 5000 ml/gram of tissue/day, is substantially higher than other tissues. By comparison, blood flow to

the brain is about 1500 ml/gram of tissue/day. Of the total renal blood flow, approximately 60,000 ml of fluid becomes the glomerular filtrate daily (200 ml/min) in a 30-lb dog. Only 1% or 600 ml (ml/lb/day) of urine are excreted daily. Although the fluid load imposed upon the kidneys through glomerular filtration is great, most of the fluid is reabsorbed. A 30-lb dog has an approximate blood volume of 1200 ml. If the PVC were 50, then the plasma volume is 600 cc. The plasma is filtered approximately 100 times a day, and the urine excreted is approximately equivalent to one plasma volume daily.

Blood entering the glomerulus is subject to glomerular filtration. The glomerular filtrate is an *ultrafiltrate* of blood plasma. The filtrate is devoid of blood cells and contains only trace amounts of albumin. Molecules with molecular weights in the range of 5000 filter through the glomerulus as easily as water. Molecules with molecular weights of 70,000— a molecular weight equivalent to albumin—have a permeability that is about 1/200 the permeability of water. Molecules of this size, therefore, are filtered minimally. Small molecular-weight compounds occur in the flitrate in approximately the same concentration that they occur in the interstitial fluid; the filtrate is *isosmotic* with the interstitial fluid. The barrier that selectively excludes large particles may be perceived as a molecular sieve. Whereas the endothelial cells and podocytes exclude the passage of large particulate matter, their fenestrations and filtration slits, respectively, do not exclude all substances. The effectiveness and selectivity of the barrier

to various substances is dependent upon the properties of the endothelial cells, basal lamina and filtration slits.

The formation of the glomerular filtrate *(capsular urine)* is dependent upon energy expended by the cardiovascular system without the expediture of energy by the cells of the renal corpuscle. The principles that govern the formation of tissue fluid (Chapter 6) in other parts of the body apply to glomerular filtrate formation.

Various factors influence glomerular filtration rate (GFR): permeability and surface area of the glomerular filtration surface, blood and tubular hydrostatic pressure, blood colloid osmotic pressure. The permeability of the basal lamina may be altered in disease processes in which high molecular weight compounds (immune complexes, mucosubstances, immunoglobulins) are deposited on or within the barrier; the GFR decreases in this circumstance. The failure to develop and/or maintain the number and size of the renal corpuscles may result in a decreased GFR. Increasing tubular hydrostatic pressure (urinary obstruction) or increasing the colloid osmotic pressure of the blood also decreases the GFR. Increasing blood hydrostatic pressure or decreasing blood colloid osmotic pressure increases the net driving force and increases the GFR.

Tubular Reabsorption. Neither the entire volume nor all the constituents of capsular urine become the final excretory product. Substances are reabsorbed selectively in different parts of the uriniferous tubules. Some (glucose, amino acids, sodium) are reabsorbed by active transport mechanisms, whereas others (water, urea) are reabsorbed passively. Most active transport mechanisms have maximal reabsorption limits. Beyond these limits, substances that are usually absorbed will be excreted in the urine. Some hormones (parathormone, aldosterone, antidiuretic hormone [ADH]) also influence the reabsorption process. Passive tubular reabsorption processes are dependent upon the same mechanisms that govern the formation of tissue fluid and its constituents.

Glucose, passing freely through the filtration barrier, is part of the capsular urine; however, 100% of filtered glucose is reabsorbed by an active transport mechanism in the proximal convoluted tubule. Glucose appears in the urine *(glucosuria)* when the capacity of the carrier molecule in the brush border of the lining cells is exceeded. The *glucose threshold* for tubular reabsorption is not exceeded until blood glucose levels reach twice normal levels or 180–200 mg%.

Amino acids are transported actively by three distinct mechanisms for different groups of amino acids.

Other substances reabsorbed by the tubular system include Na^+ K^+, $HPO_4^=$, Ca^{++}, ketone bodies (acetoacetate, β-hydroxybutyrate), ascorbic acid, and water. Whereas most of the active transport mechanisms are part of the proximal convoluted tubule, other components of the uriniferous tubules participate also.

Sodium, the most important extracellular ion in terms of blood volume and osmolality, is 98% reabsorbed in the proximal convoluted tubule and loop of Henle. The remaining 2% in the distal convoluted tubule and collecting duct is reabsorbed under the influence of aldosterone. Potassium, magnesium, bicarbonate, and sulfate are almost completely reabsorbed in the proximal tubules of the nephron. *Calcium* and phosphate ions are filtered and reabsorbed by the proximal convoluted tubule.

Urea, formed as a consequence of nitrogen metabolism, passes freely across the diffusion barrier. Its concentration in the glomerular filtrate is isosmotic with the plasma. Urea is absorbed passively by the proximal part of the uriniferous tubules. The concentraion of urea increases in the tubules as water is reabsorbed; thus, urea passes out of the tubules down its concentration gradient into the interstitium and vasa recta. The rate of urine flow and the extent of water reabsorption influence the amount of urea in the urine. Most of the urea (about 70%) is reabsorbed under conditions of low flow rate and the formation of a concentrated urine. High flow rates and dilute urine formation may reduce urea reabsorption to 10% of that which is filtered.

The amount of urea in the blood is expressed often as *blood urea nitrogen (BUN)*. Whereas glomerular filtration is the prime mechanism of urea clearance, the amount of urea cleared by the kidneys is never equal to the amount filtered because of tubular reabsorption. An increased BUN may indicate abnormal kidney function; however, other factors may cause an increased BUN—increased dietary protein intake, increased protein catabolism, decreased renal perfusion, postrenal obstruction.

Urea tends to concentrate in the renal interstitium especially at the apex of the pyramids. The graded concentration of urea within the medullary pyramids contributes to the ability of the kidney to concentrate other solutes in the urine.

Despite the urine being an ultrafiltrate of plasma, small amounts of low molecular weight *proteins* (albumin) are constituents of the filtrate (approximately 0.03%). Most of the filtered protein is reabsorbed by the tubular epithelial cells. Protein in the urine *(proteinuria)* may result from a decreased capacity of tubular resorption or tubular damage, but most proteinuria is a consequence of altered glomerular filtration.

Tubular Secretion. Tubular secretory mechanisms complement the clearance of substances that are filtered at the glomerulus. The substances secreted include not only those compounds produced endogenously (creatinine, histamine, and metabolic products of hormones) but also exogenously administered compounds and their metabolic products (antibiotics, aspirin, various other drugs). Additionally, water, various cations (H^+, K^+, Na^+) and anions (HCO_3^-, $HPO_4^=$) pass into the tubular lumen by active or passive mechanisms.

Whereas separate mechanisms are utilized by the kidney for the reabsorption of various substances, only two distinct processes are used for the tubular secretion of organic compounds. Both processes are part of active transport mechanisms by the proximal convoluted tubular epithelium. One system secretes *organic acids* and the other system secretes *organic bases*. Each system has a maximal capacity, and compounds within each group compete with each other.

The role of the kidneys in calcium and phosphate metabolism is discussed in Chapter 9.

The movement of water, ammonia, sodium, chloride, potassium, bicarbonate, urea, and hydrogen ions is an essential component of countercurrent and/or acid/base mechanisms.

Countercurrent Mechanism. The *countercurrent mechanism* is predicated upon the maintenance of an osmolality gradient that is established from the base of the pyramid to the apex of the pyramid (papilla) (Fig. 23.19). The base of the pyramid (interstitium, tubules, and vasa recta) is *isosmolar* with the blood (300 mOsm), whereas the apex of the pyramid is approximately four times more concentrated *(hyperosmolar)* or 1200 mOsm. The loop of Henle, the *countercurrent multiplier*, establishes the gradient by virtue of its permeability characteristics, juxtaposition of descending and ascending components, and the direction of the flow of urine within the tubules. The inflow in the descending limb runs parallel and counter to the outflow in the ascending limb. The operation of the countercurrent mechanism is explained by various theories; the following satisfies many of the observations made. The descending limb of the loop of Henle, although, relatively impermeable to most solutes, permits the movement of water into the interstitium. The ascending limb of Henle's loop is impermeable to water but allows free movement of sodium into the interstitium. This relationship, alone, establishes an increasing tonicity toward the hairpin loop in the descending limb and interstitium and a decreasing tonicity from the hairpin loop up the ascending limb and interstitium. The transport of sodium, linked to the active transport of chloride in the thick segment of the ascending limb, produces a hypotonic tubular fluid in this segment. Sodium may be actively transported out of the distal convoluted tubule and collecting duct. Sodium also may be passively transported out of the collecting duct, whereas water moves passively into the interstitium in the distal convoluted tubule and collecting duct.

Urea also contributes to the concentration gradient. Urea concentration increases toward the apex of the loop of Henle, both within the tubules and the medullary interstitium. The gradient is dependent upon the recirculation of urea from the collecting duct into the interstitium and then into the ascending and descending limbs of Henle's loop. The dynamic and constant circulation of urea assures a high concentration of the compound in the urine and aids in increasing the sodium and chloride concentrations of the inner medulla.

The vasae rectae contribute to the countercurrent mechanism as *countercurrent exchangers*. Water diffuses out of the arteriolae rectae, while sodium and urea move down their concentration gradients into the vessels. Conversely, water diffuses into the venae rectae, while solutes (sodium, urea) move into the interstitium. The fluids within the tip of the vasa recta are in equilibrium with the hairpin loop of Henle and interstitium. The recirculation phenomenon maintains the tubular, vascular, and interstitial gradient. The meager and retarded flow of blood through the medulla assists in the maintenance of these gradients.

The establishment of the medullary gradient, a tubular function, occurs passively and is attributed to the selective permeability of the tubular epithelium. Evidence exists that the passive movement of sodium occurs with the active transport of chloride in the ascending thick segment of Henle's loop. The maintenance of the gradient, a vascular function, occurs passively.

The maintenance of proper tissue fluid and blood osmolality is essential for proper cellular function. Hyperosmolar tissue fluid and blood draw fluids from cells, thereby decreasing cellular volume. Hypotonic extracellular fluids cause fluids to move into cells, increasing cellular volume. Both situations impair cellular function. The countercurrent multiplier and exchanger mechanisms provide vehicles for the conservation of water and sodium, both of which are essential for proper fluid volume and tonicity. The reabsorption of water in the proximal convoluted tubule accounts for approximately an 80% recovery of the filtered fluid volume; the loop of Henle reabsorbs another 5% of the filtered fluid. Another 14% is reabsorbed in the distal convoluted tubule and collecting ducts under the influence of ADH. The remaining 1% becomes the fluid volume of the excreted urine.

The imbibition of excessive quantities of water increases extracellular fluid volume and results in cellular swelling. Hypotha-

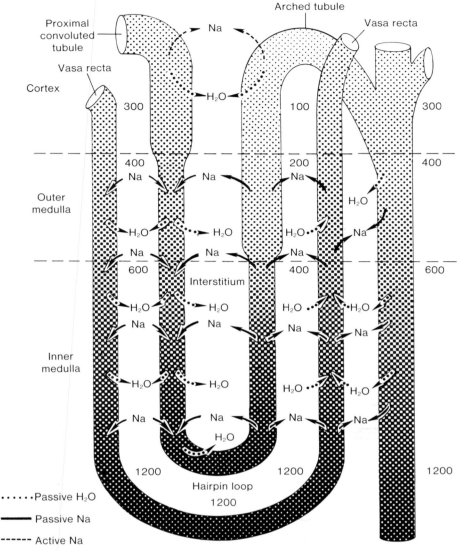

Figure 23.19. A simplified diagram depicting the movement of water and sodium as it relates to the countercurrent mechanism. The concentration of urine within the collecting tubules, as illustrated, occurs under the influence of ADH. Other solutes, notably urea, contribute to the gradient. The gradient, as depicted, 300–1200 milliosmoles, is not the same in all species; however, the relationships are similar. The gradient within the interstitium is similar to that noted for the tubules and vessels. Tubular urine becomes progressively more concentrated toward the hairpin loop, decreases to a hypotonic urine in the thick segment of the ascending limb and becomes hypertonic in the collecting duct system under the influence of ADH.

metabolic product, results in the formation of acid accordingly:

$$CO_2 + H_2O \rightleftharpoons H_2CO_3 \rightleftharpoons H^+ + HCO_3^-$$

Other acids are components of the diet or result from metabolism (sulfate, phosphate, lactate, hydrochloric acid, β-hydroxybutyrate). Various mechanisms are utilized to neutralize excess acids and bases. The lungs rid the body of excess carbon dioxide. Buffer systems (carbonate, phosphate, protein, hemoglobin) serve to neutralize excess acids and bases. Also, the kidneys function to excrete or conserve acids and bases. The normal pH of the urine varies between species and among individuals of a given species. The normal pH of the urine of carnivores is acidic, whereas that of herbivores is alkaline; the pH of the urine of omnivores (swine, man) may be acidic or alkaline. Numerous factors—diet, metabolism, disease—can alter urinary pH.

The proteins of the body are the most powerful buffers. These amphoteric substances are capable of releasing acids or bases in response to microenvironmental pH changes. The pKs of some of the proteins are close to the microenvironmental pH, 7.4. These proteins, then, have a high buffering capacity.

The phosphate buffer system is operational close to one of its pKs. Accordingly, the system affords a high potential for buffering. The extracellular fluid space does not contain high concentrations of phosphate compounds; their role is important within cells and renal tubules.

The bicarbonate system is not a powerful buffer, because the interstitial fluid pH is more alkaline than the effective pK of this system. The efficacy of the bicarbonate buffer system, however, accrues from the ability to regulate the constituents. The lungs regulate carbon dioxide and the kidneys regulate bicarbonate ion.

Deviations from normal blood pH occur under various circumstances. The amount of carbon dioxide in body fluids affects the pH. **Increased concentrations of CO_2 in the body fluids decrease the pH, whereas decreased concentrations of CO_2 in the body fluids increase the pH.** Since carbon dioxide is a continuous product of tissue metabolism, the tendency is for the body fluids to become progressively more acidic. The rate at which CO_2 is removed from the body via expiration must be matched to the rate at which it is produced by the tissues. An increased metabolic rate produces an increased amount of carbon dioxide in the tissue fluid that must be accompanied by an increased respiratory rate. The converse is true with a decreased metabolic rate.

The respiratory rate, independent of the metabolic rate, affects the amount of car-

lamic cells *(osmoreceptor cells)* respond to the increased fluid volume by decreasing ADH secretion. In the absence of ADH, the distal convoluted tubule and collecting duct become impermeable to water, resulting in the excretion of a dilute (hypotonic) urine. Conversely, a decreased fluid volume, resulting in the release of ADH, is characterized by a low volume and hypertonic urine. Animals with *diabetes insipidus* are unable to produce ADH or are unable to produce proper quantities of this hormone; they characteristically produce large volumes of dilute urine *(polyuria)*. To compensate for the urinary fluid loss, they must ingest large quantities of water *(poly-*

dipsia). Polyuria is not always characterized by a hypotonic urine. The retention of osmotically active substances within the tubules causes the retention of water also. Exceeding the glucose threshold, as occurs in *diabetes mellitus*, results in a hypertonic, high volume urine. Glucose causes an *osmotic diuresis*, whereas ADH insufficiency results in a *water diuresis*; however, polydipsia is a compensatory mechanism for both.

Acid/Base Balance. Deviations from normal pH alter metabolic processes by accelerating or depressing enzymatic activity. Animals are exposed to large quantities of acids daily. Carbon dioxide, the primary

bon dioxide in the tissue fluids. The carbon dioxide concentration within the tissues is inversely proportional to alveolar ventilation. Under circumstances of a constant metabolic rate, a decreased ventilation results in an increaed accumulation of CO_2. Increasing ventilation to twice the normal rate—blowing off CO_2—raises the pH by about 0.2 pH units. Conversely, decreasing ventilation to one-quarter of the normal rate—retaining CO_2—depresses the pH by about 0.4 pH units. *Hyperventilation*, the excessive loss of carbon dioxide through the lungs, causes a *respiratory alkalosis*, whereas *hypoventilation*, the inadequate elimination of carbon dioxide through the lungs, results in *respiratory acidosis*.

Metabolic acidosis may result from various conditions that cause a loss of base: diarrhea, vomiting, or an increased production of acid (ketoacidosis). *Metabolic alkalosis* may result from vomiting in which only gastric contents are lost. Similarly, metabolic alkalosis may result from the sequestration of acids in the stomach as occurs in abomasal displacement and other abomasal disorders.

Excursions away from the normal concentration of H^+ are accompanied by renal and pulmonary compensatory mechanisms. Pulmonary compensation of metabolic acidosis is an increased ventilation that results in the rapid decrease of CO_2 in the tissue fluids. This increases the pH toward normal. The pulmonary compensatory mechanism in metabolic alkalosis is the opposite to that just described. Metabolic alkalosis induces a decreased pulmonary ventilation that results in retention of CO_2. This retention increases the H^+ concentration of the tissue fluids.

Renal compensation of pulmonary acidosis is the secretion of excess hydrogen ion. Secretion of H^+ is accompanied by bicarbonate moving into the interstitium (base conservation). Just the opposite constitutes the renal compensation for respiratory alkalosis.

A *paradoxical aciduria* does accompany some metabolic alkalotic conditions (canine vomiting, bovine abomasal displacements). The need to conserve electrolytes (Na^+, K^+, Cl^-) may be considered a more important renal function than the conservation of H^+ under these circumstances.

The renal secretion of hydrogen ion is achieved by the epithelium of the proximal and distal convoluted tubules in a manner similar to that used by the parietal cell (Fig. 23.20). The active transport (secretion) of H^+ is associated with the passive uptake of Na^+. The secretion of one H^+ is linked to the movement of a Na^+ into the interstitium and K^+ into the cell (Na^+-K^+ pump); a bicarbonate moves out of the cell into the interstitium for each H^+ secreted also.

Although the transport mechanism for H^+ is active, a limiting concentration exists

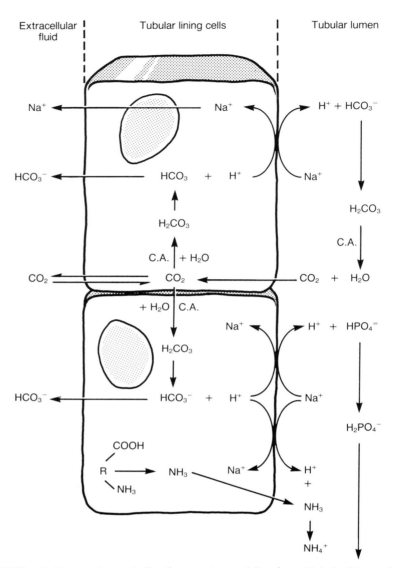

Figure 23.20. A diagram demonstrating the secretory activity of renal tubular lining cells. *C.A.*, carbonic anhydrase.

beyond which the transport mechanism does not work. Free hydrogen ions are removed from the urine by reacting with HCO_3^-, $HPO_4^=$ and NH_3 (ammonia). Hydrogen ions react with tubular HCO_3^- to form carbonic acid (H_2CO_3). Carbonic anhydrase on the brush borders of the proximal tubular epithelial cells catalyzes the conversion of carbonic acid to carbon dioxide and water and effectively removes hydrogen from the tubular fluid. Carbon dioxide diffuses into the cells and becomes part of the available CO_2 to form more H_2CO_3 under the influence of carbonic anhydrase. The intracellular H_2CO_3 dissociates into HCO_3^- and H^+. The HCO_3^- diffuses into the extracellular fluid and the H^+ is secreted actively into the tubular lumen. Combination of H^+ with $HPO_4^=$ in the distal convoluted tubules and collecting ducts removes H^+ from the tubular urine.

Finally, ammonia (NH_3) is formed within all of the tubular epithelial cells by the activity of enzymes associated with the removal of amines from amino acids. The NH_3, because of its lipid-solubility, flows freely across the plasmalemmal barrier into the lumina of the tubules. Once within the tubular fluid, NH_3 reacts with H^+ to form NH_4^+ (ammonium ion). Because of its charge, NH_4^+ remains in the tubular urine. The amount of NH_4^+ in the urine depends upon the amount of H^+ secreted. Ammonium concentration is high in acidic urine. These mechanisms facilitate the secretion of H^+ by the kidneys.

Although the mechanisms described previously account for H^+ secretion, the reactivity of H^+ with HCO_3^-, HPO_4^-, and NH_3^- are important mechanisms for base conservation. During periods of excess H^+ secretion, an increase in detectable (titratable) urinary acids (H⁺, $H_2PO_4^-$, NH_4^+) occurs at a time that the body has a need for more HCO_3^- to neutralize the excess acidity. The formation of H_2CO_3 within the tubule, its conversion to CO_2 and H_2O and subsequent reabsorption of the CO_2 by the tubular cells returns the base (HCO_3^-) to the somatic pool. The formation of titratable urinary acids also serves to conserve sodium. The ammonium ion replaces Na⁺ that may be exchanged while a H⁺ is secreted.

Urinary Passages

Renal Pelvis. The inner surface of the renal pelvis is continuous with the epithelial lining of the papillary ducts. The epithelium becomes a thin transitional lining that becomes thicker toward the pelvis. The lamina propria-tunica submucosa is composed of areolar connective tissue. In equids, branched, tubuloalveolar, mucous glands occur in this region and extend into the ureter. These glands account for the frothy appearance of the urine of these species. The tunica muscularis may be composed of three layers of muscle that are arranged in bundles. The layers, however, are not always distinct. The contraction of these muscle bundles tends "to milk" urine from the kidney.

Ureters. The ureters are lined by a lamina epithelialis mucosa of transitional epithelium (Fig. 23.21). Goblet cells may be present in these structures in the horse. The lamina propria-tunica submucosa consists of areolar connective tissue. Mucous glands may be present in some species (Fig. 23.22). The tunica muscularis is present and three layers of muscle may be apparent. The tunica adventitia, also, is present and typical. Part of the ureters is covered by a tunica serosa (peritoneum).

Urinary Bladder. The ureters open obliquely into the bladder near its neck, and the longitudinal coat of the tunica muscularis of the ureters continues into the bladder wall. There is very little circularly oriented muscle at this junction. Pressure within the bladder tends to close the orifice. The contractions of the ureteral musculature tend to squirt urine into the bladder. The mural elements of the bladder are similar to those of the ureters.

The tunica mucosa of the ureters and the bladder may be highly folded. At this time, the lamina epithelialis mucosae is thick (Fig. 5.16). Upon distention of the bladder, the transitional epithelium is reduced in thickness and the mucosal folds are effaced (Fig. 5.17).

Urethrae. The urethrae are discussed with their respective reproductive systems.

Micturition. *Micturition (urination)*, the passage of urine from the bladder to the exterior of the body, is a spinal reflex that may be facilitated and/or inhibited by

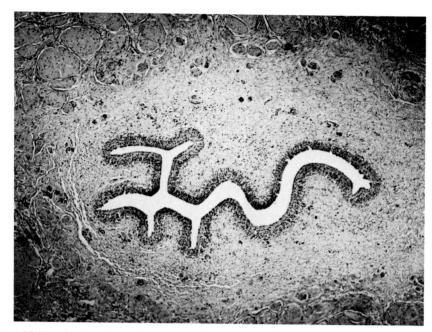

Figure 23.21. Canine ureter. The ureter is lined by transitional epithelium. The lamina propria-submucosa is extensive and surrounded by smooth muscle. ×4.

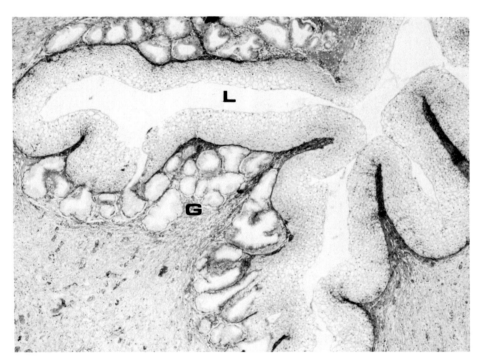

Figure 23.22. A section of part of an equine ureter. The lumen *(L)* is lined by transitional epithelium. Note the mucous glands *(G)* in the lamina propria. ×25.

higher brain centers. Damage to the sacral segments of the spinal cord may result in an *autonomous bladder* that is devoid of extrinsic stimulatory innervation and sensation. Voluntary control of bladder function is lost, and urine flow results from bladder overflow. Residual bladder volume is high in this condition. An *automatic bladder* results from damage occurring to the nervous system cranial to the sacral spinal segments. The reflex arc remains intact, but voluntary control of bladder function is lost. Residual bladder volume is low.

References

Andrews, P. M. and Porter, K. R.: A scanning electron microscope study of the nephron. Am. J. Anat. *140*:81, 1974.

Barajas, L.: The ultrastructure of the juxtaglomerular apparatus as disclosed by three dimensional reconstructions from serial sections. J. Ultrastruct. Res. *33*:116, 1970.

Barajas, L.: The juxtaglomerular apparatus: anatomical considerations in feedback control of glomerular filtration rate. Fed. Proc. *40*:78, 1981.

Beeuwkes, R. and Bonventre, J. V.: Tubular organization and vascular tubular relations in the dog kidney. Am. J. Physiol. *229*:695, 1975.

Calhoun, M. L.: Comparative histology of the ureters of domestic animsls. Anat. Rec. *133*:365, 1959.

Christensen, G. C.: Circulation of blood through the canine kidney. Am. J. Vet. Res. *13*:236, 1952.

Dalton, A. J. and Haguenau, F. (eds.): *Ultrastructure of the Kidney*, Vol. 2, Academic Press, New York, 1967.

Dicker, S. E.: *Mechanisms of Urine Concentration and Dilution in Mammals.* Arnold, London, 1970.

Fisher, E. R. : Lysosomal nature of juxtaglomerular granules. Science. *152:1752*, 1966.

Gans, J. H. and Mercer, P. F.: The kidneys. *In:* Swenson, M. J. (ed.), 9th edition. *Duke's Physiology of Domestic Animals.* pp. 463–492, Comstock Publishing, Ithaca, 1977.

Gingerich, D. A. and Murdick, P. W.: Paradoxic aciduria in bovine metabolis acidosis. J. Am. Vet. Med. Assoc. *166:227*, 1975.

Grahame, T.: The pelvis and calyses of the kidneys of some mammals. Brit. Vet. J. *109:51*, 1953.

Jorgensen, F.: Electron microscopic studies of normal visceral epithelial cells. Lab. Invest. *17:225*, 1967.

Kaneko. J. J. and Cornelius, C. W.: *Clinical Biochemistry of Domestic Animals.* Vol. 2, 2nd edition, Academic Press, New York, 1971.

Latta, H.: The glomerular capillary wall. J. Ultrastruct. Res. *32*:526, 1970.

Latta, H., Johnson, W. H. and Stanley, T. M.: Sialoglycoproteins and filtration barriers in the glomerular capillary wall. J. Ultrastruct. Res. *51:*354, 1975.

Monis, B. and Zambrano, D.: Transitional epithelium of urinary tract in normal and dehydrated rats. Z. Zellforsch. *85:*165, 1968.

Osawa, G., Kimmelsteil, P. and Seiling, V.: Thickness of glomerular basement membranes. Amer. J. Clin. Path. *45:*7, 1966.

Osborne, C. A., Low, D. G. and Finco, D. R.: *Canine and Feline Urology.* W. B. Saunders, Philadelphia, 1972.

Pease, D. C.: Electron microscopy of the tubular cells of the kidney cortex. Anat. Rec. *121:*723, 1955.

Rhodin, J.: Anatomy of kidney tubules. Int. Rev. Cytol. *7:*485, 1958.

Sullivan, L. P. and Grantham, J.J.: *Physiology of the Kidney.* Lea & Febiger, Philadelphia, 1982.

Walker, F.: The origin, turnover and removal of glomerular basement membrane. J. Pathol. *110:*233, 1973.

Woodburne, R. T.: The sphincter mechanism of the urinary bladder and the urethra. Anat. Rec. *141:*11, 1961.

24: Respiratory System

General Characteristics

Form and Function. The respiratory system *conducts* and *exchanges* gases. This system may be subdivided into three components: conductive, transitional, and exchange components (Fig. 24.1). The *conductive components* extend from the external nares to the bronchioles. A *transitional component* is present in some animals and consists of respiratory bronchioles—structures that conduct and exchange gases. The *exchange component* consists of alveolar ducts, alveolar sacs, and alveoli.

Numerous ancillary functions are accomplished by the respiratory system: *phonation, olfaction, body temperature regulation, excretion,* and *acid/base balance.* Also, *blood pressure* is influenced by the activation of angiotensin I to angiotensin II by a converting enzyme within the lung and other organs. Numerous active substances (histamine, prostaglandins E and F, kallikrein) are produced by the lungs for release into the circulation. Similarly, other active substances (prostaglandins E and F, serotonin, bradykinin, norepinephrine) are removed from the pulmonary circulation by the lungs. The respiratory system also has *protective* functions. Inhaled dry air is humidified by glandular secretions and cooled or warmed by the erectile tissue of the upper respiratory tract. Hairs trap large foreign particles at the external nares, whereas those that gain entrance to the respiratory tract are moved to the nasopharynx by the numerous cilia of the epithelium of the "upper" respiratory tract and lung—mucociliary apparatus. Finally, alveolar macrophages are scattered throughout the lung.

Respiratory Tract

Conductive Components

General Remarks. Besides the *conduction* of air, this portion of the system is also responsible for *cleansing, humidifying,* and either *cooling* or *warming* the air. Specific portions of the tract are responsible for *olfaction* and *phonation.*

Nasal Cavity

The nasal cavity is divisible into three histologically distinct regions: vestibular, respiratory, and olfactory regions.

Vestibular Region. The extent of the *vestibular region* is species-variable. It is the point of transition from the integument to the cutaneous mucous membrane of the nasal cavity. The lamina epithelialis mucosae is not keratinized. Pigment cells may be present. The typical lamina propria-tunica submucosa blends with the underlying fascial covering of muscle or the fibrous layer of the associated investments of bone or cartilage. Hairs (vibrissae), sweat glands, and sebaceous glands occur in the cutaneous part. Branched, tubuloalveolar glands (serous and mixed) may also be present. These glands assist in humidifying the air.

Respiratory Region. The vestibular cutaneous mucous membrane changes to the mucous membrane of the *respiratory region* (Fig. 24.2). The latter comprises the bulk of the nasal cavity. The lamina epithelialis mucosae, a pseudostratified ciliated columnar epithelium with goblet cells, humidifies and cleanses the air. The lamina propria-tunica submucosa is typical. Numerous, branched, tubuloalveolar, mixed glands, *nasal glands*, which are predominantly serous, are scattered throughout this layer. *Erectile tissue* may also be present. Erectile tissue, consisting of vascular cavities that are lined by endothelium, is continuous with the blood vessels of a particular region. Although the erectile tissue is usually collapsed, it becomes engorged with blood under proper neural stimulation. The glandular tissue humidifies the air, whereas the engorged erectile tissue cools or warms it by using the mucous membrane as a heat transfer device. The connective tissue of this region is continuous with the underlying connective tissue associated with the bone or cartilage.

Olfactory Region. The *olfactory region* is a specialized region for olfaction that is positioned on the ethmoturbinates, adjacent dorsal turbinates, and the nasal septum (Fig. 24.3). The lamina epithelialis mucosae, which consists of pseudostratified columnar epithelium, is thick; as many as 15 strata of nuclei may be apparent in section. This region has three cell types. *Sustentacular cells* are tall with broad apices and narrow bases. Oval, vesicular nuclei are positioned toward the apex. Pigment granules responsible for the color of the region grossly are contained within these cells. Basal cells are typical of those that occur in this type of epithelium. The *olfactory cells* are modified bipolar neurons, the basal processes of which continue to the brain as axons of the first cranial nerve. The apex of the cell is modified as a bulb-like projection, the *olfactory vesicle*, from which modified cilia, *olfactory hairs*, project. The hairs are the receptors for olfactory stimuli. The round, vesicular nucleus is positioned centrally or basally. The underlying lamina propria mucosae is typical and contains branched, tubuloalveolar serous glands (Plate II.8). These glands, *Bowman's glands*, are responsible for cleansing the olfactory surface and for solubilizing odor-producing substances.

Paranasal Sinuses. The *paranasal sinuses* are spaces within the maxillary, frontal, ethmoid, and sphenoid bones of the skull that are continuous with the nasal cavity. The epithelium may be cuboidal, squamous, or thin pseudostratified ciliated columnar. Goblet cells and nasal glands occur less frequently than in the nasal cavity proper. Erectile tissue is not present. The remaining connective tissue/osseous relationships are similar to those of the nasal cavity proper. Because of the intimate relationship of the mucosa to the underlying bone, these structures are referred to collectively as a *mucoperiosteum.*

Vomeronasal Organ. The *vomeronasal organ* or Jacobson's organ is a paired, tubular structure that is located parallel to the base of the rostral part of the nasal septum. The organ is partially enclosed by hyaline cartilage (vomeronasal cartilage). The organ opens into the incisive duct, which connects the nasal and oral cavities.

The rostral part of the vomeronasal organ is lined by respiratory epithelium, whereas the caudal part is lined by respiratory epithelium along its lateral wall and olfactory epithelium along its medial wall.

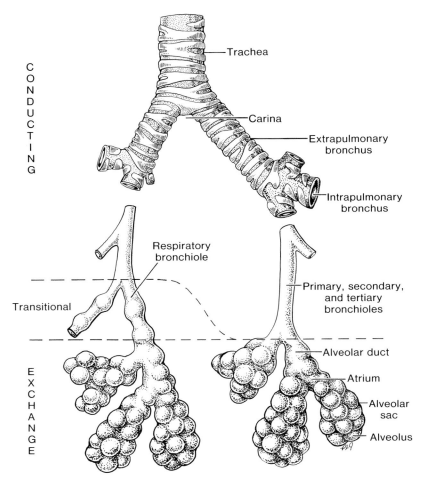

Figure 24.1. A diagram of airways from the trachea to the alveoli. The transitional zone is not present nor equally developed in all species.

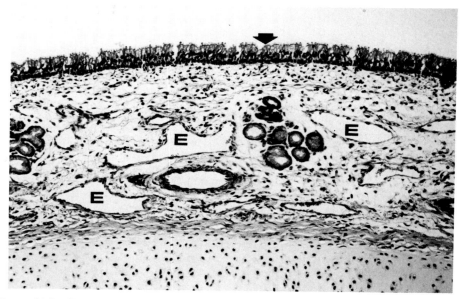

Figure 24.2. Respiratory mucosa. The lamina epithelialis mucosae *(arrow)* is pseudostratified ciliated columnar epithelium with goblet cells. The lamina propria mucosae contains serous glands and erectile tissue *(E)*. The connective tissue of the lamina propria mucosae is continuous with the fibrous perichondrium of the underlying cartilage. ×40.

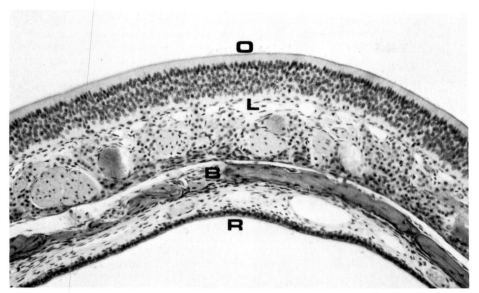

Figure 24.3. Olfactory and respiratory mucosal covering of an osseous portion of a turbinate. The olfactory mucosa (O) is a nonciliated pseudostratified columnar epithelium that is thicker than the respiratory epithelium (R). The lamina propria (L) contains numerous serous glands and bone (B). ×40.

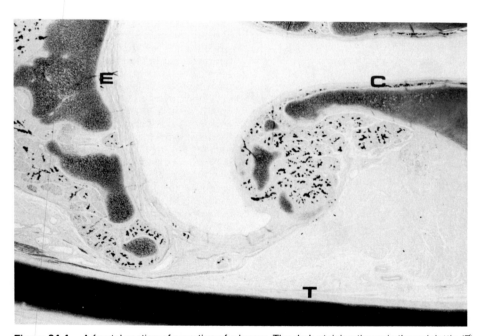

Figure 24.4. A frontal section of a portion of a larynx. The dark-staining tissue is the epiglottic (E), cricoid (C) and thyroid (T) cartilages. ×4 (Aldehyde fuchsin).

Although the olfactory epithelium has some unique ultrastructural features, this accessory lining essentially resembles typical olfactory epithelium. The lamina propria-submucosa is typical. Serous, mucous, and seromucoid glands have been noted in association with the organ.

The position of the organ permits sampling of substances that are volatilized easily from licking and/or inhalation. This organ may be the sensory receptor for stimuli that lead to behavioral patterns associated with specific substances. The receptor may recognize specific pheromones and induce mating behavior.

Nasopharynx

The *nasopharynx* is that portion of the nasal cavity dorsal to the soft palate that connects the nasal cavity with the oropharynx. The lamina epithelialis mucosae is pseudostratified ciliated columnar epithelium with goblet cells. The lamina pro-

pria-tunica submucosa is typical with numerous diffuse and aggregated lymphatic tissue and tonsils. Elastic fibers are prominent in the connective tissue space. Branched, tubuloalveolar glands (mucous, serous, mixed) are present. The tunica muscularis is composed of skeletal muscle in various orientations. The tunica adventitia is continuous with the fascia of this region.

Larynx

The *larynx* connects the pharynx with the trachea. It is an irregularly shaped, cartilage-reinforced, muscular tube (Fig. 24.4). The lamina epithelialis mucosae varies at specific foci within the larynx. The lining tissues may be stratified squamous or pseudostratified ciliated columnar epithelia. Taste buds may be present on the epiglottis of some species (carnivores, swine, ruminants, man). The lamina propria-tunica submucosa is typical with various amounts of elastic fibers. Diffuse and nodular lymphatic tissue is present. Branched, tubuloalveolar glands are predominantly mucoid, but serous and mixed glands are present also.

The tunica muscularis does not consist exclusively of striated muscle fibers. Rather, cartilage replaces some of the muscle mass in a specific manner that accounts for the recognition of specific laryngeal cartilages and skeletal muscle masses at the gross level of examination. Although hyaline cartilage predominates, elastic cartilage is present also. The tunica adventitia is typical loose connective tissue.

Trachea

This tubular organ extends from the larynx to the primary extrapulmonary bronchi (Fig. 24.5).

The lamina epithelialis mucosae is composed of pseudostratified ciliated columnar epithelium with a variable number of goblet cells. The lamina propria-tunica submucosa is typical; elastic fibers are prominent and are believed to replace the lamina muscularis mucosae. Mucosal glands are branched, coiled, tubuloalveolar mucous glands that extend into the submucosal region between and peripheral to the tracheal cartilage.

The tunica muscularis is reduced to a dorsally positioned, transversely oriented mass of smooth muscle (trachealis muscle) that extends between the open ends of the horseshoe-shaped cartilage. The actual attachment of the muscle to the cartilage is species variable. The smooth muscular mass may also be perforated and interrupted by the mucosal glands. The tunica adventitia is areolar connective tissue that blends with the surrounding connective tissue of the cervical fascia or thoracic mediastinum.

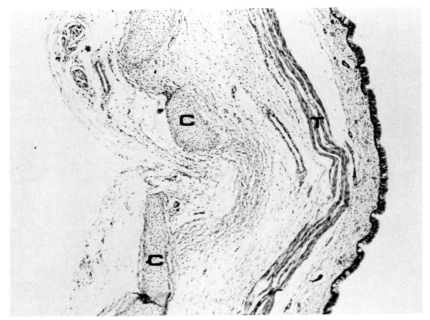

Figure 24.5. A section of a porcine trachea. The cartilage rings (C) are incomplete and connected by connective tissue. The trachealis muscle (T) is internal to the cartilage. The epithelial lining of the mucosa is typical pseudostratified cilited columnar epithelium with goblet cells. ×16.

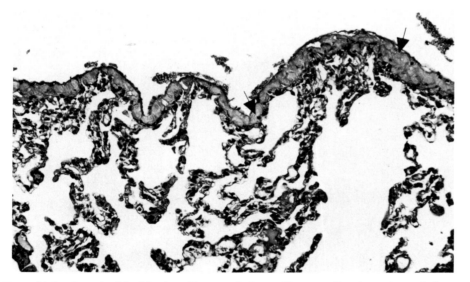

Figure 24.6. Capsule of the feline lung. The capsule (arrows) is covered by a layer of mesothelium—visceral pleura. ×40.

Extrapulmonary Bronchi

The *extrapulmonary* or *primary extrapulmonary bronchi* arise from the bifurcation of the trachea at the carina and are structurally similar to the trachea.

Lung

Conductive Components

General Remarks. The lung may be considered a compound, tubuloalveolar gland that secretes carbon dioxide across the alveolar surface in exchange for the uptake of oxygen. This exchange is facilitated by the elastic properties of the lung. An extensive network of elastic fibers accounts for part of its contractility in response to an alteration in the size of the thoracic cavity.

The lung consists of two *half-lungs*. Each half-lung, often referred to simply as a lung, is subdivided into various numbers of *lobes* (species variable). Lobes are subdivided into *lobules*. The lobular subdivisions are apparent on the lung surface in ruminants and pigs. In horses and man, lobular subdivisions are not very distinct; they are absent in dogs and cats.

The lung is covered by a serous membrane *(visceral pleura)*. The subserosal connective tissue consists of a thin layer of coarse areolar connective tissue that is rich in elastic fibers (Fig. 24.6). This serous membrane follows the surface contours of the lobes. The interlobular connective tissue is loose connective tissue rich in elastic fibers. The intralobular or interstitial space is occupied by reticular connective tissue. Elastic fibers may be present also.

Development. The development of the lung requires contributions from the endoderm and the mesoderm. The endoderm gives rise to the parenchyma of the lung as a diverticulum from the foregut. The parenchyma is the lining epithelium of the conductive, transitional and exchange components of the lung. The mesoderm gives rise to all other interstitial pulmonary structures. The formation of the lung may be divided into three disinct yet continuous stages of development: the *glandular stage (pseudoglandular stage)* of development is characterized by the extensive arborization of the single diverticulum from the foregut, the *laryngotracheal groove*. This stage establishes the basic branching patterns that characterize lung structure. The conductive airways and most of the presumptive transitional and exchange components are established. During this stage, the compound, tubuloalveolar organizational pattern of the lung is obvious. The glandular stage of development is characterized by two epithelial features—*established airways* and *terminal buds*. The terminal buds are lined by actively mitotic cells that continually invade into the mesenchyme, expanding the pulmonary airways. The *canalicular stage* is characterized by the onset of attenuation of the lining cells of the exchange components. Airways and capillaries grow toward each other attenuating the epithelial lining of the lung during the process. This process is responsible for presumptive alveolar lining attenuation and the establishment of the intimate juxtaposition of the capillaries to the parenchyma of the lung. The differentiation of two alveolar lining cells—type I and II pneumonocytes—occurs during this stage also. The *alveolar stage (terminal sac stage)* of development is the period during which the structural and functional relationships of the blood-air boundary are established. Complete lung development extends into the immediate postnatal period.

Intrapulmonary Bronchi

General Features—Mural Organization. The intrapulmonary duct system is a continuation of the extrapulmonary bronchi. The elastic fibers of the extrapulmonary bronchi become integral components of the lamina propria mucosae in intrapulmonary bronchi. The smooth muscle fibers of the trachealis muscle become positioned as the lamina muscularis mucosae. The cartilage, however, remains in the position normally occupied by the tunica muscularis.

Intrapulmonary bronchi are subdivided into *primary*, *secondary*, and *tertiary bronchi* based upon their branching, luminal size, and mural constituents. A gradual continuum of change occurs from the primary to the tertiary bronchi. Intrapulmonary primary bronchi are continuations of extrapulmonary primary bronchi. Their mural constituents are similar (Fig. 24.7).

The lamina epithelialis mucosae is pseudostratified ciliated columnar epithelium with goblet cells. The lamina propria mucosae is typical but contains numerous elastic fibers. A lamina muscularis mucosae is present and disposed in a helical manner similar to that of the elastic fibers. These spiral configurations result in a highly folded tunica mucosa. The tunica submucosa also consists of areolar connective tissue and contains branched, tubuloalveolar, mucous, or seromucous glands. Usually,

these glands diminish in number toward the tertiary bronchi. In cats, however, they may extend into the primary bronchioles. In some species, they are present only in the extrapulmonary bronchi or may extend only a short distance into the lung. The cartilaginous rings of the larger bronchi diminish in size, become cartilaginous plaques, and eventually do not occur at the transition from tertiary bronchi to primary bronchioles (Fig. 24.8).

Bronchial Glands. The *bronchial glands*

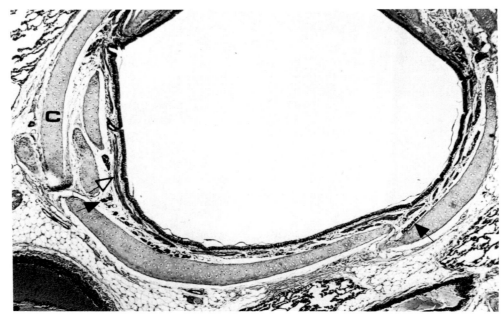

Figure 24.7. Primary bronchus (feline lung). The cartilage *(C)* is disposed as plates. A lamina muscularis mucosae *(open arrow)* and mucous glands *(solid arrows)* are present. ×10.

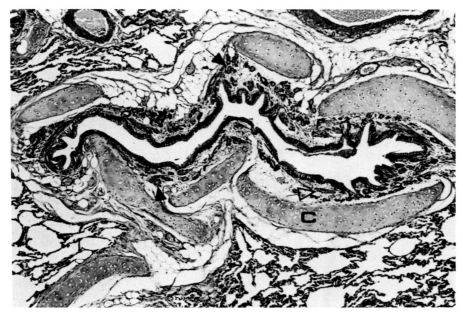

Figure 24.8. Small bronchus (feline lung). Cartilage plates *(C)*, mucous glands *(solid arrow)*, and smooth muscle *(open arrow)* are present, but the luminal diameter is reduced. ×16.

are a mixture of serous and mucous cells. The serous cells are typical in appearance; they are responsible for watery and protein-rich secretory products. The mucoid cells, morphologically similar to mucous cells throughout the body, produce different types of mucoid materials. The *mucins* are glycoprotiens consisting of more than 50% carbohydrate. The number and types of the secretory cells, as well as the nature of the products is subject to species variation. Additionally, numerous other factors—stress, infection, surface irritation—influence the number, distribution, and secretory characteristics of the cells.

Bronchial fluid is the secretory product of all of the cells of the laryngobronchial surface. Bronchial fluid is an admixture of secretory and transudative materials that includes: mucins, serum proteins, lactoferrin, immunoglobulins, and numerous glycoproteins.

The mucinous component is generally composed of two types. *Sulfomucins* are glycoproteins that are rich in sulfated amino sugars and uronic acids. *Sialomucins* are rich in sialic acid. Numerous other glycoproteins are present, but they have not been characterized. Additionally, some serum proteins filtered from the blood are characteristic of this fluid.

Lactoferrin is an iron-binding protein that contributes to nonspecific immune protection against Gram-positive and Gram-negative bacteria. Many bacteria require iron for their metabolism. Lactoferrin binds the available iron; the growth of the iron-requiring bacteria is retarded by this effective bacteriostatic agent.

Surface protection is afforded at all mucous membranes—gastrointestinal, urogenital, and respiratory surfaces—through *secretory immunoglobulins*. Immunoglobulin A (IgA) mediates this surface protection. The B cells of the gut-associated lymphatic tissue (GALT) are responsible for producing IgA. These cells migrate from the GALT to the connective tissue of the mucous membranes mentioned previously. The IgA produced by the plasma cells diffuses through the epithelial lining and attaches to a proteinaceous *secretory piece* produced by the epithelial cells. The secretory piece and IgA form *secretory IgA (SIgA)*. The SIgA seems to prevent adherence of bacteria and viruses to epithelial surfaces. In the ox, IgA_1 is the major secretory immunoglobulin. Immunoglobulin G (IgG) may occur in bronchial fluid also. If antigens gain access to the mast cells associated with the mucous membranes, then a type I hypersensitivity reaction may occur. The resulting increased vascular permeability can flood the region and mucosal surface with IgG.

Neuroendocrine Cells. These cells are discussed subsequently with respiratory bronchioles.

Bronchioles

Mural Organization. The bronchioles are the smallest divisions of the conductive components (Fig. 24.9). The lamina epithelialis mucosae consists of simple cuboidal or columnar epithelium devoid of goblet cells. The lining cells are ciliated in the *primary bronchioles*. The cilia diminish in the more distally positioned bronchioles and do not occur in the tertiary bronchioles. **Cilia extend further down the respiratory tree than do glands.** This relationship minimizes the potential for secretions being trapped in the transitional and exchange portions of the lung. The glands and cilia comprise the protective *mucociliary apparatus*. The lamina propria mucosae consists of fine collagenous and elastic fibers. The lamina muscularis mucosae is continuous. The peripheral connective tissue is similar to the lamina propria mu-

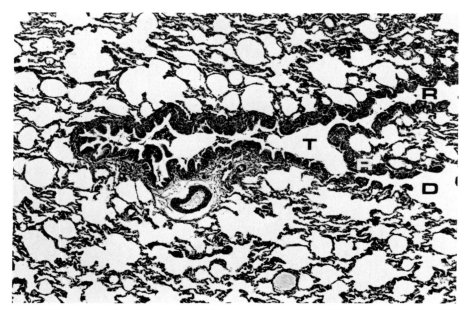

Figure 24.9. Bronchioles of a feline lung. The walls are devoid of cartilage. The terminal bronchiole *(T)* has divided into two respiratory bronchioles *(R)*. An alveolar duct *(D)* is present also. ×16.

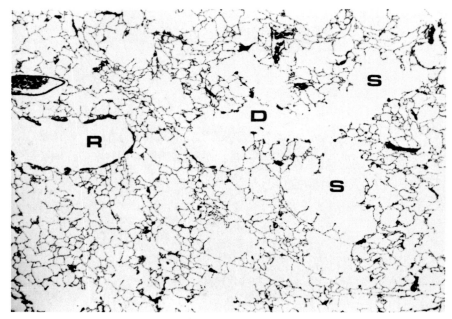

Figure 24.10. Distal airways of a canine lung. A respiratory bronchiole *(R)* continues as an alveolar duct *(D)*, which then continues as two alveolar sacs *(S)*. The atrium is the common opening of the alveolar sacs. ×40.

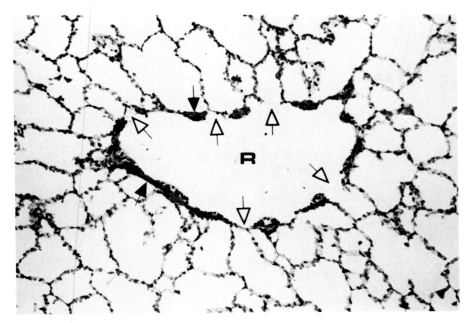

Figure 24.11. Respiratory bronchiole *(R)* of a canine lung. The lamina epithelialis mucosae is underlaid by smooth muscle *(solid arrows)*. The epithelial lining is interrupted by alveoli *(open arrows)*. ×40.

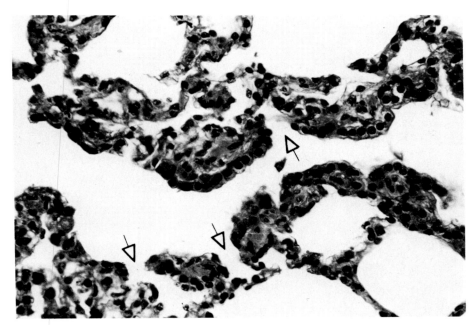

Figure 24.12. Lining of a feline respiratory bronchiole. The cuboidal epithelium is interrupted by alveoli *(arrows)*. ×100.

cosae but is not extensive. No cartilage is present. The tertiary or *terminal bronchioles* are the primary conducting pathways into a secondary lobule. The terminal bronchioles divide into several respiratory bronchioles, if the latter are present in the lung.

Bronchiolar and Neuroendocrine Cells. These cells are discussed subsequently with respiratory bronchioles.

Transitional Components

Respiratory Bronchioles

Organization. *Respiratory bronchioles* are components responsible for conduction and exchange of gases (Fig. 24.10). The lamina epithelialis mucosae consists of cuboidal cells, some of which may be ciliated (Fig. 24.11). The cuboidal cells are not a continuous lining but are interrupted by alveoli that protrude from the walls of this bronchiole (Fig. 24.12). The lamina propria mucosae is indistinct, but fine collagenous and elastic fibers support the lining cells. Smooth muscle is present, but it is organized loosely beneath the cuboidal epithelium.

Species Differences. Respiratory bronchioles are neither equally developed nor present in all species. They are observed infrequently in ruminants and swine, poorly developed in horses and man, well developed in monkeys and carnivores and absent in mice. In those species in which they are absent, the terminal bronchiloles open directly into several alveolar ducts (Fig. 24.13).

Bronchiolar Lining Cells. Two major cell types comprise the lamina epithelialis mucosae of bronchioles—ciliated and nonciliated cells. The ciliated cells are predominant in the larger bronchioles and are typical ciliated cells. The nonciliated cells increase in frequency in the small branches of the bronchioles becoming the characteristic cell of the terminal and respiratory bronchioles, if the latter are present.

The nonciliated cells, *bronchiolar cells (Clara cells)*, are cuboidal cells with dome-shaped apices that protrude into the lumen. Ultrastructural studies confirm that these serous-appearing cells contain apically positioned, membrane-bound vesicles. Basally, the cells have numerous rough endoplasmic reticular profiles. Additionally, numerous profiles of smooth endoplasmic reticulum occur apically and in a supranuclear position. Their morphological features, coupled with information obtained from studies of the incorporation of tritiated-labeled precursors, confirm their ability to secrete proteinaceous, lipid and carbohydrate products. The role of these cells, especially based upon the presence of an extensive smooth endoplasmic reticulum, needs further clarification. The synthesis of nonprotein products and biotransformation of atmospheric contaminants have been attributed to these cells. Still, they may secrete proteolytic or mucolytic enzymes that minimize bronchiolar obstruction due to the accumulation of cellular detritus and mucus in the small airways.

Neuroendocrine Cells. *Neuroendocrine cells* extend from the larynx to the *bronchioloalveolar portals*. (The latter are the points of transition between the cuboidal bronchiolar epithelium and the squamous alveolar lining cells.) These small-granule cells are part of the APUD (Amine Precursor Uptake and Decarboxylation) series of cells. The APUD cells of the respiratory system occur singly or as small aggregates *(neuroepithelial bodies)* within the mucosal lining.

The cells are not visible with routine preparation and staining techniques. Fluo-

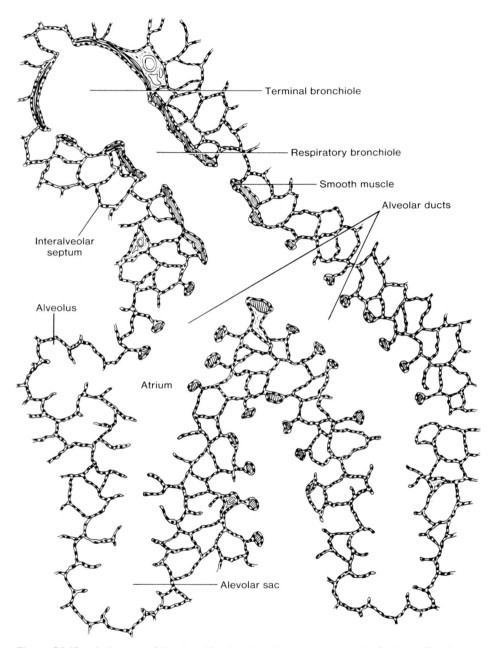

Labels on figure: Terminal bronchiole, Respiratory bronchiole, Smooth muscle, Alveolar ducts, Interalveolar septum, Alveolus, Atrium, Alevolar sac

Figure 24.13. A diagram of the transitional and exchange components of a lung. Respiratory bronchioles do not exist nor are they equally developed in all domestic species.

rescence techniques and special stains are effective methods of demonstration. The presence of dense-core cytoplasmic granules is the identifying feature of electron microscopy.

Some of the cells are innervated. Whether they are innervated by sensory or motor nerves is not clear. The precise role of these cells needs further clarification. Different classes of these cells have been described based upon staining characteristics and ultrastructural features. The cells are juxtaposed intimately to the smooth muscle of the conducting airways and the pulmonary capillaries of the bronchioloalveolar portals. Additionally, hypoxia seems to induce degranulation of these cells. The establishment of a local regulatory function for these cells seems inevitable.

Exchange Components

Alveolar Ducts, Saccules, and Alveoli

The respiratory bronchiole of a lobule or the terminal bronchiole of a lobule divide into numerous *alveolar ducts* (Fig. 24.14).

These tubules are completely lined by alveoli. Smooth muscle may be present along the luminal border at the apices between adjacent alveoli. Alveolar ducts divide and expand peripherally into *saccules* (sacs) that are completely lined by alveoli (Fig. 24.15). The common opening of the saccules is referred to as the *atrium*.

The alveolar lining consists of two types of cells: membranous pneumonocytes and granular pneumonocytes.

Membranous Pneumonocytes. This lining cell has various names: *membranous pneumonocyte, agranular pneumonocyte, squamous alveolar epithelial cell, type I pneumonocyte, small alveolar cell, and pulmonary epithelial cell.* The membranous pneumonocyte is the primary lining cell of the alveoli (Fig. 24.16). The cell is a squamous cell with a prominent perinuclear region that thins immediately to attenuated processes (Fig. 24.17). The nucleus protrudes into the alveolar lumen and is the only part of the cell that is visible with the light microscope.

The ultrastructural features and metabolic activities of these cells are not indicative of special metabolic needs. Typical organelles are not conspicuous and those that are present are scattered throughout the cell. As the primary lining cell, the main function appears to be the maintenance of the interface between the air and blood to allow the passage of gases.

Granular Pneumonocyte. This cell has various names, too: *granular pneumonocyte, type II pneumonocyte, great alveolar cell, large alveolar cell, alveolar cell.* The granular pneumonocyte is the secretory cell of the alveolar lining epithelium. The cell is visible with the light microscope as a round or cuboidal cell that projects into the

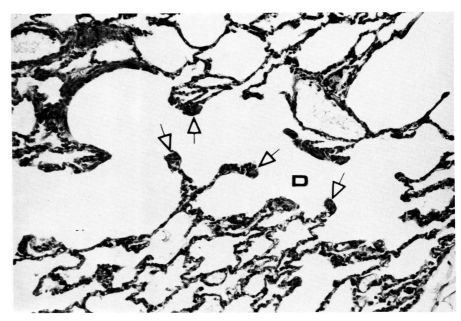

Figure 24.14. Alveolar duct of a feline lung. The alveolar duct *(D)* is lined by alveoli. Smooth muscle overlaid with attenuated lining cells *(arrows)* occupies the apices of septa between adjacent alveoli. ×40.

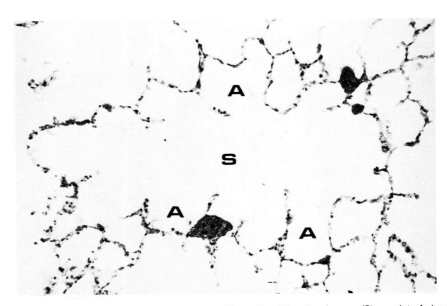

Figure 24.15. An alveolar sac of a canine lung. The walls of the alveolar sac *(S)* consist of alveoli *(A)*. The interalveolar septa are devoid of smooth muscle. ×40.

alveolar lumen (Fig. 24.18). Although the cells have a limited occurrence (one to several per alveolus), their foamy cytoplasm makes them a conspicuous feature of the lining.

As part of the alveolar lining, these cells are joined to the type I cells by tight junctions. Ultrastructural features confirm the role of this cell in secretory functions. Well-developed mitochondria are complemented by granular endoplasmic reticular profiles, an extensive Golgi apparatus, and *lamellar bodies.* Numerous multivesicular

bodies are present also. The lamellar bodies are the diagnostic features of these cells when they are examined with the electron microscope (Fig. 24.19). Also, these cells retain their potential for mitosis. They are believed to be the source of both type I and II pneumonocytes.

Surfactant and Surface Tension. Pulmonary *surfactant* is the secretory product of type II pneumonocytes. The secretion is derived from lamellar bodies. Surfactant is a detergent that consists of various substances: dipalmitoyl phosphatidylcholine,

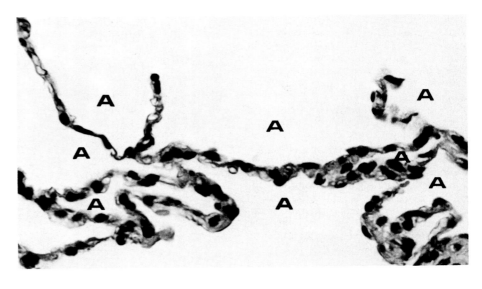

Figure 24.16. An alveolus of a bovine lung. Alveoli *(A)* are adjacent to each other and are separated by capillaries and a minimal amount of connective tissue. Some of the alveoli are collapsed from processing. ×160.

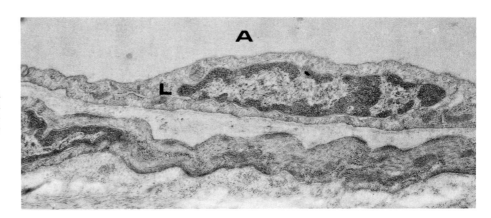

Figure 24.17. An electron micrograph of a membranous (agranular) pneumonocyte from a bovine lung. The squamous lining cell *(L)* lines the alveolus *(A)*. A fibroblast is subjacent to the lining cell. ×18,000. (Courtesy of G. P. Epling).

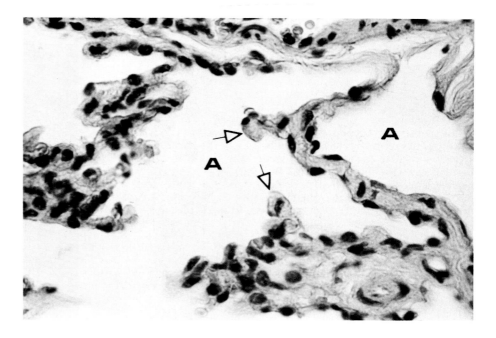

Figure 24.18. Type II lining cells. The predominant cell of the alveoli *(A)* is the membranous pneumonocyte. Type II cells *(arrows)* are scattered along the lining. The distinguishing feature of these cells is their vacuolated cytoplasm; however, they are difficult to identify in light microscopic sections. ×160.

phosphoglycerol, cholesterol, protein and carbohydrate. Most of the substance consists of phosphotidylcholine, a surface tension-reducing agent.

Surface tension is the attractive force between molecules at the interface between dissimilar substances. Because alveoli may be considered bubbles attached to tubes (bronchioles), the insights of Laplace are applicable. The surface tension (T) in the wall of a spherical bubble tends to contract the bubble, whereas the air pressure (P) inside the bubble tends to expand it. At equilibrium, the forces tending toward expansion, P, and those tending toward contraction, T, are related accordingly:

$$P = 2T/r,$$

where r is the radius of the sphere. If the surface tension were to remain the same independent of the radius, then the pressure required to inflate the sphere increases as the radius decreases. Conversely, the pressure required to inflate the sphere decreases as the radius increases.

The significance of these relationships is exemplified by the following example: Two bubbles of unequal size are formed independently as depicted in Figure 24.20.

When the stopcock of the connecting tube is opened, the smaller bubble empties into the larger bubble. This system is easily demonstrated with balloons or soap bubbles. Importantly, these relationships apply to the pulmonary alveoli. The lung, through its millions of alveoli, is unstable. Based upon Laplace principles, numerous small alveoli would tend to empty into larger ones until the lung consisted of one large alveolus. Similarly, small alveoli would require greater pressure (and more work) to overcome surface tension during inspiration.

Surfactant interdigitates itself between the water molecules in the aqueous phase of the alveolar surface film. This interdigitation reduces the cohesive properties of the molecules and reduces the surface tension. As alveoli become smaller and the surfactant becomes more concentrated in the aqueous phase, the surface tension is reduced. Conversely, as the alveoli become larger, surfactant is spread more thinly; surface tension increases. Surfactant, then, stabilizes the alveoli and insures that they remain a uniform size. Additionally, surfactant reduces the work of inspiration by reducing alveolar surface tension. Alveoli

with surfactant are able to fill and expand at lower alveolar pressures than alveoli without surfactant.

The initial inflation of the lungs at birth is relatively easy because of the presence of surfactant. An absence of surfactant at birth due to a type II pneumonocyte deficiency in humans (respiratory distress syndrome) is characterized minimally by labored inspiratory efforts.

Alveolar Pores. Adjacent alveoli are sometimes connected by pores. These pores are believed to distribute the gases and resulting pressure equally among alveoli. They may also serve for the interalveolar transmission of fluids, particulate matter, bacteria, and alveolar macrophages.

Pulmonary Macrophages. The lung is exposed constantly to insult from inspired foreign materials. Various methods are used to cleanse the conductive airways and exchange surfaces. The protective substances within bronchial fluid and the mucociliary apparatus are complemented by the activity of the pulmonary macrophages.

Two populations of macrophages have been identified within the lung. The macrophage of the pulmonary connective tissue space, *septal cell*, is a typical macrophage. Materials that reach the alveolar surface and traverse the alveolar wall are subject to clearance by the phagocytic activity of these cells.

The second population of macrophages undergoes *transalveolar migration*. These are the cells called *alveolar macrophages*. These cells may protrude into the alveolar lumen between lining cells, reside upon the lining cells or be free in the lumen (Fig. 24.21). They are observed rarely as a constituent of the alveolar lining in residence upon the basal lamina.

Upon gaining access to the alveoli, the macrophages scavenge the surface ingesting

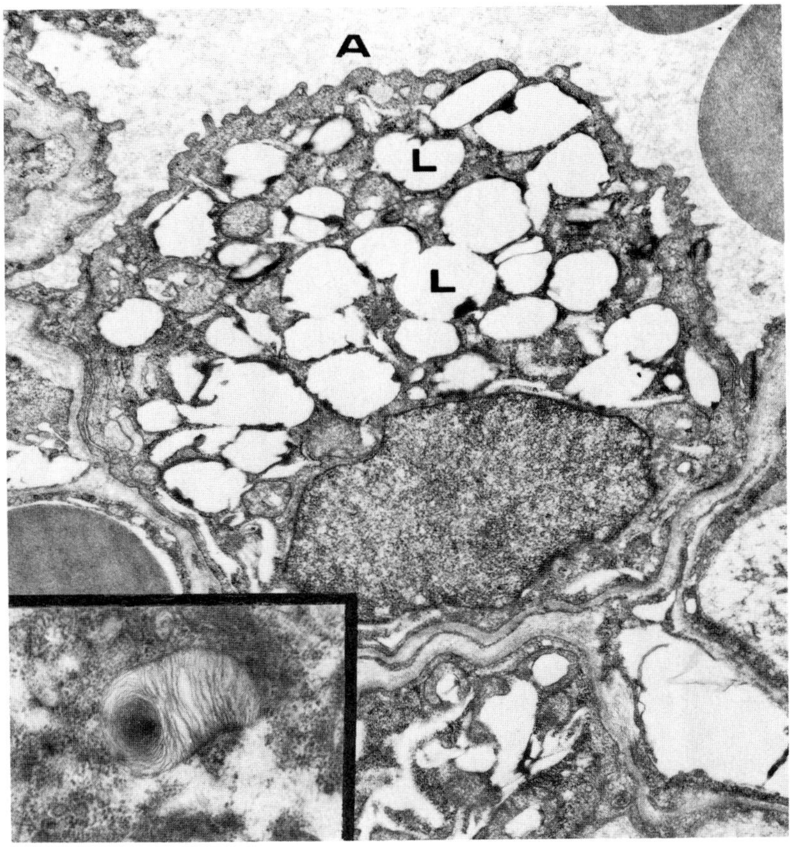

Figure 24.19. An electron micrograph of a granular pneumonocyte. The cytoplasm protrudes into the alveolus *(A)*. Pale areas *(L)* are lamellar bodies; their dissolution was a result of the processing. ×14,000. (Courtesy of G. P. Epling). *Inset*: A typical lamellar body of a granular pneumonocyte. ×17,000.

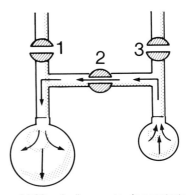

Figure 24.20. A diagram to demonstrate the significance of surface tension to luminal diameter. The balloons are filled separately and unevenly while stopcock 2 is closed. With stopcocks 1 and 3 closed, the smaller balloon will empty into the larger balloon when stopcock 2 is opened. Without surfactant, alveoli would react similarly.

Figure 24.21. An alveolar macrophage *(M)* in the alveolar lumen of a canine lung. The transalveolar migration of these cells is a significant protective mechanism. ×160.

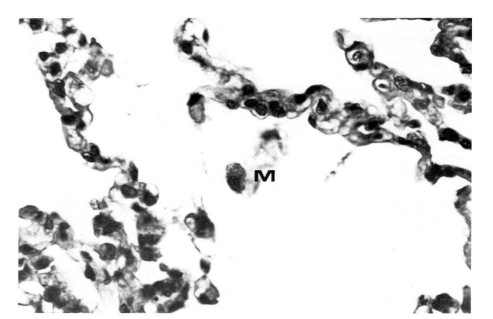

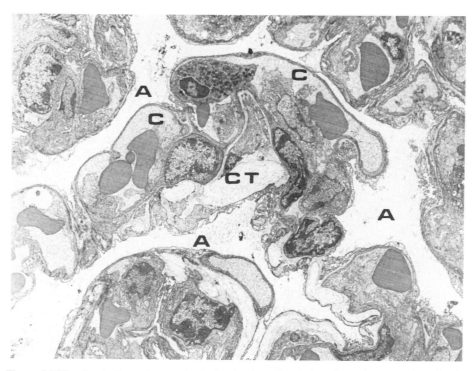

Figure 24.22. An electron micrograph of a bovine lung. Capillaries *(C)* are juxtaposed to alveolar lining cells. These components and the interdigitated basal lamina comprise the blood-air barrier. Alveoli *(A)* are collapsed. Small amounts of connective tissue *(CT)* comprise the septa areas. ×4000. (Courtesy of G.P. Epling).

foreign material. Their orad movement is accelerated once they encounter a ciliated surface. The migration of these cells toward the mouth culminates in their being swallowed or expectorated.

Macrophages from the bone marrow are seeded in the lung early in fetal development. This intrapulmonary pool of cells is capable of sustaining itself with appropriate mitotic activity. The bone marrow, however, is the adult extrapulmonary source of cells that augments the intrapulmonary pool.

Blood-Air Barrier

The lining cells, both type I and II, are supported by a basal lamina and fine collagenous, reticular and/or elastic fibers. Adjacent alveoli clearly delimit a distinct, but greatly reduced, interstitial or *septal space* that contains the aforementioned fibers, fibroblasts, macrophages, and blood capillaries.

The blood-air barrier consists of: *alveolar lining cell, alveolar basal lamina, septal space, endothelial-associated basal lamina and endothelial cell* (Fig. 24.22). The thickness of the barrier, however, is variable. Minimally, it is composed of: *alveolar lining cell, fused basal laminae, and endothelial cell* (Fig. 24.23). This is the thinnest and most efficient diffusion pathway.

Stromal Elements

Vasculature, Lymphatics, and Nerves. The vascular supply to the lung is achieved by the *pulmonary artery* and *bronchial artery* (Fig. 24.24). This circulatory pattern represents a division of functional and nutritional blood supply, respectively. The pulmonary artery and its peripheral subdivisions follow the distribution of the airways to the level of the respiratory bronchioles at which point they are continued as an extensive capillary bed associated with the alveoli. In carnivores and monkeys, this artery also supplies the pleura. In ruminants, swine, horses, and man the bronchial artery supplies the pleura.

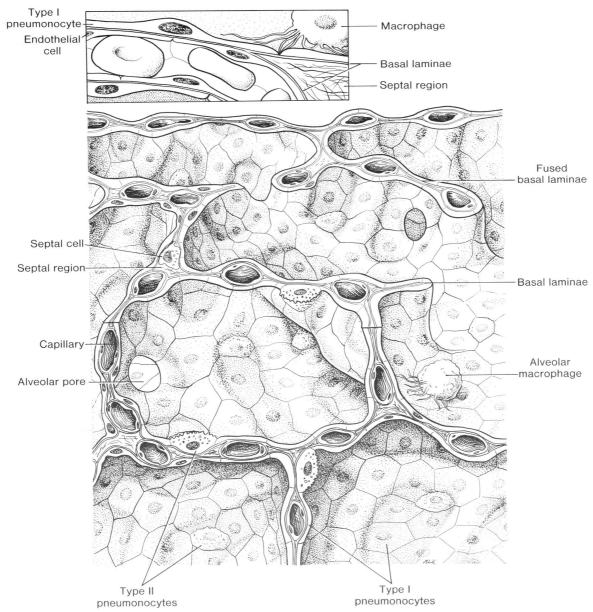

Figure 24.23. A diagram of alveoli. The inset is a drawing of the blood-air barrier. The entire lung surface is lined by a continuous layer of epithelial cells.

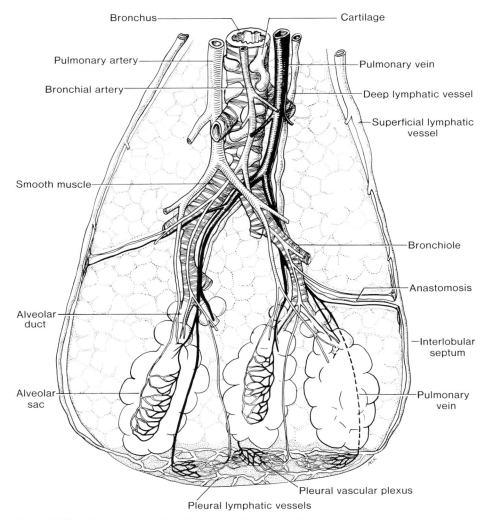

Figure 24.24.   A diagram depicting the relationships of arteries, veins, and lymphatics to the distal airway in a bovine lung.

The position of the pulmonary veins is species-variable. In some species, the interlobular pulmonary vein receives blood from adjacent lobules. In others, it is intralobular and requires that each lobule has its own pulmonary vein.

The bronchial arteries, which may supply the pleura (horses, man, ruminants, and swine) as well as the alveoli (horses), are the primary blood supply for the walls of the bronchi and bronchioles. Although bronchial veins are present, most of the bronchial arterial blood is returned to the heart via the pulmonary veins. The pulmonary vein of the ox has a thick and disrupted tunica media. This imparts a sphincter-like appearance to the vessel when it is cut in cross section.

Two sets of lymphatic vessels drain the lungs: *superficial vessels* and *deep vessels* (Fig. 24.24). The lymphatic capillaries of the superficial drainage originate in the pleural connective tissue and drain toward the hilus in the interlobular septa. The deep vessels originate at the level of the respira-

tory bronchioles or terminal bronchioles and follow the path of the bronchial tree to the hilus of the lung. The deep vessels anastomose with the superficial drainage in the interlobular septa. Lymphatic vessels have not been demonstrated in the interalveolar septa.

General visceral efferent fibers from the vagus and thoracic segments of the sympathetic trunk innervate the smooth musculature of the airways. The parasympathetic nerves stimulate *bronchoconstriction*, whereas the sympathetic nerves cause *bronchodilation*. General visceral afferent fibers, carried primarily by the vagus nerve, originate from stretch receptors within the lung substance and from nerve endings within the epithelium that lines the conductive airways.

Histophysiology of the Lung

Exchange of Gases

General Remarks. Oxygen delivered to the blood-air barrier must traverse the bar-

rier, enter the blood, and be transported to the tissues. The oxygenation of blood within the pulmonary capillaries is dependent upon varied factors: *the amount of oxygen in inspired air, the integrity of the blood air barrier, the amount of blood flowing within the pulmonary circulation, the quantity of O_2 dissolved in the blood, the amount of hemoglobin in the blood, and the affinity of the hemoglobin for O_2.*

Oxygen and Hemoglobin. The partial pressure of oxygen (P_{O_2}) in dry air, based upon 20% of 760 mm Hg at sea level, is approximately 150 mm Hg. After the addition of water, the P_{O_2} within alveoli is 100 mm Hg. The P_{O_2} of venous blood (Pv_{O_2}) is approximately 40 mm Hg. Oxygen moves down its pressure gradient, traverses the blood-air barrier and is carried by the blood. Some of the oxygen dissolves in the plasma and is carried to the tissues in this form; however, the amount of dissolved oxygen within the plasma amounts to about 0.3 ml% due to solubility limitations. Most of the oxygen is carried by the hemoglobin of the erythrocytes. Hemoglobin increases the oxygen-carrying capacity of blood about 70 times, to approximately 20 ml%. Each hemoglobin molecule contains 4 porphyrins, *heme*, each with a *ferrous iron atom*. The oxygenation of hemoglobin occurs progressively in four steps and is summarized by the following equation:

$$Hb_4 + 4\ O_2 \rightleftharpoons Hb_4(O_2)_4$$

The reversible reaction, which proceeds to the right in the pulmonary capillaries, occurs in less than 10 msec within the lungs. Each of the heme moieties has a different affinity for O_2. The affinity increases with each oxygenation, so the last heme has a much greater affinity for O_2 than the first heme. The oxygen-carrying capacity of the blood is maximized at atmospheric pressure, and most of the oxygen is attached to hemoglobin. Whereas *hemoglobin saturation* or 100% of its oxygen-carrying capacity may be achieved experimentally, hemoglobin saturation in vivo at an alveolar P_{O_2} of 100 mm Hg is only 97% of saturation. Bronchial venous drainage achieved via the pulmonary veins, dilutes the saturation percentage.

Oxygen-Hemoglobin Dissociation. Once carried to the level of the tissues, oxygen must dissociate from the hemoglobin, move across the capillary wall into the tissue fluid and diffuse into the cells. The P_{O_2} within the tissues is generally less than 30 mm Hg and may be much less than 10 mm Hg, while the P_{O_2} of arterial blood is between 40 and 100 mm Hg. Oxygen then dissociates from the hemoglobin, moves into the plasma and then into the tissues. The dissociation of oxygen from hemoglobin follows a characteristic sigmoid curve *(oxygen-hemoglobin dissociation curve)* that relates to the varying affinities for oxygen by the heme moieties (Fig. 24.25). At rest, about 27% of the oxygen is released to the tissues; venous blood contains hemoglobin at 70% saturation. Various factors influence the dissociation of oxyhemoglobin: P_{CO_2}, temperature, pH. **Active tissues produce high quantities of CO_2, elevate local temperature, and increase hydrogen ion concentration ([H$^+$]); more oxygen dissociates from hemoglobin and is available to the tissues. The converse occurs when CO_2, temperature, and [H$^+$] are decreased.**

Oxygen Delivery to the Tissues. The nature of the oxygen-hemoglobin dissociation curve tells much about hemoglobin and the manner in which O_2 is delivered to tissues. The P_{O_2} of blood is due to the small amount of dissolved O_2 in the plasma, approximately 0.3 ml%. But 70 times this amount is carried by the hemoglobin. As more dissolved O_2 leaves the plasma, more O_2 dissociates from hemoglobin. The dissociation and/or saturation of hemoglobin is dependent upon the P_{O_2} of dissolved oxygen in plasma. The shoulder of the curve between a P_{O_2} of 40–100 mm Hg is the normal range of arterial blood. A large change in the P_{O_2} (100–40) is accompanied by a small decrease in percent hemoglobin saturation. In the resting organism, much more oxygen is carried by the blood than is needed by the tissues. The normal P_{O_2} of venous blood is considered to be 40 mm Hg. Metabolically active tissues have high oxygen requirements. As more oxygen diffuses to them, the P_{O_2} of the blood decreases. Hemoglobin is less able to hold its O_2 and dissociation occurs rapidly below 40 mm Hg. A small drop in P_{O_2} below 40 mm Hg. delivers a large quantity of O_2 to the tissues from dissociated hemoglobin. The flat portion of the curve between 100–70 mm Hg is associated with a minor change in hemoglobin saturation, from 97 to 93%. Accordingly, animals are able to live at altitudes higher than sea level (P_{O_2} = 150 mm Hg) without reducing markedly the O_2 carrying-capacity of the blood.

Carbon Dioxide. The partial pressure of CO_2 (P_{CO_2}) within the tissues is approximately 50 mm Hg, whereas the P_{CO_2} of arterial blood is 40 mm Hg. Carbon dioxide moves down its pressure gradient from the tissues into the blood. Within the blood, the transport of CO_2 is achieved in three ways: *dissolved in the plasma (8%), carried in the red blood cell (RBC) as a carbaminohemoglobin (27%) and carried in the plasma as bicarbonate (65%).* Some of the carbon dioxide reacts chemically with reduced hemoglobin to form the carbaminohemoglobin molecule. Most of the CO_2 that enters the RBC is converted to carbonic acid (H_2CO_3) by the enzyme carbonic anhydrase. (Some of the plasma-dissolved CO_2 slowly forms HCO_3^- and H^+.) The subsequent dissociation of H_2CO_3 forms HCO_3^- and H^+ within the RBC. The HCO_3^- diffuses out of the RBC into the plasma wherein it is carried for exchange in the pulmonary circulation. The P_{CO_2} of venous blood is approximately 46 mm Hg, whereas that of the alveolar air is 40 mm Hg. Within the pulmonary vessels the reverse reactions occur. Carbon dioxide diffuses down its pressure gradient from the plasma and bicarbonate, diffusing into the RBC, is converted back to CO_2 by carbonic anhydrase. More CO_2 leaves the RBC, enters the plasma, and is exchanged. Similarly, the carbamino CO_2 separates from the hemoglobin and is replaced by O_2.

The chemical events of gas exchange are summarized in Figure 24.26.

Acid/Base Balance. The bicarbonate system comprises a significant buffer system for the body. Carbon dioxide produced by the tissues reacts according to the following equation under the catalytic influence of *carbonic anhydrase*:

$$CO_2 + H_2O \rightleftharpoons H_2CO_3 \rightleftharpoons H^+ + HCO_3^-$$

Carbonic acid, a weak acid, dissociates to hydrogen ion and bicarbonate ion, the latter being the conjugate base of carbonic acid. With excess H^+, the equilibrium shifts to the left accordingly:

$$H_2CO_3 \leftarrow H^+ + HCO_3^-$$

In the presence of excess base (OH^-), the equilibrium shifts to the right accordingly:

$$OH^- + H_2CO_3 \rightarrow H_2O + HCO_3^-$$

The function of the carbonate buffer system is not to prevent pH changes with excess acid or base but to minimize the changes that result.

The amount of CO_2 in the blood greatly influences these relationships. Increased carbon dioxide shifts the equilibrium to the right:

$$\uparrow CO_2$$
$$\therefore CO_2 + H_2O \rightarrow H_2CO_3$$
$$\downarrow$$
$$H^+ + HCO_3^-$$

The inability of the lungs to eliminate CO_2, as in *hypoventilation*, results in an increased CO_2 and a decreased pH (increased [H$^+$])—*respiratory acidosis*. Renal secretion of excess H^+ and conservation of HCO_3^- are compensatory mechanisms—*compensated respiratory acidosis*.

A decreased amount of CO_2 shifts the equilibrium to the left:

$$\downarrow CO_2$$
$$\therefore CO_2 + H_2O \leftarrow H_2CO_3$$
$$\uparrow$$
$$H^+ + HCO_3^-$$

The elimination of too much CO_2, as in *hyperventilation*, causes a decreased CO_2 and an increased pH (decreased [H$^+$])—*respiratory alkalosis. Compensated respiratory alkalosis* results as the kidneys conserve H^+ and excrete HCO_2^-. Respiratory acidosis and alkalosis are not only associated with changes in blood CO_2 but result from these changes.

Ventilation and Perfusion. *Ventilation* is the oxygenation of blood within the pulmonary capillaries, whereas *perfusion* is the movement of blood through the capillaries.

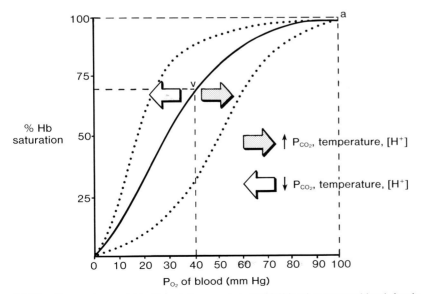

Figure 24.25. Oxygen-hemoglobin dissociation curve. *a*, arterial blood; *v*, venous blood. An alveolar P_{O_2} of 100 mm Hg results in 97% hemoglobin saturation. Arterial blood varies from 100 to 40 mm Hg P_{O_2}. Venous blood has a P_{O_2} of ≤40 mm Hg. Active tissues cause a shift to the right, whereas inactive tissues cause a shift to the left.

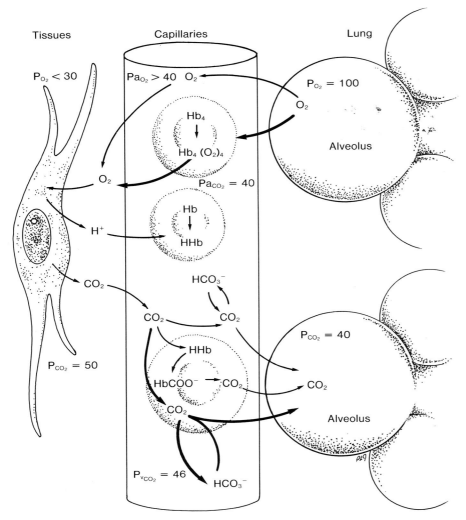

Figure 24.26. A diagram of the chemical events resulting in the exchange of gases within the lung and somatic tissues.

The proper exchange of gases occurs at the blood-air barrier when alveolar ventilation ($\dot{V}$) is matched appropriately to pulmonary perfusion ($\dot{Q}$) and is expressed as the $\dot{V}/\dot{Q}$ ratio. The $\dot{V}/\dot{Q}$ ratio for the entire lung averages about 1.0 under normal circumstances; however, not all aveoli have a $\dot{V}/\dot{Q}$ ratio of 1.0. In quadrupeds, dorsally positioned alveoli are usually underperfused and ventrally positioned alveoli are overperfused. Underperfused alveoli represent wasted ventilation; air is moved (inspired and expired), but exchange either does not occur or is insufficient. An increased amount of pulmonary dead space exists. Overperfusion represents wasted circulation to the lung, because more blood is flowing to the alveoli than air. The $\dot{V}/\dot{Q}$ ratio may be altered by changes in both ventilation and perfusion.

Changes in the $\dot{V}/\dot{Q}$ ratio that affect the entire lung appreciably alter arterial P_{O_2}. *Anoxia* (reduced P_{O_2}) and *cyanosis* (blue mucous membranes) result. Whereas perfusion may be adequate, ventilation is decreased. Various lung problems (asthma, bronchitis, pneumonia) result in low $\dot{V}/\dot{Q}$ ratios. A high $\dot{V}/\dot{Q}$ ratio is characterized by an increased arterial P_{CO_2}, whereas arterial P_{O_2} may not reflect changes. Vascular problems (pulmonary stenosis, pulmonary emboli, right-to-left cardiac shunts) generally account for high $\dot{V}/\dot{Q}$ ratios.

Regulation of Respiration

Integrated Activity. Pulmonary regulation is integrated with cardiovascular regulation, because the control of both is essential for appropriate ventilation and perfusion. Metabolic demands are accompanied by alterations in respiratory and cardiovascular activity. Increased metabolic demands require an augmented delivery of O_2 to the tissues as well as an increased ability to remove CO_2. Such metabolic activity is accompanied by increased ventila-

tion and perfusion. The converse is true also.

Neuronal Control. Breathing is accomplished through the rhythmic activity of neurons located in the brain stem (pons and medulla oblongata). The automatic discharge of specific neuronal pools within the brain stem is modulated by information from conscious centers (cerebrum) and afferent information transmitted to respiratory centers from the periphery. Whereas the central regulatory neuronal pools are referred to as *respiratory centers*, little agreement exists concerning the nature, extent, distribution, location, subdivision, and discreteness of the centers. Classically, a region within the medulla oblongata has been called the *respiratory center*, a region consisting of dorsal and ventral neuronal pools that are responsible for rhythmic inspiratory and expiratiory activity. The dorsal neuronal pool controls the discharge of the phrenic nerve to the diaphragm, whereas the ventral neuronal pool controls the intercostal and accessory respiratory musculature. Two additional respiratory centers occur within the pons. The *pneumotaxis center*, located in the rostral pontine region, prevents apnea (respiratory arrest), whereas the caudally positioned *apneustic center* causes apnea. The pontine centers, which respond to afferent information from the periphery, probably mediate their influence upon respiration through the medullary respiratory center.

Chemical Influences. Chemical alterations of the blood influence respiratory activity. Arterial P_{O_2}, P_{CO_2} and pH are monitored by central and peripheral chemoreceptors (Chapter 18). The peripheral chemoreceptors (carotid and aortic bodies) are sensitive to altered P_{O_2}, P_{CO_2} and pH. A decreased arterial P_{O_2}, increased P_{CO_2} and increased [H^+], translated into general visceral afferent impulses in the vagus and glossopharyngeal nerves, result in an augmented ventilatory effort. The central chemoreceptors located within the medulla are sensitive to the P_{CO_2} and [H^+] of cerebrospinal fluid or the fluid within the brain interstitium. The hydration of CO_2 within the cerebrospinal fluid or brain interstitium produces H^+. The increased [H^+] causes an increased respiratory activity.

Although the chemoreceptors respond to P_{CO_2} and P_{O_2}, increased P_{CO_2} *(hypercapnia)* is a stronger influence on respiration than is decreased P_{O_2} *(hypoxia)*. Arterial P_{O_2} must decrease to about 60 mm Hg before the hypoxic drive is evident. Also, a decreased P_{O_2} depresses neuronal activity.

Avian Respiratory System

Upper Respiratory Tract. The upper respiratory tract of birds includes all those structures described for mammals with the addition of the syrinx. These organs function in a manner similar to those in mammals.

The *nasal cavity* is lined by the same types of epithelia characteristic of the mammal. The vestibular region is lined by a stratified squamous epithelium which, from surface view, has a beaded appearance. The basal and intermediate cell layers are oriented vertically. They consist of large cells with centrally located nuclei. These rows are covered by a thin double layer of cornified cells. The remaining respiratory and olfactory epithelia are typical. Intraepithelial glands typify the respiratory epithelium (Fig. 5.20). The lamina propria mucosae is areolar connective tissue with diffuse and aggregated lymphatic tissue. It is continuous with the underlying connective tissue investments of bone or cartilage.

The *trachea* of the bird is similar to that of the mammal. The following differences, however, are apparent. The typical epithelium contains intraepithelial mucous glands that may protrude slightly into the typical lamina propria mucosae. Mucosal and submucosal glands are of variable occurrence. The cartilaginous rings are hyaline cartilage and are complete. They are an hour-glass shape in lateral view. The diameters of these rings vary so that a narrow part of one ring fits into the wide part of an adjacent ring. This imparts an overlapping pattern to the tracheal rings. Ossification of these supportive rings is common in some species (goose, duck). Longitudinally oriented striated muscle is located at the periphery of the trachea in a lateral position.

The primary bronchi are similar in structure to the trachea. The hyaline, cartilaginous rings, however, are gradually replaced by dense white fibrous connective tissue (DWFCT), and smooth muscle may connect the free surfaces of the cartilage.

The *syrinx* is located at the junction of the trachea and bronchi. It is an inverted Y-shaped structure. At the bifurcation of the trachea, a cartilaginous bar with a mucosal-submucosal fold constitutes the *median vocal fold*. By drawing the bronchi toward each other, two *lateral vocal folds* are produced at the level of the median vocal fold. The combination of these folds is responsible for phonation.

The lamina epithelialis mucosae of the syrinx consists of either a bistratified squamous or a columnar epithelium. Mucosal glands as well as diffuse and nodular lymphatic tissue are present in the lamina propria mucosae.

Lung. The lungs of birds are very different from the lungs of mammals. Compared to the size of the thoracic cavity, the lungs are extremely small. Moreover, they do not change volume during inhalation and exhalation. The structures that do change volume are the air sacs, which are continuous with the duct system of the lung.

The duct system bears no similiarity to the one in mammals (Fig. 24.27). The *primary bronchi* enter the lung and expand as the *vestibulum*. This continues through the lung as the *mesobronchus* and is connected to the *abdominal air sac*. Secondary bronchi and air sacs arise from the vestibulum and mesobronchus. Secondary bronchi are described as *dorsal bronchi, ventral bronchi,* or *lateral bronchi* on the basis of their gross orientation. Secondary bronchi give rise to *tertiary bronchi (parabronchi)* that are then continuous with other secondary bronchi. Thus, a complete air-conducting loop is formed. The parabronchi are analogous to the alveolar ducts of mammals. *Air vesicles (atria)* project radially from the parabronchi. These atria are continuous with the *air capillaries (air cells)*. The air capillaries are continuous loops that open back into the atria. The air capillaries are the structures responsible for the actual exchange of gases with the closely associated vascular capillaries.

Air Sacs. The air sacs associated with the avian lung aid in the movement of air through the lung. They are membranous structures that do not contribute to the

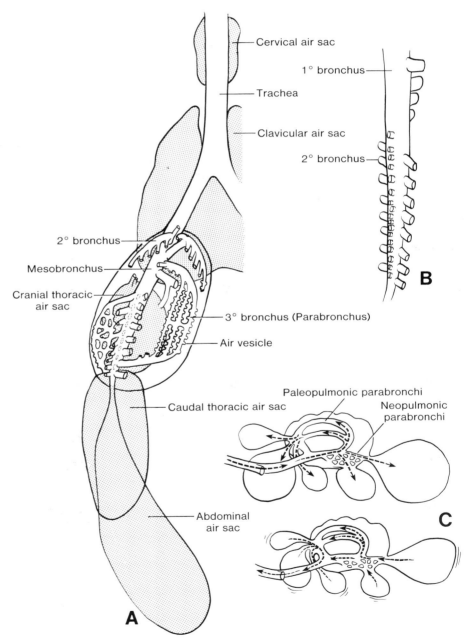

Figure 24.27. A diagram depicting the major portion of the avian respiratory system. *A,* The trachea, lung, and air sacs are depicted. *B,* Primary and secondary bronchial relationships are shown. *C,* The movement of air through the lung and air sacs is shown.

exchange of gases. Most birds have nine air sacs: *unpaired cervicals, paired claviculars, paired cranial thoracics, paired caudal thoracics, paired abdominals.* The air sacs occur free in the body cavities and send diverticula into the bones with which they are associated. *Recurrent bronchi* extend from the air sacs and attach to the parabronchi. *Recurrent bronchi* are involved in the return of the air from the air sacs to the lung proper.

Pulmonary Histology. The *intrapulmonary primary bronchi* are extensions of the bifurcated trachea and are similar in structure to their extrapulmonary counterparts. The lamina epithelialis mucosae consists of pseudostratified ciliated columnar epithelium with goblet cells and intraepithelial mucous glands. The lamina propria mucosae is areolar connective tissue with numerous diffuse and aggregated lymphatic tissue. Lymph nodules, however, are rarely present. The lamina muscularis mucosae is disposed primarily as a circularly or spirally oriented mass of muscle with some longitudinal bundles as well. Hyaline cartilaginous rings are present in the initial portions of these bronchi but are replaced by plaques of cartilage. The latter are not present within the vestibulum. The tunica adventitia blends with the surrounding interstitial connective tissue.

The mural elements of the *vestibulum*, except for the previously mentioned differences in the cartilage, are similar to those of the intrapulmonary primary bronchi. The vestibulum, however, is an enlarged portion of the primary conductive pathway through the lung that is continued caudally by the *mesobronchus*. The latter is a continuation of the primary conductive pathway. Its morphology is similar to the vestibulum. The luminal diameter of this tubule, however, is smaller than those described previously.

Secondary bronchi, whether they are lateral, dorsal, or ventral, have a similar morphology (Fig. 24.28). The lamina epithelialis mucosae is composed of columnar or cuboidal cells and is devoid of goblet cells. The lamina propria mucosae is composed of areolar connective tissue that is usually devoid of lymphatic tissue. The lamina muscularis mucosae is interrupted and multidirectionally oriented. Cartilage is not present. Numerous interruptions of the mural elements are encountered commonly due to the occurrence of parabronchi and, in some regions, air vesicles. Because of the latter, portions of the secondary bronchi may be considered analogous to mammalian respiratory bronchioles.

The mucosal lining of *parabronchi* is interrupted by the laterally projecting air vesicles (Fig. 24.29). Between the interruptions, the parabronchi are lined by a cuboidal or squamous epithelium. The reduced lamina propria mucosae is composed of a

fine areolar connective tissue. The lamina muscularis mucosae is confined to the region beneath the ridges of the lamina epithelialis mucosae as separate bundles of smooth muscle.

The *air vesicles* are lined by a simple squamous epithelium and are supported by a fine interstitial connective tissue (Fig. 24.30). The epithelium of the air vesicles is

continuous as a simple squamous lining of the *air capillaries*. The air capillary-blood capillary relationship is similar to that described for mammals.

Ventilation of the Lung. The lung of the bird is divided into two phylogentically distinct units. The *paleopulmon* is well-developed in all groups of birds and is especially well-developed in the domestic fowl. The

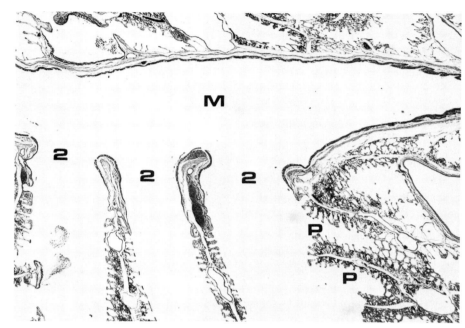

Figure 24.28. A section of an avian lung. *M*, mesobronchus; *2*, secondary bronchi; *P*, parabronchi (3° bronchi). ×4.

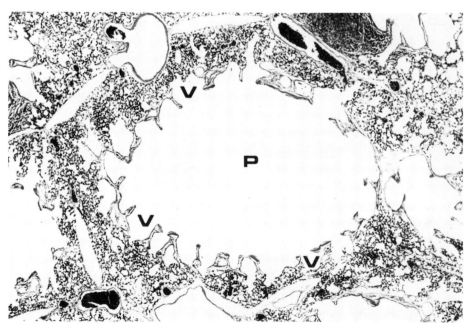

Figure 24.29. A parabronchus of the avian lung. The parabronchus *(P)* has numerous air vesicles *(V)* in its wall. ×16.

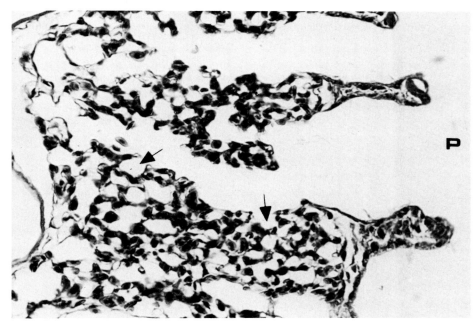

Figure 24.30. Air vesicles of the avian lung. The air vesicles comprise the walls of the parabronchi *(P)*. The air vesicles are composed of air capillaries *(arrows)* and blood capillaries. ×100.

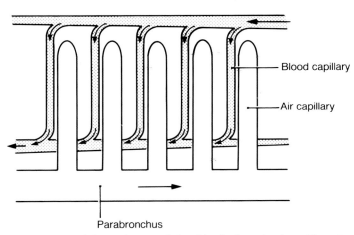

Parabronchus

Figure 24.31. A diagram of the exchange relationships in the avian lung. The orientation of the blood and air capillaries establishes a countercurrent relationship.

laries and air capillaries is that of a *countercurrent-type exchanger*. Mixed venous blood enters a blood capillary and flows adjacent and opposite to the flow in an air capillary. The blood flow in the capillary exits at the point in which parabronchial air enters. The relationship may facilitate gaseous exchange and enhance gaseous equilibration between blood and air capillaries.

References

Respiratory Tract—Conductive

Ali, M. Y.: Histology of the human nasopharyngeal mucosa. J. Anat. *99*:657, 1965.
Amoare, J. E., Hohnston, H. W. and Rubin, M,: The stereochemical theory of odor. Sci. Amer. *210*:43, 1964.
Arstila, A. and Wersall, J.: The ultrastructure of the olfactory epithelium of the guinea pig. Acta Otolaryngol. *64*:187, 1967.
Baradi, A. F. and Bourne, G. H.: Gustatory and olfactory epithelia. Int. Rev. Cytol. *2*:289, 1953.
Bojsen-Moller, F.: Topography and development of the anterior nasal glands in pigs. J. Anat. *101*:321, 1967.
Frisch. D.: Ultrastructure of mouse olfactory mucosa. Amer. J. Anat. *121*:87, 1967.
Hansell, M. M. and Moretti, R. L.: Ultrastructure of the mouse tracheal epithelium. J. Morph. *128*:159, 1969.
Rhodin, J. and Dalhamn, T.: Electron microscopy of the tracheal and ciliated mucosa in rat. Z. Zellforsch. *44*:345, 1956.

Mammalian Lung

Banks, W. J., Jr. and Epling, G. P.: Differentiation and origin of the type II pneumocyte: An ultrastructural study. Acta Anat. *78*:604, 1971.
Bertalanffy, F. D.: Respiratory tissue: structure, histophysiology and cytodynamics. I. Review and basic cytomorphology. Int. Rev. Cytol. *16*:233, 1964.
Bowden, D. H., Adamson, I. Y. R., Grantham, G. and Wyatt, J. P.: Origin of the lung macrophage: Evidence derived from radiation injury. Arch. Pathol. *88*:540, 1969.
Comroe, J. H. Jr.: *Physiology of Respiration: An Introductory Text.* Year Book Medical Publishers, Chicago, 1965a.
Comroe, J. H. et al.: *The Lung: Clinical Physiology and Pulmonary Function Tests.* 2nd edition. Year Book Medical Publishers, Chicago, 1965b.
Epling, G. P.: Electron microscopy of the bovine lungs: Lattice and lamellar structures in the alveolar lumina. Amer. J. Vet. Res. *25*:1424, 1964.
Engel, S.: *Lung Structure.* Charles C Thomas, Springfield, 1962.
Engel, S.: *The Prenatal Lung.* Pergamon Press, New York, 1966.
Karrer, H. E.: The ultrastructure of mouse lung. The alveolar macrophage. J. Biophys. Biochem. Cytol. *4*:693, 1958.
King, R. J.: The surfactant system of the lung. Fed. Proc. *33*:2238, 1974.
Krahl, V. E.: Current concept of the finer structure of the lung. Arch. Intern. Med. (Chicago) *96*:342, 1955.
Krahl, V. E.: Anatomy of the Mammalian Lung. In *Handbook of Physiology. Sect. 3, Respiration.* Vol. 1, Chapter 6, Fenn, W. O and Rahn, H. (eds.).American Physiological Society, Washington, D. C. Williams & Wilkins, 1964.
Krahl. V. E.: *The Human Lung* (translation of *Die Menschliche Lunge* by H. van Hayek, Springer Verlag, Berlin, 1953). Hafner, New York, 1960.
Loosle, C. G. and Porter, E. L.: Pre- and postnatal development of the respiratory portion of the human lung. Amer. Rev. Resp. Dis. *80*:5, 1959.
Low, F. N.: Electron microscopy of the rat lung. Anat. Rec. *113*:437, 1952.

paleopulmon lies dorsal and medial to the primary bronchus. A *neopulmon* lies ventral and lateral to the primary bronchus; the degree of its development is species variable. Whereas paleopulmonic parabronchi are hightly organized in parallel arrays, the neopulmonic parabronchi form a highly anastomotic network.

Ventilation of the avian lung is achieved by the air sacs functioning as bellows without any alteration to the volume of the lung. The bird is an abdominal breather. Inspiratory muscle movements increase the size of the air sacs, decrease pressure, and cause air to move inwardly. The reverse occurs during expiration. Air movement through the avian lung is unidirectional and bidirectional during inspiration and expiration (Fig. 24.27). Air moves in a bidirectional pattern through neopulmonic parabronchi to and from the caudal air sacs during inspiration and expiration. Inspiratory and expiratory effort is characterized by the unidirectional flow of air through the paleopulmonic parabronchi. The ventilation flow pattern through the lung permits the bird to extract more oxygen from a specified volume of inspired air than its mammalian counterparts (Fig. 24.31). The axes of the parabronchi are at right angles to the axes of the blood capillaries within the lung *(cross-current exchanger)*. The relationship of these structures permits gas exchange independent of direction of flow. The relationship between the blood capil-

Meyrick, B. and Reid, L.: The alveolar brush cell in rat lung—a third pneumocyte. J. Ultrast. Res. *23:*71, 1968.

Miller, W. S.: *The Lung.* 2nd edition. Charles C Thomas, Springfield, 1950.

Plopper, C.G., Mariassy, A.T. and Hill, L.H,: Ultrastructure of the nonciliated bronchilar epithelium (Clara) cell of mammalian lung. II. A comparison of horse, steer, sheep, dog and cat. Exp. Lung Res. *1:*155, 1980.

Sorokin, S. P.: A morphologic and cytochemical study of the great alveolar cell. J. Histochem. Cytochem. *14:*884, 1966.

Tobin, C. E.: Lymphatics of the pulmonary alveoli. Anat. Rec. *120:*625, 1954.

Tyler, W. S., Gillespie, J. R. and Nowell, J. A.: Modern functional morphology of the equine lung. Eq. Vet. J. *3:*84, 1971.

Avian Lung and Associated Structures

Akester, A. R.: The comparative anatomy of the respiratory pathways in the domestic fowl, pigeon and domestic duck. J. Anat. *94:*488, 1960.

Cover, M. S.: The gross and microscopic anatomy of the respiratory system of the turkey. I. The nasal cavity and infraorbital sinus. Amer. J. Vet. Res. *14:*113, 1953.

Cover, M. S.: The gross and microscopic anatomy of the respiratory system of the turkey. II. The larynx, trachea, syrinx, bronchi and lungs. Amer. J. Vet. Res. *14:*230, 1953.

Cover, M. S.: Gross and microscopic anatomy of the respiratory system of the turkey. III. The air sacs. Amer. J. Vet. Res. *14:*239, 1953.

Freeman, B.M. (ed.): *Physiology and Biochemistry of the Domestic Fowl.* Vol. 4 Academic Press, New York, 1983.

McLeod, W. M. and Wagers, R. P.: the respiratory system of the chicken. J. Amer. Vet. Med. Assoc. *95:*59, 1939.

Sturkie, P. D. (ed.): *Avian Physiology.* 3rd edition. Springer-Verlag, New York, 1976.

25: Endocrine System

General Characteristics

Introduction. The glands of the endocrine system are the *ductless glands* or *glands of internal secretion*. Their development was described (Fig. 5.21). The glands may be distinct organs (pituitary, adrenals, thyroid, etc.) or parts of organs (islets of Langerhans, interstitial cells of the testes, follicles, and corpora lutea of the ovary).

These glands may be encapsulated, lack an extensive stroma, are highly vascularized, and possess cells in varied configurations. The configurations may be *single cells, cell clusters, cell cords,* or *cell follicles*. The cells are intimately associated with capillaries or sinuses into which they secrete their products.

The *hormones* secreted may be proteins, glycoproteins, polypeptides, steroids, or catecholamines. A gland may secrete one or several hormones. These hormones may be synthesized and immediately secreted (adrenal cortex), synthesized and temporarily stored as presecretory granules (islets of Langerhans) or synthesized and stored in a follicle (thyroid). Once these products have been secreted into the bloodstream, they may have an effect upon the entire organism, selected organs, or a specific organ. Although the entire organism may be affected, one organ or group of organs may respond specifically. The latter is termed the *target organ* or *target organs*; i.e., some organs have a sufficiently low threshold to a specific hormonal stimulation that their response is measured readily.

Nature and Function of Hormones. Hormones are chemical substances secreted by various cells into the body fluids exerting an influence upon other cells of the body. Communication between cellular constituents is an essential feature of integrated activities. Various chemical substances serve as messengers that influence the activities of target cells. *Neurocrine cells* release neurotransmitters that affect target cells through directed and nondirected synapses. *Paracrine cells* (e.g., neuroendocrine and enteroendocrine cells) release their messengers into the interstitial fluid and affect adjacent target cells. *Endocrine cells* secrete messengers that are carried by the blood to distant target organs. Hormones

are regulatory substances that function to alter the rates at which existing reactions occur without contributing mass nor energy to the reaction. These substances are significant contributors to homeostasis, because they influence metabolic reactions, cellular differentiation, as well as developmental, maturation and aging processes. Hormones influence cell function by either activating cyclic adenosine monophosphate (protein and polypeptide hormones) within cells or by activating specific genes within cells (steroid hormones).

Regulatory Mechanisms. Hormones affect cellular activity and regulate various substances that contribute to homeostasis. The activities and substances regulated by specific hormones vary; also, the specific mechanisms utilized in regulation differ. Despite the diversity, some generalizations about the mechanisms are possible. The regulation of a substance *(regulated system)* requires the participation of a receptor, regulator, and effector. The *receptor*, perceiving alterations in the level of a particular substance, informs the *regulator*. The regulator sends signals to the *effector*, which initiates the appropriate response, thereby changing the level of the regulated substance. The most important regulated systems in the animal body are *negative feedback systems* or *loops*—the effector reverses the initiating event. If a controlled substance were to increase, then the effector decreases the substance (Fig. 25.1). The converse is true also. Although the simplified scheme represents the essence of a negative feedback loop, variations exist. The receptor and regulator may be combined; more than one regulator and effector may be involved.

Positive feedback loops amplify or intensify the initiating event in a regulated system. They are not common in the normal organism; however, such systems may be operational in various disease conditions.

Hypophysis Cerebri

Organization and Development. The *pars tuberalis* and *pars distalis* constitute the *anterior lobe* or *anterior pituitary*. The *pars intermedia* and the *infundibular process* constitute the *posterior lobe* or *posterior*

pituitary. The *pars tuberalis* and the *infundibular stalk* comprise the *hypophyseal stalk*. The terms anterior and posterior pituitary are not totally applicable to all mammalian species (Fig. 25.2). In some species, the posterior pituitary is actually dorsal to the anterior pituitary, whereas in other species the anterior pituitary totally surrounds the posterior pituitary.

The development of the pituitary gland is dependent upon contributions from the buccal cavity (ectoderm) and the floor of the diencephalon (neuroectoderm). *Rathke's pouch*, an outgrowth of the roof of the oral cavity, grows toward the base of the brain (Fig. 25.3). This pouch is responsible for the differentiation of the *adenohypophysis*. As it grows and contacts the infundibulum from the floor of the diencephalon, its connection with the oral cavity disintegrates. That portion of Rathke's pouch that contacts the neurohypophysis differentiates into the pars intermedia. The rostral portion becomes the pars distalis, whereas the dorsal extension of the pars distalis that comes in contact with the infundibular stalk becomes the pars tuberalis. The *residual lumen* of Rathke's pouch may persist as a separation between the anterior and posterior pituitary.

The infundibular stalk is an outgrowth of the median eminence. The median eminence is the ventral boundary of the third

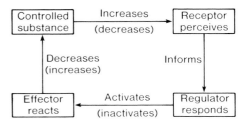

Figure 25.1. A flow chart that depicts the relationships of the components of a regulated system. A negative feedback loop is the common servomechanism of the body. Alterations of a regulated substance or activity results in a reversal of the initiating event by various effector tissues or organs. If the level of a substance or activity were to increase, then the effectors decrease the level of the substance or activity. The converse occurs also.

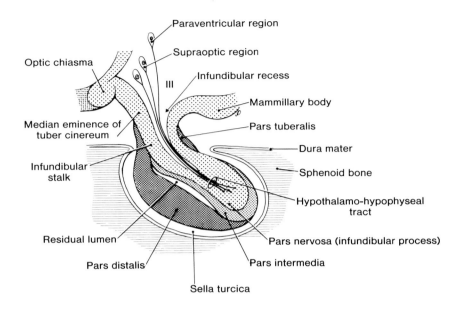

Figure 25.2. A drawing of the hypophysis cerebri of a pig. The hypophysis cerebri is a ventral evagination of the diencephalon that occupies a recess, the sella turcica, within the sphenoid bone.

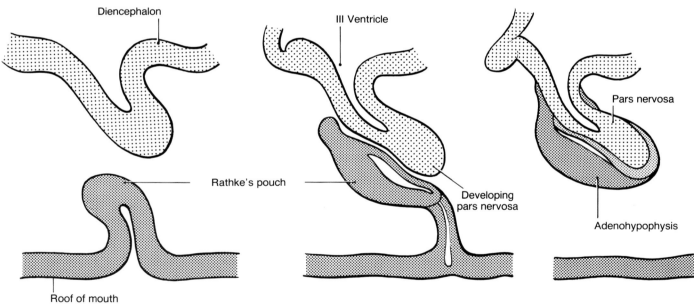

Figure 25.3. A series of diagrams illustrating the formation of the pituitary gland. The ectoderm of the roof of the mouth evaginates as Rathke's pouch and becomes associated with an evagination of the diencephalon.

ventricle in this region. As the infundibular stalk grows, part of the third ventricle is carried with it as the *infundibular recess*. In most species, the recess is confined to the region of continuity of the infundibular stalk with the median eminence (Fig. 25.4). In others (pig and cat especially), the infundibular recess extends into the infundibular process.

Adenohypophysis

The adenohypophysis consists of a *pars distalis, pars intermedia*, and *pars tuberalis*.

Pars Distalis

The *pars distalis* comprises the greatest bulk of the adenophypophysis (Fig. 25.5). It is covered by a fibrous capsule of dense white fibrous connective tissue (DWFCT) that is continuous with the reticular fibers of the stroma. The parenchyma consists of cellular cords or clusters that are intimately associated with sinuses. The cells of the pars distalis may be divided into two groups: *chromophobic cells* and *chromophilic cells*.

Chromophobic Cells

Chromophobic cells are called *chief cells, principal cells, reserve cells, C cells,* or *γ cells*. These small round cells have a scant amount of cytoplasm. Granules, as evidence of secretory activity, are not evident with light microscopy (Fig. 25.6). They have very little affinity for stains. These cells are usually clustered and may form the center of a cord of cells. Electron microscopic studies have demonstrated that these cells contain small granules. The chromophobic cells may be chromophilic cells in a state of partial degranulation. Some of the chromophobic cells, however, may be undifferentiated, nonsecretory cells.

Chromophilic Cells

Acidophils. *Chromophils* are divisible into *acidophils* and *basophils*. The acidophils include *α cells* and *ε cells*. These cells contain granules that are periodic acid-Schiff (PAS)-negative but stain with eosin, acid fuchsin, orange G, and azocarmine. *Acidophils*, generally, are much larger than chromophobes, possess a granular cytoplasm that is acidophilic and may be polarized (Fig. 25.6). Specific staining techniques permit the subdivision of the acidophils into two distinct groups. The α cell has granules about 300 nm in diameter. These granules also stain positively with orange G; thus, they are also referred to as *orangeophils*. The ε cells, however, have granules that range between 100 and 900 nm. These granules specifically stain with the azocarmine dye. These cells are referred to as *carminophils*.

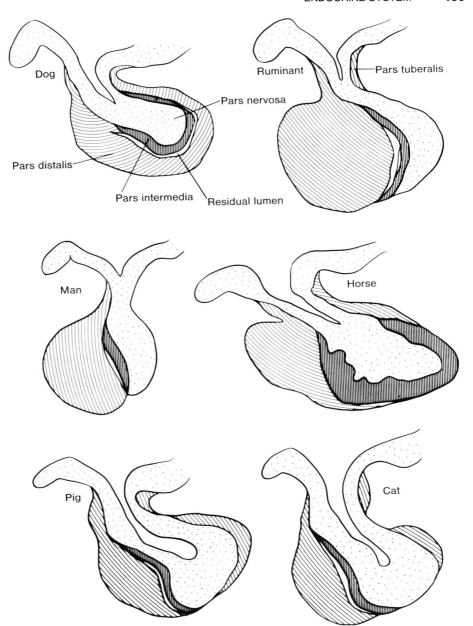

Figure 25.4. A diagram of the hypophysis cerebri of selected species. The pituitary glands are not drawn to scale.

Basophils. *Basophils* contain granules that are PAS-positive because of the glycoprotein nature of the secretory products (Fig. 25.6). They are larger cells than the acidophils. The granules of the basophils range from 150 to 200 nm in diameter. Although all of the basophilic granules are PAS-positive, the cells are subdivided into *β* and *δ cells* on the basis of specific staining. Beta-cell granules are alcianophilic and aldehyde fuchsin-positive. Delta-cell granules are aldehyde fuchsin-negative, alcianophilic and fast green-positive. Additionally, the cells responsible for corticotropin and

melanocyte-stimulating hormone are weakly PAS-positive. They, too, are basophils.

Routine Staining Characteristics. With routine staining (hematoxylin and eosin) only three cell types are identifiable: *chromophobes* (agranular and unstained), *acidophils* (granules that are eosinophilic), and *basophils* (granules with an affinity for hematoxylin). The proportion of cell types varies according to the age, species, sex, and physiological conditions. Generally, 50% are chromophobes 40% are acidophils and 10% are basophils.

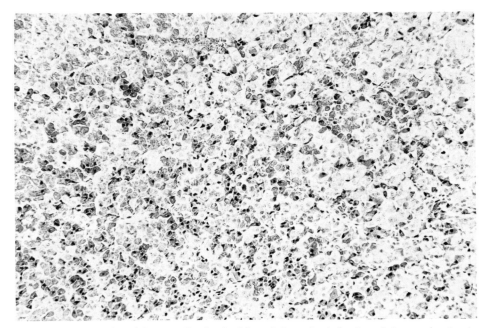

Figure 25.5. A section of the pars distalis of a feline pituitary gland. Cords and clumps of variously stained cells are associated intimately with sinusoids. ×10.

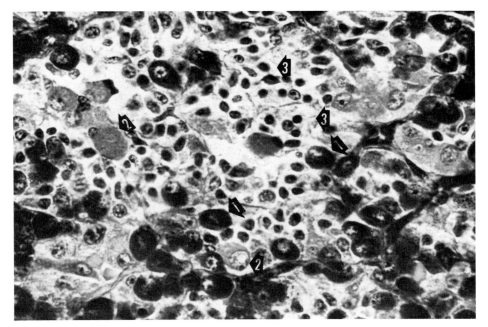

Figure 25.6. A section of an equine pars distalis. Three different cells are identifiable within this Azan-stained specimen: acidophils *(1)*, basophils *(2)* and chromophobes *(3)*. Fine connective tissue septa delineate clumps of cells. ×160.

Pars Tuberalis

Form and Function. The *pars tuberalis* consists of weakly basophilic cuboidal cells (Fig. 25.7). Granules, if present, are small. The cells are disposed in cords or clusters or as follicles. The function of the pars tuberalis has not been established.

Pars Intermedia

Form and Function. The *pars intermedia* is not well-developed in man but is well-developed in domestic animals (Fig. 25.8). This portion of the pituitary is adjacent to, but separated from, the neurohypophysis by a discontinuous connective tissue sheath. Migration of cells of the pars intermedia into the pars nervosa is common. The predominent cell type of this region is a nonspecific basophil (Fig. 25.8). Although these cells are usually disposed as cords or clusters of cells, follicles are encountered. Cells in the pars intermedia secrete *melanocyte-stimulating hormone (MSH, intermedin)*.

Histophysiology of the Adenohypophysis

Vascular Relationships. Whereas the origin and specific course of the vessels that supply the adenohypophysis vary among the domestic species, the common feature is the formation of an *hypophyseal portal system (hypothalmo-hyopohyseal portal system)*. *Rostral hypophyseal arteries* form an arterial ring around the median eminence and give rise to arterioles that supply the hypothalamus, including the infundibular stalk. These vessels, however, do not extend into the infundibular process. The pars distalis is supplied indirectly by the rostral hypophyseal arteries.

Arteriolar branches terminate as *primary capillary loops* within the median eminence and infundibular stalk. *Short primary capillary loops* supply the external portion of the median eminence, whereas *long primary capillary loops* supply the inner portion of the median eminence. The primary capillary loops coalesce to form veins that descend into the pars distalis via the pars tuberalis. The veins divide into a second set of capillaries or sinuses throughout the pars distalis. The hypophyseal portal system, formed by primary capillary loops, veins, and secondary capillary plexuses, comprises the major blood supply to the pars distalis. Small neurosecretory neurons *(parvicellular neurons)* of hypothalamic nuclei influence the activity of the pars distalis by releasing neurosecretory substances into the primary capillary loops of the hypophyseal portal system.

Somatotrophic Hormone. *Somatotrophic hormone (somatotropin, STH, GH, growth hormone)*, produced by the α-cell population, causes hypertrophy and hyperplasia in somatic cells. The effects of growth hor-

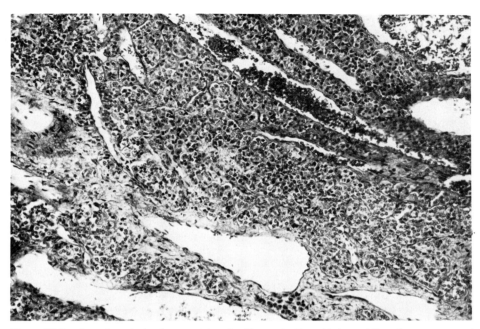

Figure 25.7. A section of a bovine pars tuberalis. The cords of weakly basophilic cells are separated by large vessels. ×40.

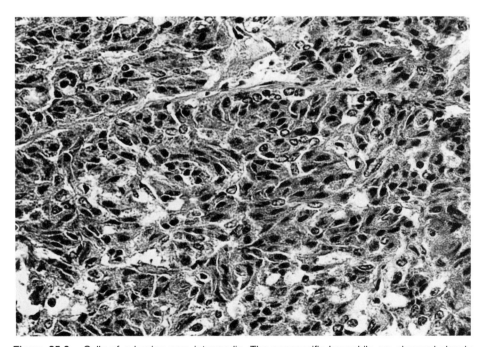

Figure 25.8. Cells of a bovine pars intermedia. The nonspecific basophils are clumped closely. Although not apparent in this section, follicles may be present. ×100.

mone are manifested and mediated through a group of polypeptides collectively called *somatomedin*. At least five different somatomedins have been isolated, each manifesting slightly different metabolic effects. Somatomedin is derived from liver, kidney, and probably muscle also. Without the mediation of somatomedin, the direct effects of GH are only manifested at excessive hormonal concentrations.

Metabolic processes are altered by the secretion of GH. Protein synthesis is enhanced by the augmented cellular uptake of amino acids, the decreased catabolism of proteins, the reduced utilization of amino acids as energy sources, and the increased formation of ribonucleic acid. Glucose utilization is decreased and glycogen storage is enhanced. The increased blood levels of glucose associated with GH secretion are sufficient to identify the hormone as *diabetogenic*. Under stimulation from GH, animals mobilize lipid stores and utilize them as sources of energy. Excessive lipid metabolism may result in the formation of many ketone bodies; therefore, STH is also *ketogenic*.

The control of GH release is regulated by two hypothalamic hormones: *growth hormone releasing factor (GHRF) and growth hormone inhibitory factor (GHIF)*. The inhibitory factor is also called *somatostatin*. Although most of the control of GH is probably mediated through the releasing factor, somatostatin is capable of influencing the release of GH and other secretions. Somatostatin is also produced by the δ cells of the pancreatic islets. Its secretion inhibits insulin and glucagon secretion as well as GH.

Despite the depletion of circulating amino acids being a weak stimulant for GH secretion, additional studies are necessary to clarify the circumstances or stimuli that lead to GH release. Acutely, hypoglycemia is a strong stimulus for release. Increased concentrations of some amino acids stimulate the release of GH. Chronically, the depletion of cellular protein is a strong stimulus for GH secretion.

The response of skeletal tissues to abnormal STH levels throughout life may be marked by dramatic changes. An oversecretion during adolescence causes *gigantism*, whereas an undersecretion in adolescence causes *dwarfism*. After the closure of the growth plates, an oversecretion of the hormone results in *acromegaly*. GH has an indirect effect, through somatomedin, upon osseous, cartilaginous, and muscular growth.

Prolactin. *Prolactin (luteotrophic hormone, LTH, lactogenic hormone)* is secreted by the ε cells of the pars distalis. Mammary gland development occurs under the combined influence of prolactin, estrogen, and progeterone. Prolactin causes the secretion of milk after the development of the mammary gland. Murine and ovine prolactin has luteotrophic activity. In columbiform birds, prolactin is responsible for the secretory activity of the crop associated with the formation of "crop milk."

Adrenocorticotrophic Hormone. The *adrenocorticotrophic hormone (ACTH, corticotropin)* is secreted by basophils. The primary effects of ACTH are manifested upon the adrenal glands to effect the secretion of *glucocorticoids*. Whereas small amounts of ACTH (permissive effect) are required for the secretion of *mineralocorticoids*, aldosterone secretion is regulated by other mechanisms. As a trophic hormone affecting glucocorticoid release, the effects of ACTH are manifested as those of glucocorticoids.

The regulated release of ACTH is mediated by circulating levels of glucocorticoids manifesting a negative feedback influence.

Corticotropin release and the subsequent increase in circulating glucocorticoids is affected by emotional and physical stress. Additionally, circulating levels of glucocorticoids are subject to the circadian rhythm of hypothalamic and adenohypophyseal secretion. This circadian activity is manifested as a sine wave-type rhythm in which maximal ACTH and glucocorticoid levels occur in the morning.

Follicle-Stimulating Hormone. *Follicle-stimulating hormone (FSH)* is the secretory product of specific δ cells (gonadotropes). The hormone is responsible for the growth and development of ovarian follicles. It also activates the testes to produce spermatozoa. The combined activities of FSH and LH (luteinizing hormone) are responsible for the maturation of ova, ovulation, and the development of the corpus luteum.

Luteinizing Hormone. *Luteinizing hormone (LH)*, also a secretion of δ cells, promotes the conversion of ruptured follicles into corpora lutea. The combined activity of FSH and LH was mentioned previously. In the male, LH is also called *ICSH (interstitial cell-stimulating hormone)*. The hormone stimulates the secretion of testosterone by *testicular interstitial cells (cells of Leydig)*.

Thyrotrophic Hormone. *Thyrotrophic hormone (TSH, thyroid-stimulating hormone)* is responsible for the stimulation and maintenance of the secretory activity of the thyroid gland.

Melanocyte-Stimulating Hormone. *Melanocyte-stimulating hormone (MSH, intermedin)* is a secretory product of the pars intermedia that is responsible for the dispersion of melanin in melanocytes. Although this activity has been well-established in lower vertebrates (amphibians), the precise role of MSH in mammals has not been documented.

Lipotropins. Two polypeptide hormones called *β-lipotropin(βLPH) and γ-lipotropin (γLPH)* have been isolated from the adenohypophysis. In some species, these substances have the ability to mobilize fats. Beta-lipotropin is a precursor to *β-endorphin*.

Within the pars distalis, a single basophil is responsible for the production of ACTH and LPH. Accordingly, these cells are called ACTH/LPH cells. A common precursor molecule in these cells is cleaved to form ACTH, βLPH and γLPH. Within the pars intermedia, βLPH is metabolized to yield *βMSH and β* endorphin, whereas ACTH is metabolized to yield *α melanocyte-stimulating hormone (αMSH)*.

Regulation of the Adenohypophysis

Adenohypophyseal secretions are regulated by *releasing* and *inhibitory factors* that are secreted by the parvicellular neurons of the hypothalamus. The primary

capillary loops of the hypophyseal portal system and the telodendria of the neurons comprise the *neurohemal organs* (Chapter 14). Hypothalamic hormones released into the portal system include:

> *Growth hormone releasing factor—GHRF,*
> *Growth hormone inhibitory factor—GHIF,*
> *Prolactin releasing factor—PRF,*
> *Prolactin inhibitory factor—PIF,*
> *ACTH releasing factor—CRF,*
> *FSH releasing factor—FRF,*
> *LH releasing factor—LRF,* and
> *TSH releasing factor—TRF.*

Specific excitatory or inhibitory events—body temperature, blood glucose concentration, cellular protein levels, circulating levels of certain general hormones or trophic hormones—exert an influence upon the secretory activity of hypothalamic neurons. The hypothalamic hormones adjust the activity of the adenohypophysis. The trophic hormones, besides mediating their influence upon target organs, may function in a short negative feedback loop to affect the secretion of the hypothalmic cells. The involvement of more than one regulator generally assures the precise regulation of a particular substance or event.

Neurohypophysis

General Structure. The *neurohypophysis* is a ventral evagination of nervous tissue of the hypothalmus (Fig. 25.4). It includes the *median eminence* of the *tuber cinereum*, *infundibular stalk*, and *infundibular process* (Fig. 25.9). Numerous unmyelinated neurons comprise the *hypothalamohypophyseal tract*, the cell bodies of which are located in the supraoptic and paraventricular nuclei of the hypothalamus. These *magnocellular neurons* are neurosecretory. Their *neurosecretions* move along the axons and accumulate in the nerve fibers as *Herring bodies* (Fig. 25.10). Numerous *pituicytes* and neuroglial elements are scattered among the nerve fibers.

Neurohypophyseal Hormones and Neurophysins. The secretory products of magnocellular neurons of the supraoptic and paraventricular nuclei include *oxytocin*, *vasopressin*, and *neurophysins*. Neurophysins are cystine-rich, proteinaceous, intracellular carrier molecules for the prohormonal forms of the neurosecretory substances. Specific neurophysin for each hormone is packaged into each secretory granule with a prohormone and a converting enzyme. Neurophysins are linked to the prohormones in a 1:1 molar ratio. *Neurophysin I* is associated with antidiuretic hormone (ADH) and *neurophysins II and III* are associated with oxytocin. The specificity of the neurophysins is so precise that

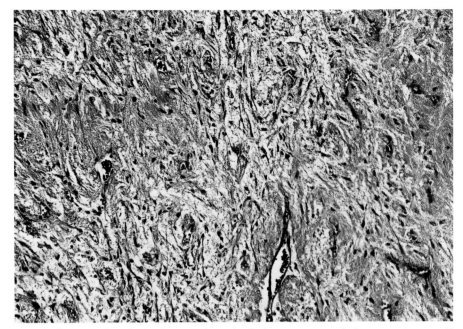

Figure 25.9.   A section of a bovine neurohypophysis. It appears as typical nervous tissue. ×40.

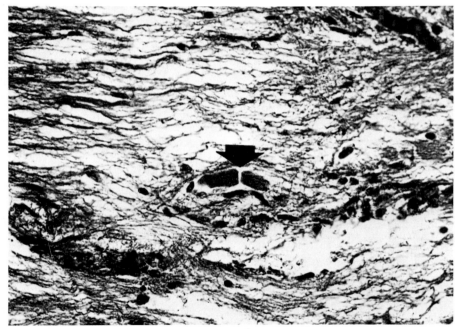

Figure 25.10.   Herring bodies. The neurosecretory products and carrier molecules of specific hypothalamic nuclear regions are transported along axons as Herring bodies *(arrow)*. ×100.

they may be used to separate these hormones from pituitary extracts. The secretory granules move by rapid axoplasmic flow to the neurohemal interface. An action potential, triggered by the cell body in response to some excitatory events, causes a change in cell membrane permeability, an increase in intracellular calcium and the exocytotic release of the hormones and neurophysins.

Oxytocin. *Oxytocin*, produced primarily within the paraventricular nucleus, affects the reproductive organs. Milk letdown is mediated by oxytocin in response to suckling. The afferent stimulation reaches the hypothalamus, causing the release of the hormone. The hormone has a stimulatory effect upon the myometrium. Oxytocin-induced contractions facilitate the ascent of spermatozoa into the oviduct. During pregnancy, oxytocin is secreted by the maternal hypophysis under the influence of fetal and placental estrogens and prostaglandins. The release of oxytocin stimulates myometrial contractions and accelerates parturition. As the fetus passes through the dilated cervix, point pressure of the fetus upon the vaginal wall stimulates additonal oxytocin release and the marked abdominal contractions characterizing labor. These cascading events are irreversible. Oxytocin can be used to induce parturition in the mare.

Antidiuretic Hormone. *Antidiuretic hormone (ADH, vasopressin)*, produced primarily within the supraoptic nucleus, manifests its antidiuretic properties on the lining cells of the distal convoluted tubules and collecting ducts of the kidneys. Blood osmolality and fluid volume are the stimuli for ADH secretion. Osmoreceptors within the hypothalamus respond to the osmolality of the fluid bathing them and influence the magnocellular neurons responsible for ADH secretion. An increased blood osmolality increases the activity of the osmoreceptors and results in the release of ADH. The kidney, responding to ADH by increasing the tubular resorption of water, excretes a low volume, hypertonic urine. The converse is true when blood osmolality decreases.

The extracellular fluid (ECF) volume of the body influences ADH release. An increased ECF volume decreases ADH secretion, whereas a decreased ECF volume increases ADH secretion. Changes in ECF volume effect changes in blood volume. Low pressure, venous baroreceptors located in the great veins of the heart, atria, and pulmonary vessels monitor blood volume and influence ADH release. The venous baroreceptors probably influence ADH greater than the high pressure, arterial baroreceptors, because subtle changes in blood volume are not always associated with arterial pressure changes. The marked reduction of blood volume, as resulting from hemorrhage, involves the arterial baroreceptors (carotid and aortic sinuses) in the regulation of ADH release. The attendant fall in blood pressure causes an increased release of ADH.

The vasopressive activity of ADH is manifested by the exogenous administration of the hormone at dosages exceeding physiological levels. Even after hemorrhage, it is dubious that ADH will manifest sufficient vasopressive activity to alter blood pressure.

Epiphysis Cerebri

Form and Function. This organ is also referred to as the *pineal gland*. It is a dorsal evagination of the roof of the diencephalon. An understanding of the functional significance of the pineal body has been slow to evolve. In lower vertebrates, it is a photoreceptor organ, the *third eye* or *pineal eye*. Despite its position in the mammalian cranium, it is a light-sensitive organ. Information from the optic system is carried to the midbrain and thence to the thoracic region of the spinal cord wherein sympathetic nerves carry the information to the apex of the pineal body.

Melatonin and *serotonin* are secretory products of this gland. Under continuous light stimulation, the pineal gland decreases in activity, melatonin production decreases, and gonadal activity increases. Pineal body tumors result in delayed puberty. It is not clear, however, whether the pineal gland mediates its influence through the hypothalamus (releasing factors), pars distalis, or directly upon the gonads. The gland is probably the biological clock that sets circadian rhythms associated with estrous cycles and seasonal breeding characteristics of some species.

Histology. The pineal body is covered by the connective tissue of the pia mater (Fig. 25.11). Septation and lobulation of the organ is accomplished by invasion of the connective tissue elements. The primary cellular components are *astrocytes* and *pinealocytes* (epithelioid cells). Typical connective tissue cells (plasma cells, fibroblasts, mast cells, and macrophages) may also be present. The *pinealocytes (chief cells)* are large cells with a large, round, open nucleus set in an acidophilic cytoplasm (Fig. 25.11). The *astrocytes* are typical and are interdigitated between the vascular supply and the pinealocytes. These are often called *interstitial cells.*

The pineal gland contains concretions called *corpora arenacea (acervuli, brain sand, psammona bodies).* These deposits appear to be glial or stromal in origin and have the structure of hydroxyapatite crystals. Although they tend to increase with age, their increased frequency is not associated with a diminution of pineal activity.

Thyroid Gland

Development. The thyroid gland is an outgrowth from the floor of the buccal cavity that subsequently loses its cellular connection *(thyroglossal duct)* with the pharyngeal endoderm. This glandular mass fuses with cellular masses from each fifth pharyngeal pouch *(ultimobranchial body).* Endodermal evaginations from the third and fourth pharyngeal pouches (parathyroid glands) also become intimately associated with or are embedded within the mass of thyroid tissue. The thyroid gland eventually assumes a dorsolateral relationship with the trachea in the region of the larynx.

Histology. The capsule of the two lobes of the thyroid gland consists of areolar connective tissue. Connective tissue septa of similar tissue support the organ. Perifollicular connective tissue consists of extensive quantities of reticular fibers.

The structural unit of the thyroid gland is the *thyroid follicle* (Fig. 25.12). Follicles are hollow spheres that are variable in size. Individual follicular size is a function of the activity of the lining cells. The center of the follicle is filled with a gel-like material called *colloid.* This is the storage from of the follicular epithelial secretory products. The lining epithelium varies from low cuboidal to high columnar (Fig. 25.13). The height of the cells within a given follicle, however, is uniform.

The thyroid epithelium actually consists of: *follicular lining cells* that comprise at least 90% of the cellular population and *light cells (parafollicular cells, C cells).* Follicular lining cells are acidophilic with a basally positioned nucleus (Fig. 25.13). A pale-staining Golgi area may be apparent in a supranuclear position. There may be colloid droplets adjacent to the luminal surface. Parafollicular cells may occur in a parafollicular position or they may occur within the lining of the follicle wherein they occasionally reach the luminal surface (Fig. 25.14). They are surrounded by a basal

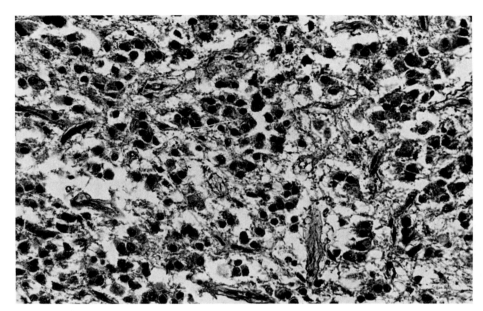

Figure 25.11.   Cellular components of an ovine pineal body. ×90.

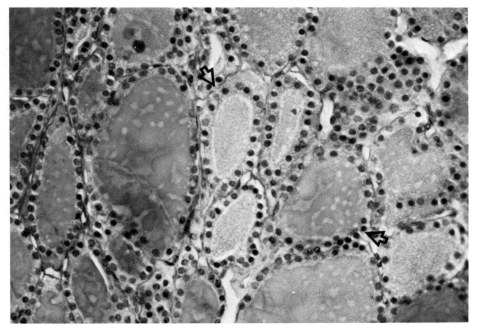

Figure 25.12.   A section of a canine thyroid gland. The parenchyma is disposed as follicles *(arrows)* surrounding colloid. ×100. (PAS).

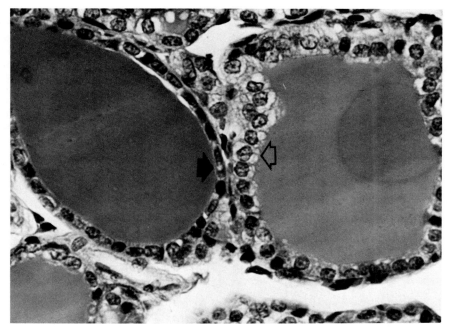

Figure 25.13. Thyroid follicular epithelial cells and follicles. The lining cells may vary from low cuboidal *(solid arrow)* to columnar *(open arrow)*, depending upon the level of activity of the gland and individual follicles. ×160.

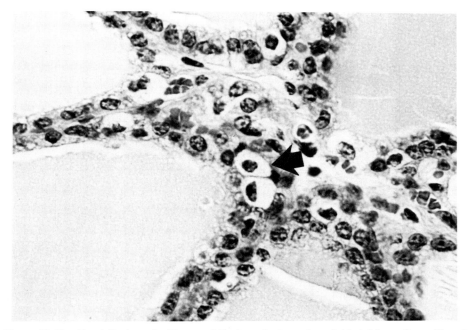

Figure 25.14. Parafollicular cells. The parafollicular cells *(arrow)* are light-staining cells positioned at the edges of the follicles. ×160. (PAS).

lamina that delimits the follicle from the connective tissue space. They are cells with a pale-staining cytoplasm.

Colloid, which contains proteins, glycoproteins, and enzymes, is usually acidophilic. The glycoprotein is PAS-positive. In an active follicle, the colloid has peripheral irregularities and vacuoles as well as a strong acidophilia. In an inactive follicle, the colloid is slightly basophilic or even acidophilic. The periphery has a smooth profile and vacuoles are not present. The size of the follicles as well as the height of the epithelium are also indicators of follicular or glandular activity. The activity of a follicle is approximately inversely proportional to the diameter of the follicle. **Small follicles usually have a high epithelium (and the appropriate colloid characteristics) and are active. Large follicles usually** have a low epithelium and the appropriate colloid characteristics, and they are less active than small follicles. In inactive follicles, the follicular epithelium may even be squamous.

Synthesis and Storage of Thyroid Hormones. The simplicity of thyroid follicular morphology is barely indicative of the complex mechanisms involved in the synthesis, storage, mobilization, and subsequent secretion of its hormones—T_4 *(thyroxine or tetraiodothyronine)* and T_3 *(triiodothyronine).*

The synthesis of T_3 and T_4 is dependent upon thyroid-stimulating hormone (TSH) and the availability of iodide. Iodide (I^-) is actively transported across the basal cell membrane under the influence of TSH. The iodide pump permits the concentration of iodide within the thyroid follicular cell. Moving through the epithelial cell to the apical border, iodide is oxidized or activated to its reactive form, iodine (I_2). A *peroxidase* located in the microvilli of the cell may cause the activation of the halogen. Concomitantly, amino acids that enter the cell permit the synthesis of a polypeptide within the rough endoplasmic reticulum. Glycosylation of the polypeptide within the Golgi apparatus results in the formation of a *glycoprotein* contained within a secretory vesicle that is transported across the apical cell border into the colloid. The *iodination* or *organification* of the glycoprotein occurs within or on the apical surface of the cells as the glycoprotein is secreted. Organification results in the formation of *thyroglobulin,* a glycoprotein with a molecular weight in excess of 650,000. Thyroglobulin contains some carbohydrates (galactose, mannose, N-acetylglucosamine, sialic acid) and *iodoamino acids.* The iodoamino acids are 3-monoiodotyrosine *(MIT),* 3,5-diiodotyrosine *(DIT),* 3,5,3'-triiodotyrosine *(T_3)* and 3,5,3',5'-tetraiodotyrosine *(T_4, thyroxine).*

The iodination of tyrosyl residues attached to thyroglobulin and the formation of MIT and DIT is the key to the formation of T_3 and T_4. The DIT moieties of adjacent thyroglobulin molecules, probably under the influence of a peroxidase, attach to each other to form T_4. Similarly, DIT and MIT on adjacent thyroglobulin molecules attach to each other to form T_3. The coupling of DIT with DIT and DIT with MIT may occur under the influence of TSH.

The synthesis of thyroglobulin conforms to the typical cellular mechanisms utilized to produce a glycoprotein. The organification process is a unique feature of thyroid follicular epithelial cells. Moreover, the storage of the secretory products within the thyroglobin of colloid is a unique feature of this endocrine gland. The mobilization of thyroblobin is essential for the secretion of T_3 and T_4. Thyroglobulin must move back into the cell and be digested before release of T_3 and T_4 is achieved.

Mobilization of Thyroid Hormones. After stimulation by TSH, follicular epithelial cells undergo morphological changes linked to the transport of thyroglobulin back into the cell. The tall columnar epithelial cells increase in height and acquire numerous microvillous projections along their apical borders. The microvilli move in and out of colloid. The foamy and serrated appearance of the colloid at the apical border/colloid interface of active cells is indicative of the mobilization of colloid. The endocytotic movement of thyroglobulin into the cells is manifested as numerous colloid-containing vesicles within the apical margins of the cells. These vesicles, which may be considered phagosomes, migrate toward the basal border and fuse with a primary lysosome. The secondary lysosome, with its activated complement of hydrolases, digests the thyroglobulin molecule. T_3 and T_4 are secreted across the basal cell border, while MIT and DIT, also released by the protease activity, are recycled within the cell as free tyrosyl and iodide. Under normal conditions, thyroglobulin never occurs outside of the thyroid follicle.

Effects of Thyroid Hormones. The thyroid hormones manifest numerous effects upon the cells, tissues, and organs of the body. Whereas the specific activities of the hormones are diverse, most of them involve energy metabolism, growth, and differentiation. The hormones increase the consumption of O_2 by metabolically active tissues and effect the increased production of energy. Because heat is lost during this process, it is often termed the *calorigenic effect*. The thyroid hormones increase the rates of carbohydrate and lipid metabolism, effects consistant with a generalized increase in basal metabolism. Increased absorption of glucose from the intestines, gluconeogenesis, and glycogenolysis occur under the influence of these hormones. Although the peripheral utilization of glucose is increased, a transitory rise in blood glucose, even to the point of exceeding the renal threshold, may occur in response to T_3 and T_4 secretion. Additionally, the rate of synthesis and secretion of cholesterol, as well as a total body loss of the substance occurs in response to thyroid hormone stimulation. Although the thyroid hormones generally stimulate protein synthesis, protein catabolism may occur when metabolic demands require energy supplementation from gluconeogenesis. Similarly, excessive quantities of the thyroid hormones are accompanied by protein catabolic processes. Numerous other specific effects are manifested by T_3 and T_4 upon other tissues and organs of the body.

The thyroid hormones influence growth and developmental processes. They are essential for the normal development of most organs and systems within the animal body. The nervous system and skeletal system especially manifest altered development and growth in the absence of these hormones. The mechanisms utilized by the thyroid hormones to influence the normal progression of growth and development are not understood.

Regulation of Thyroid Hormones. Some iodine occurs free in the plasma, but most of it occurs as *protein-bound iodine (PBI)*, of which the majority is attributable to T_4 and T_3. Protein binding is achieved primarily by a *thyroxine-binding globulin (TBG)*. The free hormones, in equilibrium with those bound to TBG, diffuse into the tissues to manifest their varied influences upon metabolic processes. The precise biological relationships between T_4 and T_3 have not been clarified. T_4 has a greater binding affinity for protein, a more prolonged action, and a longer half-life than T_3. Although some investigators believe that both hormones are active, some believe that T_4 is a prohormone that undergoes deiodination to the more rapidly active T_3.

Three mechanisms are used to metabolize the iodothyronines (T_4 and T_3): *conjugation, deamination/transamination*, and *deiodination*. Conjugation with a glucuronide occurs within the liver followed by the excretion of the conjugated hormones in the bile. Hydrolysis of the conjugated product within the intestines may result in the reabsorption of the hormones via the enterohepatic circulation. As amino acids, the iodothyronines are subject to deamination/transmination reactions within the liver and kidneys. The most important deactivation process is the deiodination of the hormones within the target cells.

The release of T_4 and T_3 by the thyroid gland is regulated by secretion of the TSH by the pars distalis. The release of TSH is controlled by the hypothalamic secretion of TRF. The thyroid hormones have a negative feedback influence upon the pars distalis and hypothalamus. Exposure to cold ambient temperatures stimulates the hypothalamus to secrete TRF. Emotional stress also has an effect upon TRF release; however, such stress, usually associated with sympathetic discharge and increased metabolic activity, inhibits the release of TRF.

Alterations in thyroid gland activity may be manifested as a decreased secretory activity *(hypothyroidism)*. Hypothyroidism may be manifested as a primary or secondary condition. Primary hypothyroidism, a condition in which the thyroid gland is unable to respond to TSH stimulation and produce appropriate quantities of the thyroid hormones, may result from various disease processes that affect the thyroid gland. Without the appropriate T_3 and T_4 hormones to influence the hypothalamus and pars distalis, the thyroid gland is subjected to constant stimulation by TSH; thyroid enlargement *(goiter)* may result. Iodine-deficient diets manifest this type of change in the thyroid gland. Secondary hypothyroidism is a condition that results from a defect in the hypothalamic or pituitary portion of the control axis. Although the thyroid gland is capable of producing T_3 and T_4 under these circumstances, the gland does not have appropriate stimulation. Thyroglobulin, normally sequestered within the follicles of the thyroid gland, may be exposed to immune system components subsequent to damage to the thyroid gland. Upon exposure, thyroglobulin functions as an antigen; an immune-mediated (autoimmune) hypothyroid condition may result. *Hyperthyroidism* may result from excessive stimulation of the gland or from a thyroid tumor.

The role of calcitonin in calcium regulation is discussed in Chapter 9.

Parathyroid Glands

General Considerations. The parathyroid glands are derived from the third *(external parathyroids)* and fourth *(internal parathyroids)* pharyngeal pouches. The position of the external parathyroids may vary from cranial to the thyroids to the level of the thoracic inlet. The internal parathyroids may be missing (bird, pig) or may be embedded within, upon, or close to the thyroid gland.

Histology. The capsule of the external parathyroids is areolar connective tissue that blends with the surrounding fascia. The internal parathyroids do not have a capsule per se but are surrounded by the areolar connective tissue of the interstices of the thyroid gland. The parenchyma of the organ consists of cords, clusters, strands, sheets, or rosettes of secretory cells. Occasionally, follicles may be present (Fig. 25.15). These cells are supported by a stroma of reticular fibers with numerous capillaries. The primary cell types of the organ include *chief* and *oxyphil cells*. The *chief* or *principal cells* may be subdivided into *clear* or *light chief* and *dark chief cells*. Chief cells are more abundant than the oxyphilic cells.

Dark and *light chief cells* represent different physiological states of the same cell. The light chief cell is the inactive cell that has a light-staining acidophilic cytoplasm and a large vesicular nucleus (Fig. 25.16). This cell predominates in the parathyroid glands of domestic animals and man. These cuboidal cells have an electron-transparent cytoplasm that contains few organelles and few secretory granules. Lipid droplets and lipofuscin inclusions may be present in the ox, as well as glycogen (man, felids). The dark chief cells or active cells occur less frequently than their inactive counterparts in most species. The small, vesicular nucleus is surrounded by an acidophilic cy-

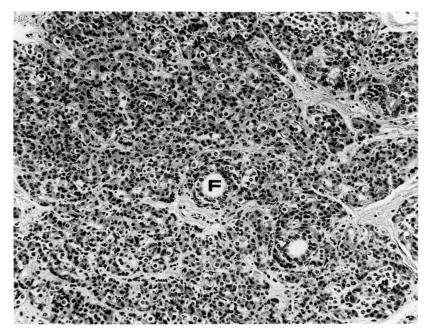

Figure 25.15. A section of a bovine parathyroid gland. Cords or clumps of cells characterize the parenchyma. Follicles *(F)* may occur also. ×40.

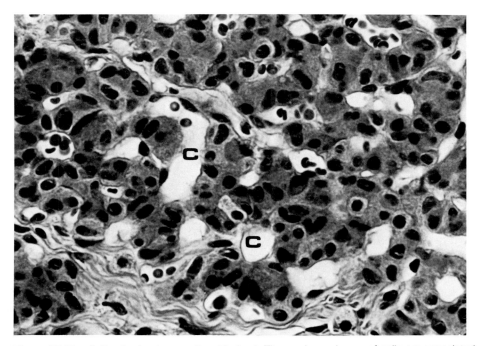

Figure 25.16. Cells of a bovine parathyroid gland. The cords or clumps of cells are associated closely with capillaries *(C)*. ×160.

toplasm with numerous secretory granules. Stimulation of the parathyroid gland results in the release of the secretory products and a lightening of the cytoplasm. Constant stimulation converts these cells to light principal cells that may become vacuolated and eventually clear (water-clear cells). Water-clear cells represent exhaustion atrophy of the chief cells.

The *oxyphil cells* occur in oxen, horses, and man, but they do not occur regularly in other domestic species. They are large cells with a granular, acidophilic cytoplasm. Their nuclei are small and dark-staining. These cells usually occur in small clusters. It is presumed that chief cells give rise to these cells. The precise function of these cells has not been determined.

Parathyroid Hormone. The role of parathormone in calcium regulation is discussed in Chapter 9.

Adrenal Glands

Introduction. The *adrenal glands* or *suprarenal glands* are small organs situated at or near the cranial poles of the kidneys. Embryologically, the adrenal glands are derived from two germ layers: *mesoderm* and neural crest *ectoderm*. The mesenchyme between the root of the mesentery and the developing gonad proliferates and differentiates into the *fetal* or *primitive adrenal cortex*. Neural crest cells develop within the middle of the fetal cortex to form the adrenal medulla. Subsequently, other mesenchymal cells invade the developing gland, proliferate, and develop into the *definitive* or *adult cortex*. After birth, the fetal cortex regresses, except for its innermost region, which becomes the reticular zone. In mammals, a distinct cortex and medulla are apparent despite the striking interdigitations that may occur (Fig. 25.17). In birds, the cortical and medullary tissue is intermixed (Fig. 25.18). Auxiliary cortical adrenal tissue is a common occurrence in some species. In some rodents, auxiliary adrenal tissue is contained within the epididymis.

The organ is enclosed within a capsule of DWFCT. The trabeculae of areolar connective tissue invade the parenchyma to the level of the medulla. The supportive stroma consists of fine collagenous and reticular fibers.

Vascular, Lymphatic, and Neural Relationships. The adrenal glands are highly vascularized organs. The main arteries branch before entry into the gland giving rise to numerous arterioles. Three primary circulation patterns arise from the arteriolar supply. A subcapsular capillary plexus branches throughout the subcapsular region and drains into subcapsular veins. The second pattern is the blood supply to the cortex, which drains through veins into the medulla. Lastly, arterioles traverse the cor-

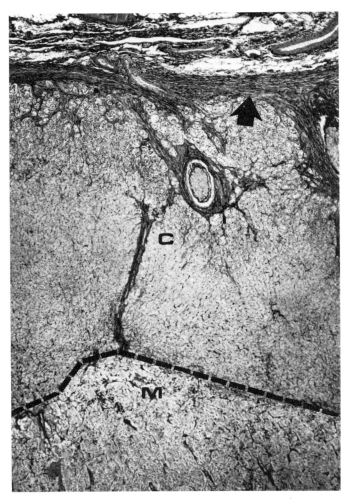

Figure 25.17. Bovine adrenal gland. The adrenal gland capsule *(arrow)* is continuous with connective tissue septa. The gland is divided into a cortex *(C)* and medulla *(M)*, which are delimited clearly *(dashed line)*. ×10. (Azan stain).

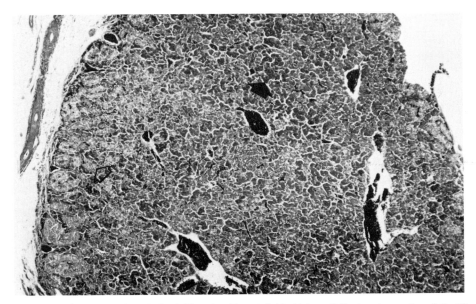

Figure 25.18. Avian adrenal gland. The gland is not divided into a distinct cortex and medulla. The medullary tissue *(solid arrow)* is dark-staining and is interspersed among the light-staining cortical tissue. ×9. (Azan stain).

tex to supply the medulla and drain into medullary veins.

Nerves of the parasympathetic and sympathetic nervous systems innervate the cortex and medulla; however, little information is known about the function of the parasympathetic innervation of the gland. Most of the nerve fibers are preganglionic, sympathetic fibers to the adrenal medulla.

Lymph vessels occur in the connective tissue of the capsule and interstitial tissue of the gland.

Adrenal Cortex

Zonation and Cellular Features. The adrenal cortex consists of polyhedral, secretory cells that are organized into cords, usually two cells thick. The cords are oriented radially from the medullary region (Fig. 25.19). The orientation of the cords and some cytological differences permit the identification of cortical subdivisions: *zona glomerulosa, zona fasciculata, zona reticularis.*

The *zona glomerulosa* is also referred to as the *zona arcuata* and the *zona multiformis* (Fig. 25.20). This subcapsular zone (Fig. 25.21) consists of curved cords or arcades (horses, carnivores, pigs), or clustered groups of glomeruli (ruminants, man). The cells of this zone are columnar (man, horses, carnivores, pigs) or polyhedral (other species) (Fig. 25.22). The parenchyma is closely associated with an extensive vascular network. The cytoplasm is more evenly acidophilic and less foamy than the cells of the adjacent zone. The nuclei of the cells of the zona glomerulosa are smaller and darker than those of the adjacent zone. The occurrence of fine lipid inclusions is usually linked with an increased cellular activity. In man and ruminants, basophilic granules may be observed in the cytoplasm. A *zona intermedia*, consisting of undifferentiated cells is interdigitated between the zona glomerulosa and the zona fasciculata of most domestic animals

The *zona fasciculata* is the widest zone of the cortex (Fig. 25.23). It consists of cuboidal or polyhedral cells that are arranged in radial cords. Each cord consists of one or two cells separated from adjacent cords by an extensive sinus network. The large cells of the outer two-thirds of this zone contain a large, vesicular nucleus (binucleations are common) within a very foamy cytoplasm (Plate II.3). These cells are often called *spongiocytes* (Fig. 25.24). The inner third of this zone contains cells that are free of lipids and have a more basophilic cytoplasm.

The *zona reticularis* consists of cells that are disposed as freely anastomosing cords (Fig. 25.25). The cells are very similar to the cells of the zona fasciculata. The cells of the zona reticularis contain less lipid and their nuclei and cytoplasm are darker stain-

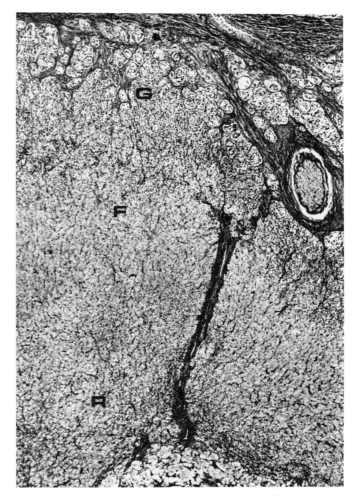

Figure 25.19.   Bovine adrenal cortex. *G*, zona glomerulosa; *F*, zona fasciculata; *R*, zona reticularis. ×16. (Azan stain).

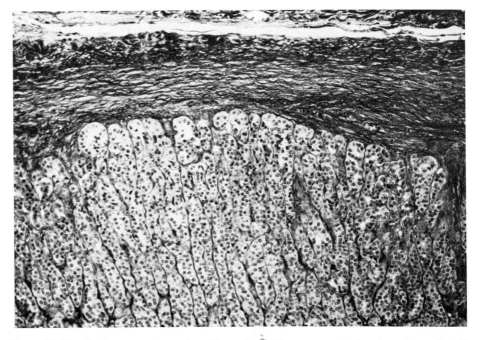

Figure 25.20.   Bovine zona glomerulosa. The cells of this zone are clustered as glomeruli. ×40. (Azan stain).

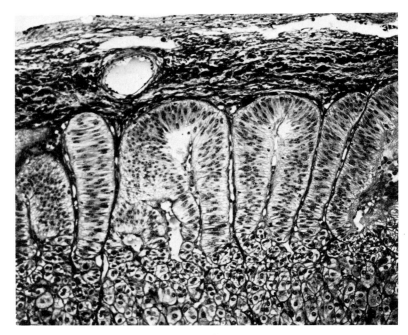

Figure 25.21. Equine zona arcuata. Arcades of cells characterize the outermost zone in this species. ×40. (Azan stain).

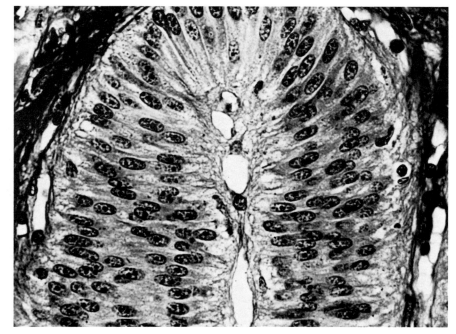

Figure 25.22. Columnar cells of the zona arcuata of the equine adrenal gland. ×160. (Azan stain).

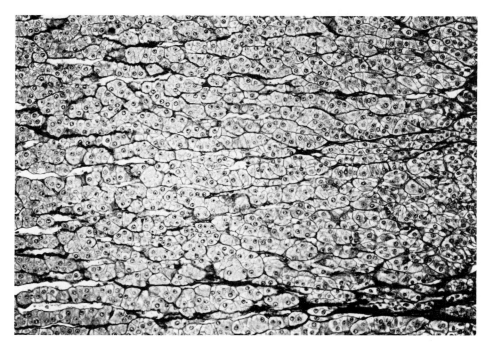

Figure 25.23. Zona fasciculata of an equine adrenal gland. Polyhedral cells arranged as cords characterize this zone. ×40. (Azan stain).

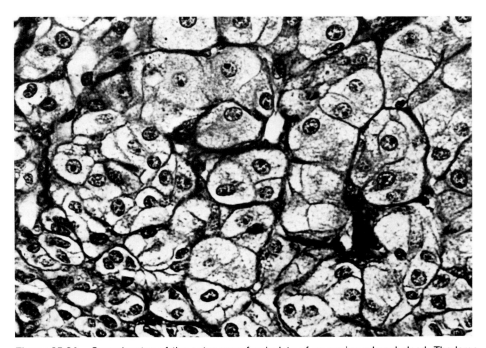

Figure 25.24. Spongiocytes of the outer zona fasciculata of an equine adrenal gland. The large cells have a foamy cytoplasm and vesicular nuclei. ×160. (Azan stain).

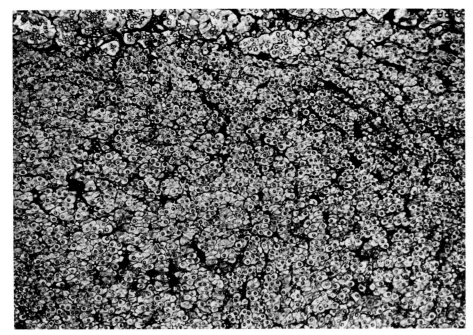

Figure 25.25. Zona reticularis of the equine adrenal gland. The cells are disposed as freely anastomosing cords. ×25. (Azan stain).

ing than the cells of the peripherally adjacent zone. Lipofuscin pigments are commonly encountered.

The adrenal cortex is required for life because its hormones influence numerous essential somatic processes. Although numerous steroid hormones have been isolated from the cortical tissues, they are readily grouped accordingly: *mineralocorticoids, glucocorticoids,* and *sex hormones.*

Some evidence exists that the zona glomerulosa may be responsible for the proliferation and differentiation of cells within the cortex. Cells may proliferate within the zona glomerulosa and differentiate into the characteristic cells of the zona fasciculata. The cells appear to move through the cords eventually degenerating within the zona reticularis.

Histophysiology—Mineralocorticoids. The *mineralocorticoids,* primarily from the activity of the cells of the zona glomerulosa, exert an influence upon ECF electrolytes—especially sodium and potassium. The most important mineralocorticoid is *aldosterone;* however, other corticosteroids have mineralocorticoid activity (corticosterone, cortisol, desoxycorticosterone). The most important activity of aldosterone is the increased tubular resorption of Na^+ by the kidneys. Aldosterone exerts a similar effect upon the sweat glands, salivary glands and intestines.

Numerous secondary effects are related to this Na^+ conservation mechanism under the influence of aldosterone. The reabsorption of Na^+ is linked to the secretion of K^+ and H^+. Potassium wasting and a slight metabolic alkalosis can result. Decreased

K^+ levels can result in muscular weakness, muscular paralysis, and cardiac arrhythmias. The metabolic alkalosis that results from aldosterone is usually transitory and can be corrected by acid/base regulating mechanisms.

Increased Na^+ retention also increases the retention of water, causing an increased ECF and blood volume that is compounded by polydipsia. The increased fluid volume increases the amount of work that must be accomplished by the heart. Polyuria also occurs as a compensation for the increased fluid volume.

The reverse effects occur in the absence of aldosterone. Hyponatremia (decreased Na^+), hyperkalemia (increased K^+), and decreased fluid volume can be anticipated without the proper release of aldosterone. The cardiovascular system is unable to function properly because of the decreased fluid volume (hypovolemia), and cardiac activity decreases in response to the decreased fluid volume and increased levels of K^+. *Hypovolemic shock* (insufficient tissue perfusion) and death can result.

The regulated maintenance of Na^+ and K^+ levels within the body is essential to minimize an increase or decrease of these ions. Aldosterone is essential for this balance. The secretion of aldosterone is regulated by the concentration of K^+ and Na^+ in the ECF and the renin-angiotensin system (Chapter 23). Insufficient adrenocortical secretions of mineralocorticoids (and glucocorticoids) are characteristic of *hypoadrenocorticism (Addison's disease).* Although *Cushing's syndrome (hyperadrenocorticism)* may manifest effects associated

with excessive secretions of aldosterone, the primary effects are those manifested by the excess glucocorticoids. The chemotherapeutic approach to Cushing's syndrome, if not monitored carefully, can produce an Addisonian animal.

Histophysiology—Glucocorticoids. The glucocorticoids are secreted primarily by the zona fasciculata of the adrenal cortex. Although other corticosteroids possess glucocorticoid activity (corticosterone, cortisone), the most important glucocorticoid is *cortisol.* Cortisol transported in the blood bound to a plasma globulin, *transcortin* or *cortisosteroid-binding globulin (CBG),* has diverse effects upon the tissues of the body.

Cortisol causes an increased blood glucose *(hyperglycemia)* and a decreased peripheral utilization of glucose. Glycogenesis and gluconeogenesis complement the increased release of hepatic glucose. Cortisol is diabetogenic. Whereas the glucocorticoids stimulate the synthesis of hepatic proteins, the synthesis of proteins in other tissues is inhibited. The role of cortisol in lipid metabolism is not well understood. Whereas cortisol is lipolytic and causes an increased release of free fatty acids from adipose tissue, excessive quantities of the hormone result in excessive lipid deposition. The stimulation of insulin release by cortisol may account for increased lipid deposition, because insulin promotes lipogenesis and increased amounts of adipose tissue.

The anti-inflammatory properties of the glucocorticoids are significant functions. These hormones stabilize lysosomal membranes, decrease collagen synthesis, increase collagen degradation, and inhibit the proliferation of fibroblasts. Glucocorticoids exert numerous other effects upon the body that are related to the reduction of peripheral protein synthesis—depressed immunocompetency, delayed wound healing, quantitative osteopenia. Gastric ulceration can result from excessive glucocorticoids; the precise mechanism of parietal cell stimulation is not understood. Glucocorticoids, released in response to stress, help to maintain ECF volume and decrease vasodilatation associated with shock. Cortisol and similar drugs exert an influence on mental status. Mental depression associated with glucocorticoid insufficiency may progress to euphoria after the administration of glucocorticoids. Cortisol also possesses permissive properties that complement the functioning of other hormones (GH, glucagon, catecholamines). Glucocorticords also manifest antiallergic properties by preventing the release of histamine associated with the type I hypersensitivity reaction.

The synthesis and release of glucocorticoids from the adrenal cortex are regulated by the secretion of ACTH from the pars distalis. The hypothalamic secretion of CRF controls the activity of the pars distalis. Circulating levels of glucocorticoids exert a negative feedback influence upon the hypothalamus and pars distalis. Notwithstanding the significance of the servomechanism, other factors influence glucocorticoid release. The circadian rhythmicity of ACTH and glucocorticoid release is probably influenced by cerebral cortical and limbic system activity. Similarly, the emotional influence upon circulating levels of glucocorticoids is probably mediated through the limbic system. Trauma, perhaps triggering activity in the limbic and reticular-activating systems, stimulates the increased release of glucocorticoids. Stress is a significant stimulus of glucocorticoid secretion.

Adrenal insufficiency (Addison's disease) is marked by the inability of the adrenal glands to produce mineralocorticoids and glucocorticoids. Cushing's syndrome results from the excessive secretion or administration of glucocorticoids.

Sex Hormones. The only sex hormone produced in any quantity under normal circumstances is a moderately active adrenal androgen called *dihydroepiandrosterone*. This substance can be metabolized to other sex hormones (testosterone and estradiol).

Adrenal Medulla

Histology. The corticomedullary junction may be a sharply delineated junction or may be highly interdigitated (Fig. 25.26). The primary constitiuents of the medulla include *glandular cells, ganglion cells, venules,* and *capillaries.* The aforementioned cells are derived from neural crest ectoderm. The secretory cells are part of the APUD (Amine Precursor Uptake and Decarboxylase) system.

The *glandular cells* are large columnar or polyhedral cells that possess a large, vesicular nucleus (Fig. 25.27). The cells are polarized; one pole is apposed to a capillary and the other is apposed to a venule. The cytoplasm is basophilic and contains fine, chromaffin-positive granules (Fig. 25.28). The resulting pigments are sometimes referred to as *adrenochromes.* As a result of this chromaffin reactivity, the glandular cells are also called *chromaffin cells* or *pheochrome cells.* This reactivity is due to the presence of the *biogenic amines* (catecholamines), *epinephrine* and *norepinephrine.* The reaction of the catecholamines with chromic acid produces a brown reaction product. The chromaffin cells secrete one or the other of the catecholamines. In most species, these cells are randomly distributed throughout the medulla. In the ox, however, an outer lamina of epinephrine-producing cells is distinct from an inner lamina of norepinephrine-producing cells.

Sympathetic ganglion cells are randomly scattered throughout the medulla.

Histophysiology. The function of the ad-

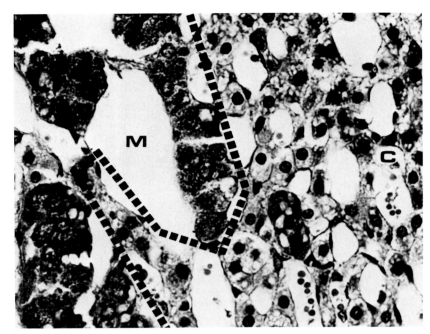

Figure 25.26. Adrenal medulla and zona reticularis of a porcine adrenal gland. The corticomedullary junction *(dashed line)* is irregular. The medulla *(M)* consists of dark-staining cells, whereas the zona reticularis of the cortex *(C)* consists of light-staining cells. ×160. (Chromaffin stain).

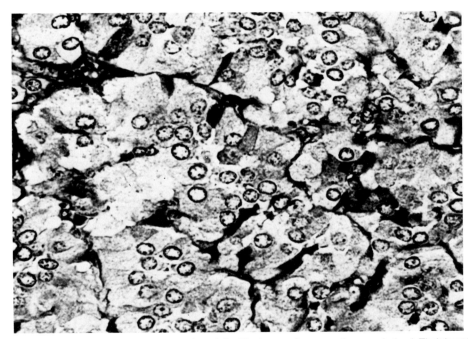

Figure 25.27. Cells of a bovine adrenal medulla. The large columnar cells are polarized. Their basal borders are associated with capillaries. ×160. (Azan stain).

renal medulla and its relationship to the autonomic nervous system are discussed in Chapter 17.

Chromaffin System. Besides the occurrence of chromaffin cells in the adrenal medulla, there are numerous small bodies *(paraganglia)* associated with the abdominal aorta in a retroperitoneal position. The paraganglia include two large bodies, the *glands of Zuckerkandl.* The cells of the paraganglia contain chromaffin-positive granules. The paraganglia plus the adrenal medulla comprise the chromaffin system. Naturally, the paraganglia are part of the APUD system of cells. *Pheochromocytomas,* tumors of the adrenal medullary tissue, commonly involve all of the chromaffin system.

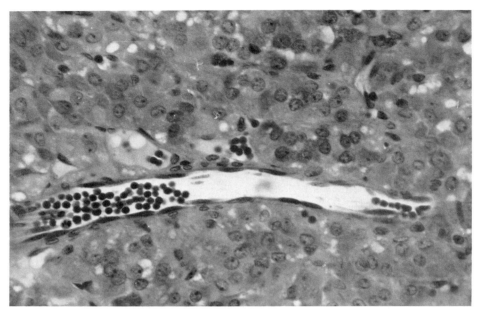

Figure 25.28. A plastic section of a canine adrenal medulla. The cellular detail is excellent. All of the medullary cells in the field are glandular cells. A sinusoidal capillary traverses the center of the field. ×100. (Glycol methacrylate-embedded, 2-μm section).

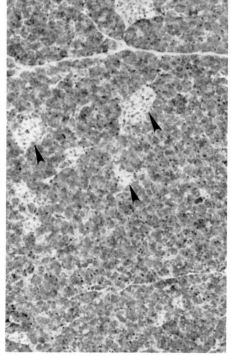

Figure 25.29. A plastic section of a canine pancreas. The pancreatic islets are scattered throughout the substance of the gland. ×10. (Glycol methacrylate-embedded, 2-μm section).

Endocrine Pancreas

General Remarks. The organization of the pancreas reflects its duplicity of function as an exocrine and endocrine organ. The endocrine portions are the *islets of Langerhans* that are randomly scattered throughout the organ (Fig. 25.29). Developmentally, the cells of the islets, as well as those of the acini, are derived from endoderm. The islet cells detach from the developing duct system and are established as endocrine cells.

Histology. The islets are scattered masses of pale-staining cells that are supported by reticular connective tissue (Fig. 25.30). Large sinuses separate the cords or clusters of cells. The basic cell types of the islets are *α cells* and *β cells*. C cells and δ *(D) cells* have been identified also.

The *alpha (A, α) cells* are polygonal cells with a nucleus that has a coarse distribution of heterochromatin. The granules of the α cells are insoluble in alcohol, stain pink or red with the Gomori aldehyde fuchsin technique, and stain red with the Mallory-Azan stain.

The *beta (B, β) cells* are structurally similar to the α cells. Their granules, however, are soluble in alcohol, stain dark purple with the Gomori aldehyde fuchsin technique, and stain orange with the Mallory-Azan stain.

C cells do not contain granules. Delta (D, δ) cells stain blue with the Mallory-Azan technique. Enterochromaffin-like cells also have been identified in the islets.

The B cells are the predominant cells and may comprise more than 75% of the islet cellular population in the dog. The B cells secrete *insulin*, whereas A cells secrete *glucagon, cholecystokinin (CCK), gastric inhibitory protein*, and *ACTH-endorphin*. The functional significance of C cells, which have been identified in the guinea pig pancreas, has not been clarified. Some investigators believe that the C cell may be a progenitor of the A cell; others believe that the C cell may be a resting or exhausted A or B cell. The C cells comprise a small percentage of the cell population. Immunofluorescent studies have shown that the D cell produces *somatostatin* and *vasoactive intestinal peptide (VIP)*. Because somatostatin exerts a potent inhibitory influence upon A and B cell activity, it has been postulated that the D cells may serve as local inhibitors for insulin and glucagon secretion. Enterochromaffin cells are believed to secrete *serotonin, motilin*, and *substance P*.

Histophysiology. *Insulin* is the *hypoglycemic factor* secreted by the B cells of the pancreatic islets. *Glucagon*, the *hyperglycemic factor*, is secreted by the A cells.

Proinsulin is synthesized as an inactive, single polypeptide with a molecular weight of approximately 9000. Activation occurs within the secretory granules of the cell during which time proinsulin is cleaved by the action of a trypsin-like enzyme into *insulin* and a cleavage fragment (connecting segment). Insulin is a dipeptide with a molecular weight of approximately 6000.

Glucagon is a single polypeptide with a molecular weight of approximately 3500. Whereas most of the glucagon is produced by the A cells of the pancreatic islets, some glucagon *(enteroglucagon)* is secreted by cells of the gastrointestinal mucosa. The functional significance of enteroglucagon is not understood completely.

Insulin and glucagon regulate carbohydrate metabolism within the body. Insulin release is achieved in response to increased levels of blood glucose *(hyperglycemia)*, whereas glucagon is secreted in response to decreased blood glucose concentrations *(hypoglycemia)*. The A and B cells are the receptors and regulators of the servomechanism that responds to blood glucose levels, whereas numerous tissues of the body serve as effectors to maintain homeostatic levels of blood glucose and insure an ample supply of energy for the body.

Insulin exerts numerous and varied influences upon the cells and tissues of the body. The generalized effect of insulin upon carbohydrate metabolism is the facilitation of cellular uptake of glucose. This effect reduces blood glucose levels while making glucose available for cellular metabolic processes. The brain, liver, proximal convoluted tubules of the kidney, intestinal mucosa, and red blood cells do not require insulin for the uptake of glucose.

Muscle metabolism is affected by insulin. Glucose uptake is increased and the metabolism of glucose is enhanced. Glycogenesis and glycolysis are increased. Amino acid uptake is increased and protein synthesis is enhanced, whereas fatty acid utilization is decreased.

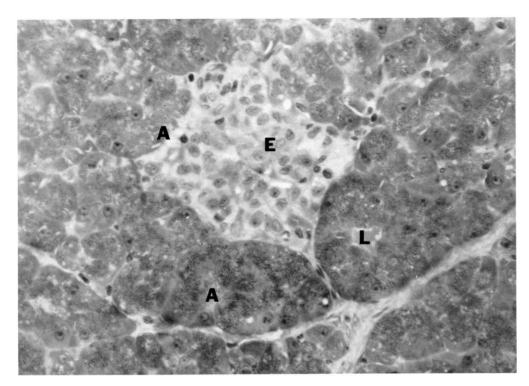

Figure 25.30. A plastic section of a canine pancreas. The endocrine *(E)* portions of the gland—pancreatic islets—are surrounded by pancreatic acini *(A)*. Zymogen granules are evident in the apical cytoplasm. L, lumen. ×100. (Glycolmethacrylate-embedded, 2-μm section).

Insulin also increases the glucose uptake by adipocytes. The augmented transport of glucose increases the utilization of glucose as a source of energy, enhances the storage of glucose as glycogen, and favors lipogenesis from carbohydrates. Blood levels of free fatty acids and triglycerides decrease in response to insulin.

Although insulin does not exert a direct effect upon the uptake of glucose by the liver, the hormone increases hepatocytic metabolism of glucose. Gluconeogenesis decreases under insulin stimulation. Lipogenesis, amino acid uptake, and protein synthesis increase within hepatocytes under the influence of insulin.

Insulin is one of the most important anabolic hormones of the body. It facilitates the utilization of glucose as an energy source and enhances the storage of glucose as glycogen for future use. It increases the storage of triglycerides and diminishes their use as an energy source. Moreover, amino acids are incorporated into proteins instead of being used as a source of energy. Insulin also has an effect upon intracellular and extracellular K^+. The uptake of glucose is accompanied by the movement of K^+ into cells.

Insulin is inactivated by a group of enzymes, collectively called *insulinases*, that are present in many cells of the body (liver, kidneys, skeletal muscle). The rapid turnover of insulin—the plasma half-life is approximately 10 minutes—requires the continual secretion of insulin to maintain proper metabolic activities.

The absence or insufficient secretion of

insulin by the B cells causes *diabetes mellitus*. Glucose levels are high and exceed the renal threshold; therefore, glucosuria is a significant feature of the disease. The osmotic diruesis from glucose in the urine causes a polyuria accompanied by polydipsia. Animals suffering from diabetes mellitus are literally "starving in a sea of plenty." Glucose levels are high, but the animal is unable to utilize glucose as an energy source. *Complicated diabetes mellitus* is characterized by ketoacidosis. Excessive mobilization of lipids overwhelms the metabolic capacity of the liver and ketone bodies form. The excess release of H^+ from the dissociation of ketone bodies causes an acidosis. Diabetic coma and death follow if uncorrected. Hypoglycemia occurs under various circumstances; an islet cell tumor *(insuloma)* causes the excessive and unregulated release of insulin.

Glucagon, as the antagonist of insulin, is glycogenolytic, gluconeogenic, and lipolytic. The hormone ensures the availability of glucose as an energy source. Hepatocytes respond to glucagon stimulation by increasing the release of glucose, the availability of free fatty acids, the oxidation of amino acids and ketone body formation. Adipocytes release free fatty acids in response to glucagon. Although most of the effects of glucagon are manifested in the liver, the limited effects of this hormone are sufficient to counterbalance the effects of insulin. Glucagon inactivation results from the enzymatic degradation of the polypeptide; however, little is known of the precise mechanism.

Miscellaneous Endocrine Glands

Introduction. Numerous cells of the body perform endocrine functions that may be adjunctive activities of the organs with which they are associated. Although the organs of which these cells are a part may not be considered endocrine organs, the functional significance of their contribution to endocrine regulatory mechanisms is no less important than the classic endocrine organs.

Secretion of Chemical Messengers. The maintenance of integrated cellular activity is dependent upon intercellular communication. This communication is achieved through the use of chemical messengers that talk to and influence the behavior of target cells. Classically, the nervous and endocrine systems were considered the communication systems of the body. Currently, however, other cells have been identified as cells that secrete chemical substances for the purpose of intercellular communication. The means by which these chemical messengers are delivered to target cells is the basis for three general categories of these cellular communicators: neurocrine, paracrine, and endocrine cells.

The *endocrine cells* secrete their chemical messengers into the interstitial space. These messengers move into the blood and are distributed subsequently to target cells some distance from the site of origin. These intercellular messengers, once called hormones, are now referred to as *general hormones*. The general hormones are steroids, proteins, and glycoproteins. Based upon its method of delivery to target cells, epinephrine, a catecholamine, may be considered a general hormone.

Neurocrine cells secrete intercellular messengers from cells that are juxtaposed intimately to the target cells. The communicating neurons are the classical neurocrine cells. Directed synapses are the typical examples of this method of communication. The neurotransmitters, then, are the chemical messengers. A nondirected synapse, as exemplified by the postganglionic sympathetic varicosities, could be considered a type of paracrine secretory vehicle.

Paracrine cells secrete their chemical messengers into the interstitial fluid and influence surrounding target cells. Eicosanoids, endogenous polypeptides (angiotensin, kinins), and biologically active amines qualify as *local hormones* or *autacoids*.

APUD System. Certain secretory cells of the mucosal lining of the gastrointestinal tract and respiratory system, thyroid gland, and endocrine pancreas have the ability to secrete polypeptides and biologically active amines as local hormones. These cells are able to concentrate and store biogenic amines as well as synthesize them from requisite precursors. Accordingly, these cells have high quantities of amino acid decarboxylase—an enzyme essential for the synthesis of biogenic amines. Their ability to incorporate and decarboxylate amine precursors accounts for the name *APUD cells (Amine Precursor Uptake and Decarboxylase cells)*.

These cells, believed to be derived from neural crest ectoderm, are scattered diffusely, aggregated in small groups or clustered as small glands throughout the body. Over 30 different cell types—all capable of polypeptide and amine synthesis and secretion—have been described. These include:

1. Cells that secrete gastrointestinal hormones.
2. C cells (parafollicular cells) from the ultimobranchial body that secrete calcitonin.
3. Pancreatic islets cells.
4. Some adenohypophyseal cells.
5. Adrenal medullary cells.
6. Cells of the respiratory tract.

Tumors formed by these cells are called *apudomas*. These include gastrin-secreting tumors of the Zollinger-Ellison syndrome and calcitonin-producing tumors of the parafollicular cells.

Any attempt at classifying biological entities is usually fraught with problems. The classification of chemical messenger-secreting cells is no exception. Neurocrine cells, especially those associated with nondirected synapses could be easily classifed as paracrine cells. Many paracrine cells are actually APUD cells involved in the secretion of local hormones. But some APUD cells produce general hormones. Similarly, postganglionic sympathetic neurons are derived from neural crest ectoderm, secrete biologically active amines (norepinephrine), and are classified as neurocrine cells. Reasonable justification could be offered for their being classified as paracrine or APUD cells. A coherent classification scheme relating to these messenger-producing cells will have to await additional insights.

Reproductive Hormones. The *ovary* and *testes* are responsible primarily for the production of gametes, but these organs synthesize and secrete hormones that affect reproductive as well as other somatic structures and functions. The ovaries secrete *estrogens* and *progestins* at various stages of the estrous cycle. *Relaxin* is produced by the ovaries in those species that require functional ovaries throughout gestation. The testes, through their population of interstitial cells, produce *androgens*. *Estrogens* are produced by the Sertoli cells of the testes, especially in the stallion. The *placenta* is an essential reproductive structure in eutherian mammals. Among its numerous functions, it is also an endocrine organ. The placentas of many mammals secrete *estrogens, progesterone, placental gonadotropins,* and *prostaglandin $F_{2\alpha}$*.

Gastrointestinal Hormones. Numerous cells scattered throughout the gastrointestinal system secrete polypeptides and biogenic amines. Various names are applied to these cells: *gastrointestinal endocrine cells, enteroendocrine cells, argentaffin cells, argyrophilic cells, and enterochromaffin cells*. Since these cells occur throughout the stomach, intestine and pancreas, they are also appropriately called *gastroenteropancreatic cells (GEP cells)*. These cells do not comprise a homogeneouis cellular population. Twelve ultrastructurally distinct gut endocrine cells are known to secrete more than 20 hormones, suspected hormones and neurotransmitters. Some of these cells have a narrow luminal pole with a tuft of microvilli that opens to the surface ("open cells"); others reside upon the basal lamina and do not reach the luminal surface ("closed cells"). The open cells may be sensory cells that are responsive to the dynamic chemical changes that occur within the lumen.

Some of the GEP cells are appropriately called argentaffin cells, because their secretory granules stain with silver. Others stain with dichromates and are called enterochromaffin cells. These characteristics, however, are not applicable to all GEP cells. Argentaffin and enterochromaffin cells comprise two subsets of the GEP cellular populations.

Most of the GEP cells are APUD cells that permit the local modulation of neurogenic regulation of the gastrointestinal system.

Numerous peptide hormones have been isolated from the gastrointestinal tract and characterized: *gastrin, secretin, CCK, gastric inhibitory peptide (GIP), VIP, motilin, substance P, enteroglucagon,* and *somatostatin* have been isolated from the gastrointestinal mucosa. A summary of the physiological actions of these hormones is given in Table 25.1.

Although the activity and origin of gastrointestinal hormones are confined generally to this system, one hormone somatostatin, is produced in a number of locations. *Somatostatin (GHIF)* is secreted by the hypothalamus, D cells of the pancreatic islets, and gastrointestinal mucosa.

Eicosanoids. *Eicosanoids* are a family of compounds that are derivatives of *arachidonic acid* (eicosatetraenoic acid) This is a fatty acid that contains 20 carbons (eicosa = 20 carbons) and four (tetra) unsaturated bonds (enoic = double bonds). Subsequent metabolism of arachidonic acid results in the formation of biologically active lipids that include the following: prostaglandins (PG), thromboxanes (TX), hydroperoxyeicosatetraenoic acid (HPETE), hydroxyeicosatetraenoic acid (HETE) and leukotrienes (LT).

Eicosanoids are generated from perturbations to the plasma membranes of many cells of most organs in varying amounts and kinds. Ater stimulation, arachidonic acid is released from its esterified position in the glycerophospholipids of the lipid bilayer (Fig. 25.31). *Phospholipase A_2* or a combination of *phospholipase C* and *diglyceride lipase* mediate the release. Upon release, arachidonic acid activates a *cyclooxygenase* that converts this acid to unstable endoperoxide intermediates—*prostaglandin G_2 and prostaglandin H_2*. The prostaglandins are compounds that consist of prostanoic acid—a pentane ring with two aliphatic side chains. Subsequent isomerase and reductase activities produce other prostaglandins. Nine groups of prostaglandins exist and have been designated by the letters A through I. They differ from each other by various substitutions at the nine and 11 positions on the pentane ring.

The biological effects of prostaglandins are manifested locally, because the liver and lungs rapidly deactivate the substances. The prostaglandins exert their influence upon the organ in which they are produced or downstream upon an organ associated with the venous drainage from the organ or tissue of origin.

PGA_2, PGE_1, and PGE_2 are vasodilators. Bronchodilation, sodium/water diuresis, and increased gastrointestinal motility are mediated by PGE_2. Also PGE_2 may stimulate renin release and inhibit gastric secretion. The vasopressor activity of $PGF_{2\alpha}$ is well documented. It is also a bronchodilator and luteolytic compound. $PGF_{2\alpha}$ is produced in the endometrium and transported to the ovary by a utero-ovarian vein. The mechanism of transfer to the ovarian artery has not been determined. The regression of

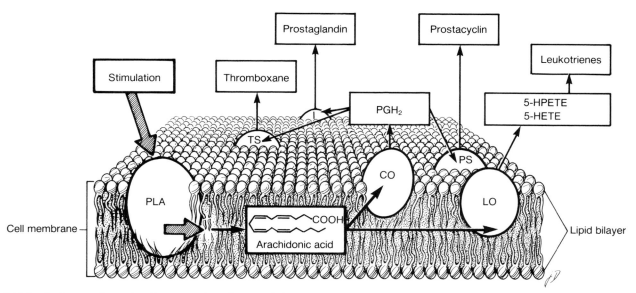

Figure 25.31. A diagram illustrating the generation of extracellular messengers derived from arachidonic acid. Minor damage to cell membranes causes the release of arachidonic acid from the fatty acid chains of the lipid bilayer through the action of phospholipase A *(PLA)*. Subsequent enzyme activity converts this substance to various eicosanoids. *CO*, cyclo-oxidase; *LO*, lipoxygenases; *PS*, prostacyclin synthase; *I*, isomerase; *TS*, thromboxane synthase; *PGH₂*, prostaglandin H_2; *5-HPETE* and *5-HETE* are hyroxy fatty acid intermediates in the leukotriene pathway.

Table 25.1
Selected Gastrointestinal Hormones

Hormone	Target	Action
CCK	Stomach	↑ Motility
	Small intestine	↑ Motility
	Pancreas—acini	↑ Secretion
Gastrin	Stomach	↑ HCl secretion
		↑ Enzyme secretion
		↑ Motility
	Small intestine	↑ Motility
Secretin	Pancreas—ducts	↑ HCO_3^- secretion
	Liver	↑ HCO_3^- secretion
	Small intestine	↓ Motility
GIP	Stomach	↓ HCl secretion
Motilin	Stomach	↑ Motility
Substance P	Stomach	↑ Motility
	Small intestine	↑ Motility
Somatostatin	Pancreas—islets	↓ Insulin secretion
	Pancreas—acini	↓ Secretion
	Stomach	↓ Gastrin secretion
VIP	Stomach	↓ HCl secretion
		↓ Enzyme secretion
		↓ Motility
	Pancreas—ducts	↑ HCO_3^- secretion
	Pancreas—acini	↑ Enzyme secretion
Enteroglucagon	?	?
Histamine	Stomach	↑ HCl secretion

the corpus luteum occurs under the influence of $PGF_{2\alpha}$. The luteolytic activity of the compound terminates the luteal phase of the estrous cycle and permits the next wave of follicles to mature. The luteolytic function has been documented in the mare, ewe, cow and sow. *Prostacyclin (PGI₂)* is a vasodilator that also inhibits platelet aggregation *(antithrombotic agent)*.

The thromboxanes are produced from the endoperoxide intermediates by the action of *thromboxane synthase*. *Thromboxane (TXA₂)* is a vasoconstrictor that also stimulates platelet aggregation *(thrombogenic)*. The interaction of TXA_2/PGI_2 at the endothelial-blood interface may serve as mediators in the maintenance of vascular homeostasis in health and disease.

Arachidonic acid is converted by a lipooxygenase to *hydroperoxyeicosatetraenoic acids (HPETEs)*. The HPETEs are converted either to *hydroxyeicosatetraenoic acid (HETEs)* or the *leukotrienes (LT)*. The HETEs can cause bronchial smooth muscle contraction with a potency comparable to histamine.

The LTs are designated A through E. These substances cause the contraction of vascular and respiratory smooth muscle. Also, the activity attibuted to the slow reacting substance of anaphylaxis (SRS-A) is known to be caused by LTC_4 and LTD_4 (Chapter 19).

Miscellaneous Hormones. Although the primary function of the kidneys is excretion, the organ is involved in endocrine functions also. *Erythrogenin* is essential for the generation of erythropoietin (Chapter 20). Some scientists consider *vitamin D* and its active metabolites to be hormones (Chapter 9).

References

Pituitary Gland

Brahms, S.: The development of the hypophysis of the cat *(Felis domestica)*. Amer. J. Anat. *50*:251, 1932.
Conklin, J. L.: The identification of acidophilic cells in the human pars distalis. Anat. Rec. *156*:347, 1966.
Goldberg, R. C. and Chaikoff, I. L.: On the occurrence

of six cell types in the dog anterior pituitary. Anat. Rec. *112*:265, 1953.

Harris, G. W. and Donovan, B. T. (eds.): *The Pituitary Gland.* University of California Press. Perkeley, 1966.

Herlant, M.: The cells of the adenohypophysis and their functional significance. Int. Rev. Cytol. *17*:299, 1964.

Knigge, K. M., Scott, D. E. and Weindl, A. (eds.): *Brain Endocrine Interaction. Median Eminence: Structure and Function.* S. Karger, Basal. 1971.

Lederis, K.: An electron microscopical study of the human neurohypophysis. Z. Zellforsch. *68*:847, 1965.

Nakane, P. K.: Classification of anterior pituitary cell types with immunoenzyme histochemistry. J. Histochem. Cytochem. *18*:9, 1970.

Page, R. B., Munger, B. L. and Bergland, R. M.: Scanning microscopy of pituitary vascular casts. Am. J. Anat. *146*:273, 1976.

Pelletier, G. Robert, F. and Hardy J.: Identification of human pituitary cell types by immunoelectron microscopy. J. Clin. Endocrinol. *46*:534, 1978.

Share, L. and Grosvenor, C. E.: The neurohypophysis. *In* Guyton, A. C. and McCann, S. M. (eds.). *International Review of Science, Endocrine Physiology.* Series 1, Vol. 5 pp. 1–30. Butterworth & Co., London, 1974.

Zambrano, D.: Ultrastructural changes of the neurohypophysis of the rat after castration. Z. Zellforsch. *86*:14, 1968.

Pineal Body

Anderson, E.: The anatomy of bovine and ovine pineals: Light and electron microscope studies. J. Ultrastruc. Res. Suppl. *8*:1, 1965.

Axelrod, J.: The pineal glands: A neurochemical transducer. Science *184*:1341, 1974.

Cardinali, D. P.: Melatonin. A mammalian pineal hormone. Endocrine Rev. *2*:327, 1981.

Herbert, J.: The pineal gland and light-induced oestrus in ferrets. J. Endocr. *43*:625, 1969.

Jordan, H. E.: The histogenesis of the pineal body of the sheep. Amer. J. Anat. *12*:249, 1911.

Reiter, R. J. (ed.): *The Pineal Gland.* CRC Press, Boca Raton, FL, 1981.

Snyder, D. L., Cowan, R. L. and Kavanaugh, J. F.: The effect of pineal gland removal on nutrition, antler growth and hormone levels in male white-tailed deer. *In* Brown, R. D. (ed.). *Antler Development in Cervidae.* p 467. Caesar Kleberg Wildlife Research Institute, Kingsville, 1983.

Wurtman, R. J., Axelrod, J. and Kelly, D. E.: *The Pineal.* Academic Press, New York, 1968.

Thyroid Gland

Ekholm, R.: Thyroglabulin biosynthesis in the rat thyroid. J. Ultrastruct. Res. *20*:103, 1967.

Ekholm, R. and Ericson, L. E.: The ultrastructure of the parafollicular cells of the thyroid gland in the rat. J. Ultrastruct. Res. *23*:378, 1968.

Kingsbury, B. E.: ultimobranchial body and the thyroid gland in the fetal calf. Amer. J. Anat. *56*:445, 1935.

Klinck, G. H., Oertel, J. E. and Winship, I.: Ultrastructure of normal human thyroid. Lab. Invest. *22*:2, 1970.

Martin, J. B.: Regulation of the pituitary—thyroid axis. *In*: Guyton, A. C. and McCann, S. M. (eds.): *International Review of Science, Endocrine Physiology.* Series I, Vol. 5 pp. 1–30. Butterworth & Co., London, 1974.

Sobel, H. J.: Electron microscopy of I-irradiated thyroid. Arch. Path. *78*:53, 1964.

Welsch, U., Flitney, E. and Pearse, A. G. E.: Comparative studies of the ultrastructure of the thyroid parafollicular C cells. J. Microscop. *89*:83, 1969.

Parathyroid Glands

Capen, C. C. and Rowland, G. N.: The ultrastructure of the parathyroid glands of young cats. Anat. Rec. *162*:327, 1968.

Gaillard, P. J., Talmage, R. V. and Budy, A. M. (eds.): *The Parathyroid Glands.* University of Chicago Press, Chicago, 1965.

Godwin, M. C.: The development of the parathyroids in the dog with emphasis upon the origin of accessory glands. Anat. Rec. *68*:305, 1937.

Gray, T. K., Cooper, C. W. and Munson, P. L.: Parathyroid hormone, thyrocalcitonin and the control of mineral metabolism. *In*: Guyton, A. C. and McCann, S. M. (eds.): *International Review of Science, Endocrine Physiology.* Series I, Vol. 5 pp. 239–278. Butterworth & Co., London, 1974.

Nakagami, K., Yamazaki, Y. and Tsunoda, Y.: An electron microscopic study of the human fetal parathyroid gland. Z. Zellforsch. *85*:89, 1968.

Adrenal Glands

Bloodworth, J. M. B., Jr. and Powers, K. L.: The ultrastructure of the normal dog adrenal. J. Anat. *102*:457, 1968.

Brenner, R. M.: Fine structure of adrenocortical cells in adult male rhesus monkeys. Amer. J. Anat. *119*:429, 1966.

Elfvin, L. G.: The development of the secretory granules in the rat adrenal medulla. J. Ultrastruct. Res. *17*:45, 1967.

Hopwood, D.: Adrenal medullary basophilia in ox, pig and sheep: A histochemical, immunohistochemical and cell fractionation study. Histochemie *11*:268, 1967.

Merklin, R. J.: Suprarenal gland lymphatic drainage. Am. J. Anat. *119*:359, 1966.

Migally, N.: The innervation of the mouse adrenal cortex. Anat. Rec. *194*:105, 1979.

Mulnix, J. A.: Adrenal cortical disease in dogs. Vet Scope. *19*:12, 1975.

Rhodin, J. A. G.:The ultrastructure of the adrenal cortex of the rat under normal and experimental conditions. J. Ultrastruct. Res. *34*:23, 1971.

Thorn, G. W. (ed.): *Steroid Therapy: A Clinical Update for the 1970's.* Upjohn Company. Kalamazoo, 1974.

Whitehead, R. H.: The histogenesis of the adrenal in the pig. Amer. J. Anat. *2*:349, 1903.

Wood, J. G.: Identification of and observations on epinephrine and norepinephrine containing cells in the adrenal medulla. Amer. J. Anat. *112*:285, 1963.

Endocrine Pancreas

Greider, M. H., Howell, S. L. and Lacy, P. E.: Isolation and properties of secretory granules from rat islets of Langerhans. J. Cell Biol. *41*:162, 1969.

Lacy, P. E.: Electron microscopy of the beta cells of the pancreas. Amer. J. Med. *31*:851, 1961.

Like, A. A.: The ultrastructure of the islets of Langerhans in man. Lab. Invest. *16*:937, 1967.

Machino, M.: On the substructure of secretory granules of the chick beta islet cell. J. Ultrastruct. Res. *31*:199, 1970.

Unger, R. H.: The pancreas as a regulator of metabolism. In: Guyton, A. C. and McCann, S. M. (eds.): *International Review of Science.* Endocrine Physiology. Series 1, Vol. 5 pp. 179–204. Butterworth & Co., London, 1974.

Miscellaneous Hormones

Bell, T. G. et al.: Biologic interaction of prostaglandins, thromboxane, and prostacyclin: Potential nonreproductive veterinary clinical applications. J. Am. Vet. Med. Assoc. *176*:1195, 1980.

Goldyne, M. E.: Prostaglandins and other eicosanoids. *In*: Katzung, B. G. (ed.): *Basic and Clinical Pharmacology.* p 196. Lange Medical Publishing, Los Altos, 1982.

Hightower, N. C. and Janowitz, H. D.: Gastrointestinal hormones. *In*: Brobeck, J. R. (ed.): *Best and Taylor's Physiological Basis of Medical Practice.* 10th edition, pp. 20–23. Williams & Wilkins, Baltimore, 1979.

Kindahl, H.: Prostaglandin biosynthesis and metabolism. J. Am. Vet. Med. Assoc. *176*:1173, 1980.

Seguin, B. E.: Role of prostaglandins bovine reproduction. J. Am. Vet. Med. Assoc. *176*:1178, 1980.

Welbourn, R. B. et al: The APUD cells of the alimentary tract in health and disease. Med. Clin. North. Am. *58*:1359, 1974.

26: Male Reproductive System

General Characteristics

Introduction. The male reproductive system consists of the *testes, excretory (genital) ducts, accessory glands,* and *penis.* The constituent organs contribute to the primary function—*reproduction.* The *production* and *transport of spermatozoa, secretion* of fluids, and the *placement* of semen in the female tract are complementary functions. The intermittent copulatory organ also functions to *transport urine* to the external environment.

Testes

General Remarks. These organs are contained within a specialized pouch of the skin, the *scrotum* (Chapter 20.) The testes are combined exocrine and endocrine organs. The exocrine portion is a compound, coiled tubular gland that produces spermatozoa as its holocrine secretory product. The endocrine portion is repesented by the interstitial *cells of Leydig* and the sustentacular *cells of Sertoli.*

Testicular Investments. The testes are enclosed by a capsule, the *tunica albuginea,* which is composed of dense white fibrous connective tissue (DWFCT) (Fig. 26.1). This capsule is covered by a tunica serosa, the connective tissue of which blends insensibly with the tunica albuginea.

A *stratum vasculare* (vascular layer) is present in the tunica albuginea of most species. It is superficial in dogs and rams; it is deep in stallions and boars. Smooth muscle fibers may be present in the tunica albuginea of horses.

The tunica albuginea is continuous with the areolar connective tissue of the *mediastinum testis,* in most species, at the anterior pole of the testis (Fig. 26.1). It surrounds the *rete testis.* Although the mediastinum of the stallion is atypical and inconspicuous, it exists as a true mediastinum. The rete testis of the stallion is extratesticular and penetrates the tunica albuginea to unite with the efferent ducts.

The tunica albuginea also is continuous with areolar connective tissue of the *septuli testis* (Fig. 26.1). These septa effectively divide the testis into lobules *(lobuli testis).* The tubules of the lobule *(tubuli contorti* and *tubuli recti)* are surrounded by areolar connective tissue with numerous reticular fibers.

Seminiferous Tubules. The parenchyma of the organ consists of the lining cells of the seminiferous tubules and their ducts, as well as the *cells of Leydig.* The *seminiferous tubules (tubuli contorti)* are the exocrine portions of the gland (Fig. 26.2). The tu-

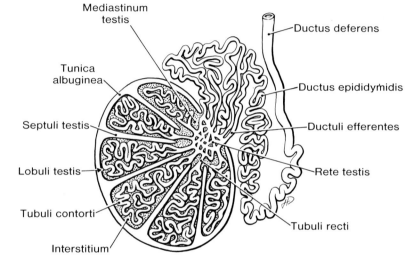

Figure 26.1. A drawing of the testis and associated structures. The connective tissue investments of the extratesticular ducts are not shown.

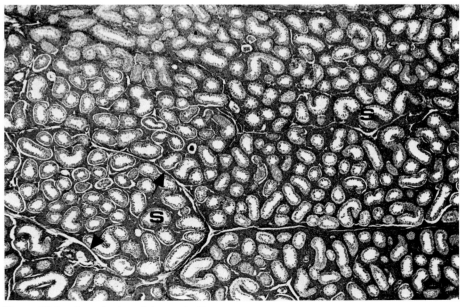

Figure 26.2. Organization of the testis. The seminiferous tubules *(S)* occur within lobules that are separated from each other by connective tissue septa *(arrows).* ×4.

489

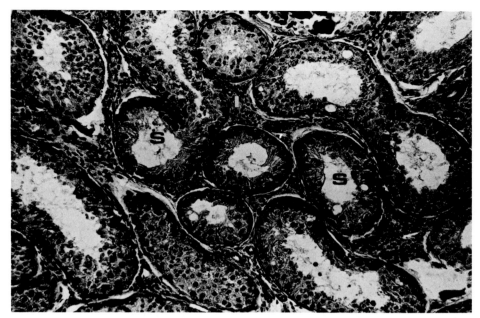

Figure 26.3. Seminiferous tubules of a cervine testis. The seminiferous tubules *(S)* are separated by connective tissue and interstitial cells *(I)*. ×40.

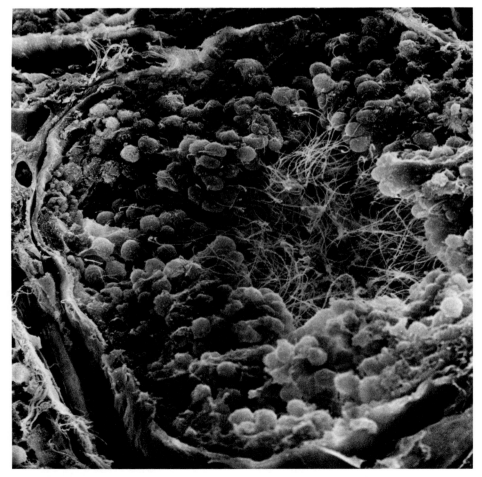

Figure 26.4. A scanning electron micrograph of a freeze-fractured sample of a canine seminiferous tubule. Numerous cells comprise the stratified epithelium. The tails of developing spermatozoa protrude into the lumen of the tubule. ×670. (Negative courtesy of C. J. Connell).

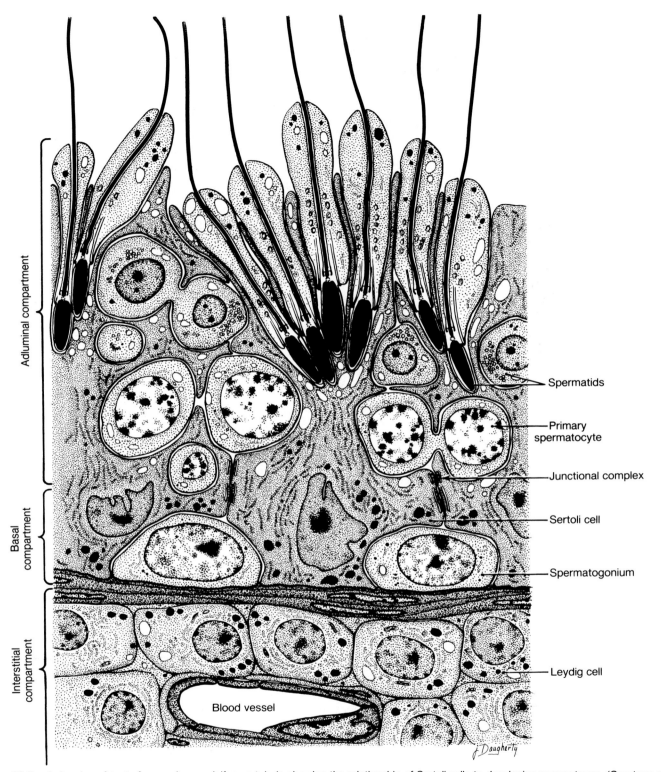

Figure 26.5. A drawing of part of an equine seminiferous tubule showing the relationship of Sertoli cells to developing spermatozoa. (Courtesy of R. P. Amann.)

bules radiate from the mediastinum testis as coiled, tubular adenomeres (Fig. 26.3). The tubules are lined by stratified epithelia that consist of basal, intermediate, and superficial zones. The presence and constitu-ents of the zones are dependent upon the spermatogenic activity of the tubules. Al-though the epithelium is stratified, it is not typical stratified epithelia (Fig. 26.4). The stratified cells consist of *spermatogonia,* *primary spermatocytes, secondary sperma-tocytes, spermatids,* and *spermatozoa* (Fig. 26.5).

Leydig Cells. *Leydig cells* are the endo-crine component of the testes and are re-

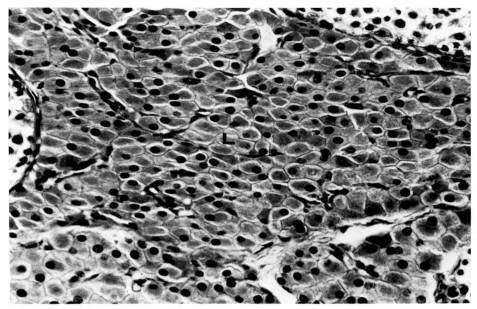

Figure 26.6.   Interstitial cells of a porcine testis. The Leydig cells *(L)* have an acidophilic and foamy cytoplasm. ×100.

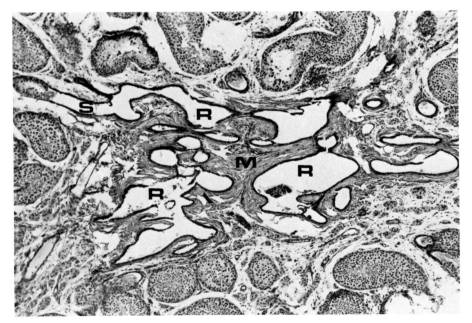

Figure 26.7.   Mediastinum of a feline testis. The mediastinum *(M)* contains the rete testis *(R)*. Straight tubules *(S)* connect the rete testis with the seminiferous tubules. ×10.

sponsible for the elaboration of *testosterone* (Fig. 26.6). The cells, which are located in the septal connective tissue, are polyhedral with a large spherical nucleus and a distinct nucleolus. Their acidophilic cytoplasm contains numerous lipid droplets and granules, but these are lost during routine processing (Plate II.1). As a result, the cells are foamy. These cells are abundant in boars and bulls.

Tubuli Recti and Rete Testes. The sem-iniferous tubules are continuous with the *straight tubules (tubuli recti)* and the passages of the *rete testis* (Fig. 26.7). These regions are lined by a squamous, cuboidal, or columnar epithelium. In bulls, the rete testis may be lined by a bistratified cuboidal epithelium. These two regions are similar to each other and are best identified by position within the testis. Whereas the tubuli recti are straight tubules, the rete testis consists of randomly anastomotic tubules

(Fig. 26.8). In boars, the apical borders of the lining cells may possess blebs that have been interpreted as apocrine secretory activity. Some believe that the lining cells of these regions actually represent a continuation of the Sertoli cell population of the tubuli contorti.

Genital Ducts

Ductuli Efferentes. The *ductuli efferentes* connect the rete testis with the ductus epididymidis (Fig. 26.9). The efferent ductules vary from six to 20 coiled ducts lined by intermittently kinociliated columnar epithelium (Fig. 26.10). The current created by the movement of the cilia assists in the movement of spermatozoa toward the larger ducts. Some nonciliated cells are secretory; others are absorptive—their apical surface has microvilli. The surrounding lamina propria mucosa blends with the other connective tissue of the region, and some smooth muscle cells are present. The widened and tightly convoluted portions of these tubules that connect with the ductus epididymidis constitute the head of the organ.

Ductus Epididymidis. This is the coiled tube that, with associated connective tissue and muscle, forms the *head, body*, and *tail* of the epididymis (Fig. 26.11). The latter continues as the ductus deferens.

The lamina epithelialis mucosae is pseudostratified stereociliated columnar epithelium (Fig. 26.12). The basal cells contain lipid droplets, whereas the columnar cells are long and slender, contain lipids, and have apical modifications in the form of stereocilia (Fig. 26.13). These processes are nonmotile and serve to increase the absorptive and/or secretory surface of the lining. They are usually heavily matted together by their secretory products. The nature and significance of these products is not known. The lamina propria mucosae consists of a highly vascularized areolar connective tissue. The lamina muscularis mucosae is arranged in a circular array and becomes thicker toward the tail of the epididymis. The tunica submucosa is areolar connective tissue centrally and DWFCT peripherally that is continuous with the tunica albuginea. Numerous spermatozoa are stored within the lumen of the ductus epididymidis during which time they mature.

Ductus Deferens. The ductus deferens is the continuation of the ductus epididymidis (Fig. 26.14). The lamina epithelialis mucosae consists of a pseudostratified columnar epithelium. There is, however, a gradual transition from the lining epithelium of the ductus epididymidis to that of the ductus deferens. The lamina propria-submucosa consists of areolar connective tissue. The mucosal glands of this duct comprise the ampulla. The tunica muscularis is thick and varies from two distinct inner and

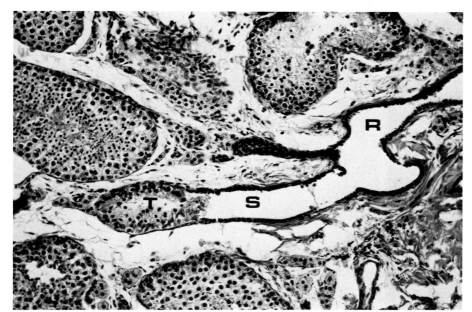

Figure 26.8. Rete testis and tubuli recti of a feline testis. The tubule contorti *(T)* are connected to the rete testis *(R)* by the tubuli recti (S). ×40.

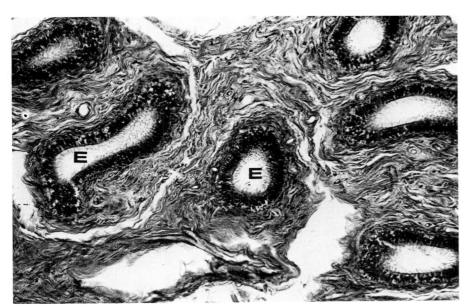

Figure 26.9. Ductuli efferentes. The tubules *(E)* connect the rete testis to the ductus epididymidis. ×40.

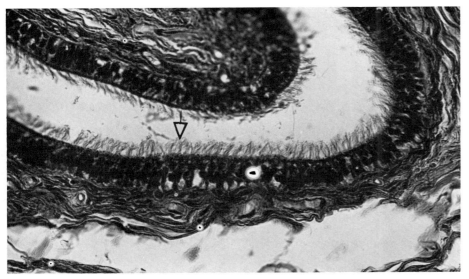

Figure 26.10. Lining cells of the efferent ducts. The columnar epithelial cells are kinociliated *(arrow)*. ×100.

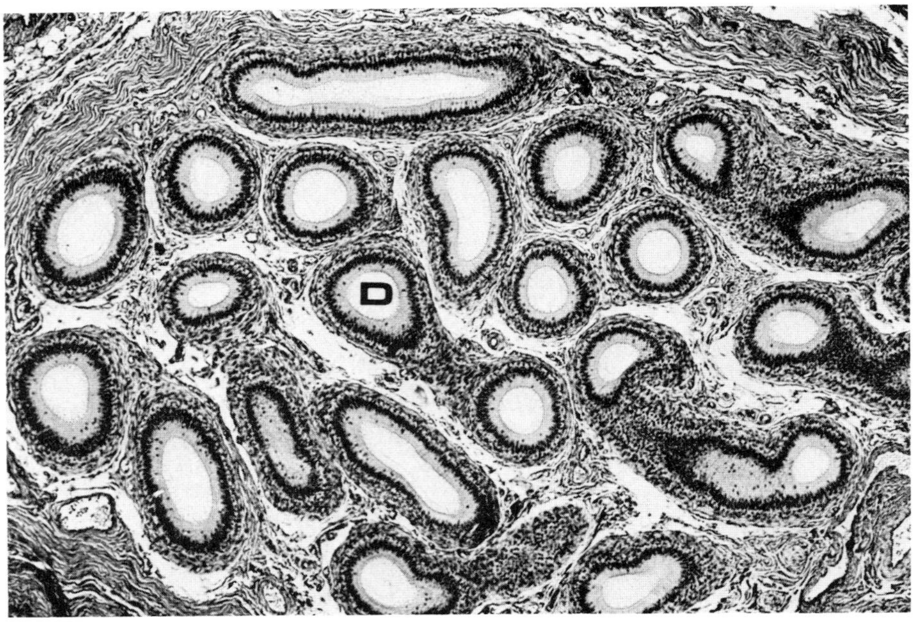

Figure 26.11. A portion of the epididymis. The ductus epididymidis *(D)* is the tubular portion of the organ. ×20.

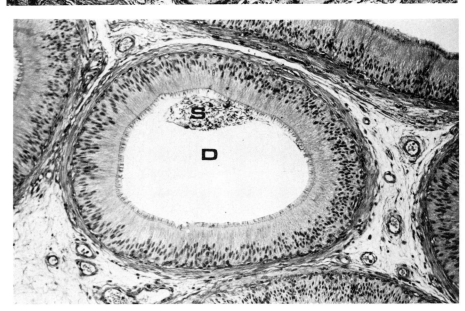

Figure 26.12. Lining cells of the ductus epididymidis. The tubules *(D)* contain spermatozoa *(S)* and are lined by stereociliated epithelium. ×10.

Figure 26.13. Stereocilia of the ductus epididymidis. The lining cells are stereociliated *(open arrow)*. Terminal bars *(solid arrows)* are apparent. ×100.

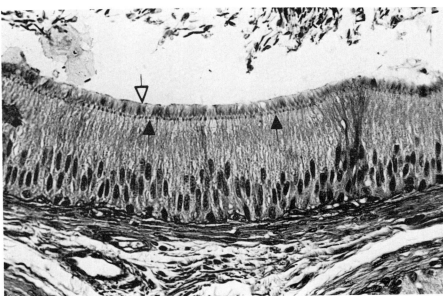

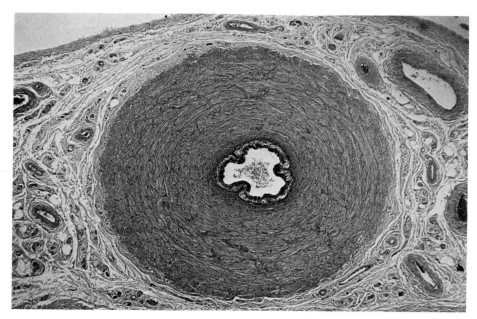

Figure 26.14. Ductus deferens. The duct is a continuation of the ductus epididymidis. Note the extensive amount of smooth muscle peripheral to the lumen of the organ. The ductus deferens is the tubular portion of the vas deferens. ×10.

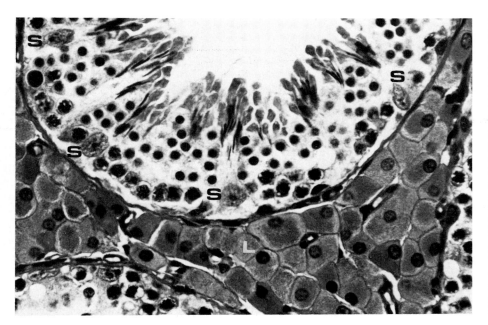

Figure 26.15. Sertoli cells of the porcine testis. The Sertoli cells *(S)* are triangular cells with triangular nuclei that are positioned basally. The developing gametes are associated intimately with the Sertoli cells. *L*, Leydig cells. ×160.

Three distinct periods are characteristic of the spermatogenic process: *mitotic, meiotic,* and *metamorphic.* Not all seminiferous tubules are in the same period of activity, nor are different portions of the same tubule characterized by cells with the same degree of differentiation. Although there are species variations, the spermatocytogenic process is described as occurring in helical waves down the tubule contorti to the straight tubules.

Sertoli Cells. *Sertoli cells* of the seminiferous tubules are sustentacular or nurse cells for the developing gametes (Fig. 26.15). Sertoli cells are tall columnar or triangular cells the cytoplasm and cellular margins of which are difficult to distinguish with light microscopy (Plate II.2). Developing gametes are embedded within invaginations of the Sertoli cell cytoplasm. They are the only cells of the seminiferous tubules that extend from the basal lamina to the tubular lumen. The oval nucleus is usually positioned basally. It is vesicular and has a distinct nucleolus. A characteristic longitudinal fold in the nuclear membrane may be visible.

Electron microscopy was required to clarify the nature of the intimacy between gametes and Sertoli cells. Developing gametes are contained within invaginations along the margins of the Sertoli cells that may totally enclose the gametes (Fig. 26.16). Smooth endoplasmic reticular profiles are extensive along the basal border of the cell. The presence of this organelle has been interpreted as a priori evidence of the ability of the Sertoli cell to synthesize steroids. The Golgi apparatus is extensive. An *androgen binding protein* (ABP), secreted into the seminiferous tubular lumen, is degraded in the ductus epididymidis. Numerous cytofilaments are scattered throughout the cell. The cytofilaments are obvious especially along the lateral margins of the cell where they are oriented parallel to the long axis of the cell and aggregated in bundles. The movement of developing gametes from the basal border to the apical margin is dependent upon changes in the Sertoli cell probably attributable to alterations in the cytofilaments. Lysosomes in various stages of activity are conspicuous. The presence of lysosomes correlates with the removal, phagocytosis, and digestion of residual cytoplasmic droplets from developing spermatozoa.

The basilar regions of the lateral cell membranes of adjacent Sertoli cells are joined by tight (occluding) junctions. The tight junctions effectively divide the seminiferous tubule into two distinct regions—basilar and apical compartments. The *basilar compartment,* located peripherally between the tight junctions and the basal lamina, is the location of the spermatogonia. The spermatogonia are influenced by substances that move across the basal

outer layers to intermingled fibers. The tunica serosa is present and typical.

Spermatogenesis

Introduction. *Spermatogenesis* occurs within the tubuli contorti and ductus epididymidis. The former are responsible for the production of gametes; whereas, the latter aid in their maturation process. The sequence of events involves a series of nuclear and cytoplasmic changes that result in haploid cells that are highly motile and suited to survive for short periods outside the body. The progression begins with *spermatogonia* and terminates with *spermatozoa.* These cells, with *Sertoli cells,* comprise the stratified lining. The most primitive cells are located near the periphery of the tubule; whereas, the more developmentally advanced cells are located on the luminal border.

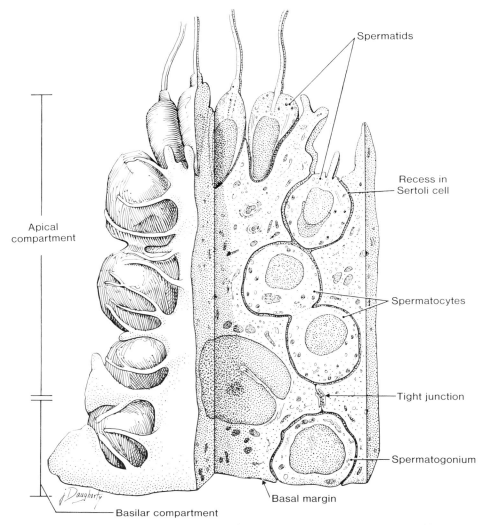

Figure 26.16. A three-dimensional drawing of the electron microscopic appearance of adjacent Sertoli cells. Spermatogonia occupy the basilar compartment and are exposed directly to influences from the interstitium. Spermatocytes occupy the apical compartment and are insulated from direct influences by the blood-testis barrier.

lamina from the testicular interstitium. Exchange between the basal border of the Sertoli cell and the surrounding interstitial vasculature is facilitated by the relationship. The *apical compartment*, located between the tight junctions and the apical border, contains the developing gametes. Whereas the Sertoli cell is influenced by direct exchange from the surrounding vasculature, the developing gametes are "insulated" from direct influences by the Sertoli cell. The tight junctions and contiguous Sertoli cells form an effective *blood-testis barrier*.

The Sertoli cell provides physical support, protection, and probably nutrition for the developing gametes. The Sertoli cell may participate actively in the centripetal movement, development, and release of the gametes, because alterations in Sertoli cell morphology correlate with events in the spermatogenic cycle. The intimacy of the relationship implies that the Sertoli cell is a metabolic regulator. Additionally, damaged gametes are phagocytized by the Sertoli cells.

The Sertoli cells also secrete estrogens. Sertoli cell tumors, which are common in dogs, may be accompanied by the development of secondary female sex characteristics.

Stage of Multiplication. The *stage of multiplication* or *mitotic stage* is characterized by an increase in the number of spermatogonia. Through successive mitotic divisions, numerous spermatogonia undergo changes that result in spermatozoa—all derived from one cell. If one spermatogonium differentiated into subsequent cell types, then only four haploid gametes would be produced. As a result of the mitotic stage, the number of spermatogonia is increased greatly. Accordingly, the number of potential spermatozoa increases also. Not all spermatogonia differentiate simultaneously. Some are retained as stem cells for future differentiation. If complete differentiation were to occur, the potential for gamete production would diminish rapidly and eventually terminate.

Spermatogonia actually represent many generations of cells. These include: A cells, intermediate cells (I_1 and I_2), and B cells. *A spermatogonia* are the stem cells for this process. The cells are round with a large, round nucleus that contains finely dispersed chromatin and an eccentrically positioned nucleolus. Upon mitotic division, one cell remains as a stem cell whereas the other divides and its progeny differentiate into *intermediate (I) spermatogonia*. I spermatogonia are oval cells with an oval nucleus. The nucleus contains peripheral-positioned, coarsely clumped chromatin and two or three nucleoli. Subsequent divisions of intermediate spermatogonia give rise to *B spermatogonia*. These cells are round and small. The oval nucleus contains coarsely clumped chromatin. Subsequent division of these spermatogonia leads to the differentiation of *primary spermatocytes*. As many as 16 primary spermatocytes are derived from a single A spermatogonium. Incomplete cytokinesis is characteristic of the mitotic process that results in B spermatogonia.

Spermatogonia occur adjacent to the basement membrane, either singly or in clusters. They do not form a complete basal layer and may be difficult to find.

Spermatocytogenesis. This stage of the spermatogenic process involves the *spermatocytes*. These are the largest cells of the spermatogenic epithelium that comprise the intermediate zone. Type B spermatogonia differentiate into *primary spermatocytes*. These cells have rather long lives (approximately 16 days in the bull) and usually are easy to find and identify. Although their interphase nuclei contain a fine chromatin network, they are often observed in the first division of meiosis. They also have a long premeiotic prophase. Therefore, the nucleus may be coarsely granulated or chromosomes may be visible.

The end of the first division of meiosis marks the differentiation of the *secondary spermatocytes*. These cells are haploid (1N number of chromosomes). These cells are smaller than primary spermatocytes and are difficult to find, because they enter the second meiotic division almost immediately and form *spermatids*. Their life-span varies from minutes to one hour. Throughout these divisions, cytokinesis is incomplete and the cells are joined by numerous intercellular bridges.

Spermiogenesis. The *spermatids* that result from the division of the secondary spermatocytes are haploid (1N number of chromosomes). These cells, spermatids, comprise the most developed, most numer-

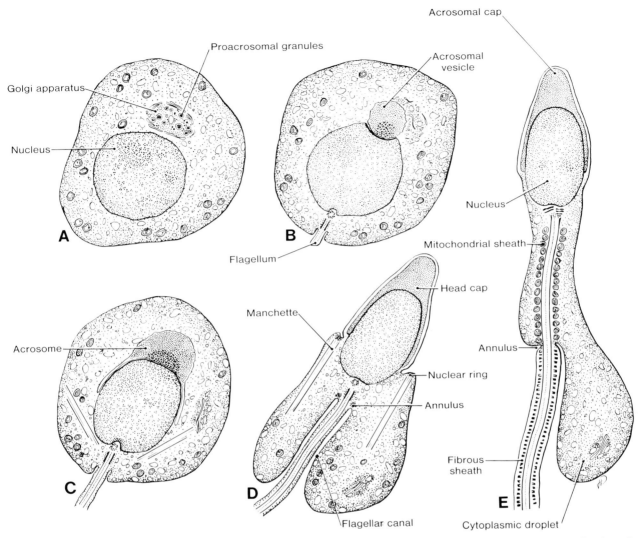

Figure 26.17. A diagram of the successive stages in the differentiation of a spermatid during spermiogenesis. (Redrawn and modified from Clermont, Y. and Leblond, C. P.: Amer. J. Anal. *96:229*, 1955).

ous, and largest layer of the seminiferous tubular epithelium. The luminal zone in which they are located is referred to as the *zone of metamorphosis*. The process by which spermatids are converted to spermatozoa is referred to as *metamorphosis* or *spermiogenesis*. As spermatogenesis ensues, the spermatids move in a centrifugal direction (toward the basement membrane) then in a centripetal direction toward the lumen. The primary organelles involved in the spermiogenic process are the nucleus, Golgi apparatus, and centrioles (Fig. 26.17).

Small granules *(proacrosomal granules)* appear in the vesicles of the Golgi apparatus. These small vesicles coalesce to form a single large *acrosomal vesicle* that contains the *acrosome*. The acrosome results from a coalescence of proacrosomal vesicles. The acrosomal vesicle migrates to the nucleus and contacts the outer nuclear membrane at the acrosome.

The acrosomal vesicle enlarges and extends itself over half the nucleus and collapses to form the *head cap*. At the same time, the centrioles migrate to the periphery of the cell in a position opposite the acrosome. Residual Golgi apparatus also migrates to this general region.

The acrosome becomes indistinguishable from the head cap. The nucleus becomes dense and begins to elongate. At this time the centrioles and developing *flagellum* migrate toward and come in contact with the nuclear membrane. A *caudal sheath* or *manchette* develops at the caudal edge of the head cap. This sheath is composed of microtubules. At the same time, the spermatid elongates.

A small dense ring condenses around the proximal centriole. This *anulus* is attached to the inner lamina of the plasmalemma. It slides down the flagellum. At the same time, the mitochondria orient themselves

in a helical pattern between the proximal centriole and the anulus. Nine longitudinal fibers develop in a position between the flagellar doublets and the mitochondria. This structure comprises the *middle piece*.

The *principal piece* is composed of a flagellar core, dense fibers, and a fibrous sheath.

The irregularly arranged flagellar microtubules comprise the *end-piece*.

As the formation of these entities occurs, the remaining cytoplasm is displaced distad along the tail and eventually lost as the *residual body*.

The mature spermatozoon, therefore, consists of the following: *head, neck, middle piece, principal piece*, and *end-piece* (Fig. 26.18). The *head* is covered by the head cap on the rostral and lateral surfaces and the calyx on the lateral and caudal surfaces. The *neck* has a depression (fossa) in which the centriole is located. Longitu-

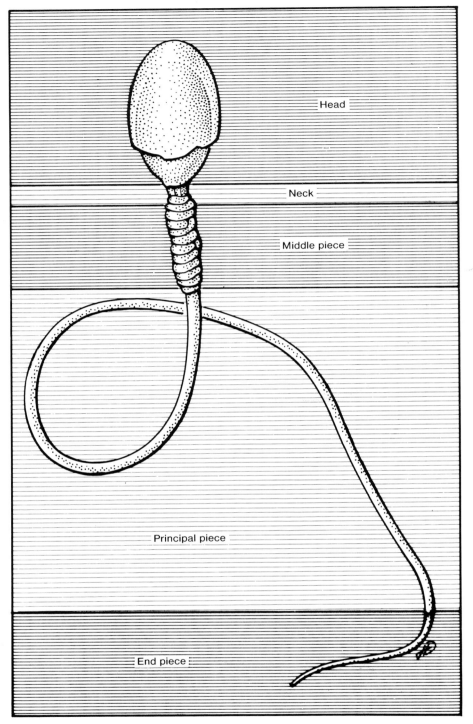

Figure 26.18.   A drawing of a typical spermatozoon.

gions of the same tubule are in the same stage of development (Fig. 26.19). The activity is cyclic, may occur in a helical pattern within a seminiferous tubule, and is referred to as a *spermatogenic wave*. Various combinations of cells are always associated with each other during the developmental process. In the bull, for example, eight stages have been identified. Stage 1, from basal to luminal border would include the following: *spermatogonia, pachytene primary spermatocytes,* and *round spermatids*. Stage 8, however, would include: *spermatogonia, zygotene primary spermatocytes, secondary spermatocytes, round spermatids,* and *spermatozoa*. The six remaining stages involve other permutations of the basic cell types. Various stages, the number of stages, as well as the overall duration of the stages are species variable. The *spermatogenic wave* or *cycle*, therefore, is the sequence of cellular events that occurs between two successive identical stages (Fig. 26.20).

In some species, from a spermatogenic point of view, the male is always capable of spermiation; i.e., the ejection of viable sperm from the testes. In seasonal breeders, the epithelium of the seminiferous tubules is incapable of producing spermatozoa except during specific periods of the year, the breeding season (Fig. 26.4). Examination of tubuli contorti during the nonbreeding season would reveal the presence of scattered spermatogonia and Sertoli cells. Few other cells would be present. Also, the tubules would be involuted and replaced by connective tissue.

Testicular Secretions

The testes are responsible for the production of gametes and the elaboration of steroid hormones. Both are secretory functions; gamete secretion is a holocrine-type secretory activity, whereas steroid hormone secretion is an endocrine function. The seminiferous tubules produce the gametes and the interstitial cells of Leydig are responsible primarily for steroid hormone synthesis and secretion. Spermatogenesis and testicular steroidogenesis are integrated and associated activities. Regulation of testicular function is achieved through the hypothalamopituitary-gonadal axis. The axis is separated into a hypothalamo-interstitial cell axis and a hypothalamo-tubuli contorti axis for convenience. The functions of both axes are related intimately.

Hypothalamo-Interstitial Cell Axis. The hypothalamus is the first regulator of the axis by virtue of its synthesis and secretion of gonadotropin releasing factors—*luteotropin releasing factor (LRF)* and *follicle-stimulating hormone releasing factor (FRF)*. The secretion of LRF and FRF from the hypothalamus is subject to modulation by external influences. The effects

dinally segmented columns connect the head to the tail. The *middle piece* consists of a flagellar core in a 9 + 2 arrangement, fibers that are continuous with those of the neck, a helical arrangement of mitochondria, and an anulus that is attached to the plasmalemma. The *principal piece* contains a flagellar core in a 9 + 2 arrangement,

fibers of various sizes that end in this segment and a fibrous sheath. The *end-piece* consists of a flagellar 9 + 2 core that terminates in a random fashion. Naturally, the entire spermatozoon is enclosed with a plasmalemma.

Spermatogenic Cycle. As mentioned previously, not all seminiferous tubules or re-

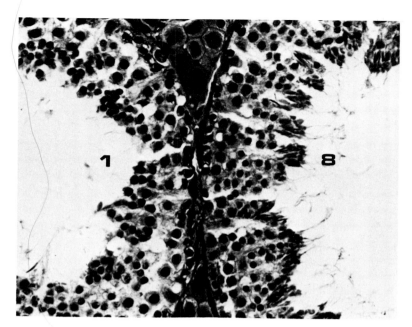

Figure 26.19. Different developmental stages in adjacent seminiferous tubules. Stages *1* and *8* represent different degrees of development of spermatozoa. ×100.

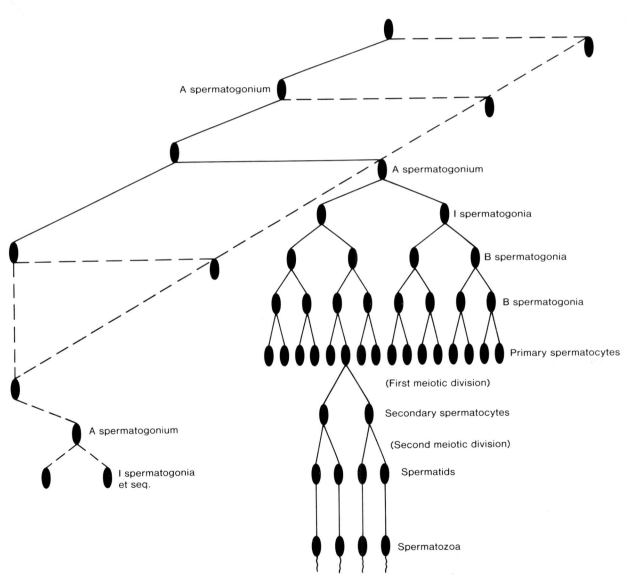

Figure 26.20. A diagram of the sequential and repetitive stages of spermatogensis.

of temperature upon testicular activity may be directed upon the testes or mediated through the hypothalamus. Light is probably the most important influence upon the axis. The seasonal breeding activity of deer, animals that have a rutting season, is responsive to decreasing amounts of light in the photoperiod. Some domestic animals (goat) increase testicular activity with decreasing daylength, whereas others (horse) manifest increased activity with increasing daylength. The tonic activity of the hypothalamus also accounts for the maintenance of testicular activity. Additionally, hypothalamic secretory activity is subject to regultion by the negative feedback influence of testicular hormones.

The secretion of LRF and FRF initiates secretory activity by specific basophilic cells of the pars distalis and the release of *luteinizing hormone (LH)* and *follicle-stimulating hormone (FSH)*. Luteinizing hormone and *interstitial cell-stimulating hormone (ICSH)* are identical; the term LH is now used for both the male and female. LH is the tropic hormone that regulates the secretory activity of the Leydig cells. The function of FSH is discussed with the hypothalamo-tubuli contori axis. *Prolactin* also exerts an influence upon the male reproductive tract by potentiating the effect of LH upon the Leydig cells. Additionally, prolactin and testosterone increase the secretory activity of the prostate and vesicular glands. Cells responsive to androgens have membrane receptor sites for prolactin.

Testosterone, the steroid hormone of the Leydig cells, is synthesized from acetate or circulating cholesterol. Although other androgens occur in the male, testosterone is the most important of these hormones. Small amounts of testosterone occur free as active hormones within the blood; however, most of the hormone is bound to a *testosterone-estradiol-binding globulin (TeBG)*, a β-globulin distinct from that used for cortisol binding. Upon entry into a cell from the active pool within the blood, testosterone may be converted to a more active form (dihydrotestosterone) or inactivated to metabolites characterized as *17-ketosteroids*. The 17-ketosteroids are the primary excretory products of testosterone, although the liver participates in testosterone inactivation by converting the hormone to sulfates and glucuronides that are secreted in the bile. Other tissues inactivate testosterone by converting it to *estradiol*, a potent estrogen.

Actions of Testosterone. Although testosterone exerts a significant influence upon the gonads, accessory sex glands, and those organs responsible for secondary male sex characteristics, the hormone affects almost every cell in the body. During development, the elaboration of testosterone by the forming of testes within the genital ridge is responsible for the development of the external genitalia, accessory sex glands, and the descent of the testes into the scrotum. The external genitalia and accessory sex glands grow under the influence of this hormone. Secondary sex characteristics also develop in response to testosterone. The effects of testosterone upon the reproductive organs, accessory sex glands, and the organs responsible for secondary sex characteristics are the *androgenic effects* of the hormone. The effects upon somatic tissue generally are described as the *anabolic effects* of the hormone.

The anabolic properties of testosterone are expressed in many cells and tissues. Testosterone has a positive influence upon basal metabolic rate, electrolyte balance, red blood cell production, nitrogen retention, skeletal muscle mass, bone development and bone maintenance.

Hypothalamo-Tubuli Contorti Axis. The seminiferous tubules are subject to the regulatory activity of the hypothalamus and pars distalis. The secretion of LH and FSH by the pars distalis, controlled by the secretion of hypothalamic releasing factors, is essential for development of the tubuli contorti. Although FSH manifests a direct effect upon the seminiferous tubules, the effects of LH are manifested through testosterone. Testosterone and FSH stimulate the synthesis of ABP by the Sertoli cells. FSH initiates spermatogenic events, but testosterone is required for the maturation of the spermatozoa. The mechanisms that regulate the release of FSH need further clarification. Testosterone does not exert a negative feedback influence upon FSH secretion; however, experimental evidence indicates that steroid-free extracts of testicular tissue suppress FSH secretion. This extract contains the hormone *inhibin* that is secreted by the Sertoli cell. Inhibin has a negative feedback influence upon the pars distalis and FSH secretion.

Accessory Glands

Introduction. The accessory genital glands of the male include *ampullary glands, vesicular glands, prostate gland, bulbourethral glands*, and *urethral glands*. They elaborate serous and mucous secretory products that subserve various functions. Together these secretory products may serve to nourish the spermatozoa, activate the spermatozoa, clear the urethral tract before ejaculation, serve as a vehicle for the transport of the spermatozoa within the female tract, as well as plugging the female organs to help ensure fertilization.

All of the glands are generally described as branched tubular or branched, tubuloalveolar glands that are arranged into lobular units. Each lobular unit may drain into a dilated collecting sinus. These sinuses are not present in all the glands of all species, however. They are absent in equine vesicular glands and in porcine and ruminant pars disseminata prostatica. The glandular epithelium and that of the collecting sinus (when present) consist of a simple columnar lining that is continuous with the pseudostratified or transitional epithelium of the excretory ducts. The glands of a given species may be readily distinguished from one another, but extreme care must be taken when making interspecific comparisons. There is much variation among the domestic species.

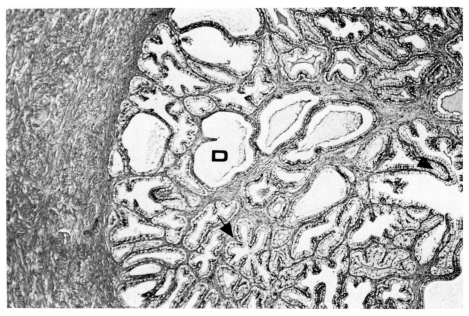

Figure 26.21. A section of a bovine ampullary gland. The glands are branched *(arrows)*, tubular glands that have sac-like dilations *(D)*. ×10.

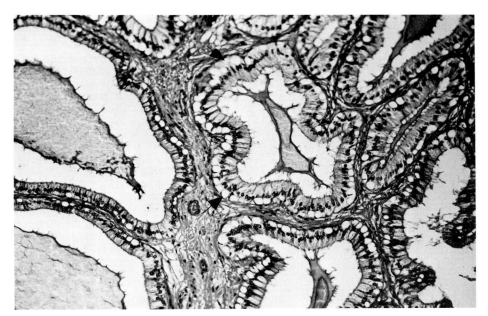

Figure 26.22. Lining cells of a bovine ampullary gland. Columnar epithelial cells contain basal lipid deposits *(arrows)*. ×40.

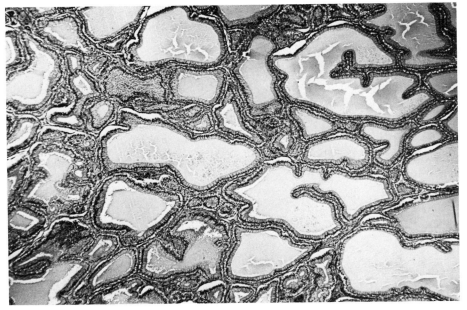

Figure 26.23. A section of bovine seminal vesicle. ×10.

Ampullary Glands. The *ampulla* is an enlargement of the terminal portion of the ductus deferens. The glands are branched, tubular structures with sac-like dilations (Fig. 26.21). Some authors describe them as branched, tubuloalveolar glands. These glands are lined by a simple columnar epithelium (Fig. 26.22). In bulls, basal accumulation of lipid droplets may be apparent. There is no special excretory duct system.

The ampulla, present in ruminants, horses, and dogs, contains typical glands in the lamina propria-submucosa. Glands are absent in the ampulla of cats, and they are not well developed in porcine ampullae.

The ampullary glands secrete a white serous fluid the precise function of which is unknown. The secretory product is similar to that of the vesicular gland. The large lumina and openings of the glands are capable of storing viable spermatozoa.

Vesicular Glands. The *vesicular glands* are also referred to as the *seminal vesicles* (Fig. 26.23). The glandular epithelium is simple columnar (Fig. 26.24). Infranuclear lipid droplets may be apparent in the bull.

The main excretory ducts are lined by a stratified columnar epithelium. The overall configuration of the gland is that of a pinnately arranged structure; i.e., a central duct is present from which radially branching secretory endpieces emanate. Lobular subdivisions are present.

The lamina propria-submucosa is typical. The tunica muscularis may consist of inner circular and outer longitudinal layers or may be entirely intermingled. A tunica adventitia or a tunica serosa are typical when present.

The vesicular glands are absent in carnivores. The glands of horses are true vesicular outpocketings, whereas those of ruminants and swine are compact glandular structures.

Seminal fluid, as well as the secretory products of other accessory sex glands, provide a vehicle for the transport of spermatozoa. The white, gelatinous secretory product aids in the formation of the vaginal plug in some rodents. The secretory product contains large quantities of fructose that is used as an energy source by ejaculated spermatozoa.

Prostate Gland. This organ consists of two parts, the *corpus prostatae* and *pars disseminata*. The gland is a compound, tubuloalveolar structure that is lined by secretory cells in a cuboidal or low columnar configuration (Figs. 26.25 and 26.26). Secretory cells have apical blebs that indicate an apocrine-type secretory activity. Acidophilic granules and lipid droplets may be present. The duct system, initially lined by a cuboidal or columnar epithelium, is lined by transitional epithelium at the entrance to the urethra.

The body of the gland is surrounded by a capsule of DWFCT that is continuous with the areolar connective tissue of the lamina propria-submucosa in which the adenomeres are located. The disseminate portion is surrounded by the areolar connective tissue of the lamina propria-submucosa.

The pars disseminata is best developed along the dorsal surface of the urethra and extends laterad and ventrad to encompass the urethra totally. The disseminate portion is continuous with both laterally oriented lobes of the body of the gland. Although the disseminate portion is usually confined to the pelvic urethra, it is not unusual to find isolated portions of the gland in the wall of the penile urethra.

The body and disseminate portions of the prostate gland are not developed equally in all domestic species. The body of the prostate, which is located peripheral to and surrounds part of the pelvic urethra, is well-developed in carnivores and horses. The disseminate portion is better developed than the body in bulls and boars. Rams do not have a distinct corpus prostatae.

The gland is basically a serous gland with

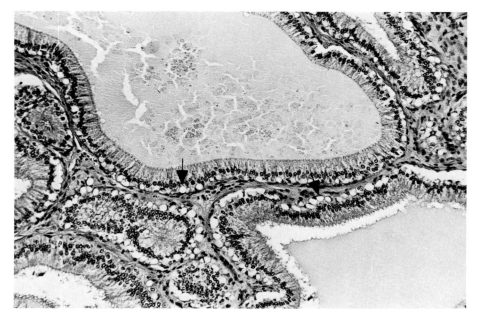

Figure 26.24. Lining cells of a bovine seminal vesicle. The columnar lining cells have infranuclear lipid deposits *(arrows)*. ×40.

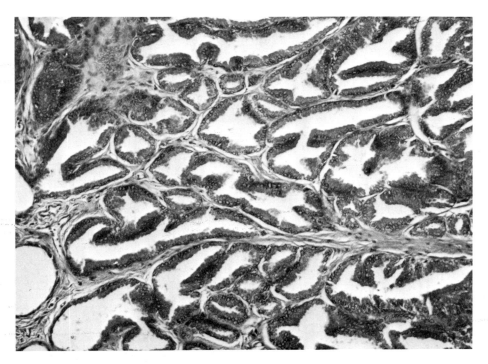

Figure 26.25. A section of a canine prostate gland. ×40.

occasional mucous end-pieces. It is, however, a seromucoid gland in bulls and a serous gland in dogs. Concretions of these secretory products may be present in the alveoli and duct system. Its secretory activity is known to increase the motility of spermatozoa, as well as contribute to the formation of the vaginal plug. In the bull, the secretory fluid contains high quantities of fructose and citric acid. Little else is

known of the functional significance of this secretory product.

Bulbourethral Glands. These glands are also referred to as *Cowper's glands*. These glands are paired structures that are located dorsolaterally to the pelvic urethra. The bulbourethral glands are compound, tubuloalveolar glands (Fig. 26.27). The lining cells of the adenomeres are columnar or pyramidal (Fig. 26.28). They have a baso-

philic cytoplasm and a basally displaced nucleus that is rounded or flattened. The duct system is lined by columnar, pseudostratified, or transitional epithelium.

The capsule of the organ is DWFCT that may contain some smooth muscle. Striated muscle from the bulbocavernosus and urethralis muscle is associated with the capsule. The capsular connective tissue is continuous as septal components (areolar connective tissue) of the lamina propria-submucosa. Diffuse and nodular lymphatic tissue is encountered commonly.

Bulbourethral glands occur in all domestic species except dogs.

The mucus secreted by these glands serves to clear the urethra of urine and to lubricate the urethra and vagina with a preejaculatory fluid. The mucus may serve as a source of energy for ejaculated spermatozoa.

Urethra

General Remarks. The male urethra is the continuation of the duct system that arises at the urinary bladder and opens to the outside. It serves the dual function of transporting urine as well as semen and spermatozoa. Secretory products involved in reproduction gain access to the pelvic urethra at the *colliculus seminalis*. It is in this region that the *deferent ducts, vesicular glands*, and some *prostatic ducts* gain access to the urethra. The urethra is divided into *pelvic* and *penile portions* that contain erectile tissue along the entire length. The urethra also contains branched, tubular, mucous glands, *glands of Littré* or *urethral glands*, along its length (horses, cats). The occurrence and distribution of these glands, however, is species-variable. They are obliquely oriented and are especially numerous along the dorsal surface of the urethra.

Pelvic Urethra. The pelvic urethra is lined by a transitional epithelium. The surrounding lamina propria-submucosa consists of areolar connective tissue, numerous glandular elements, and erectile tissue *(stratum cavernosum)*. A tunica muscularis with three muscle layers is present in the neck of the bladder, but these are replaced by a striated *urethral muscle*. An inner and outer layer (superficial and deep to the musculus urethralis), however, may be present throughout the extent of the pelvic urethra. A tunica adventitia is present. This portion of the urethra generally has more glands but less erectile tissue than the penile urethra.

Penile Urethra. The penile urethra is lined by a transitional epithelium (Fig. 26.29). Stratified cuboidal, stratified columnar, and simple columnar epithelium may be observed also. This epithelium changes to stratified squamous epithelium before or at the urethral opening. Glands

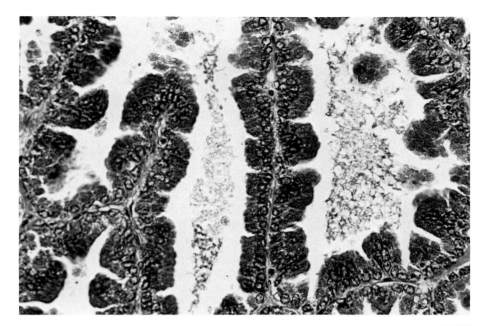

Figure 26.26. Columnar lining cells of a canine prostate gland. ×100.

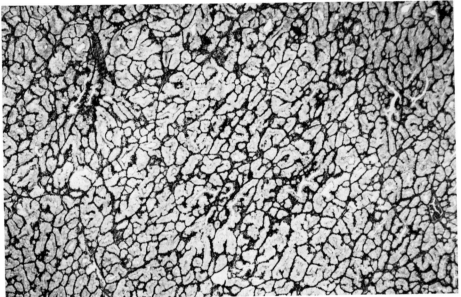

Figure 26.27. A section of a bovine bulbourethral gland. The compound, tubuloalveolar gland secretes mucus. ×10.

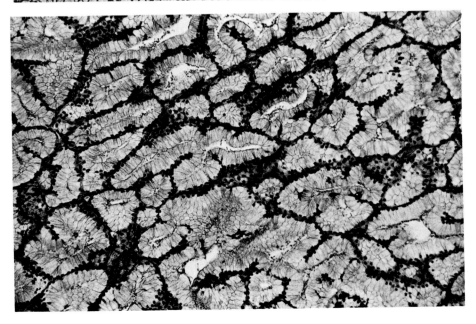

Figure 26.28. Lining cells of a bovine bulbourethral gland. The lining cells are columnar and basophilic. Nuclei are positioned basally. ×40.

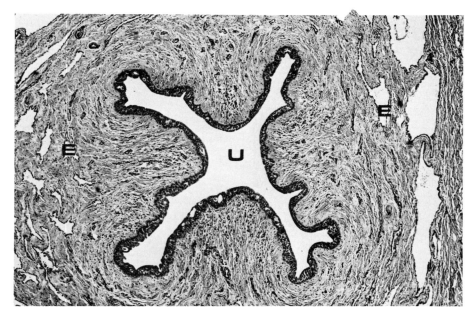

Figure 26.29. A cross section of a canine penile urethra. The urethra *(U)* is lined by transitional epithelium. Erectile tissue *(E)* is peripheral to the lumen of the urethra. ×16.

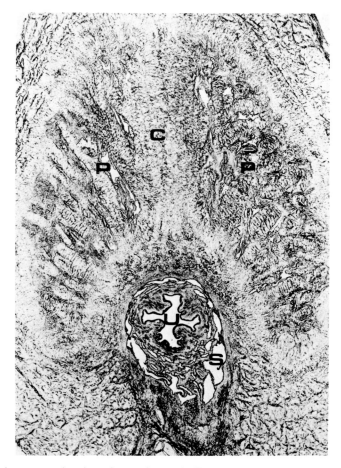

Figure 26.30. A cross section through a canine penis. The urethra *(U)* is surrounded by erectile tissue of the corpus spongiosum *(S)*. Dorsally, the two corpora cavernosa penis *(P)* are separated by connective tissue *(C)* that is continuous with the peripherally positioned tunica albuginea. ×4.

may be present in the lamina propria-submucosa, especially in the stallion and boar. The tunica muscularis returns to being composed of smooth muscle. Cavernous tissue *(corpus cavernosum urethrae)* is also present in the subepithelial connective tissue space.

Copulatory Organ

Penis. The penis is the organ that serves as the common outlet for urine and the copulatory ejaculate (semen and spermatozoa). It is, therefore, a part of the urinary system as well as serving as an intermittent copulatory organ.

Although the histological components of the penis are similar among most mammalian species, the organizational differences are too numerous to be able to cite a configuration as being absolutely typical. Moreover, a section from one part of the structure may differ appreciably from a section through a different part. This variability is due to the differential distribution of some component parts along the length of the organ.

The following description applies to the general configuration and component parts. The penis is divided into: *roots, body* and *glans.* The structure of each root and the body of the penis are similar. The body consists of a capsule, erectile tissue *(corpora cavernosa penis, corpus cavernosum urethrae,* or *corpus spongiosum)*, smooth muscle *(retractor penis muscle)*, skeletal muscle *(bulbocavernosus muscle)*, and urethra (Fig. 26.30).

The body of the penis is enclosed by the DWFCT of the tunica albuginea that is especially well-developed in those species with a fibrous-type penis (boar, ruminants). Connective tissue septa originate from the capsule and continue as the fibrous coverings of the erectile tissue components. These components may include elastic fibers and smooth muscle. Erectile tissue consists of DWFCT rich in elastic fibers and sinuses. These are capable of being engorged with blood during erection. In the vascular-type penis (horse, carnivores, man), this erectile tissue is well-developed.

The glans penis is well-developed in primates, horses, and dogs. It is covered by the penile portion of the prepuce, which is actually a reflection of the integument. The reflected portion is, therefore, a mucous membrane. The glans penis may contain erectile tissue (vascular penis), bone *(os penis* of carnivores), cartilage, and DWFCT (bulls). The bulk of this portion of the penis consists of highly vascularized areolar connective tissue. The free portion of the penis is covered by stratified squamous epithelium.

Erectile Mechanism. The primary blood supply of the penis, under erotic stimulation, is directed through *helicine arteries* that open into the cavernous tissue. These vessels, as well as the cavernous tissue, become engorged with blood. The peripherally located, thin-walled veins are occluded against the tunica albuginea. This further enhances rigidity. The cavernous tissue of the corpus spongiosum (corpus cavernosum urethrae) is not as thickly encapsulated as the other cavernous tissue. This permits expansion without occluding the urethra.

During the period of *detumescence*, the helicine arteries contract and regain their initial tone. The resulting diminution of blood supply results in a decreased pressure against the compressed veins. The blood is gradually removed from the erectile tissue and normal blood flow through the penis is resumed.

References

Testes and Associated

Amann, R. P.: A review of anatomy and physiology of the stallion. J. Equine Vet. Sci. May/June, p 83, 1981.

Amann, R. P., Johnson, L. and Pickett, B. W.: Connection between the seminiferous tubules and the efferent ducts in the stallion. Amer. J. Vet. Res. *38*:1571, 1977.

Bawa, S. R.: The fine structure of the Sertoli cell of the human testis. J. Ultrastruc. Res. *9*:459, 1963.

Belt, W. D. and Cavazos, L. F.: Fine structure of the interstitial cells of Leydig in the boar. Anat. Rec. *158*:333, 1967.

Christensen, A. K. and Fawcett, D. W.: The fine structure of the interstitial cells of the mouse testis. Amer. J. Anat. *118*:551, 1963.

Elftman, H.: Sertoli cells and testis structure. Amer. J. Anat. *113*:25, 1963.

Fawcett, D. W. and Burgos, M. H.: Studies on the fine structure of the mammalian testes. II. The human interstitial tissue. Amer. J. Anat. *107*:245, 1960.

French, F. S. and Ritzen, E. M.: A high affinity androgen binding protein (ABP) in rat testis: Evidence for secretion into efferent duct fluid and absorption by epididymis. Endocrinology *93*:88, 1973.

Krestser, D. M. D.: The fine structure of the testicular interstitial cells in men of normal androgenic status. Z. Zellforsch. *80*:594, 1967.

Ladman, A. J.: The fine structure of the ductuli efferentes of the opossum. Anat. Rec. *157*:559, 1967.

Nagano, T. and Suzuki, F.: Freeze-fracture observations on the intercellular junctions of Sertoli cells and of Leydig cells in the human testis. Cell Tiss. Res. *166*:37, 1976.

Roberts, S. J.: *Veterinary Obstetrics and Genital Diseases.* 2nd edition. Edwards Brothers, Ann Arbor, 1971.

Spermatogenesis

Amann, R. P.: Spermatogenesis in the stallion: A review. J. Equine Vet Sci. July/Aug, p 131, 1981.

Amann, R. P.: Endocrine changes associated with onset of spermatogenesis in Holstein bulls. J. Dairy Sci. *66*:2606, 1983.

Clermont, Y.: The cycle of the seminiferous epithelium in man. Amer. J. Anat. *112*:35, 1963.

Curtis, S. K. and Amman, R. P.: Testicular development and establishment of spermatogenesis in Holstein bulls. J. Anim. Sci. *53*:1645, 1981.

Fawcett, D. W. and Ito, S.: The fine structure of bat spermatozoa. Amer. J. Anat. *116*:567,1965.

Goldvieg, S. A. and Smith, A. U.: The fertility of male rats after moderate and after severe hypothermia. J. Endocr. *14*:40, 1956.

Heller, C. G. and Clermont, Y.: Kinetics of the germinal epithelium in man. Recent Progr. Hormone Res. *20*:545, 1964.

Kehlstrom, J. E.: A sex cycle in the male. Experientia *22*:630, 1966.

Rattner, J. B. and Brinkley, B. R.: Ultrastructure of spermiogenesis. J. Ultrastruct. Res. *32*:316, 1970.

Roosen-Runge, E. C.: The process of spermatogenesis in mammals. Biol. Rev. *37*:343, 1962.

Steinberger, E.: Hormonal control of mammalian spermatogenesis. Physiol. Rev. *5*:1, 1971.

Swiestra, E. E. and Foote, R. H.: Duration of spermatogenesis and spermatozoan transport in the rabbit based on cytological changes, DNA synthesis and labeling with triated thymidine. Amer. J. Anat. *116*:401, 1965.

Accessory Glands

Bharadwaj, M. and Calhoun, M. L.: Histology of the bulbourethral gland of the domestic animals. Anat. Rec. *142*:216, 1962.

Brandes, D.: The fine structure and histochemistry of prostatic glands in relation to sex hormones. Int. Rev. Cytol. *20*:207, 1966.

Fisher, E. R. and Jeffrey, W.: Ultrastructure of human normal and neoplastic prostate. Amer. J. Clin. Path. *44*:119, 1965.

Hirsch, E. W.: Comparative anatomy of prostate gland. J. Urol. *25*:669, 1931.

Kainer, R. A., Faulkner, L. C. and Abdel-Raouf, M.: Glands associated with the urethra of the bull. Amer. J. Vet. Res. *30*:963, 1969.

McDonald, L. E.: *Veterinary Endocrinology and Reproduction.* Lea and Febiger, Philadelphia, 1969.

Riva, A.: Fine structure of human seminal vesicle epithelium. J. Anat. *102*:71, 1967.

Young, W. C. (ed.): *Sex and Internal Secretions.* Williams & Wilkins, Baltimore, 1961.

Penis and Associated

Bharadwaj, M. and Calhoun, M. L.: The histology of the urethral epithelium of domestic animals. Amer. J. Vet. Res. *20*:841, 1959.

Bharadwaj, M. G. and Calhoun, M. L.: Mode of formation of the preputial cavity in domestic animals. Amer. J. Vet. Res. *22*:764, 1961.

Hart, B. J. and Kitchell, R. L.: External morphology of the erect glans penis of the dog. Anat. Rec. *152*:193, 1965.

27: Female Reproductive System

General Characteristics

Form and Function. The female reproductive system includes male counterparts, various organs that contribute directly to or complement the primary function of *reproduction*. Among the varied functions are *production* of ova, *transport* of male and female gametes for fertilization, *accommodation* and *nourishment* of the developing organism, *parturition* at the appropriate time, and *secretion* of hormones. Portions of the system also complement the function of the urinary system. The organs of the reproductive system include *ovary, oviduct, uterus, vagina*, and *vulva*. Although the mammary gland is included with the integument, this gland is also considered part of the reproductive system.

Cyclic activity is an integral part of female reproductive organs. These changes are more pronounced in the female than the male and have an effect on more organs than in the male.

Ovary

General Remarks. The ovaries are paired structures that are the female counterparts of the testes. The ovary performs an endocrine as well as an exocrine function. The former involves the production of estrogen and progesterone, whereas the latter is concerned with the production of *female gametes, ova*.

Histological Organization. The ovary is covered by a *surface epithelium* that is a modification of the visceral peritoneal covering of the ovary and is continuous with the *mesovarium* (Fig. 27.1). During early development of the ovary and oogenesis, the epithelium is cuboidal. It changes with age to a squamous lining. Underlying the surface epithelium is a capsule of dense white fibrous connective tissue (DWFCT) that may have a lamellar configuration—*tunica albuginea ovarii*. It is similar to but thinner than the male counterpart.

The ovaries of most animals, the mare excepted, consist of two distinct zones: *cortex* or *zona parenchymatosa* and *medulla* or *zona vasculosa* (Fig. 27.2). In the mare, the cortex and medulla are reversed. The cortex is confined to the deep zone of the ovary and only reaches the surface at the

ovulation fossa. The surface epithelial covering of the ovulation fossa continues over the rest of the ovary as a typical tunica serosa.

The cortex contains numerous *follicles* in various stages of development, *corpora lutea*, as well as interstitial cells and stromal elements. The cortical stromal connective

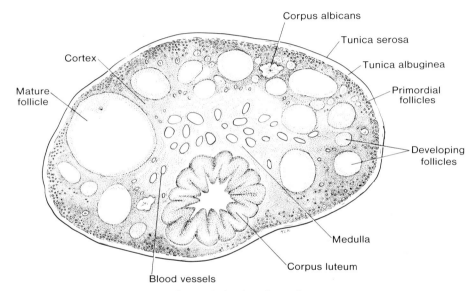

Figure 27.1. A drawing of a canine ovary.

Labels: Corpus albicans, Tunica serosa, Tunica albuginea, Primordial follicles, Developing follicles, Medulla, Corpus luteum, Blood vessels, Mature follicle, Cortex

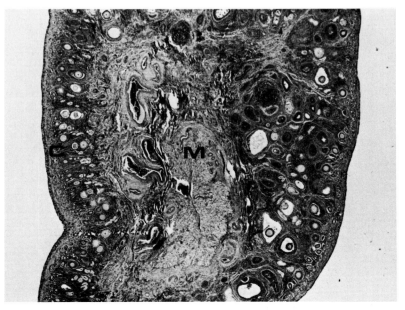

Figure 27.2. A section of a canine ovary. The ovary has a distinct cortex *(C)* and medulla *(M)*. ×4.

tissue must be considered a specialized tissue. Various cells typical of areolar connective tissue are present. However, this tissue is hyperplastic and dense aggregates of "fibroblasts" are present. They may be parallel to the surface or in an orderly arrangement around the follicles or vessels with which they are associated. The fibroblasts of this region are not ordinary fibroblasts. They are adaptive and pleomorphic. They even assume epithelioid characteristics as follicular theca and interstitial gland cells in association with follicles.

The *medulla* is characterized by large vessels, lymphatics, nerves, and some embryonic remnants. It is an areolar connective tissue rich in elastic and reticular fibers. The medullary constituents are continuous with the mesovarial attachment. The embryonic remnants are parts of the *rete ovarii*, the female homologue of the rete testis. They are short, solid cords of epithelial cells.

Vascular, Neural, and Lymphatic Relationships. The ovarian artery enters the organ at the hilus and is distributed to the medulla. Branches of the vessel continue to the corticomedullary junction and form an extensive plexus from which vessels that supply the cortex arise. The cortical vessels supply stromal elements, the thecae of developing and growing follicles, and corpora lutea. Capillaries form a complete spherical network around developing follicles. As corpora lutea develop, nascent branches from the peripherally positioned capillary bed form an extensive vascular network within the corpora lutea. Blood is shunted readily within the cortex. The venous drainage from the cortex is similar to the arterial supply. An extensive medullary venous plexus may form before the exit of the vessels at the hilus.

The cortex contains numerous lymphatic vessels that are associated intimately with the theca externa of developing follicles. The vessels coalesce, pass radially through the medulla, exit at the hilus, and drain through the lumbar lymph nodes.

The majority of the unmyelinated nerves of the ovary are vasomotor nerves; however, some sensory nerves have been observed. Whereas ganglion cells have been noted within the medulla of the organ, the precise relationships of the parasympathetic nervous sytem to the ovary are obscure.

Ovarian Cycle

Regulation. The ovary undergoes cyclic changes that are influenced by the effects of trophic hormones secreted by the pars distalis. Activity of the pars distalis, as in the male, is regulated by hypothalamic releasing factors—*luteinizing hormone releasing factor (LRF)* and *follicle-stimulating hormone releasing factor (FRF)*. Control of hypothalamic activity is subject to

regulatory influences similar to those manifested in the male. Optic and olfactory stimuli modulate activity within the *hypothalamo-ovarian axis*. Induced ovulators (cat, mink, lagomorphs) respond to the mechanical stimulation of coitus by ovulating approximately 24–48 hours postcoitus. Tonic secretory activity of the hypothalamus and negative feedback from ovarian hormones influence the cyclic reproductive activity of the female.

The release of FSH and LH from the pars distalis is the specific regulator of ovarian activity. FSH causes the growth and maturation of ovarian follicles as well as being responsible for the secretion of estrogens by these structures. Ovarian follicle rupture, ovulation, and the development of corpora lutea occur under the influence of LH. Some LH may be necessary for FSH to manifest its trophic influence upon the follicles. Prolactin manifests luteotrophic properties upon the ovary in rodents and sheep.

The combined influence of FSH and LH

(and prolactin in some species) regulates the cyclic activity of the ovary. The cyclic activities include *differentiation of ova, development of follicles, ovulation, formation of the corpus luteum, degeneration of follicles*, and *degeneration of the corpus luteum*.

Oogenesis. *Oogenesis* is the formation and development of the ova. The differentiation of ova occurs in two stages that are similar to the development of male gametes: *stage of mitosis* and *stage of meiosis*. During the stage of mitosis or multiplication, *oogonia* proliferate from *primordial germ cells* that had migrated to the germinal ridges from the yolk sac endoderm (Fig. 27.3). The oogonia divide and give rise to several generations of identical cells. In some species, the differentiation and multiplication of oogonia occur within the developing fetus long before parturition occurs (ruminants, rodents, swine, man). In others (carnivores, lagomorphs), the differentiation is prolonged into the immediate postnatal period. Oogonia, entering into the prophase of the first meiotic division,

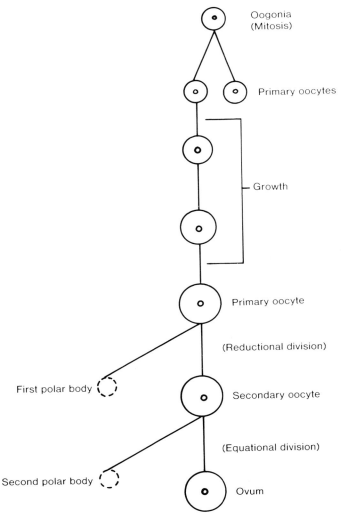

Oogonia (Mitosis)

Primary oocytes

Growth

Primary oocyte

(Reductional division)

First polar body

Secondary oocyte

(Equational division)

Second polar body

Ovum

Figure 27.3. A diagram showing the events of oogenesis. Compare this process to spermatogenesis in Figure 26.20.

become primary oocytes before or shortly after birth in most species. *Primary oocytes are arrested in prophase until sexual maturity is achieved.* Further development of primary oocytes is synchronized with the development and maturation of follicles. The *first meiotic division (reductional division)*, with the consequent conversion of a primary oocyte to a *secondary oocyte*, occurs just before ovulation in most species and is accompanied by the formation and expulsion of the *first polar body*. In the horse and dog, secondary oocyte formation occurs postovulation and may be delayed for 48 hours in the canid. In most species, other than the horse and dog, the *second meiotic division (equational division)* is accomplished when a spermatazoon penetrates the zona pellucida and "activates" the secondary oocyte. The *second polar body* is extruded at this time.

Follicular Development. An *ovarian follicle* is a spherical aggregation of cells that contains the developing gamete. The growth and development of follicles is accompanied by changes in the associated gametes. The cyclic continuum of follicular development is characterized by the identification of specific follicles—*primordial follicle, primary follicle, secondary follicle, mature follicle* (Fig. 27.4). Follicular growth and maturation occur under the influence of gonadotropins from the pars distalis (Plates I.6 and I.7).

Concomitant with the differentiation of primary oocytes, a single layer of flattened mesodermal cells, *follicular cells*, becomes associated with and surrounds the primary oocyte. At this stage, the complex is referred to as a primordial follicle. A *primordial follicle*, therefore, contains a *primary oocyte*. These are also referred to as *quiescent follicles* (Fig. 27.5). They occur singly or in clusters in the periphery of the cortex.

The activation of the primordial follicle results in a *primary follicle* (Fig. 27.5). This activation involves alterations in the primary oocyte, follicular cells, and other stromal elements. An accumulation of yolk granules is noted within the primary oocyte. The follicular cells become cuboidal or columnar. **The primary follicle still contains a primary oocyte.**

The *secondary follicle* is identified by an increase in the follicular cell population associated with the primary oocyte and the development of a zona pellucida between the primary oocyte and follicular cells (Figs. 27.6 and 27.7). The follicular cells are active mitotically and are now referred to as the *membrana granulosa*. They are separated from the primary oocyte by a periodic acid-Schiff (PAS)-positive, amorphous material, the *zona pellucida*. This is actually a very thick basement membrane. Stromal cells differentiate into two layers: *theca folliculi interna* and *theca folliculi externa*. The thecal cells are separated from the

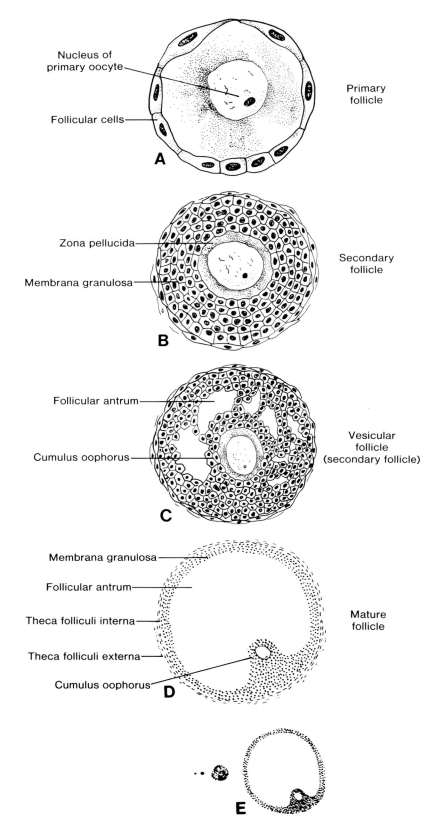

Figure 27.4. A diagram of the stages of folliculogenesis from primary to mature follicle formation. Drawings *A, B, C* and *D* are not drawn to scale. The approximate scale is indicated in *E*.

membrana granulosa cells by a basement membrane. The theca folliculi interna consists of large, epithelioid cells and an exten-

sive vascular network. The theca folliculi externa is a fibroblastic layer of cells. The growth of the follicle and the development

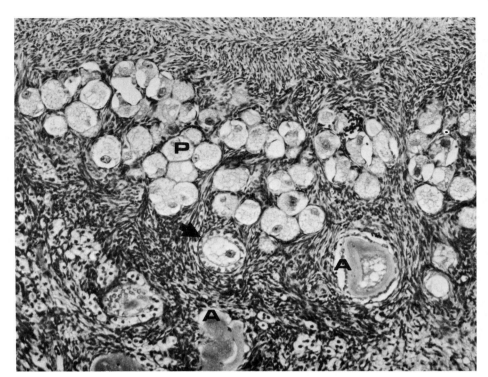

Figure 27.5. Immature follicles of a feline ovary. Primordial *(P)* and primary follicles *(solid arrow)* are present. Atretic follicles *(A)* are apparent also. Note the high cellularity of the interstitial connective tissue. ×40.

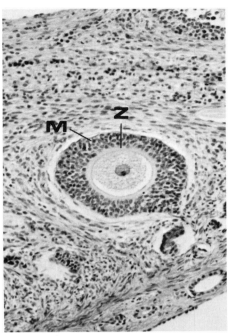

Figure 27.6. A small secondary follicle from a canine ovary. The follicular cells have proliferated and are called the membrana granulosa *(M)* at this stage of development. A zona pellucida *(Z)* separates them from the primary oocyte. The development of a thecal cone is apparent in the 4 o'clock position of the follicle. ×40.

of multilaminar thecal investments is accompanied by the secondary follicle moving away from the cortical surface. Part of the sheath of thecal cells is directed toward the surface as a *thecal cone*. The cone appears to displace superficially positioned follicles away from the deeply positioned, expanding follicle.

The development of a *tertiary follicle (vesicular follicle)* results from the secretory activity of the granulosa cells (Fig. 27.8). Small, fluid filled, PAS-positive spaces between granulosal cells, *Call-Exner bodies*, are apparent during antral development. These small lakes or intercellular clefts filled with *liquor folliculi* become confluent and form the *follicular antrum*. The Call-Exner bodies are believed to be the precursors of liquor folliculi. This is accompanied by the continued growth of the follicle. The primary oocyte is still surrounded, however, by a cluster of granulosa cells that is continuous with the peripherally displaced membrana granulosa. The mound of cells is referred to as the *cumulus oophorus*. Granulosa cells of the cumulus oophorus immediately adjacent to the primary oocyte become columnar cells that are oriented radially as the *corona radiata*. These cells have cytoplasmic processes that penetrate the zona pellucida and contact microvilli from the ovum. The cells of the corona radiate probably provide nutritional support for the oocyte. The cells of the cumulus oophorus constitute a visceral

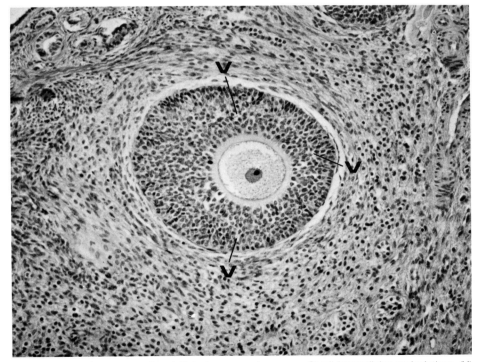

Figure 27.7. A large secondary follicle from a canine ovary. Small intercellular vesiculations *(V)* have begun to form. They will coalesce to form the antrum. ×40.

layer of granulosal cells separated by the follicular antrum from the parietal layer of granulosal cells. The parietal layer forms a multilayered aggregation of polyhedral cells called the *stratum granulosum*. The basal layer of this stratum resides upon a base-

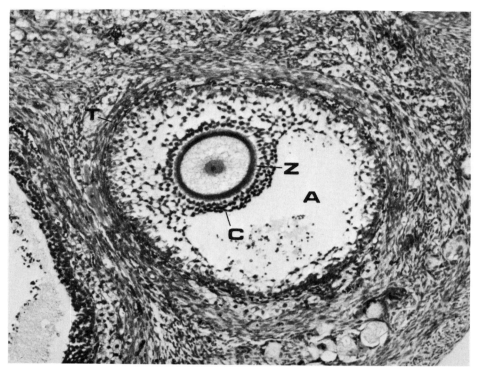

Figure 27.8. A vesicular follicle from a feline ovary. The follicular antrum *(A)* has formed. *C,* cumulus oophorus; *Z,* zona pellucida; *T,* thecal cells. ×40. (Lendrum's phloxine-tartrazine stain).

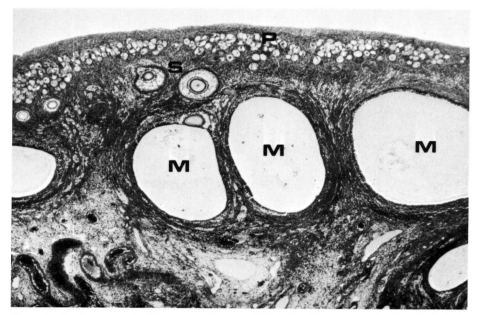

Figure 27.9. A section of a feline ovary. *P,* primordial follicles; *S,* secondary follicles; *M,* maturing vesicular follicles. Note the size difference. ×10. (Lendrum's phloxine-tartrazine).

ment membrane that separates these cells from those of the theca folliculi interna. **Despite the developmental changes associated with the granulosal and thecal cells, a vesicular follicle still contains a primary oocyte.**

Preovulatory follicles are also called *mature follicles or Graafian follicles*. They are greatly enlarged structures (Fig. 27.9). They extend from a protrusion at the surface to the depths of the cortex. The antrum is large and its attenuated wall still consists of the previously mentioned cellular and intercellular components.

Ovulation. *Ovulation* is the rupture of the follicle and the release of the oocyte.

The precise mechanism of ovulation has not been determined. Deterioration of the follicular wall through the enzymatic hydrolysis of connective tissue components by LH-induced *collagenase, protease,* or *plasmins* may be contributory. An increased intrafollicular fluid pressure is not associated with the ovulatory process. The thecal investments of the follicle and the cortical components (tunica albuginea) become thin and the follicle protrudes from the surface of the ovary. The protrusion, *follicular stigma,* is the site of rupture. The liquor folliculi released upon ovulation probably assists in the transport of the oocyte from the ovarian surface to the infundibulum.

The oocyte upon ovulation is surrounded by the zona pellucida and the *corona radiata.* The corona radiata is several layers of cells intimately associated with the oocyte that comprised the innermost zones of the cumulus oophorus. The oocyte and its associated cells may provide a sufficient mass that can be picked up by the fimbria. The corona radiata, however, is lost at the time of ovulation in the cow. In other species, the corona radiata remains intact until spermatozoa are present.

Follicular Atresia. Not all of the developing follicles terminate in ovulation. Many follicles undergo *follicular atresia* (degeneration). The degeneration of follicles may occur at any point in their developmental sequence (Fig. 27.10). During the primordial follicular stage, the dissolution of the ovum and granulosa cells is not characterized by remaining scar tissue. It simply disintegrates. Polyoocytic follicles are common and are destined to become atretic.

Follicular atresia during advanced stages of follicular development results in degeneration that is followed by the formation of a scar, the *corpus atreticum.* The degenerative process includes the oocyte and associated cells. The oocyte liquefies, the zona pellucida becomes thickened and folded, and the associated cells degenerate. The walls of the follicle collapse. This is accompanied by a connective tissue, phagocyte and vascular invasion of the follicle. The basement membrane between the granulosal and thecal cells thickens and the cells of the theca folliculi interna may hypertrophy and undergo changes similar to their conversion to theca lutein cells. (See Corpus Luteum.) The hypertrophic follicular cells are arranged as cords around the degenerating central components. Phagocytic activity from associated macrophages and fibrotic activity from fibroblasts complete the transition to a corpus atreticum.

Interstitial Gland. The *interstitial gland* of the ovary consists of polyhedral, epithelioid cells within the ovarian stroma that have the characteristics of steroid-producing cells. They are similar to the theca lutein cells of the corpus luteum. The origin

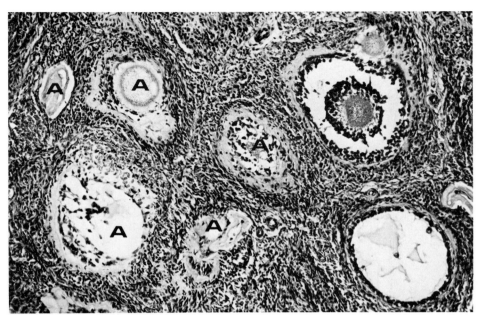

Figure 27.10. Atretic follicles from a canine ovary. Not all follicles reach maturity. Many undergo atresia *(A)*. ×40.

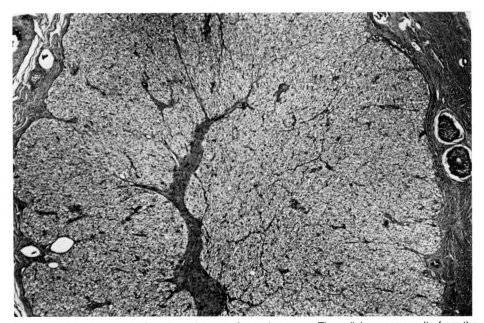

Figure 27.11. A section of a corpus luteum of a canine ovary. The cellular mass results from the transformation of membrana granulosa and theca interna cells. ×10.

of the interstitial gland cells is believed to be the theca folliculi interna cells from atretic follicles. The presence of these glandular structures in prepuberal animals supports this belief.

These glands may supply the estrogens necessary for the development of secondary sex characteristics in prepuberal animals. After puberty, the differentiation of interstitial glands is linked to the ovarian cycle and the cyclic atresia of follicles associated therewith. These cells may be a source of estrogens during the postovulatory period of the ovarian cycle. The complete function of these glands requires further clarification.

Cells located at the hilus of the ovary, *hilus cells*, have features that are similar to the interstitial cells of the testes. Tumors or hyperplasia of these cells results in masculinization in women.

Corpus Luteum. After the rupture of the ovarian wall and associated mural elements of the follicle, the ovum is ejected and passes into the oviduct. The remaining portions of the follicle do not degenerate but undergo pronounced changes that lead to the formation of the *corpus luteum* (Fig. 27.11).

The follicular walls collapse upon themselves and the granulosa cells protrude into the residual lumen. The hemorrhage that accompanies ovulation eventually clots and the resulting transitory structure is referred to as a *corpus hemorrhagicum*. The granulosa cells proliferate, hypertrophy, and are transformed into *granulosa lutein cells* (Fig. 27.12). In the mare, cow, bitch, queen and woman, the accumulation of a yellow lipid pigment *(lutein)* and other lipids marks the transition to granulosa lutein cells. Although lutein does not accumulate in the ewe and sow, the accumulation of other lipids marks the transition from membrana granulosa cells to granulosa lutein cells.

The invasion of this region by stromal cells and vasculature removes the clot, results in reticular fiber deposition, and converts this region into a highly vascularized gland.

The cells of the theca folliculi interna are also converted to lipid-producing cells, the *theca lutein cells*. These cells are smaller than the granulosa lutein cells and are dispersed peripherally or as septal-like clusters intimately associated with the other cell type that is predominant. In some species (ox), the two types of lutein cells cannot be distinguished easily. The process by which granulosa and theca cells are converted to luteal cells is called *luteinization*. Hypertrophy, hyperplasia, and the accumulation of pigment are essential factors in the process.

Whether lutein is present or absent, the resulting structure is referred to as the *corpus luteum (yellow body)*. The fate of the corpus luteum is dependent upon the reproductive success or failure of the individual. If fertilization does not occur, the *corpus luteum cyclicum* slowly degenerates *(corpus luteum regressum)* and is replaced by connective tissue. The corpus luteum, therefore, is converted to a *corpus albicans*.

If fertilization does occur, the *corpus luteum graviditatis* is persistent and active for a variable amount of time throughout the pregnancy. Retrogressive changes similar to the aforementioned characterize the degeneration of this structure. In some species, the corpus luteum graviditatis is required throughout the entire pregnancy. In others, it may be removed at various time periods without any detrimental effects upon the gravid uterus.

Ovarian Hormones. The production of ova by the ovary is complemented by its functions as an endocrine organ. The ovarian hormones are *estrogens* and *progesterone*. The ovary performs its endocrine functions under the influence of the adenohypophyseal hormones FSH and LH.

Under the influence of LH, the theca interna cells produce two androgens, *androstenedione* and *testosterone*. Under the

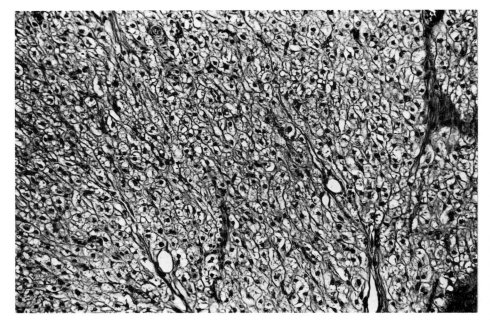

Figure 27.12.   Cells of the corpus luteum. The large, clear cells are granulosa lutein cells. ×40.

influence of FSH, the membrana granulosa cells produce estrogens, primarily *estradiol-17β*. The thecal androgens reach the granulosal cells wherein aromatizing enzymes convert the androgens to estrogens. The estrogens reach the developing antrum and induce the proliferation of more granulosal cells and the growth of the follicle. The interstitial gland is a source of estrogens also.

Additionally, the granulosa cells produce a protein hormone, *folliculostatin*, that has a negative feedback influence upon FSH production.

Progesterone is produced primarily by the granulosa lutein cells of the corpus luteum. The corpus luteum also produces a polypeptide hormone *relaxin* that functions to relax the ligaments associated with the pubic symphysis before parturition.

The steroidal hormones, responding to the influence of the gonadotropins upon the ovary, are synthesized, released and exert a negative feedback influence upon the hypothalamus and pars distalis. Estrogens are responsible for the receptive behavior of the female during estrus. The development of female secondary sex characteristics is due partially to estrogens. Mammary gland development is influenced by this hormone also. The normal development and function of the female reproductive tract are dependent upon estrogens. Estrogens also potentiate the effects of oxytocin and prostaglandins upon uterine smooth muscle contraction. Estrogens influence various functions of the body beside those associated with reproduction—skeletal growth, bone maintenance, sebaceous gland activity, electrolyte balance, calcium and phosphate retention,

and fat deposition. Estrogens are anabolic steroids.

Progesterone is the primary ovarian hormone of the luteal stage of ovarian activity. The main source of the hormone is the corpus luteum. Progesterone assists estrogens in eliciting the characteristic sexual behavior associated with estrus. The hormone inhibits uterine smooth muscular contraction while promoting uterine gland development; progesterone is required for maintenance of pregnancy. The hormone

exerts a negative feedback influence on the hypothalamus and pars distalis. Progesterone also enhances the development of the secretory and excretory portions of the mammary gland. Additionally, progesterone exerts a minor catabolic influence upon somatic proteins and may influence electrolyte balance.

Uterine Tubes

General Remarks. The uterine tubes are extensions of the uterus that serve for the transport of the male and female gametes. Fertilization occurs within the oviducts. This structure is subdivided into *infundibulum, ampulla,* and *isthmus.*

Histology of the Oviduct. The lamina epithelialis mucosae consists of intermittently ciliated columnar cells in most species (Fig. 27.13). In the sow and cow, however, it may be pseudostratified intermittently ciliated columnar epithelium. Kinocilia are especially prominent in the cranial portion of the oviduct wherein they assist in the movement of ova along the highly folded tunica mucosa (Fig. 27.14). Some of the lining cells are devoid of cilia. Ciliogenosis occurs in response to circulating levels of estrogen. The nonciliated, secretory cells become taller under the influence of progesterone and may nourish the ova as well as capacitate the spermatozoa for fertilization.

The lamina propria-submucosa consists of areolar connective tissue and is devoid of glands. The tunica mucosa of the ampulla is highly folded. Primary, secondary, and tertiary folds may be apparent in some species. The tunica muscularis is best de-

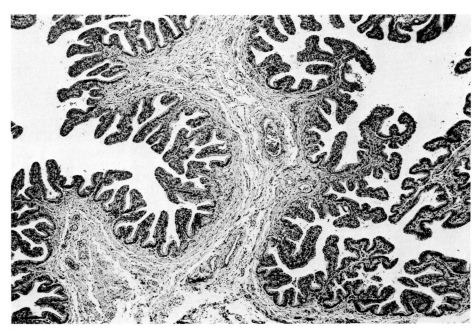

Figure 27.13.   A section of an equine oviduct. The lining consists of intermittently ciliated columnar epithelium. ×16.

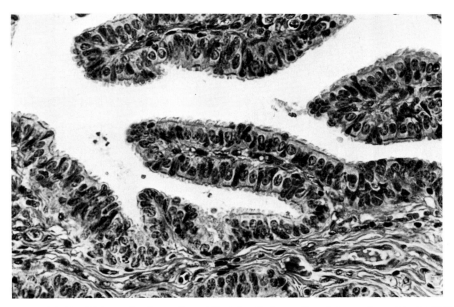

Figure 27.14. Lining cells of a section of the infundibular portion of the equine oviduct. ×100.

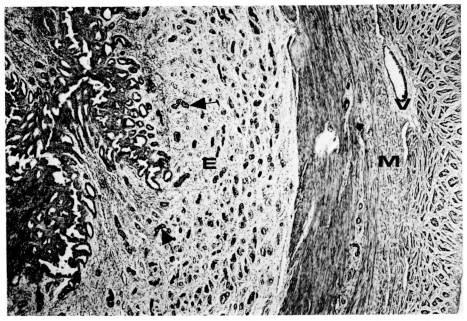

Figure 27.15. A section of a gravid canine uterus. The tubular glands *(arrows)* are branched and coiled. *E*, endometrium; *M*, myometrium; *V*, vessels of the stratum vasculare. ×40.

veloped in the isthmus. The smooth muscle is disposed in longitudinal and circular arrays. The tunica serosa is present and typical. Numerous blood vessels occur within the tunica serosa and form a distinct vascular layer.

Uterus

General Remarks. The *uterus* performs functions that are essential to reproduction. In the horse, semen is deposited in the uterus; in swine, semen is deposited in the cervix. In other species (ruminants, cat,

dog, lagomorphs, man), insemination is vaginal. Uterine contractions are essential for transport of the spermatozoa. Finally, the uterus is the site of development for the embryo and fetus. The uterus consists of a *body (corpus uteri), uterine horns (cornua uteri),* and *cervix (neck, cervix uteri).*

The form of the uterus is species-variable. Most domestic species have a *bicornuate uterus,* a uterus with a body and two prominent horns with a single cervix. Primates have a *simple uterus,* an organ with a prominent body, two small uterine horns, and a single cervix. Lagomorphs, mono-

tremes, and marsupials have a *duplex uterus.*

Capacitation, a process by which the spermatozoa achieve the ability to penetrate the corona radiata and zona pellucida to accomplish fertilization, occurs after exposure of the spermatozoa to the female reproductive tract. The uterus and oviducts play a role in the process. The need for capacitation has been determined in a few species but is suspected in others.

The wall of the uterus is divided into three distinct regions: *endometrium, myometrium,* and *perimetrium* (Figs. 27.15, 27.16, and 27.24). Although the terminology applied to the mural elements of this tubular visceral organ differs from that presented in Chapter 15, the mural elements and their organization is similar to those that occur in other tubular viscera. The morphology of the uterus changes in synchrony with the estrous cycle. A general description of the uterus follows; the changes associated with the estrous cycle are discussed subsequently.

Endometrium. The *endometrium* is the tunica mucosa (Fig. 27.16). The lamina epithelialis mucosae is simple columnar epithelium. Patches of pseudostratified columnar epithelium may be encountered in the sow and cow. Isolated foci of cuboidal epithelium may occur also. *Uterine glands* are simple or branched tubular glands (Fig. 27.17). Their distal ends have a variable degree of coiling that is species-dependent. The secretory products of the lining and glandular epithelia include mucus, lipids, glycogen, and proteins. These glands extend into the lamina propria-submucosa.

The lamina propria-submucosa is a hyperplastic, areolar connective tissue superficially that consists of numerous protective cells—mononucleated and polymorphonucleated cells. In ruminants, regions of the lamina propria-submucosa are highly vascularized and devoid of glands. These *caruncles* are devoid of uterine glands and are the eventual sites at which the maternal tissues make contact with the extraembryonic membranes (Fig. 27.18). The peripheral connective tissue of the lamina propria-submucosa is less cellular than that which is subepithelial. Many melanophores are present in the connective tissue of the caruncular regions of the ewe.

Myometrium. The *myometrium* is the tunica muscularis. This layer consists of a thick inner circular and thinner outer longitudinally oriented coat of smooth muscle that continues into the mesometrium (Fig. 27.15). A *stratum vasculare* occurs between the two layers of smooth muscle.

Perimetrium. The *perimetrium* or tunica serosa is typical, although a large number of lymphatic vessels may be present.

Cervix. The *cervix uteri* serves as a valve to close off the uterine lumen from the vagina. In the sow, the cervix is a thin-walled structure, whereas in the cow it is

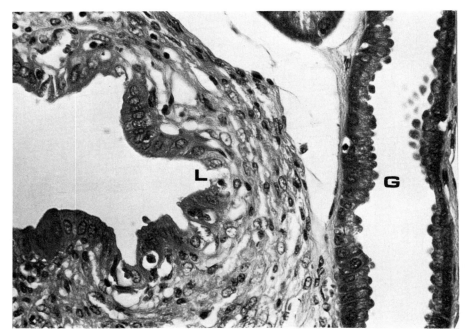

Figure 27.16. Lining and glandular cells of a bovine metestrous uterus. The lining cells *(L)* are columnar. The glandular cells *(G)* are columnar and have apical blebs. ×100.

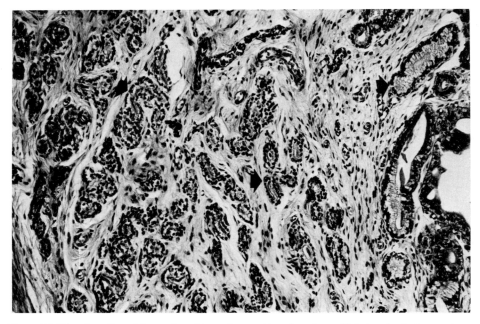

Figure 27.17. A section of the endometrium of a gravid canine uterus. Tubular glands *(arrows)* are branched and coiled. ×40.

extremely well-developed. The lining cells of the cervix of the cow are highly glandular. Their secretory activity varies with the stages of the estrous cycle and pregnancy. A clear mucus is secreted during estrus and a thick cervical seal is produced during pregnancy. Numerous longitudinal folds impart the impression that the cervix is glandular. The lamina epithelialis mucosae of the canine cervix, however, is lined by stratified squamous epithelium that is un-

derlaid by a glandless lamina propria-submucosa.

The lamina epithelialis mucosae of the cervical canal of the cow is composed primarily of goblet-like cells, but some kinociliated columnar cells may be present in some species. Also, some simple, tubular glands may occur in some species. The lamina propria-submucosa varies from loose connective tissue to DWFCT during various stages of the estrous cycle. The

tunica muscularis is well-developed and rich in elastic fibers.

Vagina

The lamina epithelialis mucosae is a stratified squamous lining that is usually nonglandular (Fig. 27.19). In the cow, isolated foci of goblet cells are present in the cranial portion of the organ. In the bitch, intraepithelial glands have been observed during estrus. The tunica mucosa and tunica submucosa are highly folded.

The underlying connective tissue of the lamina propria-submucosa is areolar or DWFCT and possesses scattered lymphatic nodules.

The tunica muscularis consists of two or three layers: an inner longitudinal (variable), middle circular, and an outer longitudinal. A tunica serosa is present cranially and is continued caudad as a tunica adventitia. Some smooth muscle *(muscularis serosae)*, as a continuation of that of the broad ligament, may also be observed in the subserosal space.

Vulva

The vulva consists of the *vestibule* and *labia*. The *clitoris* is part of the vestibule and the *urethra* opens into the vestibule.

Vestibule. The structure of the *vestibule* is similar to the caudal portion of the vagina. The lamina epithelialis mucosae is nonkeratinized stratified squamous epithelium with an extensive lymphocytic infiltration. The lamina propria-submucosa consists of loose and dense connective tissue that is rich in elastic fibers. *Vestibular glands* are present. *Major vestibular glands* (ewe, cow, queen) are compound, tubuloalveolar, mucous glands that are embedded within the constrictor vestibuli muscle. *Minor vestibular glands* are branched, tubular, mucous glands that are scattered throughout the vestibule in most domestic species. In the cow, they are concentrated near the clitoris. The major vestibular glands are homologues to the male bulbourethral glands, whereas the minor vestibular glands are homologous to the male urethral glands.

The tunica muscularis consists of an inner longitudinal and outer circular layer. The outer layer comprises two distinct muscles, *constrictor vestibuli* and *constrictor vulvae*. The tunica adventitia is typical.

Clitoris. The clitoris is homologous to the male penis. It consists of a body, glans, and preputial covering. The body contains cavernous tissue *(corpus cavernosa clitordis)*, adipose tissue, and smooth muscle that is surrounded by a sheath of DWFCT. The *glans clitoridis* may contain cavernous tissue (bitch, mare) or areolar connective tissue that is highly vascularized. The *preputial* covering is an aglandular and hairless

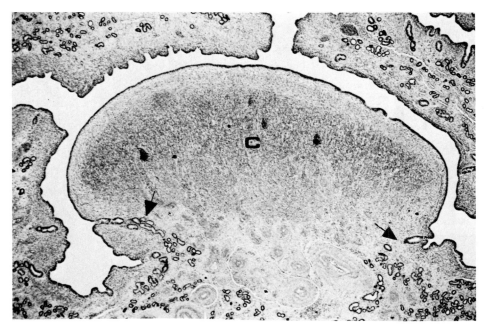

Figure 27.18. A section of a bovine caruncle. The caruncle (C) is devoid of uterine glands *(arrows)*. ×5.

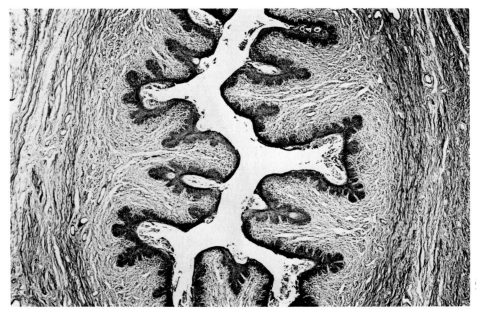

Figure 27.19. A section of a feline vagina. The tunica mucosa is highly folded and lined by stratified squamous epithelium. ×10.

reflection of the cutaneous mucous membrane of the vestibule that is rich in sensory nerve endings.

Urethra. The female *urethra* is lined by transitional epithelium that is continuous with the cutaneous mucous membrane of the vestibule. The change from transitional epithelium to stratified squamous epithelium occurs close to the external orifice. Before the transition, bistratified cuboidal or bistratifies columnar epithelia may be apparent. The lamina propria-submucosa varies from DWFCT to areolar connective tissue that contains cavernous sinuses. The distribution and extent of the cavernous tissue is subject to species variation. The tunica muscularis is composed of two or three layers of smooth muscle cranially. The fibers of smooth muscle become intermixed with skeletal muscle fibers caudally. The amount, distribution, and relative amounts of these tissues are subject to species variation.

Labia. The *labia* are folds of the integument that are comprised of typical integumentary structures.

Cyclic Changes

Introduction. The female reproductive tract is subject to greater periodic changes than that associated with the male. Moreover, female cyclic activity is manifested microscopically and grossly, as well as behaviorally. These various states of morphology, function, and behavior are related directly with the estrous cycle. The estrous cycle, or period of varying reproductive activity, is under the influence of the trophic hormones of the adenohypophysis. This cycle is subdivided into five distinct but continuous stages: *proestrus, estrus, metestrus, diestrus, and anestrus.*

Proestrus is that period of the cycle characterized by the acceleration of follicular growth under the influence of FSH. The follicle begins to secrete estrogen, which in turn influences the genital organs. The increasing levels of estrogen suppress the declining levels of progesterone. *Estrus* is marked by the genital organs being under the full influence of estrogen. This is the period of *heat* in which the female will accept the male. *Metestrus* is a transitional stage in which the declining levels of estro-

Table 27.1.
Characteristics of the Reproductive Cycles of Selected Domestic Animals*

Animal	Type of Cycle	Length of Cycle	Duration of Estrus	Time of Ovulation	Pregnancy Length
Cow	Polyestrus (nonseasonal)	21 days	16 hours	13 hours proestrus	285 days
Ewe	Polyestrus (seasonal)	17 days	1 day	End of estrus	145 days
Mare	Polyestrus (seasonal)	21 days	6 days	Day 5 of estrus	335 days
Sow	Polyestrus (nonseasonal)	21 days	2–3 days	Day 2 or 3 of estrus	113 days
Bitch	Monestrus	7–8 months	4–14 days	Day 2 or 3 of estrus	63 days
Queen	Polyestrus	15–21 days	10–14 days†	Induced	63 days

* The averages and ranges included are subject to individual and breed variation.
† If mating is achieved, then the duration is reduced to 4–6 days.

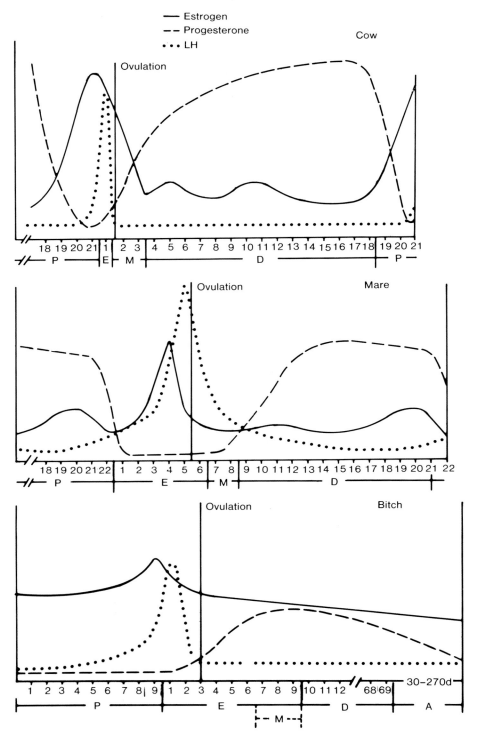

Figure 27.20. Diagrams of the comparative estrous cycles of the cow, mare, and bitch. A prolonged anestrus is an unique feature of the canine estrous cycle.

Animals are either *monestrous* or *polyestrous*. In monestrous species (dog), one estrous cycle (proestrus, estrus, metestrus, diestrus) is followed by a long period of anestrus. In polyestrous animals (cow, sow, rodents), one estrous cycle terminates in a period of diestrus that merges as the proestrus in the succeeding estrus cycle. In seasonally polyestrous animals (mare, queen, ewe), the terminal diestrus continues as a period of anestrus before the next estrous cycle. The anestrous period in these animals is appreciably shorter than that which occurs in monestrous animals.

Blood hormone levels vary throughout the length of the estrous cycle. The levels of hormones at various stages of the reproductive cycle are subject to species variation also. The hormone levels of the cow, mare, and bitch are compared non-parametrically in Figure 27.20. Cyclic changes in the ovaries, uterus, and vagina are synchronized with the cyclic secretion of gonadotropins and ovarian hormones.

Ovarian Changes. During *proestrus*, the ovaries are influenced by the gonadotrophin, FSH. This results in the rapid growth of the follicles and the initiation of estrogen secretory activity.

During *estrus*, the follicle (or follicles) reaches maturity and estrogen secretory activity is maximal. FSH secretion begins to drop, while LH secretion is initiated. This results in ovulation. Ovulation may be considered a transitory period between estrus and metestrus or part of the metestrous stage.

During *metestrus*, the development of the corpus luteum occurs and the secretion of progesterone is initiated.

The *diestrus* is characterized by a maximal development of the corpus luteum and a maximal productivity of progesterone. If pregnancy is not achieved, the latter part of diestrus is characterized by an involution of the corpus luteum and its degeneration into a corpus albicans. If pregnancy does occur, the corpus luteum continues its maximal secretory activity.

In *anestrus*, the ovary is relatively quiescent. The corpus luteum continues its involution and follicular development is arrested.

Uterine Changes. During *proestrus* the lining epithelium hypertrophies, while the uterine glands remain relatively straight (Fig. 27.21). There is an increasing vascularity and congestion in the connective tissue space, as well as occasional hemorrhage. Heterophils begin to invade the epithelial lining.

During *estrus* the epithelial and glandular proliferation is continued and is more apparent (Fig. 27.22). Secretory activity of the cells is marked, whereas agranulocytic infiltration of the epithelium continues. The connective tissue space is marked by maximal congestion, edema, and hemorrhage.

gen are counterbalanced by the increasing levels of progesterone. *Diestrus* is the period of the cycle that is under the sole influence of progesterone. Fertilization of the ova and subsequent pregnancy results in a prolonged diestrus. If fertilization is not accomplished, the *anestrus* period may follow. This is a period of variable length in which the reproductive organs are relatively quiescent.

Species Differences

The stages of the estrous cycle are of varying lengths in domestic species. Table 27.1 summarizes the characteristics of the estrous cycle of selected domestic animals.

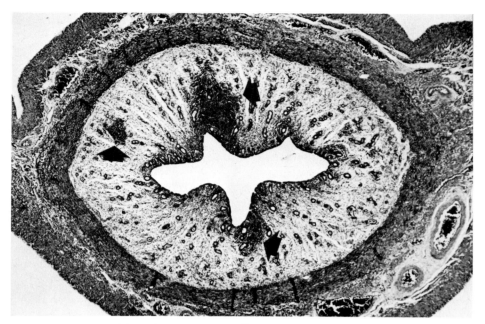

Figure 27.21. A cross section of a canine proestrous uterus. The uterine glands are straight and hemorrhage is apparent *(arrows)* in the lamina propria mucosae. ×10. (Note: the magnifications of Figures 24.19 and 24.21—24.24 are the same.)

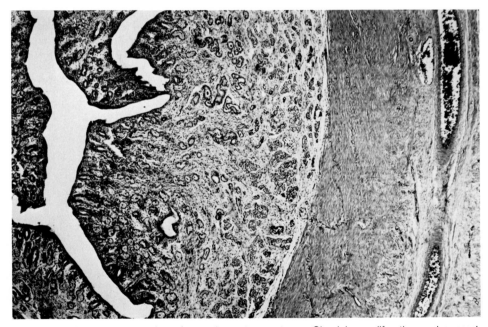

Figure 27.22. A cross section of a canine estrous uterus. Glandular proliferation and general enlargement of the uterus are apparent. ×10.

Metestrus is characterized by a continuation of glandular hyperplasia through which the coiling of glands is achieved (Fig. 27.23). The high secretory activity continues, whereas the edema of the connective tissue space declines or disappears.

In *diestrus* maximal glandular hyperplasia is achieved and the glands are coiled extensively. If fertilization occurs, maximal secretory activity is maintained. If fertilization does not occur, the vascularity de-creases, the secretory activity is arrested and the lining cells and glands involute.

During *anestrus* the endometrium is thin and lined by simple cuboidal epithelium (Fig. 27.24). Uterine glands are sparse, and they assume a simple or branched, tubular configuration.

Vaginal Changes. The vaginal changes associated with the estrous cycle are discussed in Chapter 29.

Menstrual Cycle Compared. The men-strual cycle of primates includes two phases: *follicular phase, luteal phase* (Fig. 27.25). The *follicular phase* is characterized by those events that occur in proestrus and estrus in other species. The phase is under the influence of FSH and estrogen. It is sometimes referred to as the proliferative phase. The *luteal phase* is also referred to as the *progestational* or *secretory phase.* The events are similar to those of metestrus and diestrus.

Changes associated with the endometrium are referred to as the *ischemic* or *premenstrual phase* and *menstrual phase.* Necrotic endometrial changes occur under the declining influence of progesterone and culminate with hemorrhage and the loss of part of the endometrium. Endometrial repair is achieved through proliferation of epithelium from the uterine glands and stromal elements of the lamina propria mucosa.

Comparative Placentology

Introduction. The female reproductive tract of mammals is designed to facilitate internal fertilization. Subsequent to that, the system permits the development of the fertilized egg within the uterus. Complex relationships are developed within the uterus between fetal and maternal tissues that ensure nutrition, respiration, removal of waste materials, and protection. Besides the important aforementioned functions, the placenta is also an endocrine organ that is responsible for the production of progesterone and relaxin. These functions are ensured by the formation of the *placenta,* a complex structure formed by the union of fetal membranes with the endometrium.

The endometrium was prepared for pregnancy during the metestral and diestral stages of the estrous cycle.

Not all mammals, however, are placental. Nor do all mammals bear live young. The classification of mammals is predicated upon the nature of fetal and maternal relationships. The *prototherian mammals* or *monotremes* include the platypus and echidna. These are egg-laying mammals. The *methatherian mammals* or *marsupials* include such animals as the kangaroo and opossum. These animals form a transitory "yolk sac placenta." There is no intimate contact between the fetal membranes and the uterine mucosa; they do not form a true placenta.

The remaining extant mammals comprise the *eutherian* subclass. These are the true *placental mammals.* The fetal membranes (chorion, amnion, yolk sac, and allantois) and the endometrium contribute to the formation of the placenta. This is accomplished individually or in specified combinations.

Classification. Various means have been devised to classify or characterize certain placental characteristics. These include the

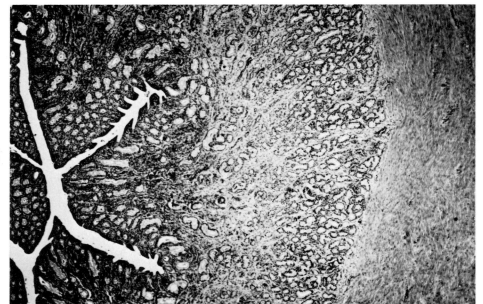

Figure 27.23. A cross section of a canine metestrous uterus. The uterine glands and uterus are larger than the estrous uterus. ×10.

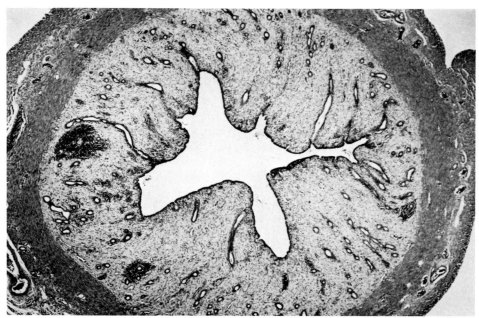

Figure 27.24. A cross section of a canine anestrous uterus. The uterine glands are reduced in number and the endometrium is reduced in size. ×10.

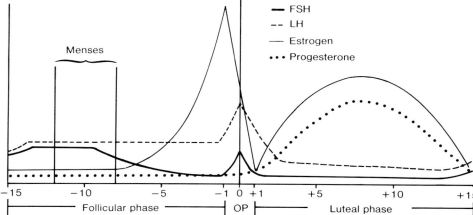

Figure 27.25. A diagram of the primate menstrual cycle. *OP*, short ovulatory phase between the two major phases of the menstrual cycle.

distribution of contact, the contributing extraembryonic membranes, the degree of implantation, the configuration of the chorionic attachment, and the combination of fetal and maternal tissues that comprise the placenta. These classifications are not mutually exclusive. Rather, they may be used in combination to describe the placenta of a particular species.

Distribution of Chorionic Villi

General Remarks. The chorion is in close contact with the uterine mucosa. Highly vascularized regions, *villi*, project from this extraembryonic membrane and form intimate contact with the endometrium. These projections may occur singly or in groups. The subsequent descriptions refer to the chorioallantoic type of placenta.

Diffuse Placentation. In the *diffuse placenta*, the chorionic villi are present over the entire surface of this membrane. The entire chorion, therefore, is attached to the endometrium. This type of placenta is typical of the mare and sow.

Cotyledonary Placentation. The *cotyledonary placenta* or *placenta multiplex* is a multiple structure. The villi are grouped as cotyledons, whereas the intercotyledonary space is smooth (devoid of villi). The cotyledons attach themselves to the *caruncles* of the endometrium. The *fetal cotyledon* and the *maternal caruncle* comprise the *placentome*. This type of placenta is typical of the cow, ewe, and doe.

Zonary Placentation. In the *zonary placenta* the villi are grouped in a region that circumscribes the midportion of the chorion. This type of placenta is characteristic of the dog and cat.

Discoidal Placentation. The *discoidal placenta* is characterized by villi being grouped in one or two disc-shaped regions. This placentation is characteristic of rodents and primates.

Extraembryonic Membrane Contributions

Chorionic Placenta. The *trophoblast* is the outer layer of the blastocyst. During *nidation*, this layer invades the uterine mucosa and serves as a nonvascularized point of attachment. This layer serves to nourish the blastocyst by obtaining nutrients from the uterus until the definitive placenta is formed.

Choriovitelline Placenta. There are two types of yolk sac placenta: *nonvascularized* and *vascularized*. In the *yolk sac, nonvascularized placenta*, the differentiated *yolk sac endoderm*, and the *trophoderm* (the trophoblast following the differentiation of the germ layers, chorion) fuse. These layers serve to transport nutrients to the embryo from the uterine mucosa.

In the *yolk sac, vascularized placenta*, the yolk sac endoderm, and trophoderm are separated by a layer of mesoderm that

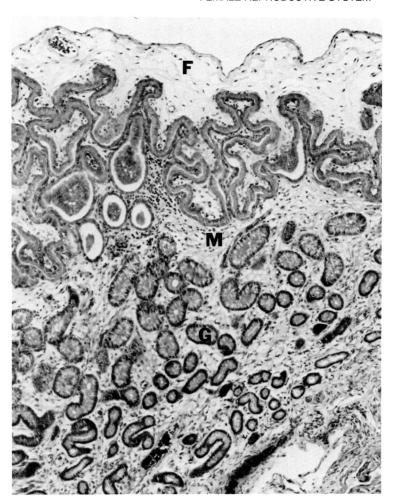

Figure 27.26. A section of the epitheliochorial placenta of a mare. The fetal *(F)* and maternal *(M)* contributions interdigitate with each other. G, uterine glands. ×10.

contains blood vessels. This is a transitory method of utilizing the embryonic circulation for physiological exchange between fetal and maternal tissues. It is a transitory structure in most eutherian mammals but persists for some time in the horse. This type of exchange organ is the definitive placenta of metatherian mammals.

Chorioallantoic Placenta. The *chorioallantoic placenta* is the definitive or "true" placenta of eutherian mammals. It is formed by the fusion of the *allantoic mesoderm* with the *chorionic mesoderm*. A vascular invasion accompanies the allantoic mesoderm, whereas the allantoic vesicle may be extensively large or vestigial in size.

Trophoblastic cells from the developing allantochorionic placenta invade the endometrial connective tissue in the mare (Fig. 27.26). The cells form dense aggregations of trophoblastic cells among scattered uterine glands (Fig. 27.27). The large aggregates, *endometrial cups*, may have a 5-cm diameter. The endometrial cup cells are large polyhedral cells that may be binucleated (Fig. 27.28). The cells are responsi-

ble for the synthesis and secretion of *equine chorionic gonadotropin (ECG)*.

The lymphocytic and eosinophilic infiltration of the endometrial cups and the vast lymphatic channels associated with them ensure their ultimate rejection by the maternal immune system. The endometrial cups are maximally developed by the 50th gestational day, begin to regress by the 60th day, and are rejected by the 150th day of gestation. After the immune events of rejection, the degenerative, detached endometrial cups become encapsulated by components of the chorion as pendulous *hippomanes*.

Degree of Implantation

General Remarks. The degree of implantation generally defines the extent of the relationship between the fetal and maternal tissues. Through the relationships so established, the shedding or nonshedding of maternal tissues at parturition is established. In those placentas in which a minimal amount of tissue is eroded during the formation of the organ, the placenta is non-

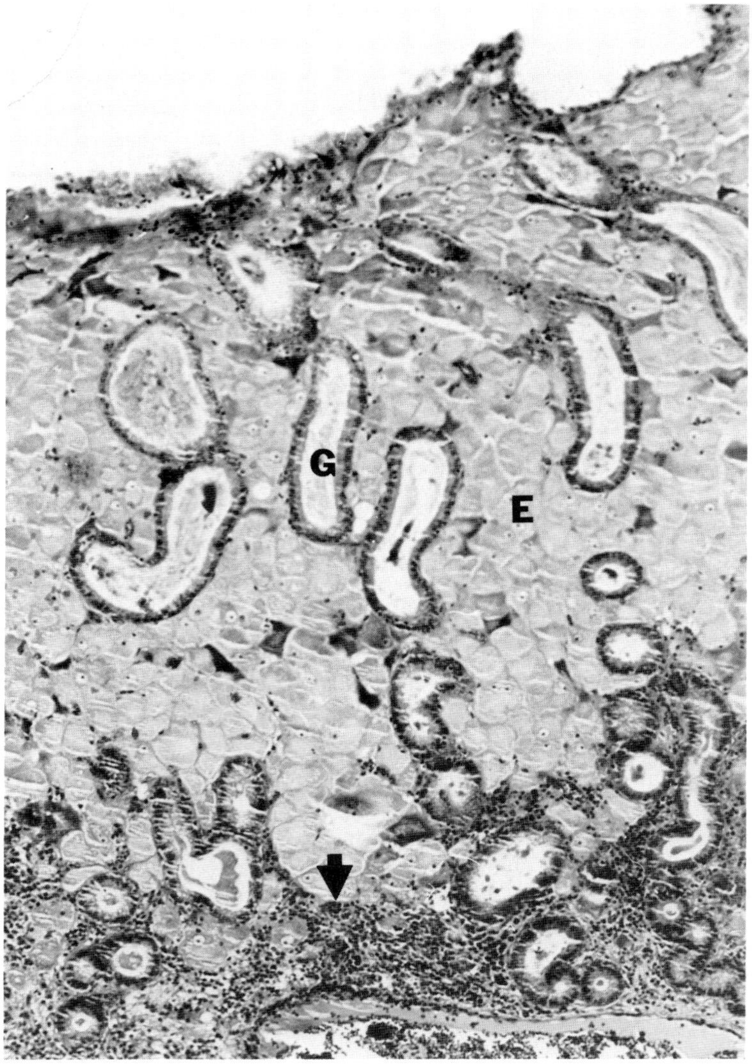

Figure 27.27. A section of endometrial cups of an equine uterus. The cells of the endometrial cups *(E)* are a prominent feature of the lamina propria mucosae. Uterine glands *(G)* are present also. The *solid arrow* indicates the advancing front of a mass of infiltrating lymphocytes. ×25.

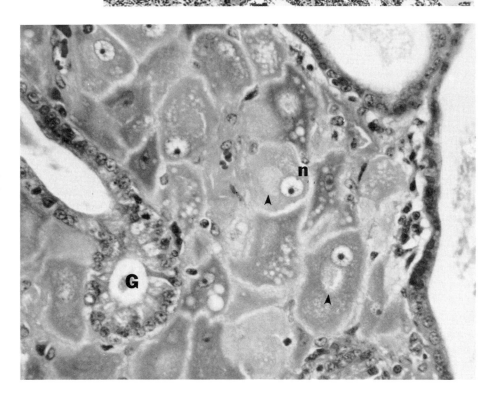

Figure 27.28. Cells of the endometrial cups of an equine uterus. The nuclei *(n)* are vesicular with a prominent nucleolus. A large negative-staining Golgi region is apparent *(arrowheads)*. G, uterine gland. ×100.

deciduate. In those in which an extensive erosion of tissues accompanies the implantation, the placenta is termed deciduate. Maternal tissues are not shed at parturition in a nondeciduate placenta as they are in a deciduate placenta.

Nondeciduate Placenta. The terms *nondeciduate placenta, apposed placenta, semiplacenta,* and *superficial nidation* are used synonymously. The fetal and maternal tissues may be interdigitated and are fused or in apposition to one another. There is, therefore, minimal erosion of the contributing tissues. No uterine mucosal elements are lost at parturition.

Deciduate Placenta. The *deciduate placenta* is also referred to as a *conjoined pla-*

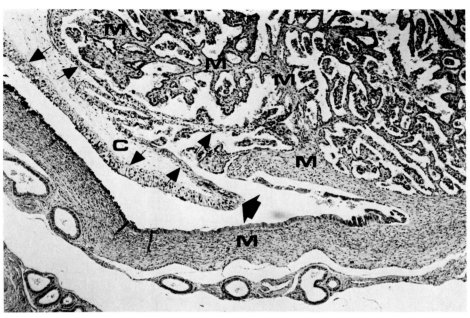

Figure 27.30. A section of a bovine epitheliochorial placenta. The chorioallantois *(C)* of the fetus *(small arrows)* interdigitates with the maternal villi *(M)*. The fetal membrane is reflected away from the placentome *(large arrow)*. ×13.

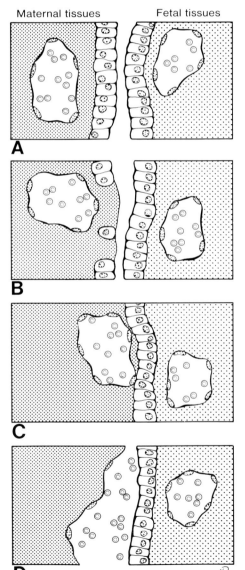

Figure 27.29. A diagram of four types of placentation. The fetal tissues remain intact in the placental relationships depicted. *A*, epitheliochorial; *B*, syndesmochorial; *C*, endotheliochorial; *D*, hemochorial.

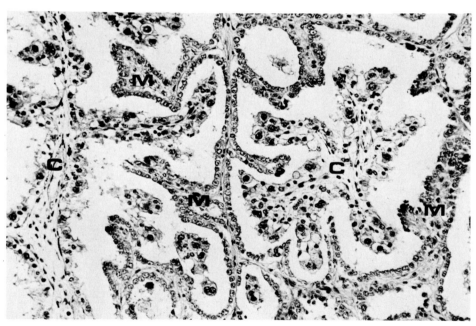

Figure 27.31. Fetal and maternal tissue relationships in a bovine placentome. The maternal tissue *(M)* is lined by uterine epithelium. The chorioallantois *(C)* of the fetus is lined by trophoblastic cells. The separation between the tissues is artifact. ×50.

centa or a *placenta vera. Interstitial nidation* also refers to the formation of this type of placenta. In the formation of this type of placenta, the uterine mucosa and chorion are eroded to varying degrees and subsequently fuse. At parturition, therefore, some maternal tissue is lost.

Decidual cells are maternal, connective tissue, stromal cells that have various shapes, sizes, and cytoplasmic inclusions in different animals. They occur in the dog, cat, and human. The precise function of these cells is not known. They may serve a nutritive function, delineate a cleavage zone at parturition, protect the uterine mucosa against the invading trophoblast or form placental gonadotrophins. These cells are typical of most eutherian mammals but occur minimally or not at all in carnivores and ungulates.

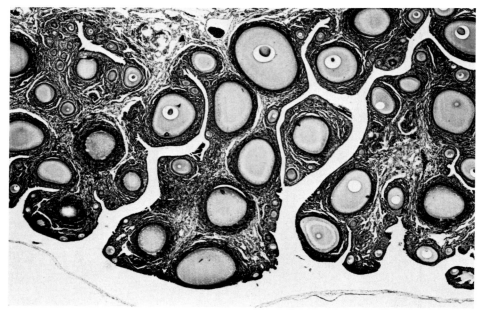

Figure 27.32. A section of an avian ovary. The ovary is a pendulous structure suspended from the abdominal wall. ×10.

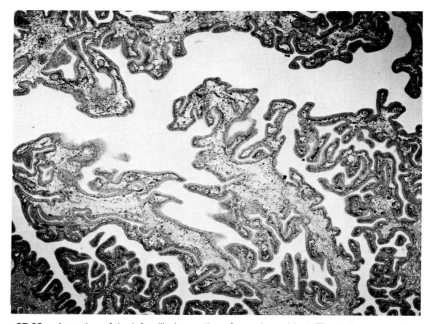

Figure 27.33. A section of the infundibular portion of an avian oviduct. The tunica mucosa is highly folded and devoid of glands. ×10.

Configuration of Chorionic Attachments

Folded, Villous, and Labyrinthine Attachments. The fetal and maternal tissues are opposed, fused, or intimately interdigitated to facilitate physiological exchange. Three types of fetal and maternal contact are defined: folded, villar, labyrinthine. In the *folded type*, undulations of both contributing tissues are interdigitated. In the *villous*, chorionic protrusions interdigitate with corresponding maternal crypts. The *labyrinthine placenta* represents a fusion of chorionic villi.

Fetal and Maternal Contributions

General Remarks. When considering the barriers across which physiological exchange must occur, all the components between the fetal and maternal capillaries must be included. The maximal barrier for this exchange includes the following: *uter-ine endothelium, uterine connective tissue, uterine epithelium, chorionic epithelium, chorioallantoic connective tissue, and allantoic endothelium.* Various placentas are formed by the intact relationship of these components or by the deletion of one or more of these components. On this basis, five types of placenta are defined (Fig. 27.29): *epitheliochorial, syndesmochorial, endotheliochorial, hemochorial, and endothelioendothelial.* In the formation of these compound names, the first term refers to the maternal component, whereas the second term refers to the fetal component.

Epitheliochorial Placenta. In this type of placenta all six layers are present (Fig. 27.30). The chorionic and uterine epithelia are in contact with one another (Fig. 27.31). This configuration is nondeciduate and is typical of the sow, mare, cow, ewe, and doe.

Syndesmochorial Placenta. In this type of placenta the chorionic epithelium is in direct contact with the uterine connective tissue, the uterine epithelium having been eroded. This configuration is also nondeciduate. This type of placentation occurs focally in ruminants after the establishment of an epitheliochorial placenta and in pathological circumstances.

Endotheliochorial Placenta. This type of placentation is characterized by the intimate contact of the chorionic epithelium with the uterine capillaries. Therefore, the uterine epithelium and connective tissue have been eroded. This is a deciduate type of placentation characteristic of the queen and bitch.

Hemochorial Placenta. In hemochorial placentation, the chorionic epithelium is in direct contact with the maternal blood. This is achieved by the erosion of the uterine epithelium, connective tissue, and endothelium. Further subdivision of this type of placentation is predicated upon the number of cell layers of the trophoderm in contact with the maternal blood. Thus, *hemomonochorial, hemodichorial,* and *hemotrichorial* placentation is recognized.

Hemochorial placentation occurs in primates and rodents.

Endothelioendothelial Placenta. This type of placentation is characteristic of the ewe. The fetal endothelium is separated from the maternal endothelium by a thin layer of discontinuous throphoblast cells. Although functionally this type of placentation has a reduced transport barrier, anatomically it may be considered an endotheliochorial placenta.

Species Differences. The following unified classification is based upon the previously discussed characteristics:

Swine: diffusely folded, epitheliochorial, nondeciduate placenta
Horse: diffusely villous, epitheliochorial, nondeciduate placenta

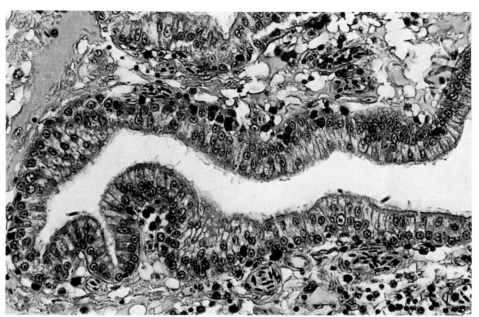

Figure 27.34. Lining epithelium of an avian infundibulum. The lining epithelium is pseudostratified cilliated. Goblet cells may be present, but multicellular glands are absent. ×125.

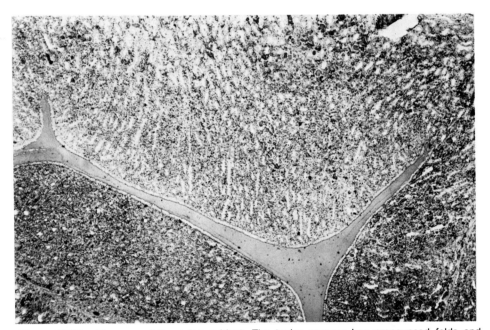

Figure 27.35. Magnum of the avian oviduct. The tunica mucosa has pronounced folds and numerous branched tubular glands. ×10.

Ruminants: cotyledonary villous, epitheliochorial, nondeciduate placenta
Carnivores: zonary labyrinthine, endotheliochorial, deciduate placenta
Man: discoidal villous, hemochorial, deciduate placenta.

Avian Reproductive System

General Remarks. The avian reproductive system is designed to facilitate internal fertilization as in the mammal. The oviduct and uterus, however, are modified to ensure the survival and development of the offspring outside the body. These structures, therefore, supply the necessary nutrients and enclose the offspring within a protective shell.

Only the left ovary and oviduct are retained in the adult as functional entities.

Ovary. The ovaries of birds are not as compact as those in mammals. Rather, the ovary consists of finger-like projections that are suspended pendulously from the abdominal wall by the mesovarium (Fig. 27.32). A cortex and medulla are distinguishable, but the latter is not well-developed and is diffuse. The cortex consists of "follicles" in various stages of development. Actually, the term follicle is a misnomer because an antrum does not develop. The oocytes and accompanying cells are extremely large structures. The follicle contains a primary oocyte, a single layer of membrana granulosa cells, a theca folliculi interna, and a theca folliculi externa. The primary oocyte reaches a diameter, in some domesticated species, of approximately 30 mm. Ovulation is not followed by the development of a corpus luteum.

Oviduct. The avian oviduct is divided into five regions: *infundibulum, magnum, isthmus, shell gland* (uterus), and *vagina.* The formation of the egg involves the elaboration of albumin, the formation of the shell membranes, the "plumping" of the egg, and the secretion of materials for the shell. Only the vaginal portion of the oviduct is not involved in these formative processes.

The *infundibulum* is the funnel-like cranial extension of the oviduct. The tunica mucosa is highly folded and well vascularized caudally (Fig. 27.33). Cranially, the mucosal folds are low. The cranial aspects of the infundibulum are lined by nonsecretory, ciliated cells. Progressing caudad, the epithelial lining cells are secretory and epithelial grooves of the tunica mucosa are replaced by tubular glands at the junction of the infundibulum with the magnum. The lining epithelium of the infundibulum is pseudostratified columnar (Fig. 27.34). The amount of ciliated cells decreases caudally. The secretory lining cells and those of the tubular glands secrete mucoid materials. The histochemical properties of their secretory products differ.

The lamina propria-submucosa is areolar connective tissue. Diffuse lymphatic tissue is commonly encountered. The tunica muscularis and tunica serosa are typical.

This portion of the oviduct receives the ova and propels them toward the caudal part of the organ. Fertilization occurs within the infundibulum before the secretion of the enveloping mass of albumen by the magnum. Infundibular glands may store excess spermatozoa.

The *magnum* is responsible for the deposition of the majority of the egg white (Fig. 27.35). The lamina epithelialis mucosae consists of ciliated and nonciliated columnar cells (Fig. 27.36). The lamina propria mucosae contains numerous branched, tubular glands that are lined by a cuboidal or columnar epithelium. Secretory granules are present along the apical border. The passage of the forming egg through the magnum probably serves as the mechanical stimulation for the release of albumin. The magnum may store enough protein to envelope two eggs.

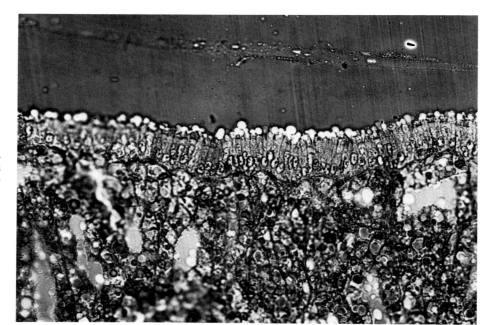

Figure 27.36. Lining cells of the avian magnum. The lumen is filled with a proteinaceous secretory product. The lamina epithelialis consists of ciliated columnar cells. ×125.

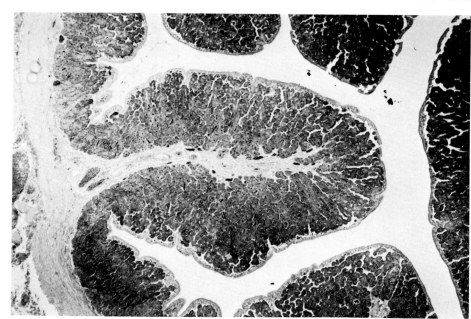

Figure 27.37. Isthmus of the avian oviduct. The tunica mucosa has pronounced folds. Numerous mucosal glands *(dark areas)* comprise part of the tunica mucosa. ×10.

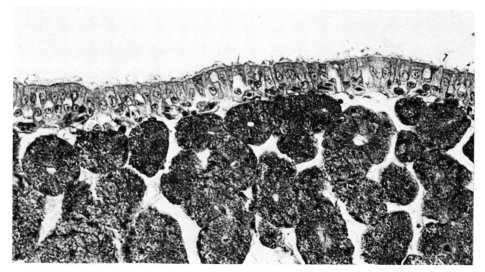

Figure 27.38. Lining and glandular epithelium of the avian isthmus. Ciliated columnar epithelial cells line the lumen of the organ. Mucosal glands *(dark areas)* are branched and tubular. ×100.

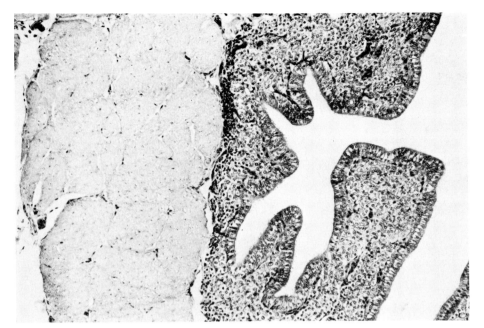

Figure 27.39. A section of the avian uterus. The tunica mucosa is highly folded. This organ produces the shell of the egg. ×50.

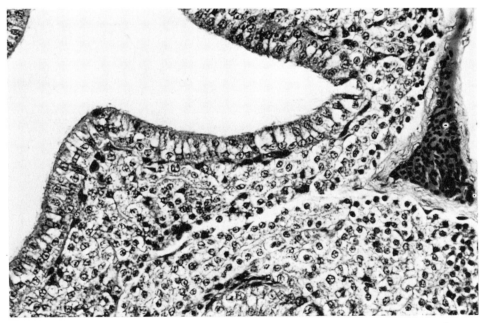

Figure 27.40. Lining cells of the avian uterus. The lamina epithelialis mucosae consists of pseudostratified intermittently ciliated coumnar epithelium. ×125.

Although three types of cells (A, B, and C cells) have been identified within the tubular glands, the A and C cells are probably the same cells in different stages of their secretory cycle. Ovalbumin appears to be derived from A cells, whereas B cells seem to be the source of lysozyme. Surface lining cells may be the source of ovomucin and avidin. Goblet cells within the caudal aspect of the magnum stain positively for acidic glycosaminoglycans.

The connective tissue of the lamina propria-submucosa is areolar with much diffuse lymphatic tissue. The tunica muscularis and tunica serosa are typical.

The *isthmus* is lined by a ciliated and nonciliated columnar epithelia (Fig. 27.37). Numerous branched, tubular glands extend into the lamina propria (Fig. 27.38). The remaining layers are similar to those of the magnum. This portion of the oviduct is responsible for the formation of the shell

membranes. It may be responsible for the secretion of albuminoids also.

Unlike the mammalian uterus, the avian *uterus* is not designed for the implantation of the fertilized ova. Rather, the avian uterus is the *shell gland* (Fig. 27.39). Its secretory activity is responsible for the formation of the egg shell, as well as for the dilution of the albuminoids. The uterus is divisible into two regions—*tubular shell gland* and *shell gland pouch*. Eggs are "plumped" by the addition of water to thinned albuminoids before shell deposition. Plumping activity may be initiated in the isthmus and completed in the shell gland pouch.

The lamina epithelialis mucosae consists of intermittently ciliated pseudostratified columnar epithelium (Fig. 27.40). Coiled, tubular glands project into the underlying connective tissue. The glandular cells have a centrally placed nucleus, whereas the cytoplasm may contain apically positioned granules or vacuoles. The remaining portions of the wall are similar to the aforementioned structures.

The *vagina* is the region that follows the shell gland. The tunica mucosa is characterized by short mucosal folds. Ciliated and nonciliated lining cells are characteristic of this epithelium, the surface cells of which are taller than those of the shell gland. This portion of the oviduct is glandless except at the junction with the shell gland pouch. The glands at the pouch-vagina junction are simple, tubular glands lined by columnar epithelial cells that contain lipids and PAS-positive material that is not glycogen. These glands, called *sperm host glands*, appear to nourish and store the sperm. The sperm are released upon mucosal distention that accompanies oviposition.

References

Ovary

Amsterdam, A., Linder, H. and Groschel-Stewart, U.: Localization of actin and myosin in the rat oocyte and follicular wall by immunofluorescence. Anat. Rec. *187*:311, 1977.

Anderson, E. and Albertini, D.: Gap junctions between the oocyte and companion follicle cells in the mammalian ovary. J. Cell Biol. *71*:680, 1976.

Baca, M. and Zamboni, L.: The fine structure of human follicular oocytes. J. Ultrastruct. Res. *19*:354, 1967.

Bjersing, L.: On the ultrastructure of the granulosa lutein cells in porcine corpus luteum. Z. Zellforsch. *82*:187, 1967.

Blanchette, E. J.: Ovarian steroid cells. II. The lutein cell. J. Cell. Biol. *31*:517, 1966.

Grandy, H. G. and Smith, D. E. (eds.): *The Ovary*. Williams & Wilkins, Baltimore, 1963.

Hadek, R.: Morphological and histochemical study on the ovary of the sheep. Amer. J. Vet. Res. *19*:873, 1958.

Hope, J.: The fine structure of the developing follicle of the Rhesus ovary. J. Ultrastruct. Res. *12*:592, 1965.

Phemister, R. D., et. al.: Time of ovulation in the Beagle bitch. Biol. Reprod. *8*:74, 1973.

Richardson, G. S.: Ovarian physiology. N. Engl. J. Med. *274*:1008, 1966.

Seguin, B. E.: Role of prostaglandins in bovine reproduction. J. Amer. Vet. Med. Assoc. *176*:1178, 1980.

Weakley, B. C.: Differentiation of the surface epithelium of the hamster ovary. An electron microscopic study. J. Anat. *105:*129, 1969.

Uterus and Associated Structures

Abdalla, O.: Observations on the morphology and histochemistry of the oviducts of the sheep. J. Anat. *102:*333, 1968.

Archibald, L. F., Baker, B. A., Clooney, L. L. and Godke, R. A.: A surgical method for collecting canine embryos after induction of estrus and ovulation with exogenous gonadotropins. Vet. Med. Sm. Anim. Clin. *75:*228, 1980.

Bal, H. S. and Getty, R.: Changing morphology of the uterine tubes of the domestic pig. *(Sus scrofa domesticus)* with age. J. Geront. *25:*347, 1970.

Dessouky, D. A.: Electron microscopic studies of the myometrium of the guinea pig. Amer. J. Obstet. Gynec. *100:*30, 1968.

Ferenczy, A., Richart, R. M., Agate, F. J., Jr., Purkerson, M. L. and Dempsey, E. W.: Scanning electron microscopy of the human fallopian tube. Science *175:*783, 1972.

Ginther, O. J.: Utero-ovarian relationships in cattle. Physiological aspects. J. Amer. Vet. Med. Assoc. *153:*1656, 1968.

Hook, S. J. and Hafez, E. S. E.: A comparative anatomical study of the mammalian uterotubal junction. J. Morph. *125:*159, 1968.

Huszar, G. and Roberts, J. M.: Biochemistry and pharmacology of the myometrium and labor: regulation at the cellular and molecular levels. Am. J. Obstet. Gynecol. *142:*25, 1982.

Pineda, M. H., Kainer, R. A. and Faulkner, L. C.: Dorsal median postcervical fold in the canine vagina. J. Amer. Vet. Med. Assoc. *34:*1487, 1973.

Schultz, R. H., Burcalow, H. B. and Fahning, M. L.: A karyometric study of epithelial cells lining the glands of the bovine endometrium. J. Reprod. Fertil. *19:*169, 1969.

Younes, M. S., Robertson, E. M. and Bencosme, S. A.: Electron microscope observations on Langerhans cells in the cervix. Amer. J. Obstet. Synec. *102:*397, 1968.

Cyclic Changes in the System

Adams, E. C. and Hertig, A. T.: Studies on the human corpus luteum. I. Observations on the ultrastructure of development and regression of the luteal cells during the menstrual cycle. J. Cell. Biol. *41:*696, 1969.

Adams, E. C. and Hertig, A. T.: Studies on the human corpus luteum. II. Observations on the ultrastructure of luteal cells during pregnancy. J. Cell. Biol. *41:*716, 1969.

Akins, E. L. and Morissette, M. C.: Gross ovarian changes during estrous cycle of swine. Amer. J. Vet. Res. *29:*1953, 1968.

Fowler, E. H., Feldman, M. K. and Loeb, W. F.: Comparison of histologic features ofovarian and uterine tissues with vaginal smears of the bitch. Amer. J. Vet. Res. *32:*327, 1971.

Fowler, E. H., Loeb, W. F. and Wilson, G. P.: Vaginal cytologic examination of intact and ovariohysterectomized bitches with mammary meoplasia. Amer. J. Vet. Res. *32:*51, 1970.

Hatch, R. D.: Anatomic changes in the bovine uterus during pregnancy. Amer. J. Vet. Res. *2:*411, 1941.

Holst, P. A. and Phemister, R. D.: Onset of diestrus in the Beagle bitch: Difinition and significance. Amer. J. Vet. Res. *35:*401, 1974.

Johnston, S. D.: Diagnostic and therapeutic approach to intertility in the bitch. J. Amer. Vet. Med. Assoc. *176:*1335, 1980.

King, B. F.: Ultrastructure of the nonhuman primate vaginal mucosa; epithelial changes during the menstrual cycle and pregnancy. J. Ultrastruct. Res. *82:*1, 1983.

McDonald, L. E.: *Veterinary Endocrinology and Reproduction,* Lea and Febiger, Philadelphia, 1969.

Peters, H. and Levy, E.: Cell dynamics of the ovarian cycle. J. Reprod. Fertil. *11:*227, 1966.

Sanger, V. L., Engle, P. H. and Bell, D. S.: The vaginal cytology of the ewe during the estrous cycle. Amer. J. Vet. Res. *19:*283, 1958.

Schutte, A. P.: Canine vaginal cytology. II. Cyclic changes. J. Sm. Anim. Pract. *8:*307, 1967.

Wagner, W.: Bovine parturition. Compend. Cont. Ed. Pract. Vet. *II:*517, 1980.

Comparative Placentology

Allen, W. R., Hamilton, D. W. and Moor, R. M.: The origin of equine endometrial cup: Anat. Rec. *177:*485, 1973.

Amorosa, E. C.: Histology of the placenta, foetal and neonatal physiology, Brit. Med. Bull. *17:*2, 1961.

Anderson, J. W.: Ultrastructure of the placenta and fetal membranes of the dog. I. The placenta labyrinth. Anat. Rec. *165:*5, 1969.

Ashley, C. A.: Study of the human placenta with the electron microscope. Arch. Path. Chicago *80:*377, 1965.

Bjorkman, N.: The fine structure of the ovine placentome. J. Anat. *99:*283, 1965.

Bjorkman, N.: Fine Structure of the fetal-maternal area of exchange in the epitheliochorial and enotheliochonial types of placentation. Act. Anat. Suppl. 1, *86:*1, 1973.

Bjorkman, N. H.: Fine structure of cryptal and trophoblastic giant cells in the bovine placentome. J. Ultrastruc. Res. *24:*249, 1968.

Bjorkman, N. H.: Light and electron microscopic studies on cellular alterations in the normal bovine placentome. Anat. Rec. *163:*17, 1969.

Bjorkman, N. H.: *An Atlas of Placental Fine Structure.* Williams & Wilkins Co., Baltimore, 1970.

Davies, J. and Glasser, S. R.: Histological and fine structural observations on the placenta of the rat. Acta Anat. *69:*542, 1968.

Enders, A. C.: A comparative study of the fine structure of the trophoblast in several hemochorial placentas. Amer. J. Anat. *116:*29, 1965.

Wimsatt, W. A.: Some aspects of the comparative anatomy of mammalian placentome. Amer. J. Obstet. *84:*11, Part 2, 1962.

Avian Reproductive Tract

Brambell, R. W. R.: The oogenesis of the fowl *(Gallus bankiva).* Phil. Trans. Toyal Soc. (B). *214:*113, 1926.

Fell, H. F.: Histological studies of the gonads of the Fowl. II. The histogenesis of the so-called "luteal" cells in the ovary. Brit. J. Exp. Biol. *1:*293, 1924.

Fertuck, H. C. and Newstead, J. D.: Fine structural observations on magnum numosa in quial and hen oviducts. Z. Zellforsch. *103:*447, 1970.

Freeman, B. M. (ed.): *Physiology and Biochemistry of the Domestic Fowl.* Vol. 4. Academic Press, New York, 1983.

Hewitt, E. A.: The physiology of the reproductive system of the fowl. J. Amer. Vet. Med. Assoc. *95:*201, 1939.

Kohler, P. O., Grimley, P. M. and O'Malley, B. W.: Estrogen-induced cytodifferentiation of the ovalbumin-secreting glands of the chick oviduct. J. Cell Biol. *40:*8, 1969.

Narbaitz, R. and DeRobertis, R. M., Jr.: Postnatal evolution of steriodogenic cells in the chick ovary. Histochemie *15:*187, 1968.

Nevalainen, T. J.: Electron microscope observations on the shell gland mucosa of calcium-deficient hens *(Gallus domesticus).* Anat. Rec. *164:*127, 1969.

Sturkie, P. D. and Mueller, W. J.: Reproduction in the female and egg production. *In:* Sturkie, P. D. (ed.): *Avian Physiology.* 3rd edition, pp. 302-330, Springer-Verlag, New York, 1976.

28: Eye and Ear

General Characteristics

Introduction. Receptors or receptor organs that are classified apart from the somatic receptors comprise the *special sensory system*. The *special somatic afferent (SSA) system* includes the eye and ear. The SSA receptors are responsive to visual *(eye)* and auditory *(cochlea)* information. The vestibular apparatus *(semicircular canals and saccules)* is a special proprioceptive apparatus that responds to linear and angular acceleration. The *special visceral afferent (SVA) system* consists of receptors that are responsible for gustatory and olfactory sensations (Chapters 21 and 24).

Eye

General Remarks. The eyeball *(bulbus oculi)* is a globe-shaped structure that is flattened slightly along the optic (rostral-caudal) axis. Light enters the globe through the rostrally positioned, transparent *cornea*. The light continues through the aperture *(pupil)*, the peripheral margins of which are defined by an adjustable diaphragm, the *iris*. Light then passes through a biconvex *lens* that is suspended from the *ciliary body*. Focusing of light upon the *retina* is accomplished usually by changing the curvature of the lens through the contraction and relaxation of *ciliary muscles*. Photosensitive cells *(rods and cones)* located within the retina transduce the photon energy into usable information. Neural activity resulting from photoreceptor cell responsiveness is processed by the central nervous system as vision.

Development. Ectoderm, neurectoderm, and mesoderm contribute to the structure of the eye. After closure of the neural tube, lateral evaginations of the diencephalon, *optic vesicles*, grow toward and make contact with the ectoderm of the presumptive skin (Fig. 28.1). The optic vesicle maintains its continuity with the neurectoderm of the diencephalon through an *optic stalk*. The optic stalk and vesicle are hollow structures. The continued growth of the optic vesicle causes an elongation of the optic stalk. The optic stalk serves as a guide for the ingrowing nerve fibers of the retina that form the optic nerve. The optic vesicle grows and invaginates to form a double-layered *optic cup* (Fig. 28.2). The invagination continues along the ventral border of the optic stalk as the *choroid fissure (optic fissure)*. The inner and outer layers of the wall of the optic cup are separated by a space, *intraretinal space*. The outer layer develops into the *pigment epithelium* of the retina, whereas the inner layer becomes the *neural retina*.

As optic cup development progresses, the portion of the optic cup in contact with the surface ectoderm continues to grow and induces the formation of a *lens placode* in the surface ectoderm (Fig. 28.1). The lens placode invaginates, grows, and pinches away from the surface ectoderm as a *lens vesicle* (Fig. 28.2). The lens vesicle, located within the "mouth" of the optic cup, is separated from the inner walls of the optic cup mesoderm. The space is destined to become the *vitreous body* (Fig. 28.3). A cavitation develops in the anterior part of the mesodermal space, and this space is lined by epithelial cells *(mesenchymal epithelium)*. The mesenchymal epithelium forms the *iridopupillary membranes*. The anterior portion of the iris, however, is devoid of epithelium, whereas the posterior portion is covered by a pigmented and nonpigmented epithelium derived from the inner (neural) and outer (pigmented) layer of the optic cup.

The *sclera* is derived from the mesoderm peripheral to the developing eye and is homologous to the *dura mater* (Fig. 28.3). The sclera is dense connective tissue that encircles the eye and is continuous with the *stroma* or *substantia propria* of the *cornea*. The cornea from without inward consists of epithelium (surface ectoderm), substantia propria, and mesenchymal epithelium that is reflected from the rostral surface of the iris (Fig. 28.3). The cavity between the caudal surface of the cornea and the rostral surface of the iris is the *anterior chamber*. It is continuous through the *pupil* with the *posterior chamber*—the space between the caudal surface of the iris and the rostral surface of the lens.

The mesoderm between the developing sclera and the outer wall of the developing eye is homologous to the *leptomeninges*. This mesoderm develops into the *vascular coat* or *uveal tract. The uveal tract includes the choroid, ciliary body, and iridial stroma.* The choroid is associated intimately with the pigment epithelium. The ciliary part of the retina—the pigment epi-

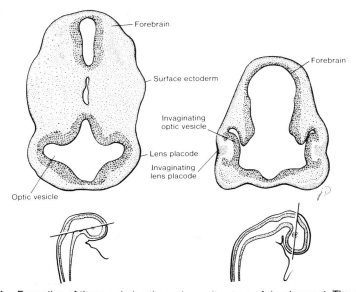

Figure 28.1. Formation of the eye during the early somite stage of development. The optic vesicle evaginates from the neural tube, contacts the surface ectoderm, and then begins to invaginate.

527

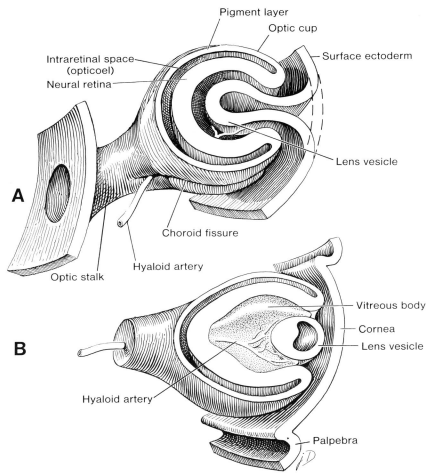

Figure 28.2. Progression in the development of the eye. *A.* The optic cup has formed and is joined to the diencephalon by the optic stalk. The lens placode has invaginated to form a lens vesicle. The hyaloid artery has become associated with the choroid fissure. *B.* The lens vesicle has separated from the surface ectoderm.

thelium and nonpigmented epithelium—cover the ciliary body. The iridial part of the retina—two layers of pigmented cells—covers the caudal surface of the iris. The lens is suspended from the ciliary body by a delicate *suspensory ligament.*

The *optic retina (pars optica retinae)*—derived from the inner and outer walls of the optic cup—undergoes differential growth. The outer lamina of the cup remains a single layer of cells, *pigment epithelium,* separated by the *intraretinal space (cavity of the optic cup, opticoel)* from the inner wall or *neural retina.* The neural retina grows and differentiates into a structure characterized by numerous layers of cells. The photoreceptor cells comprise the outermost portion of the inner lamina of the cup. They and the pigment epithelium are homologous to *ependyma.* The remaining cellular layers of the neural retina are homologous to the *mantle* and *marginal layers* of the neural tube. The neural retina and pigment epithelium are "attached" to each other at the region the axons from the neural retina emerge from the caudal pole

at the *optic disc.* They are also attached to each other at the junction with the ciliary retina, the *ora ciliaris retinae.*

The innermost portion of the neural retina is adjacent to the *hyaloid membrane,* the peripheral lining of the vitreous body. A remnant of the *hyaloid artery,* the blood supply to the caudal aspect of a developing lens, may be apparent within a fold of the hyaloid membrane in the mature eyes in some species, notably the ox. The hyaloid artery gained access to the vitreous body and caudal aspect of the lens during the formation of the *choroid* or *optic fissure.* The portion of the hyaloid artery within the optic nerve is retained as the *central artery of the retina* in humans but not in domestic animals.

Retinal detachment is related to the development of the pigmented and neural components of the retina. The intraretinal space is a potential space that may reappear after trauma. *Persistent iridopupillary membranes* may remain as a complete covering over the pupil; however, they are observed most commonly as fibrous

strands attached to the rostral surface of the lens and/or iris. A *coloboma,* a cleft-like defect, may occur in the iris, ciliary body, retina, choroid, and optic nerve from the incomplete closure of the choroid fissure. Colobomas of the iris *(coloboma iridis),* optic nerve, and optic disc are observed readily upon ophthalmic examination.

Organization. The wall of the eye is composed of three layers (tunics) that surround and enclose the refractive or dioptric components (Fig. 28.4). The three tunics of the globe are: *fibrous layer (tunica fibrosa bulbi), vascular layer (tunica vasculosa bulbi),* and *nervous layer (tunica interna [sensoria] bulbi).* The outermost fibrous layer consists of the *sclera* over most of the eye and the *cornea* rostrally. The vascular layer *(uvea)* is comprised of the *choroid, ciliary body* and *iris.* The innermost layer, *nervous tunic,* consists of the *retina.* The pigment epithelium and non-neural epithelium of the neural portion of the retina contribute to the formation of the ciliary body *(pars ciliaris retinae)* and iris *(pars iridica retinae).*

The *dioptric media* of the eye include the *cornea, aqueous humor, lens, vitreous body,* and *retina.*

The eye is divisible into an *anterior compartment*—positioned rostrally between the lens and cornea—and a *posterior compartment* occupied by the vitreous body. The anterior compartment is divided into an *anterior chamber* and *posterior chamber.* The anterior chamber occurs between the cornea and iris. The point at which the iris and cornea are in contact is the *filtration angle.* The posterior chamber is the space between the lens and iris. The posterior chamber communicates with the anterior chamber through the pupil.

Fibrous Tunic

The fibrous tunic consists of the *sclera* and *cornea.*

Sclera

The *sclera* is composed of dense white fibrous connective tissue (DWFCT) that is rich in elastic fibers (Fig. 28.5). It is divisible into an *episcleral zone, a sclera proper,* and a *lamina fusca.* The connective tissue of the sclera maintains the shape of the bulb. Alterations of the sclera that affect bulb size can have devastating effects upon vision by altering the optic axis.

Episclera. The outermost *episclera* is a transparent fibroelastic connective tissue that is attached loosely to the sclera proper. The episcleral blood vessels supply the outer, relatively avascular portion of the sclera proper. The episclera, which unites with the sclera and cornea in the rostral portion of the eye, is adjacent to but separated from a peripherally positioned thin layer of dense fibrous connective tissue,

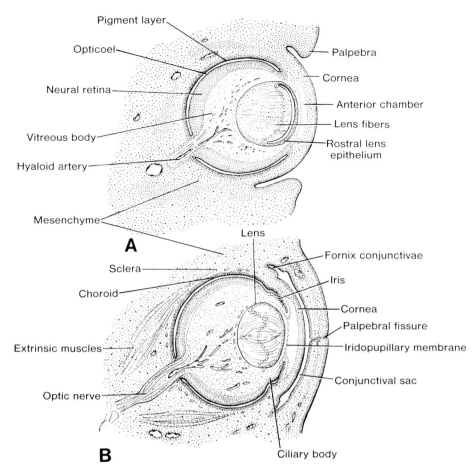

Pigment layer
Opticoel
Neural retina
Vitreous body
Hyaloid artery
Mesenchyme
Palpebra
Cornea
Anterior chamber
Lens fibers
Rostral lens epithelium

A

Lens
Sclera
Choroid
Extrinsic muscles
Optic nerve
Fornix conjunctivae
Iris
Cornea
Palpebral fissure
Iridopupillary membrane
Conjunctival sac
Ciliary body

B

Figure 28.3. Continued development of the eye. *A.* The lens is contained within the optic cup and the entire bulb is enclosed by mesenchyme. *B.* Anterior chamber has formed and the iridopupillary membrane is apparent. The fibrous and vascular tunics have begun to differentiate.

Tenon's capsule, by *Tenon's space.* Tenon's capsule is the fascial covering of the globe *(fascia bulbi).* It is difficult to see grossly.

Sclera proper. The *sclera proper* is a dense fibroelastic connective tissue that is vascularized minimally. It continues rostrally as the connective tissue of the cornea. This point of transition is termed the *corneoscleral junction* and contains blood vessels and lymphatics. The edge of the cornea at this junction is termed the *limbus.*

The fibrous components of the sclera—collagen and elastin—comprise successive layers of flattened laminae that are wider than they are thick (Fig. 28.5). The laminae radiate in all directions around the globe and interlace with each other. Rostrally, the fibers are oriented in a circular direction around the optical axis, affording firm attachment points for the insertion of the extraocular muscles.

Lamina Fusca. The *lamina fusca* is a fibroelastic connective tissue that is especially rich in elastic fibers. Pigment cells impart a brown coloration to this lamina.

Area Cribrosa. The *area cribrosa* is a fenestrated modification of the sclera near the posterior pole. This area permits the exit of axons through the bulb. The nerve fibers pass through this area like filaments through a sieve. This area of the sclera is weaker than the rest of the sclera. Increased intraocular pressure *(glaucoma)* may manifest itself as an outward bowing or cupping of the optic disc.

Cornea

The *cornea* is the transparent extension of the sclera. The transition from opaque sclera to transparent cornea occurs crisply at the *corneoscleral junction (limbus).* The corneal edge of the junction is overlapped by the sclera. The scleral vessels extend to the limbus but do not cross the corneoscleral junction normally.

The cornea consists generally of five layers (Fig. 28.6): *anterior epithelium, Bowman's membrane, substantia propria, Descemet's membrane,* and *posterior epithelium (endothelium).*

Anterior Epithelial layer. The *anterior epithelium* of the cornea is a nonkeratinized stratified squamous epithelium. The epithelial covering of the cornea is continuous with the *bulbar conjunctival epithelium.* It continues as the *palpebral conjunctival epithelium* at the *fornix conjunctivae.* The bulbar conjunctival epithelium and its associated connective tissue comprise a cutaneous mucous membrane called the *bulbar conjunctiva.* The *palpebral conjunctiva* is constituted similarly and is a cutaneous mucous membrane.

The corneal epithelium varies in thickness but contains basal, intermediate, and superficial cells. The epithelium is richly endowed with numerous naked nerve endings.

Bowman's Membrane. *Bowman's membrane* is a combination of the basement membrane and a feltwork of fine collagenous fibers. It is most clearly evident in primates but is defined vaguely in other species.

Substantia Propria. The *substantia propria* forms the bulk of the cornea. It consists of collagenous fibers (Type I and II) disposed in plate-like configurations. Flattened fibroblasts *(keratoblasts)* are present. The ground substance consists of *mucosubstances* (chondroitin sulfate, keratan sulfate, hyaluronic acid) that are essential for the maintenance of proper corneal hydration. Numerous unmyelinated nerve fibers are present; blood vessels are not present. Vascularization of the cornea occurs during repair processes from vessels at the corneoscleral junction. Subsequent to repair, the vessels will have withdrawn to the junction.

Caudal Limiting Membrane. The *caudal limiting membrane (Descemet's membrane)* separates the substantia propria from the endothelium. Although considered to be a basal lamina, electron microscopic investigations have revealed it to consist of two poorly defined layers. The region adjacent to the substantia propria consists of Type II collagen arranged in an orderly manner. This region of Descemet's membrane thickens with age. The region subjacent to the posterior epithelium consists of typical basal laminar materials. The caudal limiting membrane is a nonmetachromatic, periodic acid-Schiff (PAS)-positive structure that stains positively for elastic fibers also.

Posterior Epithelium. The caudal border of the cornea is covered by *mesenchymal epithelium.* The mesenchymal epithelial lining of the cornea *(posterior epithelium)* is commonly termed *endothelium.* These cells are not similar morphologically to true endothelial lining cells of blood and lymphatic vessels. The corneal endothelium consists of large squamous or low cuboidal cells that form a tightly interdigitated cellular covering over the caudal margin of the cornea, separating the cornea proper from the aqueous humor of the anterior chamber. The endothelium of the cornea is continuous with the endothelial lining cells of the venous plexus through which

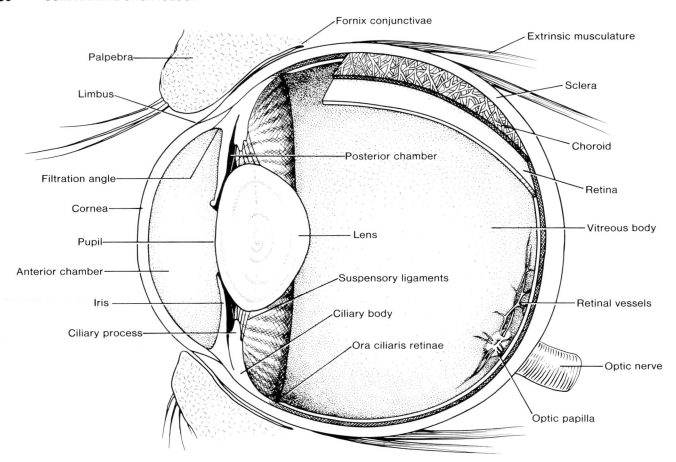

Figure 28.4.   A diagram of a parasagittal section of a bovine eye.

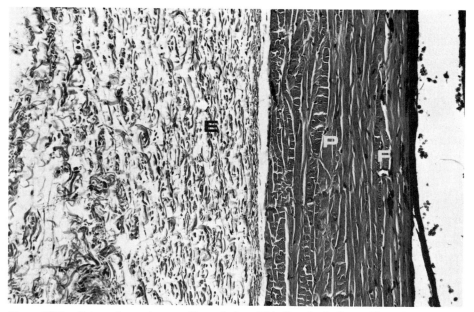

Figure 28.5.   Sclera of a canine eye. The episclera *(E)* is fibroelastic tissue. The sclera proper *(P)* is dense fibroelastic tissue that is vascularized minimally. The lamina fusca *(F)* is fibroelastic tissue that is pigmented. X40.

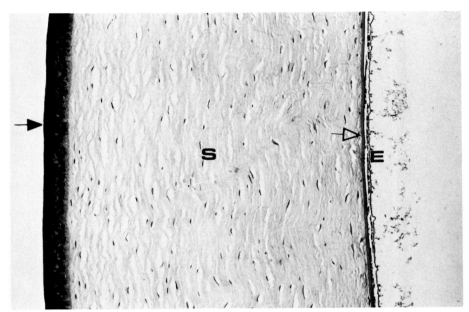

Figure 28.6. Cornea of a canine eye. The rostral epithelium *(solid arrow)*, substantia propria *(S)*, Decemet's membrane *(open arrow)* and endothelium *(E)* are indicated. Bowman's membrane, a light microscopic feature of primate eyes, is not apparent. The endothelium is artifactually displaced from the cornea. X40.

aqueous humor is returned to the circulation.

Functional Correlates. Various structural modifications of the cornea are characteristic among domestic animals. The cornea of nocturnal animals may comprise 35% of the surface of the globe; whereas the relative surface area of the cornea of domestic animals ranges from 17 to 30%. The thickness of the cornea is species variable, and individual corneas, except in man, are not a uniform thickness. The thickness of the cornea of most domestic animals ranges between 0.56 and 1.0 mm. The centers of the bovine, canine, feline and porcine corneas are thicker than the periphery, whereas the reverse occurs in the horse.

Corneal transparency is attributable to the orderly arrangement of its constituent collagenous fibers, which are arranged in laminae that parallel the corneal surface. Intralaminal fibers are parallel to each other and the surface, but contiguous laminae are oriented in different directions. By comparison, the random arrangement of collagenous fibers in the sclera contributes to its opacity. The degree of hydration of the substantia propria also contributes to corneal transparency. Edema of the cornea is characterized by various degrees of corneal opacity that ranges from a minor opacity *(nebula)*, light grey opacity *(macula)* to a dense white opacity *(leukoma)*. The intact and normally functioning stratified squamous epithelium and endothelium are essential barriers that prevent the imbibition of water and resultant corneal opacity.

The avascular cornea is dependent upon diffusion of metabolites, including O_2, from three sources: peripherally positioned limbic capillaries, aqueous humor, and the tear film. Although the tear film may not be a primary source of metabolites, it is a major source of dissolved O_2.

Repair. The cornea is modified skin. The most common congenital lesion of the cornea is a *dermoid growth (choristoma)*—the development of long (ox, dog) or short (horse) hairs and some adipose tissue within the cornea. The principles governing repair of the integument apply.

Superficial wounds involving the anterior lining epithelium heal rapidly by epithelial basal cell migration and subsequent mitosis; however, a simple, *superficial scratch* heals by cellular migration without mitosis.

Deep wounds into the substantia propria are characterized by inflammation. The cornea, devoid of its superficial epithelial lining, swells and becomes cloudy. Migration and mitosis of basal epithelial cells account for epithelial repair. Because the formation of the basement membrane occurs at a slower rate than epithelial cell replacement, new lining cells are attached loosely to the cornea and are sensitive to reinjury. Neovascularization from the limbic blood vessels occurs within 3–6 days of injury. Fibroblasts, which accompany the nascent blood vessels, and regenerating keratoblasts deposit collagen randomly, accounting for the resulting corneal scar. Complete resolution of the repair process may result in minimal scarring and a loss of the neovascularization.

Penetrating wounds into the anterior chamber disrupt all corneal components, including the endothelium. Fibrin originating from the aqueous humor plugs the defect. The repair of such a wound requires the resolution of the fibrin clot, regeneration of the endothelium, and the other events described previously.

Species differences characterize the susceptibility of the cornea to injury and the repair of the cornea subsequent to injury. Ruminant corneas are the least sensitive to injury and heal rapidly. Feline corneas are not characterized by extensive neovascular-

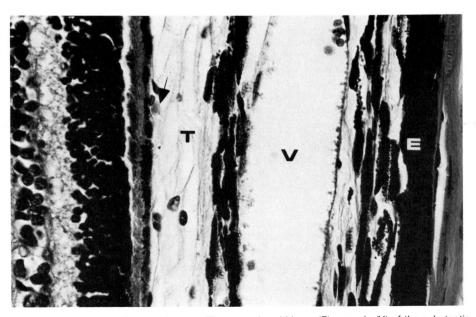

Figure 28.7. Choroid of the canine eye. The suprachoroid layer *(E)*, vessels *(V)* of the substantia propria, cellular tapetum lucidum *(T)* and choriocapillary layer *(solid arrow)* are indicated. The pigment epithelium is incompletely pigmented. This region, therefore is a transition region between tapetal and nontapetal regions. Compare with Figure 28.9. X 160.

ization and heal slowly with minimal scarring. Conversely, canine corneas develop extensive neovascularization. The equine cornea is the most sensitive cornea, reacts severely to injury, heals slowly, and culminates in extensive cicatrization.

Allographic corneal transplant is an effective method of repair of certain types of corneal injuries. The cornea, devoid of blood and lymphatic vessels is a "privileged site" that may protect the transplant from the host's immunological response.

Corneoscleral Junction. The *corneoscleral junction* is the transition from opaque sclera to transparent cornea. Scleral blood vessels terminate at this point, and the region contains the apparatus for the return of aqueous humor to the general circulation. The limbus is the point of gradual transition from rostral corneal epithelium to bulbar conjunctival epithelium. Bowman's membrane terminates at the limbus. The conjunctival stroma, interdigitated between the conjunctival epithelium and rostral attachment of Tenon's capsule, contributes to the *limbic conjunctiva*. The limbic conjunctiva continues as the *palpebral conjunctiva*.

Vascular Tunic

The *vascular tunic* or *uveal tract* consists of the: *choroid coat, ciliary body*, and *iris*. The uveal tract is not continued rostrally adjacent to the cornea but is reflected as the ciliary body and iris.

Choroid

The choroid coat is subdivided into five layers (Fig. 28.7): *lamina suprachoroidea, substantia propria, tapetum lucidum, lamina choriocapillaris*, and *basal complex (complexus basalis)*.

Suprachoroid Layer. The *suprachoroid layer (lamina suprachoroidea)* is the most peripheral layer of the choroid. This layer is separated from the lamina fusca by a *perichoroidal space (spatium perichoroideale*. Collagenous fibers, however, pass through this space and attach the tunics to each other. This avascular layer consists of a loose array of collagenous fibers, chromatophores, macrophages, and fibroblasts.

Substantia Propria. The *substantia propria* is the loose connective tissue stroma of the choroid. The stromal elements of the choroid, however, are not distributed homogeneously. Numerous melanocytes, fibroblasts, blood vessels, and special tapetal components are distributed in such a way as to define specific subdivisions of the choroid.

Tapetum Lucidum. The *tapetum (tapetum lucidum)* is a fibrous or cellular layer of the choroid coat positioned peripherally to the choriocapillary layer (Fig. 28.7). The tapetum lucidum, often described as a light-reflective surface or "ocular mirror,"

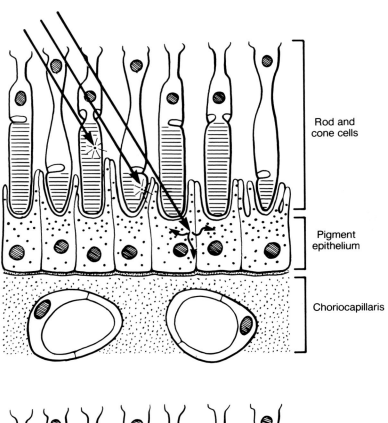

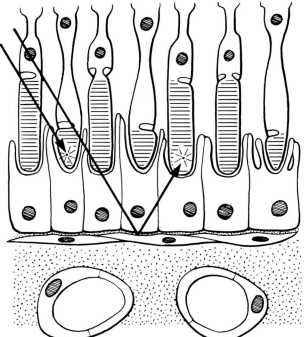

Figure 28.8. Diagrams illustrating the function of the tapetum lucidum. The upper diagram is a nontapetal region. Incoming photons excite photoreceptors; the energy is absorbed and dissipated in the pigment epithelium. The lower diagram represents a tapetal region. Incoming photons excite photoreceptors and are reflected from the tapetum lucidum to the photoreceptor cells. The pigment epithelium of these regions is devoid of pigment.

reflects light back to the photoreceptors to enhance dark-adapted *(scotopic)* vision (Fig. 28.8). The shape, size, color, and distribution of the tapetum lucidum is species-variable. The tapetum lucidum is responsible for the "eyeshine" that is obvious at

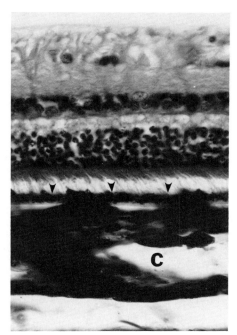

Figure 28.9. Vascular tunic of a canine eye. The choroid coat *(C)* is heavily pigmented. The pigment epithelium *(arrowheads)* is also heavily pigmented. Note that a tapetum lucidum is absent. X100.

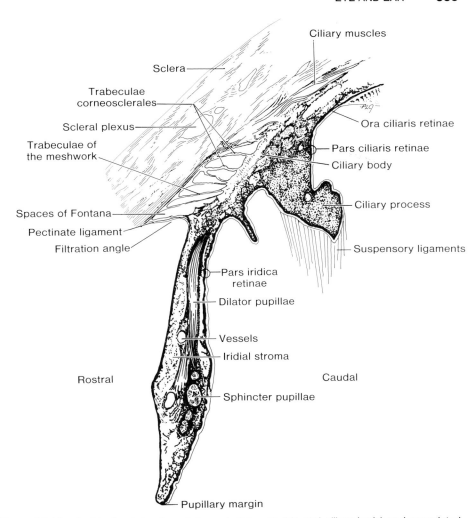

Figure 28.11. An idealized drawing of the anterior uvea (iris and ciliary body) and associated structures of a canine eye.

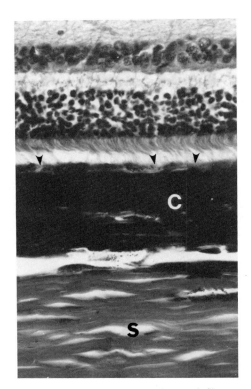

Figure 28.10. Neural, vascular, and fibrous tunics of a canine eye. The choroid coat *(C)* is peripheral to the neural tunic *(top)*. The sclera *(S)* is the most peripheral tunic. The pigment epithelium *(arrowheads)* is incompletely pigmented but is not overlaid by a tapetum lucidum. X100.

night or under reduced illumination during a fundic examination.

A *fibrous tapetum*, characteristic of many ungulates, consists of interdigitated layers of collagenous fibers, fibroblasts, smooth muscle, and melanocytes. The collagenous fibers are densely packed and their long axes are parallel to the retinal surface. Extensive fibrous lamellations are characteristic.

A *cellular tapetum* is characteristic of carnivores (Fig. 28.7). It consists of various layers of elongated, rectangular fibroblasts that have characteristic crystalline structures containing zinc *(tapetal rods)*. The tapetal cells of the dog contain high quantities of zinc cysteine hydrate, whereas feline tapetal cells contain high concentrations of riboflavin. The admixture of typical melanin granules with tapetal rods in feline tapetal cells suggests a common origin of these components. A cellular tapetum varies in thickness between species as well as within different regions of the choroid. Centrally, the layers may range from 15 (dog) to 35 (cat) cells. The number of layers diminish peripherally until the tapetum lucidum is replaced by typical choroidal stromal elements. The cells of each layer are arranged in tandem, and their long axes are oriented parallel to the retina. Successive layers of tapetal cells are separated from each other by collagenous fibers, elastic fibers, a few fibroblasts, and capillaries.

The highly pigmented, nonreflective portion of the fundus is the nontapetal region of the eye (Figs. 28.9 and 28.10). A tapetum lucidum does not occur in the eyes of swine and man.

The tapetum lucidum is visible because the underlying pigment epithelium of the retina is nonpigmented in these foci. The gradual acquisition of pigment by these cells is accompanied by the gradual diminution of the tapetum lucidum and its ultimate replacement by typical elements of the substantia propria. So, nontapetal regions of the ocular fundus are not overlaid by a peripherally positioned tapetum lucidum.

Choriocapillary layer. The *choriocapillary layer (lamina choroidocapillaris)* is rich in capillaries. These vessels not only supply nourishment to choroidal elements but provide the nourishment for the pigment epithelium of the pars optica retinae.

The choriocapillary vessels are juxtaposed intimately to the pigment epithelium. These vessels and their perivascular components are polarized. The endothelial cells adjacent to the retinal component are thin and fenestrated. The fenestrations are covered by membranous diaphragms. The endothelium on the scleral side of the choriocapillary layer is thick. Also, perivascular elements are confined to the scleral side of the vessels. These ultrastructural characteristics and relationships support the premise that fluid transport occurs between the choriocapillary layer and the pigment epithelium. These vessels, then, are one part of the dual vascular supply to the pars optica retinae. The other part is supplied by the retinal vessels.

Basal Complex. The *basal complex* is the interface between the choriocapillary layer of the choroid and the pigment epithelium of the pars optica retinae. Maximally, the basal complex of the rostral part of the bulb consists of collagenous and elastic fibrils sandwiched between two basement membranes, one associated with the pigment epithelium and the other underlying the endothelial cells of the choriocapillary layer. Minimally, the basal complex of the caudal aspect of the bulb consists of a fenestrated layer of elastic fibers through which the separate basement membranes fuse with each other. The basal complex is also called Bruch's membrane, elastic membrane, or glassy membrane.

Ciliary Body and Process

The *ciliary body* is the anterior continuation of the choroid (Fig. 28.11). It consists of contributions from the choroid and retina. The ciliary body begins at the *ora ciliaris retinae*, the point at which the neural portion of the retina stops (Fig. 28.12). The pigmented epithelium and a non-neural columnar cell extension of the retina continue rostrally to cover the ciliary body.

Histological Organization. The bulk of the ciliary body consists of areolar connective tissue rich in elastic fibers, an extensive capillary network, and smooth muscle (Fig. 28.13). The smooth muscle, *ciliary muscle*, consists of three layers that arise from the ciliary tendon that is attached to the sclera. Ciliary muscles of domestic animals are generally not well developed and result in poor accommodation potential.

The mass of smooth muscle, areolar connective tissue, and vasculature is bounded by an *elastic lamina*. This is the anterior continuation of *Bruch's membrane*. Inter-

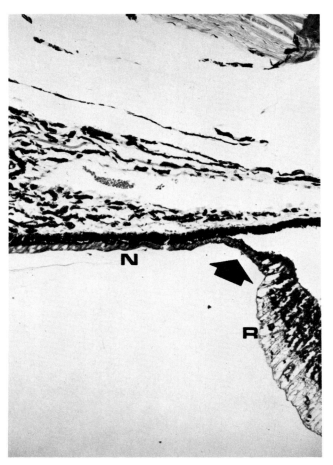

Figure 28.12. Ora ciliaris retinae of the canine eye. The ora ciliaris retinae *(arrow)* is the rostral continuation of the nonneural retina *(N)* as the double-layered epithelial covering of the ciliary body, ciliary processes, and caudal aspect of the iris. *R, pars optica retinae.* X40.

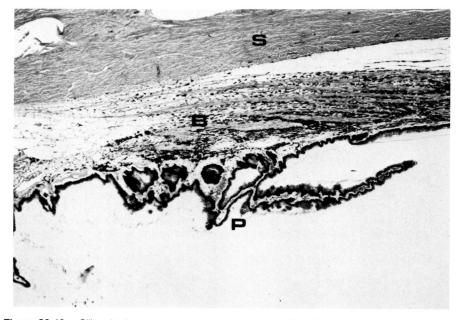

Figure 28.13. Ciliary body and processes of a canine eye. The ciliary body *(B)* and processes *(P)* are internal to the sclera *(S)*. The ciliary body and processes are part of the anterior uveal tract. The choroid comprises the posterior uvea. X10.

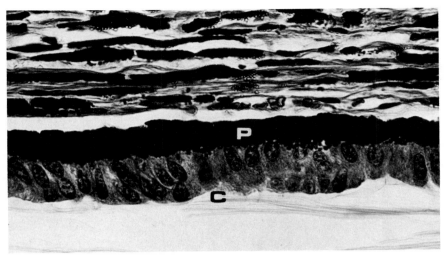

Figure 28.14. Pars ciliaris retinae of a canine eye. This double layer of cells consists of pigment epithelium *(P)* and the nonneural epithelial continuation *(C)* of the neural retina. X160.

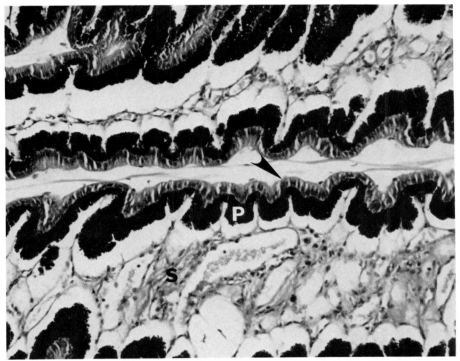

Figure 28.15. Ciliary process from an equine eye. The ciliary processes are evaginations from the ciliary body that are lined by a double layer of epithelium, the pars ciliaris retinae. The more peripheral layer consists of heavily pigmented cells *(P)* underlaid by nonpigmented epithelial cells *(arrow)*. S, stroma. X100.

sponsible for the elaboration of aqueous humor into the posterior chamber of the anterior compartment.

Functional Correlates. Contraction of the ciliary musculature does not stretch the lens and accommodate it for distant vision. Rather, contraction of the muscle fibers causes the sclera to indent slightly. This relieves tension on the suspensory fibers, causing the lens to thicken for close vision. When these muscle fibers are relaxed the elasticity for the supporting coat flattens the lens for distant vision.

Iris

The *iris* is the extension of the choroid coat into the anterior compartment (Figs. 28.11 and 28.16).

Histological Organization. The free margin of the radially oriented iris defines the *pupil*. The rostral border of the iris is not covered by a distinct limiting epithelial or endothelial lining. Rather, fibroblasts, melanocytes, and connective tissue fibers form

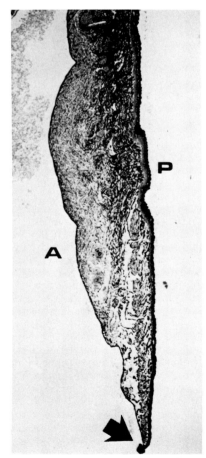

Figure 28.16. Iris of an ovine eye. The pars ciliaris retinae is continued on the caudal surface of the iris as the pars iridica retinae. A corpus nigrum *(arrow)* is obvious along the pupillary margin of the iris. *A,* anterior chamber; *P,* posterior chamber. X10.

nal to this membrane is the *basal lamina* of the *pigmented epithelium* of the retina that is continued rostrally. Internal to this cellular layer is the *ciliary epithelium*. This layer of columnar cells is the rostral continuation of nonpigmented, non-neural cells that began at the *ora ciliaris retinae*. This bilayered sheet of cells—pigmented and nonpigmented epithelia—comprises the *pars ciliaris retinae* (Fig. 28.14). The *internal limiting membrane* is a peripheral fibrillar condensation of the vitreous body. It covers the retina and ciliary body, continues rostrally and blends with the fibers that extend from the ciliary process to the lens.

The *ciliary process* is the most rostral extension of the ciliary body at the base of the iris (Fig. 28.15). Zonular fibers extend from it as suspensory fibers of the lens. The extensive capillary network of the ciliary process and associated epithelium are re-

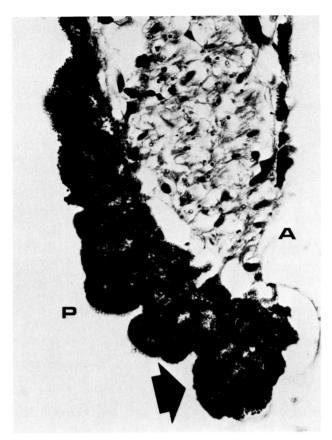

Figure 28.17. Corpus nigrum of an ovine iris. The corpus nigrum *(arrow)* is a proliferative mass of pigment epithelium and iridial stroma along the pupillary margin of the iris. *A,* anterior chamber; *P,* posterior chamber. X160.

a discontinuous lining interface with the anterior chamber. These elements constitute a *stratum avasculosum.* The spongy iridial stroma is continuous with the fluid space of the anterior chamber. Collagenous and reticular fibers often protrude directly into the anterior chamber. The *iridial stroma* consists of areolar connective tissue, blood vessels, chromatophores, and smooth muscle. The presence, absence, and distribution of iridial melanin determines iridial coloration. A blue iris is essentially devoid of stromal melanin. The blue color results from light being reflected from the pigmented component of the pars iridica retinae. Increasing the number of melanin-bearing cells in the iridial stroma changes the iridial color from blue to gray to brown. The iridial coloration of albinos is due to the vasculature.

The *pupillary sphincter* consists of a mass of circumferentially oriented smooth muscle fibers along the pupillary border of the iris. The *pupillary dilator* consists of radially oriented fibers along the caudal border of the iris.

The caudal border of the iris is covered by the same cells as the ciliary body. The cells include the anterior extension of the pigmented epithelium of the retina and the

continuation of the nonpigmented ciliary epithelial cells. These two layers of cells form the *pars iridica retinae.*

Iridial granules occur along the pupillary margin of the iris in horses and ruminants (Fig. 28.16). Iridial granules are well vascularized and proliferative extensions of the iridial stroma and pigment epithelium (Fig. 28.17). The cyst-like structures vary in size among ungulates and are most prominent along the dorsal border of the equine pupil. The corpora nigra of ruminants may be of equal size along the dorsal and ventral margin of the pupil. The iridial granules may function in the elaboration of aqueous humor, as well as occluding the central portion of the pupil when the pupillary sphincter contracts.

Functional Correlates. The iris and ciliary body comprise the *anterior uvea.* (The choroid is the *posterior uvea.*) Inflammatory changes of one of the components of the anterior uvea *(anterior uveitis)* usually affects the other because of their intimate relationship to each other.

The iris lies in direct contact with the lens, and alterations of lens curvature or position are reflected as altered iridial curvatures. Iridial pigmentation differences are characteristic of domestic animals. The dis-

tribution of iridial pigment in the dog normally imparts a two-toned *(heterochromia)* distribution of brown pigment. The feline iris is usually a single color or mixture of pigment without pigmentary zonation. The irides of ungulates are characterized by an even distribution of pigment. Hyperpigmentary changes in the iris are suggestive of chronic inflammation. Hypopigmentation of the iris is apparent in subalbinotic and albinotic animals.

Because of the method of development of the anterior chamber, varying degrees of *persistent pupillary membranes* may be observed (Fig. 28.18). Although complete obliteration of the pupil may occur, most commonly fibrous strands originating from the iris may project into the anterior chamber or attach to the iris, lens, and/or cornea.

The pupillary sphincter receives its innervation from the parasympathetic fibers originating in the Edinger-Westphal nucleus of the oculomotor nerve. The pupillary dilator receives its sympathetic innervation from postganglionic fibers originating in the cranial cervical ganglion of the sympathetic trunk. The integrity of the innervation of the two muscle masses is essential for maintaining proper muscle tone and pupillary diameter. The sympathetic innervation of the eye and periorbita maintain the smooth muscular tone of the periorbita, pupillary dilator, tarsus, and third eyelid (cat). This normal tone is manifested as normal eyeball protrusion, pupillary dilation, width of the palpebral fissure, and third eyelid retraction. Disruption of the sympathetic innervation of the eye and periorbita *(Horner's Syndrome)* may be man-

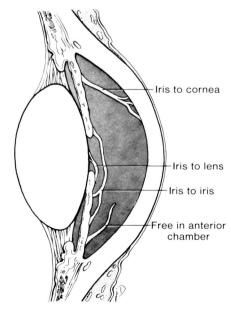

Figure 28.18. A drawing depicting the relationships of persistent iridopupillary membranes to other structures that are associated with the anterior and posterior chambers.

ifested as a: sunken eyeball *(enophthalmus)*, drooping superior palpebra *(ptosis)*, small pupil *(miosis)*, and protrusion of the third eyelid.

The parasympathetic innervation of the pupillary sphincter is the efferent limb of a II–III reflex called the *pupillary reflex.* The pupillary aperture decreases in size in response to light stimulation. Because of the cross-over of optic nerve fibers between the pretectal nuclei and the cross-over of fibers within the parasympathetic nucleus of the oculomotor nerve, the reflex contraction of the pupillary sphincter is manifested as a *direct* and *indirect (consensual)* response to light stimulation. The stimulation of one eye with light results in the contraction of the pupillary sphincter in both eyes.

Compartments of the Eye

The eye is divided into an *anterior* and *posterior compartment* by the lens, suspensory ligament, and ciliary process.

Anterior Compartment

Anterior and Posterior Chambers. The anterior compartment is delimited by the lens, suspensory ligaments, ciliary processes, ciliary body, iris, and cornea (Fig. 28.4). The anterior compartment is subdivided into *anterior* and *posterior chambers.* The posterior chamber, the region into which aqueous humor is "secreted," is bounded by the iris rostrally and the lens and its associated structures caudally. The posterior chamber communicates with the anterior chamber through the pupil. The anterior chamber, the chamber through which aqueous humor must pass before being returned to the circulation at the *filtration angle,* is bounded by the iris and cornea.

Iridial Angle. The *iridial angle (iris angle, filtration angle, iridocorneal angle)* is the peripheral margin of the anterior chamber at the region of the limbus (Fig. 28.19). The filtration angle, formed between the base of the ciliary body and iris as well as the initial caudal portion of the cornea, is filled by a triangular mass of spongy tissue, the *meshwork of the iridial angle* (Fig. 28.20). The meshwork is comprised of solid trabeculae separated by fluid spaces, the *spaces of Fontana.* The trabeculae of the meshwork consist of cores of collagenous and elastic fibers surrounded by a basement membrane upon which endothelial cells reside. The trabecular meshwork is continuous peripherally with a fine meshwork of trabeculae called the *trabeculae corneosclerales,* which are subjacent to the inner surface of the sclera. Adjacent to the anterior chamber, the trabecular meshwork coalesces as *pectinate ligaments.* The pectinate ligaments of the horse are visible at the filtration angle by direct examination, because the corneoscleral junction does not completely overlap the filtration angle.

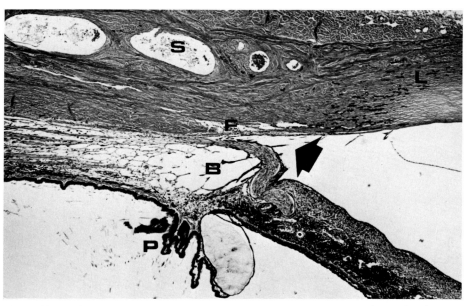

Figure 28.19. Filtration angle of a canine eye. The filtration angle *(arrow)* is located at the angle formed by the junction of the cornea, iris and ciliary body *(B).* The spaces of Fontana *(F)* are continuous with the scleral plexus *(S). L,* limbus; *P,* ciliary processes. X10.

Aqueous humor passes from the anterior chamber through the spaces between the pectinate ligaments into the spaces of the trabecular meshwork. The fluid continues through the spaces associated with the trabeculae corneosclerales to a scleral venous plexus and exits the eye via the scleral veins. The *canal of Schlemm* is a modified vein in the filtration angle that is part of the outflow tract for aqueous humor. The canal occurs in man.

Whereas aqueous humor passes freely through the filtration angle, particulate matter is trapped within the trabecular meshwork. Plugging of the meshwork with debris, as can occur in inflammation, may retard or stop the egress of aqueous humor and result in an increased intraocular pressure—*glaucoma.*

Aqueous Humor—Blood/Aqueous Barrier. Aqueous humor carries nutrients and oxygen to the lens, cornea, and retina as well as being the medium through which metabolic waste is removed from the intraocular spaces. Also, aqueous humor is the means by which intraocular pressure is maintained to ensure proper spatial relationships of ocular components. The fluid is formed by the ciliary body as an ultrafiltrate of the blood. The principles of fluid filtration are applicable, in part, to aqueous humor formation; however, the lining cells of the ciliary body utilize active transport mechanisms to secrete certain substances. The clear, watery and slightly alkaline fluid has a chemical composition similar to cerebrospinal fluid (CSF). The mechanisms involved in aqueous humor formation are similar to those utilized in CSF formation. Because of the selective nature of the epi-

thelial lining of the ciliary body in forming a fluid that differs from plasma, the boundary is called the *blood-aqueous barrier.* The actual barrier is probably comprised of the epithelial cells and their tight junctions.

Posterior Compartment

Vitreous Body. The *vitreous body (vitreous humor)* occupies the space between the lens and the retina (Fig. 28.4). The posterior compartment is filled by the vitreous body. (The posterior compartment and posterior chamber are not synonymous.) The vitreous body consists of water, some hyaluronic acid, and collagenous fibers that impart a gelatinous consistency. Despite its gelatinous nature, aqueous humor freely percolates through the vitreous body. The peripheral limit of the vitreous body is defined by the inner limiting membrane of the retina. This membrane, actually the basal lamina of the supportive cells of the retina, has collagenous fibers and fibroblast-like cells *(hyalocytes)* adjacent to it. The hyalocytes may be responsible for the synthesis of vitreous body components.

The vitreous body adheres tightly to the *optic papilla, ora ciliaris retinae, orbicularis ciliaris* (darkly pigmented and ridged portion of the ciliary body), and *posterior lens capsule.* A hyaloid canal passing through the vitreous body somewhat parallel to the optical axis is the remanant of the hyaloid artery.

Lens

The lens is one of the *dioptric* or *refractive media* of the eye. The dioptric media include all entities through which incoming

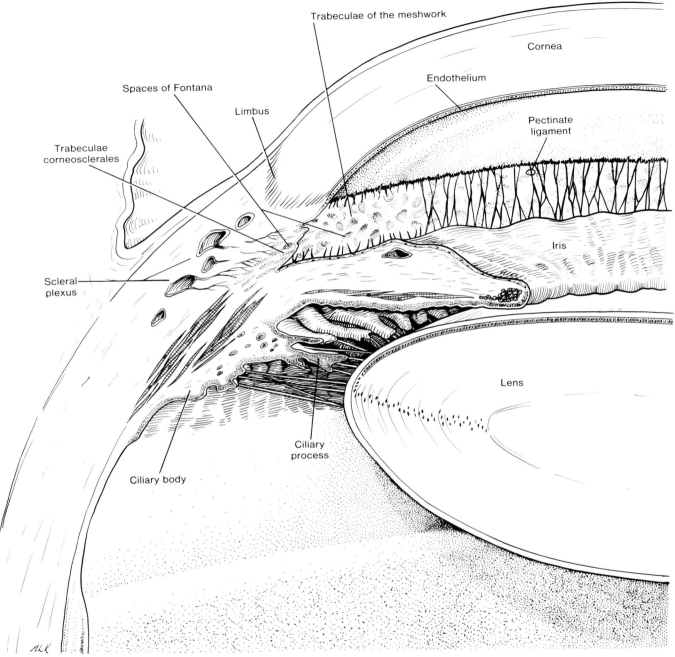

Figure 28.20. A three-dimensional drawing of the filtration angle and associated structures.

light rays must pass to reach the photoreceptor cells—cornea, aqueous humor, lens, vitreous body, and retina. The cornea and lens are the most important refractive media and exert the greatest influence upon incoming light rays. The lens is responsible for focusing light rays on the retina. The components of the lens are the *capsule, lens epithelium,* and *lens fibers.*

Capsule. The *lens capsule* completely envelopes the lens and consists of a basement membrane and fine reticular fibers (Fig. 28.21). The transparent capsule does not

have a uniform thickness; it is thicker near the equator and thin at the rostral and caudal poles. The caudal part of the capsule is thinner than the rostral component. The capsule, as the site of insertion of the suspensory ligaments, influences the shape of the lens. Metabolites must pass through the capsule as they move between the lens and the aqueous humor.

Epithelium. The *lens epithelium* of the adult lens is confined to the rostral surface beneath the capsule. The caudal lens epithelium, present during development, was

converted to lens fibers during early lens development. The rostral epithelium is cuboidal at the pole and becomes elongated at the equator forming the *lens bow* as the cells are converted to *lens fibers.* The lens fibers are elongated, modified cells that are oriented meridionally in concentric laminae around the lens. The most primitive lens fibers located at the periphery in the lens *cortex* contain nuclei. Progressive differentiation results in their conversion to typical anucleated fibers. The shape of the lens fibers in section and the nature of their

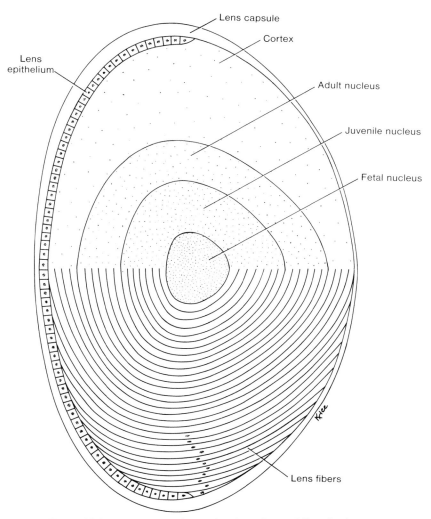

Lens capsule

Cortex

Adult nucleus

Juvenile nucleus

Fetal nucleus

Lens epithelium

Lens fibers

Figure 28.21. A diagram of a section through an adult canine lens.

relationships with each other varies. Large protrusions characterize the individual fibers of the lens bow. These protrusions become regularly shaped ball and socket interdigitations. Similarly, *flaps* and *imprints* characterize the interlocking processes of adult cortical lens fibers (Fig. 28.22).

The inner portion of the lens is called the *nucleus*. Fetal, juvenile, and adult nuclei may be evident as concentric zones of lens fibers. Older fibers are more dense, less transparent, and less elastic than younger fibers. The rostral and caudal apices of the elongated lens fibers contact each other at points called *sutures* (Fig. 28.23). The sutures, often called *lens stars*, are Y-shaped regions of lens fiber contact. An amorphous cementing substance binds the hexagonal-shaped lens fibers together. The amorphous material and the interdigitations of lens fibers at the rostral and caudal pole account for the formation of visible sutures.

Functional Correlates. The lens capsule is semipermeable and helps to regulate the low, glucose-based metabolism of the lens.

Most of the metabolism of the lens is anaerobic and is limited to the rostral epithelium and cortical lens fibers.

The posterior lens capsule is tightly adherent to the vitreous body (dog, horse). The adherent relationship between these two structures precludes the possibility of intracapsular delivery of a lens. In man, the limited attachment of the lens to the vitreous body via the ring-like *hyaloideocapsular ligament* permits the intracapsular removal of the lens.

The transparency of the lens is achieved through the registration and tight packing of the constituent lens fibers. The gradual hardening of nuclear lens fibers is a characteristic aging change called *nuclear sclerosis*. Other disruptions to lens fiber orientation and relationships—vacuolation, lens protein precipitation—result in a loss of transparency called *cataracts*.

Nervous Tunic

Organization of the Retina

The *retina* or *nervous tunic* is responsible

for the reception and transduction of light stimuli and the transmission of these signals in the form of nerve impulses to the appropriate portions of the brain. Cells of the retina are not confined to the photosensitive retina. The retina continues as a non-nervous (nonphotosensitive) layer of epithelial cells and pigment epithelium associated with the ciliary body and iris. The point of transition from retina to nonphotosensitive epithelial cells is called the *ora ciliaris retinae* in domestic animals and the *ora serrata* in man. At this point the nonphotosensitive epithelial cells and pigment cells of the retina are juxtaposed as a cellular bilayer. The rostral continuation of the cellular bilayer in association with the ciliary body is called the *pars ciliaris retinae*, whereas the cellular bilayer in association with the caudal iridial surface comprises the *pars iridica retinae*. An understanding of the developmental relationships within the eye serves to clarify these relationships. The inner and outer laminae of the optic vesicle were monolayers of cells. The inner lamina caudal to the ora ciliaris retinae proliferated to produce the characteristic cellular stratification of the retina. The inner lamina, rostral to the ora ciliaris retinae, remained a cellular monolayer. The outer wall, rostral and caudal to the ora ciliaris retinae retained its monolayer characteristics as the pigment epithelium. The intimate juxtaposition of these two monolayers of cells forms the characteristic bilayers rostral to the ora ciliaris retinae. The subsequent discussion is confined to the photosensitive portion of the retina.

The retina *(pars optica retinae)* is divisible into ten distinct layers (Figs. 28.24 and 28.25): *pigment epithelium, photoreceptor cell layer, external limiting membrane, outer nuclear layer, outer plexiform layer, inner nuclear layer, inner plexiform layer, ganglionic cell layer, optic nerve fiber layer,* and *inner limiting membrane.*

Pigment Epithelium. The *pigment epithelium* resides on a basal lamina adjacent to the elastic membrane of the choroid. These cells are cuboidal with a paracentrally positioned nucleus and centrally disposed pigment granules. Long cellular processes extend between the photoreceptors. Under high illumination, pigment moves into the cellular processes and prevents diffusion of the light to adjacent receptors. The intimate contact of the pigmented cells with the photoreceptors is apparently necessary for visual pigment synthesis. Current evidence suggests that the pigment epithelial cells may be a storage site for vitamin A. Additionally, the pigment epithelial cells phagocytize the continually growing and shedding outer segments of the rods and cones. *Lamellar phagosomes* and subsequent degradation products are common organelles within these cells.

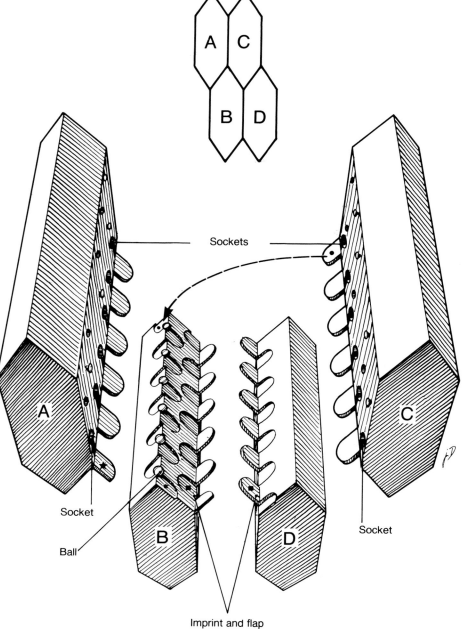

Figure 28.22. Diagrams of the relationships of lens fibers in the eye of a bird. The lens fibers are interdigitated tightly *(top)*. The exploded view *(bottom)* demonstrates the devices used for their attachment with each other. The ball on *B* fits into the socket formed by the juxtaposition of *A* and *C*. The imprint and flap *(black boxes)* on *B* and *D* fit together tightly. Similarly, the imprint an flap (★) on *A* and *B* are intimately juxtaposed to each other. Finally, the flap and imprint *(black dot)* on *C* and *B* fit together. These relationships have been simplified for clarification.

Sockets

Socket

Ball

Imprint and flap

Socket

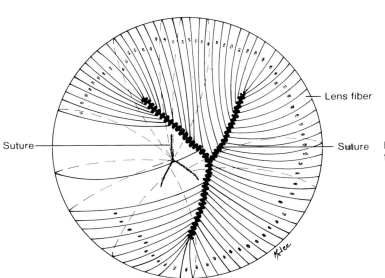

Suture

Lens fiber

Suture

Figure 28.23. A diagram illustrating the relationship of the lens fibers to the rostral and caudal sutures.

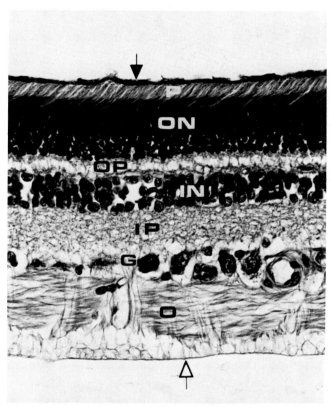

Figure 28.24. Retina of a canine eye. *Solid arrow,* pigment epithelium; *P,* photoreceptor cell layer; *ON,* outer nuclear layer; *OP,* outer plexiform layer; *IN,* inner nuclear layer; *IP,* inner plexiform layer; *G,* ganglion cell layer; *O,* optic nerve fiber layer; *Open arrow,* inner limiting membrane. The outer limiting membrane is not apparent. X100. (N.B.: The photoreceptor cell layer is positioned away from incoming light rays).

Photoreceptor Layer. The *photoreceptor layer* consists of the rods and cones. These are modified neuronal processes of the photoreceptor rod and cone cells that are described in detail after the description of the retinal layers.

Outer Nuclear Layer. The *outer nuclear layer* is comprised of the nuclei of the photoreceptor cells.

Outer Plexiform Layer. The *outer plexiform layer* consists of axons of the photoreceptor cells, the dendrites of the subjacent bipolar neurons, as well as the fibers from association neurons located in this zone or the periphery of the subjacent nucler zone.

Inner Nuclear Layer. The *inner nuclear layer* contains the cell bodies of bipolar neurons and association neurons.

Inner Plexiform Layer. The *inner plexiform layer* consists of axons of the bipolar neurons, the dendrites of subjacent ganglionic cells, and the processes of association neurons.

Ganglionic Cell Layer. The *ganglionic cell layer* consists of the cell bodies of the ganglion cells.

Optic Nerve Fiber Layer. The *optic nerve fiber layer* consists of axonal processes of the ganglion cells that are directed toward

the *optic papilla (blind spot)* and emerge from the eye as the optic nerve (Fig. 28.26).

Limiting Membranes. The *internal limiting membrane* consists of fibrillar material (basal lamina) and the conjoined processes of the supporting Müller cells. The *outer limiting membrane,* located just peripheral to the outer nuclear layer, is an incomplete structure formed by the processes of Müller cells forming junctions with the cell bodies of the photoreceptor cells. The cell bodies of these cells are located in the inner nuclear area. The peripheral processes form the external or outer limiting membrane, whereas their internal processes abut on the outer surface of the inner limiting membrane.

Despite the apparent complexity of the retina, it may be simplified by recognizing that it consists of three neurons in succession with intervening regions of synapses. Also, light must pass through the retina in order to stimulate the photoreceptor cells.

Ocular Fundus

The area of most acute vision in domestic animals is the *area centralis retinae.* Cone cells, bipolar neurons, and ganglion

cells are increased in number in this area. Although a depression *(fovea centralis)* does not occur in domestic species, this macular region is comparable to that which occurs in man.

The retina of most species is regularly curved along the posterior portion of the globe of the eye. The horse, however, has a *ramp retina.* The retina in these animals is irregularly curved along the posterior surface in such a manner as to permit different axial lengths associated with near and far vision. A rotation of the eye for near vision results in a long focal distance.

Photoreceptor Cells

The cells that comprise the retina include *pigment epithelium, photoreceptor cells, bipolar neurons, ganglionic cells, association neurons,* and *neuroglial elements.*

The *photoreceptor cells* are neuroepithelial cells modified for the reception, transduction, and transmission of visual stimuli. The cells are the *rod cells* and *cone cells.*

Rod Cells. The *rods* consist of an *outer segment, connecting cilium, inner segment, outer rod fiber, perikaryon, inner rod fiber,* and *rod spherule* (Fig. 28.27). The outer segment is an elongated process of the cell that contains numerous double-membraned lamellae and the visual pigment, *rhodopsin.* Nine doublets of microtubules (devoid of a central pair) continue through the *connecting cilium* to terminate in a typical basal body within the expanded inner segment. The inner segment narrows as the outer rod fiber. This is continuous with the perikaryon. The inner rod fiber or axon terminates in a swelling, the *rod spherule,* and synapses with the dendrite of a bipolar neuron.

Cone Cells. The *cones* are similar to the rods (Fig. 28.27). The lamellae of the outer segment are often continuous with the plasmalemma. This segment, which is larger than that of the rods, contains *iodopsin.* The connecting cilium is not constricted. The inner and outer segments, therefore, have a cone-like appearance. The nucleus of the cones does not contain as much dense chromatin as that of the rods. Also, the cell bodies are located in the outer portion of the outer nuclear layer.

The rods are generally distributed throughout the retina, whereas the cones are the predominant or only type of photoreceptor in the *area centralis retinae.* This is the region for bright light vision and is the area of most acute vision. The remaining portion of the retina, rich in rods, is for dark-adapted vision. There is wide species variation in the distribution of the type of photoreceptor cells.

Müller cells are neuroglial elements unique to the retina. *Astrocytes, oligodendroliocytes,* and *microgliocytes* are present and typical. *Amacrine cells* and *horizontal*

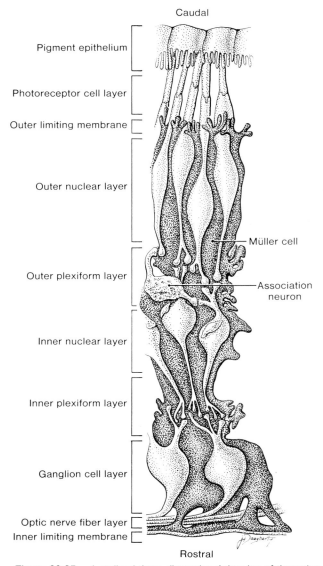

Caudal

Pigment epithelium

Photoreceptor cell layer

Outer limiting membrane

Outer nuclear layer

Müller cell

Outer plexiform layer

Association neuron

Inner nuclear layer

Inner plexiform layer

Ganglion cell layer

Optic nerve fiber layer
Inner limiting membrane

Rostral

Figure 28.25. A stylized three-dimensional drawing of the retina.

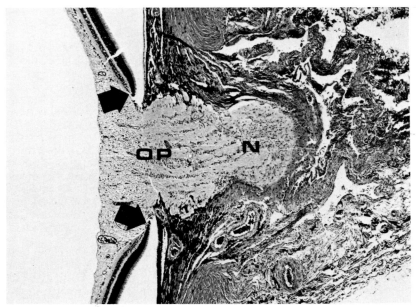

Figure 28.26. Optic papilla of a canine eye. The neural retina stops *(arrows)* and the optic nerve fibers continue into the optic papilla *(OP).* The fibers continue as the optic nerve *(N).* X10.

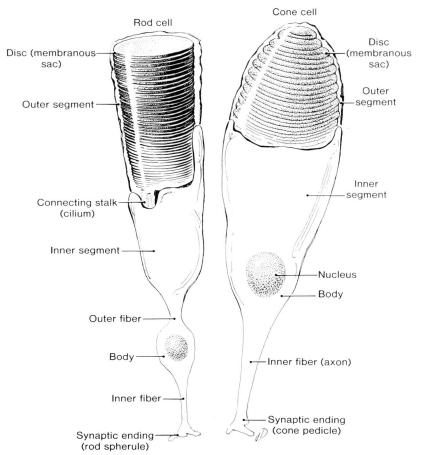

Figure 28.27.   A stylized three-dimensional drawing of rod and cone cells. The discs are folds of membranes that contain the visual pigments rhodopsin (rods) and iodopsin (cones) and are formed at the base of the outer segment. The discs of rods lose contact with the plasmalemma, whereas those of the cones remain attached to the plasma membrane of the outer segment.

cells are association neurons within the retina that serve to modify the visual stimuli from other cells of the retina. The *horizontal cells* are in contact with groups of rods. The amacrine cells are in contact with bipolar cells, ganglion cells, and other amacrine cells.

Retinal Blood Supply

Outer Layers. The outermost layers of the retina—pigment epithelium through outer plexiform layer—are devoid of blood vessels. The vessels of the choriocapillary layer are the blood supply for the outermost regions of the retina.

Retinal Arteries. The retinal artery is the viable remnant of the hyaloid artery in man. The intimate relationship of the artery to the optic nerve was established during the development of the choroid fissure. The central artery of the optic nerve is the source of the retinal artery and its branches in man. The retinal arteries and their branches are derived from posterior ciliary arteries in domestic animals. The retinal arteries supply those portions of the retina not nourished by the choriocapillary layer of the choroid coat. The distribution of retinal vessels varies among the domestic species. Most of the domestic animals (large and small ruminants, swine, carnivores), rats, mice, and primates have a *holangiotic* vascular pattern characterized by major retinal vessels emanating from the optic papilla. The horse and guinea pig have a *paurangiotic* vascular pattern characterized by a few small vessels restricted to the area of the optic papilla. A *merangiotic* vascular pattern (rabbit) is one in which only a limited portion of the retina has obvious vessels emerging from the optic papilla. The fundus of avian species and some mammals (chinchilla, armadillo, sloth, bat) is devoid of obvious vessels *(anangiotic)*.

Ocular Adnexa

Eyelids

General Structure. The eyelids *(palpebrae)* are folds of skin that cover the anterior surface of the eye (Fig. 28.28). The external surface is covered with stratified squamous epithelium and underlaid by the dermis. Fine hairs, sweat glands, and sebaceous glands are present. The glands are especially well-developed in the pig. The margin of the upper eyelid is characterized by thick hairs. Sweat and sebaceous glands are associated with them. Occasionally, sinus hairs may be present. Hairs are either small or absent (dog, pig) along the margin of the lower eyelid.

At the margin of the eyelids the skin is continued by a cutaneous mucous membrane *(palpebral conjunctiva)*. The lamina epithelialis mucosae of the internal surface *(conjuctiva)* varies throughout its distribution. It may be stratified columnar or stratified squamous with goblet cells. At the point of reflection on to the surface of the cornea, it is stratified squamous.

The DWFCT of the dermis and lamina propria mucosae fuses centrally as the *tarsus*. The tarsus consists of laminae of collagenous fibers. The extent of the tarsus corresponds to the shape of the eyeball covered by the palpebra. The tarsus is not as well-developed in domestic animals as it is in man. Anterior to the tarsus are bundles of striated muscle fibers of the *orbicularis oculi* and the *levator palpebrae superioris*. Smooth muscle is present also.

Palpebral Glands. The *tarsal glands (glands of Meibom)* are modified sebaceous

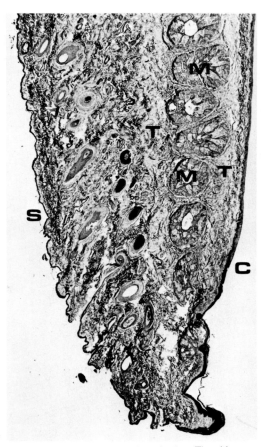

Figure 28.28.   A section of a palpebra. The skin *(S)* is reflected at the margin of the lid as the palpebral conjunctiva *(C)*. The palpebra contains Meibomian glands *(M)* within a core of DWFCT, the tarsus *(T)*. X4.

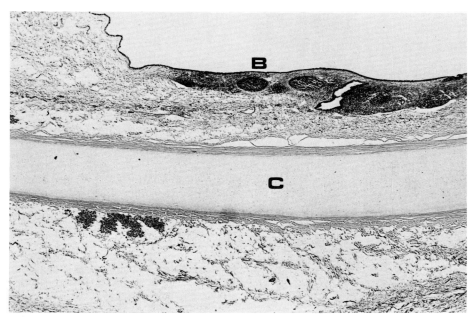

Figure 28.29. A portion of a bovine nictitating membrane. The bulbar surface *(B)* has lymphatic nodules associated with it. The core of the structure is hyaline cartilage *(C)*. X4.

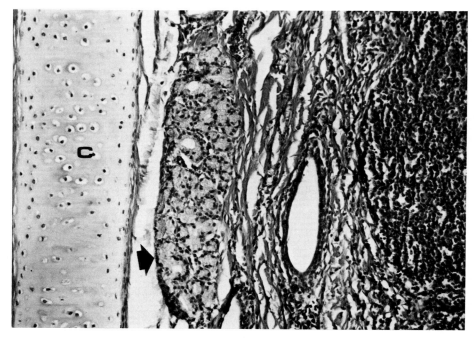

Figure 28.30. Canine nictitating membrane. The cartilage (C) is closely associated with superficial glands of the organ *(arrow)*. These are seromucoid glands. X40.

glands that open at the margin of the eyelid (Fig. 28.28). These glands are better developed in the upper eyelid than in the lower eyelid. Sweat glands open anterior to the cilia or into the follicle of the cilia. These *ciliary glands (glands of Moll)* are modified sweat glands that assume a spiral rather than a coiled configuration. These glands are a constant palpebral feature of all domestic animals, but their function is unknown. The *glands of Zeiss* are sebaceous glands associated with palpebral cilia. Serous and/or seromucoid *glands of Krause* and *Wolfring* are accessory lacrimal glands that reportedly occur in the palpebral conjuctiva of domestic animals. Their presence is not consistent. Goblet cells are often present.

Nictitating Membrane

The *nictitating membrane* or *third eyelid (palpebra tertia)* is a fold of conjunctiva

that contains hyaline cartilage (ruminants, dog) or elastic cartilage (horse, pig, cat). The areolar connective tissue may contain some smooth muscle fibers (cat). Lymphatic nodules are extensive along the bulbar surface (Fig. 28.29).

The *superficial glands* of this organ surround the cartilaginous plate (Fig. 28.30). Their secretion is serous (horse, cat), seromucoid (dog, ruminants), and mucoid (pig). The *deep gland (gland of Harder)* is a mixed gland that occurs in the pig and ox (Fig. 28.31).

Lacrimal Apparatus

Constituents. The lacrimal apparatus consists of the *lacrimal glands*, the *conjunctival sac*, and the *lacrimal passages*.

The *lacrimal glands* are located at the dorsolateral margins of the orbit (Figs. 28.32 and 28.33). In the pig, the glands are mucoid.

The fluids of the *conjunctival sac* accumulate in the medial widening of the sac, *lacus lacrimalis*, enter the *lacrimal canaliculi* through the *puncta lacrimalia*, and continue to the *lacrimal sac* and thence to the *nasolacrimal duct*. The luminal surfaces of the lacrimal sac and duct are lined by a squamous or columnar epithelium (horse).

Precorneal Tear Film. Glands that moisten the corneal and conjunctival epithelia include the lacrimal gland, nictitans gland, and accessory lacrimal glands. The *accessory lacrimal glands* include: tarsal glands, ciliary glands, glands of Zeiss, Krause, and Wolfring. These glands produce a *precorneal tear film* that is about 7-μm thick. The film is divisible into three layers that have a distinct composition—superficial, aqueous, and mucoid.

The *superficial layer* consists of lipids that are secreted by the tarsal glands and glands of Zeiss. This layer limits the evaporation of the underlying aqueous layer. Also, the superficial layer provides a binding effect for the tear film through its high surface tension.

The *aqueous layer* consists primarily of water derived from the lacrimal and nictitans glands. The middle layer of the tear film subserves various functions. It flushes foreign materials from the conjunctival sac and lubricates the palpebral/corneal interfaces. The aqueous film is the medium through which oxygen, protective cells, immunoglobulins, and non-specific protective substances reach the cornea. Also, this layer fills in corneal surface defects to provide a smooth surface for the undistorted refraction of light by the cornea.

The *mucoid layer* is the mucoproteinaceous product of conjunctival cells that is interdigitated between the aqueous layer and the cornea. The corneal surface, because it consists of cellular membranes, is lipophilic and hydrophobic. The aqueous film, however, is hydrophilic and lipopho-

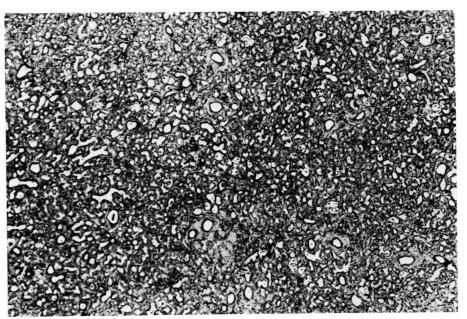

Figure 28.31. Bovine gland of Harder. This gland is seromucoid. X16.

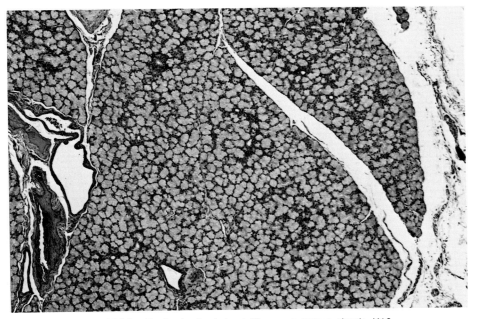

Figure 28.32. Equine lacrimal gland. These are serous glands. X16.

bic. The mucoid layer, which is probably bipolar, presents the necessary hydrophilic tail to the aqueous film and the hydrophobic tail to the corneal surface. This layer, therefore, binds the aqueous film to the cornea.

Mucous threads are accumulations of mucus at the conjunctival fornices. These threads migrate to the puncta carrying debris that collects in the conjunctival sac. Dehydrated accumulations of these threads form the "sleep" or "sand" commonly present along the nasal canthus in the morning.

Ear

General Remarks. The ear is responsible for the reception of auditory stimuli, mechanical transduction of the stimuli, and the transmission of nerve impulses to appropriate portions of the central nervous system. To accomplish these functions, the ear consists of various components: *auricle, auditory meatus, tympanic membrane, tympanic cavity with ossicles, cochlea,* and *organ of Corti.*

The ear also functions, however, as an organ of balance. The components of the vestibular portion of the inner ear include *semicircular canals, utriculus,* and *sacculus.*

External Ear

The external ear includes the *auricle* and *external auditory meatus.*

Pinna. The *auricle* or *pinna* is a sac of typical skin that contains hairs and associated glands. On the anterior surface (concave side), sebaceous glands are numerous and the frequency of hairs diminishes toward the external auditory meatus. The dermal tissue contained within the sac is typical and contains supportive structures composed of hyaline or elastic cartilage. Striated muscle associated with the movement of the ear is also contained with the fold of integument.

The pinna is the "antenna" of the auditory apparatus. In most species, it also serves the important function of "directional finding."

External Auditory Meatus. The *external auditory meatus* or canal is the tubular extension of the auricle. The surface lining of the meatus is typical skin with some hairs and numerous sebaceous and *ceruminous glands.* Ceruminous glands are modified, apocrine, tubular, sweat glands. The combined product of the ceruminous glands and the sebaceous glands, *cerumen,* is a brown waxy material that protects the canal and keeps the tympanic membrane moist and pliable.

The underlying dermis is typical and blends with the periosteum or perichondrium of the supportive bone or cartilage.

Middle Ear

The middle ear includes the *tympanic membrane, tympanic cavity, ear ossicles* and the *internal auditory meatus.* Within the middle ear, the vibrations of the air are transduced to mechanical movement of the ossicles. These, in turn, produce waves in the perilymph of the inner ear via vibrations of the membranous *oval window.*

Tympanic Membrane. The *tympanic membrane* consists of an outer and inner epithelium that covers a core of collagenous fibers. The outer epithelium *(stratum cutaneum)* is a reflection of the epithelial lining of the external auditory meatus. It is, however, hairless, glandless, and generally devoid of epidermal pegs. The core of connective tissue is divisible into two zones. A dorsally positioned region, *pars flaccida,* has few collagenous fibers. The remainder, *pars tensa,* consists of an inner circular array of collagenous fibers *(stratum circulare)* and an outer radial array of collagenous fibers *(stratum radiatum).* The perichondrial covering of the manubrium of the malleous blends with the fibers of the stratum radiatum. Peripherally, the layers of fibers are continuous with a fibrocarti-

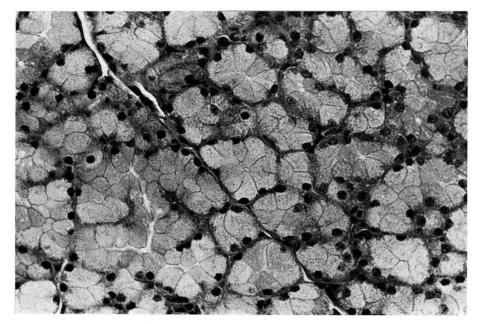

Figure 28.33. Serous lining cells of an equine lacrimal gland. X100.

laginous ring *(anulus fibrocartilagineus)* that connects the connective tissue of the tympanic membrane with the circumscribing bone. The inner epithelium *(stratum mucosum)* is a simple squamous or low cuboidal epithelium that is continuous with the lining of the tympanic cavity.

Tympanic Cavity. The *tympanic cavity* is lined by a squamous or cuboidal epithelium. At the opening of the *auditory tube (internal auditory meatus)*, ciliated columnar cells are present. The cavity contains three *auditory ossicles: malleus (hammer), incus (anvil),* and *stapes (stirrup)*. These bones are covered by a periosteum and are connected to each other by two diarthrodial joints. The handle (manubrium) of the malleus is embedded in the tympanic membrane, whereas the stapes is attached to the oval window by a fibrous joint. Two muscles are associated with these ossicles, the *tensor tympani* and *stapedius* muscles. These are striated muscles that serve to dampen the effects of high-frequency vibrations.

Auditory Tube. The *auditory tube (Eustachian tube, internal auditory meatus, pharyngotympanic tube)* connects the tympanic cavity with the nasopharynx. It is lined by respiratory epithelium—pseudostratified ciliated columnar epithelium. The lamina propria-submucosa consists of areolar connective tissue with diffuse lymphatic tissue and numerous serous and mixed glands. The connective tissue is continuous with the periosteum or perichondrium of the bone and cartilage that lines the canal. During deglutition (swallowing), the tube is opened and the air pressure within the tympanic cavity is equalized with the air pressure in the external auditory meatus.

The *guttural pouch (diverticulum tubae auditivae)* of the horse is a diverticulum of the auditory tube that is lined by a pseudostratified ciliated columnar epithelium with goblet cells. The supportive lamina propria is rich in smooth muscle fibers, elastic and collagenous fibers, serous and mucous glands, and lymph nodules.

Inner Ear

Osseous Labyrinth. The inner ear is located within the petrous portion of the temporal bone. The bone forms the *osseous labyrinth.*

Membranous Labyrinth. A *membranous labyrinth* is contained within the osseous chamber. Its shape conforms to that of the osseous labyrinth and consists of squamous epithelium throughout most of its distribution. The membranous labyrinth contains *endolymph* and is surrounded by *perilymph*. The endolymph is a peculiar extracellular fluid that has ion concentrations that are similar to intracellular fluid; i.e., it has high K^+ and low Na^+ concentrations. These concentrations contribute to a potential difference between the endolymph and the surrounding perilymph. The potential may be related to the transduction function of the hair cells associated with the membranous labyrinth.

Endolymph is believed to be produced by the *stria vascularis* of the cochlear duct. The fluid is drained into the venous sinuses of the dura mater by the endolymphatic duct.

Perilymph is probably tissue fluid that is produced by the periosteal blood vessels associated with the osseous labyrinth. The perilymph is drained into the subarachnoid space by the perilymphatic duct.

The form of the membranous labyrinth is complex, for it is divided into numerous sacs and canals that are interconnected and separated by bone. The subdivisions of the membranous labyrinth include *utriculus, sacculus, endolymphatic duct, endolymphatic sac, semicircular canals, ductus reuniens,* and the *ductus cochlearis* (Fig. 28.34). The latter is involved with auditory

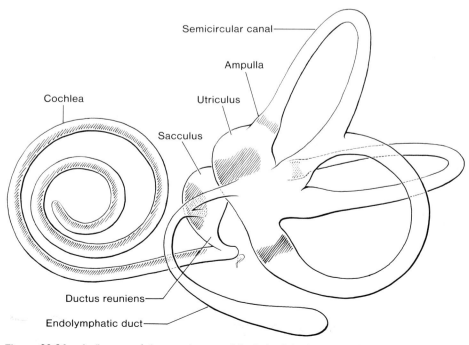

Figure 28.34. A diagram of the membranous labyrinth of the inner ear. The *hatched areas* are locations of sensory receptors.

sensations, whereas the saccule, utricle, and semicircular canals are involved in balance.

Vestibular Apparatus

General Remarks. The vestibular apparatus is that special sensory organ that is concerned with awareness of the position of the body (Fig. 28.35). Two types of sensations are involved in this sense: *static sensation* and *kinetic sensation*. Special sensory regions of the saculus and utriculus (*macula sacculi* and *macula utriculi*) contain substances that respond constantly to gravity. Other sensory areas *(cristae ampullares)* of the semicircular canals respond to movement of endolymphatic fluid and are responsible for the kinetic sensations of angular acceleration.

Hair Cells—Polarized Transducers. *Hair cells* are the specialized, non-neural, receptor cells of the vestibular and cochlear apparatus. They are the common sensory cells of the macula utriculi, macula sacculi, cristae ampullares, and the organ of Corti.

Vestibular hair cells are designated Type I and II (Fig. 28.36). *Type I hair cells* are round cells with a constricted neck. A cup-like afferent neuronal ending encircles the entire cell. Numerous efferent terminals synapse with the cup-like afferent ending probably exerting an inhibitory influence upon the ·afferent terminal. *Type II hair cells* are columnar cells the bases of which are innervated by afferent and efferent neuronal terminals. Sustentacular cells separate and support the hair cells. The apical surface of the hair cell is characterized by bundles of cilia that have a distinct polarity. Numerous stereocilia (about 40–80 per cell) become longer toward one pole. The long stereocilia are adjacent to a single kinocilium that has the typical axonemal 9 + 2 pattern.

Shearing of the cilia results in altered discharge rates associated with these cells (Fig. 28.37). As the stereocilia are sheared toward the kinocilium, the hair cells depolarize and increase their rate of discharge. As the cilia are sheared away from the kinocilium, the cells become hyperpolarized and their discharge frequency decreases. Depolarization with the resulting increased frequency discharge is excitatory, whereas hyperpolarization with its decreased frequency discharge is inhibitory. This is the means by which mechanical stimuli—movement of endolymph and otoconia—are converted into useful information.

Utriculus and Sacculus. These portions of the membranous labyrinth are lined by a squamous or cuboidal epithelium, except in the sensory regions. The sensory regions are similar to each other, but they are oriented perpendicular to each other.

The *macula utriculi* and the *macula sacculi* are responsible for the static sensations associated with balance. The epithelium of

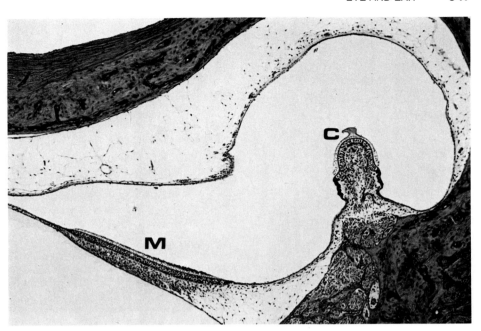

Figure 28.35. A semicircular canal and utriculus. The macula utriculus *(M)* and one of the three cristae ampullares *(C)* are apparent. X16.

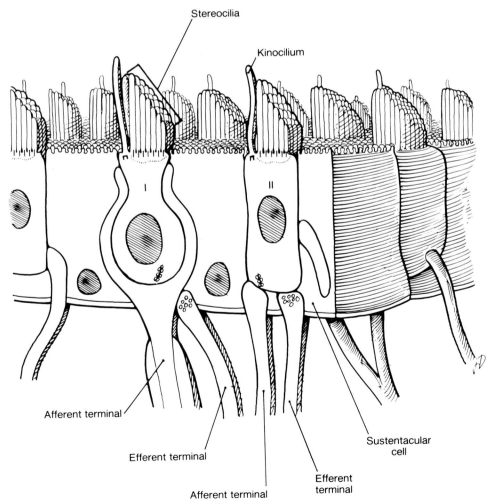

Figure 28.36. A diagram of hair cells and sustentacular cells of the vestibular apparatus. Numerous afferent and efferent terminals are associated with the vestibular hair cells.

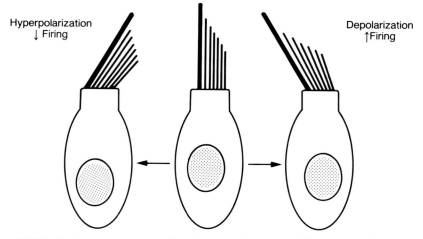

Hyperpolarization
↓ Firing

Depolarization
↑Firing

Figure 28.37. Surface shearing and alteration to discharge rate. The center configuration is the configuration associated with a resting discharge rate. Shearing away from the kinocilium *(left)* causes hyperpolarization and a decreased discharge rate. Shearing toward the kinocilium *(right)* causes depolarization and an increased discharge rate. Shearing as depicted in these drawings results from endolymphatic fluid movement within the semicircular canals.

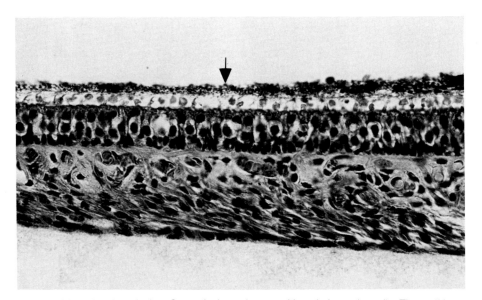

Figure 28.38. Macula utriculus. Otoconia *(arrow)* are positioned above the cells. The otoliths are embedded within a gelatinous material. X100.

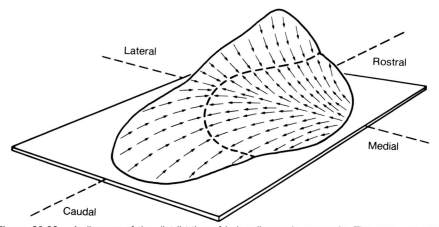

Lateral

Rostral

Medial

Caudal

Figure 28.39. A diagram of the distribution of hair cell axes in a macula. The axes are oriented toward a curvilinear region called the striola. This type of orientation ensures vestibular input for all head positions.

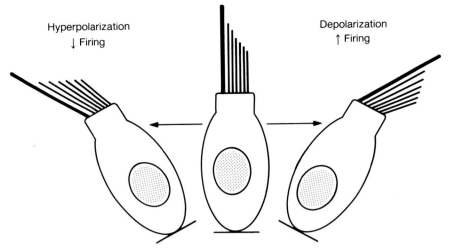

Hyperpolarization
↓ Firing

Depolarization
↑ Firing

Figure 28.40. A diagram of hair cell shearing in a macula. Head tilt achieves the same result as fluid movement. Compare with Figure 28.37.

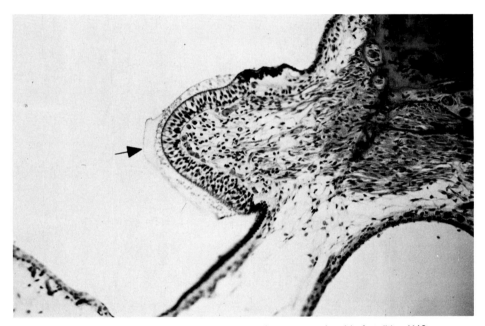

Figure 28.41. The cupula *(arrow)* is a gelatinous mass devoid of otoliths. X40.

these sensory regions consists of sensory cells and sustentacular cells (Fig. 28.36). There are two types of sensory cells in the maculae—Type I and II as described previously. The stereocilia and kinocilia of both of these cells are not free in the endolymph. Rather, they are embedded in a gelatinous matrix that contains *otoconia* or *otoliths* (Fig. 28.38). These are concretions of calcium carbonate and protein that move in response to gravity as the position of the head changes. The gelatinous material and otoliths are referred to as the *otolithic membrane*.

The hair cells of the maculae are oriented in a specific pattern that is characterized by ciliary bundles being oriented in various directions. This ensures that the cells are able to respond to various directional movements of the otolithic membrane. The orientation of the ciliary bundles is from small stereocilia to the kinocilium. This orientation is represented diagrammatically as an arrow in which the arrow head represents the kinocilium. All of the hair cells are oriented toward a curvilinear landmark called the striola (Fig. 28.39). Movement in any direction ensures that some cells are depolarized while others are hyperpolarized (Fig. 28.40). The dual signal provides an accurate monitoring mechanism of head position.

The *sustentacular cells* are nonciliated columnar cells. They support and nurture the other cells with which they are associated.

The basal margins of the sensory cells are surrounded by nerve endings that arise from the vestibular branch of the auditory nerve.

Semicircular Canals. The semicircular canals are tubules that arise from the utriculus. The three canals are oriented perpendicular to each other. There are three sensory areas, *cristae ampullares*, located at the bulbous enlargements (ampullae) of the canals close to the point of contact with the utriculus (Fig. 28.35).

The lining of the semicircular canals is simple squamous or cuboidal. In the sensory regions, the epithelium is thickened and a mound of cells is formed (Fig. 28.41). The constituent cells are similar to those described with the maculae. However, otoliths are not present in the conical mass of gelatinous material, the *cupula*.

The currents of the endolymph during movement distort the cupula and embedded hairs accounting for kinesthetic sensation.

Auditory Apparatus

General Remarks. The auditory apparatus is responsible for the reception of auditory stimuli, the transduction of the mechanical signal, the transmission of nerve impulses to the central nervous system, and the dissipation of the energy of the auditory signal. This is accomplished through the *ductus cochlearis, scala vestibuli,* and *scala tympani.*

The cochlear duct is part of the membranous labyrinth and is connected to the vestibular apparatus by the *ductus reuniens.* The scala vestibuli and scala tympani are perilymphatic spaces that surround the cochler duct. The scala vestibuli is continuous with the scala tympani at the *helicotrema.* This is the apex of the spirally arranged organ.

The movement of the stapes causes a corresponding movement in the oval window. In turn, this causes waves to move through the perilymph of the scala vestibuli. These waves ascend in the scala vestibuli, communicate with the scala tympani at the helicotrema, descend within the perilymph of the scala tympani and dissipate at the *round window.* The latter is a fibrous covering in the wall of the tympanic cavity.

Cochlea. The cochlear duct, scala vestibuli, and scala tympani are disposed in a spiral manner within the osseous labyrinth of the petrous portion of the temporal bone (Fig. 28.42). A central core of bone, the *modiolus,* and its lateral projections, the *bony spiral lamina,* support the membranous subdivisions of the *cochlea.* Fibrous connective tissue extends from the *spiral lamina* to the outer wall of the osseous labyrinth forming the *basilar membrane.* Another fibrous sheath extends from the spiral lamina and passes obliquely to the outer wall of the osseous laybrinth forming the vestibular membrane. The osseous labyrinth, therefore, is subdivided into three membranous compartments (Fig. 28.43).

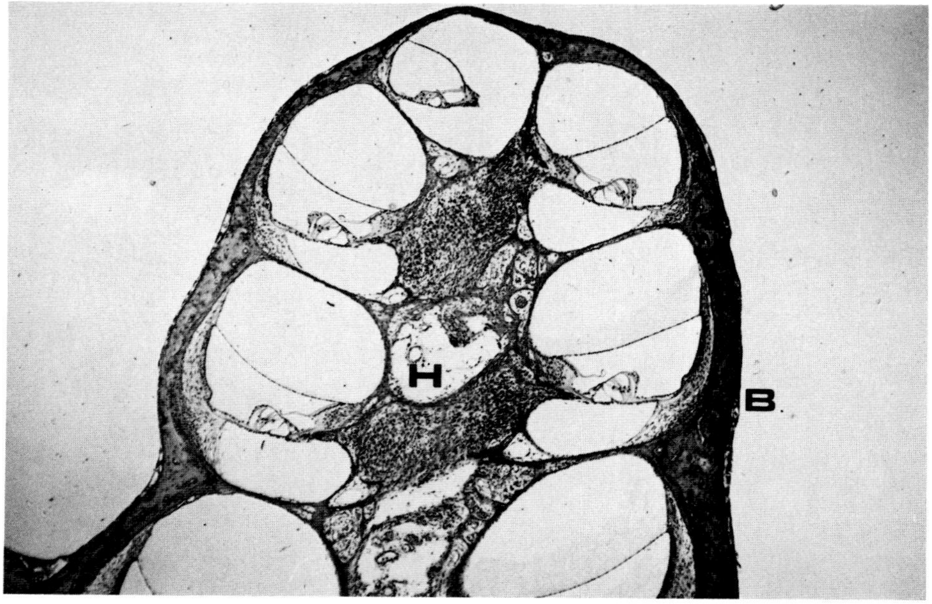

Figure 28.42. The auditory apparatus. The cochlea is embedded within the bone *(B)* of the petrous portion of the temporal bone. The modiolus *(H)* is the central core of supporting bone. X10.

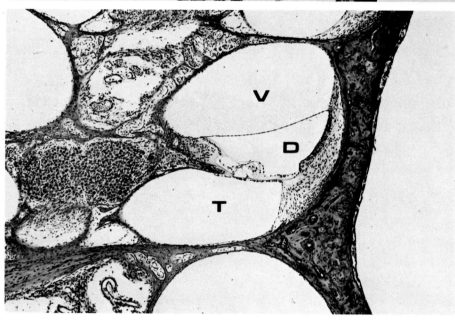

Figure 28.43. The cochlea. The cochlea is divided into compartments. *V*, scala vestibuli; *D*, cochlear duct; *T*, scala tympani. X16.

Figure 28.44. The cochlear duct. *D*, cochlear duct; *V*, scala vestibuli; *R*, Reissner's membrane; *T*, scala tympani; *B*, basilar membrane; *S*, stria vascularis; *L*, spiral ligament; *M*, tectorial membrane. X40.

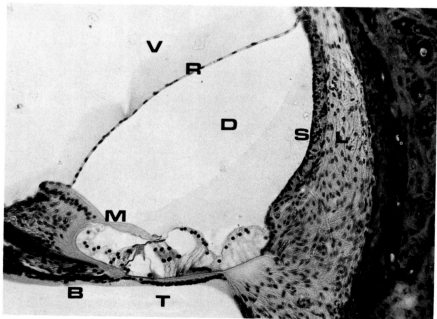

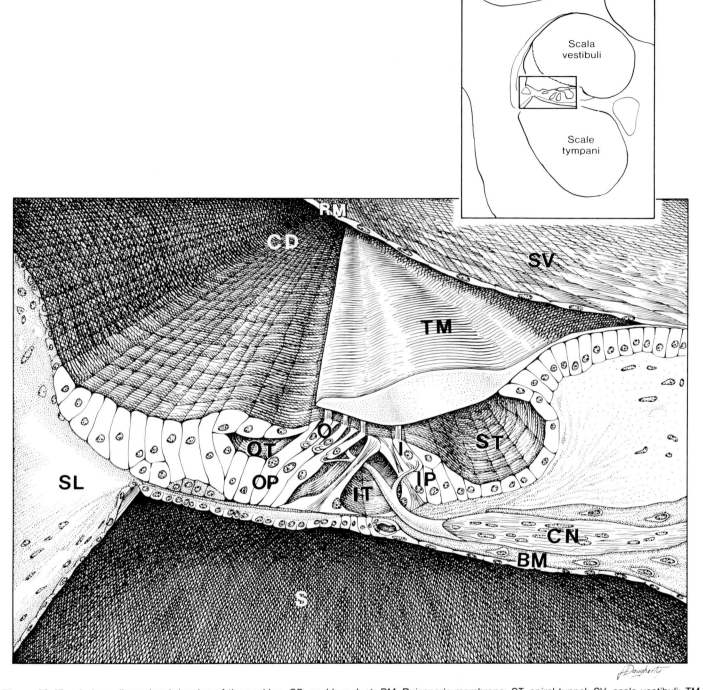

Figure 28.45. A three-dimensional drawing of the cochlea. *CD*, cochlear duct; *RM*, Reissner's membrane; *ST*, spiral tunnel; *SV*, scala vestibuli; *TM*, tectorial membrane; *O*, outer hair cells; *I*, inner hair cells; *OT*, outer tunnel; *OP*, outer phalangeal cells; *SL*, spiral ligament; *IT*, inner tunnel; *BM*, basilar membrane; *CN*, cochlear nerve; *IP*, inner phalangeal cells; *S*, scala tympani.

The dorsal compartment, *scala vestibuli*, is lined by a squamous epithelium. The middle compartment, *cochlear duct*, is lined by various epithelial types. Adjacent to the scala vestibuli, the lining is squamous. Thus, the *vestibular membrane* consists of two laminae of squamous cells and a thin central core of collagenous fibers. The lining of the ventral duct, the *scala tympani*, is similar to that of the scala vestibuli.

Nerve fibers of the auditory nerve ascend through the osseous modiolus and pass laterally to the *organ of Corti* which is contained within the cochlear duct.

The cochlear duct is an endolymphatic space continuous with the vestibular apparatus through the ductus reuniens (Fig. 28.44). The squamous cells adjacent to the scala vestibuli aid in the formation of the vestibular membrane *(Reissner's mem-*

brane). The lateral or outer wall of the cochlear duct is composed of a bistratified layer of cuboidal or columnar cells. This region is referred to as the *stria vascularis*. It is underlaid by connective tissue, the *spiral ligament*, which is highly vascularized. The stria vascularis is believed to be responsible for the productin of endolymph. The basal cells of this region continue as the *spiral prominence* and are continuous with the cuboidal lining cells of the basilar membrane.

The *basilar membrane* is the supportive structure for the *organ of Corti*. The organ of Corti consist of *sensory (hair) cells, sustentacular cells*, and a *tectorial membrane*. The hair cells have numerous stereocilia projecting from them arranged in a V pattern. In young organisms a central kinocilium is usually present at the base of the V. It is usually lost in adults. The sustentacular cells are numerous and varied. They, in conjunction with the hair cells, account for the complex morphology of the organ of Corti. The *tectorial membrane* is a fibrous and gelatinous, tongue-like structure that rests upon the hair cells. It is believed to be a secretory product of specific supportive cells, the *interdental cells*.

The following disposition of sensory and sustentacular cells accounts for the complexity of this organ. Besides the neuroepithelial cells, the organ includes: *inner* and *outer pillar cells, inner* and *outer phalangeal cells, interdental cells, border cells, cells of Hensen* and the *tectorial membrane, the outer tunnel (tunnel of Corti* and the *spiral tunnel* (Figs. 28.44 and 28.45).

The *inner* and *outer pillar* cells are narrow triangular cells with broad bases and narrow apices. Microtubules are prominent in these cells. These cells are joined at their apices and delimit the *inner tunnel.*

The *inner phalangeal cells* are medial to the inner pillar cells. They are columnar cells with a cuplike depression that almost totally surrounds the *inner hair cell.* The inner hair cell is a goblet-like cell. Nerve terminals are associated with it in the space between the hair cell and the inner phalangeal cell. The inner phalangeal cells gradually diminish in size and are transformed into squamous *border cells* which, with the

tectorial membrane and inner phalangeal cells, define the spiral tunnel.

The border cells are continuous with columnar cells, *interdental cells*, which probably secrete the tectorial membrane.

The *outer phalangeal cells* are adjacent to the outer pillar cells. They are columnar cells with a cup-shaped depression which supports the outer hair cells. A cytoplasmic process of the outer phalangeal cells reaches the apex of the columnar outer hair cells. Microtubules extend from the base to the apex of the outer phalangeal cells. A smooth border is formed, therefore, above which the stereocilia of the hair cells project to touch the tectorial membrane.

Columnar and polygonal cells, the *cells of Hensen*, are lateral to the outer phalangeal cells. There is a space, the *outer tunnel*, between these cells. Toward the *spiral prominence* the cells are reduced in size to cuboidal cells, the *cells of Claudius.*

Vibrations of the perilymph within the scala vestibuli are transmitted to the vestibular membrane. This causes the endolymph to vibrate. The basilar membrane vibrates accordingly. These vibrations cause a distortion of the hairs that are resting against the tectorial membrane. This distortion results in the transduction of the stimulus and the generation of a nerve impulse. This is carried via the auditory branch of the eighth cranial nerve to the spiral ganglia, which are contained within the osseous labyrinth, and then to appropriate centers in the brain.

References

Eye

Aguirre, G., Rubin, L.F. and Bistner, S.I : The development of the canine eye. Am. J. Vet. Res. *33*:2399, 1972.

Aguirre, G. D. and Gross, S. L.: Ocular manifestations of selected systemic diseases. Compend. Cont. Ed. Pract. Vet. *II*:144, 1980.

Anderson, B.G. and Anderson, W.D.: Vasculature of the equine and canine iris. Am. J. Vet. Res. *38*:1791, 1977.

Bedford, P. G. D.: Gonioscopy in the dog. J. Sm. Anim. Pract. *18*:615, 1977.

Bill, A.: The drainage of aqueous humor. Invest. Ophthalmol. *14*:1, 1975.

Bok, D. and Young, R. W.: The renewal of diffusely distributed protein in the outer segments of rods and cones. Vision Res. *12*:161, 1972.

deLahunta, A.: *Veterinary Neuroanatomy and Clinical Neurology*. W. B. Saunders, Philadelphia, 1977.

Gelatt, K.N. (ed.):*Textbook of Veterinary Ophthamology*. Lea and Febiger, Philadelphia, 1981.

Jakus, M. A.: *Ocular Fine Structure*. Churchill, Ltd., London, 1964.

Pedler, C. M. H. and Tilly, R.: The fine structure of photoreceptor discs. Vision Res. *7*:829, 1967.

Prince, J. H., Diesem, C. D., Eglitis, I. and Ruskell, G. L.: *Anatomy and Histology of the Eye and Orbit in Domestic Animals*. Charles C Thomas, Springfield, IL., 1960.

Shively, J.N. and Epling, G.P.: Fine structure of the canine eye: Iris. Amer. J. Vet. Res. *30*:13, 1969.

Shively, J. N. and Epling, G. P.: Fine structure of the canine eye: Cornea. Amer. J. Vet. Res. *31*:713, 1970.

Slatter, D.H.: *Fundamentals of Veterinary Ophthalmology*. W.B. Saunders Co., Philadelphia, 1981.

Tripathi, R. C.: Ultrastructure of Schlemm's canal in relation to aqueous outflow. Exp. Eye Res. *7*:335, 1968.

Villegas, G. M.: The ultrastructure of the human retina. J. Anat. *98*:501, 1964.

Young, R. W.: The renewal of photoreceptor cell outer segments. J. Cell Biol. *33*:61, 1967.

Young, R. W.: Visual cells and the concept of renewal. Invest. Ophthalmol. *15*:700, 1976.

Ear

Bredberg, G., Lindemann, H. H., Ades, H. W. and West, R.: Scanning electron microscopy of the organ of Corti. Science *170*:861, 1970.

Hinojosa, R. and Rodriguez-Echandia, E. L.: The fine structure of the stria vascularis of the cat inner ear. Amer. J. Anat. *188*:631, 1966.

Iurta, S.: *Submicroscopic Structure of the Inner Ear*. Pergamon Press, Oxford, 1967.

SECTION V:

EXFOLIATIVE CYTOLOGY

29: Introduction to Exfoliative Cytology

Introduction

General Considerations. Cytology is the study of individual cells without regard to the architectural patterns that characterize the tissues of origin. Cytology provides a rapid and simple means of diagnosis that occasionally precludes the need for histopathological examinations. Cytology may be superior to histopathology in the evaluation of bone marrow and certain types of tumors. Cytological examinations require exfoliated cells. Some cells exfoliate spontaneously into body cavities or are components of inflammatory exudates; others have to be exfoliated mechanically by techniques such as scraping, aspirating, or washing.

Abnormal cytology associated with various disease processes is included as a means of comparison with normal cytology. **The cellular descriptions are based upon staining properties seen with Romanowsky stains.**

Cytology of Selected Organs and Systems

Nervous System

General Considerations. Examination of cells in cerebrospinal fluid (CSF) is often a useful aid in obtaining a neurological diagnosis. Additionally, total cell counts and quantitative protein determinations are helpful. Cells in CSF degenerate rapidly; consequently, total cell counts should be performed immediately after sampling. Normal CSF contains less than 5 cells/mm³. Cell concentration techniques such as membrane filtration or cytocentrifugation are utilized to facilitate evaluation.

Cytology. The cells in normal CSF are primarily small lymphocytes and other occasional mononuclear cells. The blood cells observed approximate the morphological and staining characteristics of those observed in a peripheral blood smear. An increase in the number of nucleated cells *(pleocytosis)* in CSF occurs with many neurological diseases. The pleocytosis of viral infections is due to an increase in lympho-cytes and some plasma cells. Bacterial and mycotic infections are characterized by an increase in neutrophils. Macrophages occur in viral and bacterial infections. In animals with central nervous system trauma, a slight increase in neutrophils may be accompanied by occasional macrophages. Numerous erythrophagocytes and macrophages containing hemosiderin pigment may be seen in animals with hemorrhage in the central nervous system (Plate VII.6). Tumor cells and inflammatory cells (neutrophils, macrophages) may be present in animals with central nervous system neoplastic diseases.

Hemic-Lymphatic System

The cytology of blood, bone marrow, lymph nodes, and related structures is a valuable diagnositic procedure, because tissue architecture is less important in these organs than in many other structures.

Bone Marrow Aspiration Biopsy. *Aspiration biopsy* is indicated when it is impossible to confirm a diagnosis by the history, phsyical examination, and careful examination of the peripheral blood. Cases of unexplained nonregenerative anemias, leukocytic dyscrasias, thrombocytopenias, myeloproliferative disorders, lymphosarcomas, and abnormalities of immunoproteins are justifications for aspiration biopsies. *Punch biopsy* is indicated when attempts to obtain an aspirate have been unsuccessful. Abnormalities of the structural architecture of bone marrow may be evaluated by punch biopsy. A bone marrow biopsy is generally contraindicated when an animal is sufficiently ill or anemic that restraint further endangers its life.

The most common sites for bone marrow biopsy in the cat and dog are the iliac crest and the proximal end of the femur. The ribs or sternabrae are preferred sites in the horse and ox.

Lymph Node Aspiration Biopsy. Selection of a lymph node for biopsy should be made on the basis of clinical findings. Lymph node enlargement, whether localized or generalized, is an indication for lymph node aspiration biopsy.

Cytology of Lymph Nodes. Cytological evaluation of excised lymph nodes can be performed by gently touching a cut surface of a node to a dry microscope slide. Cell types encountered in normal lymph nodes include mature lymphocytes, lymphoblasts, neutrophils, macrophages, plasma cells, and mast cells.

Mature *lymphocytes* are similar to the mature lymphocytes of the peripheral blood (Plate VII.7). The nuclear chromatin is coarsely clumped. The cytoplasm, generally scant, is a narrow rim around the nucleus. The mature lymphocyte is the primary cell type of normal and hyperplastic nodes.

The nuclear chromatin in *lymphoblasts* is fine and diffuse (Fig. 29.1). A nucleolus may be seen. Lymphoblasts are approximately 1 1/2 to 3 times the size of mature lymphocytes, and may possess a broad or narrow rim of cytoplasm. Lymphoblasts are present in normal and hyperplastic lymph nodes but usually do not exceed 15% of the total cell population.

Any lymph node involved in inflammatory processes contains many neutrophils.

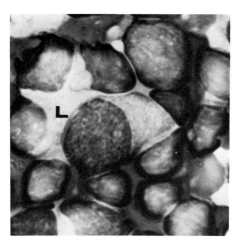

Figure 29.1. A lymphoblast from a normal canine lymph node. The lymphoblast *(L)* is surrounded by distorted lymphocytes. Note the fine chromatin pattern and extensive cytoplasm. ×400.

These may appear healthy and intact if the inflammatory process is nonseptic (Fig. 29.2). Degenerative changes in the nucleus (karyolysis, karyorrhexus) of the neutrophil indicate septic inflammation. Bacteria may be observed within the cytoplasm of the neutrophils. Monocytes and macrophages,

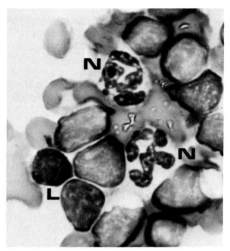

Figure 29.2. Small lymphocytes *(L)* and normal neutrophils *(N)* within a canine lymph node. ×400.

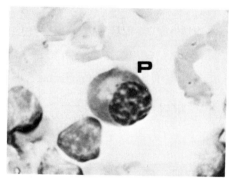

Figure 29.3. A plasma cell *(P)* within a canine lymph node. The negative Golgi zone and eccentrically positioned nucleus are identifying features. ×400.

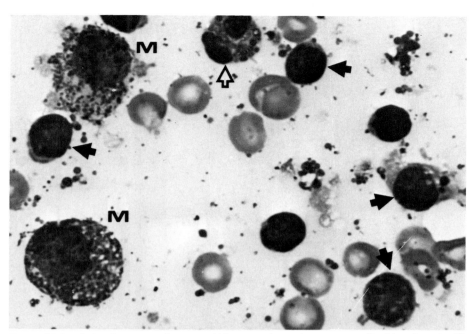

Figure 29.5. Cells of a mast cell tumor within an aspirate of a canine popliteal lymph node. The mast cells *(M)* had metastasized to the lymph node. Particulate matter scattered throughout the aspirate are granules from ruptured mast cells. *Solid arrows*, lymphocytes; *open arrow*, eosinophil. ×400.

observed in certain chronic inflammatory conditions, may contain cellular debris. Plasma cells may be present (Fig. 29.3). Plasma cells containing packets of immunoglobulin, *Mott cells*, may be observed in antigen-stimulated lymph nodes (Fig. 29.4, Plate VII.7). A few mast cells occur in all lymph node aspirates; however, increased numbers may indicate mast cell neoplasia with metastatic involvement of the lymph node (Fig. 29.5).

Neoplastic cells, such as carcinoma cells, may be present in lymph nodes involved in metastatic processes (Fig. 29.6). The presence of cells that are not part of the normal cell population of the lymph node should be obvious. (Be certain that a structure such as a salivary gland was not aspirated inadvertently.) Malignant cells are usually pleo-

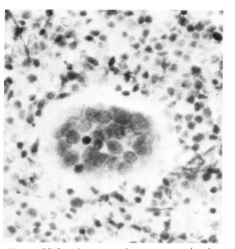

Figure 29.6. A metastatic mammary gland carcinoma within an inguinal lymph node of a dog. The carcinoma is recognizable as a cluster of epipthelial cells. ×100.

morphic with an increased nuclear/cytoplasmic ratio. The nuclei, varying in size and shape, often contain prominent multiple nucleoli. Many mitotic figures and multinucleated cells may be observed. Cytoplasmic vacuolation may be obvious. Malignant cells commonly stain more deeply basophilic than other cells.

Small flakes of cytoplasm may be intermixed with the cells of a lymph node sample. The flakes of cytoplasm, *lymphoglandular bodies*, are characteristic features of lymphoid tissue aspirates (Fig. 29.7).

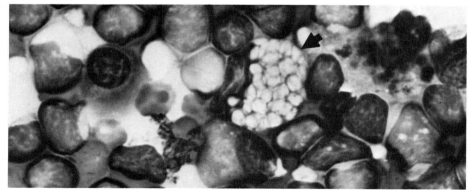

Figure 29.4. A Mott cell *(arrow)* within a canine lymph node. The large inclusions, Russell bodies, contain packets of immunoglobulins. ×400.

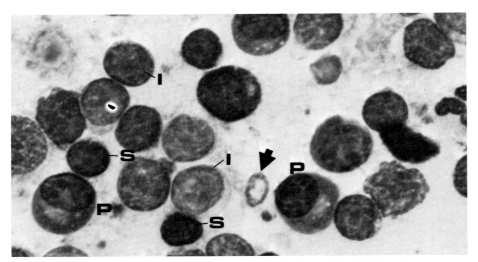

Figure 29.7. Lymphogranular body *(solid arrow)* within a reactive canine lymph node. *S*, small lymphocytes; *I*, intermediate lymphocytes. *P*, plasma cell. ×400.

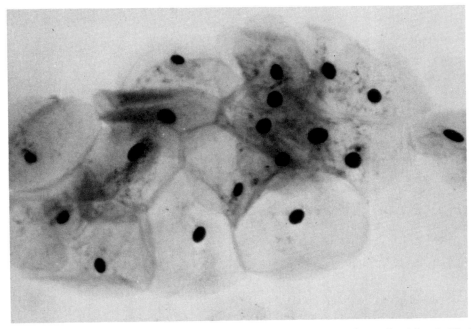

Figure 29.8. Cells from a scraping of the buccal cavity of a dog. The surface cells of the stratified squamous epithelium contain pyknotic nuclei. ×100.

The classification of lymph nodes based upon their cytologic characteristics includes the following: *normal node, inflammatory node (purulent), immunologically reactive node (benign lymphoid hyperplasia), inflammatory and reactive node (mixed), primary neoplastic node*, and *metastatic neoplastic node*, (Plate VII.8).

Mature lymphocytes are the predominant cell type in *normal lymph nodes*. Lymphoblasts do not exceed 15% of the population, whereas plasma cells and inflammatory cells are observed rarely. *Benign lymphoid hyperplasia* is characterized by increased numbers of immature and mature plasma cells (Plate VII.7).

Cytology of the Spleen. Fine needle aspiration biopsy of the spleen is a commonly rewarding diagnostic procedure; however, aspiration of the spleen is contraindicated when unruptured hemangiosarcoma is suspected. Splenic aspirates are always rich in blood. The tissue cells in the normal spleen are lymphoid cells, endothelial cells, monocytes, and macrophages.

Cytology of the Tonsil. The cytology of the normal tonsil consists of a mixture of lymphocytes and squamous epithelial cells of the buccal or pharyngeal mucosa. Cytology of reactive, inflamed and neoplastic tonsils is very similar to findings in other lymphatic tissue aspirates. Primary neopla-

sia of the tonsils include lymphosarcoma and squamous cell carcinoma.

Integumentary System

General Considerations. A cytological sample of a normal integument consists of superficial epithelial cells containing keratin. If aspirates of the full-thickness skin are made, then basilar epithelial cells or glandular epithelial cells from adnexal structures may be present. Dermal lesions are some of the most accessible lesions for cytological examination. Inflammatory (neutrophils, macrophages), cystic (sebaceous gland lining cells), and neoplastic (melanocytes, mast cells) components involving the integument are identified readily by cytology. Parasites of the skin may be observed while examining cytological specimens.

Digestive System

General Considerations. Impression smears of the oral cavity and esophagus of normal animals consists of squamous epithelial cells in various stages of maturation and a mixed population of bacteria (Fig. 29.8). Neutrophils may be present also. Inflammatory lesions of the mouth usually contain large numbers of neutrophils and bacteria (Fig. 29.9). Neoplastic lesions of the buccal cavity contain characteristic cells.

Gastric impression smears or washings consist of columnar epithelial and goblet cells. In the horse, squamous epithelial cells may be present. Chief cells may be seen occasionally. They contain metachromatic granules and resemble columnar epithelial cells.

Rectal swabs from normal animals consist of columnar epithelial cells, goblet cells, and bacteria. Aspirates of intestinal contents may consist of large numbers of various types of bacteria. Degenerating epithelial cells may be seen also.

Impression smears or aspirates may be obtained from the liver. Normal liver cells have round nuclei that contain one or two nucleoli. The abundant lavender cytoplasm may contain bile pigment (Fig. 29.10). Binucleate cells may be numerous.

Urinary System

General Considerations. The cytological evaluation of urine sediment is a useful procedure to determine the state of health or disease of the urinary system. The urinary bladder may be evaluated by cytological examination of urine sediment. Transitional epithelial cells that line the urinary bladder are encountered frequently in normal urine sediment. The cells are variable in size, have round to oval vesicular nuclei

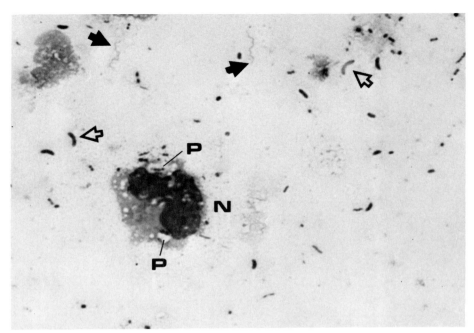

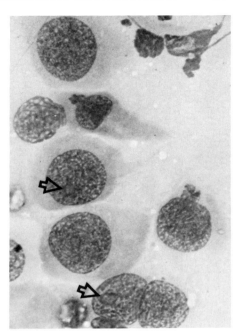

Figure 29.9. A scraping of the buccal cavity of a cat with gingivitis. Spirochetes *(solid arrows)*, fusiform bacteria *(open arrows)*, and bacilli are scattered throughout the smear. A toxic neutrophil *(N)* contains phagocytized bacteria *(P)*. ×400.

Figure 29.11. Transitional epithelial cells from the urinary bladder of a normal dog. The large nuclei contain a fine chromatin network. Nucleoli *(arrows)* are evident in some of the cells. ×250.

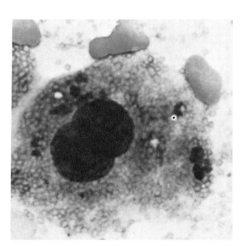

Figure 29.10. Hepatocyte from a biopsy of a canine liver. The large cell is binucleated, and the cytoplasm contains dark granules of bile pigment. ×400.

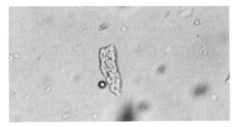

Figure 29.12. A granular cast from the urinary sediment of a dog. ×100.

casts are refractile yellow casts with broken ends.

Respiratory System

General Considerations. Transtracheal aspiration is a useful method for obtaining cells from the respiratory tract for cytological evaluation. Methods that bypass the mouth and oropharynx, avoiding normal flora that could be confused with pathogens, are best. These techniques require the percutaneous passage of a catheter that enters the trachea through the cricothyroid membrane and is passed to the carina. The instillation and immediate aspiration of fluid completes the sampling.

Cytology. Tracheobronchial epithelial cells are ciliated columnar or cuboidal cells (Fig. 29.13). Epithelial cells occur in aspirates from normal and diseased patients (Plate VII.10). Mucus-producing goblet cells may be seen also.

Neutrophils are the predominant cell type in inflammatory conditions (Plate VII.11). The appearance of the neutrophils varies with the length of time the cells were in the trachea or bronchi and depends on the degree of sepsis. If neutrophils appear toxic (nuclear swelling, nuclear membrane rupture), then bacteria may be present in the cytoplasm. If bacteria are seen, then an additional smear should be Gram-stained for bacterial characterization. *Eosinophils* occur in varying numbers in animals with allergic pulmonary conditions and dirofilariasis (Fig. 29.14). *Lymphocytes* and *plasma cells* are present in viral infections.

with one or two nucleoli (Plate VII.9). The abundant cytoplasm is lavender. Multinucleated cells are encountered frequently (Fig. 29.11). Renal epithelial cells may occur in urine sediment when renal disease is present. Desquamated renal epithelial cells may occur as components of *renal casts*. Renal casts are proteinaceous models of renal tubules. As renal epithelial cell casts degenerate, they progress from *granular casts* to *waxy casts*. Granular casts contain particles that are derived from disintegrating renal epithelial cells (Fig. 29.12). Waxy

Their numbers are increased also in other chronic inflammatory conditions. *Macrophages* are present in numerous types of inflammatory conditions (Figs. 29.15 and 29.16). They may contain phagocytized red blood cells, cellular debris, lipids, and anthracotic pigment. Macrophages may originate as alveolar phagocytes (histiocytes) or blood monocytes. *Mucus* is increased in most inflammatory conditions. It appears as a diffuse, light blue-staining and homogeneous background. *Fibrin* and other proteins may be present in inflammatory conditions. Fibrin stains pink and appears as fine whorled strands. It should not be confused with degenerating nuclear debris. *Fungal* elements (hyphae, spores) may be present in pulmonary mycoses. Fungal contaminants, such as *Alternaria sp.*, are common in aspirates from large animals. *Viral inclusion bodies* may be seen within epithelial cells. Canine distemper viral in-

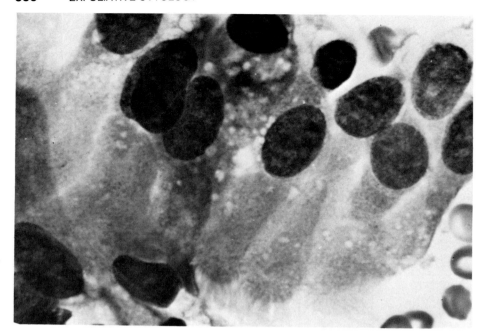

Figure 29.13. Columnar ciliated cells obtained from a tracheal wash of a normal dog. ×400.

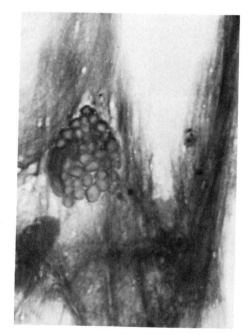

Figure 29.14. An eosinophil from an equine trancheal wash. The dark-staining background material is mucin. ×400.

clusions and canine adenoviral inclusions have been observed in tracheal aspirations.

Glandular Organs

Thyroid Gland. The cells of the normal thyroid gland are follicular epithelial cells that form pseudosyncytia in which cytoplasmic borders are indistinct (Fig. 29.17). The cytoplasm of thyroid follicular epithe-

lial cells disrupts easily, resulting in the presence of many "naked nuclei" (Plate VII.12). The nuclei are round with small inconspicuous nucleoli, whereas the cytoplasm is basophilic. A few cells may contain vacuoles or blue-black granules within the cytoplasm (Plate VIII.1).

Salivary Gland. Aspirates of normal salivary glands contain large (25 mm), foamy, glandular epithelial cells with small dense nuclei and a lavender cytoplasm filled with uniform small vacuoles (Plate VIII.2).

Reproductive System

Introduction. Cytological techniques are useful aids for evaluation of the male and female reproductive system. The utility is not confined to the diagnosis of disease.

Cytology is a significant evaluative technique used to determine the reproductive potential of the male (semen evaluation) and the stage of the estrous cycle in dogs and cats. Various techniques are employed and include ejaculation, massage, washes, aspiration biopsy, and scrapings.

Cytology of the Prostate Gland. Prostatic fluid may be obtained by prostatic massage or fine-needle aspiration biopsy. Based upon cytological findings, prostatic disease can be differentiated into five categories: *benign prostatic hyperplasia, prostatic cyst formation, prostatic inflammation (prostatitis or abscessation), prostatic neoplasia,* and *squamous metaplasia.*

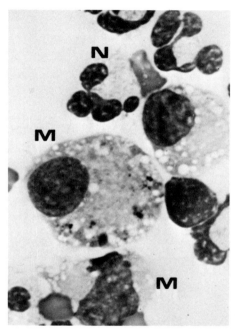

Figure 29.16. Macrophages *(M)* and neutrophils *(N)* from a canine tracheal wash. The dark material within the macrophage is hemosiderin. ×400.

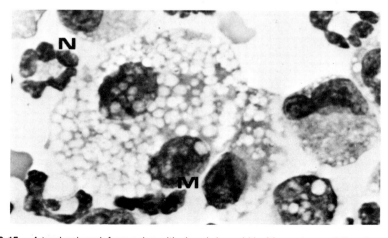

Figure 29.15. A tracheal wash from a dog with chronic bronchitis. Macrophages *(M)* and neutrophils *(N)* are apparent. ×400.

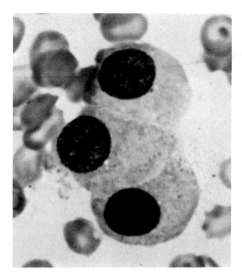

Figure 29.17. Thyroid follicular cells from a normal dog. ×400.

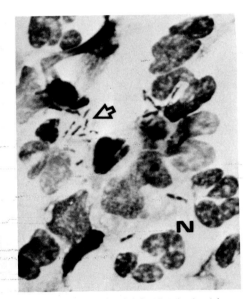

Figure 29.18. A smear of cells obtained from the urinary tract by a prostatic massage per rectum. Numerous toxic neutrophils (N) and bacteria (arrow) are present. ×400.

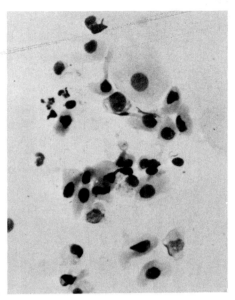

Figure 29.19. A vaginal smear from a dog in anestrus. ×100.

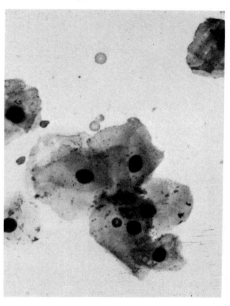

Figure 29.20. A vaginal smear from a dog in early estrus. Some erythrocytes are present. The straight edges of cytoplasmic borders of the epithelial cells are indicative of cornification. ×100.

The normal prostate has clusters of uniform cuboidal or columnar epithelial cells that vary from 10–15 μm in diameter. Nuclei are round to oval and are basilar in the columnar cells. Nucleoli are small and inconspicuous. The cytoplasm is finely granular and basophilic (Plate VIII.3). These cells can be differentiated easily from transitional epithelial cells, which are larger and lighter staining than prostatic cells.

Benign prostatic hyperplasia (Plate VIII.4), prostatic cysts, prostatitis (Fig. 29.18), prostatic abcess, and prostatic adenocarcinoma (Plate VIII.5) may be identified on the basis of the characteristics of the aspirate. Similarly, squamous metaplasia of prostatic epithelial cells may be identified (Plate VIII.6).

Vaginal Cytology. Examination of cells from the vagina of dogs and cats is a valuable aid in evaluating the stage of the estrous cycle, as well as diagnosing uterine and vaginal disease. The following descriptions refer to the dog specifically.

The wall of the anestral vagina normally is lined by epithelium that consists of two to four cell layers. As estrogen levels increase, the vaginal lining increases in thickness to about 40 cells. The increased thickening of the stratified squamous epithelium is the basis for cytological changes that are observed in the vaginal smear. Epithelial cells progress from noncornified to cornified as the thickening occurs. Neutrophils disappear during proestrus and estrus because the thickened epithelium does not allow their passage to the lumen of the vagina. Red blood cells from the uterus appear in the vaginal discharge during proestrus and estrus.

The *anestrous* vagina has many noncornified, round to oval epithelial cells that contain large, distinct and uniform nuclei (Fig. 29.19). A few neutrophils may be present. Minimal cellular debris is present.

The *proestrous* vagina is characterized by cornifying, superficial, epithelial cells. They constitute a major portion of all epithelial cells by the third day. The rounded cytoplasmic borders are replaced by straight edges. The nuclei become pyknotic and may disappear. Leukocytes are absent by the middle of proestrus. Erythrocytes may be numerous as a result of diapedesis from the underlying vascular bed. Various types of bacteria may be free, on or within epithelial cells.

The *estrous* vagina has epithelial cells that are cornified with straight cytoplasmic borders and pyknotic nuclei (Fig. 29.20 and Plate VIII.7). Late estrus is characterized by epithelial cells without nuclei. The number of erythrocytes is reduced. Various types of bacteria are present. As the epithelial cells begin to disintegrate, cellular debris becomes abundant (Fig. 29.21). Neutrophils reappear one or two days before diestrus.

In *diestrus*, neutrophils are abundant and small, round, noncornified, epithelial cells reappear. Neutrophils may occur within epithelial cells (Plate VIII.8). Debris and erythrocytes usually disappear. As diestrus progresses, neutrophils are reduced in number. Late diestrus appears cytologically similar to anestrus.

Large number of neutrophils with phagocytized bacteria are present in *vaginitis* and *pyometra*. The neutrophils may be more degenerate in pyometra than in vaginitis. A white blood sample will usually differentiate these two conditions.

Postpartum vaginal secretions contain large numbers of neutrophils, erythrocytes, and debris for approximately two weeks. Foamy endometrial epithelial cells may be present. If puppies are undergoing maceration in the uterus, muscle fibers may be present (Fig. 29.22).

Body Cavities

General Remarks. In the normal horse and ox, fluid can be aspirated from the thoracic and abdominal cavities. In the normal dog and cat, the quantity of fluid

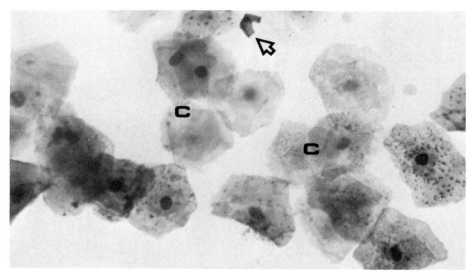

Figure 29.21. A vaginal smear from a dog in estrus. The dark granules are bacteria. Some cells *(C)* are devoid of nuclei, whereas some cells have disintegrated *(arrow)*. The nuclei are pyknotic. ×100.

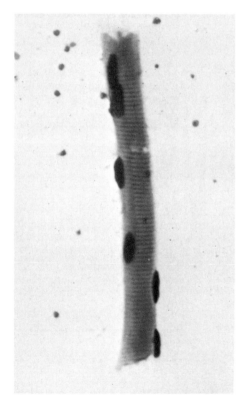

Figure 29.22. A skeletal muscle fiber within a vaginal smear from a bitch with a puppy undergoing maceration in utero. ×160.

present in the abdominal cavity is so small that attempts at sampling are usually futile. If four-quadrant paracentesis is unsuccessful, then peritoneal lavage with physiological saline may be attempted. Unfortunately, saline distorts the cells. Many abnormal conditions are characterized by

fluid accumulation. The normal equine thoracic fluid usually contains approximately 4800 nucleated cells/mm³, the majority of which are healthy neuthrophils with some large mononucleated cells and lymphocytes.

Body Cavity Effusions. Body cavity effusions are generally classified as either *transudates* or *exudates*. Transudates are capillary filtrates that accumulate in the extravascular compartment. The most common causes for the formation of *transudative effusions* are *hypoproteinemia* and *venous stasis*. Low serum albumin (<1–2 gm/dl) results in low colloid osmotic pressure and a subsequent accumulation of extravascular fluid. Hypoproteinemia may result from inadequate protein intake (starvation, inadequate protein digestion, malabsorption, parasitism), inadequate protein synthesis due to chronic liver disease (cirrhosis, congestive heart failure, portocaval shunts, neoplasia), or excessive protein loss (protein-losing glomerulonephrophthy, protein-losing enteropathy, hemorrhage, massive exudative lesions). Venous stasis may be a result of heart failure or venous or lymphatic obstruction. Venous or lymphatic obstruction may occur in disease processes such as thromboembolic disorders, neoplasia, and hepatopathies. Pure *transudates* are caused by hypoalbuminemia. They are usually colorless and clear, have a total protein of less than 1.5 gm/dl and contain fewer than 500 cells/μl.

A *modified transudate* is a transudative-type fluid that has been modified by the addition of protein and/or cells. In general, this type of fluid accumulates in patients that have venous stasis or impaired lymphatic drainage (congestive heart failure, passive congestion of the liver, neoplasia). Modified transudates contain 2–3.5 gm/dl

of protein and usually less than 5000 cells/ μl.

Exudates are formed in conditions in which an increased capillary permeability results in fluid, protein and cells leaving the capillaries at an increased rate. Increased capillary permeability is a result of an inflammatory process. The inflammation may or may not be due to bacterial infection. *Nonspecific exudates* contain no bacteria and form in conditions such as gall bladder or urinary bladder rupture, pancreatitis, presence of sterile foreign bodies, feline infectious peritonitis, neoplasia, and long-standing modified transudates. The latter may eventually initiate an inflammatory response itself. *Septic exudates* are caused by a wide variety of microorganisms.

Hemorrhagic effusions, usually caused by trauma, neoplasia, surgery, or infarction of the intestines, consist primarily of blood.

Although a clear-cut division between a transudate and an exudate does not exist, fluids are usually classified as transudates or exudates on the basis of several criteria (Table 29.1).

Physical and Chemical Evaluations. Numerous properties of fluids should be determined: volume, color, transparency, clot formation, odor, protein concentration, and occult blood (or red blood cell [RBC] count or packed cell volume). The presence of RBCs, white blood cells [WBCs], lipid and bilirubin alters the color and transparency of the fluids. Other tests, such as those for bilirubin, glucose, urea, creatinine, and amylase may facilitate a specific diagnosis.

Cytological Evaluation. A *total nucleated cell count* may be performed with an automatic counter or hemocytometer. A direct smear may be used to evaluate cellularity instead of using a nucleated cell count. *Differential cell counts* are helpful, because various types of cells occur in effusions. In cell-poor fluids, samples should be centrifuged and a smear made of the sediment. The feathered edge of the smear should always be examined; the larger cells travel to this area. Generally, smears are air dried routinely and stained with Romanowsky stains. The Papanicolaou stain is used occasionally. A Gram stain is indicated if bacteria are present.

Mesothelial cells line the pleural, pericardial, and peritoneal cavities (Fig. 29.23). When fluid accumulates in body cavities

Table 29.1
Effusion Characteristics

Property	Transudate	Exudate
Appearance	Clear	Usually cloudy
Specific gravity	1.018	1.018
Protein	<3 mg/dl	>3 gm/dl
Clot	No	Yes
Cell count	Usually low	Usually high

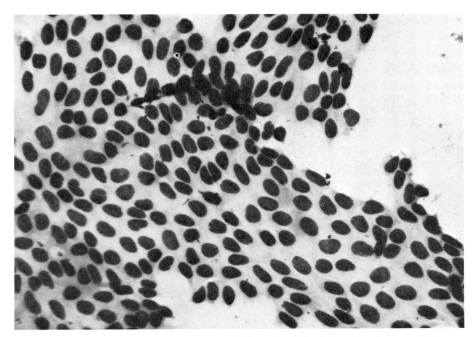

Figure 29.23. A sheet of mesothelial cells from the abdominal cavity of an ox. ×100.

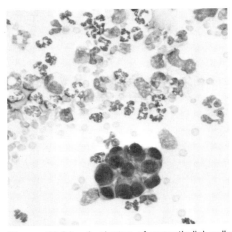

Figure 29.24. A cluster of mesothelial cells from the abdominal cavity of a horse. Macrophages and neutrophils are apparent. ×100.

these cells undergo hypertrophy and hyperplasia and eventually exfoliate into the fluid. The cells may continue to multiply after exfoliation. Mesothelial cells may appear singly or in clusters of 2, 4, 8, 16, 32, or 64 cells (Fig. 29.24). Mesothelial cells are large (12–30 μm) and have a light to dark blue cytoplasm. The nuclear-cytoplasmic ratio is high (Plate VIII.9). The nuclei are single or multiple, round to oval with one or more nucleoli. The nucleoli are generally 3 μm in diameter. Cells in mitosis may be observed. Reactive mesothelial cells should be uniform in size without nuclear molding.

Macrophages vary in diameter from 10 to 50 μm, possess one or more round to oval nuclei that may contain visible nucleoli, and have a light blue, vacuolate cytoplasm (Plate VIII.10). Macrophages phagocytize neutrophils, RBCs, lipids, cellular debris, foreign material, and certain microorganisms; however, it is unusual to observe bacteria within phagocytic vacuoles of macrophages.

Neutrophils, scarce in noninflammatory conditions, are present in large numbers in inflammatory effusions. The state of preservation of the neutrophils is an important determinant. Neutrophils in nonseptic effusions are well-preserved and appear much as they do in peripheral blood, with intact nuclear membranes and dense chromatin. As neutrophils age, they become hypersegmented and eventually pyknotic. In septic effusions, neutrophils are affected by bacterial toxins and undergo rapid degeneration and eventual rupture. Nuclear lobes become swollen, karyolysis occurs, and the chromatin becomes light pink and smudged *(chromatolysis)*. The cytoplasm becomes basophilic, vacuolated, and cytoplasmic membranes commonly rupture. Careful examination in this smeared area near the feathered edge usually reveals the presence of bacteria within the cytoplsm of the neutrophils or free in the exudate. Bacterial (all of which stain blue with Romanowsky stains) are usually discrete uniform structures that should not be confused with background protein or stain precipitate, both of which appear somewhat amorphous and dark purple. Background protein is a fine granular material seen between cells in high protein fluids. Precipitated stain, resulting from inadequate rinsing of the slide, is extremely variable in size and shape.

Other cells found in effusions include lymphocytes, plasma cells, eosinophils, mast cells, and RBCs.

Neoplastic cells may be observed in effusions resulting from a neoplastic process in a body cavity. Neoplastic cells are usually large and pleomorphic with a high nuclear-cytoplasmic ratio. Variability in nuclear size *(anisokaryosis)*, nuclear molding, multinucleation, abnormal mitotic figures, and large prominent multiple nucleoli are usually obvious. The cytoplsm usually stains quite basophilic. Incomplete cytoplasmic and nuclear division is observed commonly ("indian filing"). The most common neoplastic cells seen are lymphoblasts (lymphosarcoma) and carcinoma cells (malignant tumors of epithelial origin). Sarcoma cells (malignant tumors of connective tissue origin) rarely exfoliate into body cavity effusions.

Cytology of the Eye

The microscopic examination of conjunctival scrapings is a valuable aid in the diagnosis of external eye diseases. Samples are obtained from central palpebral conjunctiva.

Cytology. The description is based upon staining of a normal conjunctiva. Conjunctival epithelial cells occur in sheets. Deep scrapings contain parabasal cells that are round and dark staining (Plate VIII.11). Cells from the intermediate and superficial layers are flatter, appear to have more cytoplasm, and are paler staining than deeper cells. The cytoplasm is pale blue and then purple-staining nucleus is round to oval. Cytoplasmic melanin granules stain dark green to black. In some individuals, most epithelial cells contain melanin. Epithelial cells that are keratinizing have a pale lavender cytoplasm with a degenerating pyknotic nucleus. (The eyelid margin normally contains keratinized cells and care should be exercised to avoid sampling this surface, because keratinized cells are atypical in the conjunctival sac.) Goblet cells may be identified by large amounts of mucous precursors in the cytoplasm (Plate VIII.12). The nucleus is displaced to the periphery of the cell by the inclusion droplet. The mucus precursor is represented by a clear area or may stain a very light blue. Goblet cells occur normally in the fornix conjunctivae. Occasional bacteria may be present on the surface of epithelial cells. Neutrophils may be observed rarely. Inflammation of the conjunctiva may be characterized by the presence of numerous neutrophils and macrophages.

Cytology of the Musculoskeletal System

Synovial Fluid. Synovial fluid analysis is a valuable technique for determining un-

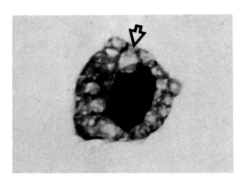

Figure 29.25. A macrophage from the joint fluid of a dog with phagocytized red bloods within the cytoplasm *(arrow)*.

derlying causes of arthritis. Synovial fluid is a dialysate of plasma and is rich in mucosubstances. Normal synovial fluid of most species contains less than 3000 nucleated cells. Approximately 90% of these cells are lymphocytes and monocytes (Fig. 29.25). The remainder are healthy neutrophils. A large amount of background protein is obvious in joint fluid smears. Various arthritides result in an increase in inflammatory cells. Viral and chlamydial infections are characterized by increased numbers of mononucleated cells, whereas bacterial infections are characterized by an increased number of neutrophils. The mononucleated and polymorphonucleated cells are typical.

References

Bach, L. G. and Ricketts, S. W.: Paracentesis as an aid to the diagnosis of abdominal disease in the horse. Eq. Vet. J. 6:116, 1974.

Beech, J.: Cyctology of tracheobronchial aspirates in horses. Vet. Pathol. 12:157, 1975.

Benjamin, M. M.: *Outline of Veterinary Clinical Pathology*, 3rd edition. Iowa State Univ. Press, Ames, Iowa, 1978.

Coles, E. H.: *Veterinary Clinical Pathology*, 3rd edition. W. B. Saunders, Philadelphia, 1980.

Creighton, S. R. and Wilkins, R. J.: Evaluation of animals using transtracheal aspiration biopsy. J. Amer. Anim. Hosp. Assoc. 10:219, 1974.

Crowe, D. T. and Crane, S. W.: Diagnostic abdominal paracentesis and lavage in the evaluation of abdominal injuries in dogs and cats: Clinical and experimental investigations. J. Amer. Vet. Med. Assoc. 168:700, 1976.

Lavach, J. D., Thrall, M. A., Benjamin, M. M. and Severin. G. A.: Cytology of normal and inflammed conjunctivas in dogs and cats. J. Amer. Vet. Med. Assoc. 170:722, 1977.

Miller, J. B. et al.: Synovial fluid analysis in canine arthritis. J. Amer. Anim. Hosp. Assoc. 10:392, 1974.

Rebar, A. H.: *Handbook of Veterinary Cytology*. Ralston Purina Company, 1979.

Soderstom, N.: *Fine Needle Aspiration Biopsy*, Grune and Stratton, New York, 1966.

Spriggs, A. I. and Boddington, M.: *The Cytology of Effusions*, 2nd edition. Grune and Stratton, Inc., New York, 1968.

Van Pelt, R. W.: Interpretation of synovial fluid findings in the horse. J. Amer. Vet. Med. Assoc. 165:91, 1974.

Van Pelt, R. W. et al.: Chronic gonitis in cattle: Clinicopathologic findings and treatment. J. Amer. Vet. Med. Assoc. 163:1378, 1973.

Vandevelde, M. and Spano, J.: Cerebrospinal fluid cytology in canine neurologic disease, Amer. J. Vet. Res. 38:1827, 1977.

Zinkl, J. L. and Keeton, K. S.: Lymph node cytology. Calif. Vet. 33:9, 1979.

Index*

A band, 190, **192**, **194–196**, 236, **237**
Aberration
  chromatic, 12
  spherical, 12
Abomasum (*see* stomach, glandular)
Acanthocytes, 168
Accessory reproductive glands
  male, 500–502
A cells
  of magnum, 525
Acervuli, 474
Acetyl
  -choline, 213, 214, 281, 311, **311**
    and muscular contraction, 193
    and autonomic nervous system, 308, **308**
  -cholinesterase, 311
  -coenzyme A, 214, **218**
Achondroplasia, 149
Acid
  acetic, 404
  acetoacetic, 404
  butyric, 404
  cholic, 426
  glaucocholic, 426
  hydrolysis, 38
    of bone, 121
  phosphatase, 36
  phosphoric, 22
  propionic, 404
  source of, 443
  taurocholic, 326
Acid/base balance
  and lung function, 461, **462**
  and renal function, 443, 444, **444**
Acidophilia, 7
Acidophils (*see* eosinophils)
  of blood, 169, **169**
  of pars distalis, 469, **470**
Acidosis
  metabolic, 444
  respiratory, 444, 461
    compensated, 461
Acromegaly, 163
Acrosomal vesicle, 497, **497**
Acrosome, 497, **497**
Actin, 70, 188, 190, 193, **199**
  fibrous, 193, **199**
  globular, 193, **199**
Active zone, 281
Addison's disease, 482
Adenine, 22
Adenohypophysis, 467, **468**, 469–472
  regulation of, 472
  vascular relationships of, 471
Adenomere, 60, 61
Adenosine
  monophosphate (AMP), 32
    cyclic (cAMP), 22, 32
  diphosphate (ADP), 22
    and hemostasis, 175
    and muscle contraction, 201, **203**
  triphosphate (ATP), 22
    and muscle contraction, 201, **203**

Adenyl cyclase, 22, 32
Adhesions, 258
  of tendons, 277
Adipocyte, **94**, 99, 105, **105, 106**
Adipose tissue, 3, 105, 106
  brown, 242, **243**
  types of (*see* specific tissue)
  yellow, 242, **243**
Adrenal
  cortex, 236, **237**
    adult, 478
    definitive, 478
    fetal, 478
    hormones of, 482, 483
    primitive, 478
    zones of, 479, **479–483**
  gland, 478–483, **478–482**
    blood vessels of, 478
    development of, 478
    functions of, 310, **310**, 311
    innervation of, 478
    lymphatics of, 478
  medulla, 310, **310**, 483, **483**
    effects of, 310, 311
    "fight or flight," 310
    innervation of, 310
    secretions of, 310
Adrenergic
  drugs, 312
  fibers, 308, **308**
  receptors 309, **309**
    distribution of, 310
    α_1, 216
    α_2, 216
    β_1, 217
    β_2, 217
    plasticity of, 217
  terminals, 214, **219**
  varicosities, **309**, 310
Adrenergics, 312
Adrenoceptors, 309, **309**
Adrenochromes, 483, **483**
Adrenocorticoids
  effects upon bone, 144
Adrenocorticotrophic hormone (ACTH), 472
  -endorphin, 484
  releasing factor, 472
Afferent, 208
  fibers, 288
  nerve terminals, 293, 294, **296, 297**
    as transducers, 293
    classifcation of, 293
    encapsulated, 294, **296, 297**
    free and diffuse, 293
    modalities, 293
    types of, 293, **296, 297**
  system
    general somatic (GSA), 288, **290**
    general visceral (GVA), 288, **290**
    special somatic (SSA), 288, **290**
    special visceral (SVA), 288, **290**
Agglutinin, 343
Agonists, 311
Agranular endoplasmic reticulum, 34, 36
Agranulocytes, 169–171 (*see* specific cells also)
  avian, 174, **174**, 175
  kinetics of, 186
Agranulocytopoiesis, 182, **182**

cells of, 182, 183 (*see* specific cells also)
cells of (*see* specific cells)
Air
  capillaries, 463, **463–465**
  cells, 463, **463–465**
  sacs, 463, **463**, 464
  vesicles, 463, **463**, 464, **464, 465**
Alanine aminotransferase (ALT), 428
Alar plate, 286, **289, 290**
Albumin, 164, **165**
  /globulin ratio (A/G), 187
Alcian blue, 86
Alcohol dehydrogenase, 426
Aldosterone, 482
Alimentary
  canal, 380
  tract, 380
Alkalosis
  metabolic, 444
  respiratory, 444, 461
    compensated, 461
Allergens, 346
Allergies, 345
Alpha cells
  of pancreas, 484
  of pars distalis, 469, **470**
Alveolar
  cell, 455
    great, 455
  ducts, 455, **455**
  macrophages, 457, **458**
  pores, 457
  sac, 455, **455**
  saccules, 455, **455**
Alveoli, 455, 457, **455–458**
Amacrine cells
  of retina, 541
Ameloblasts, 388, **388, 389**
γ-Aminobutyric acid, 213
Amine Precursor Uptake and Decarboxylase
  cells (APUD), 453, 483
  system, 486
Amino
  acids
    and renal function, 441
    essential, 427
    glucogenic, 427
    ketogenic, 427
    oxidase, 38
    sugars, 23
Aminoacyl-tRNA
  -synthetase, 33, **35**
  -complex, 33, **35**
Aminolevulinic acid synthetase, 184, **184**
Aminopeptidase, 409
β-Aminoproprionitrile (BAPN), 82
Amorphous calcium phosphate, 120
Amphicytes, 219, **223**, 236, **237**
Ampulla, 501, **501**, 512
Ampullary glands, 501, B501
Amylase, 430
Anagen, 355, **356**
Anal
  glands, 358, **359**
  sacs, 358, **360**
Anamnestic response, 343
Anaphylactic shock, 346
Anaphylatoxins, 347

*Boldface page numbers are references to illustrations.

Anaphylaxis, 345
  eosinophilic chemotactic factor of (ECF-A), 345
  slow-releasing substance of (SRS-A), 345
Anastomoses
  arteriolar-venular, **314**
Anatomy, 2
  objectives of, 2
  subdisciplines of, 2
    gross, 2
    microscopic, 2
Anchoring plaques, 190
Androgen-binding protein (ABP), 495
Androgens, 486
Androstenedione, 511
Anemia, 166–168
  definition of, 166
  hypochromic
    macrocytic, 168
    microcytic, 168
  macrocytic, 167
    true, 168
  microcytic, 168
  nonregenerative, 166
  normocytic, 167
  pseudomacrocytic, 168
  regenerative, 166, **167**
  transitory, 168
Anestrus, 516, 517
Angiotensin I, II, 439
Angiotensinogen, 439
Anisocytes, 167, **168**
Angular limb deformities
  correction of, 261, 262, **262**
Anisocytosis, 167, **168**, 187
Anisokaryosis, 561
Anisotropy, 14
Anoxia, 462
Antagonists, 311
Anterior chamber, 527, 528, **530**
Antiadrenergics, 312
Antibodies, 341
  humoral, 99
  cytotrophic, 345
Anticholinergics, 308, 311
Anticoagulants, 186, 187
Antidiuretic hormone (ADH), 208, 472, 473
Antigenic determinant, 341
Antigens, 341
Antiglobulin, 9
Antimuscarinics, 308
Antiplasmin, 177
Antithrombin III, (ATIII), 176
Antlers, 372
Anulate lamellae, 27
Anuli fibrosi, 324
Anulus
  fibrocartilagineus
    of tympanic membrane, 546
  of spermatid, 497, **497**
Anus, 410
  avian, 455
Aortic
  bodies, 325, 326
  sinuses, 326
Apneustic center, 462
Apudomas, 486
Aqueous humor, 537
Arachidonic acid, 486
Arachnoid
  granulations, 296, **298**
  villi, 296, **298**
Arachnoidea, 296, **298, 299**
Arched collecting tubules, 437
Area
  centralis retinae, 541
  cribrosa, 431, 438
    of eye, 529
  gastricae, **392**, 393
Areolar connective tissue, 101–103, **101, 102**
Argentaffin cells, 395, 405, 486
Argyrophilia, 82
Argyrophilic cells, 486
Arrector pili muscle, 351, **351**, 354
Arteries
  arciform, 438, **440**
  arcuate, 438, **440**

bronchial, 459, **460**
cutaneous
  mixed, 350
  simple, 350
distributing, 315, **316**
elastic, 322, **322**
epiphyseal, 263, **264**
helicine, 504
hepatic, 423
hyaloid, 528, **528**
medium, 315, **316**
metaphyseal, 263, **264**
nutrient, 263, **264**
periosteal, 264, **264**
pulmonary, 459, **460**
renal, 438, **440**
retinal, 543
rostral hypophyseal, 471
small, 315, **316, 317**
splenic, 335
trabecular
  of spleen, 336, **341**
Arteriolae
  rectae
    spuriae, 438, **44**
    verae, 438, **440**
Arterioles, 315, **320, 321**
  afferent, 438, **440**
  bronchial, 459, 460, **460**
  efferent, 438, **440**
  nodular, 335, **338–340**
  penicillar, 336, **340, 341**
  pulmonary, 459, 460, **460**
  red pulp, 336, **340, 341**
  sheathed, 336, **341**
  straight
    false, 438, **44**
    true, 438, **440**
  terminal, 336, **340, 341**
Arthus reaction, 347
Articular
  capsule, 270, **270, 271, 274, 275**
    fibrous, 271, **272**
  cartilage, 118, 240, **241**, 271, **271–174**
    histology of, 276
  development of, 271, **271, 272**, 274
    nutrition of, 276
  presumptive, 271, **272, 274**
  repair of, 276
  weeping of, 275
  zones of, 271, **273, 274**
Articulations, 269–275
  characteristics of, 269, 270
  composition of, 270
  classification of, 270
Artifacts, 19–20
Arylsulfatase, 36, 346
Ascending
  limb, **432**, 436, 437
  thin segment, **432**, 437
Astrocytes, 218, **220, 221**
  of pineal gland, 474
  of retina, 541
Atopy, 345
Atria, 463
Atrial granules, 205
Atrioventricular
  bundle, 324, **326**
  node, 324, **326**
Atropine, 308
Auerbach's plexus, 395
Auditory
  apparatus, 549–552
  ossicles, 546
  tube, 546
Auricle, 545
Autocoids, 486
Autoimmunity, 347
Autolysis, 38
  postmortem, 7
Autonomic nervous system (ANS), 304–312
  adrenal medulla and, 310, **310**
  characteristics of, 304, 305
  comparison of components, **307**, 308
  components of, 304
    afferent, 304

central, 304
  peripheral, 304
cranial nerves of, 306
divisions of
  parasympathetic, 306, **307**
  sympathetic, 306, **307**
drugs acting upon, 308, 311, 312
drugs and
  anticholinergic, 308
  antimuscarinic, 308
  cholinergic, 308
  muscarinic, 308
  nicotinic, 308
dual innervation by, 306, 307
effectors of, 304
functional correlates, 306, 307
homeostasis and, 304
hypothalamus and, 304, **305**
innervation ratios within, 308
nerves of
  adrenergic, 309
  cholinergic, 308
neurons of
  postganglionic, 306, **306–308**
  preganglionic, 306, **306–308**
neurotransmitters of, 308, **308, 309**
parasympathetic division (see parasympathetic nervous system)
pharmacology of, 311, 312
receptors within
  adrenergic, 308–310, **308, 309**
  choloinergic, 308, **308**
  muscarinic, 308, **308**
response, 308, 309
reflex arc and, 304, **305, 306**
  comparison of, 305, **306**
  somatic 305, 306
  visceral, 305, **305, 306**
sympathetic division (see sympathetic nervous system)
synapses of, 308
  directed, 308
  intermediate, 308
Autophagic vacuoles, 37, **39**
Autophagocytosis, 37, **39**
Autoradiography, 9, **9**
Axis cylinder, **209**, 211, **214**, 220, **223, 225, 228**
Axolemma, 220, **225**
Axon, 208
  hillock, **209**, 211, **214**
  initial segment of, 211
  terminals, 211, **218**
  transport within
    fast, 211
    slow, 211
    somatofugal, 211
    somatopetal, 211
Axoneme, 40, **40**
Axonic zone, 209, **213**
Axoplasm, 211
Azurophilic granules, 168, 187

Band fibers, **312**, 313
Barbs, 378, **378**
Barbules
  distal, 378, **378**
  proximal, 378, **378**
Baroreceptors, 326 (see aortic and carotid sinuses also)
Barr body, 28
Bars, 365, **366**
Basal
  body, 40, **40**, 41, **222**
    rootlets of, 41
  cells
    of taste buds, **385**
  complex
    of choroid, 534
  lamina, 52, **69**, 71, **72**, 92, 95
    of kidney, **433–437**, 435
  membrane, 549
  plate, 286, **289, 290**
Basic metabolic unit (BMU)
  of bone, 139, **140**, 142
Basilar membrane, 549, **550**, 551, **551**
Basket cell, 66, **68**

Basement membrane, 52, 70, 71, **71**
Basophil, 169, **170**, 244, **245**
  avian, 174, **174**
  kinetics of, 186
  of pars distalis, 469, **470**
  tissue, 98
Basophilia, 7
Basophilic
  erythroblasts, 181
  leukocyte, 169, **170**
  normoblasts, 181
  stippling, 167, **167**
B cells
  of magnum, 525
  of the pancreas, 484
Beta cells
  of pancreas, 484
  of pars distalis, 469, B470
Beta-hydroxybutyric acid, 404
Bell stage, 386, **387, 388**
Bethanechol, 311, **311**
Bicarbonate buffer, 461
Bile
  canaliculi, 421. **423–425**
  ducts, 421, **423, 425**
  salts, 426
Bilirubin, 184, **185**, 426
  conjugated, 184, **185**
  glucuronide, 184, **185**
  unconjugated, 184, **185**
  plasma bound, 184, **185**
Biliverdin, 184, **185**
Biogenic amines, 483
Biopsy
  aspiration, 554
  punch, 554
Biotransformation, 426
Bipolar neurons, 208, **212**
Birefringence, 14, **15**
Blastoid transformation, 183, **183**
Bloat, 404
Blockers
  α-, 312
  β-, 312
Blood, 164–178
  barriers (see specific barriers)
  cells of, 166–174 (see specific cells also)
    avian, 173–175
    bovine, 173
    canine, 171, 172
    caprine, 173
    counts of
      differential, 187
      red cell, 187
      white cell, 187
    destruction of, 184. 185, **185**
    developmental
      deteminants, 179, 180
      theories of, 179
        diphyletic, 179
        monophyletic, 179, **179**
        polyphyletic, 179
    equine, 172, 173
    evaluation of, 186, 187
    feline, 172
    mammalian, 166–173
    ovine, 173
    porcine, 173
    trends in development of, 180, **180**
  characteristics of, 164
  coagulation of
    factors in, 175, 176, **176**
  development of, 179–186
  functions of, 164
  general characteristics of, 179, 180
  hemoglobin and, 181
  kinetics of, 183–186
  oxygenation of, 460
  selected parameters of, **164**
  urea nitrogen (BUN), 442
    postrenal, 442
    prerenal, 442
    renal, 442
Blood-
  air barrier **458**, 459, **459**
    minimal, **458**, 459, **459**

aqueous barrier, 537
  cerebrospinal fluid barrier, 300, **302**
  brain barrier, 300, **302**
  nerve barrier, 293
  testis barrier, 496, **496**
  thymic barrier, 340, **343, 344**
Bodian classification, 208, **213**
Body
  cavities
    cytology of contents of, 559, 560, **561**
  fluids
    and ground substance, 86, 87
    mechanisms of exchange, 88, **88, 89**
  water, 86
    distribution of, 86, 87, **87**
Bone
  as an organ, 259–264
  as a tissue, 119–142
  ash content of, 259
  basic metabolic unit (BMU) of, 139, **140**
  cartilage and modeling of, 260, **262**
  cells of, 122–129 (see specific cells also)
  characterisitics of, 119
  changes of
    qualitative, 259
    quantitative, 259
  chemical composition of, 119, 120
  classification of, 119
  collagen of, 119
  comparison of cartilage to, 119
  composition of, 259
  configurations of
    cancellous, 119
    compact, 119
    spongy, 119
    trabecular, 119
  decalcification of, 121
  density, 259, **259**
    radiographic, 259
    high, 259
    low, 259
  development of, 146–163 (see ossification also)
  envelopes of, 121, **121**, 122, **122, 123**
  flexure-drift of, 260, 261, **261**
  functions of, 119
  growth of, 119
  growth plates and, 157–159
  hormonal influence upon, 142–2145
  in vivo labels of, 142, **143**
  lamellae of
    endosteal, 131, **134, 135**
    circumferential
      inner, 131, **134, 135**
      outer, 131, **134, 135**
    periosteal, 131, **134, 135**
  lymphatics of, 263
  marrow
    biopsy of, 554
    evaluation of, 187
    red, 179, 180, **181**
      compartment of
        vascular, 180, **181**
        hematopoietic, 180, **181**
    yellow, 179, 180, 181
  matrix of, 119–121
    inorganic, 119–121
    organic, 119
  metabolism and
    calcium, 142–145
  mineral content of, 119, 120
  modeling of, 262, **263**
  nerves of, 263, 264
  organization of, 131–135
  osteons of (see osteons)
  piezoelectricity and, 259, 260, **260**
  porosity, 131
  preparation of samples of
    demineralized, 121
    mineralized, 121
  properties of
    biological, 262–264
    biomechanical, 260, **260**
    compressive, 120
    dynamic, 262
    physical, 259, 260
    tensile, 120

transducer, 259, 260, **260**
remodeling of, 135–142
  ARF sequence and, 139
  histological evidence for, 139, **140**, 141
  stimuli for, 139
  sigma for, 139
  remodeling unit (BRU), 139, **140**
repair, 264–269 (see fracture repair also)
stem cells of, 119
strain and, 260
  compressive, 260, **260**
  flexural, 260
  shearing, 260
  tensile, 260
  torque, 260
stress and, 260
structural unit of, 139
subchondral, **272, 273**
tetracycline labeling of, 142, **235**
types of, 119
  fibrous, 119
  immature, 119
  lamellar, 119
  mature, 119
  woven, 119
vasculature of, 262, 263, 264, **264**
  anastomotic, 264
venous drainage of
  cortical, 263
  periosteal, 263
Bony spiral lamina, 549
Book, 403
Border
  basal, 52
  brush, 71, 74
  cells, **551**, 552
  luminal, 52
  striated, 71, **73**
Boutons, 213, **218**
  en passage, 213, **218**
  terminaux, 213, **218**
Bowl-shaped cells, 168
Bowman's
  capsule, 431, **432**, 433, **433**
    layer of
      parietal, 433, **433**, 435
      visceral, 433, **433**
  glands, 447
  membrane, 529
Bradycardia, 327
Brain, 303, 304, **304**
  development of
    three-vesicle stage and, 285, **287**
    five-vesicle stage and, 285, **287**
  sand, 474
  stem, 242, **243**, 303, **303**
Bronchi
  avian, 463, 464, **464**
  extrapulmonary, 450
    primary, 450
  fluid of, 452
  glands of, 451, **451**
  intrapulmonary, 450, 452, **451**
    primary, 451, **451**
    secondary, 451
    tertiary, 451, **451**
  recurrent, 464
Bronchial
  fluid, 452
  glands, 451, **451**, 452
Bronchiolar cells, 453
Bronchioles, 452, **452**, 453, **453**
  primary, 452
  respiratory, 453, **454**
  secondary, 452
  terminal, **452**, 453
  tertiary, 452
Bronchioloalveolar portals, 453
Bronchoconstriction, 460
Bronchodilation, 460
Brown adipose tissue, 106, **106**
Bruch's membrane, 534
Brunner's glands,
Brush border
  of osteoclasts, 129, **129, 130**
  of proximal convoluted tubules, 436, **437**

Buccal
  cavity, 380
    avian, 412, **412**
    cytology of, (*see* specific organs also)
  glands
    dorsal, 418
    ventral, 418
Buffer systems, 443
Bulbar conjunctival epithelium, 529
Bulbocavernosus muscle, 504
Bulbourethral glands, 502, **503**
Bulbs, 371
Bulbus oculi, 527, **530**
Bundle
  atrioventricular, 324, **327**
  branches
    left, 324, **326**
    right, 324, **326**
  of His, 324, **326**
Bursa of Fabricius, 183
  equivalent of, 183, **183**
Burst-forming unit—erythrocytic (BFU-E), 179, 180, 184
Butyric Acid, 404

Caeca, 415
Calamus, 378, **378**
Calciferol, 143
Calcification, 146
  dystrophic, 144
  metastatic, 146
Calcium
  as a messenger, 32
  and vitamin D, 142–145
  and renal function, 442
  complexed, 142
  diffusible, 142
  free, 142
  functions of, 142
  homeostatic
    levels of, 142
    maintenance of, 142–145
  hormonal regulation of, 142–145
  metabolism of, 142–145
  nondiffusible and protein bound, 142
  regulation of, 142–145
  regulatory system for
    PTH/CT/Vitamin D, 144, **145**
Calcitonin (CT), 142–145, **145**
  biological effects of, 143
  target organ responses to, 143, 144, **145**
Calculus, 390
Call-Exner bodies, 509
Callus, 266, 267, **267**
  formation of,
  types of
    bridging, 268
    endosteal, 267, **268**
    external, 267, **267**, **268**
    hard, 268
    internal, 267, **268**
    permanent, 268
    soft, 268
    temporary, 268
Calmodulin, 32
Calorigenic effect, 476
Canaliculi
  bile, 421, **423–425**
  bone, 119, 128, **128**, **129**
  secretory, 65, **66**
Canal
  communicating, **138**
  of Schlemm, 537
  Volkmann's, 135
Cancellous bone, 131, **133**
Capacitation, 513
Capillaries, 314, 315, **314**, B317–319
  continuous, 315, **318**
  fenestrated, 315, **318**
  lymphatic, 328
  perforated, 315, **318**
  sinusoidal, 315
  terminal arterial, 336, **341**
  venous, 322
Cap stage, 386, **387**, **388**
Capsular urine, 441

Capsule, 113
Carbachol, 311, **311**
Carbaminohemoglobin, 461
Carbohydrates, 23
Carbon dioxide, 461, **462**
Carbonic anhydrase, **398**, 399
Carboxyhemoglobin, 166
Carboxypeptidase A, B, 430
Cardiac
  glands, **394**, 395
  glycosides, 327
  inhibitory center, 326, 329
  muscle, 204–206, 242, **243**
    functional correlates of, 206
    histology of, 204, **204**, **205**
    junctional complexes of, 204, **206**
    regeneration of, 207
    repair of, 207
  output, 327, **328**, **329**
  stimulatory center, 326, **329**
  valves, 324, **326**, **327**
Cardiovascular system, 314–329
  activity of
    and pain, 328
    antidiuretic hormone and, 328
  characteristics of, 314
  components of (*see* specific components)
    comparison of, 322
    exchange, 314, **314**, 315
    pressure
      high, 315–322
      low, 322
  features of, 322, 323
  functions of, 314
  hormonal influence upon, 328
  neuroregulation of, 326, 327, **328**
  organization of, 314
    mural (*see* tunica)
Carminophils
  of the pars distalis, 469, **470**
Carotid
  bodies, 325
  sinuses, 326
Carpal glands, 365
Cartilage, 108–118
  articular (*see* articular cartilage)
  canals, 157, **157**
  cells of, 108 (*see* specific cells also)
  characteristics of, 108
  classification of, 109
  collagen of, 109, **110**
  compressibility of, 110
  electron microscopy of, 111, **112–114**
  fibers of, 109
  functions of, 108
  glycosaminoglycans of, 109, **109**, 110, **111**
  ground substance of, 109, 110
  growth of, 108
  maintenance of, 117, 118
  matrix of, 109–112
    capsular, 110, **111**
    haloes of, 111
    heterogeneity of, 111
    hydrodynamic domain of, 110
    interterritorial, 110, 111, **11–113**
    pericellular, 110, 111, **11–113**
    stability of, 109
    territorial, 110, 111, **11–113**
    volume definition of, 109, 110
  models, 153
  origin of, 108
  repair of, 117, 118
  staining of, 110, 111
  types of, 113–117 (*see* specific tissue also)
  ultrastructure of, 111, **111–113**
Caruncles, 513, **515**, 519
  maternal, 519
Casts
  granular, 557, **557**
  renal, 557
  waxy, 557
Catagen, 355, **356**
Catalase, 38
Cataracts, 539
Catecholamines, 214, 216, **219**, 493
Catechol-o-methyl transferase (COMT), 215, **219**

Caudal
  limiting membrane, 529
  sheath, 497, **497**
Caveolae, 71, 73, **73**
C cells,
  of the pancreas, 484
  of magnum, 525
  of the pars distalis, 469, **470**
  of the thyroid gland, 474, **475**
Cecum, 409, **410**
Cell
  body, 208, **209**
  coat (*see* glycocalyx)
  counts
    white blood, 187
    red blood, 187
  culture, 4, **4–5**
  cycle, 45, 46, **46**
  differentiation,
  division, 45–48, **46**, **47**
  -mediated immunity, 171
  membrane, 29
    as receptors, 32
    properties of, 31
    fluidity of, 31
    functions of, 31
    structure of, 29, 30, **30**, 31
    transport functions of
      active, 32
      passive, 32
  messengers, 32
    primary, 32
    secondary, 32
  nests, 113, **115**
  specialization, 45, 47
Cell-mediated immunity (CMI), 344, 347
α Cells
  of the pars distalis, 469, 470
  of the pancreas, 484
β Cells
  of the pars distalis, 469, **470**
  of the pancreas, 484
δ Cells
  of the pars distalis, 469, **470**
  of the pancreas, 484
ε Cells
  of the pars distalis, 469, **470**
γ Cells
  of the pars distalis, 469, **470**
Cells (*see* also specific cells)
  activities of, 23, 24
  compartmentalization within, 29
  conductivity by, 23
  contractility of, 23
  division of labor among, 23
  general characteristics of, 22–24
  growth of, 24
  internal respiration by, 23
  irritability of, 23
  maintenance of, 24
  metabolism by, 23
    anabolic, 23
    catabolic, 23
  morphological features of, 24
  nutritive inclusions of, 43, 45
  of Claudius, **551**, 552
  of Hensen, **551**, 552
  of Leydig, 489
  of Sertoli, 489
  organelles of, (*see* specific organelles also)
  properties of
    biological, 23, 24
    chemical, 22, 23
    physical, 22, 23
  reproduction of, 24
  shape of, 24, **24–27**
  size of, 24
  spatial organization of, 24, **27**
Cellular
  limits, 29
  meshwork, 94
  polarity, 24, 52
  reticulum, 94
  tubes, **312**, 313
Cement line, 135, **135**, **136**, 240, **241** (*see* reversal line also)

Cementoblasts, 389
Cementocytes, 389
Cementum, 386, **387**, 388
  acellular, 389
  cellular, 389
Centesis
  abdominal
    smear of, 248, **249**
Central
  intermediate substance, 303, **303**
  nervous system, 285–287, 294–304
Centrifugation
  differential, 5
  density gradient, 5
Centrioles, 39, **40**, 47
Centroacinar cell, 429, **429**, **430**
Centromere, 47
Centrosphere, 39, 47
Cephalic phase, 398
Cephalin, 23
Cephalization, 285, **287**
Cerebellum, **235**, 303, **304, 305**
Cerebral hemispheres, 285, **287**
Cerebrum, 303, **305**
Cerebrospinal fluid (CSF), 294, 296–302
  barrier between blood and, 300, **301, 302**
  characteristics of, 297
  circulation of, 298
  ependymal cells and, **302**
  formation of, 297, 298
  functions of, 298, 300
Ceruloplasm, 166
Cerumen, 545
Ceruminous glands, 545
Cervical
  enlargement, 303
  intumescence, 303
Cervix, 512
  uteri, 513
Chamber
  anterior, **530**, 537
  posterior, **530**, 537
Cheek, **380**, 381
Chelation, 121
Chemoreceptors, 325, 326 (see carotid and aortic bodies
    also)
Chestnut, 372
α-Chains, 77, **78, 79**
Chief cells
  of glandular stomach, 395, **395–397**
    clear, dark and light
    of parathyroid gland, 142, 476, **477**
  of pars distalis, 469, **470**
  of pineal gland, 474
Cholagogues, 429
Cholangioles, 421, **425**
Cholecalciferol, 143
  and calcium metabolism, 143–145
  1, 25-dihydroxy-, 144, 145
  24, 25-dihydroxy-, 143, 144
  25-hydroxy-, 143
Cholecyst, 428, **428**, 429
Cholecystokinin (CCK), 399, 428, 484, 487
Cholesterol, 31
Choline, 23
  acetylase, 214
Cholinergic
  drugs, 308, **308**, 311, **311**
  fibers, 308, **308**
  receptors, 308, **308**
Cholinesterase
  acetyl, 214
    inhibitors, 311
  true, 214
  specific, 214
Cholinomimetics, 311, **311**
Chondroblast, 108, 113, **114, 115**
Chondroclast, 108
  origin of, 108
  relationship to osteoclast, 108
Chondrocytes, 108, 113, **113–116**, 240, **241**
Chondrodysplasia, 149
Chondrodystrophy, 110
Chondrogenic centers, 108, **152–154**, 153
Chondroitinase, 111

Chondroitin
  -4-sulfate, 84, **85**
  -6-sulfate, 84, **85**
Chondronectin, 76, 86
Chondrones, 271
Chordae tendinae, 324
Choriocapillary layer, 534
Choristoma, 531
Choroid, 527, 528, **530–532**, 532, **533**
  fissure, 527, 528
  layers of, 532
  plexus, 219, **22**, 296, **300, 301**
Chromaffin
  cell, 483, **483**
  system, 483
Chromatids, 48
Chromatolysis, 209, 561
  retrograde, **312**, 313
Chromatin, 28
Chromatophores, 100
Chromomere, 171
Chromoprotein, 184
Chromophilic cells
  of the pars distalis, 469, **470**
Chromophobic cells
  of the pars distalis, 469, **470**
Chromosomes, 47
  homologous, 48
  replication of, 46
Chromoproteins, 23, 184
Chronotropy
  negative, 327
  positive, 217, 327
Chylomicrons, 409
Chyme, 393
Chymotrypsin, 430
Chymotrypsinogen, 430
Cilia, 39-42, **40–43**, **53**, 55, **55**, 222
  beat cycle of, 42, **43**
    stroke of
      effective, 42, **43**
      recovery, 42, **43**
  kino-, 40, **40**, **41**, 52, 73
  motility of, 42, **43**
  rootlet of, **222**
  stereo-, 39, **41**, 52, 73, **74**
Ciliary
  body, 527, **530**, **533**, 534
  epithelium, 535, **535**
  glands, 544
  muscle, 527, 534
  process, 534, 535, **535**
Circumanal
  glands, **360**, 361
  region
    glands of, **360**, 361, **361**
Cirrhosis, 428
Clara cells, 453
Clasmatocyte (see macrophage)
Claws, 371, **371, 372**
Climbing fibers, 303
Clitoris, 514
Cloaca, 415
Clonal expansion, 341
Close junction, **68**, 70, **70**
Clot
  formation, 175
  retraction, 175
CMI (see immunity)
Coagulation, 175–177
  clot formation during, 176, 177
  dissolution of clot, 177, **177**
  factors of, 175. 176
  mechanisms of, 175, 177
  pathway of
    common, 176, **176**
    extrinsic, 175, **176**
    intrinsic, 175, 176, **176**
  scheme of, **176**
  stages of, 175
  vitamin K and, 176
Coarsely bundled bone, 129
Coat
  subendocardial, 323, **324**
  subendothelial, 323, **324**

subepicardial, 323, **324**
Cochlea, 527, 549–552, **550–552**
Cochlear duct, 549, 550, **550, 551**
Codon, 33, **35**
  initiator, 33
  signal, 33
  terminal, 33
Cohnheim's fields, **192**
Collagen, 76–82
  and bone, 119
  and connective tissue, 101, 102
  axial periodicity of, **79**, 81, **81**
  basement membrane, 77, **77**
  characteristics of, 77
  disorders of, 82
  during ossification, 146
  extracellular alteration of, 80, **80**
  fibers of, 82
  fibrils of, 82
  general properties of, 76
  histologic appearance of, 77, **77**
  interstitial, 77, **77**
  of cartilage, 109
  of cornea, 529
  of proper connective tissues, 101, **101, 102**
  microfibrils of, 81
  polymerization of, **80**, 81
  posttranslational modification of, 77, **78**, **79**, 80, 82
  structure of, 77, **78, 79**
  synthesis of, 77, **77, 78**
  types of, 71, 77, **77**
  zone of
    overlap, 81, **81**
    hole, 81, **81**
Collagenase, 84, 430
  and ovulation, 510
Collar bone, **153**, 154, **155**
Collecting
  duct system, **432**, 437, 438, **439**
  tubules
    arched, 437
    straight, 437
Colliculus seminalis, 502
Colloid, 22, 29, 475, **475**
  hydrophilic, 29
  of thyroid gland, 474, **474, 475**
Coloboma, 528
  iridis, 528
Colon, 409, **411**
Colony
  -forming unit (CFU), 179, **179**, 180
    -BL (B lymphocytic), **179**, 180, 182
    -E, (erythrocytic), **179**, 180, 184
    -EO (eosinophilic), **179**, 180
    -GM (granulocytic/monocytic), **179**, 180, 182, 186
    -M (megakaryocytic), **179**, 180
    -TL (T lymphocytic), **179**, 180, 182
  inhibiting activity (CIA), 186
  stimulating factor (CSF), 186
Colostrum, 361, 409
Communicating
  canal, **124, 138**
  junction, **68**, 70, **70**
Compact bone, 131, **134**
Complement, 347
Cone cells, 541, **543**
Cones, 427
Congeners, 311, **311**
Conjunctiva
  bulbar, 529
  limbic, 532
  palpebral, 529, 532, 543, **543, 544**
  of fornix, 529
  scraping of, 248, **249**
    with keratoconjunctivitis sicca, 248, **249**
Conjunctival
  sac, 544
    cytology of, 561
Connecting
  cilium, 541, **543**
  tubules, 437
Connective tissue, 3, 92–105
  cell populations of
    resident, 94–99
    transient, 99, 100

Connective Tissue—Continued
  characteristics of, 3, 92
  classification of, **93**, 94
  dense white fibrous, 240, 241
    irregular, 103, **103**
    regular, 103, **103**
  derivation of, 3
  embryonal
    mesenchymal, 100, **100**
    mucous, 101, **101**
  extracellular material of, 76–86
  fibers of, 76–83
  fluid of, 102
  functions of, 3, 92
  matrix of, 92
  origin of, 92
  proper, 101–104
    areolar, 101, **101**, **102**, 103, 240, **241**
      hyperplastic, 240, **241**
    elastic, 104, **104**
  regeneration of, 106, 107
  repair of, 106, 107
  reticuloareolar, 405
  special (*see* specific tissue also)
    pigmented, **100**, 105
    reticular, 104
  types of (*see* specific types)
  unique relationships of, 92
Constrictor
  vestibuli, 514
  vulvae, 514
Contractions
  eructation, 404
  mass, 410
  mixing, 404
  regurgitation, 404
  segmenting, 408, 410
  slow wave, 410
Contraction zone, 200
Converting enzyme, 439
Coprodaeum, 415
Coprophagy, 410
Corium (*see* dermis)
Cornea, 527, 528, **530**, 529, **531**
  functional correlates of, 531
  repair of, 531, 532
  species differences, 531
  stroma of, 527
  transparency of, 531
Corneoscleral junction, 529, **530**, 532
Cornua uteri, 512
Corona
  of lymph nodules, 332, **333**, 334
  radiata, **508**, 509, 510
Coronary
  corium, **366**, 367, **368**, **369**
  epidermis, **366**, 367, **368**, **369**
Coronet, 365, **366**
Corpora
  amylacea, 364, **365**
  arenacea, 474
Corpus
  albicans, 511
  atreticum, 510
  cavernosa clitoris, 514
  cavernosum
    penis, 504, **504**
    urethrae, 504, **504**
  fibrosum, 511
  hemorrhagicum, 511
  luteum, 506, 511, **511–512**
    cyclicum, 511
    graviditatis, 511
    regressum, 511
  nigrum, 536, **536**
  prostatae, 501
  spongiosum, 504
  uteri, 513
Cortical labyrinth, 431, **432**
Corticomedullary junction
  of kidney, 431, **431**
Corticosteroid-binding globulin (CBG), 482
Corticotropin, 472
Cortisol, 482
Cotyledon
  fetal, 519

Countercurrent
  exchangers, 442
  mechanism, 442, 443, **443**
  multipliers, 442
  -type exchanger
    of avian lung, 465
Cowper's glands, 502, **503**
Cranial nerves, 291, 292
  organization of, 290
  reflex patterns of, 290
Craniosacral system, 306, 307
Creatine, 201, **203**
  phosphate (CP), 201, **203**
  phosphokinase (CPK), 201, **203**
Crenated cells, 168
Cristae
  ampullares, 547, **547**, 549, **549**
  mitochondriales, 36, **37**, **38**
Critical point drying, 11
Crop, 412, **413**
  milk, 412
Cross-current exchanger
  of avian lung, 465
Crown, 386, **386**
  formation of, **387**, 388, **388**, **389**
Cryotome, 8
Crypts
  intestinal, 405, **405**
  of Lieberkuhn, 405, **405**
  of tonsils, 331, **332**
Crystalloids, 22
Cumulus oophorus, **508**, 509, **510**
Cup-shaped cells, 168
Cupula, 549
Cushing's syndrome, 482
Cutaneous mucous membrane, **257**, 258, 350, **380**, 381, **381**
Cuticle
  of the root sheath, 351, **352**
  of the hair, 351, **352**
Cutting cone, **140**, **141**, 142
Cyanomethemoglobin, 187
Cyanosis, 462
Cyclic
  adenosine monophosphate (cAMP), 32
  guanidine monophosphate (cGMP), 32
Cyclooxygenase, 486
Cytochemistry, 2, 8, **8**
Cytofilament, 43, **43**
Cytogenic organs
  types of (*see* specific organs)
Cytokinesis, 48, 182
Cytology, 2
  clinical, 554–562
  ultrastructural, 2
Cytolysosomes, 37, **39**
Cytolytic reactivity, 346
Cyton, 208
Cytoplasm, 28–45
  characteristics of, 28, 29
  compartmentalization of, 29
  focal degeneration of, 37, **39**
  ground substance of, 28
  inclusions of, 43–45
    secretory, 43
    nutritive, 43–45
  membranous compartments of, 32–38
  skeleton of, 38–43
  staining of
    acidophilic, 29
    basophilic, 29
    chromophobic, 29
    neutrophilic, 29
Cytoreticulum
  of thymus, 339, **342–344**
Cytosine, 22
Cytoskeleton, 43, **43**
Cytotoxic
  effector cells, 334
  reactivity, 346

Deamination, 427
D cell
  of pancreas, 484
Decidual cell, 521

Defense system
  primary, 330
  secondary, 330
7-Dehydrocholesterol, 143, **145**
Deglutition, 380
Deiodination, 476
Delayed
  hypersensitivity, 347
  union, 268
Delta cell
  of the pars distalis, 469, **470**
Dendrites, 208, 209, 211, **212**
Dendritic
  cells, 344
    of lymph nodes, 332
    of skin, 355
  zone, 209, **213**
Dense
  bars, 281
  bodies, 37, **39**, 190, **191**
  connective tissue, **235**
  lines, **230**, 231
Dental
  arch, 386
  lamina, 386, **387**
  pad, **381**, 382
  papilla, 386, **387**
  pulp, 389
  sac, 386, **387**, 388, **388**
Dentinal
  fibers, 389, **390**
  tubules, 389, **390**
Dentin, 386, 389, **390**
  secondary, 389
Dentition (*see* teeth)
Deoxyribonuclease, 430
Deoxyribonucleic acid (DNA), 22
Deoxyribose, 22
Dermal
  network, 350
  papillae, 349, **349**, 351, **354**
Dermatan sulfate, 84, **85**
Dermatosparaxis, 82
Dermis, 348, **348**, 349, **349**, 350
  coronary, 367, **367**
  laminar, 367, **367**
  perioplic, 367, **367**, 370, 371
  zone of
    papillary, 349, **349**
    reticular, 349, **349**
Dermoid growth, 531
Descemet's membrane, 529
Descending
  limb, **432**, 436
  thin segment, **432**, 436
Desmosine, 83
Desmosomes, 52, **56**, **68**, **69**, 70, **70**
  and cardiac muscle, 204, **296**
Detumescence, 505
Dewclaws, 372
Diabetes
  insipidus, 443
  mellitus, 443
    complicated, 443, 485
Diads, 204, **205**
Diaphyseal ossification center, 154, **154**, 155, **155**
Diarthroses (*see* synovial joints)
Dicalcium phosphate dihydrate, 120
Diencephalon, 285, **287**
Diestus, 515, 517
Differential cell counts, 560
Differentiation, 47
Diffusely basophilic erythrocyte, 181
Diffuse nerve endings, 293, 294, **296**
Diffusion, 32, 87
  facilitated, 32, 409
Digestion,
  ruminant, 404, 405
Digestive system, 380–430
  avian, 412–415
  cytology of, 556, **556**, **557**
  functions of, 380
  organization of, 252–254
  organs of (*see* specific organs)
  structure of, 380
Digital

cushion, 350, 371
   pad, 350
Diglyceride lipase, 486
Dihydroepiandrosterone, 483
1, 25-Dihydroxycholecalciferol (1, 25-DHCC), 143, **145**
24, 25-Dihydroxycholecalciferol (24, 25-DHCC), 143, **145**
Dihydroxyphenylalanine (DOPA), 214, **219**
   reaction, 100
3, 5-Diiodotyrosine (DIT), 475
Dioptric media, 528, 537
Disaccharides, 23
Distal
   convoluted tubule, 431, **432**
   ossification center, **153**, 157
Diuresis
   osmotic, 443
   water, 443
Diverticulum tubae auditivae, 546
Dopamine, 213, 214, **219**, 312
   β-hydroxylase, 214, **219**
Dorsal
   columns, 303, **303**
   funiculus, 303, **303**
   grey column, 305, **306**, 289, **289–291**
   motor nucleus of vagus nerve, 326, B329
   root, 305, **306**, **289**, 291
      ganglion, 289, **289**, 290, 291
Dromotropy
   negative, 327
   positive, 327
Ductless glands, 467–488
Ducts
   common bile, 421, 423
   cystic, 421
   excretory, 61, **62, 63**
   extrahepatic, 421, **422, 425**
   intercalated, 417, **417, 418**
   intrahepatic, 421, **422, 425**
   intralobar, 63, **63**
   intralobular, 63, **63**
   lobar, 63, **63**
   lobular, 63, **63**
   mesonephric, 433
   Müllerian, 433
   of Hering, 421, **425**
   papillary, **432**, 438
   paramesonephric, 433
   striated, 417, **417, 418**
   thyroglossal, 474
   Wolffian, 433
Ductuli efferentes, 492, **493**
Ductus
   choledochus, 421, 423
   cochlearis, 549
   deferens, 492, **495**
   epididymidis, 492, **494**
   reuniens, 549
Duodenal glands, 405, **406**
Duodenum, 405, **405, 406**
Dural
   sinuses, 294
   venous sinuses, 298, **298**
Dura mater, 294, **298, 299**, 527
Dynein, 41, **42**
Dwarfism, 472

Ear
   external, 545
   inner, 546–552
   middle, 545, 546
   ossicles, 545
Eclampsia, 144, 201
Ectoderm,
   derivatives of, 52
Ectoplasm, 29
Ectopic foci, 324
Edema, 90
Effector, 467, **467**
Efferent, 208
   fibers, 288
   system
      general somatic (GSE), 288, **290**
      general visceral (GVE), 288, **290**
      special visceral (SVE), 288, **290**
Effusions, 560, 561

hemorrhagic, 560
Ehlers-Danlos syndrome, 82
Eicosanoids, 345, 486, 487, **487**
Eicosatetraenoic acid, 486
Elastase, 430
Elastic
   cartilage, 113–115, **235**, 240, **241**
   connective tissue, 104, **104**
   fiber, 82, 83, **83**
   lamina, 534
Elastin, 76, 82
Electrochemical transmission, 211–213, **216–219** (*see* synapses also)
Electrophoresis, 187
Electrotonic
   junctions (*see* ephapses)
   transmission (*see* ephapses)
Enamel, 386, 388, **389**
   organ, 386, **387–390**
   pulp, 386, **387, 389**
   rods, 389
Encapsulated nerve endings (*see* specific type or corpuscle)
Enchondral ossification (*see* endochondral)
End
   bulbs, 213, **218**
   feet, 213, **218**
Endocardium, 323, **325**
Endochondral ossification, 149–163, **152–163**
   bone shape and, 159–161
   cartilage models and, 153–159
   diaphyseal growth during, 159, 160, **161**
   epiphyseal growth during, 153, **157**, 161, **163**
   effects of hormones upon, 161–163
   functions of, 149, 153
   general features of, 149, 153
   modeling and, 153–157, **153**
   ossifications centers in, 154–161
   sequence of, **153**
   vascular invasion during, **153**, 154
Endocrine
   cells, 467, 485, 486
   glands
      miscellaneous, 485–487
      system, 467–488
         characteristics of, 467
         glands of (*see* specific glands)
         hormones of (*see* specific hormones)
      organs of (*see* specific organs)
Endocytosis, 23, 37, 71, **73**
Endoderm
   derivatives of, 52, 53
Endolymph, 546
Endometrial cup, 519, **519, 520**
Endometrium, 513, **513–515**
   phase of
      ischemic, 517
      premenstrual, 517
      menstrual, 517
Endomitosis, 182
Endomysium, 236, **237**, 276
Endoneurium, 292, **293, 294**
Endoplasm, 29
Endorphins, 395
   β-, 472
Endosteum, 119, 121, **121**, 122, **122**, 131
   characteristics of, 121, 122
   subsets of
      cortical, 121, **121, 123**
      osteonal, 121, **123**
      trabecular, 121, **121–123**
Endotenon, 277, **278**
Endothelium, 53, 314, **314–321**, 323, **325**
   of anterior chamber, 529
   of cornea, 529, **531**
Endpiece, 497, **498**
End-plate, 158, **158, 159**
   potential, 281
Enophthalmus, 537
Enterochromaffin cells, 395, 486
Enterocrinin, 409
Enteroendocrine cells, 395, 405, 486
Enteroglucagon, 395, 484, 486, 487
Enterohepatic circulation, 185, **185**, 426
Enterokinase, 430
Eosinophilia, 186

Eosinophilic chemotactic factor of anaphylaxis (ECF-A), 345
Eosinophilopoietin, 186
Eosinophils, 169, **169**, 244, **245**
   avian, 174, **174**
   hypersensitivity and, 169, 345
   life cycle of, 186
   kinetics of, 186
Ependyma, 297, **300–302**, 528
Ependymal cells, 218, **221, 222**
Ephapses, 211, **216**
Ephedrine, 312
Epicardium, 323, **326**
Epichondral ossification, **153**, 155, **155**
Epidermal pegs, 349, **349**, 350
Epidermis, 348, **348**
   coronary, 365, **367**
   laminar, 367, **367, 368**
   layer,
      intermediate, 57
      parabasal, 57
      superficial, 57
   of bars, **370**, 371
   of frog, **370**, 371
   of sole, **370**, 371
   perioplic, 365, **367**
Epididymis, 492, **493, 494**
Epidural
   anesthesia, 295, **299**
   space, 296
Epikeras, 372
Epimysium, 276
Epinephrine, 214, 216, **219**, 312, 483
   and adrenal medulla, 310, **310**
Epineural capping, 313
Epineurium, 292, **293–294**
Epiphyseal
   disk (*see* growth plate)
   plate (*see* growth plate)
Epiphyses, 240, **241**
   vascular supply to, 262–264, **264**
   tension, 261, **262**
   traction, 261, **262**
Epiphysis cerebri, 473, 474, **474**
Episclera, 528
Episcleral zone, 529
Epitendineum, 277, **278**
Epitenon, 277, **278**
Epithalamus, 285
Epithelia, 2, 52–75
   anterior
      of cornea, 529, **531**
   apical border modifications of, 71–73
   basal border modifications of, 70, 71
   cell-to-cell modifications of, 68–70
   cellular
      polarity of, 52
      density of, 52
   characteristics of, 2, 52–54
   ciliated, 66, **67**
   classification of, 53, 54
   derivation of, 2
   derivatives of (*see* specific structures)
   enamel
      inner, 386, **387–389**
      outer, 386, **387–389**
   form of, 52
   functions of, 2, 52
   glands of, 59–66 (*see* glands)
   mesenchymal, 529, **531**
   myo-, 66, **68**
   neurosensory, 66
   olfactory, 447
   origin of, 52
   pigment, 527, 528, 535, 541, **541, 542**
   posterior
      of cornea, 529, **531**
   pseudostratified, **53**, 54, **55**, 238, **239**
   regeneration of, 73, 74
   repair of, 73, 74
   respiratory, 382
   sensory, 66
   simple
      columnar, **53**, 54, **55**, 238, **239**, 246, **247**
      cuboidal, **53**, 54, **55**, 238, **239**
      squamous, **53**, 54

Epithelia—Continued
stratified
columnar, **57**, 58
cuboidal, 58, **58**
squamous, **53**, 55–57, **56**, **57**, 238, **239**
layers of, 55–57
keraninized, **56**, **57**, 57
nonkeratinized, 57, **57**
surface
of ovary, 506, **506**
transitional, **53**, 58, **58**, 59, 246, **247**
types of, 53, **53**
unique relationships of, 53, 54
Epithelial
-reticular cell, 337, 339, **342**, **344**
root sheath, **387**, 388, **388**
Epsilon cell, 469, **470**
Equine chorionic gonadotropin (ECG), 519
Erectile tissue, 504, 505
nasal cavity, 447
Ergosterol, 143
Ergot, 372
alkaloids, 312
Eructation, 404
Erythroblasts
basophilic, 181
orthochromatic, 181
polychromatophilic, 181
pro-, 181
Erythroclasia, 184, 185
Erythrocytes, 166, **166**, **167**
avian, 173, **173**, 174
basophilic stippling of, 167, **167**
counts of, 187
diffusely basophilic, 181
kinetics of, 184, **184**, 185, **185**
life
cycle of, 184
span of, **185**
orthochromic, 181
polychromatophilic, 167, 181
refractile bodies (ER) of, 167, **167**
rouleaux formation of, 166
sedimentation rate of, 187
variants of, 166–168
Erythrogen, 487
Erythrogenin, 184, **184**
Erythrophagocytosis, 244, **245**
Erythropoiesis, **180**, 181
cells of (see specific cells)
Erythropoietin (EP), 179, 183, 184, **184**, 185, **184**, 487
Esophagus
avian, 412, **413**
deglutition and the, 391
dysfunction of, 391
histology of, 390, 391, **391**, **392**
innervation of, 391
physiology of, 391
regurgitation and the, 391
repair of, 391, 393
vomiting and the, 391
Estradiol, 483
-17β, 512
Estrogens, 486, 511
and ossification, 161
effects upon bone, 144
Estrous cycle, 515, 516
changes during
ovarian, 516
uterine, 516, **517**
vaginal, 517, **518**
species differences, 516
Ethylenediamine tetra-acetic acid (EDTA), 187
Euchromatin, 27, **27**
Eustachian tube, 546
Eutheria, 517
Excitation
-contraction coupling, 193
Excitatory postsynaptic potential (EPSP), 215, 216, 308
Exfoliative cytology, 553–562
introduction to, 554–562
Exocrine pancreas, 484, 485
Exocytosis, 24, 71, **73**
External
auditory meatus, 350, 545
elastic membrane, 314

root sheath, 350, 351, **351**
Exteroception, 208
Extracellular
fluid (ECF), 92
matrix, 92
Extrafusal fibers, 281, **282**, 283
Extrinsic factor, 398
Exudates, 560
nonspecific, 560
Eye, 527–545
compartments of, 537–539
cytology of, 561
development of, 527, **527**, 528, **528**, **529**
dioptric media of, 528
filtration angle of, 528, **530**, 537, **537**
introduction to. 527
-lid, 543, **543**, 544, **544**
organization of, 528, **530**
tunics of, 528, **530**

Factor
activated, 175, 176, **176**
I, 176, **176**
II, 176
III, 175, **176**
V, 176, **176**
VII, 176, **176**
IX, 176, **176**
X, 176, **176**
XI, 175, **176**
XII, 175, **176**
Fascia, 276
bulbi, 529
Fasciae adherentes, 204
Fascicles, 292
Fat cell (see adipocyte)
Fats
emulsification of, 409
neutral, 409
Feathers, 378, **378**, 379
pulp, 378
Feedback systems
negative, 467
positive, 467, **467**
Fermentation, 404
Ferritin, 9, 184, **185**
Ferrous iron, 460
Fibrin, 164, 175, 176, **176**
split products of, 177
soluble monomers of, 176, **176**
Fibrinogen, 164, 176
Fibrinolysin, 177, **177**
Fibrinolysis, 176, 177, **177**
Fibroblasts, 94, **94**, 95, 97, **97**
Fibrocytes, 97, **97**
Fibrocartilage (see fibrous cartilage)
Fibronectin, 76, 86, **86**
plasma, 86
cellular, 86
cell surface, 86
Fibrosis, 97, 107
Fibrous
bone (see woven)
cartilage, 115–117, 240, **241**
joints, 270
lamina, 26
tunic, 528–532
Filtration
angle, 528, **530**, 537, **537**
barrier, 435
membrane, 435, **435**
slit, 435, **435**
Final common pathway, 204, 289, **291**
Fixatives
actions of, 6
additive, 6
coagulative, 5, 6
most ideal ratio for, 6
Flagella, 39, 497, **497**
Flavin oxidase, 38
Fluid
extracellular, 87 **87**
interstitial, 83, 87, **87**
intestinal
balance of, 410, 411
intracellular, 87, **87**

mosaic model, 29
tissue, 83, 87, **87**
transcellular, 87, **87**
Folded cells, 168
Follicles
antrum of, 508, **508**, 509, **510**
atresia of, 510, **511**
development of, 508–510
Graafian, **508**, 510, **510**
mature, **508**, 510, **510**
ovarian, 506, **506**508, **508–511**
primary, 508, **508**, 509
primordial, 508, **509**
secondary, 508, **508**, 509, **509**
tertiary, **508**, 509, **510**
tonsillar, 331, **332**
vesicular, **508**, 509, **510**
Follicle-stimulating hormone (FSH), 472, 498, 500
releasing factor (FRF), 472, 507
Follicular
atresia, 510, **510**
antrum, 509, **509**, 510
cells
of ovary, 508, **508–510**
lining cells
of thyroid gland, 474, **474**, 475, **475**
stigma, 510
Folliculostatin, 512
Fontanelle, 270
Foot
corium of, 371
equine, 365–371
-pads, 350
processes, 433, **433–437**
primary, 433, **433**, 434, 436
secondary, 433, **433**, 435, 436
Foramen
interventricular, 287, **287**
magnum, 287
of Luschka, 298
of Monro, 285, **287**
Formalin, 6
Fourth ventricle, 285, **287**
Fovea centralis, 541
Foveolae gastricae, 392, 393
Fracture repair
bone formation during
direct, 266, **266**
indirect, 266
contact, 266, **266**
factors influencing, 265
features of, 264, 265
gap, 266
intrinsic influences upon, 265
mechanism of
intention
primary, 265, 266, **266**
second, 265, 267–269, **267–269**
reduction and, 269
angulation, 269
displacement, 269
distraction, 269
stability and, 264
stage of
impact, 265–267
induction, 265–267
inflammatory, 265–267
remodeling, 266–268, **268**
reparative, 266–268, **268**
strength of bone during, 269
vasculature and, 264
Free nerve endings, 293, 294, **296**
Freeze fracture, 11
Frog, 365
Frontal process, 371
Fundic glands, **394**, 395, **395–397**, 397

G actin, 193, **199**
Galatose, 84
Galactosylhydroxylysyl-transferase, 77, 80
Gallbladder, 428, **428**
Gamma
-aminobutyric acid, 213
cell, 469, **470**
efferents, 282, **282**, 283
Ganglia, 290, 291, **291–293**

autonomic, 290
collateral, 305, **306**
craniospinal, 290
dorsal root, 291, **291, 292**
intramural, 290, **291**
motor, 291, **292**
parasympathetic, 291, **292**
paravertebral, 290, 305, **306**
peripheral, 305, **306**
prevertebral, 291, 305, **306**
sensory, 290
sympathetic, 291
terminal, 290, 305, **306**
vertebral, 305, **306**
Ganglion
  cell layer
    of retina, 541, **541, 542**
  cells, 291, 292
    cell sheaths and, 219, **223, 224**
  of the adrenal medulla, 483
Gap junctions, **68**, 70, **70**
  and cardiac muscle, 204
  of neurons, 211, **216**
  of smooth muscle, 190, **191**
Gastric
  acid, **398**, 399
  areas, 393
  emptying, 399
  folds, **392**, 393
  glands proper, 395, **395–397**, 398
  inhibitory peptide (GIP), 398, 399, 484, 486, 487
  juice, 398
  phase, 398, 399
  pits, **392**, 393
  secretion, 398, 399
  slow wave, 398
  ulcers, 400
Gastrin, 395, 399, 486, 487
  enteric, 399
Gastroduodenal junction, 398, **400**
Gastroenteropancreatic cells (GEP), 486
Gastrointestinal endocrine cells, 395, 486
Gating
  chemical, 32, 215, 216
  electrical, 32
Gels, 22
Gemmules, 211, **218**
General
  afferent
    somatic (GSA), 288, **290**
    visceral (GVA), 288, **290**
  efferent
    somatic (GSE), 288, **290**
    visceral (GVE), 288, **290**
  proprioception (GP), 288, **290**
Generation time, 45, **46**
Genital
  corpuscles, 294
  ducts, 492–495
Germinal
  center, **333**
  layer, 286, **289**
  matrix, 350
Giant cells, 98
  foreign body, 98, 171
  multinucleated
    of bone, 122
Gibbs-Donan equilibrium, 88
Gigantism, 163
Gingiva, **386**, 390
Gingival
  crest, 390
  crevice, 390
  sulcus, **386**, 390
Gizzard, **414**, 415, **415**
Gland
  cistern, 361, **362**
  sinus, 361, **362**
Glands
  alveolar, 61
    branched, 61, **62**
  avian
    mucosal, 412, **413, 414**
  classification of, 59
  compound, 61
    tubular, 61, **63**

acinar, 61
  tubuloalveolar, 61, **63**
  endocrine, 60, **61**
  exocrine, 60, **60**
    external secretion by,
    formation of, 60, **60**
  general features of, 59
  internal secretion by, 60, **61**
  method of elaboration, 63–65
    apocrine, 63, **64**
    holocrine, **64**, 65
    merocrine, **59**, 63
  mixed, 65, **65–67**
  mucosal, 254, **255**
  mucous, 66
  multicellular, 59
  number of cells in, 59
  of circumanal region, 360, 361, **361**
  of Harder, 544, **545**
  of Krause, 544
  of Littré, 502
  of Meibom, 543
  of Moll, 544
  of Wolfring, 544
  of Zeiss, 544
  of Zuckerkandl, 483
  serous, 66, **66**
  simple, 61
  specific (see specific glands)
  submucosal, 254, **255**, 412, **413, 414**
  subrugosal, 412, **413, 414**
  tubular
    apocrine, 238, **239**
    branched, 61, **62**
    coiled, 61, **61**
    straight, 61, **61**
  tubuloalveolar, 61
  unicellular, 59
Glans
  clitoridis, 514
Glassy membrane, 351
Glaucoma, 529, 537
Glioblasts, 285, **288, 289**
Globin, 184, **185**
Globular actin, 193, **199**
Globulins
  α-, **165**, 166
  β-, 166
  γ-, 166
  hapto-, 166
  immuno-, 166, 343, 344, **345**
  thyroxine-binding (TBG), 166
Glomerular filtration 441
  alterations to, 441
  mechanisms of, 441
  rate (GFR), 441
Glomerulus, 431, **432**, 433, **433**, 438, **440**
Glomus cells, 325
Glucagon, 484
Glucocorticoids, 472
Glucocorticosteroids, 472
  and ossification, 161
  effects upon bone, 144
Gluconeogenesis, 427
  and propionic acid, 404
Glucose
  -6-phosphatase, 34
  renal threshold of, 441
Glucosuria, 441
Glucosylgalactosylhydroxylysy-transferase, 77, 80
Glucuronate
  β-1, 3 N-acetylgalactosamine β-1, 4, 84, **85**
  β-1, 3 N-acetylglucosamine β-1, 4, 84, **85**
Glucuronyl transferase, 184, **185**, 215, **219**, 426
Glutamic acid, 213
Glycine, 213
Glycocalyx, 30, **31**, 32
  components of, 30
  functions of, 30
Glycogen, 23, 43, **45**
  alpha particles, 43, **45**
  beta particles, 43, **45**
  rosettes, 43, **45**
Glycogenolysis, 424
Glycolipids, 23
Glycol methacrylate (GMA), 9, **10**

Glycoproteins, 23, 76, 86, 119, 475
Glycopyrrolate, 311
Glycosaminoglycans (GAGs), 23, , 84, 85, **85**, 92
  polyanionic nature of, 84
  staining of, 86
Glycosidases, 38
Glycosidic linkage, 23
Glycosyltransferases, 86
Glycosylation, 35
  of collagen, **78**, 80
Glyoxylate system, 38
Goblet cells, 43, **44**, 53, 55, **55**, 235, 238, **239**, 405
  in a smear, 248, **249**
Goiter, 476
Golgi
  complex (apparatus), 34–36, **36**, **37**
    functions of, 35, 36
    structure of, 35, **37**
  endoplasmic reticulum lysosome (GERL), 36
  -Mazzoni corpuscles, 294
  tendon organ, 284, 294
  type I neurons, 208, **210**
  type II neurons, 208, **210**
Gonadal hormones, 486
  effects upon calcium metabolism, 144
Granular layer, 303, **304, 305**
Granulation tissue, 97, 373, 378
Granulocytes, 182 (see specific cells)
  avian, 174
  basophilic, 169, **170**
  eosinophilic, 169, **169**
  neutrophilic, 168, 169, **169**
  polymorphonuclear neutrophilic, 182
Granulocytopoiesis, 181, 182
  cells of, 181, 182 (see specific cells also)
Granulokinetics
  basophils, 186
  eosinophils, 186
  neutrophils, 185, 186
Granulomas, 98
Granulosa lutein cells, 511, **512**
Grey
  commissure, 303, **303**
  matter, 302, **303**
Grid, 14
Ground substance, 28, 83–86, 92
  amorphous, 83–86
  composition of, 83–86
  demonstration of, 83, 84
  properties of, 83, 84
Growth
  appositional, 108
  cartilage, 155
  hormone (GH), 471
    and ossification, 163
    effects upon bone, 145
    inhibitory factor (GHIF), 472
    releasing factor (GHRF), 472
  interstitial, 108
  plates, **235**
    angular deformities and, 260–262
    compression, 260, 261, **262**
    dual circulation to, 263, **264**
    formation of, 157–159
    mechanical forces and, 261, 262
    tension, 261, **262**
    types of, 260–262
    zones of, **153**, 157–159, **15–161**
Guanine, 22
Gustatory
  cells, 383, **385**
  sensation, 383
Gut-associated lymphatic tissue (GALT), 183
Guttoral pouch, 546

Hageman factor (XII), 177
Hair
  auxillary, 355, **356**
  beds, 351
  bulb, 351, **351–354**
  cells
    of vestibular apparatus, 547, **547**
    of organ of Corti, 552
  club, 355, **356**
  cycle, 355, **356**
  development of, 350

Hair—Continued
  follicle, 350, 351, **350–356**
    network, 350
  functions of, 350
  guard, 351, **355**
  organization, 350, 351
  principal, 351, **355**
  secondary, 351, **353**
  sensory, 355, 356
  shedding, 355
  sinus, 355, 356
  species differences, 351, 355
  tactile, 355, 356
  wool, 351, **355**
Half-desmosomes, **69**, 71, **73**
H band, **195**, 200
Haptoglobin, 166
Hassall's corpuscles, 339, **343**
Haversian
  canal (see osteonal canal)
  systems (see osteons)
Head cap, 497, **497**
Heart
  activity of, 325
  antidiuretic hormone and, 328
  autoregulation of
    homeometric, 325
    heterometric, 325
  conduction system of, 324, **325, 326**
  influences upon, 325
  neuroregulation of, 326–328
  organization of, 323, **324**
  physiology of, 324–328
  regulation of, 325–328
  sequential contraction of, 324, 325
  skeleton of, 323
  Starling's law of the, 325
  valves of, 324, 326, **326, 327**
Heat, 515
Heinz bodies, 167, **167**
Helicotrema, 549
Helper substances, 341
Hemal nodes, 334, **336**
Hematology, 164–177
Hematopoiesis, 179–186
  colony-forming units and, 179, **179**
  developmental trends in, 180, **180**
  theories of, 179, **179**
  trends during, 180, **180**
Hematopoietic inductive environment (HIM), 180
Heme, 184, **185**, 460
Hemicircumferential periosteal elevation, 262
Hemic-lymphatic system, 330, 554
  cytology of, 554, **554–556**
Hemocytometer, 187
Hemidesmosomes, **69**, 71, **73**
Hemoglobin, 23, 184, **185**, 460
  metabolism of, 184, 185, **185**
  saturation, 460
  variations of, 184
Hemoglobinometer, 187
Hemolymph nodes, 334
Hemopexin, 166
Hemosiderin, 45, 184, **185**, 246, **247**, 335
Hemostasis, 175–177
  platelet function in, 175
  vasculature in, 175
Hemostatic plug, 175
Henle's layer, 351, **352**
Heparin, 85, **85**, 98, 187
  sulfate, 85
Hepatic
  acinus, 423, 424, **427**
  lobule, 420, **421**, 423, **427**
  sinusoids, 421, **421–425**
Hepatocytes, 47, 238, **239**, 420, **421–425**, 423
Herbst corpuscle, 294
Herring
  bodies, 472, **473**
  -bone configuration, 117, **117**
Heterochromatin, 27, **27**
Heterochromia, 536
Heterophils, 168, 169, **169**, 174, **174** (see neutrophils also)
Hilus cells, 511
Hippomanes, 519

Histaminase, 345
Histamine, 98, 175, 345, 395
  and gastric secretions, 399
  as a neurotransmitter, 213
  receptors, 345
Histiocyte (see macrophage)
Histochemistry, 2, 8, **8**
Histology, 2
  definition of, 2
  gross anatomy and, 15
  history of, 2
  interpretation skills and, 15–20
  technical achievements and, 2, 4
  tools of, 2
Histopathology, 2
Hoof, 365–371
  general features of, 365, **366**
Honeycomb, 402
Homeostasis, 23
Horizontal cells, 541, 543
Hormone D (see Vitamin D)
Hormones, 66, 467
  defined, 467
  gastrointestinal, 486
  general, 485
  local, 486
  miscellaneous, 487
  nature and function, 467
  ovarian, 511
  regulation of activity by, 467, **467**
  reproductive, 486
  specific (see specific hormones)
Horn (see keratin also)
  gland, 365
  intertubular, 367, **367, 368**, 369
  laminar, 367, **367**, 370
  tubular, 367, **367, 368**, 369
Horns, 371
Horner's syndrome, 536, 537
Howell-Jolly (HJ) bodies, 167
Howship's lacuna, 129, **130**
H$_{1, 2}$ receptors, 399, 400
Humoral antibody
  response, 171, 183, 341–344
    anamnestic, 343
    B lymphocytes and, 341
    clonal expansion of, 341
    latent period of, 341
    primary, 186, 341
    secondary, 186, 343
Huxley's layer, 351, **352**
Hyaline cartilage, 113, **113–116**, 240, **241**
Hyalocytes, 537
Hyaloid
  artery, 528, **529**, 543
  membrane, 528
Hyaloideocapsular ligament, 539
Hyalomere, 171
Hyaluronic acid, 84, **85**
  of synovial fluid, 272
Hyaluronidase, 84, 111
Hydrolytic enzymes, 36
Hydroperoxyeicosatetraenoic acid (HPETE), 487
Hydroxyapatite crystal (HAP), 119, 120
β-Hydroxybutyric acid, 404
25-Hydroxycholecalciferol (25-HCC), 143, **145**
Hydroxyeicosatetraenoic acid (HETE), 487
Hydroxylase
  prolyl-, 77, 80
  lysyl-, 77, 80
3-Hydroxyproline, 77
4-Hydroxyproline, 77
Hyperadrenocorticism, 482
Hypercalcemia, 142
Hypercalcemic factor, 142
Hypercapnia, 462
Hyperglycemia, 482, 484
Hyperglycemic factor, 484
Hyperosmolarity, 442
Hyperparathyroidism
  secondary
    nutritional, 126
    renal, 126
Hyperpolarization, 215
Hypersensitivity reactions
  delayed, 347

Type
  I, 345, 346
  II, 346
  III, 346, 347
  IV, 347
Hyperthyroidism, 144
Hyperventilation, 444
Hypoadrenocorticism, 482
Hypocalcemia, 142
Hypocalcemic
  factor, 142
  tetany, 201
Hypochromasia, 168
Hypodermis, 348, 350
Hypoglycemia, 484
Hypoglycemic factor, 484
Hypophyseal
  portal system, 471
  stalk, 467, **468**
Hypophysis cerebri, 467–473
  components of (see specific components)
  development of, 467, 469
  organization of, 467, **468**, 469
Hypopolarization, 215
Hypoproteinemia, 560
Hypothalamo-
  hypophyseal
    portal system, 471
    tract, 472
  interstitial cell axis, 498
  ovarian axis, 507
  tubuli contorti axis, 500
Hypothalamus, 285
Hypothryoidism, 476
Hypoventilation, 444, 461
Hypoxia, 462
  tissue, 184, **184**
  renal, 184

I band, 190, **192**, **194–196**, 236, **237**
Icterus (see jaundice)
Ileum, 408, **408**
Immature bone, 129
Immune-mediated diseases, 347
Immune response
  cell-mediated (see cell-mediated)
  humoral antibody (see humoral antibody)
  primary, 186
  secondary, 186
Immunity, 341–347
  cell-mediated (CMI), 344
  cellular interactions in, 344, 345
  hypersensitivities and (see hypersensitivity)
  nonspecific, 341
  passive
    placental transfer and, 409
    colostrum and, 409
  specific, 341-347
Immunoblasts, 182, 183, **183**
Immunocytochemistry, 9, **9**
Immunoglobulins, 99, 341, 409, 452
  A, (IgA), 343, 452
    secretory, 343, 452
    of salivary glands, 418
  chain of
    heavy, 343, **345**
    light, 343, **345**
  D, (IgD), 343
  E, (IgE), 343
  G, (IgG), 343
  M, (IgM), 343
Implantation, 519
Incus, 546
Infraorbital gland, 365
Infundibular
  process, 467, **468, 469**, 472, **473**
  recess
    of hypophysis cerebri, **468**, 469, **469**
    of teeth, 390
  stalk, 467, 468, **468, 469**, 472, **473**
Infundibulum, 523, **523**
  of oviduct, 512
Ingluvies, 412, **413**
Inhibin, 500
Inhibiting
  factors, 208

hormones, 208
Inhibitory postsynaptic potential (IPSP), 216, 290, 308
Initial segment, 208, 211, **213**
Inner
  enamel epithelium, 396, **397–399**
  hair cells
    of organ of Corti, **551**, 552
  nuclear
    layer, 541, **541, 542**
    membrane, 26, **28**
  plexiform layer, 541, **541, 542**
  rod fiber, 541, **543**
  segment, 541, **543**
  tunnel, **551**, 552
Inotropy
  positive, 217, 327
  negative, 327
Insulin, 484
  relationship to 1, 25-DHCC, 145
Insuloma, 485
Integument (*see* also specific structures)
Integumentary system, 348–379
  avian, 378, 379
  character of, 348
  functions of, 348
  mammalian, 348–365
Intercalated
  discs, 204, **205, 206**
  ducts, 417, **417, 418**
Intercellular substance, 3, 52
  epithelial, 52
  of connective tissue, 92
Interdental cells, **551**, 552
Interdigital glands, 365
Interferon, 171
Interleukin, 334, 341
Intermedin, 471, 472
Internal
  auditory meatus, 545, 546
  elastic membrane, 314, **315, 316**
Interneuron, 304
Internuncial neuron, 304
Interoception, 208
Interstitial
  bone, 134, 135, **135, 136, 138**
  cells
    of pineal gland, 474
    of testis, 472
  cell-stimulating hormone (ICSH), 472, 500
  gland, 510, 511
Interstitium, 83
Interventricular foramin, 285, **287**
Intervertebral disc, 270, **270**
Intermediate
  filaments, 43
  junction, **68, 69,** 70
Intestinal
  crypts, 405
  fluids, 410, 412
  phase, 398, 399
  submucosal glands, 405, **406**
Intracartilaginous ossification (*see* endochondral ossification)
Intramembranous ossification, 146–149, **147–151**
Intraperiod lines, **230,** 2312
Intraretinal space, 527, 528, **528**
Intrinsic factor, 183, 398
Insulin, 484, 485
Insulinase, 485
Insulinoma, 485
Intrafusal fibers, 282, **282, 283**
Intragemmal fibers, 383
Iodination, 475
Iodoamino acids, 475
Iodopsin, 541
Iridial
  angle, 537, **537**
    meshwork of, 537, **537, 538**
  granules, 536, **536**
  stroma, 527, **530,** 536, **536**
Iridocorneal angle, **533,** 537, **537, 538**
Iridopupillary membrane, 527
  persistent, 528, 536, **536**
Iris, 528, **530,** 535, **535,** 536, **536**
  angle of, 537, **537**
  coloboma of, 528

muscles of, 536
  pigmentation of, 536
  stroma of, 536
Ischemic necrosis, 347
Islets of Langerhans, 484, **484,** 485, **485**
Isochronal rhythm, 42
Isocitrate lyase, 38
Isodesmosine, 83
Isogenous groups, 113, **115**
Isoproterenol, 312
Isosmolarity, 442
Isotropy, 14
Isthmus, 512, 523, **524,** 525

Jaundice, 185
  hemolytic, 185
Jejunum, 405, **407**
Joints, 269–276
  classification of, 270
  composition of, 270
  functions of, 270
  lubrication of, 275, 276
  tissues of, 270
  types of (*see* specific types)
Junctional complexes, **68,** 68–73
Junctions
  close, 69, 70, **70**
  communicating, 69, 70, **70**
  gap, 69, 70, **70**
    of nerves (*see* ephapses)
  intermediate, 69, 70, **70**
  neuromuscular, 281, **281**
  tight, 69
Juveniles (*see* metamyelocyte, neutrophilic)
Juxtaglomerular
  apparatus, 435, 439–441
  cells
    agranular, 439
    granular, 439
  complex, 439–441

Kallikrein, 175, 345
  -kinin system, 346, **346**
Karyokinesis, 48, 182
Karyolymph, 29
Karyolysis, 181, 182
Karyoplasm, 29
Keratanase, 111
Keratan sulfate I and II, 84, **85**
Keratin, 57, 349
  soft, 349
  hard, 349
Keratinocytes, 349
Keratoblasts, 529
Keratohyalin, 57, 349
Ketoacidosis, 485
Ketone bodies, 404, 427
17-Ketosteroids, 500
Kidney, 431–445
  acid/base balance and, 443, 444, **444**
  acids and, 443, **444**
  amino acids and, 442
  ammonia and, 444, **444**
  base conservation and, 443, 444
  bases and, 443, 444
  collecting duct system of, **432,** 437, 438, **439**
  connective tissue of, 433
  development of, 431, 433
  ducts of, 431, **432**
  filtration by, 441
  fluid
    balance and, 441
    load and, 441
  functional correlates of, 439–441
  functions of, 431
  general features of, 431
  glucose and, 441
  innervation of, 438, 439
  ions and, 441
  multilobar, 431, **431**
  multipyramidal, 431, **431**
  nephrons of, 433–437
  organization of, 431
  physiology of, 441–445
  sodium and, 442
  secretion of H$^+$, 442–444, **444,** 445

stromal elements of, 438, 439
  tubules of (*see* specific tubules)
    reabsorption by, 441, 442, **443, 444**
    secretion by, 442, **443, 444**
    ultrafiltration by, 441
    unilobar, 431, **431**
    unipyramidal, 431, **431**
    urea and, 442
    urine formation by, 441–443
  vessels of
    blood, 438, **440**
    lymph, 438
  water and, 441
Kinetic sensations, 547
Kininogenases, 345
Kinninogens, 175, 345
  high molecular weight (HMW), 346, **346**
  low molecular weight (LMW), 346, **346**
Kinins, 345
Kinocilia, 39–42
Krause's end-bulbs, 294

Labia, 514
Labial glands, 381, 418
Labyrinth
  membranous, 546, **550**
  osseous, 549, **550**
Lacrimal
  apparatus, 544, 545
  canaliculi, 544
  glands, 544, **545, 546**
    accessory, 544
  passages, 544
  sac, 544
Lacus lacrimalis, 544
Lactase, 409
Lacteals, 405
Lactiferous sinus, 361, **362, 364**
Lactoferrin, 452
Lactogenic hormone, 472
Lacunae
  of cartilage, 108, 113, **113–116**
  of osteocytes, 128, **128, 129**
Lamellar
  bodies, 455, **457**
  bone, 120, 131, **131,** 235
  phagosomes, 539
Lamina
  choroidocapillaris, 534
  densa, 71, 435
    epithelialis mucosae, **252, 253,** 254
    of choroid plexus, 297, **300, 301**
  fibrocellularis, 71
  fusca, 528, 529
  lucida, 71
  muscularis mucosae, **252, 253,** 254
  of foot, 365, **366**
    insensitive, 367, **367**
    primary, 367, **367,** 370
    secondary, 367, **367,** 370
    sensitive, 367, **367,** 370
  propria mucosae, **252, 253,** 254
  propria-submucosa, **252, 253,** 254
  rara
    externa, 435
    interna, 435
  suprachoroidea, 532
Laminar
  corium, 367, **367,** 370
  epidermis, 367, **367,** 370
Laminin, 71, 76, 86, **86**
Langerhans cells, 355, 356
Large intestine, 409–412
  absorption by, 410
  characteristics of, 409
  contractions of, 410
    mass, 410
    segmenting, 410
    slow wave, 410
  epithelium of
    replacement of, 410
    renewal of, 410
  fermentation within, 410
  motility of, 410
  organization of, 409

Large Intestine—Continued
    regions of, 409 (*see* specific regions)
    repair of, 410
    secretion by, 410
    synthesis within, 410
Laryngotracheal groove, 450
Larynx, 449, **449**
Latent period, 341
Lateral
    funiculus, 303, **303**
    ventricles, 285, **287**
Lathyrism, 82
Lecithin, 23
Lens, 537–540
    bow, 538
    capsule, 537, 538, **539**
    cortex, 538, **539**
    epithelium, 538, **539, 540**
    fibers, 538, **539, 540**
        flaps of, 539, **540**
        imprints of, 539, **540**
    functional correlates of, 539
    nucleus of, 539, **539**
    placode, 527
    star, 539, **540**
    sutures, 539, **540**
    vesicle, 527, **528**
Leptocytes, 168, **168**
Leptomeninges, 296, **298, 299**, 527
Leukocytes (*see* specific cells)
Leukocytosis
    eosinophilic, 186
    -inducing factor (LIF), 186
Leukoma, 529
Leukotrienes (LT), 345, 346, 487
Levator palpebrae superioris, 543
Leydig cells, 236, **237**, 490, **490, 491**
Ligaments, 103
    suspensory
        lateral, 364
        medial, 364
Light
    cells
        of collecting duct system, 437
        of thyroid gland, 474, **475**
    deviated, 14
    extraordinary ray of, 14
    normophasic, **13**, 14
    ordinary ray of, 14
    phase-altered, **13**, 14
    undeviated, 14
Limbus, 529, **530**
Limiting membrane
    of cornea, 529
    of retina, 541, **542**
    of vitreous body, 537
Lingual
    glands, 418
    papillae , 382, 383
        conical, **381**, 383, **383**
        filiform, 381, **382**, 383
        foliate, **381**, 383, **384**
        fungiform, **381**, 383, **384**
        lenticular, **381**, 383, **383**
Lining cells
    small intestine, 405
Lipases, 38
    enteric, 409
    lipoprotein, 98
    pancreatic, 409
Lipid
    droplets, 45, **46**
    in digestion, 409
Lipids, 23, 43, **44**
Lipofuscin, 45, 209
Lipoproteins, 23
Lipotropins (LPH), 472
    β-; (βLPH), 472
    γ- (γ-LPH), 472
Lips, **380**, 381
Liquor folliculi, 509
Liver, 238, **239**, 419–428
    biliary system of, 421, **425**
    biotransformation by, 419, 426
    cells of (*see* specific cells)
    characteristics of, 419

    development of, 420
    duct system of, 421, **422–427**
    excretion by, 424, 426
    functions of, 419
    hepatic lobules of, 423
    histology of, 420, **421–426**
    innervation of, 423
    metabolism by, 427, 428
    portal
        areas of, 420, 423
        triads of, 421, 423, **426, 427**
    physiology of, 424–428
    regeneration of, 428
    secretion by, 424, 425
    sinusoids of, 421, **421, 422**
    storage by, 428
    synthesis by, 424
    units of, 423, 424, **427**
    vessels of
        blood, **422**, 423
        lymphatic, 423
Lobuli testis, 489, **489**
Loose connective tissue (*see* areolar connective tissue)
Loop of Henle, 431, **432**, 436, 437, **438**
Lower motor neuron, 204, 289, **291**
Lumbar intumescence, 303
Lung
    acid/base balance and, 461
    avian, 463
        structure of, 464, **464, 465**
        ventilation of, **463**, 464, 465, **465**
    bronchi of, 450–452
    bronchioles of, 452, 453
    carbon dioxide exchange and the, 461, 462
    characteristics of, 450
    components
        conductive, 450–453
        exchange, 455–460
        transitional, 453–455
    development of, 450
        stage of
            alveolar, 450
            canalicular, 450
            glandular, 450
            pseudoglandular, 450
            terminal sac, 450
    gas exchange by the, 460, **462**
    general features, 450
    innervation of, 459, 460, **460**
    oxygenation of blood, 460, 461, **462**
    perfusion of, 461, 462
    physiology of, 460–462
    regulation of, 462
    species differences, 459, 460
    ventilation, 461, 462
    vessels of
        blood, 459, 460, **460**
        lymphatic, 459 460, **560**
Lutein, 511
Luteinization, 511
Luteinizing hormone (LH), 472, 500
    releasing factor (LRF), 472, 498, 507
Luteotrophic hormone (LTH), 472
Lymph, 87
    node, 331–334
        antibody synthesis and, 334
        biopsy of, 554
        B lymphocytes of, 332, 334
        cell-mediated immunity and, 334
        cells of, 332
        cytology of, 554, **554–556**
        functions of, 334
        hemorrhagic, 334
        lymph circulation through, 332, **333**
        nerves of, 332
        reactive, 246, **247**
        recirculation through, 332
        species differences, 332, 334
        structure of, 331, **333–335**
        vascular supply, 332
        zone of
            paracortical, 332, **333**
            subcortical, 332, **333**
    nodules, 183, 332, **333, 334**
        aggregated, 330, **331**
        cortex of, 332, **333, 334**

        germinal centers of, 332, **332, 334**
        primary, 332, **333, 334**
        secondary, 332, **333, 334**
        solitary, 330, 331
Lymphatic
    nodules, 183, **183**
        germinal centers of, 183, **183**
    organs, 331–341 (*see* specific organs)
    system, 330–341
        characteristics of, 330
        classification of components, 330
        form of, 330
        functions of, 330
    tissue
        avian, 330, **331**
        dense, 330, 331
            encapsulated, 330
            unencapsulated, 330
        diffuse and unencapsulated, 330, **330**
        types of (*see* specific tissues)
    vessels, 328, 329
Lymphoblasts, 182, **182**, 246, **247**
    cytology of, 554, **554**
Lymphocytes, 244, **245**, 246, **247**
    avian, 174, **174**
    B, 170, **171** 183, **183**, 341
        memory and, 334
        of lymph nodes, 334
        of spleen, 335
    cytology of, 554, **554–556**
    cytotoxic, 344
    large, 170, 182, **182**
    kinetics of, 186
    medium, 170, 182, **182**
    origin of, 183, **183**
    recirculation of, 186
    small, **182**, 183
    surface receptors of, 171
    T, 170, **171**, 183, **183**,
        memory and, 334
        of lymph nodes, 334
        of spleen, 344, 345
Lymphocytopoiesis, 182
Lymphocytosis, 186
Lymphoepithelial organ, 337
Lymphoglandular body, 246, **247**, 555, **556**
Lymphokine-producing cells, 334
Lymphokines, 171
Lymphomyeloid organs, 182
Lymphopenia, 186
β-Lysins, 341
Lysolecithin, 430
Lysosomal enzymes, 37
Lysosomes, 36–38, **39**
    and extracellular functions, 38
    active, 37, **39**
    enzymes of, 37, 38
    functions of, 37, 38
    inactive, 37, **39**
    primary, 37, **39**
    secondary, 37, **39**
Lyssa, 382
Lysyl
    -hydroxylase, 77, 80
    oxydase, 77, **80**, 81

Macrocytes, 167
Macroglia, 218
Macrophages, 97, **97**, 98
    aggregating factor (MAF), 171
    and chronic bronchitis, 246, **247**
    chemotactic factor (MCF), 171
    cytology of, 561, **561, 562**
    fixed, 97
    in a smear, 248, **249**
    in cerebrospinal fluid tap, 246, 247
    pulmonary, 457, **458**
    relationship to monocyte, 98
    system, 106, 107, **107**
    wandering, 97
Macula
    adherens, **68–70**, 70
    densa, 437
    of cornea, 531
    sacculi **546–549**, 547
    utriculi, 546, 547, **548, 549**

Magnum, 523, **524**
Malate synthetase, 38
Malleus, 546
Maltase, 409
Mammary gland
    duct system of, 361, **362**
    general features of, 361
    lactating, 361–364, **362, 363**
    nonlactating, **361**, 364, **365**
    species differences, 364
Manchette, 497, **497**
Mandibular gland, 418, **420**
Mantle
    layer
        of neural tube, 286, 289
        of spleen, 335, **338, 339**
    zone
        of spleen, 335, **338, 339**
Many plies, 403
Marginal
    folds, 89
    layer, 286, **289**
    zone, 335
Marrow cavity, 180, **181**
Marsupials, 517
Mast cells, 98, **99**
    from a metastatic tumor, 246, **247**
Mastication, 380
Matrix
    capsular, 111, **111**
    cytoplasmic, 28, 29
    extracellular, 76–86
        defined, 76
        properties of, 76
    granules, 111, **112, 113**
    interterritorial, 111, **111**, 112
    layer, 286, **289**
    nuclear, 27
    pericellular, 111, **111**
    territorial, 111, **111, 112**
    vesicles, 111, **113**, 159
Mature bone, 120
Mean corpuscular hemoglobin concentration (MCHC), 187
Mean corpuscular volume (MCV), 187
Median eminence, **468**, 472
Mediastinum testis, 489, **489**
Medullary
    cavity, 180
    cords, 331, **333, 334**
    rays, 431, **432**
Megakaryoblasts, 182
Megakaryocytes, 182
    meta-, 182
    pro-, 182
Meiosis, 48, 537
Meissner's
    corpuscles, 294, **296**, 297
    plexus, 393
Melanin, 45, 99
    granules, 100
Melanoblasts, 99
Melanocyte, 99, 100, 355, **357**
    -stimulating hormone (MSH), 471, 472
    α-melanocyte-stimulating hormone (αMSH), 472
Melanophore, 100
Melanosome
    stage I–IV, 100
Melatonin, 474
M line, **195**, 200
Membrana granulosa, 508, **508–510**
Membranous labyrinth, 546, **546, 552**
Memory cells, 171, 341, 334
Meninges, 294–296, 298, **299**
Meniscus, 117, **117**
Menstrual cycle, 516, 517
    phase of
        follicular, **516**, 517
        luteal, **516**, 517
        progestational, **516**, 517
        secretory, **516**, 517
Mental organ, 365
Merkel disks, 294
Merocrine glands, **59, 61**, 63
Meromyosin
    heavy (HMM), 193, **199**, 201

light (LMM), 193, **199**, 201
Mesangial cells, 435, **437**
    extraglomerular, 439, **440, 441**
    intraglomerular, 439, **440**
Mesaxon, 220, **225, 228, 229**
    inner, **225, 228, 229**
    outer, **225, 229**
Mesectoderm, 53
Mesencephalic aquaduct, 285, **287**
Mesencephalon, 285, **287**
Mesenchymal
    cells, 47, 92, 94, **94, 96**, 113, 236, **237**
        and bone, 122, **125**
        and cartilage repair, 117, 118
        and connective tissues, 94
        and fracture repair, 265, 267
        and perivascular space, 47
        condensation of, 108, 146, **147, 148**, 153, **153**
        function of, 94
        of perichondrium, 113, **113**
        of periosteum, 121, 122, **122**
    connective tissue, 100, **100**
    epithelium, 53, 527
Mesobronchus, 463, **463**, 464, **464**
Mesoderm
    allantoic, 519
    chorionic, 519
    derivatives of, 53
Mesonephros, 431
    duct of, 433
Mesotendon, 277, **278**
Mesothelium, 53
    in a smear, 248, **249**
    cytology of, 560, **561**
Mesovarium, 506
Messengers, 32
    chemical, 485, 486
Metachronal rhythm, 42
Metachromasia, 86
Metamegakaryocytes, 171, 182
Metamyelocyte, 182
    basophilic, 182
    eosinophilic, 182
    neutrophilic, 182
Metanephric blastema, 431
Metanephros, 431
Metaphysis, 240, **241**
Metaplasia, 94, 109
Metarterioles, **314**, 315
Metarubricytes, 167, **167, 180**, 181, 246, **247**
Metathalamus, 285
Metatheria, 517
Metencephalon, 285, **287**
Metestrus, 515, 517
Methacholine, 311, **311**
Methyl transferase, 214, **219**
Micelles, 409
Microbodies, (*see* peroxisomes)
Microcytes, 167
Microfibrils, 81
    of cartilage, 111, **112**
Microfilaments, 43
Microglia, 218, 221
Microgliocytes, 218, **221**
    of retina, 541
Microplicae, 437, 438
Microscopy
    bright-field, 12, **13**
    dark-field, 5, 13
    electron
        scanning, 9–10, 14–15, **16**
        transmission, 9, **10**, 15, **16**
    fluorescence, **6, 9**, 13
    interference, 14, **15**
    Nomarski interference phase, 14
    phase-contrast, 5, **13**, 14, **14**
    polarizing, 14, **15**
    ultraviolet, 13
Microtome
    rotary, 7
Microtubular organization center, 39
Microtubules, 38–42, **39–42, 222**
    arms of
        inner, 41, **42**
        outer, 41, **42**
    nucleation sites of, 39

occurrence of, 39
    of neurons, 209
    radial spokes of, **40**, 41, **42**
    structure of, 39, **39**
    subfiber
        A of, **40**, 41
        B of, **40**, 41
Microvilli, 52, 71, **73, 74**
Micturition, 445
Midbody, **46**
Middle piece, 498, 497, **498**
Milk fever, 145, 201
Migration inhibition factor (MIF), 171
Mineralization, 146
Mineralicorticoids, 472, 482
Minor processes
    of podocytes, 433, **434–436**
Mitochondria, 36, **37, 38**
    conformation of
        condensed, 36, **38**
        orthodox, 36, *37*, **38**
    function of, 36
    membranes of
        inner, 36, **38**
Mitogenic factor (MF), 171
Mitotic potential, 47
Mitosis, 45–48, **46, 47**
    phase of
        ana-, 47, **47**
        duplication (s), 46, **46**
        inter-, 47, *47*
        meta-, 47
        preduplication (G₁), 45, **46**
        presynthetic (G₁), 45, **46**
        pro-, 47, **47**
        postduplication (G₂), 45
        postsynthetic (G₂), 45
        telo-, 47, **47**
        vegetative, 46, **46**
Mixed glands, 65, **65, 66**
M line, **195, 198**, 200
Modiolus, 549
Molar gland, 418
Monoamine oxidase (MAO), 215, **219**
Monocyte, 171, **171**, 244, **245**, 246, **247**
    avian, 174, **174**
    kinetics of, 186
Monocytopoiesis, 183
3-Monoiodotyrosine (MIT), 475
Mononuclear phagocytic system (*see* macrophage system)
Monosaccharides, 23, 409
Monotremes, 517
Mossy fibers, 303
Motilin, 484, 486, 487
Motor
    endplate, 281, **281**
    fiber, 288, **289, 290**
    unit, 278, 281
α-Motor neuron, 204, 289, **290, 291**, 302, 305, **306**
Mott cells, 246, **247**, 555, **555**
Mucins, 76
Mucociliary apparatus, 42, 452
Mucocutaneous junction, **380**, 381
Mucoperiosteum, 447
Mucopolysaccharides (*see* mucosubstances)
Mucoproteins, 23
Mucosal glands, 254, **255**
Mucosubstances, 43, 84
    acidic, 84
    and bone, 119
    and cartilage, 109–111
    neutral, 84
    of cornea, 529
Mucous
    cells, 65, **65, 66**, 238, **238**
    connective tissue, 101, **101**
    glands, 65, **65, 66**
    membranes, **257**, 258
    neck cells, 395, **396**
    threads, 545
Müller cells, 218, 541
Müllerian duct, 433
Multilocular fat (*see* brown adipose tissue)
Multipolar neurons, 208, **209–212**
Multivesicular body, 37

Muscarine, 308
Muscarinic
  drugs, 308, **308**
  receptors, 308, **308**
Muscle
  and basal lamina, 189
  as an organ, 276–284
  cells, 188
  characteristics of, 188
  cramps, 201
  fibers, 188
  investments of, 276, 277
  involuntary, 188
  nerve relationships, 278–283
  organization of, 276, 277
  repair and regeneration of, 206, 207
  tissue, 3, 188–207
    characteristics of, 188
    classification of, 188
    derivation of, 3
    functions of, 3, 188
    types of (*see* specific tissues)
  voluntary, 188
Muscularis serosae, 514
Muscular stomach (*see* ventriculus)
Musculoskeletal system, 259–284
  characteristics of, 259
  form of, 259
  functions of, 259
Myelencephalon, 285, **287**
Myelin, **230**, 231
  lines of
    interperiod, **230**, 231
    dense, **230**, 231
Myelination, **230**, 231
  central, **230**, 231
  peripheral, **230**, 231
Myeloblasts, 181, 182
Myelocytes, 181, 182
  basophilic, 182
  eosinophilic, 182
  meta-
    basophilic, 182
    eosinophilic, 182
    neutrophilic, 182
  pro-, 181
Myeloid/erythroid ratio (M/E), 187
Myeloid tissue, 180, **181**
  compartments of
    hematopoietic, 180, **181**
    vascular, 180, **181**
Myenteric plexus, 395
Myoblasts, 207
Myocardium, 323, **325**
Myoepithelial cells, 66, **68**, 417, **417**
Myofibrils, 188
Myofibroblasts, 378
Myofilaments, 188
Myoglobin, 200
Myometrium, 512, **512**
Myoneural junction, 281, **281**
Myosin, 43, 188, 190, 193, **199**
  heavy (HMM), 193, **199**
  light (LMM), 193, **199**
Myotendinous junctions, 276

N-acetyltransferase, 426
N-acetyl
  -galactosamine, 84, **85**
  -glucosamine, 84, **85**
    β-1, 3 galactose β-1, 4, 84, **85**
  transferase,
Nasolacrimal duct, 544
Nasal
  cavity, 447, **448, 449**
    avian, 463, 463
  glands, 447
  regions of, 447, **448, 449**
Nasopharynx, 449
Nebula, 531
Neck, 386
Necrobiosis, 38
Necrosis, 38
Negative feedback loop, 467, **467**
Neostigmine, 311

Neopulmon, 465
Nephron, 433–437
  tubular components, 435–437
Nerve cells (*see* neurons)
Nerves
  adrenergic, 214
  afferent terminals of (*see* afferent)
  cholinergic, 214
  endings, 293, 294, **296, 297**
    free, 293
  encapsulated, 293, 294, **296, 297**
  fibers
    myelinated, 220, **223–230**, 242, **243**
    of Remak, 219, 220, **225**
    unmyelinated, 219, 220, **225**
  investments of, 292, 293. **293–296**
  trunks, 291–293, **293, 294**
Nervi vasorum, 314
Nervous
  system, 285–313
    autonomic, 285, 304–312
    cellular differentiation in, 285, **285**
    central (CNS), 285
    characteristics of, 285
    components of
      central, 294–304
      peripheral, 290, 294
    cytology of, 554
    development of, 285, **296–288**
    form of, 285
    functions of, 285
    integrated function of, 286–290
    organization of
      functional, 286–290
    peripheral (PNS), 285
    physiology of, 286–290
    somatic, 285
  tissue, 3, 208–231
    cells of (*see* specific cells)
    characteristics of, 285
    derivation of, 3
    form of, 208
    functions of, 3, 208
    organization of, 285
  tunic, 539–543
Net driving force, 88, **88**
Neural
  crest cells, 285, **286, 288**
  crest ectoderm, 285, **286, 288**
  groove, 285, **286**
  plate, 285, **286**
  retina, 527
  tube, 285, **286, 287**
    layer of
      mantle, 528
      marginal, 528
Neurectoderm, 285, **286**
Neurites, **312**, 313
Neuroblasts, 285, **288**
Neurocrine cells, 467, 486
Neuroendocrine cells, 452, 453, 455
Neuroepithelial bodies, 453
Neurofilaments, 209
Neuroglia, 217–231
  central, 218, 219, **220–222**
  peripheral, 219, **223**
  types of (*see* specific cells)
Neurohemal organ, 208, **210**
Neurohypophysis,
  hormones of, 472
  structure of, **468, 469**, 472
Neurokeratin, 220, **223**
Neurolemma, 220, **225–230**
Neurolemmal
  cells, 220, **225–230**
  sheath, 220, **225–230**
Neuroma, **312**, 313
Neuromuscular
  junction, **196**, 213
  spindle, 281–284, **282**, 294
    mechanisms of action of, 282, 284
Neurons, 208, 236, 237
  adrenergic, 214, 216, **219**
    terminals of, 214, **219**
  axoplasmic flow, 211
    fast, 211

retrograde, 211
slow, 211
somatofugal, 211
somatopetal, 211
bipolar, 208, **212**, 541, **542**
cell bodies of, 209, **213**
characteristics of, 208
cholinergic, 216
  terminals of, 214, **218**
classification of, 208, **210–213**
components of
  postsynaptic, 215–217, **216–219**
  presynaptic, 213–215, **216–219**
conducting, 208, **211**
degeneration of
  primary, **312**, 313
  secondary, **312**, 313
development of, 208
Golgi type I, 208, **210**
Golgi type II, 208, **210**
information transfer by, 211–217
investments of
  cell bodies, 219, **223, 224**
  processes, 219, 220, **223–230**
lower motor, 289, **291**
magnocellular, 471
motor, 289, **291**
multipolar, 208, **209–21**
neurosecretory, 208, **211**
parvicellular, 471
processes of, 291–294
properties of, 208, **209**
regeneration of, **312**, 313
response to injury by, 312, **312**
structure of, 209
terminals of
  afferent, 293, 294
  efferent, 294
transmission, 208, **211**
transmission by, 213–217
  electrochemical (*see* synapses)
  electrotonic (*see* ephapses)
types of, 208
ultrastructure of, 209
unipolar
  true, 208
  pseudo-, 208, **212**
Neurophysins I and II, 472
Neuropil, 218
Neurosecretory
  neurons, 208, 211
  substances, 208
Neurotendinous organs, 284
Neurotransmitters, 213
Neurotubules, 209
Neutral fats, 23
Neutropenia, 186
Neutrophil (PMN), 168, 169, **169**, 182, 244, **245**, 246, **247**
  cytology of, 561
  kinetics of, 185, 186
  in a smear, 248, **249**
  polymorphonuclear, 168, **169**
  regulation of, 186, 186
  releasing factor (NRA), 186
Neutrophilia, 186
Neutrophilic
  band cells, 182, 244, **245**, 246, **247**
  filamented, 182
  metamyelocyte, 182
  nonsegmented, 182
  PMN, 182
  polymorphonuclear, 182
  segmenter, 182
  stab cells, 182
  toxic, 246, **247**
Nexi, **68**, 70, **70**
  of neurons, 211, **216**
  of smooth muscle, 190, **191**
Nexins, 41
Nicotine, 308, **308**
  drugs, 308
  receptors, 308, **308**
Nictitating membrane, 544, **544, 545**
  glands of
    deep, 544

superficial, 544
Nidation, 519
  interstitial, 521
  superficial, 521
Nissl
  bodies, 209, **214**
  substance, 209, **214**
Nitrogenous bases, 22
Node
  atrioventricular (AV), 324, **327**
  of Ranvier, 220, **226, 227**
  sinoatrial (SA), 324, **327**
Nodular arteriole, 336, **337–341**
Nodule of Arantius, 324
Nonprotein nitrogen, 404
Nonspecific granules, 182
Nonunion, 268
Norepinephrine, 213, 214, **219**, 308, **308**, 312, 483
  and adrenal medulla, 310, **310**
  and ANS, 309
  degradation of, 214, **219**
  synthesis of, 214, **219**
Normoblasts, 181
  basophilic, 181
  polychromatophilic, 181
  pro-, 181
Normocalcemia, 142
Normochromia, 168
Normocytes, **166**, 167
Nose, 350
Nuchal ligament, 83, 240, **241**
Nuclear
  bag fibers, 282, **282, 283**
  chain fibers, 282, **282, 283**
  pore, 27, **28**
  sap, 28
  sclerosis, 539
Nucleases, 38
Nucleic acids, 22
Nucleolonema, 28, **30**
Nucleolus, 28, **28**
  chromatin of, 28
  organizers, 28
Nucleoplasm, 29
Nucleoproteins, 22, 23
Nucleotides, 22
Nucleus
  chromatin of, 28
  condensed, 28
  envelopes of, 26
  euchromatin of, 28
  ground substance of, 27
  heterochromatin of, 28
  intermitotic, 25
  interphase, 25
  matrix of, 27
  membrane of
    inner, 26, **28**
    outer, 26, **28**
  morphology of, 25, **25 26**
  mitotic, 25
  number, 25, 26
  open, 28, **30**
  pores of, 27, **28**
    anulus of, 27, **28, 29**
  position, 25, 26
  sap of, 27
  shape, 25, 26
  vesicular, 28, **30**
Numerical aperture, 12

Obligatory symbiosis, 313
Octacalcium phosphate, 120
Ocular
  adnexa, 543–545 (*see* specific structures also)
  fundus, 541
Odontoblasts, 386, **387**, 389, **390**
Oil gland, 379, **379**
Olfactory
  cells, 447
  hairs, 447
  mucosa, 236, **237**
  vesicles, 447
Oligocythemia, 168
Oligodendrogliocytes, 218, **220, 221**
  interfascicular, 218

of the retina, 541
  perineuronal, 218
  perivascualr, 218
Oligosaccharides, 23
Omasum, **394**, 400, **403, 404**
Oocytes, 508
  primary, 508, **508**
  secondary, 508
Oogenesis, 507, **507**
Oogonia, 507, **507**
Opsonins, 171, 343
Opsinization, 343
Optic
  cup, 527, 528, **528**
  disc, 528, **530**
  fissure, 527, 528
  nerve fiber layer,
  papilla, **530**, 537
  retina, 528
  stalk, 527, **528**
  vesicle, 285, **287**, 527, **528**
Opticoel, 528
Ora
  ciliaris retinae, 528, **530**, 534, **534**, 537, 539
  serrata, 539
Oral structures, 380–390
Orangeophil, 469, **470**
Orbicularis
  ciliaris, 537
  oculi, 543
Ordinary
  adipose tissue (*see* white adipose tissue)
  connective tissue (*see* areolar)
Organification, 475
Organ of Corti, 550, 551, **551**
Organophosphates, 311
Organs
  organization of, 252–258, **252**
  exteriorization of, 4
  mural elements of, 252–254
  solid, 254–258
  specific (*see* specific organs)
  tubular, 252–254, **252**
  transillumination of, 4
  transparent viewing chambers for, 4
Organelles, 29 (*see* specific organelles also)
Organology, 2
  comparative, 2
Oropharynx, 390
Orthochromic erythroblasts, 181
Os cornua, 371
Osmoreceptor cells, 443
Osseous
  drift, 262
  labyrinth, 546
Ossification
  centers, 154–161
    diaphyseal, **153**, 154, **154, 155**
    epiphyseal, **153**, 157, **157, 158**
    primary, **153**, 154, **154, 155**
    secondary, **153**, 157, **157, 158**
  dystrophic, 146
  hormonal effects upon, 161–163
  mechanisms of, 146–163
    endochondral, 149–163, **152–163**
    intramembranous, 146–149, **147–151**
  metaplastic, 146
  metastatic, 146
  modeling during, 145
  pathological, 146
  phase of
    morphogenetic, 146
    cytodifferentiation, 146
  remodeling during, 146
Osteoblasts, 122–126, 236, **237**
  active, 123, **126**
  biphasic activity of, 123, **127**
  inactive, 123, **126**
Osteoclasia, 129, 144
Osteoclasts, 108, 122, 129, 171, 236, **237**
  origin of, **125**, 129
  ruffled border of, 129, **129, 130**
Osteocyte, 119, 122, 126–129
  -osteoblast pump, 128, 144
  osteoid, 128, **128**
Osteocytic osteolysis, 144

Osteogenesis, 146–163
Osteoid, 119, 121
  seam, 123, **126, 127**
Osteomalacia, 259
Osteomyelitis, 266
Osteonal canal, 135, **136**
Osteons, 131, 135, 240, **241**
  filling, **140**, 142, **142**
  mature, **140, 142**
  primary, 135, **137**
  secondary, 135, **135–137**
Osteopenia
  qualitative, 126, 259
  quantitative, 126, 259
Osteophytes
  periarticular, 272
Osteoporosis, 126, 144, 259
Osteoprogenitor cells, 122, 123, **125**
Otitis externa, 350
Otoconia, 549
Otolithic membrane, 549
Otoliths, **549**
Outer
  glial limitans, 302, **302**
  rod fiber, 541, **543**
  segment, 541, **543**
  tunnel, 551, 552
Ovalocytes, 168
Oval window, 549
Ovary, **235**, 486
  avian, **522**, 523–525
  cycle of, 507–512
    species differences, 516
  follicles of, 508, **508–511**
    mature, 508, **510**
    Graafian, 510, **510**
    primary, 508, **508–510**
    primordial, 508, **509**
    secondary, 508, **508–510**
    tertiary, 509, **510**
  organization of, 506
Oviduct, 512, **512, 513**
Ovulation, 510
  fossa, 506
β-Oxidation, 23
  enzymes of, 38
Oxidative phosphorylation
  coupled, 36
  uncoupled, 36
Oxygen
  debt, 201
  -hemoglobin dissociation, 460, 461
    curve, 460, 461, **461**
Oxyhemoglobin, 166, 187
Oxyntic cells, 398
Oxyphil cells, 476, **477**, 478
Oxytocin, 208, 472, 473

Pacemaker cells, 206
  of the heart, 324, **326**
Pachymenix, 294, **298, 299**
Packed cell volume (PCV), 187
Palate
  hard, 381
  soft, 381
Paleopulmon, 464
Palpebra, 543, **543**, 544, **544**
  tertius, 544, **544, 545**
Palpebral
  conjunctival epithelium, 529
  glands, 543
Pancreas
  endocrine, 484, **484**, 485, **485**
  enzymes of, 430
  exocrine, **428**, 429, 430
Pancreatic juice, 430
Paneth cells, 405, **405**
Panniculus adiposus, 350
Papillary
  duct
    of kidney, **432**, 438, **438**
    of teat, 361, **362, 364**
Parabronchi, 463, **463**, 464, **464**
Paracrine cells, 467, 486
Paradoxical aciduria, 444
Parafollicular cells, 142, 474, **475**

Paraganglia, 483
Paramesonephric duct, 433
Paranasal sinuses, 447
Parasympathetic nervous system, 306, **307**
Parasympathetics, 311
Parasympathomimetics, 311
Paratendon, 277, **278**
Parathormone (PTH), 142–145, **145**, 478
Parathyroid
  glands, 476–478
    external, 476
    internal, 476
  hormone, 142–145, **145**, 478
    biological effects of, 143
    target organ responses to, 143, 144, **145**
Parenchyma, 252
Parietal cells, 395, **396, 397**, 398
Pars
  amorpha, 28
  ciliaris retinae, 528, 535, **535, 539**
  convoluta, 435, **437**
  disseminata, 501
  distalis, 467, **468**, 469, **469, 470**
  flaccida, 545
  fibrosa, 28
  granulosa, 28
  intermedia, 467, **468**, 469, **469, 471, 471**
  iridica retinae, 528, 535, **535**, 536, **536**, 539
  optica retinae, 528, **539**
  recta, 435, **437**
  tensa, 545
  tuberalis, 467, **468**, 469, **469, 471, 471**
Parturient paresis, 144
Paunch, 402
Pectinate ligament, 537, **537, 538**
Pedicle, 372
Penis, 504, 505
  erectile tissue of, 504, 505
  detumescence of, 504
Pentose sugars, 22
Peptic ulcer, 400
Peptidase, 38
  signal, 77, **78**
Peptide linkage, 22
Perfusion, 461, 462
Perianal sinuses, 358
Periarterial lymphatic sheaths (PALS), 335, **338, 339**
Perichondral ring, 161, 271, 272, **274, 275**
Perichondrium, 108, 113, **113**, 153, **153**
Perichoroidal space, 532
Pericyte, 98, **98, 99**
Peridontal
  ligament, 389
  membrane, 388, **388**
Perikaryon, 24
  of neurons, 208, **209**
  of rod cells, 541, **543**
Perilymph, 546
Perimetrium, 513
Perimysium, 276
Perinuclear
  space, 26, **28**
  cistern, 26, **28**
Perineurium, 292, **293, 294**
Periosteal
  bud, **153**, 154
  new bone formation, 121, 268, **268**
Periosteum, 119, 121, **121, 122**, 131, 154, **155**
Periople, 365, **366**
Peripheralization, 183, 340
Perisinusoidal space, 421, **423–425**
Peristalsis, 408
Peristaltic rushes, 408
Peritubular plexus, 438, **440**
Peroxidase, 9, 475
Peroxisomes, 38
Peyer's patches, 405, **408**
Phagocytosis, 24
Phagosomes, 37, **39**
Phalangeal cells
  inner, **551**, 552
  outer, **551**, 552
Pharyngotympanic tube, 546
Pharynx, 390
Phenoxybenzamine, 312
Phentolamine, 312

Pheochrome cells, 483, **483**
Pheochromocytomas, 483
Phosphagen 201
Phosphatases, 38
3'-Phosphoadenine 5'-phosphosulfate (PAPS), 86
Phosphocreatine, 201, **203**
Phosphodiesterase, 32
Phospholipase, 430
  A, 430, 486
  C, 486
  D, 346
Phospholipids, 23
Phosphoproteins, 23, 119
Photoreceptor cells, 541, **542, 543**
Physis (*see* growth plate)
Physostigmine, 311
Pia mater, 296, **298, 299**
Piezoelectricity, 259, 260, **260**
Pigmented connective tissue, **100**, 105
Pillar cells
  inner, **551**, 552
  outer, **551**, 552
Pillars, 402
Pinna, 545
Pineal
  eye, 473
  gland, 473, 474
Pinealocytes, 474, **474**
Pinocytosis, 37
Pituitary gland (*see* hypophysis cerebri)
Placenta, 486, 517
  apposed, 521
  classification of, 517
  chorioallantoic, 519
  chorionic, 519
    attachments, 522
      folded, 522
      labyrinthine, 522
      villous, 522
  choriovitelline, 519
  conjoined, 521
  contribution to
    fetal, **521**, 522, 523
    maternal, **521**, 522, 523
  cotyledonary, 519
  diffuse, 519
  deciduate, 521
  discoidal, 519
  endothelioendothelial, **521**, 522
  epitheliochorial, **521**, 522
  hemochorial, **521**, 522
  hemodichorial, 522
  hemomonochorial, 522
  hemotrichorial, 522
  multiplex, 519
  nondeciduate, 521
  semi-, 521
  species differences, **521**, 522
  syndesmochorial, **521**, 522
  true, 519
  vera, 521
  yolk sac
    nonvascularized, 519
    vascularized, 519
Placental
  gonadotropins, 486
  mammals, 517
Placentology, 517–523
Placentome, 519
Planum
  nasale, 350
  nasolabiale, 350
  rostrale, 350
Plasma, 87, **87**, 164
  -blast, **182**, 183, 246, **247**
  cells, 99, **99, 100**, 182, 183, 246, **247**
  membrane, 29, **30**
    selective permeability of, 30
    structure of, 29, **30, 31**
    transport through
      water-soluble substances and, 29
      lipid-soluble substances and, 29
Plasmalemma (*see* plasma membrane)
Plamin, 177, **177**,
  and ovulation, 510
Plasminogen, 175, 177, **177**

Platelet, 171, **171, 172**, 246, **247**
  aggregating factor (PAF), 345
  degranulation of, 175
  phospholipids (PF3), 175, 176, **176**
  plug, 175
Pleocytosis, 554
Plexus
  of skin
    cutaneous, 350
    deep, 350
    middle, 350
    subcutaneous, 350
    subpapillary, 350
    superficial, 350
Plicae gastricae, **392**, 393
Pneumonocyte
  agranular, 455, **456**
  granular, 455, **456, 457**
  membranous, 455, **456**
  type I, 455, **456**
  type II, 455, **456, 457**
Pneumotaxis center, 462
Podocytes, 433, **433–437**
Poikilocythemia, 168
Polar body
  first, 508, **508**
  second, 508, **508**
Polychromasia, 167, 187, 246, **247**
Polychromatophilic
  erythroblasts, 181
  normoblast, 181
  erythrocyte, 181
Polycythemia, 167
Polydipsia, 443
Polymorphonuclear
  neutrophilic granulocyte, 182
  leukocyte (PMN), 168, 169, **169**
Polypeptide, 23
Polysaccharides, 23, 84
Polysomes, 32, **33**
Polyuria, 443
Pool
  circulating, 185, **186**
  marginal, 185, **186**
  tissue, 185, **186**
Portal
  area, 420, 423
  canal, 423
  lobule, 423, **427**
  triad, 421, 423, **426, 427**
Positive feedback loop, 467
Postcapillary venule, 186
Posterior chamber, 527, 528, **530**
Postganglionic neurons, 305, **306**
Postparturient paresis, 201
Postprandial alkaline tide, 399
Postsynaptic membrane, 211, **217–219**
  receptor sites on, 211
Post-translational proteolysis, 36
Potassium oxalate, 187
Precapillary sphincters, **314**, 315
Precipitin, 343
Predentin, 389, **390**
Preen gland, 379, **379**
Prefibrinolysin, 177
Preganglionic
  neurons, 305, **306**
  sympathetic nerves, 310, **310**
Premucin, 59
Preputial glands, 365
Presynaptic membrane, 211, **217–219**
  sites upon
    active, 214
    release, 214
Prickle cell layer, 56
Primary
  degeneration, **312**, 313
  folds
    of omasum, 402
    of reticulum 402
  granules, 168, 182
  laminae, 403
  processes
    of podocytes, 433, **433–437**
  spongiosa, 155, **155, 156**, 159, **161**
  response, 341

Primordial germ cells, 507
Principal
    cells
        of parathyroid gland, 476, **477**
        of pars distalis, 469, **470**
    piece, 497, 498, **498**
Proacrosomal granules, 497, **497**
Pro-α-chains, 79
Procollagen, 80, **80**
    aminopeptidase, 77, 80, **80**
    carboxypeptidase, 77, 80, **80**
Proctodaeum, 425
Proelastin, 83
Proerythroblast, 181
Proestrus, 515
Progesterone, 486, 511, 512
Progestins, 486
Progranulocyte, 181
Prolactin, 472, 500
    effect upon 1, 25-DHCC, 145
    releasing factor (PRF), 472
    inhibitory factor (PIF), 472
Prolymphocyte, 182
Prolylhydroxylase, 77, **80**
Promegakaryocyte, 182
Promonocyte, **182**, 183
Promyelocyte, 181
Pronephros, 431
Pronghorn, 372
Pronormoblast, 181
Propanolol, 312
Proper
    connective tissue, 101–104
    gastric glands, **395–397**, 397
Properdin system, 341
Prophospholipase A, 430
Proplasmacyte, **182**, 183
Prorubricyte, **180**, 181
Prosencephalon, 285, **287**
Prostacyclin (PGI₂), 345, 486, 487
Prostaglandin
    E, 345
    E₁,₂, 486
    effects upon bone, 445
    F₂α, 345, 486
    G₂, 486
    H₂, 486
Prostate gland, 248, **249**, 501, **502, 503**
    adenocarcinoma of, 248, **249**
    cytology of, 558
    hyperplasia of, 248, **249**
    squamous metaplasia of, 248, **249**
Prostatic ducts, 502
Proteases, 38
    and ovulation, 510
Proteins, 22, 23
    and renal function, 442
    conjugated, 23
    core, 85, **85**, 109, **109**
    denaturation of, 23
    fibrous, 23, 76
    fixation of, 23
    α-helix of, 23
    integral, 31
    intrinsic, 31
    kinase, 32
    native, 23
    peripheral, 31
    plasma, 164, **165**
    simple, 23
    staining of, 23
    structure of
        primary, 22
        secondary, 23
        tertiary, 23
        quarternary, 23
    synthesis, 33, 34, **35**
    total, 187
Proteoglycans, 23, 76, 85, **85**, 86, 92, 109, **109**
    aggregates of, 85, 109, **109**
    binding regions of, 85, **85**
    functions of, 85
    of bone, 119
    of cartilage, 109–111
    synthesis of, 85
Proteinuria, 442

Prothrombin, 176
    activator substance, 175, **176**
Protocollagen, 80
Protofilaments, 39, **40**
Protoplasm, 22
Protoplasmic bands, **312**, 313
Protoporphyrin, 184, **185**
Protothera, 517
Protyrosinase, 100
Proventriculus, 412, **413, 414**
Proximal convoluted tubule, 431, **432**, 435, **437**
Psammona bodies, 474
Pseudounipolar neurons, 208, **212**
Ptosis, 537
Pulmonary epithelial cell, 455, **456**
Puncta lacrimalia, 544
Pupil, 527, **530,** 535
Pupillary
    dilator, 536
    sphincter, 536
Purkinje
    cells, 303, **304, 305**
    fibers, 206, **206**
Purines, 22
Pyloric glands, 238, **239**, 398, **399, 400**
Pyometra, 559
Pyramids, 431, **431**
Pyrimidines, 22
Pyroninophilic cell, **182**, 183

Quarter stagger hypothesis, **79**, 81, **81**
Quill, 378, **378**

Rachis, 378, **378**
Rathke's pouch, 467, **468**
    residual lumen of, 467, **468**
Receptors, 215
    in a regulated system, 467, **467**
    adrenergic
        α, 216
        α₁, 216
        α₂, 216
        β, 216
        β₁, 217
        β₂, 217
Reciprocal innervation, 290
Recirculation
    of lymphocytes, 186
Rectoanal junction, 410, **411**
Rectum, 410, **411**
    avian, 415
Red blood cells (RBC), 166, **166, 167,** 180, 181
Red blood corpuscles (*see* red blood cells)
Red pulp, 335, **340,** 341
    sinuses, 336, **340, 341**
    veins, 336, **340, 341**
Reflex, 289
    arc, 288–290, **291**
    arterial pressoreceptor, 289, 327, **328**
    Bainbridge, 328
    baroreceptor, 327
    carotid sinus, 327
    chemoreceptor, 328
    contributions to the, 289
    depressor, 327
    duodenocolic, 410
    enterogastric, 398, 399
    gastro-
        cholic, 410
        intestinal excitatory, 408, 409
    intestino-intestinal inhibitory, 408
    monosynaptic, 289, **291**
    multisynaptic, 290
    myenteric, 408
    polysynaptic, 289, 290
    pupillary, 537
        consensual, 537
        direct, 537
        indirect, 537
    stretch, 282, 289, **291**
    vago-vagal, 289
    withdrawal, 290
Refractive media, 537
Regulated system, 467, **467**
Regulation
    down, 32

    up, 32
Reissner's membrane, **550**, 551, **551**
Relaxin, 486, 512
Release reaction, 175
Releasing
    factors, 208
    hormones, 208
Renal
    corpuscle, 433–435
    crest, 431, **431**
    erythropoietic factor (REF), 184, **184**
    pelvis, 431, **431,** 445
    pole of
        urinary, **433,** 435
        vascular, **433,** 435
    tubules, 431, **432**
Renin, 439
    -angiotensin axis, 439
Reproductive system
    avian, 523–525
    female, 506–526
    male, 489–505
Reserve cells, 469, 470
Residual body, 37, **39,** 497, **497**
Resolution, 12
Resolving power, 12
Resorption space, 129, 131
Respiration
    regulation of, 462
        chemical, 462
        neural, 462
Respiratory
    center, 462
    system, 447–465
        characteristics of, 447
        cytology of, 557, 558, **558**
        form of, 447
        functions of, 447
        tract
            avian, 462–465
                upper, 462, 463, **463**
            components of
                conductive, 447–450
Rete
    ovarii, 507
    testis, 489, **489,** 492, **492**
Reticular
    cells, 94, **96**
    connective tissue, 104
    folds, 403
    fibers, 76, 82, **82,** 188
Reticulocytes, 167, **167,** 180, **181**
Reticuloendothelial system (*see* Macrophage system)
Reticulum, **394,** 400, 403, **403**
    cellular, 100, **100**
Retina, 527, 528, **530,** 539–543
    blood supply to,
        anangiotic, 543
        holangiotic, 543
        merangiotic, 543
        paurangiotic, 543
    cells of, 541
    layer of
        ganglionic cell, 541, **541, 542**
        limiting membrane
            internal, 541, **542**
            outer, 541, **542**
        nuclear
            inner, 541, **541, 542**
            outer, 541, **541, 542**
        optic nerve, 541, **541, 542**
        photoreceptor, 541, **541, 542**
        pigment epithelial, 539, **541, 542**
        plexiform
            inner, 541, **541, 542**
            outer, 541, **541, 542**
    neural, 528
    ramp, 541
Retinal detachment, 528
Retractor penis muscle, 504
Retrograde
    flow, 211
Reversal line, 123, 135, **135,** 142, 241
Rhodopsin, 541
Rhombencephalon, 285, **287**
Ribophorin I and II, 33

Ribose, 22
Ribonuclease, 430
Ribonucleic acid (RNA), 22
  messenger (mRNA), 22
  polymerase, 33
  ribosomal (rRNA), 22
  transfer (tRNA), 22
Ribonucleoprotein (RNP), 22, 26, 32
Ribosomal receptor proteins, 33
Ribosomes, 32
  free, 32, **33**
  poly-, 32, **33**
Rickets, 126, 259
Rigor mortis, 201
Rod
  cells, 541
  spherules, 541, **543**
Rods, 527
Rokitansky-Aschoff sinuses, 428
Root, 386
  formation of, **387, 388, 388, 389**
Rosette of Furstenburg, 361
Rouget cells, 98, **98, 99**
Rough endoplasmic reticulum, 32–34, **33, 34**
Rouleaux, 166
Round window, 549
Rubriblast, **180,** 181
Rubricytes, **180,** 181, 244, **245,** 246, **247**
Ruffini corpuscles, 294
Rugosal glands, 412, **413, 414**
Rumen, **394,** 400, 401, **402,** 403

Saccules, 547–549
Sacculus, 527
Salbutamol, 312
Saliva, 418, 419
  flow of
    conditioned reflex, 419
    unconditioned reflex, 419
Salivary glands, 248, **249,** 417–419
  cytology of, 558
  duct system of, 417
  functional correlates of, 418
  major, 417
  minor, 417
Saltatory conduction, 211
Sarcoplasmic reticulum, 34, 193, **197**
  of cardiac muscle, 204, **205**
Sarcolemma, 188
Sarcomere, 190, **192, 194–196**
Sarcotubules, 193, **197, 198**
Scala
  tympani, 549
  vestibuli, 549, **550,** 551, **551**
Scalar relationships, 12, **12**
Scent glands, 365
Schistocytes, 168, **168**
Schwann cells, 219, **223**
Sclera, 527, 528, 529, **530**
  proper, 528, 529, **530**
Scopalamine, 311
Scotopic vision, 532
Scrotum, 350, 489
Sebaceous glands, 238, **239,** 361
Secondary
  degeneration, **312,** 313
  papillae
    of reticulum, 403, **403**
  processes
    of podocytes, 433, **434–437**
  response, 343
  spongiosa, 156, 159
Secretin, 399, 430, 486, 487
Secretagogues, 399
Secretory
  end-pieces, 61
  IgA, 452
  piece, 343, 452
Sections
  examination of, 16–17
Septa
  longitudinal, 155, **155, 159, 160**
  transverse, 155, **155, 159, 160**
Septal
  cells, 457
  space, 459

Septuli testis, 489, **489**
Septum membranaceum, 324
Semicircular canals, 527, **546, 547,** 549, **549**
Seminal vesicles, 501, **502, 502**
Seminiferous tubules, 236, 237, 489, **489, 490**
  compartment of
    apical, 496, **496**
    basilar, 495, **496**
Serotonin, 98, 175, 345
  as a neurotransmitter, 213
Serine proteases, 175, 176, 345
Serotonin
  from enteroendocrine cells, 395
  from pancreas, 484
  from pineal gland, 473
Serous
  cells, 65, **65, 66,** 236, **237,** 238, **239**
  demilunes, 65, 66, **67,** 417, **417–419**
  membranes, 258, **258**
  secretion, 43, **45**
Sertoli cells, 495, **495, 496**
Serum, 164
  glutamine pyruvate transaminase (SGPT) (*see* Ala-
    nine aminotransferase)
  sickness, 347
Sex hormones, 483
Sharpey's fibers, 272, **280**
Sheath
  of Hertwig, **387, 388, 388**
  of Schwann, 220, **225–230**
  of Schweigger-Seidel, 336, **341**
Shell gland, 523
  pouch, 525
Shift
  left
    degenerative, 186
    regenerative, 186
  right, 186
Shock
  hypovolemic, 482
Sialic acid, 85
Sialomucins, 452
Sialoproteins, 119
Signal
  hypothesis, 33, 34
  peptidase, 34
  sequence, 33
Sinoatrial node (SA), 324, 326
Sinusoids, 315, **319**
Skeletal muscle, 190–204, 206, 207, 236, **237,** 242, **243**
  appearance in section, 190, **192**
  as an organ, 276–283
    organization of, 276
  atrophy of, 204
  contractile mechanism of, 193, **200**
  functional correlates of, 200–204
  histology of, 190–193, **192**
  hypertrophy of, 201
  myofibrillar organization of, 193, **199, 201**
  relaxation/contraction morphology, 192–200, **200**
  regeneration of, 206, 207
  repair of, 206, 207
  -tendon junctions, 276
  type
    I, 200, **202**
    IIa, 200, **202**
    IIb, 200, **202**
    fast-twitch
      glycolytic, 200, **202**
      oxidative-glycolytic, 200, **202**
    slow-twitch, oxidative, 200, **202**
  ultrastructure of, 193, **194–197**
Skin, 235, 348, 349
  avian, **377,** 378, 379
    specialized structures of, 379
  cytology of, 556
  development of, 348
  glands of, 357–361
    miscellaneous, 365
    sebaceous, 357, **358**
    special, 358, **359,** 361, **361**
    tubular, 357, **358**
  healing of, 372–378
    first intention, 273
    second intention, 273, **273–277,** 278
    third intention, 273

  innervation of, 350
  miscellaneous appendages of, 371, 372
  organization of, 349
  repair of, 372–378
    stages of, 372–378
  specialized
    cells of, 355, 356
    regions of, 350
  vessels of
    blood, 350
    lymphatic, 350
Sleeve bone, **153,** 154, **155**
Sliding filament hypothesis, 193
Slit diaphragm, 435, **435**
Slow reacting substance of anaphylaxis, (SRS-A), 487
Small
  alveolar pneumonocyte, 455, **456**
  intensely fluorescent cells (SIF), 214
  intestine, 405–409
    absorption by, 409
    avian, 415
    characteristics of, 405
    digestion by, 409
    histology of, 405, **405–408**
    motility of, 408, 409
    physiology of, 408, 409
    regions of, 405–408
    repair and renewal, 409
Smegma, 365
Smooth
  endoplasmic reticulum, 34, 36
  muscle, 188–190, 242, **243**
    appearance in section, 189, **190**
    contraction of
      rhythmic, 190
      tonic, 190
    functional correlates of, 190
    histology of, 188, **188, 189**
    repair of, 207
    regeneration of, 207
    types
      intermediate, 190
      multiunit, 190
      vascular, 190
      visceral, 190
    ultrastructure of, 189, 190, **191**
Sodium
  and renal function, 442
  citrate, 187
  oxalate, 187
Sole, 365, **366**
Solitary tract, 306
  nucleus of, 306
Soma, 208
Somatomedin, 471
Somatostatin, 395, 484, 486, 487, 472
Somatotrophic hormone (STH), 471
Somatotropin, 471
  -somatomedin axis, 144, 145
Space
  of Disse, 421, **423–425**
  of Fontana, 537, **537, 538**
  of Virchow-Robin, 302
Spatium perichoroideale, 532
Special
  afferent
    somatic (SSA), 288, **290,** 527
    visceral (SVA), 288, **290**
  efferent
    visceral (SVE), 288, **290**
  proprioception (SP), 288, **290**
Specific granules, 168
Spermatids, 490, **490,** 496, **496,** 498
Spermatocytes
  primary, 490, **490,** 496, **496**
    pachytene, 498
    zygotene, 498
  secondary, 490, 496, 498
Spermatocytogenesis, 495–498
  stages of, 495
Spermatogenic
  cycle, 498, 499
  wave, 498, 499
Spermatogonia, 491, **491,** 495, 498, **498**
  A, 496
  B, 496

I₁, 496
I₂, 496
intermediate (I), 496
Spermatozoa, 490
Sperm host glands, 525
Spermiogenesis, 496–498
Sphingomyelin, 23
Sphincter of Oddi, 428
Spinal
cord, 302, 303, **303**
nerves, **290**, 291
Spindle fibers, 47, **47**
Spines
of neurons, 211, **218**
Spinous cell layer, 56
Spiral
lamina, 549
ligament, 551
prominence, 551
tunnel, **551**, 552
Spleen, 334–337, **337–341**
circulation through, 335, 336, **341**
closed, 336, **341**
open 336, **341**
cytology of, 556
functions of, 335
innervation of, 336
lymph vessels of, 336
physiological correlates of, 336, 337
pulp of
red, 335, **340, 341**
white, 335, **338–340**
structure of, 334, 335, **337–341**
Splenic corpuscles, 183, 335, **337–340**
Spreading factor, 84
Splenic corpuscle
periarteriolar zone of, 183, **183**
Spongioblasts, 285, **288, 289**
Spongiocytes, 479, **481**
Squamous alveolar epithelial cell, 455, **456**
Stains
acidic, 7
alcian blue, 86
azure A, 7
azure B, 7
azure C, 7
basic, 7
eosin, 7
fluorescein isothiocyanate (FITC), 9
hematoxylin, 7
modified Romanowsky, 7
neutralization reaction and, 7
oxytetracycline, 4, **6**
periodic acid-Schiff (PAS), 7
polychromed methylene blue, 7
supravital, 4
Janus green B, 5
neutral red, 5
vital, 4
lithium carmine, 5
oxytetracycline, 4
trypan blue, 5
Stapedius, 546
Stapes, 546
Starling's law of the heart, 325
Static sensation, 547
Stellate reticulum 386, **387, 389**
Stem cells, 47
Stercobilin, 185, **185**
Sterols, 23
Stimulators
α-adrenergic, 312
β-adrenergic, 312
Stomach
compound, 400–405
characteristics of, 400
development of, 400
digestion in, 404, 405
motility of, 404
glandular, 236–238, **239**, 393–400
characteristics, 393
histology of, **392**, 393–395, **393**, **394–400**
glandular regions of, 395–400
cardiac, **394**, 395
esophageal, 395
fundic, **394–397**, 395

pyloric, 398, **399, 400**
motility of, 398
physiology of, 398–400
repair and renewal, 400
secretory activity of, 398, 399
acid, **398**, 399, 400
phases of, 398, 399
muscular, **414, 415**, 415
Straight
collecting duct, **432**, 438
tubules, 492, **492**
Stratum
avasculosum, 536
basale, 55, **56**, 349, 351, **373**, 378
cavernosum, 502
circulare
of tympanic membrane, 545
compactum, 393, **393**
corneum, 57, **57**, 349, **377**, 378
cutaneum
of tympanic membrane, 545
disjunctum, 57, **57**
externum, 365, **367**
germinativum, 56, **56**
granulosum, 56, **56**, 349, 351
of ovary, 509
intermedium
of avian skin, **377**, 378
of teeth, 386, **387**, 389
lamellatum, 367, **367, 368, 370, 371**
lucidum, 57, 349
medium 367, **367–369**
radiatum
of tympanic membrane, 545
spinosum, 56, **56**, 349, 351, **377**, 378
tectorium, 365, **367**
transitivum, **377**, 378
Stratified squamous epithelium, **235**
Streptokinase, 177
Stria vascularis, **550**, 551, 546
Striated
border, 405
ducts, 417, **417, 418**
Stroma, 252
Sub-
arachnoid space, 296, **298, 299**
chondral bone, 271, **273**
cutis, 348
dural space, 295
endocardial coat, 323, **325**
endothelial coat, 314, **315, 316**, 323, **325**
ependymal organ, 219
mental organ, 365
mucosal
glands, 254, **255**
plexus, 393
synaptic web, 213
thalamus, 285
Substance P, 484, 486, 487
Substantia propria, 532, 527
of cornea, 529, **531**
Sucrase, 409
Sulfatases, 38
Sulfation, 36
Sulfomucins, 452
Summation
spatial, 216
temporal, 216
Supracaudal gland, 365
Suprachoroid layer, 532
Suprarenal gland, 478–483
Suppressor factors, 344
Surface tension, 455, 457, **457**
Surfactant, 455, 457
Suspensory ligament
of lens, 528
Sustentacular cells
of carotid sinus, 325
of macula, 549
of olfactory region, 447
of organ of Corti, 552
of taste buds, 383, **385**
Suture, 270
Sympathetic nervous system, 306, **307**
Sympathomimetics, 312
Symphyses, 270, **270**

Synapse, 211–213, **217–219**
asymmetrical, 213, **217**
directed, 211
nondirected, 213
symmetrical, 213
Synaptic
cleft, 211, **216, 217**
delay, 211
primary, 281, **281**
secondary, 281
vesicles, 213, 281, **281**
clear, 214, **217, 218**
dense core, 214, **219**
Synaptosomes, 211
granular, 214, **219**
Synchondroses, 262, **263, 264**, 270
Syndesmoses, 270
Synostosis, 262, 270
Synovial
fluid, 272–276
analysis of, **276**
cytology of, 561, **562**
functional correlates of, 276
lubrication by, 275, 276
boosted, 275
boundary, 275
fluid film, 275
lipid, 276
mixed, 275
weeping, 275
folds, 272
joints, 270–276
origin of, 270, **270**
nature of, 270
structure of, 270, **271–275**
membrane, 271, **271**, 272
types of
adipose, 272
areolar, 272
fibrous, 272
villi, 272, **272**
nutrition from, 276
protection from, 276
Syrinx, 463

Taeniae
ceci, 409
coli, 409
Tail glands, 365
Tanycytes, 219
Tapetal rods, 533
Tapetum
cellular, **531**, 533
fibrous, 533
lucidum, **531**, 532, **532, 533**
Target cells, 168
Tarsal glands, 543, **543**
Tartar, 390
Taste
buds, 383, **384–386**
pores, 383, **385**
Tear film
precorneal, 544, 545
Teat, 361, **362, 364**
canal, 361, **362, 264**
cistern, 361, **362**, 364
sinus, 361, **362, 364**
Techniques
antibody
direct fluorescent, 9, **9**
indirect fluorescent, 9
critical point drying, 11
freeze dry, 7
freeze fracturing, 11, **11**
frozen section, 8
methacrylate, 8, **10**
paraffin, 5–7
acquisition, 5
clearing, 5
dehydration, 5
embedding, 6, 7
fixation, 5, 6
mounting, 7
sectioning, 7
shortcomings of, 7
staining, 7

Tectorial membrane, 550, **551**, 552
Teeth, 383–390
  alveolus of, 390
  brachydont, 386, **386**, 390
  characteristics, 383, 385
  complex, 386
  components of
    cellular, 388, **388–390**
    matrical, 388, **388–390**
  deciduous, 386, **387**, **388**
  development of, 386–388, **387**
  epithelial attachment of, 390
  eruption of, **387**, 388
  hypsodont, 386, 390
  milk, 386, **387**, **388**
  permanent, 386
  simple, 386, **386**
Tela choroidea, 297
Telencephalon, 285, **287**
Telodendrion, **209**, **211**
Telodendritic zone, 208, **213**
Telogen, 355, **356**
Tendon, 103, 240, **241**, 276–278
  morphology of, 276, **278**
  repair of
    extrinsic, 277
    intrinsic, 277
    stages of, 277, **278**
  synovial sheath of, 277, **278**
Tenon's
  capsule, 529
  space, 529
Tensor tympani, 546
Terminal
  bar, 68
  cisterns, 193, **197**, **198**
  degeneration, **312**, 313
  ductules of liver, 421, **425**
  web, 43, 70
Tertiary papillae
  of reticulum, 403, **403**
Testis, 236, **237**, 486
  general features, 489
  investments of, 489, **489**
Testosterone, 483, 491, 500, 511
  and bone, 144
  and ossification, 161
  effects of
    anabolic, 500
    androgenic, 500
  -estradiol-binding globulin, 500
3, 5, 3′,5′-Tetraiodothyronine (T₄), 475
Thalamus, 285
Theca
  folliculi
    externa, 508, **508**
    interna, 508, **508**
  lutein cells, 511
Thecal cone, 509, **509**
T helper cells, 334
Thiamine pyrophosphatase (TPP), 35
Third
  eye, 473
  eyelid, 544, **544**, **545**
  ventricle, 285, **287**
Thoracolumbar system, 306, 307
Thrombin, 176
Thrombocytes
  avian, 174, **175**
Thrombocytopenia, 176
Thrombocytopoiesis, 182
  cells of (see specific cells)
Thrombogenic, 487
Thromboxane (TXA₂), 487
  synthase, 487, 345
  A, 175
Thymine, 22
Thymocytes, 337
Thymopoietin I and II, 341
Thymic corpuscles, 339, **343**
Thymine, 22
Thymosin, 341
Thymus, 337–341, **342–344**
  blood
    barrier of, 340, **343**, **344**
    vessels of, 340

embryology of, 337
innervation of, 340
lymph vessels of, 340
physiological correlates of, 340, 341
structure of, 337–340, **342–344**
Thyroglobulin, 475
Thyroglossal duct, 474
Thyroid
  gland, 474–476, **474**, **475**
    cytology of, 558, **559**
    follicular cells of, 246, **247**, 248, **249**
    follicles, 474, **474**, **475**
    hormones (T₃, T₄), 475, 476
      and bone, 144, 163
      effects of, 476
      mobilization of, 476
      regulation of, 476
      storage of, 475
      synthesis of, 475
  -stimulating hormone, 472
    releasing factor, 472
Thyrotoxicosis, 144
Thyrotrophic hormone (TSH), 472
Thyroxine (T₄), 475
  binding globulin, 166
Tidemarks, 271, **273**
Tight junctions, **68**, 69, **69**, 70
Tigroid granules, 209, **214**
Tissue, 2
  basic, 2
  conscience concerning, 5
  defined, 2
  density of bone, 259, **259**
  hypoxia, 184
  fluid, 86–91, **87**
    altered exchange of, 89–91, **90**, **91**
    capillary pressure and, 87, 88, **88**
      arterial, 87, 88, **88**
      hydrostatic, 87, 88, **88**
      osmotic, 87, 88, **88**
      venous, 87, 88, **88**
    dynamics of, 87
    exchange of, 88, 89. **89**
    formation of
      factors regarding, 87–91
      interstitial pressure and, 88, **88**
    lymphatic channels and, 88, 89, **89**
      hydrostatic, 88, **88**
      osmotic, 88, **88**
    mechanisms of exchange, 88, **88**, **89**
    movement of, 87
    phospholipids, 175, **176**
    simple, 2
    thromboplastin, 175, **176**
T killer cells, 334
Tolerance phenomenon, 344
Tome's
  fibers, 389, **390**
  processes, 389
Tongue, 382, 383
Tonsils, 330, **332**
  cecal, 415
  cytology of, 556
  follicles of, 331, **332**
  with crypts, 331, **332**
  without crypts, 331, **332**
Tonofilaments, 43
Toxic complex reaction, 346
Trabeculae
  corneosclerales, 537, **537**, **538**
  of connective tissue, **256**, 258
Trachea, 449, **450**
  avian, 463, **463**
Transalveolar migration, 457, **458**
Transaminase, 428
Transitional cells, 395
Transcortin, 166, 482
Transcription, 22, 33, **35**
Transferases, 35
Transfer factors, 171
Transferrin, 166
Transition zone (see perichondral ring)
Translation, 22, 33, 34, **35**
Transneuronal reactions, 312, **312**
Transport
  active, 32

carrier-mediated, 32
Na-dependent, 32
passive, 32
piece, 343
Trans-synaptic reactions, 312, **312**
Transudate, 560
  modified, 560
Transverse
  sarcotubular system, 193, **197**, **198**
  tubules, 193, **197**, **198**, 204
Triad, 193, **196–198**
Trichohyalin, 351
Trigger zone, 208, **213**
Triglycerides, 23
Trigonum fibrosum, 324
3, 5, 3′-Triiodothyronine (T₃), 475
Trophoblast, 519
Trophoderm, 519
Tropocollagen, 77, **79**, 80, **80**, 81
Tropomysin, 43, 193, **199**, **201**
Troponin, 43, 193, **199**, **201**
True
  joints (see Synovial joints)
  unipolar neurons, 208, **212**
Trypsin, 430
Trypsinogen, 430
T-suppressor cells, 344
Tuber cinereum, **468**, **469**, 472
Tubular shell gland, 525
Tubulin, 39
Tubuli
  contorta, 489, **489**
  recti, 489, **489**, 492, **492**
Tubulis recta
  distalis, 436
  proximalis, 435, **437**
Tunica
  adventitia, 254, 314, **315**, **316**, 317
  albuginea
    of testis, 489, **489**
    ovarii, 506
  fibrosi bulbi, 528, **530**
  interna (sensoria) bulbi, 528, **530**
  intima, 314, **315**, **316**
  media, 314, **315**, **316**, 317
  mucosa, 252, **252**, **253**
  muscularis, **252**, **253**, 254
  serosa, **252**, 254, **254**
  submucosa, **252**, **253**, 254
  vasculosa bulbi, 528, **530**
Tunnel of Corti, **551**, 552
Tympanic
  cavity, 545, 546
  membrane, 545
Type I cells
  of carotid bodies, 325
Type II cells
  of carotid bodies, 325
Tyrosinase, 100
Tyrosine hydroxylase, 214, **219**

Udder, 361, 362
Ultimobranchial body, 474
Umbilicus
  distal, 378, **378**
  proximal, 378, **378**
Unit membrane concept, 29
Uracil, 22
Urea, 404
  and renal function, 442
Ureters, 445, **445**
Urethrae, 445, 502, **504**, 514
  penile, 502
  pelvic, 502
Urethral
  glands, 502
  muscle, 502
Urinary
  bladder, 445
    automatic, 445
    autonomous, 445
  system, 431–445
    cytology of, 556, 557, **557**
Urination, 445
Uriniferous
  passages, 445

tubules, 431, **431**
Urobilin, 185, **185**
Urobilinogen, 185, **185**
Urodaeum, 415
Urogenital sinus, 433
Uridine diphosphate (UDP)-galactose, 80
Uronic acid, 84
Uropygial gland, 379, **379**
Urothelium, 58
Uterine
  body, 513
  glands, 513, **513–515**
  horns, 513
  tubes,
Uterus, 513, **513–515**
  avian, 523, **525**
  bicornuate, 513
  cyclic changes of, 516, **517, 518**
  duplex, 513
  simple, 513
Utriculus, 547–549
Uvea, 527, **530**
  anterior, 536
  posterior, 536
  tract, 527, **530**

Vagina
  smear of
    early estrus, 248, **249**
    diestrus, 248, **249**
Valves
  semilunar, 324
Vagina, 514, **515**
  avian, 525
  cyclic changes of, 517
  cytology of, 559, **559**
Vaginitis, 559
Vane, 378, **378**
Vasa
  recta, 438, **440**
  vasorum, 314
Vascular
  coat
    of eye, 527, **530**
  tunic, 532–537
Vasoactive intestinal peptide (VIP), 398, 484, 487
Vasoconstriction, 308
Vasodepressor region, 326, 329
Vasodilation, 308

Vassopressin, 472, 473
Vasopressor region, 326
Vater-Pacinian corpuscles, 294, **296, 297**
Veins, 322, **323, 324**
  central, 420, **421, 422,** 423
  emissary, 263
  hepatic, 423
    portal, 423
  large, 322
  metaphyseal, 263
  nutrient, 263
  sublobular, **422,** 423
  valves of, 322, **323, 324**
Venous
  sinuses, 315
  stasis, 560
Ventilation, 461
  -perfusion ratio, 462
Ventral
  columns, **303,** 320
  funiculus, 303, **303**
  grey column, 289, **291** 305, **306**
  root, 305, **306**
Ventriculus, **414, 415,** 415
Venules, **320,** 322
Vesicles
  pinocytotic, 37, 73
  secretory, 35, **37**
Vesicular glands, 501, **501, 502**
Vestibular
  apparatus, 547–549
  glands
    major, 514
    minor, 514
  hair cells I and II, 547, **547, 548, 549**
    shearing of, 547, **548**
  membrane, 550, 551, **551**
Vestibule, 514
Vestibulum, 463, 464
Vexillum, 378, **378**
Villi, 405, **406, 407**
  of placenta, 519
Visceral
  pleura, 450
  pericardium, 323, **326**
Viscous metamorphosis, 175
Vitamin
  A, 409
  D, 142–145, 409, 487

metabolites of, 143–145, **145**
  D$_2$, 143
  D$_3$, 143
  E, 409
  K, 176, 409
Vitreous
  body, 527, **528, 529, 530,** 537
  humor, **530,** 537
Vocal folds, 463
Volatile fatty acids (VFA), 402, 404
von Ebner's glands, 418
von Kupffer cells, 421, **421**
Vulva, 514

Wallerian degeneration, **312,** 313
Water
  bound, 22
  free, 22
Waxes, 23
Wharton's jelly, 101, **101**
White
  blood cells (WBCs) (*see* specific cells)
    counts of, 187
      differential, 187
  line, **370,** 371
  matter, 303, **303**
  pulp, 335, **338–340**
Wolffian duct, 433
Wound contraction, 378
Woven bone, 129, 131, **131, 132**
  during ossification, 146, **149, 150**

Zernike condensor, 14
Z lines, 190, **192, 184–196,** 236, **237**
Zollinger-Ellison syndrome, 486
Zona
  arcuata, 479, **479, 480**
  fasciculata, 236, 237, 479, **481**
  glomerulosa, 479, **479, 480**
  intermedia, 479
  multiformis, 479
  parenchymatosa, 506, **506**
  reticularis, 479, **482**
  pellucida, 508, **508–510**
  vasculosa, 506, **506**
Zonula
  adherens, **68,** 69, 70
  occludens, **68,** 69, **69,** 70
Zymogen granules, 43, **44,** 395, **395–397**